# Microbiology and Pathology

# Microbiology and Pathology

## Alice Lorraine Smith, A.B., M.D., F.C.A.P., F.A.C.P.

Associate Professor of Pathology, The University of Texas Health Science
Center at Dallas, Texas; formerly Assistant Professor of Microbiology,
Department of Nursing, Dominican College and St. Joseph's Hospital,
Houston, Texas

*with 564 illustrations, including 2 color plates*

**ELEVENTH EDITION**

# The C. V. Mosby Company

Saint Louis 1976

**Eleventh edition**

**Copyright © 1976 by The C. V. Mosby Company**

All rights reserved. No part of this book may be reproduced in any manner without written permission of the publisher.

Previous editions copyrighted 1936, 1939, 1944, 1948, 1953, 1956, 1960, 1964, 1968, 1972

Printed in the United States of America

Distributed in Great Britain by Henry Kimpton, London

**Library of Congress Cataloging in Publication Data**

Smith, Alice Lorraine, 1920-
  Microbiology and pathology.

  First ed. published in 1936 under title: Microbiology and pathology for nurses, by C. F. Carter.
  Includes bibliographies and index.
  1. Medical microbiology. 2. Pathology. I. Carter, Charles Franklin, 1890-1957. Microbiology and pathology for nurses. II. Title. [DNLM: 1. Microbiology. 2. Pathology. QW4 S642m]
  QR46.S63 1976    616.01    75-31759
  ISBN 0-8016-4674-X

GW/CB/B  9  8  7  6  5  4  3  2  1

To

**Frederick and Ned**

# Preface

I keep six honest serving-men
  (They taught me all I knew);
Their names are What and Why and When
  And How and Where and Who.

RUDYARD KIPLING

The scientific answers to the What and When and How and Who are coming so thick and fast in these exciting days that to no one's surprise it is time for a revision of *Microbiology and Pathology*. Here then is the book reworked to give contemporary coverage in sister subjects of major importance and designed to be readily assimilated by students in health science training programs.

The unit scheme of prior editions continues, with six units for microbiology and two for pathology. In microbiology the unit pattern is in biologic orbit around microorganisms. It begins with basic concepts in the first unit, includes laboratory methods in the second, and in subsequent units develops the events of injury, indicts culprits, and emphasizes restraints.

What happens when microbes and their products contact living cells of the human body is a theme permeating this book. One full unit (Unit III) is devoted to it. This unit concentrates on defenses inherent in the body, the immune system, immunopathology, allergy, and key laboratory reactions in immunology. (Tumor immunology is reserved for the chapter on neoplasms.)

A small and fairly compact unit categorizes various agents destroying or impeding microbes. The action of antibiotics is noted, and unfavorable side effects of antibiotic administration are stressed. Technics for sterilization are compared; for example, gas sterilization with steam sterilization.

The largest unit of the book makes up the roster of significant pathogens and parasites, stressing their identity and the nature of their injury. Material pertinent to the pathology and pathogenesis of a given infection is placed in the chapter considering the causative agent. The overall pathology of infectious disease is found at the end of the chapter on inflammation.

An unusual unit, the last one for microbiology, relates the student to the microbial life of our environment. A survey, yet a practical unit, it accommodates such items as measures to safeguard food and swimming pool sanitation. Herein two chapters are paired to focus on the best available information on immunization from the United States Public Health Service, the American Academy of Pediatrics, the United States Armed Forces, and the World Health Organization (WHO). The companion chapters sort out modern biologic products, outline technics in passive immunization, tabulate latest schedules for active immunization, and give crucial guidelines for administration of biologic products.

The second part of the book bisects pathology in traditional fashion. General pathology is the overview of fundamentals to disease anywhere in the body. Special pathology fits these to major anatomic areas. Wherever possible, the changes in body fluids demonstrable in the clinical laboratory are correlated with pathologic findings in tissues.

This book in frame and substance must remain relevant to the here and now in health careers. It has been edited and updated to keep it so. There are new topics and new emphases. Topics expanded include the biologic classification of microbes, the lymphoid system's role in immunity, anaerobes in disease, concepts of immunopathology, immunologic reactions, viral hepatitis, endotoxin shock, chemical carcinogenesis, and viral oncogens. Subjects new to this edition include the serologic diagnosis of protozoan and metazoan diseases, experimental production of dental caries, practical technics to evaluate cell-mediated immunity, the scanning electron microscope, early detection of breast cancer, immunotherapy, postnecrotic cirrhosis, fetal antigens, and the Dane particle.

The classification of bacteria throughout this text is that of *Bergey's Manual of Determinative Bac-*

*teriology* (1974), with the notable exception of the arrangement of enteric bacteria according to the scheme of W. H. Ewing. For viruses, not included in the eighth edition of Bergey's Manual, the most modern classification is still that based on their properties. The revisions in the new Bergey's Manual necessitated considerable reorganization and changes in terminology. Note that rickettsias, chlamydiae (bedsoniae), and actinomycetes are now bacteria.

The illustrations have been selected to enrich the meaning of the prose. For instance, when the subject of tuberculin testing is presented, the photograph of positive skin reactions makes the impact. The first of two color plates highlights the different approaches to the laboratory study of microbes, and the second presents changes in blood cells with leukemia. Every teacher knows that tables dramatize and give quick access to information. Immunization schedules, sterilization maneuvers, incubation periods, comparative sizes, coagulation factors, metric equivalents, classification of neoplasms, coagulation sequence (the "waterfall"), mechanisms of edema, comparison of comparable diseases, differential characteristics, and biologic properties can thus be arranged effectively.

Current references are gathered at the end of a unit or after closely related chapters. Thought-provoking questions for review occupy the usual place at the end of the chapter. Sources for the glossary are found in the text, standard medical dictionaries, and Webster's unabridged dictionary.

This revision would not have been possible without the counsel, technical know-how, and cooperation of certain talented persons at The University of Texas Health Science Center at Dallas. In the Department of Pathology, I gratefully acknowledge the kindness of Dr. V. A. Stembridge, Chairman, Drs. R. C. Reynolds, B. D. Fallis, Frank Vellios, professors, Dr. C. S. Petty, Chief Medical Examiner for Dallas County and Professor of Forensic Sciences and Pathology, Mrs. Phyllis Kitterman, Secretary, Mrs. Linda Bolding, Laboratory Technical Assistant, and Mr. Donald Calhoun, photographer for the Medical Examiner's office; in the Department of Medical Illustration Services, Dr. W. R. Christensen, Chairman, R. J. Castanie, medical illustrator, and Miss Jean Gionas, medical photographer; and in the Library, Mrs. Elinor Reinmiller, Reference Librarian, and other able members of Dr. Donald Hendricks's staff. I am indebted to Mrs. Earline Kutscher, Chief Technologist, and her staff at the Bacteriology Laboratory of Parkland Memorial Hospital for invaluable assistance.

Now a special word of appreciation to teachers and students whose ever-welcome criticisms and comments have guided me: may I voice a heartfelt thanks to the many of you who have used this text and who carefully consider the new edition.

**Alice Lorraine Smith**

# Contents

# Part one
# MICROBIOLOGY

**UNIT I**

Microbiology: prelude and primer

**UNIT II**

Microbes: procedures for study

**UNIT III**

Microbes: production of infection

**UNIT IV**

Microbes: preclusion of disease

**UNIT V**

Microbes: pathogens and parasites

**UNIT VI**

Microbes: public welfare

# UNIT I

MICROBIOLOGY
prelude and primer

## CHAPTER 1

# Definition and dimension

Take interest, I implore you, in those sacred dwellings which one designates by the expressive term: laboratories. Demand that they be multiplied, that they be adorned. These are the temples of the future—temples of well-being and of happiness. There it is that humanity grows greater, stronger, better.

LOUIS PASTEUR

## Definition

*Biology* is the science that treats of living organisms. The branch of biology dealing with *microbes*—that is, organisms structured as one cell and studied with the microscope—is *microbiology* ("microbe-biology"). Microbiology considers the occurrence in nature of the microscopic forms of life, their reproduction and physiology, their participation in the processes of nature, their helpful or harmful relationships with other living things, and their significance in science and industry.

Within the province of microbiology lies the study of bacteria, viruses, fungi, and protozoa. Subordinate sciences are *bacteriology,* the study of bacteria; *virology,* the study of viruses; *mycology,* the study of fungi (unicellular and multicellular plants); and *protozoology,* the study of protozoa (unicellular animals). Many microbes are parasitic. The science dealing with organisms dependent on living things for their sustenance is *parasitology.* So closely associated with microbiology as to be considered a part of it is the science of *immunology,* the study of those mechanisms whereby one organism deals with the harmful effects of another.

Although man has lived with microorganisms from time immemorial and has used certain of their activities, such as fermentation, to his advantage, the science of microbiology is a product of only the last hundred years or so. The studies of Antonj van Leeuwenhoek in the seventeenth century had shown the existence of microscopic forms of life, but it was not until the work of Louis Pasteur toward the end of the nineteenth century (some 200 years later) that the science of microbiology really took shape. The new science stated the germ theory of disease, demonstrated patterns of communicable disease, and gave man a measure of protection he had not known in his struggle against the injurious forces in the biologic environment.* In its time this very young science has influenced practically every type of human endeavor.

## Dimension
### BIOLOGIC CLASSIFICATION

All living things are classified in a scheme of categories with breakdown into successively dependent and related groups. The highest possible levels are designated kingdoms, of which there may be two or three. For years, the traditional two were the plant and animal kingdoms. Today there are forces for change in this approach. The following terms are basic ones in classification and are listed in ascending order:

1. Species—organisms sharing a set of biologic traits and reproducing only their exact kind
   a. Strain—organisms within the species varying in a given quality
   b. Type—organisms within the species varying immunologically
2. Genus (*pl.,* genera)—closely related species
3. Family—closely related genera
4. Order—closely related families
5. Class—closely related orders
6. Phylum (*pl.,* phyla)†—related classes

The lower forms of life incorporate variably features of both plants and animals and do not show the dramatic differences of the higher forms. It is difficult to define many microbes as either plant or animal,

---

*For scientific knowledge to bring results, such as in the organization of public health programs, it must be disseminated. Such is the purpose of *health education.* To the individual it explains the mechanisms by which he can protect himself against microbial hazards. To the social group it designates the available community resources.

†In plant biology, the term *division* is used instead of phylum. In Table 1-1 (p. 5), note use of the term *division* for either of the two major classifications in the kingdom to include all procaryotes.

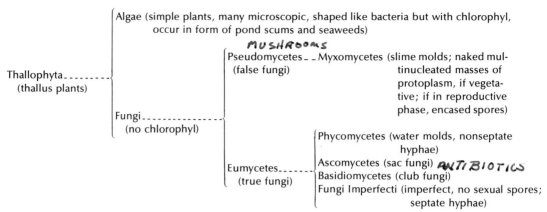

**Schema 1.** Subdivisions of Thallophyta. See also p. 326.

and as bacteria and other microbes long classified as plants have been more closely studied, the inconsistencies appear even greater. Because of this fact, a third major biological compartment with equivalent rank to the plant and animal kingdoms has been advocated to sift out the simpler units, designating them as *protists*. Basically most protists are one-cell units and remain so throughout their life history. Even if they pile cells up in large plantlike masses, their component cells remain the same and do not differentiate.

There is an alternate scheme of classification of living things, again based on complexity of structure but this time focused directly on the nucleus. It is apparent that "higher" organisms possess a true nucleus; "lower" ones do not. Thus two distinct categories emerge. The obvious nucleus in the higher forms is complete, with the expected number of chromosomes and mitotic apparatus. These organisms are termed "eucaryotic" (using the Greek word which means true nucleus). This category (or kingdom) would be one to contain some protists and the plants and animals.

In the lower forms of life, nuclear function is carried out by only a single chromosome, devoid of any membrane. Lower forms are small and less complex in other ways. For instance they do not contain such membrane-bounded organelles as mitochondria. They are designated "procaryotic," the second category to encompass all bacteria and a small group of blue-green algae (algae demonstrate plantlike photosynthesis).

Procaryotes, as a grouping, share distinctive properties. They possess certain unique components in their cell walls, and they display remarkable capabilities with regard to carbon storage, nitrogen fixation, obligate anaerobiosis, and derivation of energy from oxidation of inorganic compounds.

**Scope.** Microorganisms usually surveyed in a treatise of microbiology include bacteria (unicellular

procaryotes as indicated above), fungi, and lower forms of animal life.

Fungi are best known as plants and are gathered into Thallophyta, one of the four divisions of the plant kingdom. Thallophytes, or thallus plants (Greek, *thallos,* young shoot or branch), are defined as simple forms of plant life that do not differentiate into true roots, stems, or leaves. The term *fungi* as ordinarily used refers to molds, yeasts, and certain related microorganisms. Schema 1 gives the subdivisions of thallus plants.

Some of the most important disease-producing agents known to man are lower forms of animal life. They include the unicellular protozoa, the simplest ones, and a restricted number of the more complex multicellular or metazoan animals as well (Chapters 31 and 32).

## NAMING OF MICROBES

The scientific name of a living organism is usually made up of two words that are Latin or Greek in form. The first name begins with a capital letter and denotes the genus. The second name begins with a small letter and denotes the species. Either the genus or the species name may be derived from the proper name of a person or place or from a term describing some feature of the organism. The proper name may be that of the scientific investigator or that of the related geographic area. Biologic characteristics indicated include color, location in nature, disease produced, and presence of certain enzymes. For example, *Staphylococcus aureus* is the scientific name for bacteria of genus *Staphylococcus* (Greek, *staphylē,* bunch of grapes + *kokkus,* berry) and species *aureus* (Latin, *aureus,* golden). It indicates that the bacteria grow in typical clusters and produce a golden pigment. Honoring Sir David Bruce who discovered it, *Brucella melitensis* (pertaining to the island of Malta) by its name indicates its disease—Malta fever, or undulant

4

*Text continued on p. 16.*

**Table 1-1**

Abbreviated classification of microbes from *Bergey's Manual of Determinative Bacteriology* (1974)*

Kingdom *Procaryotae* † (highest level taxon encompassing microbes in which nucleoplasm lacks basic protein and is not bounded by nuclear membrane)

   Division I. The Cyanobacteria (blue-green algae with gliding motility, producing oxygen in light; photosynthetic procaryotes as single cells or simple or branched chains of cells; photopigments include chlorophyll *a*)

   Division II. The Bacteria (unicellular procaryotes multiplying by growth and division, usually binary; if cells remain together, arrangement classical; true branching may be seen; motility from flagella or by gliding, twitching, snapping, or darting motions; majority encased in rigid cell wall [constancy of form], most of which contain peptidoglycans; photosynthesis, if carried out, is anaerobic and bacteriochlorophylls used; chemosynthesis requires aerobic or anaerobic conditions, with some microbes facultative; endospores formed in some species, arthrospores and cysts in others, but no heterocysts)

PART 1  PHOTOTROPHIC BACTERIA‡

   Order I. *Rhodospirillales* (mostly water bacteria; gram-negative, variably shaped, all with bacteriochlorophylls and carotenoid pigments; purple-violet, purple, red, or orange-brown, brown, or green colors from photopigments in cell suspensions; some can fix nitrogen; purple [sulfur or nonsulfur] and green sulfur groups of bacteria here)

PART 2  GLIDING BACTERIA

   Order I. *Myxobacterales* (slime bacteria; gram-negative, strict aerobes with slow gliding movements found on soil and decomposing plant and animal matter; no photosynthetic pigments; chemoorganotrophs; energy-yielding mechanism respiratory, never fermentative; fruiting bodies formed from cell aggregates often brightly colored and macroscopic; bacteriolytic and cellulytic [attacking cellulose] groups here)

   Order II. *Cytophagales* (rods or filaments, gram-negative, with slow or rapid gliding; no fruiting bodies; chemolithotrophs, chemoorganotrophs, or mixotrophs)

PART 3  SHEATHED BACTERIA

   (sheath present may be encrusted with iron or manganese oxides; single cells; flagella may be found)

      Genus *Leptothrix* (gram-negative, strictly aerobic straight rods in chains within a sheath; also free-swimming as single cells, in pairs, or in motile short chains; sheaths often impregnated with hydrated ferric or manganic oxides; prevalent in iron-containing, uncontaminated, slow-running fresh waters)

      Genus *Streptothrix* (thin, gram-negative rods in chains; strictly aerobic; widely distributed in fresh water and in activated sludge; barely visible sheaths not encrusted)

PART 4  BUDDING AND/OR APPENDAGED BACTERIA

   (soil and water bacteria reproducing by budding; may have excreted appendages and holdfasts; in some a semi-rigid appendage, the prostheca, proceeds out from the cell, like the stalk of *Caulobacter* genus, extending the length of the rod, a small bit of glue at its tip)

PART 5  SPIROCHETES

   Order I. *Spirochaetales*

      Family I. *Spirochaetaceae*

         Genus I. *Spirochaeta* (motile spirals in helical form, free-living in $H_2S$-containing mud and sewage)

         Genus II. *Cristispira* (spirals with 2 to 10 complete turns; commensal in mollusks)

         Genus III. *Treponema*

            *Treponema pallidum* (syphilis)

            *Treponema pertenue* (yaws)

            *Treponema carateum* (pinta, a chronic skin disease of children endemic in South and Central America)

            *Treponema denticola* [*microdentium*]

            *Treponema* [*Borrelia*] *vincentii*

            *Species incertae sedis: Treponema buccale* [*Borrelia buccalis*]

         Genus IV. *Borrelia*

            *Borrelia recurrentis* (louse-borne epidemic relapsing fever)

            *Borrelia* species (tick-borne endemic relapsing fever)

         Genus V. *Leptospira*

            *Leptospira interrogans* [*icterohaemorrhagiae*] (leptospirosis)

---

*Based on data from Buchanan, R. E., and Gibbons, N. E., co-editors: Bergey's manual of determinative bacteriology, ed. 8, Baltimore, 1974, The Williams & Wilkins Co.

†*Eucaryotae*, the corresponding taxon at the same level, includes other protists and the plants and animals.

‡Phototrophic or photosynthetic.

*Continued.*

**Table 1-1**

Abbreviated classification of microbes from *Bergey's Manual of Determinative Bacteriology* (1974)—cont'd

PART 6   SPIRAL AND CURVED BACTERIA

Family I. *Spirillaceae*

Genus I. *Spirillum*

*Spirillum minor* (one type of rat-bite fever in man)

Genus II. *Campylobacter* (slender spiral rods found in reproductive and alimentary tracts of man and animals; some species pathogenic)

*Campylobacter* [*Vibrio*] *fetus* (abortion in sheep and cattle, infections in man)

PART 7   GRAM-NEGATIVE AEROBIC RODS AND COCCI

Family I. *Pseudomonadaceae*

Genus I. *Pseudomonas*

*Pseudomonas aeruginosa* (wound, burn, and urinary tract infections)

*Pseudomonas* [*Actinobacillus*] *mallei* (glanders and farcy in horses and donkeys; infection transmissible to man)

*Pseudomonas pseudomallei* (human and animal melioidosis)

Genus II. *Xanthomonas* (plant pathogens)

Genus III. *Zoogloea* (motile, gram-negative rods in natural waters and sewage)

Genus IV. *Gluconobacter* (ellipsoids or rods in flowers, souring fruits, vegetables, cider, wine, baker's yeast, garden soil; ropiness in beer and wort)

Family II. *Azotobacteraceae* (large, motile, aerobic gram-negative rods fixing atmospheric nitrogen; found in soil and water and on leaf surfaces)

Genus I. *Azotobacter* (nitrogen fixation)

Genus II. *Azomonas* (nitrogen fixation)

Genus III. *Beijerinckia* (nitrogen fixation)

Genus IV. *Derxia* (found in tropical soils of Asia, Africa, South America; fixation of atmospheric nitrogen)

Family III. *Rhizobiaceae* (nitrogen fixation—symbionts in root nodules of legumes; cortical overgrowths in plants)

Genus I. *Rhizobium* (nitrogen fixation)

Genus II. *Agrobacterium* (plant pathogens—tumorigenic phytopathogens; hypertrophies [galls] on stems of more than 40 plants; free nitrogen not fixed; found in soil)

Family IV. *Methylomonadaceae* (gram-negative bacteria using only one-carbon organic compounds, e.g., methane and methanol, as carbon source)

Family V. *Halobacteriaceae* (high concentration of sodium chloride necessary for growth; found in salterns, salt lakes, Dead Sea, proteinaceous material preserved with solar salt, e.g., fish, sausage casings, and hides)

Genus I. *Halobacterium* (salt-living rods)

Genus II. *Halococcus* (halophilic cocci; red colonies)

Genera of uncertain affiliation

Genus *Alcaligenes* [*Achromobacter*] (motile, aerobic rods or cocci; common saprophytes in intestines of vertebrates, in dairy products, rotting eggs, fresh water, soil; important in decomposition and mineralization processes)

*Alcaligenes faecalis* (type species; some strains denitrify)

Genus *Acetobacter* (motile, aerobic vinegar rods; oxidize ethanol to acetic acid; found on fruits and vegetables, in souring fruit juices, vinegar, alcoholic beverages)

*Acetobacter aceti* (acetic acid bacterium)

Genus *Brucella* (brucellosis)

*Brucella melitensis* (Malta fever; infection in goats, sheep, and cattle)

*Brucella abortus* (abortion in cattle; disease in man)

*Brucella suis* (usually attacks pigs; also pathogenic for other animals, man)

Genus *Bordetella*

*Bordetella pertussis* (whooping cough)

*Bordetella parapertussis* (whooping cough)

*Bordetella bronchiseptica* (found in respiratory tract of animals, sometimes man; rodent bronchopneumonia)

Genus *Francisella*

*Francisella* [*Pasteurella*] *tularensis* (tularemia)

*Francisella novicida* (experimental pathogen)

Genus *Thermus* (gram-negative, nonmotile rods and filaments; often pigmented; common in hot springs, hot water tanks, and thermally polluted rivers; unusually thermostable enzymes, ribosomes, plasma membrane)

PART 8  GRAM-NEGATIVE FACULTATIVELY ANAEROBIC RODS
    Family I. *Enterobacteriaceae*
        Genus I. *Escherichia*
            *Escherichia coli* (type species; the colon bacillus; important opportunistic pathogen)
        Genus II. *Edwardsiella*
            *Edwardsiella tarda* (type species)
        Genus III. *Citrobacter*
            *Citrobacter freundii* (type species)
        Genus IV. *Salmonella* (salmonellosis)
        Subgenus I
            *Salmonella cholerae-suis* (type species; salmonellosis)
            *Salmonella hirschfeldii* (paratyphoid C bacillus; enteritis)
            *Salmonella typhi* (typhoid fever)
            *Salmonella paratyphi-A* (paratyphoid [enteric] fever)
            *Salmonella schottmuelleri* (enteritis)
            *Salmonella typhimurium* (food-poisoning in man)
            *Salmonella enteritidis* (enteritis)
            *Salmonella gallinarum* (fowl typhoid)
        Subgenus II
            *Salmonella salamae*
        Subgenus III
            *Salmonella arizonae* (isolated from reptiles)
        Subgenus IV
            *Salmonella houtenae*
        Genus V. *Shigella* (shigellosis)
            *Shigella dysenteriae* (type species; bacillary dysentery plus effects of diffusible neurotoxin)
            *Shigella flexneri* (bacillary dysentery)
            *Shigella boydii* (bacillary dysentery)
            *Shigella sonnei* (one cause of summer diarrhea in young children; milder form of bacillary dysentery in adults)
        Genus VI. *Klebsiella*
            *Klebsiella pneumoniae* (type species; pneumonia, infections of respiratory and urinary tracts)
            *Klebsiella ozaenae* (found in ozena and chronic respiratory disease)
            *Klebsiella rhinoscleromatis* (found in rhinoscleroma, a granulomatous disorder of nose and pharynx associated with nodular induration of tissues)
        Genus VII. *Enterobacter*
            *Enterobacter cloacae* (type species)
            *Enterobacter [Aerobacter] aerogenes*
        Genus VIII. *Hafnia* (Hafnia, the old name for Copenhagen)
        Genus IX. *Serratia*
            *Serratia marcescens* (type species)
        Genus X. *Proteus* (urinary tract infections, community and hospital-acquired)
            *Proteus vulgaris* (type species; urinary tract and wound infections, rarely peritonitis, meningitis)
            *Proteus mirabilis* (most commonly encountered species in clinical specimens)
            *Proteus morganii* (one cause of summer diarrhea in infants)
            *Proteus rettgeri* (gastroenteritis)
            *Proteus [Providencia] inconstans* (urinary tract infections)
        Genus XI. *Yersinia*
            *Yersinia [Pasteurella] pestis* (plague)
            *Yersinia [Pasteurella] pseudotuberculosis* (pseudotuberculosis in animals—usually mesenteric lymphadenitis; septicemia in man)
            *Yersinia enterocolitica* (widespread; been found in sick and healthy animals and in material likely contaminated by their feces; enterocolitis in young children, mesenteric lymphadenitis, variety of other infections)
        Genus XII. *Erwinia* (plant pathogens)

*Continued.*

## Table 1-1

Abbreviated classification of microbes from *Bergey's Manual of Determinative Bacteriology* (1974)—cont'd

PART 8   GRAM-NEGATIVE FACULTATIVELY ANAEROBIC RODS—cont'd

Family II. *Vibrionaceae*

Genus I. *Vibrio*

*Vibrio cholerae* [*comma*] (type species; cholera)

*Vibrio cholerae* biotype *eltor* (El Tor vibrio; cholera)

*Vibrio parahaemolyticus* (acute gastroenteritis)

*Vibrio* [*Photobacterium*] *fischeri* (luminescent saltwater bacteria)

Genus II. *Aeromonas* (motile gas-forming rods)

*Aeromonas hydrophila* (type species; nonluminescent freshwater bacteria; infections of cold-blooded animals—red leg [bacteremia] in frogs and septicemia in snakes—and, rarely, infections in compromised host)

Genus III. *Plesiomonas* (motile rods growing mostly on mineral media containing ammonia as sole source of nitrogen and glucose as sole source of carbon; found in feces; infectious gastroenteritis reported in man)

Genus IV. *Photobacterium* (luminescent saltwater bacteria)

Genus V. *Lucibacterium* (light-emitting bacteria; luminescent saltwater bacilli; found on surfaces of dead fish)

Genera of uncertain affiliation

Genus *Chromobacterium* (soil and water bacteria producing violet pigment violacein; infections in animals; food spoilage)

Genus *Flavobacterium* (proteolytic soil and water bacteria producing yellow, orange, or red pigments; found on vegetables and in dairy products; rare infection in man by unpigmented organism)

Genus *Haemophilus*

*Haemophilus influenzae* (purulent meningitis in young children; acute respiratory infection; acute conjunctivitis)

*Haemophilus suis* (with virus, causes swine influenza)

*Haemophilus haemolyticus* (commensal in upper respiratory tract of man)

*Haemophilus parainfluenzae* (found in upper respiratory tract of man and cats)

*Haemophilus parahemolyticus* (found in upper respiratory tract of man; associated with acute pharyngitis in man; pleuropneumonia and septicemia in swine)

*Haemophilus aphrophilus* (endocarditis and other infections in man)

*Haemophilus ducreyi* (chancroid)

*Species incertae sedis*

*Haemophilus aegyptius* (Koch-Weeks bacillus; acute infectious conjunctivitis)

*Haemophilus vaginalis* (gram-variable bacilli and coccobacilli, showing metachromatic granules and arranged like *Corynebacterium*, found in human genital tract; nonspecific vaginitis and urethritis)

Genus *Pasteurella*

*Pasteurella multocida* (type species; chicken cholera; shipping fever of cattle; hemorrhagic septicemia in warm-blooded animals; in cat- and dog-bite wound infections)

*Pasteurella pneumotropica* (infections in animals; dog-bite wounds in man)

*Pasteurella haemolytica* (enzootic pneumonia of sheep and cattle; septicemia of lambs)

Genus *Actinobacillus* (actinobacillosis)

*Actinobacillus lignieresii* (actinobacillosis of cattle [wooden tongue] and of sheep)

*Actinobacillus equuli* (actinobacillosis in horses and pigs)

Genus *Cardiobacterium*

*Cardiobacterium hominis* (type species; found in human nose and throat; endocarditis in man)

Genus *Streptobacillus* [*Haverhillia*] (rods and filaments in chains, with filaments showing bulbous swellings, like a string of beads; parasites and pathogens of rats and other mammals)

*Streptobacillus moniliformis* [*Actinomyces muris-ratti*] (type species; necklace-shaped bacteria found in nasopharynx of rats; streptobacillary rat-bite fever)

Genus *Calymmatobacterium* (pleomorphic encapsulated rods like safety pins)

*Calymmatobacterium* [*Donovania*] *granulomatis* (granuloma inguinale)

PART 9   GRAM-NEGATIVE ANAEROBIC BACTERIA

Family I. *Bacteroidaceae*

Genus I. *Bacteroides* (bacteroidosis)

*Bacteroides fragilis* (type species; opportunist in visceral and wound infections; most common anaerobe in soft tissue infections)

*Bacteroides oralis* (gingival crevice of man; oral, upper respiratory, and genital infections)

*Bacteroides* [*Eikenella*] *corrodens* (part of normal flora of man and animals; opportunist in infections of respiratory and alimentary tracts)

*Bacteroides melaninogenicus* (brown to black pigment on blood agar; opportunist in infections of mouth, soft tissue, and respiratory, alimentary, and urogenital tracts)

Genus II. *Fusobacterium* (purulent or gangrenous infections)

*Fusobacterium nucleatum* (type species; wound and respiratory tract infections)

*Fusobacterium varium* (wound and serous cavity infections; intestinal contents of roaches, termites)

*Fusobacterium necrophorum* [*Sphaerophorus necrophorus*] (abscesses of man and animals)

*Fusobacterium mortiferum* (visceral abscesses and septicemia in man)

Genus III. *Leptotrichia* (oral cavity of man; not known as pathogen but found in clinical material)

*Leptotrichia buccalis* (type species)

Genera of uncertain affiliation

Genus *Butyrivibrio* (many members; biochemically versatile in rumen of most ruminants and in intestinal tract of other mammals)

Genus *Selenomonas* (gastrointestinal tract of mammals; dirty river water)

PART 10 GRAM-NEGATIVE COCCI AND COCCOBACILLI [AEROBES]

Family I. *Neisseriaceae*

Genus I. *Neisseria* (parasites of mucous membranes of mammals)

*Neisseria gonorrhoeae* (type species; gonorrhea)

*Neisseria meningitidis* (epidemic cerebrospinal fever)

*Neisseria sicca* (nasopharynx of man)

*Neisseria subflava* [*flava*] [*perflava*] (yellowish green pigment; nasopharynx of man)

*Neisseria flavescens* (xanthophil pigment)

*Neisseria mucosa* (rhinopharynx of man)

Genus II. *Branhamella* (parasites of mammalian mucous membranes)

*Branhamella* [*Neisseria*] *catarrhalis* (venereal discharges; catarrhal inflammations)

Genus III. *Moraxella* (parasites of mucous membranes of man and warm-blooded animals)

*Moraxella lacunata* (pink-eye—conjunctivitis)

Genus *Acinetobacter* (opportunist pathogens)

*Acinetobacter calcoaceticus* [*Herellea vaginicola*, acid-forming] [*Mima polymorpha*, nonacidforming] (type species; soil and water bacteria; pathogenicity uncertain)

PART 11 GRAM-NEGATIVE ANAEROBIC COCCI

Family I. *Veillonellaceae* (alimentary tract parasites of man, ruminants, rodents, and pigs)

Genus I. *Veillonella* (oral microflora; intestinal and respiratory tracts of man and animals)

*Veillonella parvula* (type species; oral microflora)

*Veillonella alcalescens* (oral microflora)

Genus II. *Acidaminococcus* (amino acid cocci—amino acids sole energy source; intestinal tract of man and pigs)

Genus III. *Megasphaera* (large cocci; rumen of cattle and sheep)

PART 12 GRAM-NEGATIVE CHEMOLITHOTROPHIC BACTERIA

a. Organisms oxidizing ammonia or nitrite

Family I. *Nitrobacteraceae* (soil and water bacteria converting ammonia to nitrite, nitrite to nitrate, and fixing carbon dioxide; nitrifying bacteria—one group oxidizes ammonia, the other nitrite)

Genus I. *Nitrobacter* (nitrate rods oxidizing nitrite to nitrate)

Genus II. *Nitrospina* (nitrate spines oxidizing nitrite to nitrate; straight, slender rods found in South Atlantic Ocean)

Genus III. *Nitrococcus* (nitrate spheres—spherical, yellowish to red cells oxidizing nitrite to nitrate; found in South Pacific Ocean)

Genus IV. *Nitrosomonas* (ellipsoidal, yellowish to red bacteria oxidizing ammonia to nitrite)

Genus V. *Nitrosospira* (nitrous spirals, yellowish to red, oxidizing ammonia to nitrite)

Genus VI. *Nitrosococcus* (nitrous spheres—spherical cells oxidizing ammonia to nitrite)

Genus VII. *Nitrosolobus* (nitrite-producing lobes; pleomorphic and lobate, yellowish to red bacteria oxidizing nitrite to nitrate; found in soils from South America, Southwest Africa, and Russia)

b. Organisms metabolizing sulfur and sulfur compounds*

Genus 1. *Thiobacillus* (sulfur rodlets—small rods in soil, sea water, fresh water, acid mine water, sewage, sulfur springs, and near sulfur deposits or where hydrogen sulfide produced)

---

*All the sulfur-metabolizing genera have not been grown in pure culture. Until then, Bergey's Manual considers them all as of uncertain affiliation.

*Continued.*

**Table 1-1**

Abbreviated classification of microbes from *Bergey's Manual of Determinative Bacteriology* (1974)—cont'd

PART 12 GRAM-NEGATIVE CHEMOLITHOTROPHIC BACTERIA—cont'd

   b. Organisms metabolizing sulfur and sulfur compounds—cont'd

      Genus 2. *Sulfolobus* (lobed sulfur-oxidizing organisms resembling mycoplasmas in solfatara areas containing hot acid environments, both soil and water)

      Genus 3. *Thiobacterium* (small sulfur rods near surface of sulfurous brackish and marine waters)

      Genus 4. *Macromonas* (large cylindrical or bean-shaped cells in fresh waters)

      Genus 5. *Thiovulum* (small sulfur egglike cells—cytoplasm at one end of cell, a large vacuole at the other—found in fresh and sea waters where sulfide-containing waters contact oxygen-containing waters)

      Genus 6. *Thiospira* (sulfur spirals in waters overlaying sulfurous muds)

   c. Organisms depositing iron and/or manganese oxides

      Family *Siderocapsaceae* (iron bacteria of iron-bearing waters)

      Genus I. *Siderocapsa* (iron bacteria of fresh water; may be attached to surface of water plants)

      Genus II. *Naumanniella* (encapsulated rods; capsule encrusted with iron compounds and manganese oxide; widespread in iron-bearing waters)

      Genus III. *Ochrobium* (bacteria yellowish from iron oxides; widespread in fresh waters bearing iron)

      Genus IV. *Siderococcus* (iron cocci in fresh water and mud)

PART 13 METHANE-PRODUCING BACTERIA

      Family I. *Methanobacteriaceae* (gram-positive or gram-negative rods or cocci, very strict anaerobes, motile or nonmotile, in a highly specialized physiologic group; to gain energy for growth, they reduce carbon dioxide forming methane (Fig. 1-1) or ferment such compounds as acetate and methanol; widespread in nature in anaerobic habitats—sediments of natural waters, soil, anaerobic sewage digestors, and gastrointestinal tract of animals and man)

      Genus I. *Methanobacterium* (methane-producing rodlets)

      Genus II. *Methanosarcina* (methane-producing sarcinae—large spherical cells in regular packets)

      Genus III. *Methanococcus* (methane cocci)

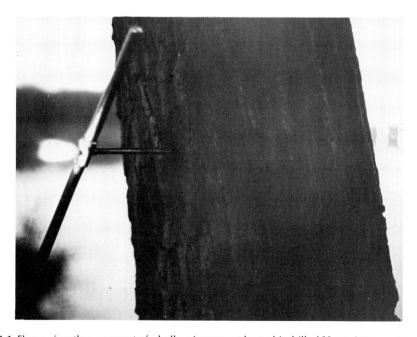

**Fig. 1-1.** Flame of methane gas out of a hollow increment borer bit drilled 20 cm. into a cottonwood growing on shore of Lake Wingra, Wisconsin. (Timed exposure at night.) (From Zeikus, J. G., and Ward, J. C.: Science **184:**1181, 1974. Copyright 1974 by the American Association for the Advancement of Science.)

PART 14  GRAM-POSITIVE COCCI
  a.  Aerobic and/or facultatively anaerobic
      Family I. *Micrococcaceae* (saprophytes and important pathogens; normal occupants of human skin and associated structures)
          Genus I. *Micrococcus* (small aerobic cocci; common in soil and fresh water and on skin of man and animals)
              *Micrococcus luteus* [*Sarcina lutea*] (type species; golden yellow pigment produced; pattern of tetrads)
          Genus II. *Staphylococcus* (primary relation to skin and mucous membranes of warm-blooded animals; wide host range; important pathogenic strains)
              *Staphylococcus aureus* (type species; type lesion: the abscess)
              *Staphylococcus epidermidis* (normal occupant of skin and mucosae of man; opportunist in stitch abscesses and other wound infections)
          Genus III. *Planococcus* (motile cocci in sea water)
              *Planococcus citreus* (type species; yellowish orange pigment produced)
      Family II. *Streptococcaceae* (saprophytic and pathogenic bacteria in chains)
          Genus I. *Streptococcus*
              *Streptococcus pyogenes* (many types of infection, usually of diffuse or spreading nature [cellulitis])
              *Streptococcus equisimilis* (upper respiratory tract infections in man and animals; erysipelas and puerperal fever)
              *Streptococcus zooepidemicus* (septicemia of cows, rabbits, and swine; wound infections of horses)
              *Streptococcus equi* (strangles in horses)
              *Streptococcus dysgalactiae* (mastitis in cows; polyarthritis, or joint-ill, in lambs)
              *Streptococcus* [*Diplococcus*] *pneumoniae* (lobar pneumonia, bronchopneumonia)
              *Streptococcus anginosus* (varied infections; alpha- and gamma-hemolytic strains formerly known as *Streptococcus* Mg relate to primary atypical pneumonia)
              *Streptococcus agalactiae* (mastitis of cows; human infections)
              *Streptococcus salivarius* (tongue, saliva, and feces of man)
              [*Streptococcus mutans*] (dental caries)
              *Streptococcus mitis* (human saliva, sputum, feces)
              *Streptococcus bovis* (alimentary canal of cows, sheep, and other ruminants)
              *Streptococcus equinus* (alimentary tract of horses)
              *Streptococcus thermophilus* (in milk and milk products; starter culture for Swiss cheese and yogurt)
              *Streptococcus faecalis* (enterococcus in intestine of man and warm-blooded animals; urinary tract infections, endocarditis)
              *Streptococcus lactis* (important in dairy industry, some strains starter cultures in manufacture of cheese and cultured milk drinks)
              *Streptococcus cremoris* (raw milk and milk products)
          Genus II. *Leuconostoc* (colorless nostoc; saprophytes found in slimy sugar solutions, on fruits and vegetables, in milk and dairy products)
              *Leuconostoc mesenteroides* (type species; used in industrial fermentation)
          Genus III. *Pediococcus* (microaerophilic saprophytes in fermenting plant material, especially spoiled beer)
          Genus IV. *Aerococcus* (microaerophilic saprophytes widely distributed in air, in meat brines, on raw and processed vegetables)
  b.  Anaerobic
      Family III. *Peptococcaceae* (occupants of alimentary and respiratory tracts of man and animals and of normal human female genital tract; found in soil and on surface of cereal grains; lesions of human female genitalia)
          Genus I. *Peptococcus* (lesions of viscera and serous cavities; postpartum septicemia; black colonies seen among species)
              *Peptococcus niger* (type species)
          Genus II. *Peptostreptococcus* (puerperal fever, pyogenic infections, septic war wounds, osteomyelitis, pleurisy, gangrene, sinusitis, dental infection, vulvovaginitis)
          Genus III. *Ruminococcus* (in rumen and cecum and colon of animals—important there in fermentation of cellulose)
          Genus IV. *Sarcina* (nearly spherical cells in packets of eight or more; found in soil, mud, surface of cereal seeds, and stomach contents of man and animals)

*Continued.*

## Table 1-1
Abbreviated classification of microbes from *Bergey's Manual of Determinative Bacteriology* (1974)—cont'd

PART 15  ENDOSPORE-FORMING RODS AND COCCI
Family I. *Bacillaceae* (saprophytic gram-positive rods, mostly; endospore formation dominant feature in defining genera)
Genus I. *Bacillus* (genus of great diversity in properties of members; several species produce antibiotics, some strains more than one; because of pattern of spore formation in nature, few species have distinctive habitats)
*Bacillus subtilis* (type species; endospores widespread, may even be in heat-treated surgical dressings and canned foods; some strains produce antibiotics)
*Bacillus licheniformis* (source of bacitracin; spores with high heat tolerance)
*Bacillus cereus* (found in foods)
*Bacillus anthracis* (anthrax)
*Bacillus thuringiensis* (microbial insecticide)
*Bacillus polymyxa* (source of polymyxin; participates in retting of flax)
*Bacillus stearothermophilus* (thermophilic; endospores highly resistant to heat)
*Bacillus brevis* (source of tyrothricin)
Genus II. *Sporolactobacillus* (bacteria like *Lactobacillus,* but sporeforming)
Genus III. *Clostridium* (strict anaerobes, motile rods; soil and water bacteria; occupants of intestinal tract of man and animals)
*Clostridium butyricum* (type species; soil, animal feces, cheese, naturally soured milk)
*Clostridium beijerinckii* (wound infections)
*Clostridium sporogenes* (wound infections; low-grade bacteremia in debilitated patients)
*Clostridium botulinum* (potent exotoxin causes botulism)
*Clostridium histolyticum* (wound infections)
*Clostridium novyi* (gas gangrene)
*Clostridium perfringens* [*Bacterium welchii*] (gas gangrene)
*Clostridium septicum* (gas gangrene)
*Clostridium tertium* (wound infections, low-grade bacteremia in debilitated patients)
*Clostridium tetani* (potent exotoxin causes tetanus)
Genus IV. *Desulfotomaculum* (sausage-shaped bacteria reducing sulfur; strict anaerobes; common soil and water saprophytes)
Genus V. *Sporosarcina* (sporeforming spherical cells; strict aerobes)
PART 16  GRAM-POSITIVE, ASPOROGENOUS, ROD-SHAPED BACTERIA
Family I. *Lactobacillaceae* (rods, nonmotile, anaerobic or facultative, highly saccharoclastic; unusual as pathogens; found in fermenting animal and plant products)
Genus I. *Lactobacillus* (found in dairy products and effluents, grain and meat products, water, sewage, beer, wine, fruits, fruit juices, pickled vegetables, sourdough, mash; some species in tooth decay)
*Lactobacillus delbrueckii* (type species; fermenting grain and vegetable mashes)
*Lactobacillus leichmannii* (compressed yeast, grain mash)
*Lactobacillus lactis* (milk, cheese; starter cultures in manufacture of cheese)
*Lactobacillus bulgaricus* (in sour milks, as yogurt)
*Lactobacillus acidophilus* (feces of infants, mouth and vagina of young human adults)
*Lactobacillus casei* (milk, cheese, dairy products, sourdough, cow dung, silage, human alimentary tract and vagina)
*Lactobacillus brevis* (milk, kefir, cheese, sauerkraut, sourdough, soils, ensilage)
Genera of uncertain affiliation
Genus *Listeria* (listeriosis)
*Listeria monocytogenes* (type species; listeriosis in man and animals)
Genus *Erysipelothrix* (parasites of mammals, birds, fish; widespread in nature)
*Erysipelothrix rhusiopathiae* [*insidiosa*] (type species; swine erysipelas, erysipeloid in man)
PART 17  ACTINOMYCETES AND RELATED ORGANISMS
Coryneform group of bacteria [not a recognized family]
Genus I. *Corynebacterium*
Section I. Human and animal parasites and pathogens (club bacteria, nonsporing, gram-positive, irregular rods; widespread in nature)
*Corynebacterium diphtheriae* (type species; diphtheria—the effect of a highly lethal exotoxin)
*Corynebacterium pseudotuberculosis* (pseudotuberculosis; chronic purulent infections in warm-blooded animals, rarely in man)
*Corynebacterium xerosis* (harmless occupant of conjunctiva; nontoxigenic)
*Corynebacterium kutscheri* (parasite and opportunist pathogen of mice and rats)

*Corynebacterium pseudodiphtheriticum* (normal in throat of man; nontoxigenic)

*Corynebacterium equi* (pneumonia of horses; nontoxigenic)

    Section II. Plant pathogenic corynebacteria

    Section III. Nonpathogenic corynebacteria (soil, water, air)

  Genus II. *Arthrobacter* (jointed gram-positive rods, strict aerobes; among dominant soil bacteria)

*Genera incertae sedis*

*Brevibacterium* (coryneform bacteria found in water, soil, dairy products, insects; widespread in nature, sewage; many of industrial import)

*Microbacterium* (small diphtheroid rods with rounded ends; found in dairy products)

  Genus III. *Cellulomonas* (coryneform bacteria with ability to attack cellulose)

  Genus IV. *Kurthia* (coryneform bacteria in fresh and putrefying meats and meat products and on working surfaces in meat plants)

Family I. *Propionibacteriaceae* (gram-positive, nonsporeforming, anaerobic, pleomorphic rods; saccharolytic members; found in skin, respiratory and alimentary tracts of most animals; some members in soft tissue infections)

  Genus I. *Propionibacterium* (nonmotile, anaerobic to aerotolerant bacteria producing propionic and acetic acids; some pathogens here)

*Propionibacterium freudenreichii* (type species; raw milk, Swiss cheese, dairy products)

*Propionibacterium [Corynebacterium] acnes* (soft tissue abscesses, wound infections; common laboratory contaminant)

  Genus II. *Eubacterium* (motile or nonmotile, obligately anaerobic rods; found in cavities of man and animals, in plant products, soil; infections of soft tissues)

*Eubacterium foedans* (dental tartar; varied infections)

Order I. *Actinomycetales* (gram-positive bacteria, mostly aerobic, forming branching filaments, which in some families develop into mycelium; some members acid-alcohol-fast; found in soil; some members pathogenic to man and animals and to plants; some species fix nitrogen as obligate symbionts in plant root nodule)

Family I. *Actinomycetaceae* (diphtheroid bacteria; no mycelium, nonacid-fast, usually facultative anaerobes; branching filaments)

  Genus I. *Actinomyces* (actinomycosis)

*Actinomyces bovis* (type species; lumpy jaw in cattle)

*Actinomyces israelii* (human actinomycosis)

*Actinomyces naeslundii* (oral cavity of man—in tonsillar crypts and dental calculus)

  Genus II. *Arachnia* (branched diphtheroid rods; gram-positive, nonacid-fast pathogens)

*Arachnia propionica* (type species; human actinomycosis)

  Genus III. *Bifidobacterium* (bifid bacteria; highly variable rods, gram-positive, nonacid-fast)

*Bifidobacterium bifidum [Lactobacillus bifidus]* (stools and alimentary tract of breast-fed and bottle-fed infants, and adults)

  Genus IV. *Bacterionema* (thread-shaped bacteria: "whip handle" cells, with filamentous branching morphology, nonacid-fast; on teeth and in oral cavity, especially in calculus and plaque deposits)

  Genus V. *Rothia* (gram-positive, nonacid-fast aerobes with filamentous branching morphology; common in normal mouth and throat)

Family II. *Mycobacteriaceae* (important acid-fast bacteria, parasitic and saprophytic; branching inconspicuous)

  Genus I. *Mycobacterium* (mycobacteriosis, chronic granulomatous disease of varied forms, tuberculosis)

*Mycobacterium tuberculosis* (human tuberculosis)

*Mycobacterium bovis* (tuberculosis in cattle, man)

*Mycobacterium kansasii* (yellow bacillus, Group I photochromogen; chronic pulmonary disease similar to tuberculosis)

*Mycobacterium marinum* (tuberculosis of saltwater fish, swimming pool granulomas in man)

*Mycobacterium scrofulaceum* (scrofula scotochromogen; suppurative cervical lymphadenitis in children)

*Mycobacterium intracellulare* (Battey bacillus; severe chronic pulmonary disease in man)

*Mycobacterium avium* (tuberculosis in birds)

*Mycobacterium ulcerans* (skin ulcers in man)

*Mycobacterium phlei* (timothy bacillus, hay bacillus; widespread in nature)

*Mycobacterium smegmatis* (smegma)

*Mycobacterium fortuitum* (mycobacteriosis in animals and in man; found in soil)

*Mycobacterium paratuberculosis* (Johne's disease in cattle and sheep)

*Myocobacterium leprae* (leprosy)

*Mycobacterium lepraemurium* (rat leprosy)

*Continued.*

**Table 1-1**

Abbreviated classification of microbes from *Bergey's Manual of Determinative Bacteriology* (1974)—cont'd

PART 17 ACTINOMYCETES AND RELATED ORGANISMS—cont'd

Order I. *Actinomycetales–cont'd*

Family III. *Frankiaceae* (symbiotic filamentous, mycelium-forming bacteria, which induce and live in root nodules of a wide variety of plants; nodules can fix molecular nitrogen)

Genus I. *Frankia* (characteristic root nodules formed and inhabited by bacteria; also free state in soil)

Family IV. *Actinoplanaceae* (soil bacteria; distinctive mycelium; shape of sporangia and spore structure make the division into genera)

Genus I. *Actinoplanes* (globose spores)

Genus II. *Spirillospora* (spiral spores)

Genus III. *Streptosporangium* (spores coiled within a sporangium)

Genus IV. *Amorphosporangium* (irregularly shaped sporangia)

Genus V. *Ampullariella* (bottle-shaped sporangia)

Genus VI. *Pilimelia* (rod-shaped spores, end to end in parallel chains; about 1000 per sporangium)

Genus VII. *Planomonospora* (single, large, motile spore in each sporangium)

Genus VIII. *Planobispora* (longitudinal pair of large spores in sporangium)

Genus IX. *Dactylosporangium* (finger-shaped sporangium)

Genus X. *Kitasatoa* (sporangia club-shaped; motile spores in single chain within sporangium)

Family V. *Dermatophilaceae* (nonacid-fast, gram-positive organisms; skin lesions of mammals)

Genus I. *Dermatophilus* (characteristic mycelium; skin pathogens)

Genus II. *Geodermatophilus* (rudimentary mycelium, tuber-shaped thallus; soil organisms)

Family VI. *Nocardiaceae* (nocardiosis; gram-positive aerobic actinomycetes; mycelium rudimentary or extensive; spore production variable)

Genus I. *Nocardia* (acid-fast to partially acid-fast, gram-positive, obligate aerobes; some strains pigmented; found in soil)

*Nocardia brasiliensis* (mycetoma)

*Nocardia asteroides* (pulmonary nocardiosis, chronic subcutaneous abscesses, mycetomas)

Genus II. *Pseudonocardia* (false nocardia; soil organisms, nonacid-fast)

Family VII. *Streptomycetaceae* (gram-positive, aerobic, primarily soil forms; well-developed branched mycelium and special spores for multiplication; many species important in production of antibiotics)

Genus I. *Streptomyces* (about 500 distinctive antibiotics from this genus; many members produce one or more antibacterial, antifungal, antialgal, antiviral, antiprotozoal or antitumor antibiotics [see Table 16-2, p. 155, for examples]; around 500 well-defined species listed)

Genus II. *Streptoverticillium* (whorled actinomycetes)

Genus III. *Sporichthya* (spores motile in water)

Genus IV. *Microellobosporia* (small spores in a pod)

Family VIII. *Micromonosporaceae* (saprophytic soil forms)

Genus I. *Micromonospora* (well-developed, branched septate mycelium, small single spores; nonacid-fast proteolytic and cellulolytic organisms; some antibiotics found here)

*Micromonospora purpurea* (source of gentamicin complex)

Genus II. *Thermoactinomyces* (heat-loving ray "fungus")

Genus III. *Actinobifida* (ray "fungus" with bifurcations)

Genus IV. *Thermomonospora* (heat-loving, single-spored organisms)

Genus V. *Microbispora* (small, two-spored organisms)

Genus VI. *Micropolyspora* (small, many-spored organisms)

PART 18 RICKETTSIAS

Order I. *Rickettsiales* (procaryotic microbes; parasitic forms related to reticuloendothelial and vascular endothelial cells or erythrocytes of vertebrates; mutualistic forms in insects; arthropods vectors or primary hosts; disease in vertebrates and invertebrates)

Family I. *Rickettsiaceae* (intracellular parasites of tissue cells, not erythrocytes; arthropod vectors important)

Tribe I. *Rickettsieae* (adaptation to existence in arthropods but can infect vertebrate hosts; man usually incidental host)

Genus I. *Rickettsia* (human pathogens; growth in cytoplasm, sometimes in nucleus, not in vacuoles of cells; not cultivated in cell-free media)

*Rickettsia prowazekii* (type species; typhus fever—man the reservoir)

*Rickettsia typhi* (murine typhus)

*Rickettsia canada* (human disease ?)

*Rickettsia rickettsii* (Rocky Mountain spotted fever)

*Rickettsia sibirica* (Siberian tick typhus)

*Rickettsia conorii* (fièvre boutonneuse and tick-bite fever)

*Rickettsia australis* (Queensland tick typhus)

*Rickettsia akari* (rickettsialpox)

*Rickettsia tsutsugamushi* (scrub typhus)

Genus II. *Rochalimaea* (like *Rickettsia* genus, but usually in extracellular position in arthropod host; can be cultured in host cell–free media)

*Rochalimaea quintana* (type species; trench fever—man primary host)

Genus III. *Coxiella* (growth in vacuoles of host cell; highly resistant outside cells)

*Coxiella burnetii* (type species; Q fever)

Tribe II. *Ehrlichieae* (minute rickettsia-like organisms; only few species; adapted to invertebrate existence; pathogens of mammals but not man)

Genus IV. *Ehrlichia* (tick-borne diseases of dogs, cattle, sheep, goats, horses)

Genus V. *Cowdria* (heartwater diseases of domestic ruminants)

Genus VI. *Neorickettsia* (helminth-borne disease of dogs, wolves, jackals, foxes)

Tribe III. *Wolbachieae* (symbionts in arthropods but not in vertebrates; miscellaneous group)

Genus VII. *Wolbachia* (associated with arthropods—seldom pathogenic for hosts)

Genus VIII. *Symbiotes* (symbiotic in insect host)

Genus IX. *Blattabacterium* (symbiotic in cockroaches)

Genus X. *Rickettsiella* (pathogenic for insect larva and other insect hosts)

Family II. *Bartonellaceae* (intracellular parasites, sometimes extracellular, in or on red blood cells of vertebrates; arthropod transmission; cultivatable on cell-free media)

Genus I. *Bartonella* (occur in or on erythrocytes and within fixed tissue cells; often have flagella; found in man and sandfly *Phlebotomus*)

*Bartonella bacilliformis* (Oroya fever, verruga peruana)

Genus II. *Grahamella* (intra-erythrocytic; no flagella; not multiply in fixed tissue cells; not found in man; grahamellosis of rodents and other mammals)

Family III. *Anaplasmataceae* (very small, viruslike particles within or on red blood cells of vertebrates; anemia main feature of disease; arthropod transmission)

Genus I. *Anaplasma* (parasites form inclusions in red cells—no appendages; anaplasmosis of ruminants)

Genus II. *Paranaplasma* (no appendages to parasitic inclusions; infections in cattle)

Genus III. *Aegyptianella* (inclusions in red cells; aegyptianellosis in birds)

Genus IV. *Haemobartonella* (parasites within or outside erythrocytes, ring forms rare; pathogens in rodents, dogs, cats)

Genus V. *Eperythrozoon* (parasites on red cells and in plasma; ring forms common; infections in various animals)

Order II. *Chlamydiales* (gram-negative parasites of vertebrates, causing various diseases; obligately intracellular reproduction typical)

Family I. *Chlamydiaceae*

Genus I. *Chlamydia [Bedsonia]* (parasites of tissue cells of vertebrates; three ecological niches: (a) man—oculourogenital and respiratory diseases; (b) birds—respiratory and generalized diseases; and (c) mammals (not primates)—respiratory, placental, arthritic, enteric diseases)

*Chlamydia trachomatis* (trachoma, inclusion conjunctivitis, lymphopathia venereum, urethritis, proctitis in man)

*Chlamydia psittaci* (ornithosis and psittacosis in birds; pneumonitis in cattle, sheep, goats; polyarthritis in sheep, cattle, pigs; placentitis in cattle and sheep)

PART 19  MYCOPLASMAS

Class *Mollicutes* (procaryotes lacking true cell wall; sometimes ultramicroscopic; saprophytes, parasites, or pathogens for animals, possibly arthropod-borne plant pathogens)

Order I. *Mycoplasmatales*

Family I. *Mycoplasmataceae* (sterol required for growth)

Genus I. *Mycoplasma* (pleuropneumonia group; tiny, very pleomorphic, delicate saprophytes and pathogens)

*Mycoplasma mycoides* (type species; contagious pleuropneumonia of cattle)

*Mycoplasma gallisepticum* (diseases in poultry)

*Mycoplasma neurolyticum* (rolling disease in mice and rats, epidemic conjunctivitis in mice; common in healthy as well as diseased mice)

*Mycoplasma pulmonis* (infectious catarrh and pneumonia of mice and rats)

*Mycoplasma canis* (inhabitants of upper respiratory and genital tracts of dogs)

*Mycoplasma hyorhinis* (arthritis in swine)

*Continued.*

**Table 1-1**

Abbreviated classification of microbes from *Bergey's Manual of Determinative Bacteriology* (1974)—cont'd

PART 19  MYCOPLASMAS—cont'd

Class *Mollicutes–cont'd*

  Order I. *Mycoplasmatales–cont'd*

    Family I. *Mycoplasmataceae–cont'd*

      Genus I. *Mycoplasma–cont'd*

        *Mycoplasma pneumoniae* (cold-hemagglutin–associated primary atypical pneumonia of man)

        *Mycoplasma agalactiae* (mastitis of animals)

        *Mycoplasma arthritidis* (purulent polyarthritis of rats)

        *Mycoplasma orale* [*pharyngis*] (common parasites of human oropharynx)

        *Mycoplasma salivarium* (gingival crevice of man; possible role in periodontal disease)

        *Mycoplasma hominis* (common parasites of lower genitourinary tract in humans; potential pathogens in postpartum fever and in pelvic inflammatory disease)

        *Mycoplasma fermentans* (possible role in rheumatoid arthritis)

        *Species incertae sedis:* "T-mycoplasmas" (common mucous membrane parasites in urogenital tract of man and animals)

    Family II. *Acholeplasmataceae* (sterol not required for growth)

      Genus I. *Acholeplasma* (free-living saprophytes; mammalian and avian parasites; wide host range; possible pathogens)

        *Acholeplasma laidlawii* (type species; saprophytes from sewage as well as parasites in animals)

---

fever—and the geographic area where first recognized.

Whether a term indicates a class, order, or family may be determined from its ending. Classes end in *etes,* orders end in *ales,* and families end in *aceae.* For instance, Phycomyc<u>etes</u> is the name of a class, Spirochaet<u>ales</u> is the name of an order, and Bacil<u>laceae</u> is the name of a family.

### CLASSIFICATION OF BACTERIA

The classification of bacteria is difficult. This applies both to the separation of bacteria into groups and to the placing of certain organisms into the proper group. Biologic classification is based largely on morphology, but the morphology of bacteria as a whole is so uniform that it is useful only in dividing bacteria into comparatively large groups. Shape has been an important factor in general classification, but for more exact identification such criteria as staining reactions, cultural characteristics, biochemical behavior, and immunologic differences must be used.

In this book we adhere to the scientific classification embodied in *Bergey's Manual of Determinative Bacteriology* with certain important exceptions. This is the one most generally accepted in the United States. Table 1-1 presents in abbreviated form an overall survey of Bergey's classification of the microorganisms designated as bacteria.*

Bacteria that live in or about the human body have been much more completely studied than have those from animals or source in nature. Of these, the ones producing disease are most familiar. Discussions in subsequent chapters will necessarily be limited largely to those microorganisms significantly related to human disease.

## Questions for review

1 What is biology? Microbiology?
2 State the purpose of health education.
3 Give the divisions of microbiology. Briefly define each.
4 List the basic units used to classify both animals and plants.
5 How is the scientific name of an animal or plant derived?
6 What is the difference between thallophytes and other plants? Do all forms of plant life contain chlorophyll?
7 Give the word ending that indicates reference to a class, order, or family. Carefully spell out three examples.
8 Make pertinent comments regarding classification of bacteria. What classification is most generally used at present?
9 What is the American Type Culture Collection?

**References on pp. 48 and 49.**

---

*The American Type Culture Collection, located outside Washington, D.C., in Rockville, Md. 20852, maintains and distributes for research or other purposes authentic cultures of practically all known microorganisms. This nonprofit, independent agency grew out of the Bacteriological Collection and Bureau for the Distribution of Bacterial Cultures, established in 1911, at the American Museum of Natural History in New York, N.Y. There are over 16,000 strains of bacteria, fungi, algae, protozoa, viruses, and animal cell lines in this collection. Each year it supplies thousands of cultures of bacteria, fungi, and viruses to industrial and educational institutions such as medical schools, breweries, wineries, oil companies, pharmaceutical houses, and food processors.

# CHAPTER 2
# The basic unit

## The cell

Every living thing, plant or animal, is made up of one or many cells. In the lowest forms of life the whole organism is but a single cell, one in which are carried on all the processes associated with life. Such is a *unicellular organism.* In the higher forms of life multiplied millions of cells arrange themselves into groups of different type cells in order to meet the varied physiologic needs of that organism. Such an organism with a division of labor is *multicellular.*

Regardless of how simple or complex the organism, the unit of structure is the *cell.* Cells are the bricks with which living organisms are built. Not only is the cell the structural unit, but it is also the operational unit. One living cell, be it ever so small, is a dynamic biologic unit, and the performance of the organism or of any of its parts is the sum of the functions of the constituent cells, acting singly or in groups. The science of the cell is *cytology.*

## Anatomy of the cell

**Protoplasm.** A cell is composed of a colorless, translucent, viscid substance of colloidal nature known as *protoplasm* (Greek, first formed) that forms the physicochemical basis of life. Protoplasm is a complex but dynamic system incorporating units of varying size, physical nature, and chemical composition. Although adapted to cells of specific types, protoplasm presents basic features in all cells. It is made up principally of water (up to 90%). Contained therein are inorganic mineral ions and organic chemical compounds of varying complexity and physiologic significance—proteins (including enzymes), carbohydrates, fats, nucleic acids (Table 2-1), hormones (usually either protein or lipid or derivatives), and vitamins (chemically heterogeneous compounds).

Certain of the organic compounds in the protoplasm of the cell have special biochemical significance in determining the form and biologic properties of the cell. Designated *macromolecules,* they are composed of organic chemical building blocks linked together in characteristic fashion. Important examples of protoplasmic macromolecules of the cell are certain carbohydrates (polysaccharides), proteins, enzymes, and nucleic acids. Most of the unique qualities of protoplasm stem from its contained macromolecules.

**Shape.** In keeping with their location inside the body of an organism and the work that they do, cells

**Table 2-1**
Outline of chief protoplasmic compounds

| | BIOCHEMICAL COMPOUNDS | | | |
|---|---|---|---|---|
| | CARBOHYDRATES | LIPIDS | PROTEINS | NUCLEIC ACIDS |
| Composition (building blocks) | Simple sugars, some with amino groups | Triglycerides of fatty acids<br>Phosphorus in phospholipids | Amino acids (at least 5 elements here); most complex; can be very large | Pentose nucleotides<br>Complex combinations with protein are nucleoproteins |
| Role in cell | Synthesis of cell wall<br>Essential fuel for all living organisms<br>Mostly found as glycogen (storage form of glucose) | Phospholipids important to cell membrane<br>Large part of energy needs met by these fuels | Most are enzymes<br>Synthesis of organelles and other parts of cell | DNA—primary function in heredity; the genetic code for cell structure and function<br>RNA—protein synthesis |

*1 in. = 2.5 cm.*
*review*

### Table 2-2
Equivalents in the metric system

| UNIT SYMBOL | SYMBOL | METER m. | CENTIMETER cm. | MILLIMETER mm. | MICRON $\mu$ | MILLIMICRON m$\mu$ | ANGSTROM Å |
|---|---|---|---|---|---|---|---|
| Meter | m. | 1.0 | 100.0 $10^2$ | 1000.0 $10^3$ | 1,000,000.0 $10^6$ | 1,000,000,000.0 $10^9$ | 10,000,000,000.0 $10^{10}$ |
| Centimeter | cm. | 0.01 $10^{-2}$ | 1.0 | 10.0 | 10,000.0 $10^4$ | 10,000,000.0 $10^7$ | 100,000,000.0 $10^8$ |
| Millimeter | mm. | 0.001 $10^{-3}$ | 0.1 $10^{-1}$ | 1.0 | 1000.0 $10^3$ | 1,000,000.0 $10^6$ | 10,000,000.0 $10^7$ |
| Micrometer | $\mu$m. | 0.000001 $10^{-6}$ | 0.0001 $10^{-4}$ | 0.001 $10^{-3}$ | 1.0 | 1000.0 $10^3$ | 10,000.0 $10^4$ |
| Nanometer | nm. | 0.000000001 $10^{-9}$ | 0.0000001 $10^{-7}$ | 0.000001 $10^{-6}$ | 0.001 $10^{-3}$ | 1.0 | 10.0 |
| Angstrom | Å | 0.0000000001 $10^{-10}$ | 0.00000001 $10^{-8}$ | 0.0000001 $10^{-7}$ | 0.0001 $10^{-4}$ | 0.1 $10^{-1}$ | 1.0 |

vary in shape, being spherical, oblong, columnar, six sided, or spindle shaped.

**Size.** Cells are of microscopic size, except the eggs of various animals (an ostrich egg is several inches around), striated muscle cells under certain conditions, and the cells of the pith, stem, and flesh of some pulpy fruits. Some cells are so small as to be barely visible with the highest magnification of the ordinary compound microscope.

For a living object of such small dimensions as the cell, a special unit of measurement is needed. For a long time this has been the micromillimeter, or *micron*, designated by the Greek letter mu ($\mu$). A micron is 1/1000 of a millimeter or 1/25,000 of an inch in length. (The paper on which this book is printed is about 100$\mu$ thick.) A *millimicron* (m$\mu$), a term also well known, is 1/1000 of a micron. Today many scientists prefer and are using the equivalent terms *micrometer* ($\mu$m.) for micron and *nanometer* (nm.) for millimicron. See Table 2-2 for metric equivalents. The average diameter of the human red blood cell is 7.5 $\mu$m. Cells show considerable variation in size, but most range in diameter from 10 to 100 $\mu$m. Individual variations in the size of multicellular organisms of the same species depend on the number, not the size, of their cells.

The information gained through the study of cells by the compound light microscope in a little over 100 years has contributed significantly to the development of modern medicine. However, the nature of light is such that it is not possible to get a clear image in the light microscope when the magnification of the object for study is greater than 2000 times. Hence

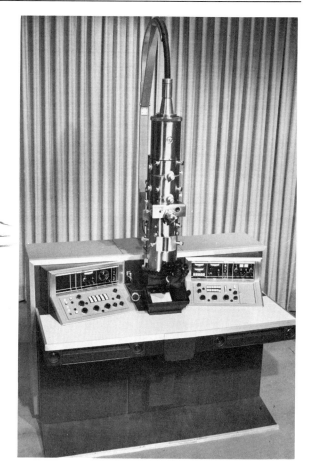

**Fig. 2-1.** Electron microscope. In this instrument, particles one ten-millionth of an inch in diameter may be visualized. (Courtesy Forglo Corp., Sunbury, Pa.)

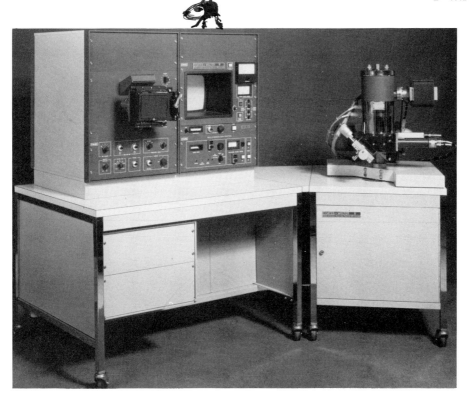

**Fig. 2-2.** Scanning electron microscope. (Courtesy Coates & Welter Instrument Corp., Sunnyvale, Calif.)

many minute (submicroscopic) structures within the cell were not visualized until the electron microscope was directed to cytologic study.

*Electron microscope* (Fig. 2-1). The electron microscope, one of our most powerful research tools, differs from the compound microscope. In the latter, rays of ordinary light pass from the object being examined to the eye to be focused there, whereas in the electron microscope, electrons pass through the specimen to be focused on a viewing screen from which a photograph is made—an *electron micrograph.* With the most modern electron microscopes the dimensions of the object under observation may be magnified 1 million times. If careful photographic technics are used, a further enlargement can be accomplished, so that today a magnification of several million times is possible. (With this magnification, a human hair viewed in its entirety in the electron microscope would appear twice the size of a California redwood.)

The *scanning* electron microscope (Fig. 2-2) provides a three-dimensional quality to study of specimens at magnifications up to 100,000 times actual size. It sweeps a very narrow beam of electrons back and forth across a specimen, revealing its surface features rather than its internal structure.

A unit even smaller than the micrometer must be

used in designating the size of objects too small to be visualized in the light microscope. This unit is the *angstrom* (Å). In Table 2-3 the sizes of *microscopic* and *ultramicroscopic* objects are compared. An ostrich egg and the mature human ovum are added to illustrate the magnitude of the size discrepancy.

**Structure.** If we magnify and examine a typical cell (Fig. 2-3), we see that there are two main parts. The central portion is occupied by a more densely arranged and usually compact structure known as the *nucleus.* The *nuclear membrane* separates the *nucleoplasm* (protoplasm of the nucleus) from a zone of less dense, spongy protoplasm surrounding and suspending the nucleus, known as the *cytoplasm.* Generally, the cytoplasm of the cell (1) aids in cell multiplication, (2) assimilates and stores food, (3) eliminates waste products, and (4) secretes enzymes* and other products of physiologic significance. The cytoplasm varies in different cells, for enzymes and enzyme systems may be possessed by only one specific kind of cell.

The nucleus (1) rules over the growth and de-

---

*Enzymes enable metabolites in the cell to be transformed at a rate and temperature unattainable in manmade laboratories.

**Table 2-3**
Comparative sizes of biologic objects

| | | BIOLOGIC OBJECT | DIAMETER | | |
|---|---|---|---|---|---|
| | | | MICROMETER (μm.) | NANOMETER* (nm.) | ANGSTROM UNIT (Å) |
| | HUMAN EYE | Ostrich egg | 200,000 | 200,000,000 | 2,000,000,000 |
| | | †Mature human ovum | 120 | 120,000 | 1,200,000 |
| LIMIT OF RESOLUTION | LIGHT MICROSCOPE | Erythrocyte (red blood cell) | 7.5 | 7500 | 75,000 |
| | | *Serratia marcescens* (bacterium) | 0.75 | 750 | 7500 |
| | | *Rickettsia* | 0.475 | 475 | 4750 |
| | | *Chlamydia psittaci* | 0.27 | 270 | 2700 |
| | ELECTRON MICROSCOPE | *Mycoplasma* | 0.15 | 150 | 1500 |
| | | Influenza virus | 0.085 | 85 | 850 |
| | | Genetic unit (Muller's estimation of largest size of a gene) | 0.02 × 0.125§ | 20 × 125§ | 200 × 1250§ |
| | | Poliomyelitis virus | 0.027 | 27 | 270 |
| | | Tobacco necrosis (plant virus) | 0.016 | 16 | 160 |
| | | Egg albumin molecule (protein molecule) | 0.0025 × 0.01§ | 2.5 × 10§ | 25 × 100§ |
| | | Hydrogen molecule | 0.0001 | 0.1 | 1 |

*Millimicrons (mμ).
†Limit of resolution of human eye is 0.1 mm. or 100 μm.
‡Limit of resolution of compound light microscope is 0.2 μm.
§Width × length.

velopment of the cell, (2) controls the metabolic processes that go on inside the cell, (3) transfers the hereditary characteristics of the cell, and (4) controls reproduction. In short, the nucleus is the center or initiating point for all the vital activities of the cell, and a cell without a nucleus is dead.* One particularly important activity is protein synthesis. It is carried on in the cytoplasm but regulated by the nucleus.

The pattern of intracellular organization is not the same in all cells, and many cells do not show all the typical structures to be given.

*Cytoplasm.* Within the ground substance of the cytoplasm are (1) numerous small, purposeful configurations of living substance called *organelles* and (2) stores of lifeless materials, sometimes transient, referred to as *inclusions.* Organelles include the plasma membrane (plasmalemma), centrosome, centrioles, mitochondria, endoplasmic reticulum, ribosomes, Golgi apparatus, lysosomes, microtubules, and several kinds of filaments and fibrils. Inclusions may be starch granules, glycogen, fat globules, proteins, pigment granules, secretory products, and crystals. Certain organelles and inclusions were well known to the cytologist, but with the electron micro-

scope to reveal the complexities of cell architecture, others were seen for the first time.

Encasing the cytoplasm is the *plasma membrane* (Fig. 2-4). This is a delicate film limiting the cytoplasm and presiding as a physiologic gatekeeper over the exchange of food materials, metabolic waste products, and various other chemicals. Between the cell and its surroundings, numerous biologic events take place on or in the plasma membrane. A three-layered membrane 80 to 100 Å thick, it is formed chemically by a precise association of protein, fat, and carbohydrate molecules. Carbohydrate makes up less than 10%, lipids about 40%, and the balance is protein. About the plasma membrane in certain vegetable cells and adherent to it is the *cell wall,* made of cellulose; this wall is absent or indistinct in animal cells. The many thin, filamentous projections of cytoplasm seen along the free border of certain cells are the *microvilli.*

The *cell center* or *centrosome* is a cytoplasmic region of altered texture usually adjacent the nucleus. It is occupied by a pair or more of rod-shaped *centrioles.* In electron micrographs centrioles are seen as hollow cylinders 300 to 500 nm. long and 150 nm. wide, placed at right angles to each other. Although the function of the centrosome is poorly understood, it is thought to play an important role in cell division.

The powerhouse of the cell is the *mitochondrion* (*pl.,* mitochondria), the site of many important biochemical reactions. A cell may contain a thousand or more. Barely visible through the light microscope

---

*The human red blood cell, with no nucleus, cannot divide and is limited in its metabolic behavior.

*STARCH - ONLY FOUND IN PLANT*
*CELLS*

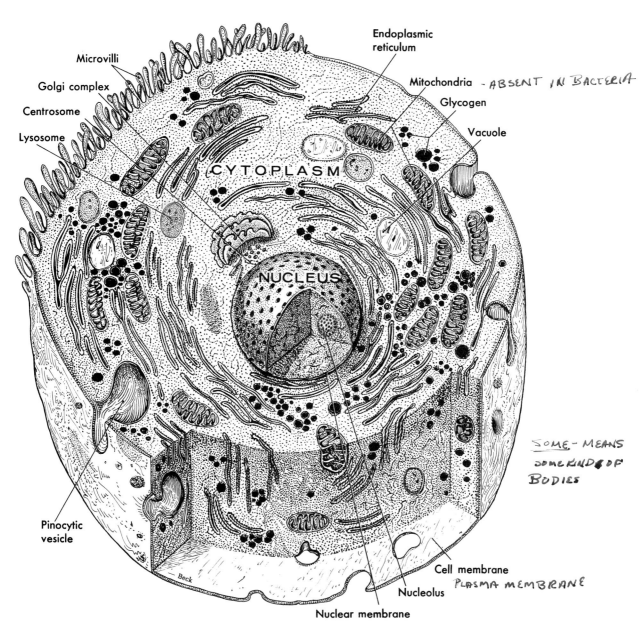

Microvilli

Golgi complex

Centrosome

Lysosome

Endoplasmic
reticulum

Mitochondria *- ABSENT IN BACTERIA*

Glycogen

Vacuole

CYTOPLASM

NUCLEUS

*SOME - MEANS*
*SOME KINDS OF*
*BODIES*

Pinocytic
vesicle

— Beck

Cell membrane
*PLASMA MEMBRANE*

Nucleolus

Nuclear membrane

**Fig. 2-3.** The cell. Diagram of structure observed in electron micrograph. (See text.) Note pinocytic vesicle representing a droplet of watery fluid going into cytoplasm. *Pinocytosis* (cell drinking) indicates uptake of certain substances in solution by the cell. (From Anthony, C. P., and Kolthoff, N. J.: Textbook of anatomy and physiology, ed. 9, St. Louis, 1975, The C. V. Mosby Co.)

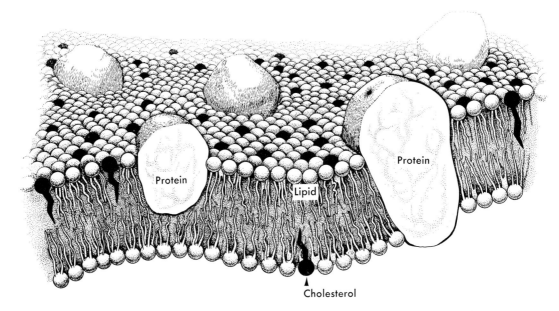

**Fig. 2-4.** Plasma membrane. Note globular (potato-like) proteins in this model, embedded in bimolecular layer of lipids (including cholesterol). Proteins make up membrane's "active sites."

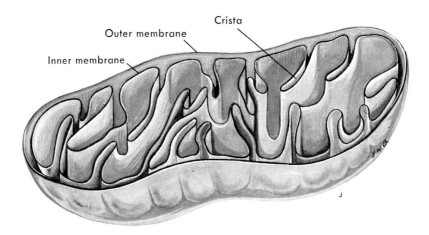

**Fig. 2-5.** Mitochondrion. Cutaway sketch to show inner and outer membranes and cristae. (From Schottelius, B. A., and Schottelius, D. D.: Textbook of physiology, ed. 17, St. Louis, 1973, The C. V. Mosby Co.)

as a threadlike form (0.2 to 3 $\mu$m.), the mitochondrion through the electron microscope is an intricate oval or elongated structure consisting of a double membrane, the inner layer of which is a system of folds called *cristae* (Fig. 2-5). The mitochondria house the bulk of chemicals (enzymes) that provide energy for cell activities; they are the principal sites at which the energy in food materials is released to the cell. (Biochemically, mitochondria can generate this energy for the cell because they contain cytochrome chains that are linked by the Krebs cycle.) With

special technics in isolated mitochondria, the necessary enzymes and coenzymes required for the complex chemical reactions can be located primarily on the membranes. A mitochondrion may contain anywhere from 50 to 50,000 such enzymes, depending on the type of cell and its functional state.

The *endoplasmic reticulum* (the cytoskeleton), seen only by electron microscopy, is an elaborate pattern of channels with a secretory function. Its membrane-bound tubules measure 400 to 700 Å in diameter. Endoplasmic reticulum may be *granular*

SaidOF A word ~ASE — ENZYME WHICH ACTS, ON THE PREFIX

(rough surfaced) or agranular (smooth surfaced). Many tiny, uniform, beadlike granules called ribosomes, which are also found free in the cytoplasmic matrix, are adherent to the outer surface of the membranes of the granular reticulum. Ribosomes are rich in ribonucleic acid (RNA) and represent the places in the cell where proteins are formed. A single cell may contain billions of them. Granular reticulum is highly developed in glandular cells that elaborate protein secretions. If the secretory product is an export from the cell, the ribosomes must be closely associated with the endoplasmic reticulum, for it is through the pathways of the reticulum that the product is transported to the Golgi region for packaging. The secretory product, stored as droplets or granules for a while in the cytoplasm, is released in time from the cell surface. Agranular endoplasmic reticulum is related to other metabolic functions of cells; in the liver cell it is involved in lipid and cholesterol metabolism, and in the cells of the gonads it is related to the production of steroid hormones.

Placed near one pole of the nucleus, the *Golgi apparatus* is made up of aggregates of flat saccules in parallel fashion, with vesicles and vacuoles clustered about. Although it still remains somewhat of a mystery, it does play an important role in cell secretion. The polysaccharide fraction of certain complex secretions is known to be formed in the Golgi complex and there to be bound to protein supplied from other organelles of the cell.

Greatly variable in different cells are small, dense particles, *lysosomes*, limited by a membrane. Lysosomes are rich in lytic enzymes, including deoxyribonuclease and ribonuclease. They are also known as "suicide bags," for their potent enzymes could digest the cell containing them if they were released from the organelle. A prime function of lysosomes is tied in with the engulfment of foreign material in the body, and they are abundant in phagocytic cells (p. 94). Close by and related to the centrioles are *microtubules*, cytoskeletal elements helping to maintain cell shape. These are straight tubules 200 to 270 Å in diameter with a dense filamentous wall 50 to 70 Å thick. *Filaments* and *fibrils* are commonly seen in the cytoplasmic matrix of many cells. Filaments enable muscle cells to contract, but for many cytoplasmic filaments the biologic significance is undetermined. A newly described cytoplasmic organelle is the *peroxisome*. It is thought to play a role in carbohydrate metabolism. It contains a heavy concentration of peroxidase. Peroxisomes (protoplasmic microbodies) are called the "microkitchens" of the cell.

Cellular inclusions may serve as stores of energy for the cell—for example, deposits of glycogen, the polysaccharide storage form of carbohydrate, and

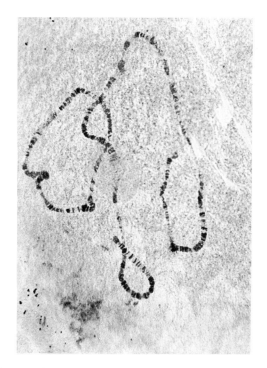

**Fig. 2-6.** Chromosomes from salivary gland of fly (species unidentified), prepared by "squash" technic. Note structure in low-power photomicrograph. (From Brown, W. V., and Bertke, E. M.: Textbook of cytology, St. Louis, 1969, The C. V. Mosby Co.)

fat (triglycerides of fatty acids). The enzymatic breakdown of the glucose derived from glycogen supplies energy to the cell and short-chain carbon skeletons to be reused in cell protoplasm. *Melanin*, the brown pigment of the skin and hair, is an example of an intracellular pigment. Certain *crystalline* inclusions visible by light and electron microscopy are assumed to be protein but are poorly understood. Tears, hydrochloric acid, mucus, milk, and digestive enzymes are well-known secretory products of cells. Mucus is one such product that may be easily visible microscopically as a droplet in the cytoplasm of the cell elaborating it.

*Nucleus.* The executive nucleus, usually found near the center of the cell, presides over the functional activities of that cell. Commonly a spherical body, it is made up of a framework of fibrils or threads on which are located the *chromatin granules*, which unite to form the *chromosomes* during cell division. For the time that cell is not dividing, the chromosomes are in an extended state and cannot be counted. Early in cell division the chromosomes begin to contract, and by metaphase (Fig. 2-6) the small rod-shaped bodies appear distinctly. The number and size of the chromosomes depend on the species and are constant for each species.

Structurally, a chromosome consists of coiled threads, each made up of a large number of strands of the giant molecule deoxyribonucleic acid, DNA. A chromosome is the unit of organization for DNA. In a way not fully understood, it represents a binding together of DNA, ribonucleic acid, histone (low molecular weight basic protein), and a more complex acidic residual protein.

In DNA three smaller chemical molecules—organic nucleotide bases, a pentose sugar (deoxyribose), and phosphoric acid—are fastened together in a characteristic spiral pattern. Two sugar-phosphate ladders with every so many paired nucleotide rungs—

that is, two identical, unbranched, rigid, intertwining, spiral chains—are thus formed. These are at least 1500 times as long as they are wide and are twisted in opposite directions about a central shaft (Fig. 2-7).

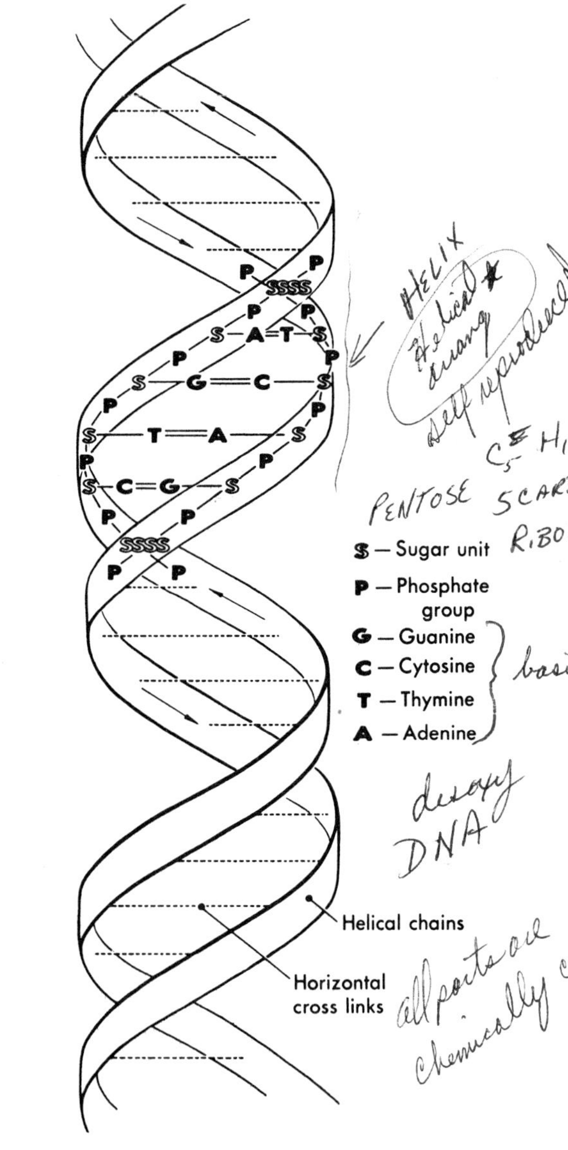

Every living organism must possess somewhere in its makeup a master plan that formulates all aspects of its appearance and behavior. For even simple organisms such a master plan encompasses vast amounts of biologic information that, to be stored efficiently, must be converted to some sort of code. Because of its vantage point in the cell, deoxyribonucleic acid is just right to do this biochemically. Its building blocks are linked in such a way that the four nucleotide bases (adenine, thymine, cytosine, and guanine) can serve as letters of a four-character code alphabet. Words can be formed in a biochemical and genetic language.* In the language of life the four characters are expressed in linkages of three, called triplet codes. There are sixty-four such triplet codes with so many possible arrangements that they can describe easily nearly 4 billion human beings populating the world. For a given organism the specifications for its every structure and life process are contained in specific chemical sequences in its DNA.

---

*The Morse or International telegraphic code, composed of the dot and dash, is a two-character code.

**S** — Sugar unit
**P** — Phosphate group
**G** — Guanine
**C** — Cytosine
**T** — Thymine
**A** — Adenine

**Helical chains**

**Horizontal cross links**

**Fig. 2-7.** DNA molecule. Note relation of purine and pyrimidine bases (**G, C, T, A**) to helical structure.

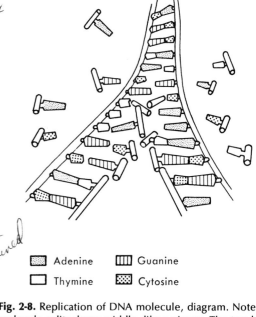

Adenine    Guanine
Thymine    Cytosine

**Fig. 2-8.** Replication of DNA molecule, diagram. Note that molecule splits down middle, like a zipper. The two bases of each rung of the ladder snap apart. Free nucleotides within nucleus move to halves of splitting ladder and reconstitute it according to precise specifications of genetic code. Shortly thereafter, there are two exact copies of original molecule.

The chromosome, then, is a biologic document. From it can be transcribed biologic messages in code, over and over again, even the same message. The chromosomes carry the particular hereditary pattern for the given organism. The hereditary pattern for each of the 100 million million tiny cells of the human body is carried in each cell in its chromosomes.

An unusual property of the DNA molecule is its ability to reproduce itself (Fig. 2-8), that is, to replicate itself into two exact copies. (Replication occurs before cell division.) Because of this the hereditary biochemical pattern or *genetic code** may be passed from one generation to the next. (Think of the thou-

sands of billions of times the DNA of the fertilized human ovum replicates itself to form the myriads of cells of the mature human being.)

If the chromosomes of the nucleus are compared to two measuring tapes side by side, when the spirals are straightened, each point, or locus, marks the position of a *gene,* which is paired with a matching gene on the corresponding tape. The majority of the life processes within the cell are carried on by enzymes, which are mostly protein. Since a gene physiologically is responsible for the development of a single protein,* collectively the influence of genes on the sum total of enzymatic action makes unicellu-

---

* The DNA of the ova resulting in the entire earth's human population would fit into a 1/8-inch cube. One-tenth of a trillionth of an ounce of DNA is present in one fertilized human egg, although the number of DNA molecules it contains is astronomically large and virtually incalculable.

*A given protein (such as an enzyme) is made up of hundreds or thousands of amino acid building blocks. The biologic property of the protein molecule is completely dependent on genes acting to align the amino acids precisely in the protein molecule.

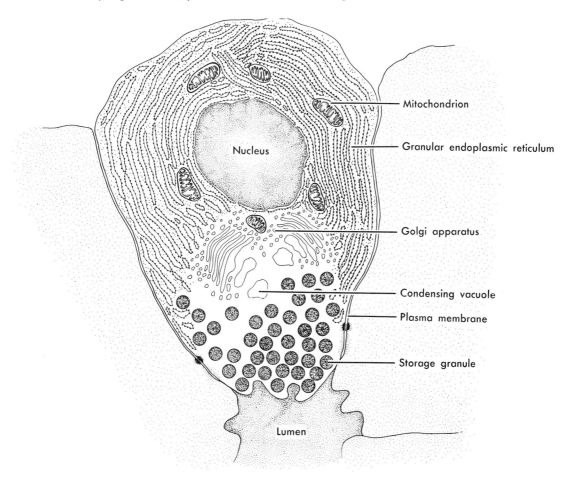

**Fig. 2-9.** Pathways in glandular cell elaborating secretion. Specifications are passed from nucleus to granular endoplasmic reticulum where product is synthesized. From there it moves to Golgi apparatus for packaging into condensing vacuoles. These ripen to storage granules that at appropriate time empty contents into lumen.

lar and multicellular organisms what they are biologically.

The other nucleic acid of physiologic significance, *ribonucleic acid* or *RNA*, is similar to DNA chemically except that its sugar is a different pentose, ribose, and its chemical pattern is laid out as a *single* coil, not a double one. About 10% of the cell's quota of RNA is found in the nucleolus, the rest in the cytoplasm. Between cell divisions the nucleus transfers information coded in the chromosomes into specific sequences of amino acids in messenger RNA, which then passes out of the nucleus to transmit instructions to the ribosomes. These structures can decipher a sequence of several thousand words (in the biochemical language) to map out complex protein patterns. (Cells of bacteria, plants, and animals contain both the nucleic acids; viruses contain either, but only one of the two.)

Within the nucleus is usually found one spherical *nucleolus* (little nucleus), sometimes more, which is incorporated with the chromosomes into the background material of the nucleus, the *nuclear sap*. There is no membrane about it. The nucleolus disappears during cell division but reforms in the daughter cells. It plays a key role in nucleic acid metabolism and protein synthesis and is itself composed largely of RNA. It is prominent in rapidly growing embryonic cells.

The outer boundary of the nucleus, the *nuclear membrane*, is seen in the electron micrograph to be made up of two membranes, each 75 Å thick, separated by a space 400 to 700 Å wide. The nuclear membrane is similar in its makeup to the endoplasmic reticulum and is thought to be derived from it. The canals of the endoplasmic reticulum appear to open into small pores along the course of the nuclear envelope, and there may be numerous ribosomes on its cytoplasmic surface.

Interesting lines of communication are set up between the inner part of the nucleus and the outer portions of the cytoplasm, extending through to the outside of the cell. These pathways go from the pores of the nuclear membrane along the channels of the endoplasmic reticulum, incorporate the membranes of the Golgi apparatus, and end with the plasma membrane (Fig. 2-9).

## Division of the cell

Every cell owes its existence to the division of a preexisting cell. Cells divide by the process of *mitosis* (Fig. 2-10), or indirect cell division, in which cleavage of the cell is preceded by a series of complicated nuclear and cytoplasmic changes. Mitotic division is characteristic of the higher animals and plants and may be seen in the lower forms as well.

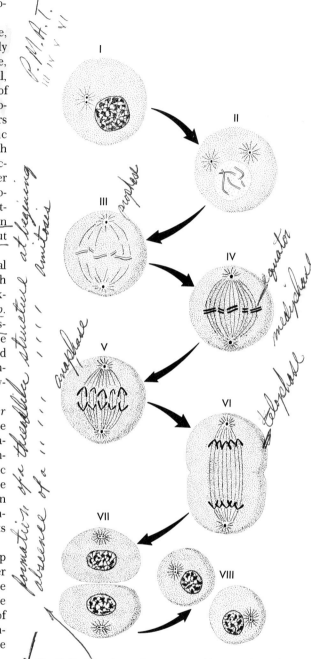

**Fig. 2-10.** Mitosis, various stages. Note nuclear changes, appearance of chromosomes, and loss of nuclear membrane. Chromosomes take shape in cell II, are divided in cell III, and are aligned on mitotic spindle in cell IV. By cell V they are separated along spindle. Cytoplasmic indentation in cell VI precedes appearance of daughter cells VII and VIII.

# Questions for review

1 Define protoplasm, cytology, mitosis, macromolecule, nanometer.
2 Outline the parts of a typical cell and give the function of each.
3 In your own words, define the cell.
4 What structure controls and regulates vital activities in the living cell?
5 What instruments are used to study cells and unicellular organisms?
6 Give the unit of measurement for cells and unicellular organisms. State why it is used.
7 How are the hereditary characters of a cell transmitted?
8 What cells may be seen with the unaided eye?
9 What is DNA? Why is it important? Where does it occur?
10 State the function of a gene.
11 What is RNA? Where is it found in the cell? What is its physiologic significance?
12 Briefly characterize the important biologic molecules in protoplasm.

**References on pp. 48 and 49.**

# CHAPTER 3

# The bacterial cell

*Gugl*

*All bacteria show a cell wall. Therefore bacteria are plants. all plants show a cell wall. Animal cells do not have a cell wall.*

## Definition

Bacteria (*sing.*, bacterium) are minute unicellular microorganisms that ordinarily do not contain chlorophyl and may be able to move about independently in their environment.

**Classification** (p. 5). In the early days of microbiology it was thought that bacteria belonged to the animal kingdom, but then for a period of years, it seemed more suitable to classify them with plants. Today we classify them as procaryotes. They are the smallest microorganisms having all the necessary protoplasmic equipment for growth and self-multiplication at the expense of available foodstuffs. They can start with rather simple substances and synthesize them into complicated organic moieties. They use food materials only in solution and excrete waste products in fluids that must diffuse outward. There is no special structure for intake of solids for digestion or for release of solid particles to the environment. Bacteria are morphologically simpler than the cells of the higher organisms, and as is true for procaryotes, they lack an organized nucleus. In spite of their relative simplicity, they have an elaborate and complicated life history.

**Distribution.** Bacteria are widely distributed in nature. They have adapted to every conceivable habitat. They are found within and upon our bodies and in the food we eat, the water we drink, and the air we breathe. They are plentiful in the upper layers of the soil,* and no place on earth, except possibly the peaks of snow-capped mountains, is free of them. They are found in frozen Antarctica and in the hot water of the geysers in Yellowstone Park. Our skin has a large bacterial population, and bacteria make up a generous portion of the contents of the alimentary tract. There are thousands of species of bacteria; of this number, about 100 produce disease in man. The ratio is given as 30,000 nondisease-producing bacteria to 1 disease producer. Some of the bacteria that produce disease in man also produce disease in the lower animals.

Others produce disease in the lower animals only, and still others attack only plants. The majority, however, do not attack man, lower animals, or living plants and either do not affect animals and plants at all or are actually helpful to them. In fact, if the activities of bacteria were to cease, all plant and animal life would soon become extinct. Bacteria that cause disease are spoken of as *pathogenic;* those that do not cause disease are *nonpathogenic.*

## Morphology

**Shape.** Bacteria occur in three possible shapes (Figs. 3-1 and 3-2):

1. Spherical—coccus*
2. Rod shaped—bacterium or bacillus
3. Spiral shaped—vibrio, spirillum, spirochete

Cocci are not necessarily round but may be elongated, oval, or flattened on one side. Some bacilli are long and slender, whereas others are so short and plump as to be mistaken for cocci. These short, thick, oval-shaped bacilli are known as *coccobacilli.* The ends of bacilli are usually rounded but may be square or concave. A *vibrio* is a curved organism shaped like a comma. A *spirillum* is a spiral organism whose long axis remains rigid when it is in motion. A *spirochete* is a spiral organism whose long axis bends when it is in motion.

*Acetic Colors* (handwritten margin note)

When bacteria, especially cocci, divide, the manner in which they do so and their tendency to cling together often give them a distinct arrangement. Cocci that divide so as to form pairs are known as *diplococci.* The opposing sides of diplococci may be flattened (examples, gonococci and meningococci). Cocci that divide and cling end to end to form chains are known as *streptococci.* Those that divide in an

---

*The following are singular and plural forms:

| Singular | Plural |
|----------|--------|
| Coccus | Cocci |
| Bacillus | Bacilli |
| Spirillum | Spirilla |
| Bacterium | Bacteria |
| Medium | Media |

---

*Take a pinch of ~~dirt~~ *Earth* Hold it between the thumb and forefinger. You may be holding as many as 200 million bacteria.

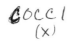
Cocci
(x)

Coccou
(k)

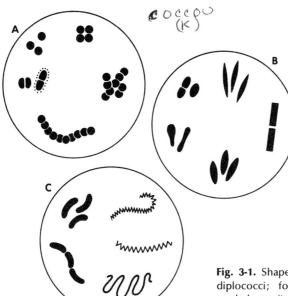

**Fig. 3-1.** Shapes of bacteria. **A,** Spherical—coccus (pair, diplococci; four, tetrad; chain, streptococci; cluster, staphylococci). **B,** Rod shaped—bacillus (including coccobacilli). **C,** Spiral shaped—vibrio, spirillum, and spirochete.

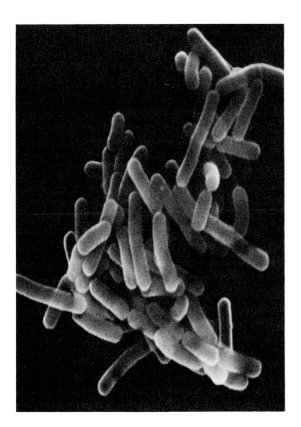

**Fig. 3-2.** Bacilli (*Lactobacillus* species), scanning electron micrograph. Note three-dimensional effect from this instrument. (Courtesy Dr. R. C. Reynolds, The University of Texas Health Science Center at Dallas.)

irregular manner to form grapelike clusters or broad sheets are known as *staphylococci*. Other characteristic arrangements of cocci are in groups of four *(tetrads)* and cubical packets of eight *(sarcinae)*. No pathogenic cocci are found in the latter group. Bacilli that occur in pairs are known as *diplobacilli* and those that occur in chains as *streptobacilli*. The diplobacillus and streptobacillus arrangements are not common. When some bacilli divide, they bend at the point of division to give two organisms arranged in the form of a V. This is known as *snapping*. In other cases they tend to arrange themselves side by side. This is known as *slipping*.

**Size.** Bacteria are so small (no larger than 1/50,000 of an inch) that the highest magnification of the ordinary compound microscope must be used to study them.* Cocci range from 0.4 to 2 $\mu$m. ($\mu$) in diameter. The smallest bacillus is about 0.5 $\mu$m. in length and 0.2 $\mu$m. in diameter. The largest pathogenic bacilli are seldom greater than 1 $\mu$m. in diameter and 3 $\mu$m. in length; the average diameter and length of pathogenic bacilli are 0.5 and 2 $\mu$m. respectively. Nonpathogenic bacilli may be larger, reaching a diameter of 4 $\mu$m. and a length of 20 $\mu$m. The spirilla are usually narrow organisms and are from 1 to 14 $\mu$m. in length. Different species of bacteria show marked variation in size, and there is some variation within a species, but as a rule the size of each species is fairly constant.

*A cubic inch would hold 10 trillion medium-sized bacteria, or as many as there are stars in 100,000 galaxies.

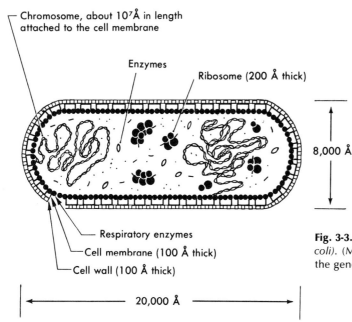

Chromosome, about $10^7$Å in length attached to the cell membrane

Enzymes

Ribosome (200 Å thick)

8,000 Å

Respiratory enzymes

Cell membrane (100 Å thick)

Cell wall (100 Å thick)

20,000 Å

**Fig. 3-3.** Ultrastructure of young bacterial cell *(Escherichia coli).* (Modified from Watson, J. D.: Molecular biology of the gene, New York, 1970, W. A. Benjamin, Inc.)

**Structure.** Bacteria, always unicellular, are so tiny and transparent (about the density of water) and so slightly refractile that unless stained with dyes, they are difficult to see even with the compound light microscope. When stained, they appear homogeneous or slightly granular. With the electron microscope, however, microbiologists can visualize minute details of bacterial structure.

The shape of the bacterial cell is maintained by a rigid *cell wall* (Fig. 3-3). The protoplasmic substance of bacteria exerts such a high osmotic pressure, equivalent to that of a 10% to 20% solution of sucrose, that in ordinary environments the cell wall is necessary to prevent the cell from bursting. If the bacterial cell is placed in a suitable hypertonic medium and the cell wall dissolved, the remainder of the bacterium is converted into a spherical protoplast. In an isotonic environment protoplasts remain viable and grow. The stability of the cell wall is derived from its chemical makeup; this varies in the two major groups of bacteria (p. 56). In gram-positive bacteria, the chief component is mucopeptide—a polymer of the amino sugars *N*-acetylglucosamine and *N*-acetylmuramic acid and short peptide linkages of amino acids. Sometimes teichoic acids or a mucopolysaccharide complex of amino sugars and simple monosaccharides may be present. In gram-negative bacteria, a mucopeptide inner layer is chemically bound to two outer layers of lipopolysaccharide and lipoprotein. There are no teichoic acids.

The cell wall is so narrow that it cannot be seen with the ordinary compound light microscope. In ultrathin sections it is revealed by the electron microscope as a well-defined structure surrounding a distinct layer, the cell membrane or *plasma membrane,* which separates it from the cytoplasm of the bacterial cell. The plasma membrane is the site of important enzyme systems, including the respiratory enzyme system (cytochrome enzymes). In fact, in bacteria it corresponds to the mitochondria of higher organisms.* In regulating the passage of food materials and metabolic by-products between the interior of the cell (where metabolic activities are carried on) and the surroundings, it functions osmotically both as a barrier and as a link. It blocks the entry of certain substances and catalyzes the transport of others into the cell.

Surrounding many bacteria is a mucilaginous envelope or *capsule* (Fig. 3-4, *A*). Indistinct in most bacteria, it is well developed in few (examples: *Streptococcus pneumoniae, Clostridium perfringens,* and *Klebsiella pneumoniae* ). The capsule is formed by an accumulation of slime excreted by the bacterium. This material is usually a complex polysaccharide. If it is present about the cell in only small amounts, a distinct capsule does not appear.

Capsule formation is most prominent in organisms taken directly from the animal body, for when grown on artificial media, the same organisms often lose their ability to form capsules. A capsule does not stain with the ordinary bacteriologic dyes but may appear as a clear halo around the bacterium,

---

*Bacteria do not contain mitochondria.

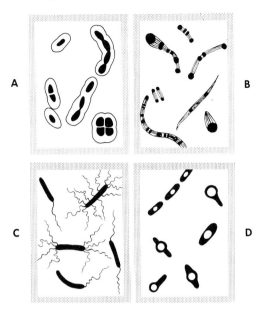

**Fig. 3-4.** Special features of bacteria. **A**, Capsules; **B**, metachromatic granules; **C**, flagella; **D**, spores. Note pleomorphism in **B**.

*virulence - amount of disease producing.*

even two or three times as broad as the bacterium. It is stained by special methods. The presence of a capsule appears to increase the virulence of an organism by protecting it against phagocytosis, and in some cases the capsule gives the organism its specific immunologic nature. For instance, relative to the nature of their capsules, pneumococci are divided into at least 82 types. The specific antigenic nature of a capsule depends on its carbohydrate content.

Within some bacteria (such as *Corynebacterium diphtheriae*) at the ordinary magnification of the light microscope are seen granules that stain more deeply than the remainder of the cell. They are known as *metachromatic granules* (Fig. 3-4, *B*) and are enzymatically active. They are thought to be reserves of inorganic phosphate stored as polymerized metaphosphate (volutin). Sulfur-oxidizing bacteria convert excess hydrogen sulfide from the environment into intracellular granules of elemental sulfur. In some species granules are arranged irregularly within the cell, whereas in others they are located in one or both ends of the cell and are known as *polar bodies*.

Electron microscopy reveals a dense packing of ribosomes in bacterial cytoplasm and the presence of spherules and various submicroscopic granules. The ribosomes, as would be expected, play an important role in protein synthesis. The submicroscopic granules are known to be biochemically complex and active; they may represent stores of food materials or even

elimination products. There seems to be no relation of these granules to the ability of the bacteria containing them to produce disease.

As special staining methods designed to visualize the chemical substances making up the nucleus in the higher forms of life were applied to the study of bacteria, it became evident that bacteria contained nuclear material. This was seen in electron micrographs as a distinct and relatively transparent structure of rounded proportions with no detectable nuclear membrane. The nuclear material in bacteria consists essentially of deoxyribonucleic acid (DNA) present as a single chromosome, which if unfolded would stretch approximately 1 mm. It is hooked at one point to an infolding of the plasma membrane known as a *mesosome*. Many bacteria possess one chromosome, but in young, actively dividing cells, two or more may be seen. As it is for all cells, the nuclear material is precisely the governing force for the bacterial cell, and vital activities cannot be carried on in a bacterial cell without it.

**Chemical composition.** Even in a unit such as the bacterial cell, 500 times smaller than the average plant or animal cell, the chemical composition is exceedingly complex. To gain an idea as to the chemical makeup of any bacterial cell, let us look at one that, since it is easily grown and manipulated in the laboratory, is undergoing almost as intensive study today as man. This is the colon bacillus, *Escherichia coli* (Fig. 3-3). *ORGANISM FOUND IN LARGE INTESTINE OR COLON*

Biochemically, this microbe contains perhaps 3000 to 6000 different types of molecules (Table 3-1). Of these, specific proteins account for 2000 to 3000 kinds. The amount of DNA present is postulated to be that required to code for the necessary amino acid sequences in these proteins. About the DNA are 20,000 to 30,000 spherical ribosomes composed of protein (40%) and RNA (60%). Water, water-soluble enzymes, and a large number of various small and less complex molecules are associated with these nucleic acids.

**Motility.** Many bacilli and all spirilla are motile when suspended in a suitable liquid at the proper temperature.* True motility is seldom observed in cocci. The organs of bacterial locomotion are fine hair-like appendages known as *flagella* (little whips) that spring from the bacterial cell and cause it to move along by their wavelike, rhythmic contractions (Figs. 3-4, *C*, and 3-5). Some spirochetes aid the action of their flagella with a sinuous motion of the

---

*True motility, in which the organism changes its position in relation to its neighbors, should not be confused with *brownian motion,* a peculiar dancing motion possessed by all finely divided particles suspended in a liquid.

### Table 3-1
Chemical makeup of a single, young, actively dividing, colon bacillus (*Escherichia coli*)*

| COMPONENT | AVERAGE MOLECULAR WEIGHT | ESTIMATED NUMBER OF MOLECULES | NUMBER OF DIFFERENT KINDS OF MOLECULES | PERCENT TOTAL CELL WEIGHT |
|---|---|---|---|---|
| Proteins | 40,000 | 1,000,000 | 2000 to 3000 | 15 |
| Carbohydrates and precursors | 150 | 200,000,000 | 200 | 3 |
| Lipids and precursors | 750 | 25,000,000 | 50 | 2 |
| Nucleic acids | | | | |
|   DNA | 2,500,000,000 | 4 | 1 | 1 |
|   RNA | 25,000 to 1,000,000 | 461,000 | More than 1000 | 6 |
| Amino acids and precursors | 120 | 30,000,000 | 100 | 0.4 |
| Nucleotides and precursors | 300 | 12,000,000 | 200 | 0.4 |
| Other small molecules (breakdown products of food molecules) | 150 | 15,000,000 | 200 | 0.2 |
| Inorganic ions ($Na^+$, $K^+$, $Mg^{++}$, $Ca^{++}$, $Fe^{++}$, $Cl^-$, $PO_4^{--}$, $SO_4^{--}$) | 40 | 250,000,000 | 20 | 1 |
| Water | 18 | 40,000,000,000 | 1 | 70 |

*From J. D. Watson: Molecular biology of the gene, second edition. Copyright 1970, W. A. Benjamin, Inc., Menlo Park, Calif.

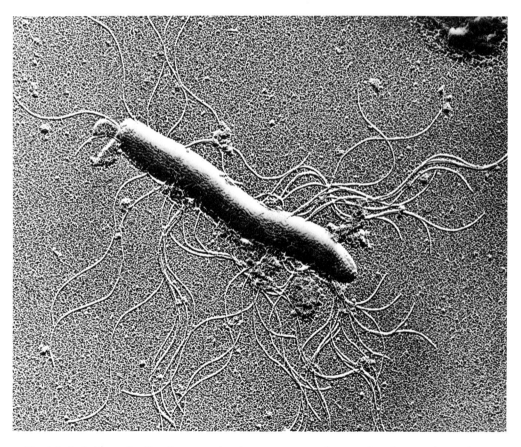

**Fig. 3-5.** Peritrichous bacillus from mouth, electron micrograph. Note flagella—number and arrangement. In preparation specimen shadowed with gold. (×28,000.) (Courtesy Dr. J. Swafford, Arizona State University, Tempe; from Brown, W. V., and Bertke, E. M.: Textbook of cytology, ed. 2, St. Louis, 1974, The C. V. Mosby Co.)

entire cell body. A bacterium may have one flagellum (monotrichous), a few, or many flagella in a tuft (lophotrichous), and the flagella may be attached to one end, both ends, or all around the organism (peritrichous) (Fig. 3-4, *C*). Flagella, which chemically are elastic proteins, do not take the ordinary bacteriologic dyes but have to be stained by special methods.

Bacteria may be motile when grown on one medium and nonmotile when grown on another. Also, they may be motile at one temperature and nonmotile at another. Different organisms travel at different rates of speed. The rod-shaped organism that causes typhoid fever *(Salmonella typhi)* is able to progress at a rate of 2000 times its own length per hour.

*Pili* (Latin, hairs) are surface projections like flagella found in gram-negative bacteria (Fig. 3-6). However, they are shorter and finer and do not propel the cell. Also called *fimbriae*, they may be part of the attachment of cells in conjugation; but otherwise their purpose is unknown.

**Endospores.** Under certain poorly understood conditions, some species of bacteria (examples: species in genera *Bacillus* and *Clostridium*) form, within their cytoplasm, bodies that are resistant to influences

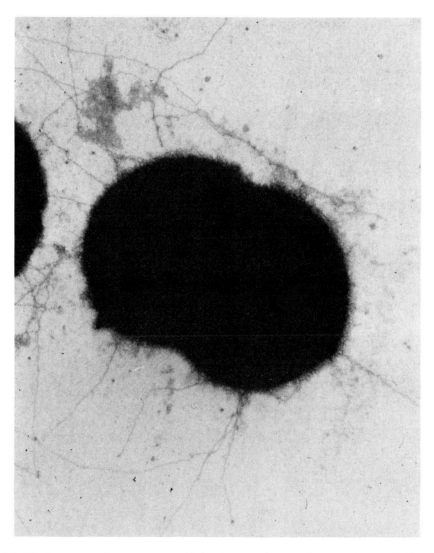

**Fig. 3-6.** Pili of gram-negative gonococcus *(Neisseria gonorrhoeae)*, electron micrograph. Negative staining with 2% uranyl acetate (p. 33). (×88,020.) (Courtesy Janice C. Bullard and Dr. Stephen J. Kraus, Venereal Disease Research Unit, Center for Disease Control, Health Services and Mental Health Administration, Department of Health, Education and Welfare, Atlanta.)

adverse to bacterial growth. These bodies are known as *spores* *(endospores)* (Fig. 3-4, *D*). Spore formation seems to be a characteristic of bacilli, being exceedingly rare in cocci and spirilla. Among bacilli about 150 species, most of which are nonpathogenic, form spores. The important pathogenic, sporeforming bacteria are those that cause tetanus, gas gangrene, botulism, and anthrax.

Since spores seem to form when conditions for bacterial growth are unfavorable, spore formation may be a protective mechanism, but in the life of certain species of bacteria it seems to be a normal phase. Bacteria that do not form spores and sporebearing bacteria in which spores are not forming are known as *vegetative bacteria*. Those in which spores are forming are *sporulating* bacteria. When conditions suitable for bacterial growth are established, the spore converts itself back to the actively multiplying form (germinates). The germinating spore becomes the vegetative form of the bacterium.

There is a temperature for each species at which spore formation is most active, and spore formation is preceded by a period of active vegetative reproduction. Some species form spores only in the presence of oxygen; others form spores only in its absence. Some observers regard the spore phase as a period of rest, or hibernation, for the organism. Spore formation is not a reproductive phenomenon because a spore forms but a single bacterium, and a bacterium forms but a single spore.

Sporulation occurs in the following manner. The bacterial cell forms within its substance a round or oval, highly refractile body surrounded by a capsule. This body increases in size until it is as broad or broader than the cell. The portion of the cell that remains gradually disintegrates, leaving only the spore. Spores from which the remainder of the cell has disappeared are *free* spores. In the electron microscope a spore has a structural pattern: a coat, a cortex, and a nuclear core of chromatinic material.

Spores do not take the ordinary bacteriologic dyes but may be stained by special methods. Ordinary stains of sporulating organisms may show the spore as a clear, unstained area situated in the end of the bacterium (terminal), near its center (central), or in an intermediate position (subterminal) (Fig. 3-4, *D*). In shape, spores may be spherical, ellipsoidal, or cylindrical. In anaerobic bacteria the spore is broader than the remainder of the bacterial cell, causing the bacterium to assume a spindle shape if the spore is central and a club shape if it is terminal or subterminal. The shape and position of the spores help to identify certain bacteria.

Although spores are especially resistant to heat, chemicals, and drying, the vegetative forms are no more resistant to these or other adverse influences than nonsporebearing bacteria. An idea of the value of the protection of spores can be drawn from the observation that some spores withstand boiling for hours, whereas the temperature of boiling water kills vegetative bacteria within 5 minutes. On the one hand, spores resist tremendous pressures, but on the other hand, they can persist in a vacuum approaching the emptiness of space. Spores have also been known to resist the temperature of liquid air ($-190°$ C.) for 6 months. Their resistance is probably the result of the membrane about them and of the concentrated, water-free nature of their substance. Although only a few species of bacteria produce spores, these spores are everywhere. This means that *spore-killing* methods in bacteriologic and surgical sterilization and in the canning industry are absolutely necessary.

## Reproduction

**Cell division.** The typical mode of bacterial reproduction, an asexual process, is by simple transverse division (binary fission) (Figs. 3-7 and 3-8). Bacteria do not divide by mitosis—there is no mitotic spindle. In preparation for division the nuclear chromosome of the dividing cell replicates to produce equal division of nuclear material into two sister chromosomes. Replication initiates active membrane synthesis at the periphery, and a transverse membrane is formed that moves into the bacterium. The membrane, along with a new cell wall, constricts the bacterium along its short axis and, partly because of the presence of the mesosome, pushes the sister chromosomes apart and into each of two daughter cells formed by the deepening constriction. Each newly separated cell soon elongates to full size and in turn divides. A newborn bacterium requires from 15 to 30 minutes to reach adult size and divide. Reproduction is always specific; for example, staphylococci always reproduce staphylococci.

**Production of L-forms.** In certain species of bacteria (examples: *Proteus* species, *Bacteroides* species, and some of the coliforms) a normal cell may swell to a large entity only to disintegrate into numerous particles approximately 0.2 $\mu$m. in diameter, known as L-forms. This kind of change may occur without known stimulus or with a well-defined one, such as a drug. Although these forms possess distinguishing characteristics, they are not only akin to the parent cell but also can revert to it.

## Variation

Living organisms, or the aggregate of living organisms, are seldom, if ever, exactly the same. Microbes are no exception. The deviation from the parent form

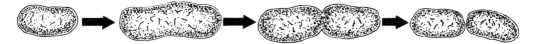

**Fig. 3-7.** Simple transverse division (binary fission). The young bacterium on left becomes full-grown and divides into two young ones, seen on right.

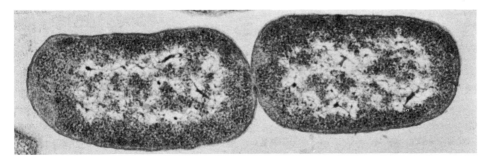

**Fig. 3-8.** Transverse fission of bacterium *(Escherichia coli),* electron micrograph. Two microorganisms are still attached in one area along line of division. (From Councilman, M., and others: J. Bacteriol. **93:**1987, 1967.)

in bacteria of the same species growing under different or identical conditions is known as *variation.*

Variation may be caused by external or internal influences. Environmental factors include the kind of culture medium, the temperature of growth, the length of time grown artificially, and the event of exposure to chemicals or to radiant energy (x rays, for example). Variation may also result from factors inherent in the bacteria themselves.

**Observed variations.** Variation may affect all the biologic properties—size, shape, biochemical nature, colonial characteristics, and physiologic activities—of bacteria and may be temporary or permanent.

*Dissociation.* A change in the kind of colony formed on a semisolid culture medium as an example of bacterial variation is termed bacterial (or microbial) *dissociation.* Although a pure culture of an organism is used to streak the surface of a culture medium, the resultant colonies may present contrasting appearances. There may be *smooth* or *mucoid* colonies: regular in outline, round, moist, and glistening—the *S-type* colonies. At the other extreme are the *rough* colonies: larger, irregular in outline, indented, and wrinkled—the *R-type* colonies. Between the two are intermediate forms. By proper laboratory manipulation organisms forming S-type colonies can be made to form R-type colonies and vice versa. Usually organisms forming S-type colonies are more vigorous in their disease-producing capacities than those forming R-type colonies. This variation offers some explanation as to the rise and fall of epidemics.

*Morphologic variants.* Bacteria of the same species, growing under most favorable conditions, may show considerable variation in size, shape, and appearance. This is *pleomorphism.* Growing under unfavorable conditions (for example, in old cultures), the members of some species assume irregular bizarre shapes and stain irregularly. These swollen, shrunken, or granular aberrant (or abnormal) variants are known as *involution* or *degenerative forms.* In this instance variation in morphology probably reflects the presence of many dying as well as dead cells in the culture medium and the injurious effect of the accumulation therein of metabolic by-products.

Organisms that are surrounded by a capsule when grown in the animal body often lose their capsule when grown artificially. In some cases capsule formation may be restored by return of the organism to a susceptible animal. Capsule formation is pronounced in anthrax bacilli infecting a susceptible animal, but from the artificial media of the laboratory there is hardly a sign of a capsule for the very same organism. Bacteria with capsules tend to form smooth colonies, and those with none tend to produce rough colonies.

**Adaptation.** One of the attributes of living cells is their power to adapt themselves to their surroundings. This is probably truer of bacterial than of many other types of cells. For instance, certain bacteria that require specially prepared media to sustain their continued growth when first isolated from the animal body gradually acquire the ability to grow on media devoid of the growth-promoting and enriching materials necessary for their early growth. They may also be grown artificially in a gradually changing environment until at last they are able to grow under conditions of food supply, temperature, moisture, and oxygen supply far different from those in which they originally grew best.

Those variations (changes in bacterial makeup) that represent physiologic adjustment to the environment are designated by the term *adaptation*.

*Plasmids* are extrachromosomal genetic elements widely seen among bacteria and not essential to viability. They determine bacterial traits crucial to adaptation.

*Attenuation.* An important form of adaptation is *attenuation* (an important concept in immunology), which indicates a loss in disease-producing ability of a given organism. An organism whose virulence is decreased is attenuated. A highly pathogenic organism may be rendered temporarily or permanently nonpathogenic if repeatedly subcultured on artificial laboratory media. For example, by cultivation of a strain of bovine tubercle bacilli on media containing bile until the strain had lost its ability to cause disease, a suitable preparation (BCG vaccine) was developed for vaccination against tuberculosis. Virulence, although artificially eliminated, may often be restored by animal passage, that is, the serial injection of microorganisms into and their recovery from susceptible animals.

**Genetic factors.** Certain internal factors operative in bacterial variations pertain to changes in the genetic makeup of the bacteria.

*Mutations.* Mutations in bacteria are analogous to those in the higher forms of life. Since the specific intracellular enzyme (protein) is regulated biochemically by a specific gene positioned on the chromosome of the cell, the related structure (and function) of the cell must depend on the integrity of that gene. Within the gene, the significant component is the sequence of the nucleotide bases, with any change in this pattern projecting an effect on the cell. Such a change constitutes a *mutation* and is inheritable.

Rearrangement of the nucleotide sequence of a gene can result from an error in replication or from a breakage of the sugar-phosphate backbone of the DNA molecule. Mutations occur spontaneously or are induced by certain mutagenic agents that can alter the nucleotide bases in such a way as to promote replication errors. The most effective mutagens are certain alkylating agents and forms of radiant energy.

*Intermicrobial transfer.* Variations resulting from the passage of nuclear material from one bacterium to another are easily demonstrated. If two bacterial strains, variants in a single species, are incubated together under special circumstances, such a transfer is borne out by the appearance in the culture of new organisms displaying qualities of both original strains. When genetic material (nuclear DNA) is

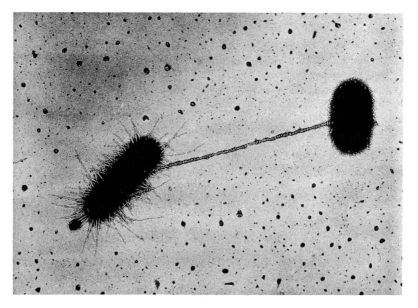

**Fig. 3-9.** Conjugation in bacteria: passage of genetic material by means of a long thin filament between bacterium of one species and that of a different species (both in family Enterobacteriaceae). A factor inducing resistance to certain antibiotics is known to be so transferred (p. 158). Note pili on surface of microbe on left. (Courtesy Dr. C. C. Brinton, Pittsburgh.)

transferred from one cell to another, the receiving cell does not gain the full complement of chromosome but only a portion. Immediately after the event of transfer, this portion must be matched to the corresponding segments of the chromosome in the cell, and genetic material exchanged and eliminated. From this rearrangement a newly formed chromosome emerges, containing DNA from two bacterial cells. This is the *recombinant chromosome,* shaped by the process of *recombination.*

*Conjugation* is a process effecting transfer of genetic material in a special way. Recent studies indicate that on occasions a type of sexual reproduction occurs in bacteria wherein hereditary material is passed from one organism to the other on a transient physical contact. In fact, in an electron micrograph (Fig. 3-9) two individual bacterial cells are seen to unite by means of a cytoplasmic bridge extending between them. Even male and female mating types have been defined for the closely related groups of enteric (gram-negative) bacteria in the family Enterobacteriaceae that have been studied. Conjugation can occur between any two members of the family, not just within a given genus. However, there is no new cell as a consequence. The progeny of the cell receiving the nuclear material are produced in the usual way, by binary fission of the parent.

*Transformation* is a process of direct transfer of nucleic acid. Certain species of bacteria release DNA into the medium in which they are growing, such as certain species of *Neisseria* that release it in their extracellular slime. A small number of bacteria in a given population, referred to as *transformable* bacteria, can pick up this DNA. How they do it is not known. Within the bacterial cell the DNA is integrated with the DNA already present, and what is left over is degraded. The net effect is the replacement of a *short* region of the chromosome with a new portion of genetic material.

*Transduction* is a special form of indirect transfer of genetic material. A bacterial virus or bacteriophage carries a small fragment of the chromosome from the bacterial cell in which it was produced to the bacterium it invades. Transduction occurs in certain coliforms, enteric pathogens, and staphylococci.

The above-mentioned internal factors may pertain to changes in the genetic substance of bacteria. When nuclear material (DNA) is transferred from one bacterium to another (transformation), there is alteration of some property in the recipient.

**Drug-fastness.** A microbial variation with considerable therapeutic importance is one that arises through a mutation or other genetic mechanism giving the organism an increased tolerance for an antimicrobial drug. This tolerance for the drug is termed *drug resistance* or *drug-fastness.* An organism that becomes resistant to a drug used in the treatment of disease is said to be drug-fast. Strains of bacteria are always emerging resistant to one or more antibiotics, a resistance usually acquired when clinical infectious disease has been inadequately treated with the given antibiotic.

Bacteria may become tolerant of more than one antimicrobial drug. This *cross-resistance* is noted especially in the case of closely related antibiotics.

## Questions for review

1 Define bacteria. Indicate their distribution.
2 Discuss the function of the cell wall. Of what is it composed?
3 Name and describe three forms of bacteria.
4 What is the function of the plasma membrane?
5 Give two characteristics of bacteria at least partly dependent on the capsule.
6 How do bacteria move about in a fluid medium?
7 How do bacteria reproduce?
8 What are spores? Comment as to their formation and purpose.
9 Give examples of bacterial variation.
10 Discuss adaptation.
11 State the importance of drug-fastness and cross-resistance.
12 Briefly discuss the bacterial chromosome.
13 List significant contributions of the electron microscope to our knowledge of the bacterial cell.
14 Briefly define L-forms, conjugation, mutation, transformation, transduction, attenuation, recombination.

**References on pp. 48 and 49.**

# CHAPTER 4

# Bacteria
## biologic needs

*[handwritten annotations: "basic", "obligatory – lives on living things"]*

## Environmental factors

For bacteria to grow and multiply most rapidly, certain requirements must be met: (1) sufficient food of the proper kind must be present; (2) moisture must be available; (3) the temperature must be that most suitable for the species; (4) the proper degree of alkalinity or acidity must be present; (5) the oxygen requirements of the species must be met; (6) light must be partially or completely excluded; and (7) by-products of bacterial growth must not accumulate in great amounts. Significant departure from any of these requirements will modify bacterial growth, although bacteria generally possess a greater degree of resistance to unfavorable conditions in the environment than do plants and animals.

Food materials prepared for the growth of bacteria in the laboratory are known as *culture media.* Some bacteria will grow on practically any properly prepared culture medium. Others grow only on especially nutritious ones, and a few will not grow on any artificial medium.

**Nutrition.** The protoplasm of the bacterial cell is composed of numerous organic compounds, including proteins, fats, and carbohydrates, as well as various inorganic components containing sulfur, phosphorus, calcium, magnesium, potassium, and iron. Proteins comprise about 50% of the dry weight of the cell (each species has a type of protein peculiar to itself), and bacterial nitrogen makes up 10%. In some species carbohydrates are plentiful, and some of the important traits of the species depend on these compounds.

*Nutrition* is the provision of food materials (that is, chemical substances) to bacteria so that they can grow, maintain their constituents, and multiply. For their nourishment bacteria require sources of carbon and nitrogen, growth factors, certain mineral salts, and sources of energy. With the exception of some saprophytic species, all bacteria derive their carbon and nitrogen from organic matter. A number of minerals are required, the most important of the salts

being those of calcium, phosphorus, iron, magnesium, potassium, and sodium. Certain minerals are important in the activation of enzymes.

Many microorganisms can synthesize all the organic compounds of their complex makeup if supplied with the basic nutrients. Many cannot, however, since they require vitamins and certain organic growth factors (a growth factor is utilized as the intact substance) for their activities. In this respect microorganisms resemble rather closely higher forms of life. In fact, such vitamins as nicotinic acid; pantothenic acid, para-aminobenzoic acid, biotin, and folic acid—requirements for animal nutrition—were first studied and identified as substances necessary for the growth of microorganisms.

*Kinds of organisms.* Organisms that obtain their nourishment from nonliving organic material are known as *saprophytes.* Those that depend on living matter for their nourishments are *parasites. Facultative saprophytes* usually obtain nourishment from living matter but may obtain it from dead organic matter. *Facultative parasites* usually obtain nourishment from dead organic matter but may obtain it from living matter. Some pathogenic bacteria can exist only on living material (for example, the spirochete of syphilis cannot be grown outside a living organism). Most, however, are capable of leading either a parasitic or a saprophytic existence. A few pathogenic bacteria, usually saprophytic, may adapt themselves to a parasitic existence (example: bacteria that cause gas gangrene). The organism on which a parasite lives is known as a *host.*

Organisms that obtain their nourishment by breaking down organic matter into simpler chemical substances are *heterotrophic.* Those that obtain their food by building the organic compounds in protoplasm from the simpler inorganic substances are *autotrophic.* All pathogenic bacteria and many nonpathogenic ones are heterotrophic.

**Moisture.** Water is necessary for the growth and

38

multiplication of bacteria. Not only is water a major component of the bacterial cell cytoplasm (on an average, 75% to 80% of the bacterial cell is made up of water), but it also dissolves the food materials in the environment of the bacterial cell so that they can be absorbed.

Drying is highly detrimental to bacterial growth. Delicate bacteria such as the gonococcus resist drying for only a few hours, and even highly resistant bacteria such as the tubercle bacillus succumb to drying within a few days. Spores, however, may resist drying for years. As a rule, bacteria with capsules are more resistant to drying than those with none.

**Temperature.** For each species of bacteria there is a minimum, optimum, and maximum temperature, meaning respectively the lowest temperature at which the species will grow; the temperature at which it grows best, and the highest temperature at which growth is possible (Fig. 4-1). The optimum temperature for a species corresponds to the average temperature of its usual habitat. For instance, bacteria that naturally live in or attack the human body live best at 37° C.* (the normal temperature of the body). These are *mesophiles*. The lowest temperature at which any of these species will continue to multiply is around 20° C. (Celsius). and the highest is from 42° to 45° C.

Many bacteria will not grow at a temperature more than a few degrees above or below their optimum. Some pathogenic bacteria die off rapidly at only 38° C. The majority of saprophytic bacteria (mesophiles) grow best between 25° and 30° C., but some *thermophiles*, or heat-loving species, grow at a temperature above 45° C. and high as 65° C. A few *psychrophiles*, or cold-loving species, grow at temperatures just above the freezing point (20° C. or less). They proliferate slowly in the refrigerator. Many psychrophilic organisms have red pigments. Where they grow on the surface of ice and snow, they color it to give a red snow.

Cold retards or stops bacterial growth, but when the bacteria are later exposed to a temperature favorable for their growth, multiplication is resumed. Refrigeration (4° to 6° C.) is one of the best methods of preserving bacterial cultures, since bacteria are generally resistant to low temperatures and even to freezing. Prolonged freezing, however, destroys them.

High temperatures are much more injurious to bacteria than low ones and are used effectively in

*The temperature scale called centigrade in America has been known in many other countries as Celsius after Anders Celsius (1701-1744), the Swede who originated it in 1742. According to the Eleventh General Conference on Weights and Measures (1960), the term centigrade is inexact and the name Celsius replaces it; with the capital C retained.

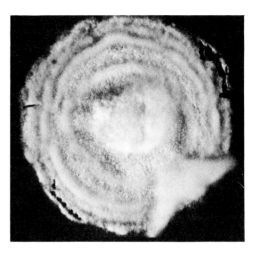

**Fig. 4-1.** Variation in growth rate from changes in temperature. Note rings of rapid and slow growth in giant colony of fungus *(Histoplasma capsulatum)*. One sector of mutant growth is seen in lower right-hand corner. (Courtesy Dr. R. H. Musgnug, Haddonfield, N.J.)

practical situations where bacteria and their spores must be destroyed. (See Chapter 15.)

**Reaction.** For each species of bacteria there is a certain degree of alkalinity or acidity (a certain pH), at which growth is most rapid. The reactions of culture media must be carefully adjusted to the desired hydrogen ion concentration. The best growth of most microorganisms is found in a narrow pH range of not less than 6 or more than 8. Most pathogens grow best in a neutral or slightly alkaline medium. Regardless of the influence of the environment, the reaction of the interior of the cell is just at the neutral point (pH 7).

**Oxygen.** Organisms that grow in the presence of free atmospheric oxygen are known as *aerobes*. If an organism cannot develop at all in the absence of free oxygen, it is an *obligate aerobe*. Those that cannot grow in the presence of free oxygen but must obtain it from oxygen-containing compounds (inorganic sulfates, nitrates, and carbonates or certain organic compounds) are *anaerobes*. Few of the pathogenic organisms are anaerobic. Of these, the organisms of tetanus and gas gangrene are notable. Organisms adaptable to either the presence or absence of atmospheric oxygen are *facultative*. Organisms growing best in an amount of oxygen less than that contained in the air are known as *microaerophiles*, whereas organisms vulnerable to free oxygen are *obligate anaerobes*. The enzyme systems of obligate anaerobes are inactivated by the oxygen of the atmosphere.

Organisms designated *capnophiles* need a 3% to 10% increase in carbon dioxide in the environment to initiate growth.

**Light.** Violet, ultraviolet, and blue lights are highly

destructive to bacteria,* green light is much less so, and red and yellow lights have little bactericidal action. Because of its content of ultraviolet light, direct sunlight kills most bacteria within a few hours. Bright daylight has an effect similar to that of sunlight but one of less potency.

A few species of saprophytic bacteria containing chlorophyl can utilize sunlight to build up the compounds of which they are composed. This bacterial chlorophyl is scattered throughout the cytoplasm, unlike the chlorophyl of plant cells, which is contained in their chloroplasts.

**By-products of bacterial growth.** If it were not for inhibitory influences, bacteria could completely submerge the whole world. It is estimated that the progeny from the unrestricted growth of a single bacterium would be 280 trillion at the end of only 24 hours. In cultures, bacterial reproduction is so rapid that bacteria soon exhaust their food supply and release products that inhibit further bacterial growth, Notable are organic acids from carbohydrate metabolism that inhibit growth by changing the reaction of the medium. The practical application of this is found in the pickling industry, where the acid medium is used to prevent bacterial contamination.

**Electricity and radiant energy.** By itself, electricity does not destroy bacteria, but it causes heat and

_____
*The use of ultraviolet light in sterilization is discussed on p. 144.

changes that may be lethal in the medium in which the bacteria are growing. Electric light inhibits bacterial growth, but the inhibition is an effect of the light, not of electricity.

The effects of roentgen rays are generally harmful to most bacteria, being about a hundred times more effective in their action against bacteria than ultraviolet light. There are, however, notable exceptions.

**Chemicals.** Certain chemicals destroy bacteria, and others inhibit their growth (p. 146). Some attract bacteria (*positive chemotaxis*), whereas others repel them (*negative chemotaxis*).

**Osmotic pressure.** The bacterial cell is encased in a membrane said to be *semipermeable* because it allows water to pass freely in and out of the cell but gives a varying degree of resistance to dissolved substance in the fluid medium in which the cell is suspended. This makes the cell a small osmotic unit responsive to changes in its fluid environment (Fig. 4-2).

Under normal conditions there is a higher concentration of dissolved substances within the cell than without it. The greater osmotic pressure inside the cell keeps the protoplasm of the cell firmly against the cell wall, and the cell is said to be *turgid*. If a bacterial cell is placed in solutions having varying concentrations of dissolved substances, changes take place. In a solution with a high concentration of dissolved substances (*hypertonic* solution), water leaves the interior of the cell and the cell begins to shrink. If

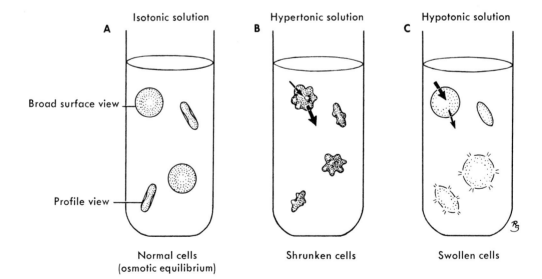

Fig. 4-2. Effect of osmotic pressure on cells. Observe the red blood cell in the following fluids. **A,** With same amount of dissolved substance as cell protoplasm (isotonic solution), water does not transfer, and red cell does not change size or shape. **B,** With more dissolved substance (hypertonic solution), water passes from cell to surrounding fluid, and cell shrinks. **C,** With less dissolved substance (hypotonic solution), water moves into red cell, and it swells and bursts.

the difference in concentration between the interior and the exterior of the cell is not too great, the cell may be able to adjust to the hypertonic solution, regain its turgor, and continue its growth. If not, the cell continues to shrink and finally dies (*plasmolysis*).

If a cell is placed in a solution with a low concentration of dissolved substances or in distilled water (*hypotonic* solution), water passes into the cell, the cell swells, and it may burst (*plasmoptysis*). A solution containing that concentration of dissolved substances in which the cell neither swells nor shrinks is said to be *isotonic*.

Most bacteria resist small changes in osmotic pressure but are killed or inhibited by high concentrations either of salt (as used in brines) or of sugar. This fact is utilized in the preservation of foods such as syrups and jellies and in the preservation of meats in brine. That some microorganisms can adjust to a high concentration of sugar is seen in molds on jellies. To preserve foods safely, higher concentrations of sugar must be used than of salt.

That a few species of bacteria (*osmophiles*) do well in a hypertonic solution, is seen from the bacterial life of the oceans. Even the Dead Sea with its high salt content supports a bacterial population (*halophiles*). A small amount of various salts in the fluid medium for bacteria is beneficial to bacterial growth. Traces of such salts are furnished by natural foods such as meat extracts.

## Interrelations

**Symbiosis.** Certain species of bacteria grow well together, and the associated species accomplish harmful or beneficial results that neither does alone. For instance, staphylococci and influenza bacilli multiply more rapidly when grown together than either does when grown alone. This is known as *synergism*.

*Symbiosis* refers to the relation of mutual benefit existing between two organisms. For example, there is the beneficial relation between the leguminous plants and the nitrogen-fixing bacteria living in the root nodules of these plants (p. 373). *Commensalism* is the term applied when two organisms live together without benefit or injury to each other.

**Antagonism.** Sometimes the presence of certain species of bacteria inhibits the growth of others. For instance, growth of the gonococcus is inhibited by the presence of almost any other species of bacteria. This is *antagonism*. Theories put forth to explain antagonism are (1) that one organism secretes a substance toxic to the growth of the other and (2) that one organism promotes a defense mechanism of the animal body against the other. The appearance of certain infections after the administration of antibiotics may be explained in terms of an antagonistic relationship between two organisms, only one of which succumbs to the action of the antibiotic. Released by the antibiotic, the other microorganism can now become quite aggressive.

## Questions for review

1 Name at least five requirements for bacteria to grow and multiply.
2 Classify bacteria from the standpoint of food requirements. Name elements required for the nourishment of bacteria.
3 Define host, autotrophic, heterotrophic, facultative, obligate, hypertonic, hypotonic, isotonic.
4 How are bacteria affected by heat and cold?
5 Classify bacteria from the standpoint of oxygen requirements.
6 What are the effects of light on bacteria?
7 What is the difference between negative and positive chemotaxis? Plasmoptysis and plasmolysis?
8 Consult outside sources and briefly discuss semipermeable membranes.
9 What is commensalism? Synergism? Symbiosis? Antagonism?
10 What is the preferred designation of the scientific temperature scale?
11 What are psychrophiles? Halophiles? Thermophiles? Osmophiles?

**References on pp. 48 and 49.**

# CHAPTER 5

# Bacteria
## biologic activities

Bacteria engage in a complex of biologic activities of varying importance. Of prime consideration are those relating to the growth and integrity of the microorganism. Those resulting in the elaboration of toxins and substances harmful to other living cells have special significance in the production or aggravation of disease. Other events in the life of the bacterial cell, although striking in their manifestations, are not vital and are of secondary importance.

## Major metabolic events

Bacteria first drew attention to their very existence by the dramatic changes resulting from their metabolic activities. Today their biochemical capabilities are obvious when one considers the phenomena of fermentation (p. 69), putrefaction (p. 70), decay, soil fertility (p. 372), and infectious disease (p. 83).

Much of the general body of information concerning metabolism in creatures more complex than bacteria has come from studies of comparable processes in bacteria and other microorganisms. Because bacteria multiply rapidly, we can learn much about their activities in 2 days. To obtain comparable information about man would require 200 years or more.

The bacterial cell makes two biologic demands of its environment: it must obtain therein the chemical ingredients with which it can build and maintain itself, and at the same time it must derive therefrom the energy necessary to do its work. *Metabolism* encompasses all biochemical reactions occurring within the bacterial cell by which these two requirements are met.

**Enzymes.** Enzymes are essential, very efficient ingredients in the complex maze of metabolic activity. Life is not possible with them.* The term *enzyme* is of

Greek origin and means "leavened" (*en*, in; *zyme*, leaven).

*Characteristics.* Enzymes are catalysts* and, being proteins, are therefore organic catalysts. Although produced by a living cell, an enzyme operates independently of that cell. Its activity is not lessened when it is separated from the cell that produced it.

Over a thousand enzymes have been identified among living cells. Well-known ones in animals include ptyalin of the salivary glands, pepsin from the glands of the stomach, and trypsin elaborated in the pancreas. Bacteria produce enzymes that are remarkably like those produced by the organs of higher forms of life.

In the cell a protein is a key component and functional unit that is made up of a characteristic chain of some 200 amino acids. Twenty distinct amino acids compose proteins, and the identity of a given protein is largely the result of different patterns of these amino acids, the number present, and the sequence in which they are placed. There is an almost infinite number of proteins belonging to different animals and plant species. A given organism, however, builds only a certain number.

Of the multitude of proteins built by living cells, the majority function as enzymes. A bacterium contains, on an average, about 2000 enzymes. Elaboration of proteins and therefore enzymes within a cell is under the direction of the DNA of the bacterial nuclear apparatus. For 2000 enzymes there would be a corresponding 2000 control positions (genes) on the bacterial chromosome (the one gene—one enzyme hypothesis).

Enzymatic action (Fig. 5-1) is specific; that is, each enzyme causes only its own peculiar type of

---

*In space exploration, the enzyme phosphatase, common to most forms of life on this planet, is considered a good indicator for the presence of life or prelife if detected in even trace amounts in outer space.

*A catalyst is a substance that accelerates a chemical reaction which otherwise would occur either very slowly and ineffectively or not at all. In the reaction the catalyst is not chemically altered. It contributes nothing to the end product and does not furnish energy.

chemical change on its specific substrate.* Enzymes represent large protein molecules of special chemical configuration. The specific activity of the enzyme comes from its particular shape and the shape of the molecules reacting with it. The enzyme molecule is a kind of template into which the reacting compound can fit. Once the chemical reaction is complete, a new compound is released. However, the enzyme by

---

*Substrate* is the term designating the material acted on by the enzyme.

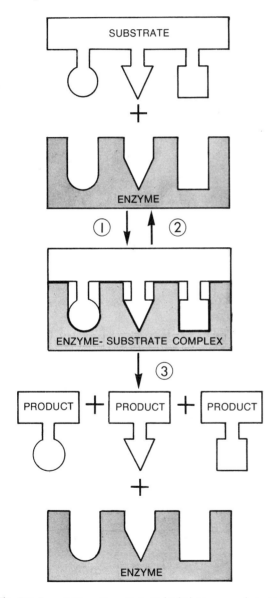

**Fig. 5-1.** Enzymatic action. Note tight fit between substrate and enzyme molecule to form enzyme-substrate complex. (From Tuttle, W. W., and Schottelius, B. A.: Textbook of physiology, ed. 16, St. Louis, 1969, The C. V. Mosby Co.)

definition remains intact. Enzymatic action can result in separation as well as combination of molecules. For the activation of an enzyme, a small molecule, usually an inorganic metallic ion such as magnesium, manganese, zinc, or iron, may be needed. The molecular *activator* does not participate in the process.

Very small amounts of enzyme can bring about most extensive chemical changes. One molecule of enzyme can catalyze the reaction for 10,000 to 1 million moles* of substrate per minute. Although the enzyme is not destroyed during the chemical reaction, its activity may be inhibited by the end products formed. The accumulation of end products may also block the formation of more enzyme. This is spoken as *negative feedback control*.

Enzymes are most active at temperatures from 35° to 40° C. and within a limited pH range. They are delicate structures; a temperature of 60° destroys them within 10 to 30 minutes (heat denaturation). Freezing retards their action but does not destroy them. A medium that is too acid or too alkaline inhibits their action or destroys them. Since the biochemical reactions occurring in bacteria are complicated and interrelated ones, enzymes may function in a group or as an *enzyme system*, with several enzymes being responsible for closely related chemical changes.

A *coenzyme* is a nonprotein organic compound that may be necessary for enzymatic activity. It serves to position the substrate to the enzyme. Some coenzymes are tightly bound to their enzymes; others are less so. Although it is changed during the catalytic reaction, the coenzyme reappears at the end of the reaction in its original form. Many coenzymes come from dietary vitamins.

It is possible for enzymes performing the same chemical function to exist with different molecular structures. The physiologic equivalent for a given enzyme is an *isoenzyme*. An enzyme may have one or more isoenzymes. The enzyme lactic dehydrogenase has five.

*Classification.* From the standpoint of a given cell, enzymes may be *exoenzymes* or *endoenzymes*. The former are elaborated within the cell and are diffused through the plasma membrane into the surrounding medium, where they are active. Endoenzymes are liberated only by the disintegration of the cell that produced them. Exoenzymes are more important; some have been separated and crystallized. Enzymes are also related to the type of chemical reaction catalyzed or to the particular substrate affected. They are named by adding the suffix *ase* to the name of their substrate or to the name of the reaction influenced.

---

*One mole is one gram-molecular weight of substrate in one liter solution.

In 1964, the Commission on Enzymes of the International Union of Biochemists adopted a classification separating enzymes into six major categories according to their type reaction:

1. *Oxidoreductases* catalyze oxidation-reduction reactions (include oxidases and dehydrogenases).
2. *Transferases* catalyze the transfer of a specific group from one substrate to another (as in transamination or transmethylation). Examples are transaminases, transacetylases, and kinases.
3. *Hydrolases* catalyze hydrolytic reactions. Here are found digestive enzymes (proteinases, lipases, amylases) that break down large molecules to smaller, readily assimilated ones. Others include peptidases, esterases, and phosphatases.
4. *Lyases* (nonhydrolytic enzymes) catalyze the removal of specific groups from given substrates, as, for example, when bonds are split between carbon atoms (decarboxylases) and between carbon and oxygen atoms (carbonic anhydrase). Others are deaminases and aldolases.
5. *Isomerases* catalyze the interconversion of two compounds of the same atomic composition but with different structure and properties. An isomerase is an important component of the glycolytic pathway.
6. *Ligases* catalyze the joining together of two molecules, coupled with the breakdown of adenosine triphosphate (ATP) or a similar energy-yielding triphosphate. Ligases are also known as synthetases and as "activating" enzymes.

**Chemosynthesis.** The plant cell, possessing chlorophyl, obtains energy from the environment in the form of light (photosynthesis). Microorganisms with no cholorophyl must gain their energy from the chemical alteration of the substances at hand, a process termed *chemosynthesis.* Because of the complexity of their metabolic enzymes, most bacteria can break down the proteins, fat, carbohydrates, and other organic compounds they contact. Organisms utilizing inorganic matter as their source of energy are *lithotrophs.* Those utilizing organic matter are *organotrophs.* Most bacteria are organotrophs.

A series of enzymatic steps characterizes the chemical changes involved in chemosynthesis. The starting point is bacterial *digestion;* the end point is *biologic oxidation.*

*Digestion.* The principal sources of energy for bacteria in their environment are mostly complex molecules too large for the bacterial cell to deal with directly. They must be reduced to workable particle size.

To accomplish this, bacteria rely on certain enzymes (hydrolases), which they release into the medium to split the large molecules chemically by a process that includes the addition of water. This is *hydrolysis.* The hydrolytic enzymes are examples of exoenzymes. Briefly, digestion is the exoenzyme-catalyzed hydrolysis of a large molecule to secure fragments small enough for passage into the bacterial cell.

*Absorption.* After the bacterial cell has reduced the large molecules into smaller particles, it must next absorb them. There are two ways of doing this. Because of the osmotic pressure gradient, the cell can passively allow the molecules to move in by diffusion. This is slow and inefficient at best. On the other hand, the cell can actively participate to speed the movement. The manner in which this is brought about is referred to as *active transport.* As would be expected, the mechanisms of active transport, including the enzymes required, are located on the cell membrane, and their activity constitutes a "pump."

*Oxidation.* Some of the molecules that the cell pulls into itself from without are ready for the sequences of biologic oxidation. Most are not, and these must be prepared, that is, changed into a form that can be oxidized. If a phosphate group is attached to the molecule (phosphorylation), a very significant chemical bonding is made. When this phosphorylated compound is oxidized, the chemical bond of the phosphate group traps energy not only in a form suitable for later use but also in large amounts. Phosphorylation is the most important preliminary sequence to oxidation, but other chemical reactions may be encountered at this step.

Biologic oxidation is the chemical setup whereby a cell is provided with energy that it can use biologically. The complicated reactions contributing to it, many of them chain reactions, are carried out notably by enzymes (oxidases, dehydrogenases, or oxidoreductases), coenzymes, and hydrogen acceptors or carriers. *Oxidases* act on a substrate to cause it to undergo oxidation, that is, a reaction wherein electrons are removed from a substrate with accompanying hydrogen ions. Enzymes making possible the removal of hydrogen (or electrons) are called *dehydrogenases.* As the hydrogen ions are removed, there must be a suitable compound to receive them, a *hydrogen acceptor* or *carrier,* which in so accepting becomes reduced. Hydrogen acceptors or carriers, which can be oxidized and reduced, function in the transport of hydrogen (or electrons) from tissue metabolites to oxygen or some other end product. Transfer of electrons constitutes oxidation and reduction, and the end results must include an oxidized product, a reduced one, and energy liberated or trapped.

**Storage of energy.** There is no dissipation of heat

in biologic oxidation. The energy released is held in the chemical bond between an organic molecule and a phosphate group. Bacteria store this energy-rich bond solely on the organic molecule adenosine diphosphate, ADP. When a phosphate group is transferred to ADP, there is formed adenosine triphosphate, ATP, from which energy-rich reserves are available.

**Classes of biologic oxidation.** If the ultimate and final hydrogen acceptor is molecular oxygen, the events (aerobic) of biologic oxidation to generate energy are those of *respiration*. If it is an inorganic nitrate, sulfate, or carbonate, the metabolic processes are those of *anaerobic respiration*. The sulfate- and carbonate-reducing organisms are obligate anaerobes relying exclusively on these compounds for energy. The denitrifying bacteria are facultative aerobes using nitrate only in the absence of oxygen.

If the final hydrogen acceptor is an organic compound, the processes of biologic oxidation are those of *fermentation*. Fermentation, then, is metabolism utilizing organic compounds as both electron donors and electron acceptors. Many organic compounds can be fermented, and many microorganisms, including disease producers, can live anaerobically to satisfy their energy needs through fermentation reactions. Seven different biochemical types have been elucidated.

Using microbial metabolism of glucose, let us compare respiration (aerobic) with fermentation (anaerobic). In the presence of molecular oxygen, respiration takes place in all animal cells and in microbes, and glucose is changed in a biochemical sequence to carbon dioxide and water. In the absence of oxygen, microbes ferment the glucose but with different end products. Among bacteria generally, incomplete oxidation of this nature is the rule, and a wide variety of end products accumulate. The most commonly occurring sequence for glucose degradation is the Embden-Meyerhof glycolytic pathway, in which glucose is changed to pyruvate.

Respiration is a much more efficient process than fermentation. Many more intermediate steps mean much more energy generated. The potential from complete oxidation of glucose is far greater than that from its conversion to alcohol and carbon dioxide; for instance, respiration yields over 30 molecules of ATP (the energy source) as compared to the net of only 2 for each mole of sugar fermented.

Microbial fermentation reactions however are of great value to man because of the many by-products of practical worth to home and industry. They are also useful in the laboratory study of microbes.

**Macromolecular synthesis.** In a microbial cell physiologic phenomena are geared primarily for growth, that is, an orderly increase in mass or number of its constituents, most of which are macromolecules. Macromolecules are found in the protein-synthesizing groups of the cytoplasm, on membranes of organelles, in chromosomes, in the cell wall, and in the various enzyme systems, The metabolic activities of the cell revolve around these large molecules, and one of the crucial functions of the cell is their biosynthesis. To put together a macromolecule, two things are needed: (1) the subunits for linkage and (2) the energy to do the work. The energy to induce linkage comes from the cellular reserves of ATP. The subunits must come from either the environment or the metabolic activities of the cell and depend on the chemical nature of the unit complex. For proteins these are amino acids; for carbohydrates, simple sugars; for lipids, glycerol (or other alcohols) and fatty acids; for nucleic acids, nucleotides; and for phospholipids, such substances as choline. The alignment of subunits in the macromolecule is determined in one of two ways. In nucleic acids and proteins, it is template directed: DNA serves as template for its own synthesis and for the synthesis of the types of RNA. Messenger RNA serves as template for the synthesis of proteins. In carbohydrates and lipids the arrangement of subunits is entirely enzymatic.

Although many metabolic activities are universally the same, some are unique to bacteria, for example, the biochemical pathway by which the mucopeptide of the cell wall is structured. This provides a chemical basis for the design of an antimicrobial compound with a selective effect on one of the steps in the biosynthesis of the cell wall. Since bacterial protoplasm is under greatly increased osmotic pressure in relation to the isotonicity of the host cells, weakening the cell wall jacketing the bacterium can easily explode it.

## Medically related activities

**Toxins.** Practically all species of bacteria produce poisonous substances known as *toxins*. The capacity to elaborate toxins is *toxigenicity*. In some the toxin is almost entirely responsible for the specific action of the bacteria. Toxins are of two types: *exotoxins*, diffused by the bacterial cell into the surrounding medium, and *endotoxins*, liberated only when the bacterial cell is destroyed. Some bacterial exotoxins are more deadly than any mineral or vegetable poison. Among the comparatively few bacteria (mostly gram-positive) noted for their exotoxin production are *Corynebacterium diphtheriae*, *Clostridium tetani*, and *Clostridium botulinum*. In disease caused by *Corynebacterium diphtheriae* (diphtheria) and *Clostridium tetani* (tetanus), the bacteria grow restricted to a superficial area in the body. Within themselves these organisms produce little effect, but the soluble exotoxins elaborated at the site of growth are ab-

45

sorbed into the body to cause serious and often fatal illness. Such illness is better thought of as chemical poisoning rather than as disease induced by growth of bacteria.

It is interesting to note that some bacteria are harmful only when they are diseased. Evidence is accumulating that the above-mentioned organisms make exotoxin only because they are infected with bacterial virus (bacteriophage). The virus initiates (codes for) the production of toxin. (See also p. 242.)

Exotoxins are proteins in composition and are antigenic and specific. When a small amount of a toxin is injected into an animal, it stimulates the production of *antitoxin*. The *specificity* of exotoxins refers to the fact that diphtheria bacilli elaborate a toxin that causes diphtheria and nothing else and tetanus bacilli elaborate a toxin that causes tetanus and nothing else. When an exotoxin is inactivated with formaldehyde, it no longer causes disease but still can produce an immunity to the disease. Such modified toxins are known as *anatoxins* or *toxoids*. Toxoids are used to produce a permanent immunity to diphtheria and tetanus.

Substances contained in the seeds of certain plants and some of the secretions of animals resemble exotoxins. Among these are crotin, derived from the seed of the croton plant; ricin, from the castor bean; and the venoms of snakes, spiders, and scorpions.

Endotoxins are complex lipopolysaccharides that are an integral part of the cell wall of most gram-negative bacteria. Endotoxins are not found in the surrounding medium when bacteria are grown in a liquid. They do not effectively promote the formation of antitoxins, do not possess the specificity of exotoxins, and cannot be converted into toxoids. The lipid fraction of the complex is related to the numerous biologic manifestations of endotoxin — fever, circulatory disturbances, certain immunologic effects, and so on. (See Table 5-1.) Noteworthy for their production of endotoxins are *Salmonella typhi*, the cause of typhoid fever, and *Shigella flexneri*, one of the causes of bacillary dysentery.

The biochemical mechanisms by which toxins injure cells and produce disease are poorly understood.

**Harmful metabolic products.** Bacteria produce a number of enzymatic substances not directly toxic but related significantly to disease. *Hemolysins* are substances that cause the lysis (dissolution) of red blood cells. There are many types, among which are immune hemolysins, hemolysins of certain vegetables, hemolysins contained in venoms, and bacterial hemolysins. The bacterial hemolysins are of two types: (1) those that may be separated from the bacterial cells by filtration (filtrable hemolysins) and (2) those that are demonstrated about the bacterial colony on a culture medium containing red blood cells. The filtrable hemolysins are named after the bacteria that give rise to them (examples: *staphylolysin*, derived from staphylococci, and *streptolysin*, derived from streptococci). The filtrable hemolysins have a certain degree of specificity; that is, a given hemolysin may act on the red blood cells of one species of animal but not on those of another species. They are protein and inactivated by exposure to a temperature of 55° C. for 30 minutes. In the body of an animal they induce the formation of antibodies against themselves.

## Table 5-1
Distinguishing features of toxins

| FEATURE | EXOTOXINS | ENDOTOXINS |
|---|---|---|
| Location | Gram-positive bacteria | Gram-negative bacteria |
| Relation to cell | Extracellular | Closely bound to cell wall (release with destruction of cell) |
| Toxicity | Great | Weak |
| Tissue affinity | Specific (examples: nerves—tetanus toxin; heart muscle, adrenals—diphtheria toxin) | Nonspecific (local reaction—injection site; systemic reaction—fever, shock) |
| Chemical nature | Protein | Lipopolysaccharide complex |
| Stability | Unstable (denatured with heat, ultraviolet light) | Stable |
| Antigenicity | High (neutralizing antibodies) | Weak |
| Conversion to toxoid | Yes | No |
| Diseases where action is important | Diphtheria | Salmonelloses |
| | Tetanus | Asiatic cholera |
| | Gas gangrene | Brucellosis |
| | Staphylococcal food poisoning | |
| | Botulism | |

Staphylococci, streptococci, pneumococci, and *Clostridium perfringens* are important producers of these hemolysins. An organism may have more than one filtrable hemolysin; for instance, streptococci produce two hemolysins known respectively as streptolysin O and streptolysin S.

The hemolysins detected when bacteria are grown on a culture medium containing blood are of two types, *alpha* and *beta*. Beta hemolysins give rise to a clear colorless zone of hemolysis around the bacterial colony. Alpha hemolysins give rise to a greenish zone of partial hemolysis. The relation existing between filtrable hemolysins and those detected by growing the bacteria on a culture medium containing blood is not known. The relation between hemolysin production and virulence is obscure. As a rule, the hemolytic strains of pathogenic bacteria have greater capacities to cause disease than the nonhemolytic strains. On the other hand, certain nonpathogenic bacteria produce hemolysins. Hemolysins probably contribute to the invasive capacity of some bacteria.

*Leukocidins* destroy polymorphonuclear neutrophilic leukocytes. The leukocytes, or white blood cells, take an active part in the battle of the body against infection. Leukocidins are produced by pneumococci, streptococci, and staphylococci. Their relation to immunity is not known. It is likely that they enhance virulence. Certain hemolysins and leukocidins appear to be identical.

*Coagulase* is elaborated by bacteria to accelerate the coagulation of blood and under suitable laboratory conditions causes oxalated or citrated blood to clot. Coagulase formation appears to be confined to the staphylococci. The *coagulase test,* performed by mixing a culture of staphylococci with a suitable amount of oxalated or citrated blood under specified conditions, is used to differentiate pathogenic and nonpathogenic staphylocci. Because the former cause the blood to coagulate, they are said to be *coagulase-positive*. The role of coagulase in immunity is not known. Possibly it protects organisms against the destructive action of leukocytes (phagocytosis). The coagulum from plasma that has leaked into the tissues forms a barrier between the bacteria and the white blood cells.

The *bacterial kinases* act on certain components of the blood to liquefy fibrin. Kinases interfere with coagulation of blood, since a blood clot is made up of red blood cells enmeshed in interlacing strands of fibrin. Kinases liquefy clots already formed. There seems to be a relation between the kinases and virulence because kinases destroy blood or fibrin clots that form around a site of infection to wall it off. The most important kinase is *streptokinase*, also known as *fibrinolysin*, elaborated by many hemolytic streptococci.

Staphylococci and certain other bacteria also produce kinases. Streptokinase has been used in certain locations in the body to dissolve clots and to prevent the formation of adhesions that would be laid down on the fibrin precipitated in the body cavities.

*Hyaluronidase* is secreted by certain bacteria to make the tissues more permeable to the bacteria elaborating it. It hydrolyzes hyaluronic acid, a constituent of the intercellular ground substance of many tissues that helps to hold the cells of the tissue together. Hyaluronidase was formerly spoken of as the "spreading factor." It is produced by pneumococci and streptococci.

*Bacteriocins* are bacterial protein or polypeptide substances produced by strains of a family of microbes and active only on certain other strains in the given family. *Colicins* are those produced by strains in the family Enterobacteriaceae. They are highly specific and seem to be directed chiefly against the bacterial membrane. Nearly twenty different ones have been described and grouped by their bactericidal specificity.

## Other effects

**Pigment production.** So far as is known, pigment production has no relation to disease and no importance other than in identification of pigment-producing organisms. Yellow pigments are most prevalent, but pigments of almost any color occur. The red and yellow pigments belong to the same chemical group as those in turnips, egg yolk, and fruits. Pigments are produced by both parasitic and saprophytic bacteria, but most species of bacteria do not produce any pigment. Common pigment producers are *Staphylococcus aureus,* with a golden pigment, and *Pseudomonas aeruginosa,* with a bluish green pigment. *Serratia marcescens* produces a red pigment. Pigment-producing or *chromogenic* bacteria lose that property when grown under unfavorable conditions.

**Heat.** During the growth of all bacteria, heat is produced but in such small amounts that it can be detected in ordinary cultures only by most delicate methods. The heating of damp hay is in part the result of bacterial action.

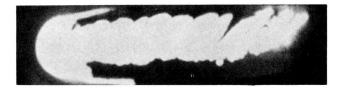

**Fig. 5-2.** Luminescent bacteria *(Vibrio fischeri)*. Photograph made in total darkness to show light produced by culture. (Courtesy Carolina Biological Supply Co., Burlington, N.C.; from Noland, G. B., and Beaver, W. C.: General biology, ed. 9, St. Louis, 1974, The C. V. Mosby Co.)

**Light.** A few species of bacteria have the ability to produce light without emitting heat (bioluminescence) (Fig. 5-2). Most of them live in salt water, and some live a parasitic existence on the bodies of salt-water fish. Fox fire, seen on decaying organic material especially in the woods, is from luminescent bacteria. None of the light-producing bacteria is pathogenic.

**Odors.** Certain odors are characteristic of some species of bacteria. Some arise from the decomposition of the material on which the bacteria are growing.

## Questions for review

1 Briefly discuss bacterial metabolism. What are the two main functions of metabolism?
2 Define enzymes. Give salient features.
3 Differentiate an exoenzyme from an endoenzyme. Give an important example of an exoenzyme.
4 Classify enzymes. Give examples.
5 What are toxins? Classify them and define each class.
6 Explain chemosynthesis, digestion, phosphorylation, oxidation-reduction, fermentation.
7 Name three species of bacteria important as exotoxin producers and two producers of endotoxins.
8 What are toxoids? For what are they used?
9 Define hemolysin, leukocidin, coagulase, streptokinase. Name an organism that produces each.
10 Classify bacterial hemolysins. What is meant by alpha and beta hemolysis?
11 What is hyaluronidase? Why is it sometimes called the "spreading factor"? In infections with what organisms is it important?
12 Discuss pigment production by bacteria.
13 Give an example of heat production by bacteria.
14 What is the importance of the coagulase test?
15 Define catalyst, substrate, macromolecule, colicins.

**REFERENCES** (Chapters 1 to 5)

American Type Culture Collection, ASM News **38:**590, 1972.
Andrew, W.: Microfabric of man: a textbook of histology, Chicago, 1966, Year Book Medical Publishers, Inc.
Bonner, J. T.: The size of life, Natural History **78:**40, Jan., 1969.
Brock, T. D.: Biology of microorganisms, Englewood Cliffs, N.J., 1974, Prentice-Hall, Inc.
Brown, W. V., and Bertke, E. M.: Textbook of cytology, ed. 2, St. Louis, 1974, The C. V. Mosby Co.
Buchanan, R. E., and Gibbons, N. E., co-editors: Bergey's manual of determinative bacteriology, Baltimore, 1974, The Williams & Wilkins Co.
Burrows, W.: Textbook of microbiology, Philadelphia, 1973, W. B. Saunders Co.
Busch, H.: The cell nucleus, New York, 1974, Academic Press, Inc.
Cairns, J.: The bacterial chromosome, Sci. Am. **214:**36, Jan., 1966.
Chedd, G.: The new biology, New York, 1972, Basic Books, Inc.
Crick, F. H. C.: The genetic code I, Sci. Am. **207:**66, Oct., 1962; III, Sci. Am. **215:**55, Oct., 1966.
Culliton, B. J.: Cell membranes: a new look at how they work, Science **175:**1348, 1972.
Dalton, A. J., and Haguenau, F., editors: Membranes (ultrastructure in biological systems), New York, 1968, Academic Press, Inc.
Dalton, A. J., and Haguenau, F., editors: Nucleus (ultrastructure in biological systems), New York, 1968, Academic Press, Inc.
Davis, B. D., and others: Microbiology including immunology and molecular genetics, New York, 1973, Harper & Row, Publishers.
Dickerson, R. E.: The structure and history of an ancient protein, Sci. Am. **226:**58, April, 1972.
Dowben, R. M., editor: Biological membranes, Boston, 1969, Little, Brown & Co.
Fawcett, D. W.: The cell: its organelles and inclusions, an atlas of fine structure, Philadelphia, 1966, W. B. Saunders Co.
Fogg, G. F., and others: The blue-green algae, New York, 1973, Academic Press, Inc.
Fox, C. F.: The structure of cell membranes, Sci. Am. **226:**30, Feb., 1972.
Frost, J. K.: The cell in health and disease. Vol. 2 in Wied, G. L., editor: Clinical cytology, a series of monographs, Baltimore, 1969, The Williams & Wilkins Co.
Gibson, W. C.: Some Canadian contributions to medicine, J.A.M.A. **200:**860, 1967.
Gray, P,: The dictionary of the biological sciences, New York, 1968, Van Nostrand Reinhold Co.
Hamburger, M.: Wall-defective bacteria, Arch. Intern. Med. **122:**175, 1968.
Horowitz, N. H., and others: Microbiology of the dry valleys of Antarctica, Science **176:**242, 1972.
Hungate, R. E.: Potentials and limitations of microbial methanogenesis, ASM News **40:**833, 1974.
Imshenetsky, A. A.: Microbiological research in space biology, ASM News **40:**518, 1974.
Jawetz, E., and others: Review of medical microbiology, Los Altos, Calif., 1974, Lange Medical Publications.
Joklik, W. K., and Smith, D. T., editors: Zinsser microbiology, ed. 15, New York, 1972, Appleton-Century-Crofts.
Klainer, A. S., and Geis, I.: Agents of bacterial disease, New York, 1973, Harper & Row, Publishers.
Kornberg, A.: The synthesis of DNA, Sci. Am. **219:**74, Oct., 1968.
Lamanna, C., and others: Basic bacteriology, Baltimore, 1973, The Williams & Wilkins Co.
Lee, L. W.: Elementary principles of laboratory instruments, ed. 3, St. Louis, 1974, The C. V. Mosby Co.
Leive, L., editor: Bacterial membranes and walls, Microbiology Series, vol. 1, New York, 1973, Marcel Dekker, Inc.
Lennette, E. H., and others, editors: Manual of clinical microbiology, Washington, D.C., 1974, American Society for Microbiology.
Lentz, J.: The age of the enzyme, Today's Health **48:**32, April, 1970.
Mayr, E.: Theory of biological classification, Nature **220:**545, 1968.
Medical news: bacterial synergism — an unexplored realm of research, J.A.M.A. **191:**25, March 8, 1965.

Metric medicine for a metric American (editorial), Ann. Intern. Med. **76:**138, 1972.

Minckler, J., and others, editors: Pathobiology: an introduction, St. Louis, 1971, The C. V. Mosby Co.

Mirsky, A. E.: The discovery of DNA, Sci. Am. **218:**78, June, 1968.

Neutra, M., and Leblond, C. P.: The Golgi apparatus, Sci. Am. **220:**110, Feb., 1969.

Noland, G. B., and Beaver, W. C.: General biology, ed. 9, St. Louis, 1974, The C. V. Mosby Co.

Norris, H. T.: Ion transport and bacterial toxins (editorial), Ann. Intern. Med. **67:**216, 1967.

Nourse, A. E.: The body (The Life Science Library), New York, 1964, Time-Life Books, Time, Inc.

Palade, G. E.: Structure and function at the cellular level, J.A.M.A. **198:**815, 1966.

Pfeiffer, J.: The cell (The Life Science Library), New York, 1969, Time-Life Books, Time, Inc.

Phillips, D. C.: The three-dimensional structure of an enzyme molecule, Sci. Am. **215:**78, Nov., 1966.

Roller-Massar, A.: Discovering the basis of life: an introduction to molecular biology, New York, 1974, McGraw-Hill Book Co.

Ryter, A.: Association of the nucleus and the membrane of bacteria: a morphological study, Bacteriol. Rev. **32:**39, 1968.

Shapiro, L., and others: Bacterial differentiation, Science **173:**884, 1971.

Sleigh, M. A., and MacDonald, A. G., editors: The effects of pressure on organisms. Proceedings of a Symposium, Bangor, North Wales, 1971, New York, 1972, Academic Press, Inc.

Smith, H.: Biochemical challenge of microbial pathogenicity, Bacteriol. Rev. **32:**164, 1968.

Stanier, R. Y., and others: The microbial world, Englewood Cliffs, N.J., 1970, Prentice-Hall, Inc.

Stimson, H. F.: Celsius versus centrigrade: the nomenclature of the temperature scale of science, Science **136:**254, 1962.

Swatek, F. E.: Textbook of microbiology, St. Louis, 1967, The C. V. Mosby Co.

Symposium on Membrane Structure and Function (editorial), J.A.M.A. **219:**1756, 1972.

Threadgold, L. T.: The ultrastructure of the animal cell, Elmsford, N.Y., 1967, Pergamon Press, Inc.

Toner, P. G., and Carr, K. E.: Cell structure; an introduction to biological electron microscopy, Edinburgh, 1971, E. & S. Livingstone, Ltd.

Trumbore, R. H.: The cell: chemistry and function, St. Louis, 1966, The C. V. Mosby Co.

Vanderkooi, G., and Green, D. E.: New insights into biological membrane structure, BioScience **21:**409, 1971.

Watson, J. D.: Molecular biology of the gene, New York, 1970, W. A. Benjamin, Inc.

Weissman, G.: The many-faceted lysosome, Hosp. Pract. **3:**30, Feb., 1968.

Whittaker, R. H.: New concepts of kingdoms of organisms, Science **163:**150, 1969.

Wischnitzer, S.: Introduction to electron microscopy, Elmsford, N.Y., 1970, Pergamon Press, Inc.

# UNIT II
MICROBES
procedures for study

## CHAPTER 6
# Visualization

## Plan of action

The microbiologist studies microbes in many ways. To visualize them, he must use an instrument of precision, the microscope. The test specimen from a contaminated site or diseased area that he inspects with the microscope may be unstained, or, as is often the case, it may be stained by one of several methods. He may make a culture from the suspect material. After the microorganisms have multiplied sufficiently to form visible growth, he may note the physical pattern of this growth, study the microorganisms in stained or unstained microscopic preparations made from the growth, and use some of it to determine their biochemical and biologic properties. He may inject microbes recovered from the test specimen into a suitable laboratory animal and observe their effect on the animal. Finally, he may apply well-known immunologic tests.

*Note:* In summary, the methods used to study microbes include (1) direct (microscopic) examination, (2) culture, (3) biochemical tests, (4) animal inoculation, and (5) immunologic reactions. They will be presented in a sequence of five chapters distributed through three units.*

Microbes must be handled with extreme caution and in accordance with well-known principles of conduct in microbiologic laboratories. *Bacteria or other disease-producing agents can be very dangerous, and accidental laboratory infections can be fatal.* In a recent survey of 1300 infections among laboratory workers, 39 ended fatally. In many cases the infections occurred in research workers and highly trained technologists.

## Tool for the study

The microbiologist has many instruments of precision at his command. Some are in constant use; others are needed only in special investigations.

---

*Discussions of the laboratory methods for identification and diagnosis of microbes are not confined to Unit II but are included in material specifically related to the different microbes throughout the book.

**The microscope.** The instrument most often used by the microbiologist and one to be handled with the greatest of care is the compound light microscope (Fig. 6-1). Needless to say, its workmanship should be of the highest quality.

*General description.* Microscopes are of two kinds, simple and compound. A *simple* microscope is little more than a magnifying lens. A *compound* microscope incorporates two or more lens systems so that the magnification of one system is increased by the other. Practically, it consists of two parts, the supporting stand and the optical system. The supporting stand includes (1) a base and pillar, (2) an arm to support the optical system and house the fine adjustment, (3) a platform (stage) on which the object to be examined rests, and (4) a condenser and mirror fitted beneath the stage. The condenser and mirror focus the light through a central opening in the stage on the object to be examined.

The optical system consists of a body tube that supports the *ocular* lenses (eyepiece) at the top end and the *objective* lenses attached to a revolving *nosepiece* at the other end. The optical system is connected to the arm of the supporting stand by an *intermediate slide* that moves up and down on the arm in response to movement of the *fine adjustment*. The intermediate slide contains the rack and pinion for the *coarse adjustment* that acts directly on the tube of the optical system. The platform of the microscope is usually equipped with a *mechanical stage* to hold firmly the microslide on which the object is mounted so that it can be moved from place to place by set screws. The advantages of this device are that the specimen can be examined systematically and, unless moved, the specimen remains in a fixed position.

The magnification of an objective is usually designated by its equivalent focal distance in inches or millimeters. By *equivalent focal distance* is meant the focal distance of a lens having the same magnification as the objective. The higher the number of the objective, the less is its magnification. American microscopes are usually fitted with 16 mm., 4 mm., and

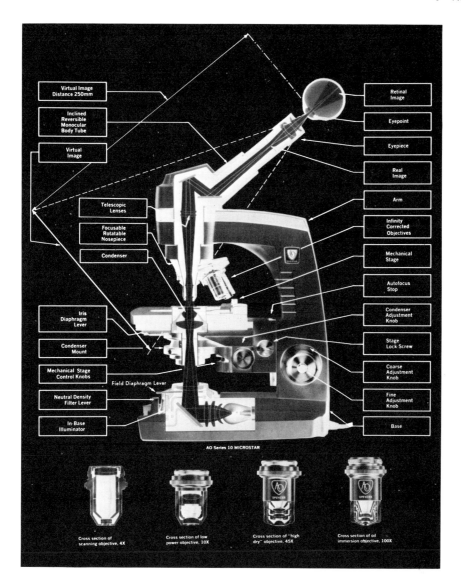

**Virtual Image Distance 250mm**

**Inclined Reversible Monocular Body Tube**

**Virtual Image**

**Telescopic Lenses**

**Focusable Rotatable Nosepiece**

**Condenser**

**Iris Diaphragm Lever**

**Condenser Mount**

**Mechanical Stage Control Knobs**

**Field Diaphragm Lever**

**Neutral Density Filter Lever**

**In-Base Illuminator**

**Retinal Image**

**Eyepoint**

**Eyepiece**

**Real Image**

**Arm**

**Infinity Corrected Objectives**

**Mechanical Stage**

**Autofocus Stop**

**Condenser Adjustment Knob**

**Stage Lock-Screw**

**Coarse Adjustment Knob**

**Fine Adjustment Knob**

**Base**

**AO Series 10 MICROSTAR**

**Cross section of scanning objective, 4X**

**Cross section of low power objective, 10X**

**Cross section of "high dry" objective, 45X**

**Cross section of oil immersion objective, 100X**

**Fig. 6-1.** Dissection of microscope—parts and optical features of monocular microscope. Note how light rays are reflected from mirror through microscope to eye of observer. This modern microscope is fitted with a movable stage whereby specimen may be focused to objective; observer need not change eye level. (Courtesy American Optical Corp., Scientific Instrument Division, Buffalo, N.Y.)

1.8 mm. objectives. The last is known as an *immersion objective* because for the best results there must be a liquid (oil or water) between the objective and the object being examined. Usually this is immersion oil. The 16 mm. objective magnifies 10 times; most 4 mm. objectives magnify 43 times; and most 1.8 mm. objectives magnify 97 times (Fig. 4-6).

The oculars of a microscope are given $6\times$, $10\times$, and similar designations to indicate that they increase the magnification of the objective 6, 10, or more times,

respectively. To obtain the magnification of any combination of ocular and objective lenses, multiply the magnification of the objective by that of the ocular. (See Table 6-1 and Fig. 6-2.) Remember that magnification refers to both the length and the width of an object; that is, a magnification of 100 means that the object is made to appear 100 times as long and 100 times as wide.

*Use of the microscope.* The following instructions are given to the student:

## Table 6-1
Magnification with lens combinations of the compound microscope

| OCULARS | OBJECTIVES | | |
| --- | --- | --- | --- |
| | 16 mm.<br>10× | 4 mm.<br>43× | 1.8 mm<br>97× |
| 6× | 60× | 258× | 582× |
| 10× | 100× | 430× | 970× |
| 15× | 150× | 645× | 1455× |

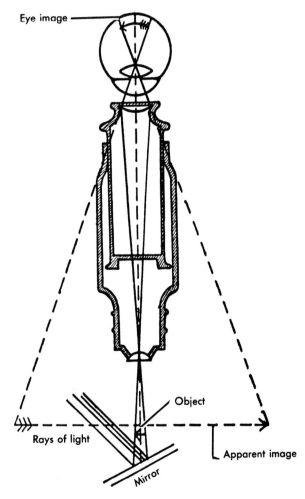

**Fig. 6-2.** Diagram to show how microscope magnifies. Apparent image is approximately 4 cm. in length. If object is 40 $\mu$m. in length, what is magnification?

1. Keep both eyes open. A very little practice will enable you to do this.
2. Avoid direct sunlight. North light is advantageous. Good results are obtained with daylight.
3. When a slide is placed on the stage, see that it lies flat against the platform. Adjust the light so that the object is evenly illuminated.
4. By means of the coarse adjustment, move the objective to be used until it nearly (but *not quite*) touches the cover glass or upper surface of the mounted specimen. Then focus *up* until the object comes plainly into view. Complete the focusing with the fine adjustment. Beginners should learn to focus with the low-power objectives (such as the 16 mm. objective). When an immersion objective is used, a drop of immersion oil must first be placed on the object before it can be clearly brought into view.
5. Keep the microscope clean and handle all parts with care. Do not touch the glass parts of the microscope. Do not allow chemicals to contact the microscope, since they may injure it. The mechanical parts may be cleaned by application of olive oil on gauze, which can be wiped off with chamois or lens paper. To remove oil from the optical glass parts, wipe with lens paper moistened with xylol. Do this as rapidly as possible to prevent injury to the optical settings.
6. Clean the microscope thoroughly when you are finished. Leave objectives with the lowest power in the working position. This precaution ensures that the least expensive objective will be injured should the optical system be jammed down accidentally. Keep the microscope covered when not in use.

**Ocular micrometer.** Microbes can be measured microscopically by means of a device known as a micrometer. The simplest type is the ocular micrometer, which consists of a scale on a glass disk that fits (scale side down) between the lenses of the eyepiece. The spaces between the lines on this scale do not represent true measurements. Real values are obtained by calibrating the ocular micrometer against a stage micrometer. This is a glass slide with a true measurement scale on it; the lines on the scale are either exactly 10 or 100 $\mu$m. ($\mu$) apart. By placing the stage micrometer in the position occupied by a smear of cells and by looking through the ocular of the microscope, one may superimpose the scale of the ocular on that of the stage micrometer. It is then easy to determine the actual unit length that the distance between the lines of the ocular micrometer represents.

**Photomicrographic camera** (Fig. 6-3). Another instrument of great value to microbiologists is the photo-

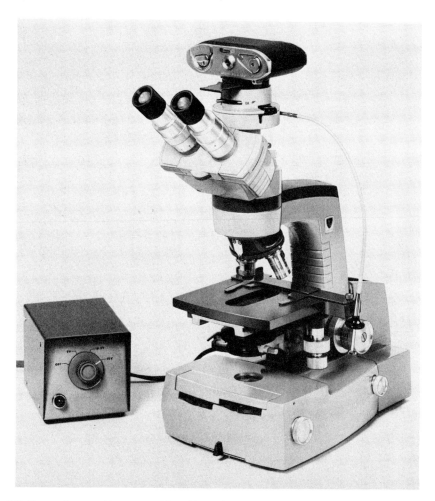

**Fig. 6-3.** Photomicrographic camera. Note binocular compound microscope fitted with camera for making photomicrographs (photographs of microscopic objects). Camera is fitted onto adaptor. (Courtesy American Optical Corp., Scientific Instruments Division, Buffalo, N.Y.)

micrographic camera, with which pictures are made of objects seen under the microscope. This gives an easily preserved visual record of microscopic findings and renders a wealth of material available for future study.

## Examination of unstained bacteria

It may be desirable to examine unstained bacteria to determine their biologic grouping, motility, and reaction to chemicals or specific sera. These characteristics may be determined in a *hanging drop* preparation. A few species of bacteria that cannot be stained by the methods to be discussed are often examined by *dark-field illumination.*

**Hanging drop preparations.** To examine bacteria microscopically in a hanging drop, one must use (1) a platinum loop for transferring the material to be ex-

amined to (2) a cover glass, and (3) a hanging drop slide.

The platinum loop (Fig. 6-4) is a piece of fine platinum wire about 3 inches in length. One end is fastened in a handle and the other end is fashioned into a loop about $1/16$ inch in diameter. Platinum is used for making wire loops because heating this metal in a flame repeatedly to sterilize it does not destroy it; the wire cools quickly after being heated.

A hanging drop slide is a thick glass slide with a circular concavity or depression as its center. A cover glass is a piece of very thin glass about $7/8$ inch square.

Make the preparation as follows: spread a small amount of petroleum jelly around the concavity of the slide. If the specimen to be examined is a culture growing on a solid medium or material such as thick

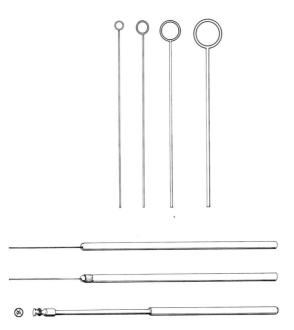

**Fig. 6-4.** Platinum wire loops and inoculating needles with holders. A length of platinum wire about 1½ inches makes a microbiologic loop. Gauge 26 or 27 wire is satisfactory for most routine inoculations; gauge 24 wire is better for stabbing.

pus, take up a loopful of specimen with the platinum loop and mix thoroughly with a drop of sterile isotonic salt solution placed in the center of the cover glass. If bacteria growing in a liquid medium are to be examined, transfer a drop of the fluid to the cover glass by means of the wire loop. Place the hanging drop slide over the cover glass in such a way that the center of the depression lies over the drop. The petroleum jelly seals the cover glass to the slide, holds it in place, and prevents evaporation. Invert the slide now so that the drop to be examined hangs from the bottom of the cover glass but does not touch the surface of the concavity at any point. The preparation is ready for microscopic examination. Examine with the 4 mm. (high dry) lens, and reduce the amount of light passing through it by partly closing the diaphragm of the substage condenser of the microscope. When hanging drop preparations are observed, brownian motion and flowing of organisms in currents should not be mistaken for true motility.

*The platinum loop must be sterilized immediately before and after each transfer of material containing bacteria* (Fig. 6-7, *D*). Since hanging drop preparations contain living bacteria, discard the slide and cover glass into a suitable container of disinfectant after the examination is finished.

The *wet mount* is similar to the hanging drop preparation except that an ordinary microslide is used instead of the thick hanging drop slide with its central

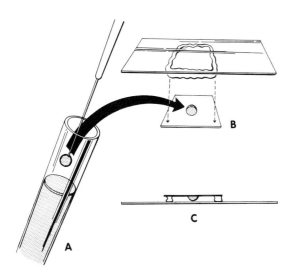

**Fig. 6-5.** Wet mount preparation. Rim clean cover glass with petroleum jelly (or make ring of it on a clean microslide). *Flame platinum loop!* Then proceed as shown in figure. **A,** Use loop to take drop of fluid specimen (either test fluid or test material in sterile isotonic saline). **B,** Place drop on cover glass. Invert cover slip onto microslide as in **C.** This simple procedure is easily carried out and readily adaptable.

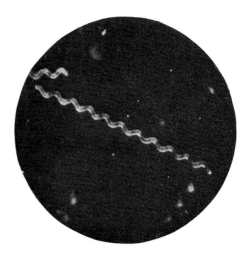

**Fig. 6-6.** Dark-field microscopy. A large spiral organism is white against black background. The dark-field microscope is an important tool in identification of various kinds of spiral microbes. This is *Spirulina jenneri,* one of the algae. (Courtesy American Optical Corp., Scientific Instrument Division, Buffalo, N.Y.)

depression (Fig. 6-5). Many of the applications are the same. (See also p. 326.)

**Dark-field illumination.** Dark-field illumination is used to examine certain delicate bacteria that are invisible in the living state in the light microscope, that cannot be stained by standard methods, or that are so distorted by staining as to lose their identifying characteristics. Its greatest usefulness is in the demonstration of *Treponema pallidum* in chancres and other syphilitic lesions, but it is of value in the examination of many other organisms (Fig. 6-6) as well.

The material to be examined is placed on an ordinary slide and covered with a cover glass. Sealing the

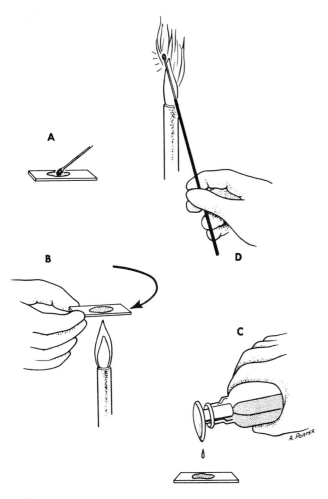

cover glass to the slide with a ring of melted pariffin prevents the cover glass from slipping and the accidental infection of the fingers. Dark-field illumination depends on the use of a substage condenser so constructed that the light rays do not pass directly through the object being examined, as is the case with an ordinary condenser, but strike it from the sides at almost a right angle to the objective of the microscope. The microscopic field becomes a dark background against which bacteria or other particles appear as bright silvery objects. A similar effect is seen when a beam of light enters a darkened room and renders visible particles of dust that cannot be seen in a better lighted room.

## Examination of stained bacteria

**Staining.** The bodies of bacteria are so small that, when examined in hanging drop preparations, little of their finer structure can be made out; to be studied more closely, they must be colored with some dye. This process is called *staining*. The dyes most often used are aniline dyes, derivatives of the coal tar product aniline. (Dye-impregnated paper strips for staining bacteria are commercially available.)

For a stained preparation, place a small amount of the material to be examined on a perfectly clean glass slide and spread out into a thin film by means of a platinum loop or a swab (Fig. 6-7). The film is known as a *smear*. After it is allowed to dry in the air, slowly pass the slide, smear side up, through a flame two or three times. *Flaming* kills the bacteria in the smear and causes them to stick to the slide. This is known as *fixing*. Other methods of fixing, such as immersion in methyl alcohol or Zenker's solution, are sometimes used, but heat is the most suitable for routine work. Apply the stain to the fixed smear and wash off with water; blot the slide dry between sheets of absorbent paper. Flame sterilization of the platinum loop is sketched in Fig. 6-7, *D*.

Three classes of stains are used in bacteriology: (1) simple stains, (2) differential stains, and (3) special stains. In addition, there is the process of *negative staining*.

*Simple stains.* A simple stain is usually an aqueous or alcoholic solution of a single dye. It is applied to the fixed smear from 1 to 5 minutes and washed off. The stain preparation is then ready for microscopic examination. Widely used simple stains are Löffler's alkaline methylene blue, carbolfuchsin, gentian violet, and safranine. The length of time that the stain remains on the smear depends on the avidity with which it acts. Sometimes a chemical to make it stain more intensely is added to the solution. Such a chemical is called a *mordant*.

Most bacteria stain easily and quickly with simple

**Fig. 6-7.** Preparation of stained bacterial smear. **A,** Spread loopful of test specimen thinly on clean glass microslide. Allow to dry. **B,** Fix specimen onto glass slide (held between fingers) by passing it through flame. **C,** Apply drops of stain from dropper bottle to slide (according to technic indicated). **D,** Sterilize inoculating loop (or needle) before and after it is used. Hold the length of wire in flame until it glows. *This is a very important step!*

stains, some do not stain so readily, and a few do not stain at all. Capsules and spores are not stained with these simple stains but may give contrast as clear *unstained* structures. Flagella cannot be stained in this way and are not seen as contrasting structures.

*Differential stains.* More complex staining methods divide bacteria into groups, depending on their reaction to the chemicals used for staining. Of these, the *Gram stain* and the *acid-fast stain* are most often used.

The method of staining introduced by Hans Christian Gram divides bacteria into two great groups: those that are *gram-positive* and those that are *gram-negative*. This method depends on the fact that, when bacteria are stained with either crystal violet or gentian violet and the smear is then treated with a weak solution of iodine (mordant), the bodies of some bacteria combine with the dye and iodine to produce a color that cannot be removed by alcohol, acetone, or aniline, whereas the color is readily removed from certain other bacteria by these solvents. Bacteria from which the color cannot be removed are spoken of as being *gram-positive,* and those from which it can be removed are spoken of as being *gram-negative.* A few bacteria that sometimes keep the stain and that at other times do not are *gram-variable.* Certain physiologic differences are generally correlated with Gram staining. Gram-positive bacteria tend to be more resistant to the action of oxidizing agents, alkalis, and proteolytic enzymes than are gram-negative ones. They are more susceptible to the acids, detergents, sulfonamides, and antibiotics, such as penicillin, than gram-negative ones. Many modifications have been devised for the original Gram's method. This method outlined below is often used. The explanations appended will apply to any technic used.

1. Make a thin smear of material for study and fix in a flame.
2. Stain with crystal violet or gentian violet (Gram I*) for 1 minute.
3. Blot thoroughly to take up excess stain.
4. Cover the smear with Gram's iodine solution (Gram II†) for 1 minute.
5. Drain and blot dry. Both gram-positive and gram-negative bacteria are now stained a dark violet or purple color.
6. Drop acetone on the smear (Gram III) until no more color flows from the smear (about 5 to 10 seconds). Blot dry. All gram-negative bacteria are completely decolorized. The gram-positive ones are not affected.
7. Cover the smear with a stain (Gram IV*) that gives a contrast in color (counterstain) for 1 minute.
8. Wash with water, blot dry, and examine.

Stains used to give contrast in color are *counterstains.* The ones most often used in the Gram stain are safranine and dilute carbolfuchsin, both of which give a red color, and Bismarck brown, which, as its name implies, gives a brown color. Gram-negative bacteria are stained with the counterstain. Gram-positive bacteria do not stain with the counterstain because they are completely stained with the stain-iodine–bacterial cell combination that gives them their gram-positive microscopic appearance.

Table 6-2 gives the reaction of the Gram stain of important pathogenic bacteria.

A method of staining known as the acid-fast or Ziehl-Neelsen stain is discussed next. When most bacteria and related forms are stained with carbolfuchsin, they stain easily, but when the smear is treated with acid, they are completely decolorized. It is difficult to stain certain other microbes with carbolfuchsin, but once stained, they retain the dye even

---

*Gram IV is usually made by mixing 10 ml. of a 2.5% alcoholic solution of safranine with 90 ml. of distilled water.

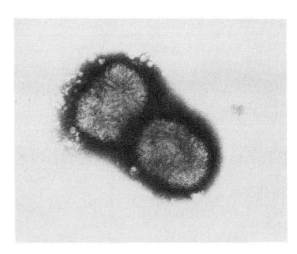

**Fig. 6-8.** Negative staining applied to study of viruses. Example here is virus of smallpox. Phosphotungstic acid provides background opaque to electrons when specimen is examined in electron microscope and one against which surface structures of viral particle are defined by contrast. (×120,000.) (Courtesy Dr. Derrick Baxby, University of Liverpool, England.)

---

*Gram I is usually a mixture of a 10% solution of crystal violet in 95% ethyl alcohol (solution A) with a 1% solution of ammonium oxalate in distilled water (solution B) in the ratio of 1 part of solution A to 4 parts of solution B (Hepler's ratio 1:8).

†Gram II is prepared by dissolving 2 gm. of potassium iodide and 1 gm. of iodine crystals in 300 ml. of distilled water; it should be stored in a brown glass bottle.

## Table 6-2
Reactions of some pathogenic bacteria to Gram staining

| GRAM-POSITIVE (DARK VIOLET OR PURPLE) *retain stain* | | GRAM-NEGATIVE (COLOR OF COUNTERSTAIN) | |
|---|---|---|---|
| Cocci | Bacilli | Cocci | Bacilli |
| Staphylococcus aureus | Bacillus anthracis | Neisseria gonorrhoeae | Bordetella pertussis *WHOOPING COUGH* |
| Streptococcus pneumoniae | Clostridium botulinum ⎫ | Neisseria meningitidis | Brucella abortus |
| Streptococcus pyogenes | Clostridium novyi ⎬ *BOTULISM* | | Brucella melitensis *GOATS, SHEEP* |
| | Clostridium perfringens ⎭ | | Brucella suis *HOGS* |
| | Clostridium septicum | | Escherichia coli *INTESTINAL TRACT* |
| | Clostridium tetani *LOCK JAW* | | Francisella tularensis *TULAREMIA RABBIT* |
| | Corynebacterium diphtheriae *DIPTHERIA* | | Haemophilus ducreyi *III V.D.* |
| | Mycobacterium leprae *LEPRASE* | | Haemophilus influenzae |
| | Mycobacterium tuberculosis *T.B.* | | Klebsiella pneumoniae |
| | | | Proteus vulgaris |
| | | | Pseudomonas aeruginosa *BLUE PUS* |
| | | | Salmonella typhi |
| | | | Shigella dysenteriae |
| | | | Shigella flexneri |
| | | | Shigella sonnei |
| | | | Yersinia pestis *PUBONIC PLAGUE* |

when treated with acid. Those that retain the stain are spoken of as being *acid-fast*. That property of being acid-fast probably derives from the presence of complex fatty substances within the bacterial cell.

The technic of acid-fast staining is as follows*:

1. Make a smear on the slide and fix.
2. Flood the slide with carbolfuchsin (red)† and gently steam over a flame (do not boil) for 3 to 5 minutes. Keep the slide covered with dye.
3. Allow the slide to cool. Wash off the excess stain with water (all bacteria are now red).
4. Dip the slide repeatedly in acid-alcohol‡ until all the red color is removed from smear. Wash with water. (At this step the acid has removed red color from all bacteria that are not acid-fast. The acid-fast organisms are unaffected and remain stained a bright red color.)
5. Apply a counterstain for 1 minute to give a contrast in color. Löffler's alkaline methylene blue§

is frequently used. (The acid-fast organisms are completely saturated with the red carbolfuchsin and therefore will not take any of the counterstain. The nonacid-fast organisms, having had all their stain removed by the acid, stain a deep blue.)

Important examples of acid-fast organisms encountered in medicine are *Mycobacterium tuberculosis, Mycobacterium leprae,* the anonymous, or atypical, mycobacteria (p. 256) and the actinomycete *Nocardia asteroides.*

*Special stains.* Important special stains are those for capsules, spores, flagella, and metachromatic granules. Stains primarily designed to demonstrate metachromatic granules are especially valuable in identifying *Corynebacterium diphtheriae* and in differentiating it from related organisms. Important stains of this type are Albert's stain, which uses toluidine blue and malachite green, and Neisser's stain, which uses methylene blue.

**Negative (relief) staining.** Microorganisms such as *Treponema pallidum,* not stained by ordinary dyes, may be made visible by the process known as negative or relief staining, in which the background, but *not* the microorganisms, is stained. The microorganisms are mixed with India ink or 10% nigrosin (both of which are black); the mixture is spread out into a thin smear and allowed to dry. The microbes appear as colorless objects against a black background. Negative staining may be done with the dye Congo red; this has been used to display spiral organisms and chlamydiae (bedsoniae). Viruses are prepared by

---

*There are several standard modifications of this method.

†The carbolfuchsin solution for the acid-fast stain is made by combining 1 part of a saturated solution of basic fuchsin in 95% ethyl alcohol with 9 parts of a 5% aqueous solution of phenol.

‡Acid-alcohol for decolorizing is 3% hydrochloric acid (concentrated) in 95% ethyl alcohol.

§Löffler's alkaline methylene blue is made by mixing 30 ml. of a saturated solution of the dye methylene blue chloride in 95% alcohol (1.5% filtered) with 100 ml. of a weak (0.01%) aqueous solution of potassium hydroxide. Modern samples of the dye have been considerably purified, and the addition of alkali may not be necessary, distilled water alone giving a satisfactory preparation for staining.

negative staining for visualization in the electron microscope (Fig. 6-8).

## Questions for review

1 Name the procedures used in the study of bacteria.

2 What are the purposes of a hanging drop preparation? How is one made?

3 What is fixing?

4 What are the three classes of stains used in microbiology? Describe each one and give examples.

5 How is a simple stain made? Do many bacteria stain with simple stains?

6 Name two very important differential stains. Give the underlying principles of each.

7 Name (a) two important gram-positive cocci, (b) three important gram-positive bacilli, (c) two important gram-negative cocci, (d) three important gram-negative bacilli.

8 Name two important acid-fast bacilli and one acid-fast actinomycete.

9 What is negative, or relief, staining?

10 Briefly describe the microscope.

11 Give the steps in the preparation of a bacterial smear.

12 When is dark-field illumination used to study microbes?

**References on pp. 81 and 82.**

# CHAPTER 7
# Cultivation
DONE IN LABORATORY

The small size and similarity in appearance and staining reactions of microbes often make identification by microscopic methods alone impossible. One of the most important ways to identify them is to observe their growth on artificial food substances prepared in the laboratory. This is cultivation of the microorganisms, or *culturing*. The food material on which they are grown is a *culture medium* (pl., *media*), and the growth itself is a *culture*. Some 10,000 different kinds of culture media have been prepared.

Cultural methods help to identify microbes and also to find organisms in test material of low microbial content. When such material is placed on a suitable culture medium, each organism present multiplies many times. Practically speaking, the smear may contain few or no organisms, whereas the culture soon produces hundreds of them.

## Culture media

**General considerations.** For the most satisfactory growth of bacteria and related forms on artificial culture media, the proper temperature, right amount of moisture, required oxygen tension, and proper degree of alkalinity or acidity (pH) must be provided. The culture medium itself must contain the necessary nutrients and growth-promoting factors and, of course, must be free from contaminating microorganisms; that is, *it must be sterile*.

Most disease-producing bacteria require complex foods similar in composition to the fluids of the animal body. Therefore the basis of many culture media is an infusion of meat of neutral or slightly alkaline pH containing meat extractives, salts, and peptone to which various other ingredients may be added.*

---

*The basic infusion can be prepared by soaking 500 gm. of fresh lean ground beef in 1 liter of distilled water in the refrigerator. After 24 hours the surface layer of fat is removed with absorbent cotton, the mixture is passed through muslin or gauze, and the meat discarded. After ingredients related to the organism under study are added and the reaction of the medium is adjusted to neutral or slightly alkaline, the infusion is heated to 100° C. for 20 minutes to remove coagulated tissue proteins and then filtered through coarse paper. At each step the volume is reconstituted to 1000 ml.

Culture media are of three types: (1) a liquid, (2) a solid that can be liquefied by heating but, when cooled, returns to the solid state, and (3) a solid that cannot be liquefied. It is often desirable that the culture medium be a solid, since bacteria and related forms can be visualized on the surface. Agar (Japanese seaweed) is a solidifying agent widely used. It melts completely at the temperature of boiling water and solidifies when cooled to about 40° C. With minor exceptions it has no effect on bacterial growth and is not attacked by bacteria growing on it. The low temperature at which agar solidifies is very important if test material must be inoculated directly into melted media before it solidifies. If agar began to solidify at a temperature high enough to kill bacteria or fungi, this could not be done. Gelatin is a well-known but less frequently used solidifying agent.

Numerous enriching materials are found in different culture media—carbohydrates, serum, whole blood, bile, ascitic fluid, and hydrocele fluid. Carbohydrates are added (1) to increase the nutritive value of the medium and (2) to indicate the fermentation reactions of microbes being studied. Serum, whole blood, and ascitic fluid are added to promote the growth of the less hardy organisms. Dyes added to culture media act as indicators to detect the formation of acid when fermentation reactions are being tested or act as inhibitors of the growth of certain bacteria but not that of others. An example of an indicator dye is phenol red, which is red in an alkaline or neutral medium but yellow in an acid one. An example of an inhibitory dye is gentian violet, which inhibits the growth of most gram-positive bacteria.

In actual practice, media making is greatly simplified by the availability of commercially prepared mixtures containing the necessary and any special ingredients for growth of bacteria or fungi in just the right proportions. Such preparations are sold in the dehydrated state as a powder or tablet, either of which may be reconstituted in water.*

---

*Dehydrated culture medium (powder) is weighed out and dispensed into a given volume of distilled water. The mixture is heated carefully over a water bath to effect solution.

Before sterilization, hydrated culture media are poured into suitable test tubes or flasks that are closed with cotton plugs.* After sterilization, some of the tubes of hot liquid media containing agar remain vertical for the agar to solidify, but some are laid on a flat surface with their mouths raised so that when the medium cools and solidifies there is a slanting surface *(agar slant)*. This gives a larger surface area for growth. Cotton plugs allow the access of moisture and oxygen but block the entrance of contaminating microorganisms; therefore the medium remains sterile until used, and microbes with which it is inoculated are not contaminated by those from the outside.

A large surface area for bacterial growth is provided when a solid culture medium partly fills a Petri dish. A *Petri dish* is a circular glass (or plastic) dish about 3 inches in diameter with perpendicular sides about 1/2 inch high. Inverted over it is a glass, metal, or plastic cover exactly like it except for a slightly greater diameter. The edges of the dishes are smooth, and a container is formed that prevents either the entrance or exit of bacteria. The Petri dish may be filled with a sterile agar medium still hot from the sterilization process, or a tube of solidified agar may be melted and poured into the dish. Until the agar has completely cooled, the lid is slightly raised on the Petri dish. When the agar is solid, the lid is lowered.

Most media are sterilized by autoclaving (p. 164). Those that contain carbohydrates may have to be sterilized by the fractional method because many carbohydrates will not withstand the high temperature of the autoclave. Enrichment materials such as serum and whole blood that are injured by even moderate heat are collected in such a manner as to be kept sterile and are mixed with the medium only after it has been sterilized and allowed to cool. In the case of agar media, these substances are added when the medium reaches 40° to 42° C., because when the temperature falls slightly lower than this, the agar begins to solidify.

Almost every species of microbe has some medium on which it grows best. A few will grow only on media specially prepared for them, but most of the pathogenic ones will grow more or less luxuriantly on certain routine or standard media (Fig. 7-1). Table 7-1 lists media suitable for the isolation and growth of important pathogenic microorganisms.

**Selective and differential media.** Media that promote the growth of one organism and retard the growth of others are *selective media*. Examples are bismuth sulfite agar and Petragnani medium. Bismuth sulfite agar, used to isolate typhoid bacilli from feces, promotes the growth of typhoid bacilli but retards the growth of bacteria normally resident in the stool. Petragnani medium promotes the growth of tubercle bacilli but retards the growth of any other organism present.

Media that distinguish organisms growing together are *differential media*. Examples are eosin–methylene blue (EMB) agar and MacConkey agar, used in the differentiation of the gram-negative bacteria of the intestinal tract. The incorporation of lactose into such differential media makes possible a sharp differentiation between the organisms that ferment this sugar and those that do not. The colonies of the lactose fermenters are deeply colored; colonies of the nonfermenters are colorless. This point is important because generally the pathogens in the intestinal tract do *not* ferment lactose, whereas the normal inhabitants, the coliforms, do (Fig. 7-2).

Selective and differential media are of great value in the diagnosis of infections in such areas of the body as the respiratory and intestinal tracts, where normally a variety of organisms reside. The presence of pathogenic bacteria in the area may not disrupt the normal bacterial pattern for the area (the normal flora); such pathogens tend to be mixed with other organisms in material taken from the site.

**Synthetic media.** The culture media just discussed are made up of components of variable composition, such as meat infusions, serum, or other body fluids. Such media are *nonsynthetic media. Synthetic media,* on the other hand, contain com-

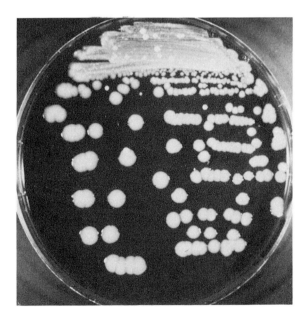

**Fig. 7-1.** Use of blood agar in Petri dish. Bacterial colonies are those of *Escherichia coli,* the colon bacillus.

---

*An electric warming jacket about the funnel keeps the culture medium in the liquid state during the tubing process.

**Table 7-1**

Microbes related to culture media

| ORGANISM | MEDIA MOST SUITABLE FOR GROWTH |
|---|---|
| *Actinomyces bovis* | Brain-heart infusion glucose broth and agar; thioglycollate broth medium (Brewer modified) (anaerobic) |
| *Bacillus anthracis* | Growth on almost all media |
| *Bacteroides* | Blood agar (anaerobic system) |
| *Blastomyces dermatitidis* | Blood agar; beef infusion glucose agar; Sabouraud glucose agar (antibiotics added to media used) |
| *Bordetella pertussis* | Glycerin-potato-blood agar (Bordet-Gengou agar) |
| *Brucella abortus, melitensis,* and *suis* | Trypticase soy broth and agar |
| *Candida albicans* | Sabouraud glucose agar; brain-heart infusion blood agar; corn meal agar; rice infusion agar |
| *Chlamydia (Bedsonia)* | Chick embryo; tissue culture |
| Clostridia of gas gangrene | Thioglycollate broth medium (Brewer modified); anaerobic blood agar; cooked meat medium under petroleum; Clostrisel agar |
| *Clostridium tetani* | Same as for *Clostridia* of gas gangrene |
| *Coccidioides immitis* | Sabouraud glucose agar |
| *Corynebacterium diphtheriae* | Löffler blood serum medium; cystine-tellurite-blood agar |
| *Cryptococcus neoformans* | Blood agar; beef infusion glucose agar; Sabouraud glucose agar |
| *Entamoeba histolytica* | *Entamoeba* medium (Difco) with dilute horse serum and rice powder |
| *Escherichia coli* and coliforms | Eosin–methylene blue (EMB) agar; Endo agar; MacConkey agar; desoxycholate agar; blood infusion agar (growth on almost any medium) |
| *Francisella tularensis* | Cystine glucose blood agar |
| Fungi, including dermatophytes | Sabouraud glucose agar with antibiotics; Littman oxgall agar |
| *Haemophilus influenzae* | Chocolate agar with yeast extract; rabbit blood agar with yeast extract |
| *Histoplasma capsulatum* | Brain-heart infusion glucose blood agar with antibiotics; Sabouraud glucose agar with antibiotics; brain-heart infusion glucose broth |
| *Mycobacterium tuberculosis* | Slow growth on special media such as Petragnani medium, Lowenstein-Jensen medium, or Dubos oleic agar; Dorset egg medium |
| *Neisseria gonorrhoeae* | Chocolate agar; Thayer-Martin medium |
| *Neisseria meningitidis* | Chocolate agar |
| *Nocardia asteroides* | Beef infusion blood agar; beef infusion glucose agar; Sabouraud glucose agar; Czapek agar; Dorset egg medium |
| *Proteus vulgaris* | EMB agar; Endo agar; MacConkey agar; desoxycholate agar; blood infusion agar (growth on almost any medium) |
| *Pseudomonas aeruginosa* | Blood agar; EMB agar; Endo agar; MacConkey agar; desoxycholate agar (growth on almost any medium) |
| *Rickettsia* | Chick embryo; tissue culture |
| *Salmonella* | Desoxycholate agar; desoxycholate-citrate agar; *Salmonella-Shigella* (SS) agar; MacConkey agar; tetrathionate broth; selenite-F enrichment medium |
| *Salmonella typhi* | Bismuth sulfite agar; SS agar; desoxycholate agar; desoxycholate-citrate agar; MacConkey agar; tetrathionate broth; selenite-F enrichment medium |
| *Shigella* | SS agar; desoxycholate agar; desoxycholate-citrate agar; MacConkey agar; tetrathionate broth; selenite-F enrichment medium |
| *Staphylococcus* | Growth on almost any medium |
| *Streptococcus* | Blood infusion agar; trypticase soy broth; tryptose phosphate broth; brain-heart infusion media |
| Viruses | Chick embryo; tissue culture |

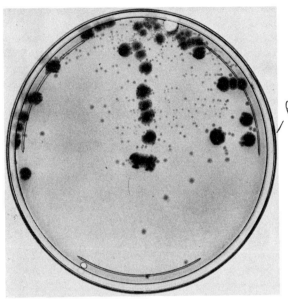

**Fig. 7-2.** Use of differential culture medium. On Mac-Conkey agar, dark (red-purple) colonies of lactose-fermenting *Escherichia coli* contrast with colorless colonies of nonlactose-fermenting *Shigella* species.

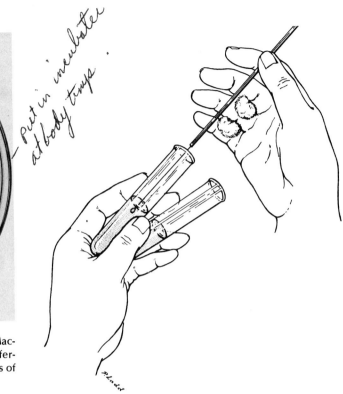

**Fig. 7-3.** Inoculating tube of liquid culture medium. Note slanting position of test tubes during maneuver. Contaminating organisms from air are less likely to drop into open tubes. Fingers of right hand are lifted away from handle of platinum loop to show how cotton plugs are held.

ponents of definite chemical composition. Used primarily in research work, such media have the advantage that, wherever prepared, their composition is the same. Therefore the results of microbial action on these media in one laboratory are strictly comparable with those in other laboratories thousands of miles away.

## Culture methods*

**Inoculation.** A culture is made or inoculated when some of the material to be cultured, such as sputum, urine, or pus, is placed into a fluid medium or is rubbed gently over the surface of a solid medium with either a sterile swab or a flame-sterilized platinum wire loop (Fig. 7-3). The inoculated medium is then incubated for a period of time, routinely 24 to 48 hours.

**Bacteriologic incubator.** The bacteriologic incubator (Fig. 7-4) consists of an insulated cabinet fitted with an electrical heating element and a thermoregulator. When the temperature reaches the point for which the thermoregulator is set, the regulating device cuts the heat off but turns it on again when the temperature falls slightly below the point. A good thermoregulator placed in a properly constructed incubator will maintain the temperature constant from

day to day to within 0.5° C. Electrically heated incubators maintain a more nearly constant temperature than those heated otherwise.

The incubator must be properly ventilated. It may be constructed so that circulation of air is brought about by the combined effects of gravity and the difference in weight of warm and cold air. Incubators are also ventilated with blowers or fans. All incubators are fitted with perforated shelves. Most are fitted with sets of double doors; the inner ones of glass allow the contents of the incubator to be viewed, and they keep out cold air.

**Inspection of cultures.** Each microbe in the medium inoculated and incubated multiplies rapidly, and within a few hours there are many more microorganisms in the culture than there were in an equal amount of the material from which the culture was made. Consequently, bacteria or fungi are found in cultures when they are found with difficulty or not at all in smears of the test material. Diphtheria bacilli can be found in throat cultures twice as often as in throat smears.

---

*Standard aseptic bacteriologic technics are implied in the discussion to follow.

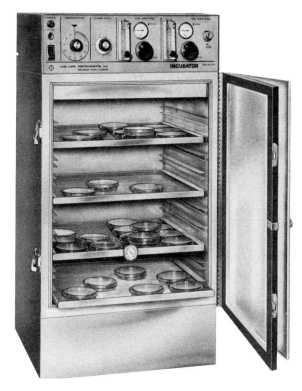

**Fig. 7-4.** Bacteriologic incubator, electrically heated with temperature kept constant by delicate thermoregulator. This one also provides measured carbon dioxide atmosphere, a feature promoting growth of certain microbes. (Courtesy Lab-Line Instruments, Inc., Melrose Park, Ill.)

When a culture is made on a solid medium, all the bacteria that grow from each bacterium deposited on the medium cling together to form a mass visible to the naked eye. This is called a *colony*. The colony has characteristics such as texture, size, shape, color, and adherence to the medium (Fig. 7-5). These are fairly constant for each species and are valuable in differentiating one species from another. Theoretically each organism should give rise to one colony, but two or more may cling together and, when planted on a medium, give rise to only one colony. If organisms that cling together are different, the colony will contain the different kinds. As a rule with *good laboratory technic* a colony contains only one kind of microorganism.

Petri dish cultures permit good observation of colonies. The large surface area favors separation of individual microorganisms. Petri dish cultures are usually spoken of as plates and the process of making them as *plating* or *streaking*.

**Pure cultures.** A *pure* culture contains only one kind of bacteria; a *mixed* culture contains two or more kinds. As a rule, infectious material contains more than one kind of bacteria. So that one kind alone can be studied, it must be separated from all other kinds and grown alone as a pure culture. Pure cultures are usually obtained by the pour plate or streak plate method. The pour plate method is as follows (Fig. 7-6):

1. Melt 3 tubes of agar in boiling water and then allow to cool to 40° or 42° C. If an enriching material that is injured by heat, such as serum

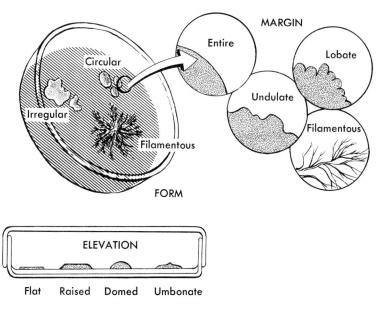

**Fig. 7-5.** Examination of colonies.

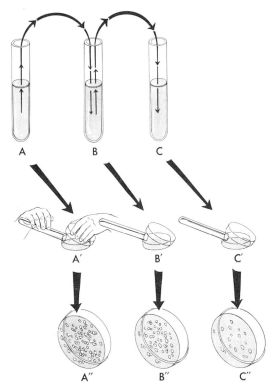

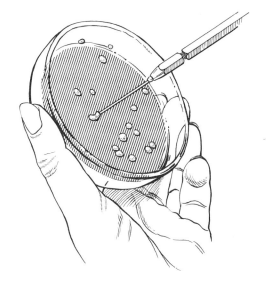

**Fig. 7-7.** Fishing a colony.

**Fig. 7-6.** Pure culture, pour plate method (see text). Step I. Inoculate tubes **A, B,** and **C,** as indicated by arrows. Step II. Transfer contents of each tube to Petri dishes **A′, B′,** and **C′,** respectively. Incubate plates. Step III. Inspect plates (**A″, B″,** and **C″**) for number and distribution of colonies. Fish representative colony for further study.

or whole blood, is needed, add it to the medium at this time.

2. Transfer to 1 tube a loopful of the test material from which one expects to obtain a pure culture. Replace the cotton plug and roll the tube between the palms of the hands to distribute the bacteria throughout the medium.
3. Flame-sterilize the loop thoroughly. Transfer 3 loopfuls of the contents of the inoculated tube to the second tube.
4. Mix the contents of the second tube with the inoculum, and sterilize the platinum loop. Transfer 5 loopfuls of the mixture to the third tube and mix.
5. Pour the contents of each tube of medium into a Petri dish and allow to solidify.
6. Incubate the Petri dishes for 24 to 48 hours. Observe the colonies carefully.

Successive dilution of the specimen in the three tubes reduces the number of bacteria and disperses them in the medium so that the colonies in the Petri

dish cultures are more likely to be distinctly separated from each other. Those that are to be studied further are removed from the Petri dish with a straight platinum wire and rubbed over the surface of one or more slants of suitable media. This is known as *fishing* (Figs. 7-7 and 7-8). If the colonies are not separated from each other, it is impossible to fish one colony without touching other colonies.

The inoculated slants are allowed to incubate for 24 to 48 hours, and these cultures are studied further (Fig. 7-9). In the majority of cases all bacteria growing on a slant will be alike because they all grew from the members of a single colony on the plate, and these in turn grew from a single bacterium in the original material. If, as may sometimes happen, the original colony on the plate contains two or more kinds of bacteria, the same two or more kinds will grow on the slant. Separation is made by suspending some of the growth from the slant in sterile salt solution and replating.

**Streak plates.** To prepare a streak plate, a single loopful of infectious material is streaked over the surface of the solid medium (agar) in a Petri dish. There are several ways to do this. The patterns illustrated in Figs. 7-10 and 7-11 are widely used and give good separation of colonies.

**Bacterial plate count.** The accuracy of the bacterial plate count (Fig. 7-12) rests on the premise that when material containing bacteria is cultured, every bacterium present develops into a colony. This statement is not strictly true, since some bacteria may fail to multiply and two or more bacteria may cling together to form a single colony. Nevertheless, the

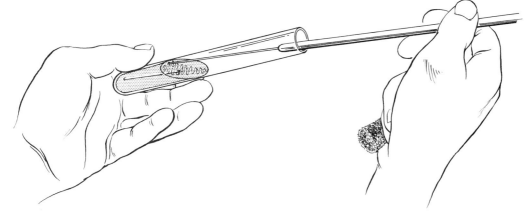

**Fig. 7-8.** Streaking agar slant.

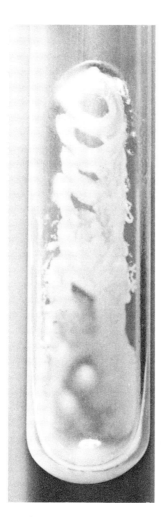

**Fig. 7-9.** Pure culture *(Staphylococcus aureus)* on agar slant. (Courtesy Ayerst Laboratories, New York.)

method is of decided value in the examination of water and milk (pp. 381 and 388).

A bacterial plate count is carried out as follows. Four tubes containing 9 ml. of sterile distilled water are needed. To the first tube, add 1 ml. of the material to be examined and mix. From this tube, transfer 1 ml. to the second tube and mix. From the second tube, transfer 1 ml. to the third tube and mix, and from the third tube, transfer 1 ml. to the fourth tube and mix. This gives 1:10, 1:100, 1:1000, and 1:10,000 dilutions of the original material. With a sterile pipette transfer exactly 1 ml. from each tube to a Petri dish and add sufficient melted agar (cooled to 42° C.). Mix the contents of each dish by rotating and allow to solidify. After incubation for 24 to 48 hours, count the colonies that have developed. Let us say that the second plate shows 200 colonies. This means that at least 200 bacteria were present in the 1 ml. of material placed in the tube, and since this was a 1:100 dilution, the original test material must have contained at least 20,000 bacteria per milliliter. More than this number of bacteria may have been introduced into the dish, since some may have failed to grow and some may have clung together in groups of two or more that developed into single colonies. In other words, the number of bacteria indicated by the count is certainly present, and more may be also.

The bacterial plate count is an important part of the microbiologic evaluation of urine from a patient with possible urinary tract infection. A measured amount of urine is handled as indicated above. A colony count is made from the bacterial growth on solid media. Quantitation helps to indicate whether bacteria recovered from urine are disease producers or contaminants. Generally, with less than 1000 to 10,000 colonies from 1 ml. of specimen, the microorganisms isolated represent normal flora of the urethra or contaminants.

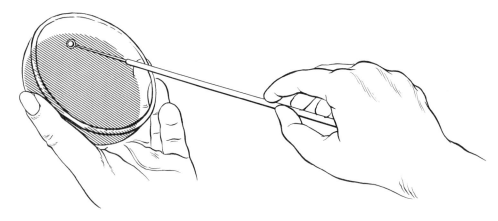

Fig. 7-10. Streaking agar plate.

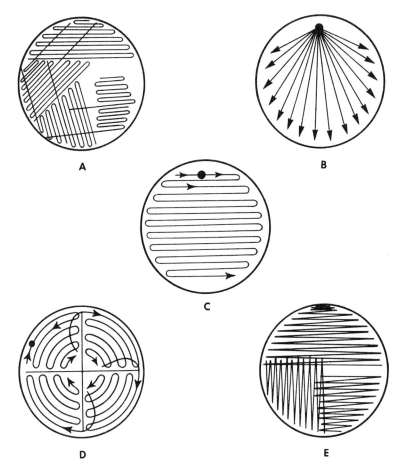

A

B

C

D

E

Fig. 7-11. Patterns for streaking agar plates. **A, D,** and **E,** Sections of plate are streaked successively. After each section is streaked, platinum loop is flame-sterilized. A bit of inoculum for next section in turn is obtained when loop is passed back into or through section just inoculated. (From Smith, A. L.: Microbiology laboratory manual and workbook, ed. 3, St. Louis, 1973, The C. V. Mosby Co.)

**Culture of anaerobic bacteria.** To grow some anaerobic bacteria, a tube of suitable culture medium about 8 inches in length and about half full of medium may be heated in a boiling water bath for several minutes to expel any oxygen present in the medium. The tube is quickly cooled and inoculated; then sterile melted petroleum jelly to make a layer about ¾ inch thick is poured onto the top of the medium, thus sealing off the culture from the air. If agar is used, the inoculation is made when the heated medium cools to a temperature of 42° C.

Thioglycollate broth, a special medium containing thioglycollic acid, supports the growth of anaerobes within the depths of a partly filled tube without special seal. Methylene blue indicator colors the upper layers of the fluid medium as oxidation occurs.

Cultures may be placed in a specially constructed glass or metal chamber from which the oxygen is either removed by some chemical reaction that is made to take place in the chamber or replaced by a gas, such as hydrogen, that does not affect the growth of the bacteria. (See Figs. 19-3 and 22-2.)

Better results are obtained with the more sophisticated methods indicated on p. 225.

**Slide cultures.** Slide cultures (p. 326) used to study fungi may be placed on the stage of the microscope and actual growth observed from time to time. The depression of a sterile culture slide may be filled with suitable medium, inoculated, and covered with a sterile cover glass. Liquid cultures may be made by inoculating a drop of medium on a sterile cover glass and proceeding as for a hanging drop preparation.

**Cultures in an embryonated hen's egg.** Important sites of growth for viruses, chlamydiae (bedsoniae), and rickettsias are the yolk sac and the embryonic membranes of the developing chick embryo (p. 288). Bacteria are occasionally grown in this way.

**Cultivation of microbes in cell (tissue) cultures.** Cell (tissue) cultures are cultures in which animal cells are growing. Cells used are from mammalian or fowl embryos or selected adult tissues such as the cornea, the kidney, and the lung. Minced tissue is placed in a suitable substrate in which cells multiply and grow. The growing cells may be supported on a solid

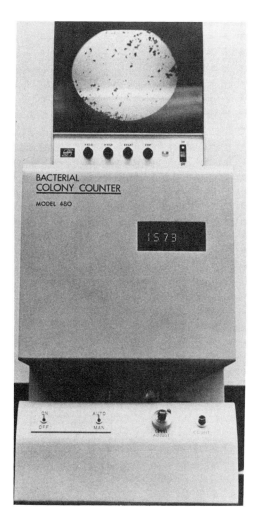

**Fig. 7-12.** Bacterial colony counter. Note Petri plate just above controls. (Courtesy Fisher Scientific Co., Pittsburgh.)

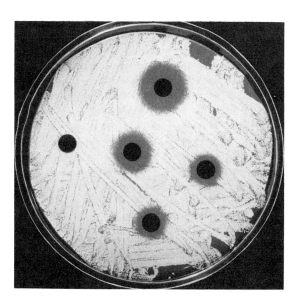

**Fig. 7-13.** Antibiotic susceptibility testing: single paper disk diffusion method. Petri dish of agar is heavily inoculated with test organisms. Disks of filter paper impregnated with different antibiotics are dropped on freshly seeded surface. Note heavy white bacterial growth with zones of inhibition about some of disks and none about one. A zone of inhibition indicates that growth of organisms would probably be limited in a patient receiving that antibiotic.

or semisolid substrate such as a fibrin, agar, or cellulose, or they may be suspended in a liquid. Certain pathogenic agents such as rickettsias, chlamydiae, and viruses, which do not grow in lifeless media, multiply with ease when incorporated into tissue cultures.

## Antibiotic susceptibility testing

The susceptibility (or resistance) of bacteria to different antibiotics may be determined by suitable laboratory tests, usually designated as *susceptibility tests*. Two methods are used: the disk susceptibility test (Fig. 7-13) and the tube-dilution method. The first employs disks of filter paper impregnated with known amounts of different antibiotics. A Petri dish is heavily inoculated with the test organisms. The disks are dropped onto the freshly inoculated surface, and the plate incubated for 24 hours. As the organisms grow, the antibiotic is diffusing out in the culture medium. If the organism is susceptible to the antibiotic, there is a zone of inhibition (no growth) around the disk. If the microorganism is unaffected by the drug, growth will cover the area around the disk. Several preparations can be tested on one plate. The method is simple and rapid, and the results correlate well with the effectiveness of the clinical treatment.

The United States Food and Drug Administration has set its stamp of approval on the standardized disk susceptibility test as precisely defined step by step in the *Federal Register* **37**(191):20527-20529, September 30, 1972. In this test Mueller-Hinton agar (beef infusion, peptone, starch, and agar at a pH of around 7.4) is used for culture of test microorganisms since it is low in interfering substances and it supports the growth of most pathogens for which testing is needed.

The second method utilizes a tube of culture medium containing both the test organism and a specified amount of a given antibiotic. The tube is incubated and the amount of growth evaluated. Since only one drug can be tested at a time, this method is laborious.

With this sort of testing, the microorganisms are reported as being susceptible or resistant to a given antibiotic. There are technics whereby the amount of certain antibiotics can be determined in the blood.

## Questions for review

1 Name important constituents of culture media.
2 Why is agar the most commonly used solidifying agent?
3 What purpose do dyes serve in culture media?
4 What advantages are there to culture by comparison with direct visualization on smears?
5 Explain differential media and selective media. Give examples.
6 Give the practicality of the Petri dish in microbiologic culture.
7 Outline the steps in making a pure culture. What is meant by a pure culture? What purpose does it serve?
8 Briefly describe how a bacterial count is made. Under what circumstances are bacterial counts made?
9 Briefly explain: cell or tissue culture, slide culture, culture on synthetic media, and culture of anaerobic bacteria.
10 How is antibiotic susceptibility testing carried out? What is its purpose?

**References on pp. 81 and 82.**

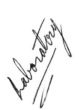

# CHAPTER 8

# Biochemical reactions and animal inoculation

## Biochemical reactions

Biochemical tests demonstrate the presence of enzyme systems within the microbial cell, such as those responsible for the fermentation of carbohydrates and the decomposition of proteins.

Miniaturization of microbiologic technics refers to the use of the commercially prepackaged test units wherein basic reagents for a given biochemical reaction are premeasured, standardized, and compacted into a tablet or onto a paper disk or filter paper strip. The test unit is applied to cultures in liquid or solid media and is chemically designed so that enzymatic action of the test organism usually results in a color change, or end point, a quick and easy observation. There are many varieties of such tests available.

**Fermentation of sugars.** Microbes ferment many organic compounds, including carbohydrates, generating in the process energy-rich chemical bonds. Simple sugars through fermentation can serve as the main source of energy for many different kinds of microbes, and in the laboratory it is practical to deal with these relatively simple test solutions. The end products of fermentation depend on the substrate, the enzymes present, and the conditions under which the reaction proceeds. For instance, the yeast enzymes that break down glucose into carbon dioxide and alcohol are without effect on sucrose (cane sugar), and certain enzymes produced by pneumococci and streptococci change glucose to lactic acid. Common products of bacterial fermentation are lactic acid, formic acid, acetic acid, butyric acid, butyl alcohol, acetone, ethyl alcohol, and the gases carbon dioxide and hydrogen.

Fermentation reactions, though varying among species of microorganisms, are quite constant and therefore of great value in differentiating species. From their specific action on a given sugar in the laboratory, bacteria (and other microbes) are classified as (1) those that do not ferment it, (2) those that do ferment it with the production of acid only, and (3) those that ferment it with the production of both acid

and gas. Media containing different sugars are inoculated with the bacteria (or other microbes) and observed for gas production and acid formation. Gas production in liquid media is detected by the accumulation of gas that displaces the fluid medium contained in the closed arm of a special tube. It may be detected in a small tube (one end of which is sealed off) placed in an inverted position within a larger tube of liquid medium, the sealed end projecting slightly above the level of the fluid. As gas is formed in the inoculated liquid, it collects in the small tube within the depths of the culture and rises toward the sealed end (Fig. 8-1).

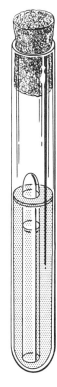

**Fig. 8-1.** Fermentation tube. Note that gas has collected in tip of smaller inverted tube.

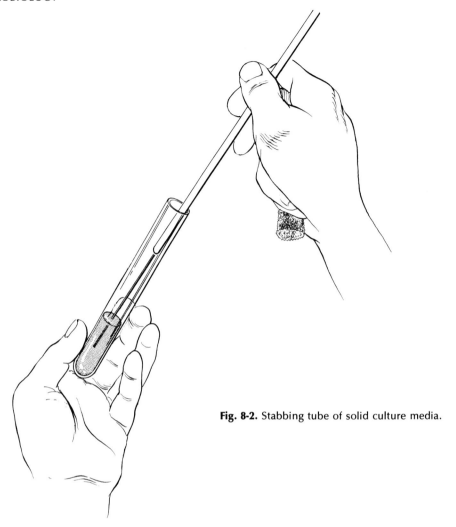

**Fig. 8-2.** Stabbing tube of solid culture media.

Solid media are inoculated for fermentation studies by plunging a straight needle carrying some of the bacteria deep into the medium. (This plunging maneuver is known as "stabbing" [Fig. 8-2].) The solid medium may be melted, cooled to 40° C., and then inoculated. Gas production in solid media is indicated by disruption of the medium by gas bubbles. Acid formation in both liquid and solid media is indicated by color changes in indicators incorporated therein.

Many carbohydrates are used in routine fermentation studies. Important sugars are glucose, lactose, maltose, sucrose, xylose, mannitol, and salicin. The fermentation of lactose is crucial in the identification of bacteria recovered from the intestinal tract, since it makes a division between the nonpathogenic coliform organisms and the pathogenic *Salmonella* and *Shigella,* those organisms that cannot ferment lactose being the pathogens (with a few exceptions).

**Hydrolysis of starch.** When microbes are grown on starch agar, a clear zone develops around the colonies of those that digest starch. If the agar is covered with a weak solution of iodine, the *undigested* starch assumes a blue color.

**Liquefaction of gelatin.*** A gelatin medium is stabbed with a wire having some of the bacteria on it, incubated at 20° C., and observed for liquefaction. It may be incubated at 37° C. (gelatin remains liquefied at this temperature) and then placed in the refrigera-

---

*The proteolytic enzymes (protein-splitting enzymes, proteinases) produced by bacteria split complex proteins into proteases, peptones, polypeptides, amino acids, ammonia, and free nitrogen. Protein decomposition is known as *putrefaction.* Some authorities restrict the term *putrefaction* to the decomposition of proteins by anaerobic bacteria, which results in the formation of hydrogen sulfide and other foul-smelling decomposition products, and they use the term *decay* for the decomposition of proteins by aerobic bacteria. The latter does not result in the malodorous decomposition products.

tor, where the unliquefied will solidify. Incubation should be continued for at least 2 weeks unless liquefaction occurs before that time, and a tube of uninoculated gelatin should be incubated as a control.

**Indole production.** Production of indole (from the amino acid tryptophan) is determined by culture of the organisms in a medium containing tryptophan. A strip of filter paper soaked with a saturated solution of oxalic acid may be hung over the culture and held in place either by the cotton plug or by the screw cap of the culture tube. A pink color on the paper indicates indole production. Important indole producers are *Escherichia coli* and *Proteus,* which avidly decompose proteins.

**Nitrate reduction.** Nitrate reduction means the removal of oxygen from the nitrate radical ($NO_3$) to convert it into nitrate ($NO_2$). The organisms are incubated in broth containing 0.1% potassium nitrate, and the broth is tested for nitrite with sulfanilic acid and alpha-naphthylamine reagents. A red color means a positive test.

**Deoxyribonuclease elaboration.** Formation of deoxyribonuclease (DNase) is demonstrated by culture of test microbes on the surface of an agar plate into which deoxyribonucleic acid has been incorporated. After 24 hours' incubation, the surface is flooded with either 1N hydrochloric acid to highlight the clear zones about the DNase-positive growth or with 0.1% toluidine blue, in which case a bright rose or pink color is the end point. Staphylococci produce this enzyme.

**Hydrogen sulfide production.** A stab culture in an agar that contains basic lead acetate is incubated for 1 to 4 days. The production of hydrogen sulfide from the sulfur-containing amino acids of the medium is indicated by the appearance of a black compound, lead sulfide, formed from the combination of the hydrogen sulfide with the lead acetate. Instead of being incorporated into the medium, the basic lead acetate may be impregnated on sterile filter paper suspended over the medium as in the test for indole production. Iron salts also may be used to detect hydrogen sulfide formation. The production of hydrogen sulfide facilitates the identification of *Brucella* species and enteric bacilli.

**Splitting of urea.** Certain microorganisms, when cultivated on media containing urea, convert it to ammonia. With phenol red as the indicator, the presence of urease is seen by the appearance of a red color. The enzyme *urease* responsible for the conversion is produced by species of the genus *Proteus.* The test separates these organisms from the urease-negative *Salmonella* and *Shigella.*

**Digestion of milk.** Bacterial growth in sterile milk may be alkaline or acid and with or without curdling. Curdling may or may not be followed by liquefaction of the curd. Excessive gas production in milk produced by *Clostridium perfringens* is stormy fermentation.

**Oxidase reaction.** The enzyme *oxidase* is produced by *Neisseria* species, and its detection is of great value in the identification of *Neisseria gonorrhoeae.* The oxidase reagent colors the positive colonies pink to red to black.

**Niacin test.** The niacin test is useful in distinguishing *Mycobacterium tuberculosis* from the anonymous, or atypical, mycobacteria. A 4% alcoholic aniline solution and a watery solution of cyanogen bromide are added to 1 or 2 ml. of emulsified bacterial growth. A yellow compound is formed when niacin or nicotinic acid, formed by the tubercle bacillus but not by atypical mycobacteria, reacts with the cyanogen bromide and a primary amine.

**Demonstration of specific enzymes.** Reagent systems for the identification of diagnostic enzymes are commercially impregnated into easy-to-use strips of paper suitable for application to bacterial cultures. Three enzymes of practical importance are so packaged: phenylalanine deaminase, cytochrome oxidase, and lysine decarboxylase.

Phenylalanine deaminase catalyzes the metabolism of phenylalanine to phenylpyruvic acid, which in turn reacts with the ferric ions present to give a brownish or gray-black color. The presence of this enzyme in cultures of *Proteus* species is responsible for the positive reaction obtained with these organisms.

$$\text{Phenylalanine} \xrightarrow{\text{Enzyme}} \text{Phenylpyruvic acid} + \text{Ferric ions} \longrightarrow \text{Color}$$

Cytochrome oxidase is produced by *Pseudomonas, Alcaligenes, Neisseria, Vibrio, Brucella,* and some *Halobacterium* species. This enzyme catalyzes a coupling reaction to give a blue color (the positive reaction) as follows:

$$\text{Dimethyl-}p\text{-phenylenediamine} + \text{Alpha naphthol} + \text{Oxygen} \xrightarrow{\text{Enzyme}} \text{Indophenol blue}$$

Lysine decarboxylase, which is formed by most of the *Salmonella* species, catalyzes the conversion of lysine to cadaverine, a more alkaline compound than lysine. In one commercial prepackaged test kit, the Prussian blue reaction is used to indicate the positive test.

$$\text{Lysine} \xrightarrow{\text{Enzyme}} \text{Cadaverine} + \text{Carbon dioxide} \longrightarrow$$
Bromthymol blue (yellow) changing to blue as pH rises

**Gas chromatography.** Gas chromatography can be used to advantage in microbiology. Under rigidly controlled conditions, a dry pellet of bacteria is subjected to pyrolysis, that is, to heat-induced breakdown of the chemical components. The gas chromatograph then separates the pyrolytic fragments, recording on a graph a constant, specific, and diagnostic pattern for the test organisms. Closely related bacteria may be similarly separated by gas-liquid chromatography, wherein analysis of certain consistent derivatives under test conditions is made, this time from hydrolysis of the given organisms, and diagnostic patterns recorded.

**Limulus test for endotoxemia.** Serum or cerebrospinal fluid from a patient (or suitable test material) is incubated with lysates derived from the blood cells (amebocytes) of the horseshoe crab (*Limulus polyphe-*

*mus*). In the presence of even minute amounts of bacterial endotoxin there is a greatly increased viscosity of the test medium (the gelation reaction), which can progress to a solid gel.

## Animal inoculation

The inoculation of suitable laboratory animals is an essential part of the study of many microbes. After an animal has been inoculated, it is observed for effects produced by the microbes. In some cases it is killed after a certain length of time and examined for evidence of disease. Smears and cultures are made, and gross and microscopic changes in the organs are noted. In other cases the animal is not killed, but

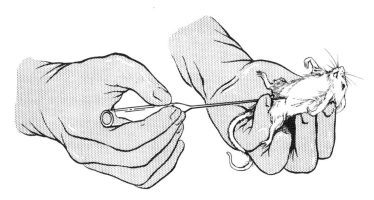

**Fig. 8-3.** Intraperitoneal inoculation of white mouse. Note point of capillary pipette directed into peritoneal cavity as mouse held firmly by nape of neck.

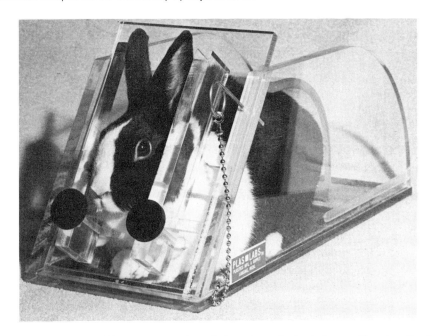

**Fig. 8-4.** Rabbit restrained for intravenous inoculation of marginal vein in ear. (Courtesy Plas Labs, Lansing, Mich.)

blood and body fluids are removed at intervals for examination. (See Figs. 8-3 and 8-4.)

The well-known laboratory animals are guinea pigs, white mice, white rats, hamsters, and rabbits. The inoculations may be given with syringe and needle subcutaneously (beneath the skin), intradermally (between the layers of the skin), intravenously (into a vein), intraperitoneally (into the peritoneal cavity), subdurally (beneath the dura of the brain), or intracerebrally (into the brain).

**Advantages.** The advantages of animal inoculation in recovery and identification of microbes are as follows:

1. Some microbes are most easily detected by animal inoculation (examples, *Francisella tularensis* and, under some conditions, *Mycobacterium tuberculosis*).
2. The virulence of microbes can be displayed (such as *Corynebacterium diphtheriae*).
3. It is sometimes the easiest way of obtaining the pure culture (*Streptococcus pneumoniae*).
4. It is often necessary in order to determine the action of drugs on microbes.
5. Microorganisms that cannot be cultured at all on artificial media can be readily recovered from suitable laboratory animals (spiral bacteria, rickettsias, and most viruses). A very few microbes can be propagated in no other way.
6. The action of pathogenic and nonpathogenic agents on the animal body can be determined experimentally.
7. Animal inoculation is basic to the manufacture of antitoxins and other antisera.

A good example of animal inoculation as the best method of detecting the microbes is the ease with which tuberculosis of the kidney is proved in a patient whose urine shows no bacteria on direct microscopic examination but whose urine produces classic disease in a guinea pig. A good example of animal inoculation being used to obtain a pure culture is seen in pneumococcal typing. Some of the sputum in which the type of pneumococcus is to be determined is injected into the peritoneal cavity of a white mouse, and within only a few hours the growth of pneumococci has outstripped that of all other organisms to such an extent that the peritoneal contents consist of practically a pure culture of pneumococci ready to be typed.

## Summary: identification of bacteria

When the various methods are applied to the study of bacteria, it will be seen that classification into comparatively large groups may be made from several standpoints, as follows (Plate 1, p. 74):

I. Direct microscopic examination
  A. Staining reactions
    1. Reaction to Gram stain
      a. Gram-positive
      b. Gram-negative
    2. Reaction to acid-fast stain
      a. Acid-fast (Plate 1, *A*)
      b. Non–acid-fast
  B. Size
  C. Shape
    1. Coccus—spherical
    2. Bacillus—rod shaped
    3. Vibrio, spirillum, spirochete—spiral shaped
  D. Presence of endospores
    1. Sporeformers
    2. Nonsporeformers
  E. Capsule formation
    1. Encapsulated
    2. Nonencapsulated
  F. Motility
    1. Motile
    2. Nonmotile
II. Culture
  A. Food requirements
    1. Saprophytes—growth on dead organic matter
    2. Parasites—growth on living matter
  B. Media most suitable for growth (Plate 1, *B*, to *D*)
    1. Growth on simple media
    2. Growth only on special media
    3. No growth on any media
  C. Appearance of growth on different media
  D. Oxygen requirements
    1. Aerobes—growth only in the presence of free oxygen
    2. Anaerobes—growth only in the absence of free oxygen
    3. Microaerophiles—growth in the presence of small amounts of free oxygen
  E. Optimum temperature for growth
  F. Characteristics of the pure culture
    1. Size, shape, texture of colonies
    2. Pigment production
  G. Production of hemolysins on blood agar
    1. Beta hemolytic—complete hemolysis of red blood cells (Plate 1, *B*)
    2. Alpha hemolytic—partial hemolysis of red blood cells
    3. Nonhemolytic
III. Biochemical relations (Plate 1, *E* and *F*)
  A. Fermentation of sugars
    1. Fermentation with acid and gas
    2. Fermentation with acid only; no gas
    3. No fermentation
  B. Fermentation of lactose
    1. Lactose-fermenters
    2. Non–lactose-fermenters
  C. Splitting of urea
    1. Urease-positive
    2. Urease-negative
IV. Animal inoculation

    A. Disease production (virulence tests)
        1. Pathogenic—disease produced
        2. Nonpathogenic
    B. Toxin production
        1. Exotoxin producers
        2. Endotoxin producers

## Questions for review

**1** How are fermentation reactions used in the study of microbes?

**2** List five sugars important in routine fermentation studies.

**3** What two observable changes may occur in the culture medium when carbohydrates are fermented?

**4** What is the importance of the fermentation of lactose?

**5** List the routine laboratory animals.

**6** State the advantages of animal inoculation.

**7** What is meant by putrefaction? Decay?

**8** Name two organisms that produce indole.

**9** What genus produces urease?

**10** Briefly outline the niacin test.

**11** How may specific enzymes be demonstrated? Name three of diagnostic value.

**12** Summarize methods used to classify and categorize bacteria.

**References on pp. 81 and 82.**

**Plate 1.** Laboratory study of microbes. 1. Smear: Acid-fast stain is made of filaments of *Nocardia asteroides* (**A**). 2. Culture: *Routine* blood agar sets off beta hemolytic zones around gray colonies of *Streptococcus* (**B**). *Differential* MacConkey agar contrasts purple colonies of lactose fermenting *Escherichia* with colorless ones of *Shigella* (**C**). *Selective* Petragnani medium favors dry buff-colored growth of *Mycobacterium tuberculosis* (**D**). 3. Biochemical tests: Key reactions for gram-negative enterics are tabulated:

| | Triple sugar iron agar (TSI) | | | | INDOL | CIT | LYS | MOT | UREA | DEX |
|---|---|---|---|---|---|---|---|---|---|---|
| **Examples** | **H₂ S** | **Lactose** | **Sucrose** | **Glucose** | | | | | | |
| *Salmonella* (**E**) | + (black) | − (red slant) | − | Obscured | − | + (blue) | + | + | − | Acid, gas (yellow) |
| *Proteus morganii* (**F**) | − | − | − | Beginning fermentation | + | − (green) | − (yellow) | + | + (red-purple) | Acid, gas (yellow) |

KEY: TSI, sugars indicated plus ferrous sulfate and phenol red indicator; sugars fermented, hydrogen sulfide produced. INDOL, tryptophan broth, Kovacs reagent (*p*-dimethylaminobenzaldehyde) added; indole produced. CIT, Simmons citrate agar, bromthymol blue indicator; citrate used as sole source of carbon. LYS, lysine decarboxylase test media, bromcresol purple indicator (p. 71). By transmitted light the positive test (alkaline reaction) is the red color seen above; the negative test (acid reaction) is yellow. MOT, semisolid nutrient agar; motile microbes grow out from stab line. UREA, see p. 71. DEX, dextrose (glucose) broth with indicator (p. 69).

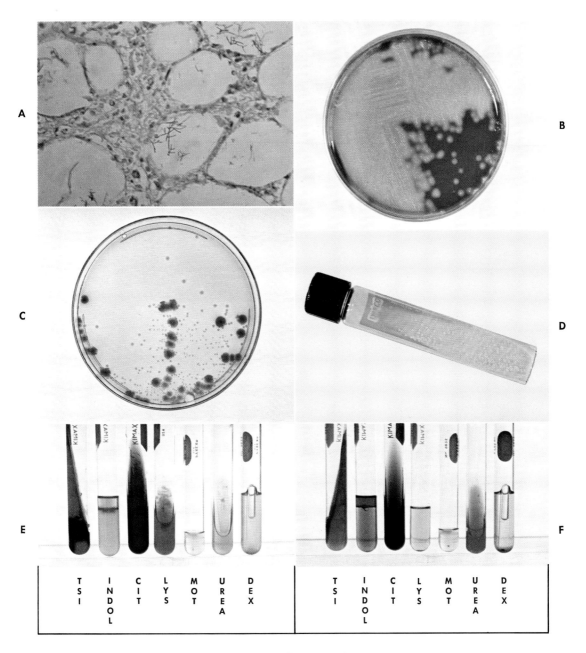

**Plate 1.** For legend see opposite page.

# CHAPTER 9
# Specimen collection

In that it defines the diagnosis and nature of disease, the microbiologic investigation determines the mode of treatment and outlook for that patient affected. In the practice of scientific medicine, specimen collection must be a crucial first step on which rests the validity of each succeeding step.

## Ground rules

In the collection of any specimen for microbiologic examination, remember the following:

1. Collect the specimen from the actual site of disease and do not contaminate it with microbes from nearby areas. For example, in making smears and cultures from ulcers in the throat, be very careful to take the material from the actual site of ulceration and not contaminate it unduly with the secretions of the mouth.
2. Always use sterile paraphernalia to collect the specimen. Place the specimen in a sterile container.
3. Sterilize material used in collecting the specimen as soon as possible after proper disposal of the specimen.
4. Collect adequate amounts of material. For instance, when pus is to be examined, collect several milliliters if possible. If it is necessary to collect the material on swabs, use more than one swab.
5. Insofar as possible, do not send specimens to the laboratory on swabs—a swab can take up a small amount of material, dry quickly, and enmesh in its fibers important cells and organisms that fail to be transferred to smears or culture media. Note that if swabs must be used, specially devised transport media are available.
6. Collect the specimen in such a manner as not to endanger others. Sputum or other excreta must not soil the outside of the container.
7. Take great care in handling specimens collected in cotton-plugged tubes. Cotton plugs can soak up a small specimen. Microbes from the environment can pass through wet plugs and contaminate the specimen.
8. Whenever possible, make smears from the original material.
9. Do not add any preservative or antiseptic to the specimen. If possible, take the specimen before the patient has received any antimicrobial drug or before his wound has had local treatment. If the patient has already received a sulfonamide or antibiotic, notify the laboratory.
10. Label the specimen properly with the patient's name, the source of specimen, and the tentative diagnosis.
11. Deliver the specimen to the laboratory immediately.

The person delivering the specimen to the laboratory may have to care for the specimen there if at the time laboratory personnel are off duty. In this event specimens already inoculated onto culture media are placed in the incubator, and those not on culture media are placed in the refrigerator. When cultures must be made without delay, the medium chosen should be that most likely to grow the suspected organisms, as well as any other that might be present. Since it supports the growth of organisms that may be present in the specimen better than any other culture medium found in the usual microbiologic laboratory, blood agar is best to use. Blood agar plates are superior to tubed media except in those instances in which the cultures must be shipped a distance to the laboratory. Plates are not easily transported.

## Clinical specimens

*Urine* for microbiologic examination may be carefully collected as a clean-voided specimen. The collection of a urine specimen with a sterile catheter has long been recommended, especially in the female, but physicians today believe that catheterization is unnecessary. No matter how carefully done, the maneuver extends infectious organisms up into the urinary tract. For most purposes a distinction can be made between infectious and contaminating micro-

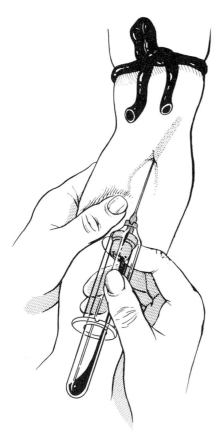

**Fig. 9-1.** Collection of blood sample by venipuncture. Note use of evacuated blood collection tube in plastic holder. (Syringe can also be used.)

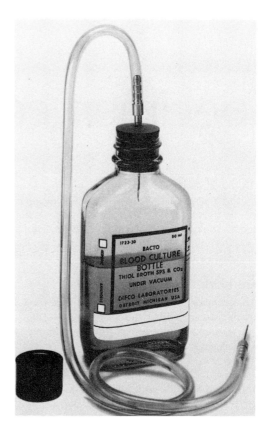

**Fig. 9-2.** Collection of blood culture. Prepared medium with sterile connections for venipuncture under vacuum is used. (Courtesy Difco Laboratories, Detroit.)

organisms in a *carefully collected,* clean-voided spec-imen. The meatus (opening) of the urethra is gently cleaned with soap (or detergent) and water. In both voided and catheterized specimens the first portion should be discarded, and the last portion should be received in a sterile container. A "clean-catch" urine specimen is one obtained during the midpart or toward the end of the act of voiding; it is received into a sterile receptacle. The sample should be promptly refrig-erated, or a suitable preservative added if laboratory examination is delayed. The urine in health is free of microorganisms.

*Blood for cultures* must be collected with special care because microbes, especially staphylococci, are present on the surface of the skin and within its super-ficial layers.

A blood culture is taken by venipuncture (Figs. 9-1 and 9-2) as follows:

1. Paint the skin over the veins in the bend of the elbow with tincture of iodine or other suitable disinfectant (70% alcohol may be used). *Note: Some persons are allergic to iodine!*

2. Remove disinfectant with 70% alcohol (or make a second application of 70% alcohol).
3. Place a 70% alcohol compress on the area.
4. Secure a tourniquet, not too tightly, around the arm just above the elbow, and ask the patient to close and open his hand several times.
5. Puncture a prominent vein with a 20- or 21-gauge needle to which may be attached a 20 ml. syringe or Vacutainer, a specially designed holder for a vacuum tube (Fig. 9-1). Remove 10 to 15 ml. of blood (or whatever amount is indi-cated for the particular laboratory test).
6. Add the blood directly to culture medium or place it in a sterile bottle containing sodium citrate to prevent coagulation and carry to the laboratory, where it is distributed to suitable culture media. To prevent contamination, re-move the needle from the syringe before ex-pelling the blood.

Bacteremia is often of short duration. If the blood culture is not collected at the proper time, the etiologic organism of the disease may not be found. Since the advent of the antimicrobial drugs, positive blood cultures are fewer. Even one dose of an antimicrobial drug before the culture is taken may mask the infection. The bloodstream in health is free of microorganisms.

*Blood for serologic examinations* (such as the precipitation tests for syphilis and various agglutination tests for the continued fevers) may be collected from a vein in the bend of the elbow. The technic is the same as that for collecting blood for culture, except that (1) the preliminary sterilization consists of scrubbing the area with 70% alcohol only and (2) the blood is placed in a chemically clean test tube and allowed to clot. Five milliliters is usually sufficient.

*Note:* Hepatitis can be conveyed to the person from whom the blood is drawn by the use of a clean *but unsterile* syringe. Use sterile *disposable needles* and preferably sterile *disposable syringes* to prevent hepatitis. (Otherwise syringes and needles must be carefully autoclaved.)

*Sputum* is often collected improperly, and samples tend to be too small. Many specimens consist of secretions from the nose, mouth, and throat and contain no sputum at all. The sputum should represent a true pulmonary secretion and should be expelled after deep coughing. It is worthwhile to instruct the patient how to bring the specimen up from the lower part of the respiratory tract. If necessary, nebulized aerosols can be used. The teeth should be carefully cleaned with toothpaste, and the mouth rinsed with sterile water before the specimen is taken. Usually more sputum is raised in the morning, and this sputum may contain *Mycobacterium tuberculosis* when specimens taken later in the day do not. Generally, sputum specimens collected for bacteriologic study are collected daily for at least 3 separate days. The ideal container for sputum is a 6-ounce widemouthed bottle (or plastic receptacle) with a tight-fitting stopper or cover.

Children swallow their sputum, and adults do also in their sleep. In children the only way to collect sputum is to aspirate stomach contents. When it is impossible to obtain a satisfactory cough specimen of sputum in adults, the stomach contents may be examined. The stomach should be aspirated early in the morning before any food or water is taken.

*Bronchial secretions* are secured by means of the bronchoscope and may be subjected to microbiologic study. After bronchoscopy, sputum specimens may be collected again for a 3-day period.

*Cultures from the nose and throat* are made many times, since sore throat and nasal discharge are frequent disorders and often part of systemic illness. To take the culture just after an antiseptic has been used is to defeat the purpose of the examination because the antiseptic retards the growth of bacteria present. (This applies to other cultures as well as to throat cultures.) When a throat culture is taken, use a good light, and insofar as possible, allow the swab to contact only the diseased area. At least two swabs are required. When cultures are taken from the nose, pass a small, tightly wound swab directly back through the nose. Avoid large loose swabs because they may slip off the applicator and lodge in the nose.

In cases of suspected diphtheria, cultures from the nose and throat are of special importance. More cases of diphtheria would be detected if cultures were made from both nose and throat instead of from the throat alone. The microbes causing diphtheria are often found in abundance in cultures after they have not been found in direct smears. Although this is true, smears should always be made when diphtheria-like lesions of the throat are encountered, since the exudate in the lesion of Vincent's angina, the causative organisms of which are detected only in smears, often bears a close resemblance to the membrane of diphtheria.

To detect meningococcal carriers, make *cultures from the nasopharynx* (the upper portion of the throat back of the soft palate). To make a swab, wrap cotton around the end of a piece of wire bent at a right angle about 1 inch from the end. When specimens from the throat and nasopharynx are obtained, take care to avoid contaminating the swabs with saliva.

*Feces* for ordinary microbiologic examination may be collected directly by the patient in a sterilized cardboard carton or other suitable container. At times it may be desirable for the patient to pass a stool into a larger, previously sterilized container, with a sterile tongue blade or spoon being used to remove a small amount to a sterile widemouthed bottle. The stool in the latter case should be examined superficially, and portions of the fecal material with mucus are preferable for microbiologic study.

Rectal swabs are very satisfactory for most microbiologic purposes and are easily obtained from both adults and children. If a disease process involves the lining of the terminal portion of the rectum, such swabs are likely to obtain material from within the focus of disease and are therefore more likely to contain disease-producing agents than is the stool of that person. Swabs are of value in testing for carriers of bacteria causing typhoid fever, dysentery, or cholera. To obtain the rectal swab clean the skin about the anus with soap, water, and 70% alcohol. Introduce a sterile cotton swab moistened with either a sterile isotonic solution or sterile broth through the anus and rotate it gently about the circumference of the lower rectum to contact a large portion of the mucosal lining. A fecal specimen may also be obtained

**Table 9-1**

The specimen and its pathogens

| SPECIMEN | IMPORTANT PATHOGENS | SPECIMEN | IMPORTANT PATHOGENS |
|---|---|---|---|
| Urine | *Brucella*<br>*Candida albicans*<br>*Escherichia coli* and other coliforms<br>Measles viruses<br>Mumps virus<br>*Mycobacterium tuberculosis*<br>*Proteus*<br>*Pseudomonas aeruginosa*<br>*Salmonella* and *Shigella*<br>*Staphylococcus aureus*<br>*Streptococcus pyogenes* and other<br>streptococci | Nose and throat secretions | Adenoviruses<br>*Bordetella pertussis*<br>*Chlamydia psittaci*<br>Coliforms<br>*Corynebacterium diphtheriae*<br>Enteroviruses<br>Fungi<br>Measles viruses<br>Mumps virus (saliva)<br>Mycobacteria<br>*Mycoplasma pneumoniae*<br>Myxoviruses<br>*Neisseria* species<br>Predominance of *Haemophilus influenzae*, *Staphylococcus aureus*, or *Candida albicans*<br>Respiratory viruses<br>*Staphylococcus aureus*<br>*Streptococcus pyogenes* and other<br>streptococci |
| Blood | Anaerobic cocci<br>*Bacteroides* species and related<br>anaerobes<br>*Brucella*<br>*Chlamydia psittaci*<br>*Coxiella burnetii*<br>*Escherichia coli* and other coliforms<br>*Francisella tularensis*<br>*Haemophilus influenzae*<br>Hepatitis viruses<br>*Leptospira*<br>*Neisseria gonorrhoeae*<br>*Neisseria meningitidis*<br>Opportunistic fungi<br>*Plasmodium*<br>*Proteus*<br>*Pseudomonas*<br>Rickettsias of spotted fevers<br>Rubeola ˉ d rubella viruses<br>*Salmonella* species<br>*Spirillum minor*<br>*Staphylococcus aureus*<br>*Streptobacillus moniliformis*<br>*Streptococcus pneumoniae*<br>*Streptococcus pyogenes* and other<br>streptococci | | |
| | | Stool (feces) | *Candida albicans*<br>Enteroviruses<br>Hepatitis virus<br>Metazoa *(Taenia,* etc.)<br>*Proteus*<br>Protozoa *(Entamoeba histolytica,*<br>etc.)<br>*Pseudomonas*<br>*Salmonella* species<br>*Salmonella typhi*<br>*Shigella dysenteriae*<br>*Shigella flexneri*<br>*Shigella sonnei*<br>*Shigella* species<br>*Staphylococcus aureus*<br>*Vibrio cholerae* |
| Sputum | *Actinomyces israelii*<br>Anaerobic streptococci<br>Atypical mycobacteria<br>*Blastomyces dermatitidis*<br>*Candida albicans*<br>*Coccidioides immitis*<br>*Cryptococcus neoformans*<br>*Histoplasma capsulatum*<br>*Klebsiella pneumoniae*<br>*Mycobacterium tuberculosis*<br>*Nocardia asteroides*<br>*Staphylococcus aureus*<br>*Streptococcus pneumoniae*<br>*Streptococcus pyogenes* | Pus, exudates,<br>wound drainages,<br>and so on | *Actinomyces*<br>Anaerobic cocci *(Peptostreptococcus, Peptococcus)*<br>*Bacillus anthracis*<br>*Bacteroides* species and related<br>anaerobic rods<br>*Blastomyces* and other systemic<br>fungi<br>*Clostridium* species<br>*Clostridium tetani*<br>Coliforms<br>*Corynebacterium diphtheriae*<br>Enterococci<br>*Francisella tularensis*<br>Mycobacteria<br>*Mycobacterium tuberculosis* |

**Table 9-1**

The specimen and its pathogens—cont'd

| SPECIMEN | IMPORTANT PATHOGENS | SPECIMEN | IMPORTANT PATHOGENS |
|---|---|---|---|
| Pus, exudates, wound drainages, and so on— cont'd | *Nocardia*<br>*Proteus* species<br>*Pseudomonas* species<br>*Staphylococcus aureus*<br>*Streptococcus pyogenes* and other streptococci | Pleural fluid | *Haemophilus influenzae*<br>*Mycobacterium tuberculosis*<br>*Staphylococcus aureus*<br>*Streptococcus pneumoniae*<br>*Streptococcus pyogenes* |
| Cerebrospinal fluid | Arboviruses<br>*Bacteroides* species<br>Coliforms<br>*Cryptococcus neoformans*<br>Enteroviruses<br>*Haemophilus influenzae*, type b<br>*Listeria monocytogenes*<br>*Mycobacterium tuberculosis*<br>*Neisseria meningitidis*<br>*Staphylococcus aureus*<br>*Streptococcus pneumoniae*<br>*Streptococcus pyogenes* | Peritoneal fluid | Coliforms<br>Enterococci<br>*Mycobacterium tuberculosis* |
| | | Fluid from conjunctiva of eye | Adenoviruses<br>*Chlamydia trachomatis*<br>*Haemophilus*<br>*Moraxella lacunata*<br>*Neisseria gonorrhoeae*<br>*Staphylococcus aureus*<br>*Streptococcus pneumoniae*<br>*Streptococcus pyogenes* and other streptococci |

from the physician's glove after digital examination of the rectum has been made.

In all cases the stool specimen should be sent to the laboratory at once because nonpathogenic intestinal bacteria may quickly overgrow the pathogenic organisms, and pathogenic amebas rapidly lose their motility if the fecal material containing them cools. In cases of suspected acute amebiasis, the warm feces should be examined immediately for pathogenic amebas showing their typical and diagnostic movement. If some delay is anticipated, receive the specimen into a vessel that has been warmed. A portion may then be placed in a small, tightly corked bottle, which may be placed in a fruit jar that has been filled with water just a few degrees above body temperature. This will keep the specimen warm for a considerable time so that it can be speeded to the nearest laboratory. In the hospital the specimen may be sent to the laboratory at once, without this special preparation. Examination for typhoid bacilli is facilitated by collecting the feces in a special brilliant green bile medium because bile facilitates the growth of typhoid bacilli and brilliant green retards the growth of many other intestinal organisms.

*Pus* from abscesses and boils may be obtained after drainage. The abscess or boil is painted with suitable disinfectant, the area is allowed to dry, and an incision is made with a sterile scalpel. Some of the contents are obtained by means of sterile swabs. If the lesion is opened widely, as much of the superficial portion should be removed as possible, and the specimen taken from the deeper part. When this is not done, the specimen is usually contaminated with surface microorganisms. Protect all specimens taken on swabs from drying. This is best done by placing the swabs in a sterile test tube containing either a drop or two of sterile physiologic salt solution or a nutrient broth that may be directly inoculated with the swabs. The swabs, which are longer than the test tube, should be placed in the test tube in such a manner that the cotton pledget is just above the salt solution and does not touch it. A cotton plug is inserted to hold the swabs in place.

*Smears for gonococci* in the female (see also p. 196) should be taken from the meatus of the urethra, the cervix uteri, and the rectum. In little girls suspected of having gonorrheal vulvovaginitis, the smears and cultures are made from the vagina because it is the vagina that is primarily attacked. In acute gonorrhea in the male the smears are obtained from the urethra. In chronic cases in the male a specimen may be obtained from the physician's massage of the prostate gland and seminal vesicles.

*Cerebrospinal fluid* is obtained by a procedure known as *lumbar puncture* (Fig. 9-3). It is carried out by the physician as follows. After the overlying skin of the lower back has been disinfected and anesthetized, a special needle with stylet is introduced slightly to one side of the midline and between the third and fourth lumbar vertebrae and passed into the spinal subarachnoid space. The strictest asepsis must be observed, and a sterile dressing placed over

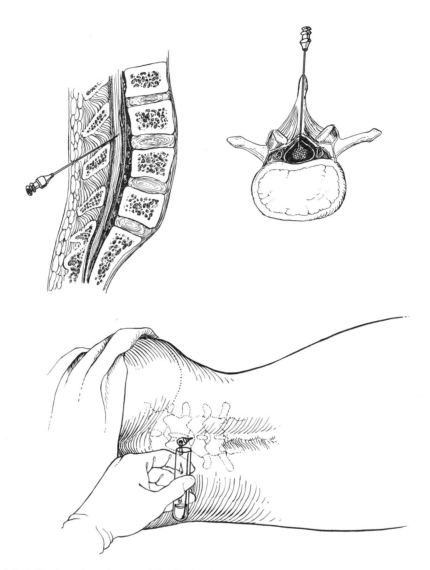

**Fig. 9-3.** Collection of cerebrospinal fluid by lumbar puncture. Note spinal needle in place in lower back. Inserts indicate anatomic position of needle in subarachnoid space.

the site of puncture. If an infant or child is seated with head and arms resting on a folded sheet, blanket, or pillow set against the abdomen, he may be held securely while the physician performs the lumbar puncture.

Cerebrospinal fluid may be obtained from the cisterna magna at the base of the brain by the skilled neurosurgeon. However, *cisternal puncture* is infrequent because of the danger at this location that the penetrating needle impale the brainstem or cervical cord. The cerebrospinal fluid is normally sterile.

*Pleural and peritoneal fluids* are obtained through the lumen of a trochar or specially designed needle inserted through the wall of the chest or abdomen.

With the trochar in place, fluid is aspirated with a syringe or freely drained into a sterile container. The strictest asepsis should be observed during this procedure, which is done by the physician.

*Smears and cultures from the conjunctiva* are made with swabs wet with sterile physiologic solution. The swabs should be handled carefully to prevent injury and spread of infection to adjacent parts of the eye or to the other eye.

*Specimens for anaerobic culture* are collected as carefully as possible: first, to avoid contamination with the abundance of anaerobes usually found in the normal flora of a given area and, second, to minimize the exposure of the specimen to the oxygen of the air.

Direct aspiration (with needle and syringe) of a given focus of disease gives a workable preparation. For example, in pulmonary infection, direct lung puncture or transtracheal aspiration is done to obtain pulmonary secretions or tissue, and in urinary tract infection, percutaneous suprapubic bladder puncture to obtain urine.

*Specimens for the viral and rickettsial laboratory,* such as blood, cerebrospinal fluid, respiratory secretions, feces, and urine should be collected with the strictest aseptic technic and placed in sterile containers. Further contamination of throat swabs, nasal washings, stools, and specimens already containing bacteria is to be avoided. Swabs may be received in tubes, in a small amount of sterile nutrient broth.

Rush all specimens to the viral diagnostic laboratory immediately after collection. Often this means that they must be transported a distance to a medical center, a large hospital, or the laboratory of a state health department. When this is the case, freeze the specimen (with the exception of blood) immediately and keep it so until shipment can be made. Refrigerate blood samples and let clot. It is desirable to separate serum from the clot. Transit is best made with specimen container packed in Dry Ice and posted airmail special delivery. A frozen shipment is likely to be a satisfactory one provided the ice or Dry Ice has not thawed out by the time the destination is reached. (Small packages in Dry Ice are likely to thaw in 8 to 12 hours or less.) To send blood samples on Dry Ice, place the clot and serum in separate tubes. Although cold shipment of fresh material is preferable most of the time, specimens may be preserved in sterile 50% glycerin solution (but *never* in formalin).

The paired samples of blood for serologic examinations in viral and rickettsial diseases (p. 289) are to be collected aseptically, the blood allowed to clot, and the serum separated from the clot. The serum is sent at once to the out-of-town laboratory by airmail.

Remember that proper labels on the outside of the package help to prevent accidental infection of laboratory personnel receiving the specimen.

## Pathogens related to specimens

In this chapter we have considered body fluids and anatomic sites in the body from which specimens for microbiologic examination are most commonly taken. Table 9-1 lists routine specimens with important pathogenic microorganisms encountered therein.

## Questions for review

1 Why is careful specimen collection stressed?
2 State the ground rules for the collection of any specimen for microbiologic examination.
3 What precautions should be taken in collecting urine specimens for microbiologic examination? Is it necessary to catheterize the female?
4 How should the skin be prepared for the collection of a blood culture? Why is this necessary?
5 What vein is commonly used as a collection site for blood specimens?
6 What are the precautions to be considered in collecting sputum specimens? In collecting stool specimens?
7 How would you handle a specimen of pus that is to be cultured?
8 Briefly discuss the collection of cerebrospinal fluid.
9 How are specimens handled that must be shipped to an out-of-town laboratory for diagnosis of viral disease?

**REFERENCES** (Chapters 6 to 9)

Alexander, E., Jr.: Lumbar puncture, J.A.M.A. **201**:316, 1967.

Bailey, W. R., and Scott, E. G.: Diagnostic microbiology, ed. 4, St. Louis, 1974, The C. V. Mosby Co.

Baker, F. J.: Handbook of bacteriological technique, New York, 1967, Appleton-Century-Crofts.

Balows, A., and others, editors: Current techniques for antibiotic susceptibility testing, Springfield, Ill., 1973, Charles C Thomas, Publisher.

Bartlett, D. I.: The survival of bacteria on swabs, Lab. Med. **1**:32, July, 1970.

Bartlett, R. C., and Carrington, G. O.: How to avoid hazards in microbiology, Med. Lab. Observer **1**:46, July, 1969.

Bartlett, R. C., and others: Blood cultures (Cumitech 1), Washington, D.C., 1974, American Society for Microbiology.

Bauer, J. D., and others: Clinical laboratory methods, ed. 8, St. Louis, 1974, The C. V. Mosby Co.

Bodily, H. L., and others, editors: Diagnostic procedures for bacterial, mycotic and parasitic infections, Washington, D.C., 1970, American Public Health Association, Inc.

Bologna, C. V.: Understanding laboratory medicine, St. Louis, 1971, The C. V. Mosby Co.

Branson, D.: Methods in clinical bacteriology, Springfield, Ill., 1972, Charles C Thomas, Publisher.

Branson, D.: Microbiology for the small laboratory, Springfield, Ill., 1972, Charles C Thomas, Publisher.

Chitwood, L. A.: Isolation and identification of Group A streptococci with commercially-available agents, Lab. Med. **2**:26, Jan., 1971.

Collins, C. H., and Lyne, P. M.: Microbiological methods, ed. 3, Baltimore, 1970, University Park Press.

Culling, C. J.: Modern microscopy, elementary theory & practice, London, 1974, Butterworth & Co. (Publishers) Ltd.

Davis, J. G.: Aspects of laboratory hygiene, Lab. Pract. **21**: 101, 1972.

Duncan, I. B. R.: Virology in a general hospital, Can. Med. Assoc. J. **98**:1050, 1968.

Elston, H. R., and Quigley, H. J., Jr.: Dye-impregnated paper strips for staining bacteria, Am. J. Clin. Pathol. **60**:476, 1973.

Finegold, S. M., and others: Rapid diagnosis of bacteremia, Appl. Microbiol. **18**:458, 1969.

Focus on the microscope, Today's Health **46**:44, Nov., 1968.

Frankel, S., and others, editors: Gradwohl's clinical laboratory methods and diagnosis, ed. 7, St. Louis, 1970, The C. V. Mosby Co.

Freeman, J. A., and Beeler, M. F.: Laboratory medicine—clinical microscopy, Philadelphia, 1974, Lea & Febiger.

Gillies, R. R., and Dodds, T. C.: Bacteriology illustrated, ed. 3, Baltimore, 1973, The Williams & Wilkins Co.

Graber, C. D.: Rapid diagnostic methods in medical microbiology, Baltimore, 1970, The Williams & Wilkins Co.

Gray, P., editor: The encyclopedia of microscopy and microtechnique, New York, 1973, Van Nostrand Reinhold Co.

Hammon, W. McD.: Human infection acquired in the laboratory, J.A.M.A. **203**:647, 1968.

Harris, A. H., and Coleman, M. B., editors: Diagnostic procedures and reagents: technics for the laboratory diagnosis and control of the communicable diseases, New York, 1963, American Public Health Association, Inc.

Heinzl, D.: Evaluation of the use of Clostrisel agar, Lab. Med. **2**:36, Oct., 1971.

Hellman, A., and others, editors: Biohazards in biological research, Cold Spring Harbor, N.Y., 1973, Cold Spring Harbor Laboratory.

Herrmann, E. C., Jr.: Experience in providing a viral diagnostic laboratory compatible with medical practice, Mayo Clin. Proc. **42**:112, 1967.

Hoskins, J. M.: Virological procedures, New York, 1967, Appleton-Century-Crofts.

Johnson, N. E.: Coping with complications of IV's, Nursing '72 **2**:5, Feb., 1972.

Joklik, W., and Smith, D. T.: Zinsser microbiology, ed. 15, New York, 1972, Prentice-Hall, Inc.

Knights, E. M.: Commercially available products for screening test, Bull. Pathol. **10**:411, 1969.

Lane-Petter, W., and Pearson, A. E. G.: The laboratory animal—principles and practices, New York, 1963, Academic Press, Inc.

Langford, T. L.: Nursing problem: bacteriuria and the indwelling catheter, Am. J. Nurs. **72**:113, 1972.

Lennette, E. H., and others: Manual of clinical microbiology, Washington, D.C., 1974, American Society for Microbiology.

Lillie, R. D., editor: H. J. Conn's biological stains, Baltimore, 1969, The Williams & Wilkins Co.

Lindberg, A., and others: Identification of gram-negative aerobic fermentors, in a clinical bacteriological laboratory, Med. Microbiol. Immunol. **159**:201, 1974.

Locatcher-Khorazo, D., and Seegal, B. C.: Microbiology of the eye, St. Louis, 1972, The C. V. Mosby Co.

Lowis, M. J.: An identification key for some aerobic bacteria, Lab. Pract. **20**:331, 1971.

MacFate, R. P.: Introduction to the clinical laboratory, ed. 3, Chicago, 1972, Year Book Medical Publishers, Inc.

Maisey, M. A.: Bacteriology, Nurs. Times **70**:142, Jan. 31, 1974.

McMennamin, A. M., and Wenk, R. E.: Use of selective media in the dip-slide method of estimating colony counts, Lab. Med. **2**:51, Jan., 1971.

McQuay, R. M.: Good parasitologic examinations depend on proper procedures, Hosp. Top. **44**:85, Oct., 1966.

Medical news: New blood culture method developed, J.A.M.A. **206**:1425, 1968.

Morgan, R. M., and Good, D. S.: Microbiology procedures: the selection and interpretation of current tests for physicians, nurses, and paramedical personnel, Springfield, Ill., 1973, Charles C Thomas, Publisher.

Needham, G. H.: The microscope: a practical guide, Springfield, Ill., 1968, Charles C Thomas, Publisher.

Nelson, D. P., and Mata, L. J.: Bacterial flora associated with human gastrointestinal mucosa, Gastroenterology **58**:56, 1970.

Nyka, W.: New techniques used to study tubercle bacilli in lungs of treated patients, Lab. Med. **3**:42, March, 1972.

Payne, J. E., and Kaplan, H. M.: Alternative techniques for venipuncture, Am. J. Nurs. **72**:702, 1972.

Pike, R. M., and Sulkin, S. E.: The laboratory as a source of infection, Bull. Coll. Am. Pathol. **22**:299, 1968.

Pike, R. M., and others: Continuing importance of laboratory-acquired infections, Am. J. Public Health **55**:190, 1965.

Portnoy, B.: Diagnosis of viral disease in the clinical laboratory, Lab. Med. **1**:38, Sept., 1970.

Provine, H., and Gardner, P.: The gram-stained smear and its interpretation, Hosp. Pract. **9**:85, Oct., 1974.

Quinn, R. W.: The positive throat culture—what does it mean? South. Med. J. **67**:1009, 1974.

Rosenzweig, A. L.: Venipuncture technique—a reappraisal, Lab. Med. **1**:36, Sept., 1970.

Short, D. J., and Woodnott, D. P., editors: The I.A.T. manual of laboratory animal practice and techniques, ed. 2, Springfield, Ill., 1971, Charles C Thomas, Publisher.

Siegelman, A. M., and Friedman, B.: Microscopy in the clinical laboratory. Part 1. Cadence Clinical Laboratory **5**:6, Sept.-Oct., 1974.

Snyder, B.: Pitfalls in the gram stain, Lab. Med. **1**:41, July, 1970.

So you're going to collect a blood specimen, Chicago, 1974, College of American Pathologists.

Stein, H. J.: Caution: biology may be hazardous to your health, BioScience **21**:80, 1971.

Stewart, J. A.: Methods of media preparation for the biological sciences, Springfield, Ill., 1974, Charles C Thomas, Publisher.

Stier, A. R., and Miller, L. K.: Reagent-water specifications and methods of quality control, Pathologist **26**:41, 1972.

Taylor, W. I.: Rapid detection of bacteria in urine, Lab. Med. **2**:29, Sept., 1971.

Tilton, R. C.: Methodologic advances in clinical microbiology, Lab. Med. **1**:54, Feb., 1970.

Ungvarski, P.: Mechanical stimulation of coughing, Am. J. Nurs. **71**:2358, 1971.

Washington, J. A., II, editor: Laboratory procedures in clinical microbiology, Boston, 1974, Little, Brown & Co.

Zabransky, R. J.: Isolation of anaerobic bacteria from clinical specimens, Mayo Clin. Proc. **45**:256, 1970.

Zugibe, F. T.: Diagnostic histochemistry, St. Louis, 1970, The C. V. Mosby Co.

## CHAPTER 10

# Role in disease

### Infection

When microbes or certain other living agents enter the body of a human being or animal, multiply, and produce a reaction there, this is an *infection.* The host is *infected,* and the disease is an *infectious* one. The reaction of the body may or may not be accompanied by outward signs of disease. Infection is differentiated from *contamination,* which refers to the mere presence of infectious material (no reaction produced). Superficial wounds in skin and mucous membranes are often the site of a large microbial population. As long as these microorganisms do not invade the deeper tissues and induce a reaction there, they are considered contaminants instead of agents of infection.

### Resident population

**Microbes normally present.** *The mere presence of microbes in the body does not mean infection, since microorganisms normally inhabit many parts of the body without invading the deeper tissues to cause disease.* Certain of the body fluids such as blood and urine are normally sterile, that is, free of the presence of microorganisms. In parts of the body other than the circulatory system and the urinary tract, the secretions or excretions are normally in contact with a resident population of microorganisms. These microbes are consistently present in varying proportions. This pattern of growth, conspicuously bacterial, is associated with the well-being of the person and in an area such as the intestinal tract is even necessary to his health. These microorganisms constitute the *normal flora of the body.* Table 10-1 gives their normal habitats in the human body.

### Invasion of body

**Source of microbes causing infections.** The microbes that cause infections fall into two classes: (1) those that can cause disease in healthy persons and reach such persons directly or indirectly from animals, persons ill of the disease, or carriers (such microbes are pathogens and cause communicable diseases) and (2) those that attack the host at a time of injury or lowered resistance or when they themselves are increased in virulence (these are ordinarily saprophytes but can be opportunists). To the second group belong both microorganisms that normally inhabit the body and produce disease only under given conditions and certain ones that are inadvertently introduced into the body by wounds, injuries, and such.

**How microbes reach the body.** According to the manner in which the causative agent reaches the body, infectious diseases may be classified as communicable and noncommunicable.

A *communicable disease* is one whose causative agent is directly or indirectly transmitted from host to host. Examples are typhoid fever and tuberculosis. The host from which the infection is spread is usually of the same species as the recipient, but not necessarily so. For instance, cattle may transmit tuberculosis and undulant fever to man.

A *noncommunicable disease* is one whose agent either normally inhabits the body, only occasionally producing disease, or resides outside it, producing disease only when introduced into the body. For example, tetanus bacilli, inhabitants of the soil, produce disease only when introduced into abrasions or wounds. Although *not* communicable, tetanus is infectious. The term *contagious* is applied to diseases that are easily spread directly from person to person.

Infectious diseases are also classified as exogenous and endogenous. *Exogenous* infections are those in which the causative agent reaches the body from the outside and enters the body through one of the portals of entry. An *endogenous* infection is one caused by organisms normally present in the body. Endogenous infections occur when the defensive powers of the host are weakened or, for some reason, the virulence of the microorganism is increased.

**How microbes enter body.** Microorganisms invade the body by several avenues, and each species has its own favored one. The way of access to the body is known as the *portal of entry,* as indicated in the areas discussed.

*Skin.* Most pathogenic organisms do not penetrate the unbroken skin or mucous membrane, but some do. Staphylococci and some of the fungi can

**Table 10-1**
Distribution of the resident population

| ANATOMIC SITE | IMPORTANT RESIDENT MICROBES | ANATOMIC SITE | IMPORTANT RESIDENT MICROBES |
|---|---|---|---|
| Skin | *Bacillus* species<br>Coliforms<br>Diphtheroids (aerobic and anaerobic)<br>Enterococci<br>Fungi (lipophilic)<br>Mycobacteria<br>*Propionibacterium acnes*<br>*Proteus* species<br>*Pseudomonas* species<br>Staphylococci<br>Streptococci | | Mycobacteria<br>Mycoplasmas<br>*Penicillium* species<br>*Proteus* species<br>*Pseudomonas aeruginosa*<br>Spirochetes<br>Staphylococci<br>Streptococci (aerobic and anaerobic)<br>Yeasts |
| Mouth (including gingival crevice) | Amebas<br>*Bacteroides* species<br>Diphtheroids<br>Hemophilic bacilli<br>Lactobacilli<br>Mycoplasmas<br>Neisseriae<br>Pneumococci<br>Spirochetes<br>Staphylococci<br>Streptococci<br>*Trichomonas* species<br>Veillonellae | Genital tract | *Bacteroides* species<br>Coliforms<br>Diphtheroids<br>Enterococci<br>*Haemophilus vaginalis*<br>Lactobacilli<br>*Mycobacterium smegmatis*<br>Mycoplasmas<br>Neisseriae<br>*Proteus species*<br>Saprophytic yeasts<br>Spirochetes<br>Staphylococci<br>Streptococci (aerobic and anaerobic)<br>Veillonellae |
| Respiratory tract | Actinomycetes<br>*Bacteroides* species<br>*Candida albicans* and other fungi<br>Diphtheroids<br>Hemophilic bacilli<br>Mycobacteria<br>Mycoplasmas<br>*Neisseria* species<br>Pneumococci<br>Spirochetes<br>Staphylococci<br>Streptococci (aerobic and anaerobic)<br>Veillonellae | Vagina<br>  Before puberty<br><br><br>  During childbearing period<br>  After childbearing period | Coliforms<br>Diphtheroids<br>Streptococci<br>Döderlein's bacilli (*Lactobacillus* species)<br>Coliforms<br>Diphtheroids<br>Streptococci |
| | | Organs of special sense<br>  Eye<br><br><br><br>  External ear | Alpha streptococci<br>Diphtheroids<br>Hemophilic bacilli<br>Pneumococci<br>Staphylococci<br>*Bacillus* species<br>Diphtheroids<br>Nonpathogenic acid-fast organisms<br>Staphylococci and certain other cocci |
| Gastrointestinal tract*<br>(mostly in lower ileum and colon) | *Alcaligenes faecalis*<br>*Bacteroides* species<br>*Clostridium* species<br>Coliforms<br>Diphtheroids<br>Enterococci<br>Enteroviruses<br>*Lactobacillus species†* | | |

*The stomach is normally free of microbial growth because of its acid content. Microorganisms are much more plentiful in the large than in the small intestine.

†A baby is born with a sterile intestinal tract, but before or with the first feeding, bacteria are introduced. If the child is breast fed, the predominating organism is said to be *Bifidobacterium bifidum* (formerly *Lactobacillus bifidus*). If the child is bottle fed, *Lactobacillus acidophilus* (bacteria of the genus *Lactobacillus* convert carbohydrates to lactic acid) predominates. In addition, other bacteria are present.

penetrate the hair follicles and cause disease in the deeper tissues of the skin. The organisms of tularemia pass through the unbroken skin, as do hookworm larvae. In their penetration of the intact skin, malarial parasites have the help of a biting insect. Many bacteria are found in the superficial layers of the skin but under normal conditions are not able to penetrate deeply. As soon as the superficial barrier is broken, infection is easily accomplished.

*Respiratory apparatus.* Pulmonary tuberculosis, pneumonia, and influenza are contracted by way of the respiratory tract, and the viruses causing measles, smallpox, and German measles enter the body this way.

*Alimentary tract.* Some of the most important pathogens gain entrance to the body by way of the digestive tract, for example, the typhoid and dysentery bacilli, cholera vibrios, and amebas of dysentery. In many cases food and drink are the vehicles. The great majority of pathogenic microorganisms enter the body via the respiratory system or the digestive tract.

*Genitourinary system.* Certain infections are acquired chiefly through the genitourinary system, notably the venereal diseases.

*Placenta.* Most microorganisms do not pass through the placenta, but the spirochete of syphilis and the smallpox virus may.

## Event of infection

**Factors influencing occurrence of infection.** The fact that microbes have entered the body in no manner indicates that infection has occurred. Whether infection supervenes depends on (1) the portal of entry, (2) the virulence of the organisms, (3) their number, and (4) the defensive powers of the host (Chapter 11).

Most pathogenic microbes have definite portals by which they enter the body, and they can fail to produce disease when introduced into the body by some other route. For instance, typhoid bacilli produce typhoid fever when swallowed but only a slight local inflammation when rubbed on the abraded skin, whereas streptococci rubbed into the skin produce an intense inflammation (cellulitis) but are generally without effect when swallowed. If streptococci are breathed into the lungs, they may cause pneumonia. A few bacteria such as *Francisella tularensis*, the cause of tularemia, can enter the body by several different routes and produce disease in each area. Usually the route of entry determines the type of disease process for a given organism.

By *virulence* or *pathogenicity* one means the ability of microbes to induce disease by overcoming the defensive powers of the host. There is a difference in virulence not only among species but also among members of the same species. As a rule, microbes are most virulent when freshly discharged from the person ill with the disease that they cause. Organisms harbored by carriers are less virulent.

Virulence may be increased by rapid transfer of organisms through a series of susceptible animals. As each animal becomes ill, the organisms are isolated from its excreta and transferred to a well animal. Herein are explained epidemics. The causative organism of the disease, by repeated passage from person to person, becomes so virulent that everyone whom it contacts is made ill.

An organism that is highly virulent for one species of animals and less virulent for another may, with repeated passage through the animal for which it is less virulent, show a *transposal of virulence;* that is, it becomes less virulent for the animal for which it was originally highly virulent and highly virulent for the animal for which it was originally less virulent. Advantage is taken of this in the production of antirabies vaccine.

The *number* of microbes is crucial to infection. If only a few enter the body, they are likely to be overcome by the local defenses of the host even though they are highly virulent. Therefore, if infection is to occur, enough microorganisms to overcome the local defenses of the host must penetrate the body.

**How microbes cause disease.** When pathogenic microorganisms enter the body, two opposing forces are set in motion. The organisms strive to invade the tissues and colonize there. The body, utilizing its defensive powers, strives to block the invasion of the microbes, destroy them, and cast them off. If the body wins the contest, the microbes are destroyed and the body suffers no ill effects. If the microbes prevail, infection occurs.

Microbes cause disease in different ways. In some cases the mechanical effects of microorganisms operate, for example, when the organisms of estivo-autumnal malaria occlude the capillaries of the brain.

In most cases, however, biochemical effects are foremost. The ability of pathogenic microorganisms to produce disease is closely tied in with certain complex chemical substances that the organisms either elaborate and release or that are a vital part of their makeup. A soluble exotoxin (p. 45) is an example of a product released into body fluids and even into the bloodstream of the host. A constituent of the bacterial cell wall may be an injurious factor. A part of the microbial cell such as its capsule, although not harmful in itself, may so protect the microbe as to enhance its virulence. The carbohydrate (polysaccharide) capsules of the pneumococci invading the lower respiratory tract protect them from the defensive cells of the lungs, thereby facilitating the development of pneumonia.

Biochemical substances implicated in pathogenicity of bacteria and other disease-producing microbes are many, and their action is not always well understood. The major effects of these are summarized as follows:

1. They interfere with mechanical blocks to the spread of infection set up in the body (bacterial kinases).
2. They slow or stop the ingestion of microbes by the phagocytic white blood cells (leukocidins).
3. They destroy body tissues (hemolysins, necrotizing exotoxins, lethal factor).
4. They cause generalized unfavorable reactions in the host, resulting in fever, discomfort, and aching (endotoxins). Such features are usually collected together under the term *toxicity*.

Most disease-producing microbes prefer a given part of the body; they have their favored site for involvement. This is *elective localization*. For instance, dysentery bacilli attack the intestines, pneumococci attack the lungs, and meningococci localize in the leptomeninges. Toxic products released by microbes also have an affinity for certain anatomic sites; the toxin of tetanus attacks the central nervous system, and the toxin of diphtheria affects not only the central nervous system but also the heart.

**Local effects.** By local effects of microbes one means the changes produced in the tissues in which they are multiplying, summed up in the process of *inflammation*. Inflammation (Chapter 44) is the body's answer to injury. Its design is to halt the invasion and destroy the invaders. The features of the inflammatory process vary greatly with the different causative organisms and are significantly related to the disease-producing capacity of the microbe.

**General effects.** There are certain host reactions found in nearly all infectious diseases. In addition, many diseases have their own peculiar features. Among the general effects are fever (p. 94), increased pulse rate (tachycardia), increased metabolic rate, and signs of toxicity. The degree of fever approximates the severity of the infection. Anemia is a result of prolonged and severe infections.

A very common effect of infection is a change in the total number of circulating leukocytes (white blood cells) and in the relative proportion of the different kinds. This is why total leukocyte and differential white cell counts are so important in the diagnosis of disease. In most infections the total number of leukocytes is increased (*leukocytosis*). In some the number is decreased (*leukopenia*), and in a few it is unchanged. If fever or leukocytosis fails

to occur in infections where either ordinarily does, a severe infection or decreased host resistance is indicated.

An important consequence of infection is the development of immunity (Chapter 12).

**How disease-producing agents leave body.** Just as they have definite avenues of entry, pathogenic agents have definite routes of discharge from the body, known as *portals of exit*, which to a great extent depend on the part of the body that is diseased. The following list gives the important ones with examples:

1. *Feces*—bacteria of salmonellosis, bacillary dysentery, and cholera; protozoa of dysentery; and viruses of poliomyelitis and infectious hepatitis
2. *Urine*—bacteria of typhoid fever, tuberculosis (when affecting the genitourinary tract), and undulant fever
3. *Discharges from the mouth, nose, and respiratory passages*—bacteria of tuberculosis, whooping cough, pneumonia, scarlet fever, and epidemic meningitis; viruses of measles, smallpox, mumps, poliomyelitis, influenza, and epidemic encephalitis
4. *Saliva*—virus of rabies
5. *Blood* (removed by biting insects)—protozoa of malaria; bacteria of tularemia; rickettsias of typhus fever and Rocky Mountain spotted fever; virus of yellow fever

## Pattern of infection

**Course of infectious disease.** The course of many infectious diseases extends over the following:

1. *Period of incubation*—interval between the time the infection is received and the appearance of disease (Table 10-2).

   In some diseases the length is constant. In others it varies greatly. The length of the incubation period depends on (a) nature of the disease-producing agent (for example, the incubation period of diphtheria is less than that of rabies), (b) its virulence, (c) resistance of the host, (d) distance from the site of entrance to the focus of action (for instance, the incubation period of rabies, which affects the brain, is shorter when the site of inoculation is about the face), and (e) the number of infectious agents invading the body.
2. *Period of prodromal symptoms*—short interval (the prodrome) that sometimes follows the period of incubation, characterized by such symptoms as headache and malaise.
3. *Period of invasion*—disease reaching its full development to maximum intensity.

   Invasion may be rapid (a few hours, as in

**Table 10-2**
Incubation periods of important infectious diseases*

| DISEASE | USUAL INCUBATION PERIOD | DISEASE | USUAL INCUBATION PERIOD |
|---|---|---|---|
| Adenovirus infections | 5 to 6 days | Meningitis, acute bacterial | 1 to 7 days |
| Amebiasis | 2 weeks (varies) | Mumps | 14 to 21 days |
| Ascariasis | 8 to 10 weeks | Mycoplasmal pneumonia | 7 to 21 days |
| Brucellosis | 5 to 30 days (varies) | (primary atypical) | |
| Cat-scratch fever | 3 to 10 days (varies) | Pertussis | 5 to 21 days |
| Chickenpox | 14 to 16 days | Pinworm infection | 2 to 6 weeks |
| Cholera | 1 to 3 days | Plague | 2 to 6 days |
| Coccidioidomycosis, primary | 1 to 3 weeks | Poliomyelitis | 7 to 14 days |
| infection | | Psittacosis | 4 to 15 days |
| Coxsackievirus infections | 2 to 14 days | Rabies† | 2 to 6 weeks |
| Diphtheria | 2 to 6 days | | (to 1 year) |
| Echovirus infections | 3 to 5 days | Rocky Mountain spotted fever | 3 to 12 days |
| Encephalitis | 2 to 21 days (varies as to type) | Rubella | 14 to 21 days |
| | | Salmonellosis | |
| Gas gangrene | 1 to 5 days | Food poisoning | 6 to 72 hours |
| Gonorrhea | 3 to 5 days | (intraluminal) | |
| Hepatitis, viral, type A | 15 to 50 days | Enteric fever | 1 to 10 days |
| (infectious) | | (extraluminal) | |
| Hepatitis, viral, type B (serum) | 6 weeks to 6 months | Typhoid fever | 7 to 21 days |
| Herpesvirus infections | 4 days | Shigellosis (bacillary dysentery) | 1 to 7 days |
| Histoplasmosis | 5 to 18 days | Smallpox | 12 days |
| Hookworm disease | 6 weeks | Streptococcal infections (scarlet | 2 to 5 days |
| Impetigo contagiosa | 2 to 5 days | fever and the like) | |
| Infectious mononucleosis | 2 to 6 weeks | Syphilis, primary lesion | 10 to 90 days |
| Influenza | 1 to 3 days | Tetanus | 3 days to 3 weeks |
| Leprosy | 3 months to 20 years (?) | Trichinosis | 2 to 28 days |
| | | Tuberculosis, primary lesion | 2 to 10 weeks |
| Leptospirosis | 2 to 20 days | Tularemia | 1 to 10 days |
| Measles (rubeola) | 10 to 12 days | Yellow fever | 3 to 6 days |

*In this table and throughout the book the length of the incubation period is usually that given in the "Red Book" of the American Academy of Pediatrics.
†Rabies incubation in dogs is 21 to 60 days.

pneumonia) or insidious (a few days, as in typhoid fever). At the onset of acute infectious disease, rigors and chills often precede the rise in temperature. The sensation of cold is difficult to explain but probably results from a difference between the temperatures of the deep and superficial tissues of the body. To conserve heat, the superficial vessels of the skin constrict and sweating stops. The skin is pale and dry. As heat loss is decreased, the temperature rises rapidly.

4. *Fastigium or acme*—disease at its height.
5. *Period of defervescence or decline*—stage during which the manifestations subside.

During this stage profuse sweating occurs. Heat loss soon exceeds heat production. As the temperature falls, the normal hue of the body returns, and sweating ceases. Defervescence

may be by *crisis* (within 24 hours) or by *lysis* (several days, with the temperature going down a little each day until it returns to normal). Fever that begins abruptly usually ends by crisis. During the stage of *convalescence* the patient regains his lost strength.

Many diseases are *self-limited*, which means that under ordinary conditions of host resistance and microbial virulence the disease will last a certain, rather definite length of time and recovery will take place.

**Types of infection.** In a *localized* infection the microbes remain confined to a particular anatomic spot (examples: boils and abscesses). In a *generalized* infection microorganisms or their products are spread generally over the body by the bloodstream or lymphatics. A *mixed* infection is one caused by two or more organisms. If a person infected with a given organism becomes infected with still another, a *primary* infection is complicated by a *secondary* one. Secondary infections of the skin and respiratory tract are quite common, and in some cases the secondary infection is more dangerous than the primary, for example, the streptococcal bronchopneumonia that often follows measles, influenza, or whooping cough. Lowered body resistance resulting from the primary infection facilitates the development of the secondary infection.

A *focal* infection is one confined to a restricted area from which infectious material spreads to other parts of the body. Examples are infections of the teeth, sinuses, and prostate gland. An infection that does not cause any detectable manifestations is an *inapparent* or *subclinical* one. An infection held in check by the defensive forces of the body but activated when the body resistance is reduced is a *latent* infection. An infection caused by the accidental or surgical penetration of the skin or mucous membranes is sometimes spoken of as an *inoculation infection.*

When bacteria enter the bloodstream but do not multiply, the condition is spoken of as a *bacteremia.* If they enter the bloodstream and multiply, causing infection of the bloodstream itself, the condition is *septicemia.* Septicemia is the layman's blood poisoning. When pyogenic bacteria (pus-formers) in the bloodstream are spread to different parts of the body to lodge and set up new foci of disease, the condition is called *pyemia.* When toxins liberated by bacteria enter the bloodstream and cause disease, the condition is *toxemia.* Diphtheria is a good example of a toxemia. Saprophytic bacteria may grow on dead tissue such as a retained placenta or a gangrenous limb and produce poisons that cause disease when absorbed into the body. This is *sapremia.* Patients with chronic wasting diseases like cancer often die from the immediate effects of some bacterial infection, especially streptococcal and pneumococcal infections. These are *terminal* infections.

A *sporadic* disease occurs as only an occasional case in a community. An *endemic* disease is one that is constantly present to a greater or lesser degree in a community. When a disease attacks a larger number of persons in the community in a short time, an *epidemic* is said to exist. Endemic diseases may become epidemic. When a disease becomes epidemic in a great number of countries at the same time, it is said to be *pandemic.*

*Epidemiology* presents the pattern of disease in a given community and is the study of those factors influencing its presence or absence. The *incidence* of disease is the number of new cases per block of population in a specific time period. The *prevalence* of the disease is the number of cases in existence at any given time in that population.

## Spread of infection

**Transmission of communicable diseases.** The etiologic agents of communicable diseases may be transmitted from the source of the infection to the recipient by (1) direct contact, (2) indirect contact, or (3) insect carriers.

*Direct contact* is the term applied when an infection is spread more or less directly from person to person or from a lower animal to man. It does not necessarily mean actual bodily contact, except with venereal diseases (p. 198), but does indicate a rather close association. *Droplet infection,* infection by microbes cast off in the fine spray from the mouth and nose during coughing, talking, or laughing, is a form of direct contact, as is placental transmission. By direct contact, blood transfusion transmits malaria and viral hepatitis. Diseases spread directly from person to person include tuberculosis, diphtheria, measles, pneumonia, scarlet fever, the common cold, smallpox, syphilis, gonorrhea, and epidemic meningitis, and from lower animals to man, rabies and tularemia. (Some of these diseases may also be transmitted by indirect contact.)

*Indirect contact* refers to the spread of the etiologic agent of a disease by conveyors such as milk, other foods, water, air, contaminated hands, and inanimate objects. Infections arising by indirect contact are usually more widely separated in space and time than those arising by direct contact. The diseases most commonly spread by indirect contact are those in which the infectious material enters the body via the mouth.

*Food,* including milk, may convey infection. Salmonellosis, bacillary dysentery, and cholera may be spread by contaminated food. Botulism is caused by the consumption of canned foods insufficiently heated. Trichinosis and tapeworm infection are contracted by eating improperly cooked pork.

*Air* is involved in the spread of infection; particles of dried secretion from the mouth or nose (*droplet nuclei*) may float in the air for a considerable time and be carried a rather long distance. Naturally, airborne transfer operates in respiratory infections.

*Contaminated fingers* are important conveyors of infection. A person with contaminated fingers may pass on infection to other people or to different parts of his own body. Fingers easily soil food and drink.

*Fomites* are inanimate objects that spread infection. The most important are items such as handkerchiefs, towels, blankets, bed sheets, diapers, pencils, and drinking cups. Money is grossly contaminated as indicated by recent studies, especially the small unit coins and paper bills that more frequently change hands. Potential pathogens were cultured from 13% of the coins and 42% of the bills collected.

*Filth* is responsible for disease, and certain diseases are primarily diseases of filth. Of these, typhus fever, as it is seen in parts of the world, is an example. However, filth plays little or no part in the spread of typhus fever in the United States. (Typhus is rare in this country.) Persons who are unclean in their personal habits are more likely to contract an infectious disease than those who are clean, and disease is more difficult to control in an unsanitary community.

*Insects* convey disease mechanically or biologically. In the *mechanical* transfer of disease insects merely hold the pathogenic organisms on their feet or other parts of their body. Flies can transfer the agents of

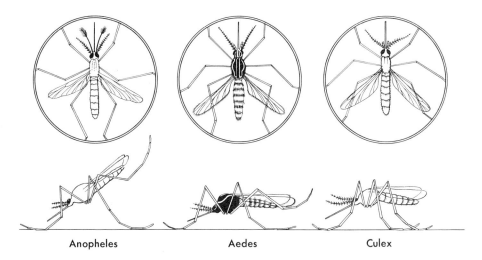

**Fig. 10-1.** Three mosquitoes as biologic vectors in spread of disease. Note typical resting positions. Mosquitoes of genus *Anopheles* transmit malaria; members of genus *Aedes,* yellow fever and dengue fever; the common house mosquito, genus *Culex,* is vector for arboviral encephalitis and filariasis.

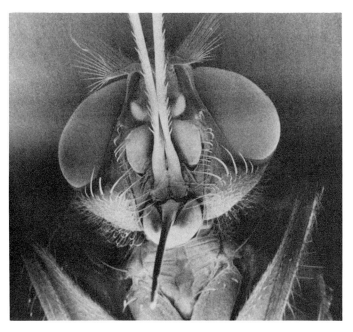

**Fig. 10-2.** Head of tsetse fly, scanning electron micrograph. (×60.) (Reproduced with permission of Eastman Kodak Company, Rochester, N.Y.)

typhoid fever and bacillary dysentery from the feces of patients to food and infect the consumer of that food. Flies act as more or less important carriers of more than twenty other diseases. The distance that flies may carry infectious agents is surprising—they have been known to travel miles in search of food.

In the *biologic* transfer of disease the insect bites a person or animal ill of a disease or a carrier and ingests some of the infected blood. The microbes taken in with the blood undergo a cycle of development within the body of the insect within a specified time. The insect can then transfer the infection to a well person, usually by biting that person. Spread in this manner are malaria, yellow fever, and encephalitis by mosquitoes (Fig. 10-1); typhus fever by lice; Texas fever (a disease of cattle) by ticks; African sleeping sickness by tsetse flies (Fig. 10-2); and plague by fleas. For diseases that are biologically transferred to be prevalent in a community, both the transmitting insect and hosts to harbor the infection must be present. As a rule, a particular infection is spread by only one species of insect, and a given insect is able to spread only one type of infection. There are, however, important exceptions.

**Sources of infection in communicable diseases.** In only few instances does the infectious agent live in lifeless surroundings outside the body long enough to maintain the source of infection. For the continuous existence of a disease there must be a *reservoir of infection*. The most important reservoirs of infection and the sources of most communicable diseases are found in practically all communities as (1) human

**Table 10-3**
Sources of infection in household pets

| DISEASE | DOGS | CATS | FARM ANIMALS | CAGED BIRDS (PIGEONS, PARRAKEETS, PARROTS, MYNA BIRDS, CANARIES, ETC.) | POULTRY | RODENTS (MICE, RABBITS, RATS, HAMSTERS, ETC.) | REPTILES (SNAKES, TURTLES, LIZARDS, ETC.) |
|---|---|---|---|---|---|---|---|
| *Viral* | | | | | | | |
| Rabies | ✔ | ✔ | ✔ | | | | |
| Encephalitides | | | ✔ | ✔ | | | |
| *Chlamydial* | | | | | | | |
| Cat-scratch disease | | ✔ | | | | | |
| Psittacosis-ornithosis | | | | ✔ | ✔ | | |
| *Rickettsial* | | | | | | | |
| Q fever | | | ✔ | | | | |
| *Bacterial* | | | | | | | |
| Salmonellosis | ✔ | ✔ | ✔ | ✔ | ✔ | ✔ | ✔ |
| Anthrax | ✔ | | ✔ | | | | |
| Brucellosis | ✔ | ✔ | ✔ | | ✔ | ✔ | |
| Tularemia | ✔ | ✔ | | | | ✔ | |
| Tuberculosis | ✔ | ✔ | ✔ | | | | |
| Leptospirosis | ✔ | | ✔ | ✔ | | ✔ | |
| *Fungous* | | | | | | | |
| Ringworm | ✔ | ✔ | ✔ | | | ✔ | |
| *Parasitic* | | | | | | | |
| Roundworm infection | ✔ | ✔ | | | | | |
| Tapeworm infection | ✔ | ✔ | ✔ | | | | |
| Toxoplasmosis | ✔ | ✔ | | | | | |

beings or animals with typical disease, (2) human beings or animals with unrecognized disease, and (3) human or animal carriers. Plants may be the reservoir in some of the fungous infections.

*Human carriers* are persons who harbor pathogenic agents in their bodies but show no signs of illness. The carrier is infected but asymptomatic. *Convalescent carriers* harbor an organism during recovery from the related illness. *Active carriers* harbor an organism for a long time *after* recovery. *Passive carriers* shelter a pathogenic organism without having had its disease. *Intestinal* and *urinary carriers* discharge the infectious agent from the body via the feces and urine, respectively. *Oral carriers* discharge infectious material from the mouth. *Intermittent carriers* discharge organisms only at intervals. (Intestinal carriers are often intermittent carriers.) Human carriers play a significant role in the spread of diphtheria, epidemic meningitis, salmonellosis, amebic dysentery, bacillary dysentery, streptococcal infections, and pneumonia.

As a rule, an actual case of a disease is more likely to spread infection to others than is a carrier. Carriers and persons with unrecognized disease keep epidemic diseases in existence during interepidemic periods. It has been found that just before the epidemic (examples: diphtheria and acute bacterial meningitis) the number of carriers increases. The prominence of carriers in the spread of a disease depends on the frequency with which people become carriers and the length of the carrier state.

*Animals* spread disease to man in a number of ways. Man may so acquire disease from (1) direct contact with an infected animal, (2) contamination of food by discharges of the animal, (3) insect or rodent vectors, (4) contaminated air or water, and (5) consumption of animal products such as milk or eggs.

Rabies is acquired by the bite of rabid dogs, cats, or other animals. Children may contract tuberculosis by drinking the raw milk of infected cows. Bubonic plague is primarily a disease of rats that is transmitted from rat to man by the flea. Undulant fever may be transmitted to man by milk, or it may be acquired when man handles the meat of infected animals. Tularemia is contracted from rodents, especially wild rabbits. Psittacosis is an infectious disease of parrots that is transmitted from the sick bird to man. Typhus fever is primarily a disease of rats that is transmitted from man to man by lice. Those handling the hides of anthrax-infected animals may contract anthrax. Tetanus may be indirectly contracted from horses because the tetanus bacillus is a normal inhabitant of the intestinal canal of the horse. This is why wounds contaminated by barnyard dirt are likely to be followed by tetanus. Shellfish such as oysters may transmit typhoid fever, hepatitis, and other enteric infections if human excreta contaminate the water in which the shellfish are grown.

All told, there are about 150 different infections that are spread from animals to man. Rats and mice carry more than fifteen different diseases, and the casualties from rodent-borne diseases are greater than those from all of history's wars.

Animals found in the home as pets may be important sources of infection (Table 10-3), since many persons live closely associated with them. The two most common household pets are cats and dogs. There are an estimated 110 million of them in the United States today. In North America the dog can transmit twenty-four diseases to man, and the cat can transmit twelve. Exotic animals that are becoming more popular as household pets may present real hazards. For example, monkeys in the home, pet shop, or even some zoos may spread such diseases to man as shigellosis, salmonellosis, and tuberculosis.

The most prevalent of the *zoonoses* (infections of animals secondarily transmissible to man) are cat-scratch disease, salmonellosis, and fungous infections. There are around 181 different diseases known to be transmitted naturally *from man to animals.*

**Spread of disease in jet age.** This is an age of travel at high speeds. More and more people are and will be traveling over the world aboard the jumbo jets or supersonic airliners and consequently exposing themselves to the infections of the geographic localities they visit. The problems in public health are enormous. Some are as follows. First, disease is so easily and quickly spread as to jeopardize public health controls. A traveler can bring back smallpox, for example, into a country that had virtually eliminated it. Second, since no two points on the earth are separated by more than 48 hours' travel time, the tourist can return home during the incubation period (feeling well), to come down with the disease days or weeks later. By this time, the diagnosis is not necessarily obvious. Third, the world sightseer may fail to take adequate precautions against a disease he inevitably contacts. The best example of this is malaria, the major risk. It is a widespread disease but nowhere is chemoprophylaxis required. The traveler must find out for himself what to do for protection. Even then, he may fail to take the suppressive drugs as required and may discontinue them after leaving an infected area, feeling they are no longer needed. Fourth, still another problem has to do with the establishment of international standards and guidelines for sanitary facilities. Maintenance of these is required for the tourist in all areas, but mandatory aboard the big jet, in the airport terminal, and in the accommodations related to it.

## Koch's postulates*

Absolute proof that an organism is the cause of a given disease rests on the fulfillment of certain requirements known as Koch's postulates. These postulates are as follows:

1. The organism must be observed in every case of the disease.
2. The organism must be isolated and grown in pure culture.
3. The organism must, when inoculated into a susceptible animal, cause the disease.
4. The organism must be recovered from the experimental animal and its identity confirmed.

---

*Robert Koch (1843-1910) stated certain principles related to the germ theory of disease with such clarity that they are known as Koch's postulates. They remain to this day the basis of the experimental investigation of infectious disease.

In exceptional cases an organism has been accepted as the cause of a disease although all of these requirements have not been fulfilled.

## Questions for review

1 Explain infection and contamination.
2 Give the routes by which microbes enter the body. Name two diseases whose causative agent enters the body by each route.
3 What is virulence? How do microbes produce disease?
4 What is one important local effect of bacterial invasion?
5 List some of the general effects of bacterial invasion.
6 What is the difference between bacteremia and septicemia?
7 Give the routes by which disease-producing agents leave the body. Name two agents eliminated by each route.
8 List five diseases spread by animals to man.
9 Define carrier. List the different kinds.
10 Name three diseases spread by carriers.
11 List important insect vectors and diseases spread.
12 State Koch's postulates.

**References on pp. 135 to 138.**

# CHAPTER 11

# The body's defense

## Protective mechanisms

If infection occurred each time infectious and injurious agents entered our bodies, we would be constantly ill. When microorganisms try to invade the body, they must first overcome certain mechanical, physiologic, and chemical barriers existing on the body surface or in the body cavity at the site of entry. The body not only reacts to the event of invasion but also is endowed with a measure of protection against that event.

**Anatomic barriers.** During his age-long struggle for existence man has developed certain mechanisms that enable him to overcome many agents of potential danger in his environment. In the first place, nature has provided him with special senses that act as watchdogs against danger. Man protects himself from major injuries by moving objects by batting his eyes and jumping aside. Although some of these acts are voluntary, they are executed as reflex movements and considered protective natural mechanisms.

The body's first line of defense is the epithelium that covers the exterior of the body and lines its internal surfaces. A condensation of resistant cells along the most superficial part of the skin offers a barrier against physical and chemical injuries or microbial invasion. Epithelium may become quite thick at a site of irritation (example: a callus or corn in the skin.) The lining cells of the mucous membranes opening on body surfaces also afford a barrier, but these cells are softer and more vulnerable to injury than are the surface cells of the skin. The hairs in the anterior nares protect the respiratory tract by filtering bacteria and larger particles from the inspired air. The respiratory passages are lined with epithelial cells from the surface of which spring hairlike appendages known as cilia that sweep overlying material from the deeper portion of the tract to the upper portion, from where it may be eliminated from the body.

Closure of the glottis during swallowing prevents food from entering the respiratory tract. Coughing and sneezing serve to expel mechanically any irritating materials from the respiratory tract. In a similar manner vomiting and diarrhea mechanically rid the intestinal tract of irritants.

**Chemical factors.** Body cavities opening onto the surface are protected by secretions that wash away bacteria and foreign materials. Body fluids such as saliva, tears, gastric juice, and bile exert an antiseptic action that reduces microbial invasion. For instance, gastric juice destroys bacteria and almost all important bacterial toxins except that of *Clostridium botulinum*. The antimicrobial action of mucus and tears is partly related to the presence of *lysozyme* (muramidase), a substance dissolving the cell walls of certain gram-positive bacteria. It is found in secretions coming from organs exposed to airborne bacteria. Lysozyme, not an antibody, was discovered by Fleming (in 1922) before he discovered penicillin. Because of their acid reaction and content of fatty acids, sweat and sebaceous secretions on the skin have antimicrobial properties.

Another internal defense is a naturally occurring substance *interferon* (not an antibody). Its target action is against viruses to block viral infection. Many cells form it quickly if so threatened.

**Physiologic reserves.** The blood supply of many parts of the body is protected by a series of *anastomoses* (connections) among the branches of the supply vessels. If a vessel is occluded, the blood is detoured around the obstruction by way of the anastomoses. A *collateral* or *compensatory circulation* is set up.

When the body becomes chilled, the superficial vessels of the skin contract to prevent heat from being dissipated at the surface, and sweating stops to slow cooling caused by evaporation. To aid in this conservation of heat, the involuntary muscles of the skin contract (gooseflesh). In animals having hair or feathers, the hair or feathers are raised to enclose in their meshes a thick layer of air, which is a poor conductor of heat. The muscular activity associated with rigor and shivering increases heat production. When the body becomes too hot, the superficial vessels dilate, and sweating occurs. Heat is dissipated from the surface, and evaporation has a cooling effect.

The functional capacities of the vital organs (organs necessary for life) extend far beyond the normal demands of life. We have much more liver, pancreas, adrenal gland, and parathyroid gland tissue than we ordinarily use. That we are able to lead a normal life after one kidney has been removed or after one lung has been collapsed illustrates the abundance of reserve possessed by our vital organs.

Vital organs (brain, heart, and lungs) are enclosed within protective bony cases, and their surfaces are bathed with a watery fluid. The fluid surrounding the brain serves as a water bed to prevent undue jarring, and the fluid that bathes the surface of the heart and lungs acts as a lubricant.

**Fever.** Fever is a condition marked by an increase in body temperature. It is usually thought to result because toxic substances arising from the disintegration of microbes and other cells in an injured (or inflamed) area gain access to the bloodstream. There are many causes, ranging from mechanical injury to microbial injury, but bacterial infection is by far the most important. Although the manifestations of fever may be disagreeable, it is primarily beneficial. If the temperature is not too high, fever accelerates the destruction of injurious agents by increasing phagocytosis and production of immune bodies (Chapter 12).

The temperature of warm-blooded animals is rather closely controlled by the temperature regulating mechanism of the brain and depends on two factors: heat production (thermogenesis) and heat dissipation (thermolysis). When less heat is dissipated, the body temperature is elevated. In fever the temperature control mechanism of the body is set to give a higher degree of heat in the body in much the same manner as the temperature of an incubator is raised by adjusting the thermoregulator.

In health the body temperature of man remains remarkably constant and, as determined by a thermometer placed in the mouth, ranges from 96.7° F. (35.94° C.) to 99° F. (37.22° C.), with an average of about 98.6° F. (37° C.). The rectal temperature is about 1° F. higher, and the temperature taken in the armpit is about 1° F. lower than the oral temperature. The rectal temperature is the most dependable because both oral and axillary temperatures are influenced by many outside factors. The temperature of the internal organs is 2° or 3° F. higher than that of the skin.

There is a close relation between pulse rate and temperature. Ordinarily an increase of around eight pulse beats per minute occurs for each 1.8° F. increase in temperature. Certain exceptions to this rule are diagnostically significant: for instance, the pulse in typhoid fever, malaria, miliary tuberculosis, and yellow fever is comparatively slow.

**Inflammation.** See Chapter 44.

## Reticuloendothelial system

The reticuloendothelial (RE) system with its widely dispersed cells constitutes one of the main organs in the body designed primarily for man's defense against both the living and the nonliving agents in his environment that harm him. The reticuloendothelial cells not only can directly fight the invader, which they do by phagocytosis, but can also clean up the debris and eliminate the cellular and metabolic breakdown products incident to the encounter. In short, they are also scavengers.

The production and regulation of the cells in the peripheral blood and bone marrow are crucial functions of the RE systems. Formation of the different blood cells (hemopoiesis) is possible because of the presence within the system of primitive nonphagocytic cells. Being multipotential cells, they give rise to the range of blood cell types found.

**Phagocytosis.** The ingestion of microbes or other particulate matter by cells is known as *phagocytosis*, and the cells that ingest such materials are *phagocytes*. Phagocytosis bears a close resemblance to the feeding process of unicellular organisms and is a universal response on the part of the body to penetration by microbes, alien cells, or other foreign particles. It is an essential protective mechanism against infection and probably plays an important part in natural immunity. Phagocytosis is a general process because the few kinds of body cells having this power can ingest many different kinds of particulate matter (bacteria, dead body cells, mineral particles, dusts, and pigments).

Study of the process has revealed that phagocytosis takes place in three phases (Fig. 11-1). First, the particle (example: a microbe) to be engulfed is isolated and incorporated into an invagination of the cell membrane of the phagocyte. The result is a phagosome, a vacuole (within the cell) surrounded by cytoplasm. Next, there is a burst of metabolic activity within the cell. The phagosome is moved into the interior of the cell, contacting its lysosomes. When hydrolytic enzymes are released into the phagosome, it becomes a *phagolysosome*. A special kind of microbicidal system is activated in preparation for the second phase. This is the killing or inactivation of the microbe, so that in the third phase it can be digested.

If, after ingesting bacteria, phagocytes fail to destroy them, the phagocytes themselves may be destroyed, with liberation of the ingested microorganisms. Relatively harmless microbes are usually completely destroyed. Sometimes the microbes will persist and even continue to multiply within the cytoplasm of the phagocyte. Virulent bacteria, especially those with capsules, are resistant to phagocytosis.

The student who wishes to see bacteria under-

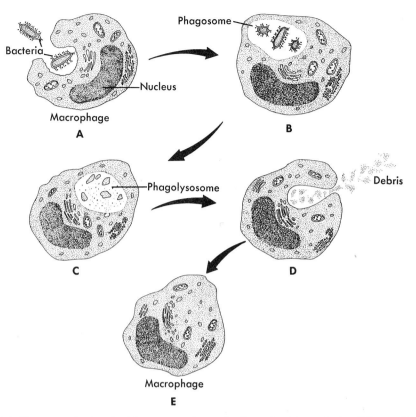

**Fig. 11-1.** Phagocytosis sketched in a macrophage. **A,** Opsonized bacteria (p. 120) engulfed by phagocyte (macrophage). **B,** Phagosome formed. **C,** Phagosome becomes phagolysosome; bacteria digested. (To this point, process of phagocytosis is comparable in either a macrophage or neutrophil, not shown.) **D,** Debris is egested. (Neutrophil would succumb here.) **E,** Macrophage returns to resting state.

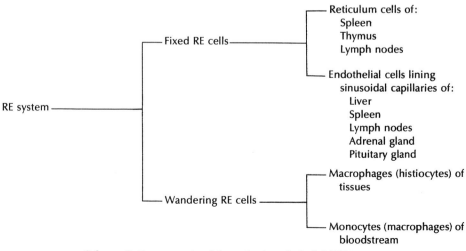

**Schema 2.** Components of the reticuloendothelial (RE) system.

going phagocytosis should stain a smear from an ordinary boil. Staphylococci can be found easily within the cytoplasm of the leukocytes. Smears from gonorrheal exudates and the cerebrospinal fluid in epidemic meningitis usually show organisms undergoing phagocytosis inside the leukocytes.

Different bacteria show differences in their susceptibility to phagocytosis. For instance, gonococci undergo phagocytosis readily, whereas tubercle bacilli are quite resistant.

Phagocytosis is not so great in the first 3 years of life as it is later on.

**Anatomy of the RE system.** The RE system is a group of cells in the body especially endowed with phagocytic powers—both the cells themselves and those to which they give rise (Fig. 11-2). In short, it is a phagocytic system. Although widespread throughout the body, these cells are concentrated in lymph nodes, spleen, bone marrow, and liver, where they are arranged as the lining cells for the peculiar kind of sinusoidal arrangement common to these organs. Although scattered, these uniform cells are spoken of collectively as the *reticuloendothelial system.* There are two main cell types: (1) the stationary or fixed (littoral) cells and (2) the free or wandering cells. The wandering cells in tissues are known as *macrophages;* in the bloodstream, as *monocytes.*

The components of the reticuloendothelial (RE) system are shown in Schema 2.

Because the macrophage moves about in body fluids and because its observed properties of phagocytosis are dramatic, it receives a lot of attention. The details of its life history, including even its exact origin, are not completely worked out. It is known by a variety of names—RE cell, histiocyte, epithelioid cell, clasmatocyte, multinucleated giant cell (if confluence of several cells)—relating it (the same cell) to different circumstances and reflecting an active participation in its diverse roles.

In *granulomatous* inflammation the disease-producing agent is dealt with directly by the reticuloendothelial system, and the main reacting cell is this wandering phagocyte or macrophage.

A most important *derivative* of the fixed cells of the RE system, also phagocytic, is the *polymorphonuclear neutrophilic leukocyte,* familiarly known as the "poly," a cell especially designed to phagocytize bacteria (microphage\*) and one of several kinds of white blood cells (leukocytes). With the majority of bacterial inflammations there is an increase in the number of these cells at the site of injury in the body and in the bloodstream (*leukocytosis*). They have been produced

---

\*A *micro*phage ingests small particles, notably bacteria; a *macro*phage, larger ones.

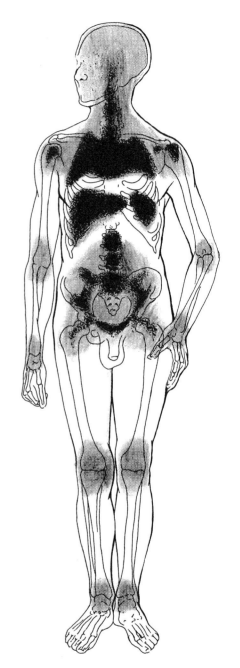

**Fig. 11-2.** Reticuloendothelial system. Note anatomic distribution of maximal activity in system, as indicated by black areas over body. To produce such an image, certain radioactive colloidal particles are given to subject, and radiation detection technics delineate tissue uptake. Note definition of liver, spleen, and active bone marrow in axial skeleton and proximal parts of long bones. (Modified from McIntyre, P. A.: Hosp. Pract. **6:**77, July, 1971.)

in the bone marrow in increased numbers in response to *chemotaxins*, products released from the inflammatory site and carried by the blood to the marrow. In conditions that produce a leukocytosis, the phagocytic power of the leukocytes is increased in patients who are doing well. Neutrophils are rich in proteolytic enzymes contained within their lysosomes. These enzymes known as leukoproteases participate in intracellular digestion of phagocytized particles.

The phagocytic cells especially related to processes of immunity (discussed in Chapter 12) are the polymorphonuclear neutrophils and the macrophages of the RE system.

## Lymphoid system (immunologic system*)

**Lymphoid tissue.** Closely interwoven with the reticuloendothelial system (the phagocytic system) and encompassed by it is the lymphoid system. This comprises the lymphoid tissues and organs of the body. The chief cells of the system are the lymphocytes, small round cells with a relatively large and darkly staining nucleus, and their constant companions, the plasma cells—slightly larger cells with

---

*Immunologic function is an important property of lymphoid tissue. Mechanisms are discussed in the next chapter.

an eccentric nucleus of distinct appearance. The lymphoid cells are packed, more or less densely, onto a spongelike support provided by a special type of cellular stroma, and collections of lymphocytes including their precursors and progeny in a well-defined, usually rounded aggregate constitutes a lymphoid nodule. A nodule may be a solitary one, or several nodules may be grouped together, as in Peyer's patches of the small intestine. If lymphoid tissue is

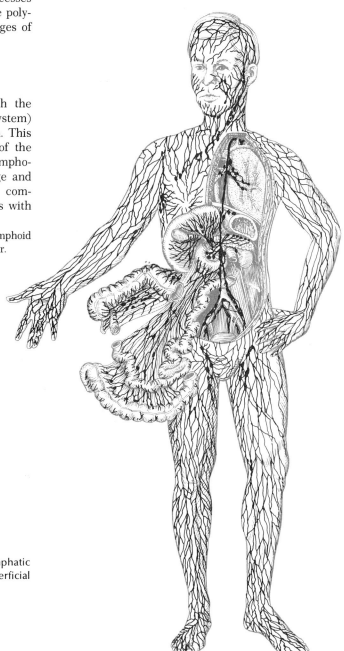

**Fig. 11-3.** Lymphoid system. Note pattern of lymphatic vessels and lymph nodes in all areas of body (superficial and deep).

organized and encapsulated, a small bean-shaped organ is formed, the lymph node (p. 102). Lymph nodes are found throughout the body, strategically placed in all major organ systems and body areas.

**Lymphatic circulation.** In the exchange of nutrients for waste products that goes on continuously between the cells and the blood of the capillaries, excess fluid leaks into the tissue spaces. From here it moves into the lymphatic capillaries, the many small thin-walled tubes of the lymphatic circulation draining the vast intercellular region of the body. The fluid circulates as lymph into successively larger vessels and ultimately pours back into the bloodstream. Along the course of the lymphatic channels at definite intervals are placed the lymph nodes in chain formations (Fig. 11-3). All the lymph of the body is filtered and strained through these chains.

**Spleen.** The largest mass of lymphoid tissue in the body is the spleen, found in the upper left abdomen. Like the lymph nodes, it is a filter, but unlike them it strains the bloodstream not the lymph stream. It functions as an important member of the reticuloendothelial system in the filtration of foreign particles from the blood, including living organisms. The fixed cells of the reticuloendothelial system line the lumens of all lymphatic channels, lymph sinuses, and splenic sinusoids. Here, there is an intimate relationship between elements designated as lymphoid and those as reticuloendothelial.

**Thymus.** The thymus, a key organ in immunologic processes, is situated in the front part of the chest just behind the breast bone. At or about the time of birth it processes certain lymphocytes, which then migrate out to colonize the spleen, lymph nodes, and other areas of the body. These in turn give rise to cells that maintain cell-mediated immunity. (See Chapter 12.)

**The lymphatic vessels in infection.** When an agent gains access to the tissues, it may sometimes be carried away from the site of entry by the lymphatic circulation and be deposited in the nearest lymph nodes. (In the lungs of persons residing in coal-burning regions, coal dust is thus deposited in the drainage nodes.) Likewise bacterial invaders may be borne from the site of disease to the regional nodes, where their presence stimulates phagocytic cells normally present to increased activity. Hopefully, these phagocytes dispose of the invaders. Should they fail to do so, the bacteria flow with the lymph stream through successive nodes in the chains into the thoracic duct, from there to be emptied into the bloodstream and disseminated throughout the body. Infection of the bloodstream (septicemia) before the days of antibiotic therapy was a rapidly fatal condition.

**RE responses in lymphoid organs.** If an infection is localized, the reticuloendothelial cells of the regional lymph nodes proliferate, and the nodes enlarge as a consequence (lymphadenopathy). Regional lymph nodes are an important second line of defense. Many injurious agents carried there are destroyed. If an infection becomes generalized, the reticuloendothlial system throughout the body responds. One notable feature of this is the enlargement of the spleen (splenomegaly) seen with such acute infectious processes as typhoid fever, malaria, and septicemia.

## Questions for review

1 List mechanisms that serve to protect the body from disease or injury and explain how each functions.
2 What is lysozyme? Who discovered it?
3 What are cilia? What is their function in the respiratory passages?
4 What is a vital organ? Name three. How are the vital organs protected in the body?
5 Define fever.
6 What is considered normal body temperature?
7 What is the relation between pulse rate and temperature?
8 Briefly describe the reticuloendothelial system. What is its chief function?
9 Briefly discuss phagocytosis. What are the three phases? Why is this an important process?
10 Outline the anatomic distribution of the reticuloendothelial (RE) system.
11 Give the component cells and organs of the lymphoid system.
12 What is meant by lymphadenopathy? By splenomegaly? With what are they associated?

**References on pp. 135 to 138.**

# CHAPTER 12
# Immunology

## Meaning of immunity

*Immunology* is the division of biology concerned with the study of *immunity*. Today the concept of immunity is hard to define. In terms of the steady progression of knowledge in the field of immunology, the meaning of the word is rapidly expanding.

Basic to an understanding of the complexity of physiologic mechanisms encompassed by immunity are the concepts of "self" and "nonself," or "foreign." For a given individual to preserve his biologic integrity (self), he must be able to recognize and deal with factors in his environment threatening it. On the one hand, there is self, which must remain intact. On the other, there are the elements it contacts, not self although perhaps of comparable makeup, and potentially harmful. Because of the many biologic parallels in nature, the distinction is a fine one. We require an arrangement whereby the cells and cell substances of our bodies are marked off as "ours" and the substances that appear on the scene are accosted as "intruders."

The scheme of things in the body that function in this discriminatory way is the machinery of immunity, and the elements making it up are collectively the *immune system*. The term *immunobiology* surveys the subject of immunity and its many ramifications in modern medicine.

*Susceptibility* is the reverse of immunity and is the result of an absence or suppression of the factors that produce immunity.

## Immunity and infection

Infectious agents such as bacteria and other microorganisms are easily "foreign" to the body (nonself), their effect detrimental, and the cause-effect relationships clear cut. The applications of immunity with infectious processes have been dramatic. The classic definition that immunity is a highly developed state of resistance has referred directly to infectious disease.

**Kinds of immunity.** Traditionally immunity has been classified as shown in Schema 3.

A *natural* immunity is a more or less permanent one with which a person or lower animal is born; that is, it is a natural heritage. It may be the heritage of a species, race, or individual. It is also known as *innate* or *genetic* immunity. *Species* immunity is that peculiar to a species (for example, man does not have distemper, nor do dogs have measles). A *racial* immunity is one possessed by a race (for example, ordinary sheep are susceptible to anthrax, whereas Algerian sheep seldom contract the disease). Species and racial immunities are more highly developed in plants than in animals. *Individual* immunity is a rare

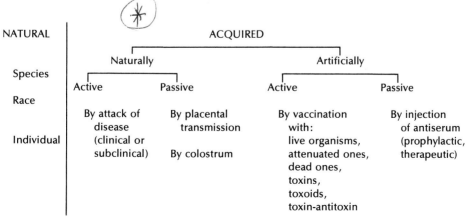

**Schema 3.** Classification of immunity.

condition, and most so-called cases are from unrecognized infections.

An _acquired_ immunity is one in which protection _must be obtained._ It is never the heritage of a species, race, or individual. It may be _naturally_ acquired when a mother transmits antibodies (protective substances) to her fetus by way of the placenta or when a person has an attack of a disease. When a person has a disease such as measles, the disease is rather severe for a time, after which recovery occurs. The person will not then contract the disease again although repeatedly exposed; he has developed a permanent immunity.

An immunity may be _artificially_ acquired by vaccination or the administration of an immune serum.

Depending on the part played by the body cells of the animal or person being immunized, acquired immunity (natural or artificial) may be classified as active and passive. If a person has an attack of measles or is vaccinated against it, his body cells respond to the presence of the agent (or its products) by producing antibodies that destroy the causative agent of the disease should it again gain access to the body. When certain body cells react to the agent or its products in this way, the naturally acquired immunity is an _active_ one. For example, if a horse is given frequent injections of diphtheria toxin, beginning with a small dose and with a gradually increased amount at each subsequent injection, the horse will eventually be able to withstand thousands of times the amount of toxin required to kill an untreated animal; it has become immune to the action of diphtheria toxin.

Immunity transferred by way of the placenta to the child from his mother is a _passive_ immunity, which the child has naturally acquired. When the serum of an actively immunized animal is injected into a nonimmune animal, the latter becomes temporarily immune. This artificially acquired immunity is _passive_ because the immunity-producing principle is introduced in the serum, and the cells of the recipient animal take no part in the process. For the first 4 to 6 months of his life an infant may have a passive immunity to measles, smallpox, diphtheria, mumps, tetanus, influenza, and certain staphylococcal and streptococcal infections because of the transfer of immune bodies from the blood of the mother to the child via the placenta. The immunity that the child receives in his mother's womb may be enhanced by the content of protective substances that he receives from his mother's milk (especially from colostrum). Naturally, the child will not receive any immunity if the mother is not herself immune. Except in newborn babies, all passive immunities are established by the administration of an immune serum (the serum of an animal that contains antibodies because the animal has been actively immunized). The production of passive immunity shows its most brilliant application in the use of diphtheria antitoxin to prevent and cure diphtheria.

Active immunity artificially acquired does not last so long as when it is naturally acquired, but active immunity always lasts longer than passive immunity. One should bear in mind that an active immunity can be established only with an attack of a given disease or with vaccination against it and that the immunity is slowly established (days or weeks) but of long duration (months or years). On the other hand, a passive immunity is ordinarily established at once by the injection of an immune serum but is of short duration (1 or 2 weeks). On these facts is based the principle of producing an active immunity when there is no immediate danger from disease and establishing a passive immunity when the danger from disease is imminent or the patient already ill.

**Level of immunity.** It seems that when an infectious disease attacks a population that has never been exposed, the attack rate is very high and many succumb to its ravages. On the other hand, when a disease endemic in a population for years becomes epidemic, the number of persons attacked and the percentage of deaths are not so great. People develop a degree of inherent resistance to a given disease through exposure for generation after generation. There is little doubt that syphilis was at one time a far more virulent disease and more often fatal than it is now. The susceptibility of aboriginal people to tuberculosis is much greater than that of people in communities in which the disease has existed for a long time.

In 1951 measles was introduced into Greenland by a recently arrived visitor who attended a dance during the onset of symptoms. Within 3 months there were more than 4000 cases, with 72 deaths. The attack rate reached the unprecedented figure of 999 cases per 1000 people. When measles was first introduced into the Fiji Islands in 1875, 30% of the population died. It has been said that the white man subjugated the American Indian more by the diseases he brought to him, to which the Indian possessed no immunity, than he did by superior knowledge or more effective weapons.

## Immune system

Immunity is important as defense against infection, but in light of current achievements it is more. Broadly speaking, immunity comprises the complexity of things that help man to maintain his structural and functional integrity and to ward off certain kinds of injury. Some of the factors in immunity are hard to define. One cannot easily measure the basic mechanisms of resistance built into all living organisms and expressed as the inflammatory process, the presence of anatomic barriers, and the effect of naturally occurring antimicrobial substances. Therefore such factors are collected loosely into the concept of *innate* or *nonspecific* immunity.

Another approach to immunity emphasizes the study of the highly developed, precisely specialized physiologic mechanisms, the topics of *specific* or *adaptive immunity*. In adaptive immunity there are two expressions of fundamental processes, both related to cells in the lymphoid system. In one there is elaboration of chemicals*—this is *humoral immunity*. In the other there is focus on less well understood activities of certain cells—this is *cell-mediated* or *cellular immunity*.

Reflecting the dual nature of the immune response, our discussion will take the twofold approach with, first, a consideration of humoral immunity and, second, a note as to the cell-mediated kind.

**Role of lymphoid tissue.** In man the lymphoid tissue is responsible for the events of specific immunity. Widely distributed in the body, it is both concentrated (lymph nodes, spleen, thymus, Peyer's patches) and scattered (lining of alimentary tract, bone marrow). The major constituent cells are lymphocytes in a mixed population that takes in plasma cells, macrophages, and their precursors (forebears). Lymphocytes circulate as single cells in the bloodstream and account for one fifth of the white blood cells present.

The cells (predominantly lymphocytes) in the different areas of lymphoid tissue look very much alike when viewed under the microscope, but in the immunologic setting they behave quite differently. At least two distinct cell populations have emerged. Both have a common origin in bone marrow stem cells, but they diverge in development of function.

One is a so-called *thymus-dependent* (processed) *system* of cells (the T cells) because its early development is influenced and its destiny fixed by the thymus gland. It is made up of small lymphocytes, T cells, that circulate in the blood and lymph. Most of the circulating lymphocytes are T cells, although these tend to congregate in certain foci within the lymphoid tissues. These cells have a very long life expectancy—many years, a decade or so—and regulate the cell-mediated immune responses (graft rejection; delayed hypersensitivity; immunologic surveillance against cancer; and those in infections from fungi, acid-fast bacteria, and viruses).

---

*Immunochemistry* is the study of the complex chemical reactions involved in immunity.

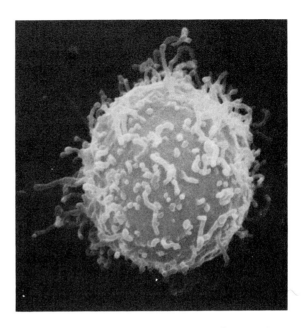

**Fig. 12-1.** B lymphocyte or B cell, scanning electron micrograph. (×16,000.) Note surface markers (fingerlike protrusions). (Courtesy Dr. Peter Andrews, The University of Texas Health Science Center at Dallas.)

The other population of lymphoid cells is a *thymus-independent system* of cells (the B cells, Fig. 12-1). It owes its differentiation to a site not as yet identified in man (possibly in the bone marrow). The small lymphocytes of this cell population are short-lived—only 1 or 2 weeks. The thymus-independent system of cells, or B cells, is responsible for the production of humoral immunity, as seen in the body's main defense against bacterial infection (as with pneumococcal, streptococcal, or meningococcal infection).

The immune system can be compartmentalized into the B-cell system and the T-cell system, although there is overlapping of the two. B-cell systems and T-cell systems can be sorted out in animals and man.

A lymph node (Fig. 12-2) shows a diffuse arrangement of lymphoid tissue well enscribed by a connective tissue capsule. In the outer part (cortex) of the node there is an orderly alignment of lymphoid aggregates, the *lymphoid follicles*. If lymph nodes are studied during the course of an immune response, definite changes may be seen within these follicles. With hormonally mediated responses, they become very active, and numerous plasma cells appear within the greatly enlarged follicles. With cell-mediated immune responses the follicles appear to be spared, but pronounced changes are found in the lymphoid tissue adjoining the cortical nodules. Within these *paracortical* areas numerous mononuclear cells containing increased amounts of RNA accumulate and

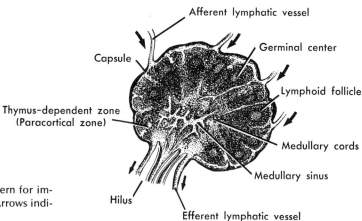

**Fig. 12-2.** Lymph node. Observe anatomic pattern for immunologically significant areas in this sketch. Arrows indicate flow of lymph.

later become small lymphocytes ready for release into the circulation.

### HUMORAL IMMUNITY

Humoral immunity is that related to antibodies.

**Antigens.** When a person or animal becomes immune to a disease, the immunity is largely the result of the development within the body of substances capable of destroying or inactivating the etiologic agent of the disease, should it gain access to the body. These substances, known as *antibodies* or *immunogens,* are produced by the body in response to a specific stimulus. Microbes and their products may stimulate the body cells to antibody production, as may also certain vegetable poisons, snake venoms, and, from an animal of a different species, red blood cells, serum, and other proteins. A substance such as any of these that elicits the production of antibodies against itself when introduced into the animal body is known as an *antigen.* To act as an antigen, it must be introduced into the body; that is, it must be a substance foreign to the body of a given individual. Antigens are usually high molecular weight substances of a protein nature, but in some cases complex carbohydrates (polysaccharides) may act as antigens. Enzymes and many hormones are antigenic. It is estimated that there are 1 million different antigens to which the human immune system can react directly.

When certain body proteins (examples: thyroglobulin and lens protein from the eye) of one animal are injected into another animal of the same species, antibodies against the proteins are produced. These antigens are called *isoantigens* (*iso*, from an individual of the same species), and the antibodies to them are *isoantibodies.* Naturally occurring isoantigens are those resident on the red blood cells and making up the blood groups (p. 111).

Comparatively simple chemical substances (certain low molecular weight lipids and carbohydrates) may be combined with the protein of an antigen to give it specificity. When separated from the protein of the antigen, these substances do not elicit the formation of antibodies but do combine with antibodies already formed against the antigen. These are known as *haptens* or *partial antigens.*

Certain chemicals that within themselves are not antigenic increase the potency of antigens. They are known as *adjuvants.* Among these are alum and aluminum hydroxide, used in preparation of toxoids. In addition to increasing the potency of the antigen they concentrate it.

**Antibodies.** As you recall, plasma is the liquid portion of the blood in which the red corpuscles and other formed elements are suspended. It is composed chiefly of water (90% to 92%), proteins (6% to 7%), and various mineral constituents. The plasma proteins are albumin, globulin, and fibrinogen.* By electrophoresis it is shown that the globulin is made up of these main fractions—alpha-1, alpha-2, beta, and gamma globulins. Antibodies migrate electrophoretically in the gamma and beta globulin regions. They are largely associated with gamma globulin, representing 1% to 2% of total serum protein. This is why this fraction (immune globulin) is used so extensively in the prevention of diseases such as infectious hepatitis, poliomyelitis, and measles.

*Serum is the fluid plasma of the blood minus the blood cells and fibrin precipitated from the plasma protein fibrinogen. To collect serum, a sample of blood is allowed to clot, the fibrin formed in the process entrapping the cells. When the clot shrinks, the fluid expressed therefrom is the serum. Practically, serum is an important source of antibodies, and in the laboratory *serology* is the study of antigen-antibody reactions in a specimen of blood serum.

*Nature.* Much is being learned of the true nature of antibodies, the specialized globulins that react precisely with the foreign molecule or antigen inducing their formation. Antibodies are better designated as *immunoglobulins* (Ig) and belong to a family of related proteins with characteristic properties when studied by special laboratory technics. They are very large and heterogeneous protein molecules and the most complex group known. Chemically, immunoglobulins adhere to a basic pattern upon which are superimposed significant variations. (See Fig. 12-3.) The basic subunit or building block is structured of four polypeptide chains in two pairs. Two of the paired chains are of greater molecular weight—heavy or H chains—and two of lower molecular weight—light or L chains. The light chains are linked to the heavy ones by single disulfide bonds. Light chains are about 200 amino acids long; heavy chains, approximately 450 amino acids.

*Classification.* The major classes of immunoglobulins as defined by the World Health Organization Committee on Nomenclature of Immunoglobulins are given in Table 12-1 with their distinguishing features; Table 12-2 indicates their immunologic capacity.

*Formation.* Antibodies (immunoglobulins) are formed in the lymphoid tissues of the body in response to a particular antigen within the body. The main anatomic sites are the spleen, lymph nodes, and bone marrow, but antibody synthesis may be shown wherever there is lymphoid tissue—*with the exception of the thymus!*

The principal cells involved are lymphocytes (B cells primarily, but T cells important), plasma cells (derivative cells of lymphocytes), and macrophages (mobile and sessile cells able to ingest fairly large particles of foreign matter).

Although B cells and T cells look alike with the light microscope, important differences on the cell surfaces can be demonstrated by special technics. Bound to the plasma membrane of the B cell are numerous (estimated 100,000) specific receptors shown to be molecules of immunoglobulin (sIg). Among these are also receptors for the third factor of complement (C3). By contrast, T lymphocytes show considerably fewer surface markers. They do possess, however, receptors for normal sheep red blood cells. In an in vitro test, sheep erythrocytes surround the T cells in characteristic "rosette" fashion, which reaction sets them apart from B cells.

When an antigen (immunogen) gains access to an appropriate lymphoid area within the body, there follows an incompletely understood sequence of events wherein the antigen is recognized, processed, and bound to an antigen-sensitive lymphocyte. Mys-

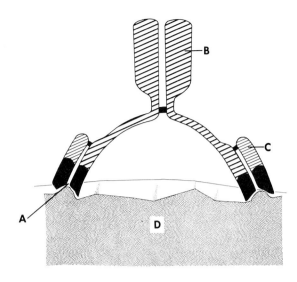

**Fig. 12-3.** Immunoglobulin molecule, IgG class. **A,** Combining site (with antigen); **B,** heavy (H) chain; **C,** light (L) chain; **D,** antigen. Note two identical light and two identical heavy chains in the diagram, united by disulfide bonds.

tery and speculation still cloud the earliest cellular changes. For antigens to attain the maximum immunologic response in production of immunoglobulin, they must induce an interaction between B and T cells with involvement of macrophages, although on occasions immunogens need affect B cells only.

On the surface of an antigen there is a special pattern of atoms designated as the *antigenic determinant,* or *marker.* The immunoglobulin resulting from the stimulus of a given antigen must be structured to make a neat fitting into the unique arrangement of the antigenic determinant.

T cells recognize the antigen in both cellular and humoral immunity and so affect and potentiate the processing of antigen by macrophages and reticulum cells of the lymphoid area. This results in changes in the antigen but not the loss of its antigenic marker. The altered immunogen is then presented to the B cells, which receive it at the specific receptor sites on their plasma membranes. The engagement of the immunogen with the membrane receptors is the signal for the lymphocyte to become immunologically active.

According to one theory of antibody formation, the given B cell, the immunologically responsive cell, responds to only one kind of antigen, a capacity in some way acquired before the encounter and most probably related to the specific nature of its surface immunoglobulin molecules. This is the "one cell—one antibody" theory. The immunogen attracted to the cell binds to a receptor on its surface because that marker is chemically built like an antibody. This starts

**Table 12-1**

Analysis of major classes of immunoglobulins (antibodies)

| W.H.O. TERM* | WHERE FOUND IN BODY | SEDIMENTATION COEFFICIENT (ULTRACENTRIFUGAL ANALYSIS)† | CHEMICAL COMPOSITION KNOWN | MOLECULAR WEIGHT |
|---|---|---|---|---|
| IgG | Serum (40% intravascular) | 7S | 4 polypeptide chains— 2 light, 2 heavy | 160,000 |
| IgA | Serum (40% intravascular) External secretions: saliva, parotid gland, gastrointestinal, respiratory tract, colostrum (secretory IgA) | 9-15S | 4 polypeptide chains— 2 light, 2 heavy | 160,000 (monomer) to 900,000 (secretory IgA: 390,000) |
| IgM | Serum (80% intravascular) | 19S | 20 polypeptide molecules of five basic 4-chain units— 2 light, 2 heavy | 1,000,000 |
| IgD | Serum (75% intravascular) | 7S | — | 180,000 |
| IgE | Serum | 8S | 4 polypeptide chains— 2 light, 2 heavy | 196,000 |

*Designation recommended by the World Health Organization Committee on Nomenclature of Immunoglobulins.
†The ultracentrifuge is an important tool in the identification of antibodies. By means of the exceedingly high gravitational forces possible in this instrument, serum protein fractions may be separated according to their molecular weights. Results are quantitated in Svedberg units (S).

the B cell on a course of immunologic activity, with formation of immunoglobulins as the net result. The B cell proliferates and soon generates a clone of differentiated and immunologically competent cells. Some of the derivative cells become plasma cells (with the influence of T cells as "helper cells"), known for a long time to synthesize and secrete antibody globulin. Others become lymphoid cells to disseminate through blood, lymph, and tissues. They establish a reservoir of antigen-sensitive cells, this time primed with a memory factor. When the same immunogen reappears on the scene, the immunologic response is enhanced and expedited.

Today we speak of lymphocytes as *immunologically competent* cells, meaning cells that can undertake an immunologic response when engaged by an antigen. During a lifetime, because of the many and varied antigens of our environments, each of us produces tens of thousands of different kinds of antibodies.

**Antigen-antibody reaction.** The antigen-antibody reaction is specific: a given antigen promotes the production of antibodies only against itself, and a given antibody acts only against the antigen promoting its development. The amino acid sequence and the three-dimensional structure of an antibody determines its specificity. The difference of even one amino acid can be detected in a specific antigen-antibody combination. A person vaccinated against smallpox is protected against smallpox only. The hemolysin in the serum of a rabbit that has been repeatedly injected with the red blood cells of a sheep dissolves the red blood cells of sheep but not those of other animals.

Within the antibody molecule there is a pattern of small areas specially designed for a close-fitting union with the antigen (like a key fitted into a lock). Most immunoglobulins are bivalent; that is, their structure allows combination with the antigen molecule at two areas.

| ESTIMATED PERCENT Ig IN POPULATION | SERUM LEVEL (gm./ 100 ml.) | CROSSES PLACENTA | BINDING OF COMPLEMENT | PERCENT CARBOHYDRATE | ELECTROPHORETIC MOBILITY (PRINCIPAL) |
|---|---|---|---|---|---|
| 75% | 1.2 | Yes | + | 2.5% | γ |
| 21% | 0.18 | No | No | 8% | Slow β |
| 7% | 0.12 | No | + | 10% | Between γ and β |
| 0.2% | 0.003 | No | No | 10% | Between γ and B |
| 0.5% | 0.0001 | ? | No | 12% | γ |

If the union of antigen and antibody occurs in such a way that the aggregation is manifest as a visible phenomenon, the antibody is said to be a *complete antibody* (Fig. 12-4). When union of an antibody occurs with a specific antigen but the antibody lacks the capacity to change the surface properties of the antigen and therefore a visible reaction does not take place, that antibody is referred to as an *incomplete* or *blocking antibody*.

*Detection of antibodies and the antigen-antibody reaction.* Discussion of this subject is found in Chapter 13.

**Complement.** Although complement (alexin) is not an antibody, its presence is necessary for the complete action of certain *lytic* antibodies, notably hemolysins, bacteriolysins, and other cytolysins, and complement or a complement-like substance enhances the action of opsonins. Basically a complex enzyme system of proteins taking part in the antigen-antibody reaction, complement is present in fresh serum (10% of globulin fraction) and is not increased by immunization. There are at least 9 distinct complement components with inhibitors in the complement system. These interact in a complicated sequence or cascade much like that in the clotting system. C3, the third component, appears to play the most significant role in disease. Complement is destroyed by exposure to room temperature for a few hours or to a temperature of 56° C. for 30 minutes. It acts only after the antigen has been sensitized (acted on) by its antibody. During the process of antigen-antibody-complement union, the complement is destroyed or at least inactivated. This is known as *complement fixation*. The activity of complement directed to cell membranes is responsible for the cytolytic effect of complement fixation reactions. The fresh serum of a guinea pig is regularly used as a source of complement because its content shows little variation in different animals and is comparatively high. Complement may be preserved by various

**Table 12-2**

Immunologic activities of the major classes of immunoglobulins

| IMMUNO-GLOBULIN | PARTICIPATION IN WELL-KNOWN ANTIGEN-ANTIBODY REACTIONS | | | | | | GENERAL REMARKS |
| | AGGLUTINATION | PRECIPITATION | COMPLEMENT FIXATION | LYSIS | NEUTRALIZATION | | |
| | | | | | VIRUSES | TOXINS (AND ENZYMES) | |
|---|---|---|---|---|---|---|---|
| IgG (gamma G) ($\gamma$G) | Weak | Strong | Strong | Weak | + | + | 1. Ones best studied<br>2. Responsible for passive immunity of newborn<br>3. Identified here:<br>  a. Certain Rh antibodies<br>  b. Bacterial agglutinins<br>  c. L.E. cell factor*<br>  d. Antitoxins<br>  e. Antiviral antibodies |
| IgA (gamma A) ($\gamma$A) | + | ± | – | – | + | ? | 1. Known to be made by plasma cells<br>2. Chief Ig in external secretions<br>3. Protective function on body surfaces exposed to environment<br>4. Identified here:<br>  a. Diphtheria antitoxin<br>  b. Blood group antibodies<br>  c. Antibodies against *Brucella* and *Escherichia coli*<br>  d. Antibodies against respiratory viruses<br>  e. Antinuclear factors in collagen disease*<br>  f. Certain other autoantibodies* (against insulin in diabetes, thyroglobulin in chronic thyroiditis) |
| IgM (gamma M) ($\gamma$M) | Strong | Variable | Weak | Strong | + | – | 1. Rapid protection here—first antibodies noted after antigen injection<br>2. Powerful agglutinins and hemolysins here (700 to 1000 times stronger than those of IgG in agglutinating red cells or bacteria)<br>3. Identified here:<br>  a. Blood group antibodies (ABO)<br>  b. Antibodies against somatic O factors of |

*For discussion of autoimmunity and autoimmune diseases see p. 501.

**Table 12-2**
Immunologic activities of the major classes of immunoglobulins—cont'd

| IMMUNO-GLOBULIN | PARTICIPATION IN WELL-KNOWN ANTIGEN-ANTIBODY REACTIONS | | | | | | GENERAL REMARKS |
|---|---|---|---|---|---|---|---|
| | | | | | NEUTRALIZATION | | |
| | AGGLUTINATION | PRECIPITATION | COMPLEMENT FIXATION | LYSIS | VIRUSES | TOXINS (AND ENZYMES) | |
| IgM—cont'd | | | | | | | gram-negative bacteria<br>c. Human anti-A isoantibody<br>d. Isohemagglutinins, cold agglutinins, rheumatoid factor |
| IgD | ? | ? | ? | ? | ? | ? | Functions not identified |
| IgE (reagin) | − | − | − | + | − | − | 1. Role in allergy—governs responses of immediate hypersensitivity (reagin activity, mast cell fixation)<br>2. Carries skin-sensitizing antibody |

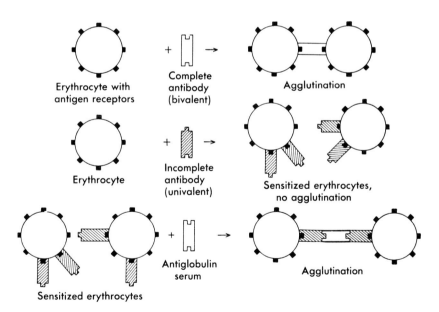

**Fig. 12-4.** Antigen-antibody reaction. Note three reactions diagrammed horizontally between antigens on erythrocytes and antibody. *Top,* Agglutination (visible clumping) results from bonding of antigens and antibody. *Middle,* Antigen-antibody complex, but without clumping. Red blood cells here are altered (sensitized). *Bottom,* In contact with antiglobulin serum (a special complete antibody, see also p. 114), sensitized red cells are clumped. (From Miale, J. B.: Laboratory medicine: hematology, ed. 4, St. Louis, 1972, The C. V. Mosby Co.)

chemical methods or by drying the fresh frozen guinea pig serum to a powder in a vacuum.

## CELL-MEDIATED IMMUNITY

In acute bacterial infections with gram-positive cocci, the mechanisms of humoral immunity in the normal individual are efficient. Persons with agamma-globulinemia, who cannot make measurable amounts of antibody globulin, do not fare well with the cocci but they do adequately resist infections caused by viruses, fungi, protozoa, and certain other bacteria. Such resistance must stem from an immunologic mechanism other than the classic antigen-antibody combination.

To the host, infection with these latter agents presents a peculiar problem in defense, since these microbes colonize the interior of host cells. There they obtain shelter from antimicrobial elements of blood and tissue fluids. Some are in danger if they pass from cell to cell, but others are unaffected in transit. The patterns of cell-mediated immunity seem designed to meet this situation.

Though much less is known of immunity related to the activities of certain cells than is known of that related to antibodies, *cell-mediated (cellular) immunity,* because of its practical implications for tissue transplantation and rejection, is a subject of considerable current interest. The notion that without demonstrable antibody cells can bring about immune responses was hard to accept for a long time.

**Comparisons.** Like humoral immunity, cell-mediated immunity is part of the body's defense. Unlike it, there is no demonstrable, clear-cut antibody. For this reason there is no equivalent of passive immunization with cellular immunity—it cannot be passed in serum. However, transfer can be made in a less predictable fashion with lymphoid cells from a sensitized host.

For the study of cellular immunity there are only a small number of immunologic procedures to match the extended list of well-standardized tests used to describe antibodies. The traditional skin test, as important as it is, depends on the subject's prior contacts with antigens and is influenced by local tissue factors. As is illustrated by the skin test, the immune responses of cellular type emerge more slowly (several days) than those mediated by antibodies, which can evolve in a matter of hours.

In both kinds of immunity, contact with antigen triggers the sequence of events, but in cell-mediated immunity the antigen does not reach the lymphoid tissues; it seems blocked peripherally. With this type of immunity, concurrence with presence of antigen is crucial. If antigen is destroyed, the immune process subsides. In tuberculin testing, for example, the

previously sensitized person has a reaction lasting until all injected tuberculoprotein is gone.

**Principal cells.** The mediating and primary reacting cells are small, *thymus-dependent* lymphocytes, T cells. Authorities think these lymphocytes possess their unique specificity for reaction with a certain antigen as a result of the prior influence of the thymus gland. When contact with that particular antigen is made, the cells become sensitized and respond immunologically.

Macrophages are secondary participants, important for their property of phagocytosis. They make up 80% to 90% of cells mobilized to the reaction site.

**The antigen.** Antigens that induce the sequence of events in cellular immunity are usually protein. The antigenic protein may be quite small or more complex, for example, the lipoprotein transplantation antigen in the mouse.

**Events.** The first step is the recognition of the antigen as "foreign" by the population of thymus-dependent lymphocytes (T cells). Then ensues blastogenesis, the transformation and enlargement of T cells into rapidly dividing blast cells, cells of an immature appearance. They elaborate and release certain factors called *lymphokines,* designed to summon macrophages to the scene and to program them for the attack. The fully equipped macrophages assemble in large numbers, primed to sequester and destroy that which does not belong. Although the activation of the macrophages by lymphocytes as an immunologic phenomenon is not well understood, it does mean that the macrophage's microbicidal faculties are enhanced.

Some of the biologically active substances include *migration inhibitory factor,* blocking movement of macrophages; *chemotactic factor,* orienting migration of macrophages into the area; *blastogenic* or *mitogenic factor,* inducing blast transformation of lymphocytes; and *lymphotoxin,* damaging or killing cells. One important substance released is *transfer factor,* recoverable as a cell-free white blood cell extract that transmits immunologic information from one person to another; the passage of sensitivity in this way is measured by skin test results. Interferon is also elaborated by T cells (p. 291).

The cytotoxic effects of the activated lymphocytes coupled with the efforts of activated macrophages result in localization and destruction of antigen or antigen carrier. Some of the progeny of the lymphocytes resume the small lymphocyte status to recirculate as memory cells.

**Manifestations.** Cell-mediated immunity is a major component of the body's resistance to viruses, fungi, and certain bacteria. Classic expressions of it are found in delayed hypersensitivity (once known as bacterial hypersensitivity), graft rejection, and graft-versus-host reactions. It is also the capacity possessed by the body to resist most forms of cancer.

## Disturbances in immunity

Considerable attention is given today to the elucidation of both normal and abnormal mechanisms in immunity. As a result immunologic disorders are better understood. Some have only recently been defined. The nature of the defect is indicated in the following listing:

1. Immunologic accidents—best example, reaction following the mismatched blood transfusion.
2. Immunologic depression (immunosuppression)—administration of immunosuppressive agents materially interfering with or inhibiting the immune system (humoral or cellular); such are the steroid hormones in huge doses, irradiation, cytotoxic chemicals (antimetabolite drugs and alkylating agents), and antilymphocytic serum (ALS).
3. Immunologic deficiency—failure or impairment of normal development of immunologically competent cells of the lymphoid system of the body, both antibody deficiencies and defects of cell-mediated immunity included.

   An absence of lymphocytes and plasma cells and hence of all immunoglobulins is termed *lymphoid aplasia*. Abnormal development of the thymus gland *(thymic dysplasia)* or a congenital absence of the thymus will result in severe impairment of immunologic mechanisms. Death comes early in infancy.

   An absence of plasma cells with very low levels of gamma globulin is either *hypogammaglobulinemia* (antibodies in greatly decreased amounts) or *agammaglobulinemia* (no demonstrable gamma globulin in the blood). An absence of or a defect in some of the immunoglobulin components of serum is *dysgammaglobulinemia*.

   Certain patients with depressed cellular immunity are peculiarly vulnerable to infections caused by *Mycobacterium tuberculosis, Pseudomonas aeruginosa,* and *Pneumocystis carinii*. An infection such as vaccinia may progress even where there is a demonstrably high titer of circulating antibodies.
4. Immunologic effects of nonimmunologic diseases—infections with bacteria, viruses, and protozoa producing striking elevations in globulin levels of serum *(hyperglobulinemia)*.
5. Allergic states—(Chapter 14).

6. Autoimmunity and autoimmune diseases—defects of immunologic tolerance* (see p. 501).
7. Immunologic aberrations secondary to malignancies of the lymphoid system—as would be expected, associated with striking abnormalities.

   The malignant prototype of the lymphoid cell can yield an abnormal type of globulin, often in large quantities. Examples of frankly abnormal globulins synthesized by malignant cells are the myeloma proteins, the macroglobulins of Waldenström, and the Bence Jones proteins. The malignancies include the leukemias, lymphomas, or other neoplastic cell proliferations arising in the reticuloendothelial tissues.

## Tissue transplantation

There are many times in medicine when it would be desirable to take normal tissue (or an organ) from a healthy person (donor) and transplant it into the body of a patient (recipient) whose corresponding tissue (or organ) is severely diseased. It is true that a piece of skin can be relocated as a graft from one site on the same body to another *(autograft)*; that a transplant of living tissue from one identical, *not* fraternal, twin will take in the other *(isograft, isogeneric* transplant†); and that in plastic surgery pieces of nonviable bone, cartilage, and blood vessel from one individual can be used in another as a framework for new growth in certain areas *(homostatic graft)*. But immunologically each of us is a rugged individual! In the natural course of things what would be lifesaving grafts of viable skin, bone marrow, kidney, and so on are cast off, rejected, because very subtle antigenic differences exist among even closely related members of the human race.

**Graft rejection.** A graft from one member to another within a noninbred species is a *homograft* or *allograft*. Without intervention of any kind this graft is characteristically rejected. For about the first week there is every indication that the graft has taken. After that time the situation changes. The circulation of blood established in the graft is cut down; the graft is infiltrated by mononuclear cells, loses its viability, and is soon cast off (Fig. 12-5).

What has happened immunologically is an expression of cell-mediated immunity. (Although antibodies may also play a part, they are not primarily

---

*Immunologic tolerance refers to the ability of the immune system to discriminate between what belongs to its host (which it tolerates) and what does not (which it attacks).
†*Heterografts* or *xenografts* are those between members of different species.

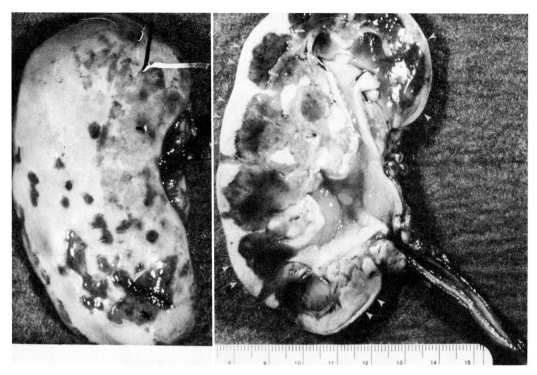

**Fig. 12-5.** Graft rejection of transplanted kidney (acute). Outer surface and cross section of kidney shown. Note diffuse death of tissue—whitish areas of outer and sectioned surfaces. Mottling is produced by hemorrhage.

implicated.) Small thymus-dependent lymphocytes detected the foreign antigen, became transformed, were sensitized in the regional lymph nodes, and were released back into the circulation as "activated" lymphocytes. They returned to the graft site to set the rejection process in motion. Although they initiated it, the actual demolition of the graft was carried out by macrophages, with the help of a few polymorphonuclear leukocytes, that the lymphocytes secured to the site.

**Transplantation antigens.** *Histocompatibility* refers to the degree of compatibility, or lack of it, between two given tissues. Of some eight to ten genetically independent systems in the body affecting graft survival or rejection, there are two that figure significantly and that are of practical importance.

The first, a very important histocompatibility factor in man, is the ABO blood group system, which is present on red blood cells and practically all tissues.

The second is determined by a complex genetic region known as the HL-A locus (histocompatibility locus-A) because it controls homograft immunity. It contains a group of antigens associated with cell membranes that are found in the majority of cells and tissues of the body, and especially in lymphoid

and blood-forming tissues (not on red blood cells, however). This complex system of at least 31 antigens, of which a person may have as many as 4, is most easily identified in leukocytes. Therefore tissue typing is commonly done with white blood cells. Practically speaking, the antigens usually referred to as *transplantation antigens* are those of the HL-A system. Part of the graft, they are the ones that mark the graft as "trespasser" to the recipient host.

**Testing for histocompatibility.** When tissue transplantation is anticipated, typing and cross-matching of blood specimens from the postulated donor and patient-recipient are done as though for blood transfusion. Any incompatibility in the ABO blood groups is an *absolute* contraindication to the use of the donor's tissue.

Tissue typing for transplantation, done with white blood cells or platelets, is partly analogous to red blood cell typing and cross matching for clinical blood transfusion. Of the various technics for tissue typing, lymphoagglutination and lymphocytotoxicity are widely used. *Lymphoagglutination* compares the clumping reactions of would-be donor and recipient lymphocytes when tested with a panel of selected antiserums. *Lymphocytotoxicity* measures the lethal effect of plasma membrane injury to presumed donor and recipient lymphocytes under similar conditions. Recipient serum can be mixed with the would-be donor's lymphocytes as a "cross match." Reaction in this indicates probability of immediate graft rejection. In evaluating the degrees of donor-recipient incompatibility for HL-A types determined from tissue typing, there are no absolute matches (except with identical twins). A "good" match still means differences, although small.

**Immunosuppression.** Various clinical and experimental technics have been designed to suppress or manipulate artificially the body's normal immune responses so that tissue transplantation would be possible. *Immunosuppression* (induction of tolerance) is the term used for the sum of approaches. Several are available. A potent antiproliferative drug such as 6-mercaptopurine (6-MP) that selectively interferes with either DNA or RNA synthesis may be used singly or combined with steroid hormones and irradiation. Depletion of lymphocytes has been attempted by drainage of the thoracic duct. Antilymphocyte globulin (ALG) has been administered to selectively eliminate the cellular population mediating the immune responses and perhaps to spare the sorely needed humoral ones. The disadvantage of immunosuppressive agents is that they concurrently impair normal host resistance. Such an individual with either subnormal or practically nonexistent immune responses is spoken of as the *compromised host*. An effort is being made experimentally to induce tolerance to the graft under conditions that do not compromise the body's normal defenses when they are needed elsewhere in the body.

**Graft-versus-host reaction.** It has been observed in animals and a few humans that at times instead of the host rejecting the graft, the graft has rejected the host. This has been found especially with transplantation of bone marrow and lymphoid tissue. In the immunologically depressed host, the graft survives. The immunologically competent lymphoid cells of the graft recognize the "foreignness" of the environment, and the stage is set for rejection. The end of it—runt disease in animals, secondary disease in man—is characterized by wasting, diarrhea, dermatitis, infection, and death.

**Present status.** Much has been accomplished in tissue transplantation. Transplantation of the kidney is established; worldwide more than 6000 recipients of a kidney transplant have survived. Transplantation of other organs is still experimental. Fallout has been considerable in terms of new knowledge in basic disciplines, control of infection, and a breakthrough in cancer immunology. It was discovered that with immunosuppression there is also a greater likelihood for the development of certain cancers. Problems are formidable still, but optimism and enthusiasm prevail.

## Immunology of red blood cell

The red blood cell is composed of a compact stromal protein that supports molecules of lipid and hemoglobin. Antigens of the blood groups are contained both in the stroma and on the surface of the red cells. On the surface exposed antigens are ready to react with specific antibodies. The spatial features of the relatively small antigenic groups out on the cell surface are such that each red cell can have a large number and variety of them.

**Agglutinins of blood.** The blood of every person falls into one of four ABO blood groups, depending on the ability of his serum to agglutinate the cells of persons whose blood is in another group. This is the result of the distribution of two agglutinins in the serum and two agglutinogens (antigens) on the red blood cells. The agglutinins are known as *anti-A* and *anti-B*. The agglutinogens are designated *A* and *B*. Agglutinin *anti-A* causes cells containing agglutinogen *A* to clump. Agglutinin *anti-B* causes cells containing agglutinogen *B* to clump (Fig. 12-6). The blood groups and their agglutinin and agglutinogen content are as follows:

Group AB: Serum contains no agglutinin; cells contain agglutinogens *A* and *B*

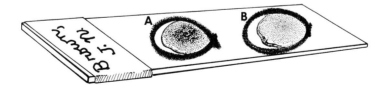

**Fig. 12-6.** Technic of blood grouping. Make suspension in isotonic saline of red blood cells from blood to be typed. Mark out two circles (wells) on microslide; label *A* and *B*. Place drop of test suspension in each. In well labeled *B*, mix in drop of serum from person of blood group A (anti-B serum); in well labeled *A*, mix in a drop of serum from person of blood group B (anti-A serum). Macroscopic agglutination of red blood cells in drop of typing serum seen in *A*. No agglutination in *B*. Well *A* contains anti-A typing serum and well *B*, anti-B. What type of blood do we have?

**Table 12-3**

Determination of blood type from agglutination of red blood cells in specific typing serum

| IF AGGLUTINATION OF RED CELLS OCCURS IN | | THEN BLOOD TYPE IS | HOW MANY PERSONS IN THE UNITED STATES WITH IT? | |
|---|---|---|---|---|
| | | | IF IT IS Rh POSITIVE | IF IT IS Rh NEGATIVE |
| Anti-A serum | Anti-B serum | | | |
| − | − | O | 1 in 3 | 1 in 15 |
| + | − | A | 1 in 3 | 1 in 16 |
| − | + | B | 1 in 12 | 1 in 67 |
| + | + | AB | 1 in 29 | 1 in 167 |

**Table 12-4**

Outline of transfusion reactions

| KIND | CAUSE | CLINICAL FEATURES |
|---|---|---|
| Hemolytic | Mismatched transfusion (example, blood type A given to patient, blood type O) | Severe chill; lumbar pain; nausea and vomiting; fever; suppression of urine (urine may be reddish brown); jaundice; death |
| Pyrogenic | Fever-producing substance in blood (sterile chemical contaminants, bacterial toxic products, antibodies to white blood cells) | Occurs 30 to 60 minutes after transfusion; flushing; nausea and vomiting; headache; muscular aches and pains; chills and fever |
| Contaminated blood | Break in aseptic technic: bacteria (usually gram-negative rods) introduced at time blood collected or with use of unsterile equipment | Chills and fever; generalized aching and pain; marked redness of skin; drop in blood pressure; shock |
| Allergic | Occurs in patients with history of allergy; cause unknown | Occurs within 1 or 2 hours of transfusion; itching of skin; hives or definite rash; swelling of face and lips; sometimes asthma |
| Sensitivity to donor white blood cells, platelets, or plasma | Multiple transfusions favor development of leukoagglutinins (those to white cells) and similar substances | Chills and fever; headache; malaise; serum may agglutinate white blood cell suspension from donor |
| Circulatory overload | Blood transfused too rapidly into person with failing circulation; likely to occur in elderly, debilitated, or cardiac patients, also in children | Difficulty in breathing; cyanosis; cough with frothy, blood-tinged sputum; heart failure |
| Embolic | Infusion of air: (1) transfusion under pressure, (2) tubing not completely filled before venipuncture | Sudden onset of cough, cyanosis, syncope, convulsions |

Group A: Serum contains agglutinin *anti-B;* cells contain agglutinogen *A*

Group B: Serum contains agglutinin *anti-A;* cells contain agglutinogen *B*

Group O: Serum contains agglutinins *anti-A* and *anti-B;* cells contain no agglutinogen (Table 12-3)

If a person whose blood belongs to one group receives a transfusion of blood from a donor whose blood belongs to another group, a hemolytic transfusion reaction is likely to occur. This is because the serum of the recipient may agglutinate the cells of the donor, or the serum of the donor may agglutinate the cells of the recipient. Reactions to transfusion of mismatched blood are associated with agglutination of red cells in the circulation, hemolysis of red cells, and liberation of free hemoglobin into the plasma; this leads to hemoglobinuria, fever, prostration, failure of kidney function, and in some cases death. A reaction is much more likely to occur if the recipient's serum agglutinates the donor's cells than if the donor's serum agglutinates the recipient's cells, since the donor's serum is considerably diluted in the circulation of the recipient. This effect tends to minimize the agglutinating capacity of the donor's serum. For the kinds of transfusion reactions see Table 12-4.

Although not a transfusion reaction, a serious complication of blood transfusion is posttransfusion hepatitis.* It is a serious concern to blood banks. The link between the disease and the Australia antigen (Au) has led in many blood banks to the routine screening of all would-be donors for its presence. The high-risk carriers of the agent (p. 318) are most likely to be the "commercial" donors from the skid row, drug addict, and prison inmate populations.

**Rh factor.** An agglutinogen with no relation to the ABO blood groups just listed is the *Rh factor.* When a guinea pig is given repeated injections of the red blood cells of a rhesus monkey, the serum of the animal acquires the ability to agglutinate the red cells of rhesus monkeys. It also agglutinates the red blood cells of a large majority of human beings (85% of the white race; more in others). The red blood cells that are agglutinated contain the Rh factor, and the person from whom the cells were removed is said to be *Rh positive.* Persons who do not have the Rh factor on their red blood cells are said to be *Rh negative.* The plasma of Rh-negative persons does not contain agglutinins against the Rh factor, but such agglutinins may develop if blood transfusions of Rh-positive blood are given to these people. Such incompatible blood transfusions, if continued, may lead to serious reactions. (See also p. 112.)

If an Rh-negative mother and an Rh-positive father have children, one or more will probably be Rh positive. The Rh-positive cells of her fetus can sometimes get into the bloodstream of the mother during gestation but usually in such small amounts that they do not induce antibody formation. It is thought that the Rh-negative mother has antibodies against the Rh factor during a given pregnancy because she was immunized in a previous one. When the Rh-positive cells of the baby enter the mother's circulation at time of delivery, they can be most effective in stimulating antibody formation. Antibodies formed against the Rh-positive cells begin to appear about 6 weeks later.

When antibodies against the Rh factor are present in the plasma of the Rh-negative mother, they freely pass through the placenta to attack the red blood cells of the fetus and destroy them. As a consequence, the child may be born with *erythroblastosis fetalis* or *hemolytic disease of the newborn.* (See also p. 543.) As to be expected, erythroblastosis seldom occurs

during the first pregnancy, but when once it happens, the condition will recur in about 80% of subsequent pregnancies.

Designated the Rh "vaccine," an immunizing agent* is available to prevent a susceptible Rh-negative mother from developing anti-Rh antibodies. It is human gamma globulin containing anti-Rh antibodies and obtained from sensitized Rh-negative mothers who have given birth to erythroblastotic babies. Injected as a single dose within 72 hours of delivery, it cancels out the antigenic effect of the Rh-positive cells that have entered the circulation. Immune mechanisms for the production of Rh antibodies are blocked. In the event of future pregnancy with an Rh-positive fetus, the immunologic basis for hemolytic disease of the newborn has been eliminated.

**Blood grouping (typing).** Human blood is routinely grouped (or typed) in modern blood bank laboratories into one of the four major blood groups, and the presence or absence of the Rh factor is determined. This means that the blood is typed to be O, A, B, or AB and as either Rh-positive or Rh-negative blood. However, the red blood cell is a very complex structure and contains many antigens or factors (at least 60) in addition to the A and B agglutinogens and the Rh factor, and new blood factors are constantly being discovered. As these antigens are studied, an attempt is made to classify them into categories containing related antigens, designated *systems.* The ABO system is made up of four blood groups, relating to the presence or absence of the agglutinogens A and B as just explained. There are today at least fifteen well-known systems of blood groups: (1) ABO, (2) MNS, (3) Rh, (4) P, (5) Lewis, (6) Kell, (7) Lutheran, (8) Duffy, (9) Kidd, (10) Sutter, (11) Vel, (12) Diego, (13) I, (14) Auberger, and (15) Xg (the only sex-linked blood group).

**Cross matching.** In routine blood grouping or typing for purposes of blood transfusion, the presence or absence of antigens in all these systems is not determined. But it is important to determine whether blood from a donor will be safe to give to a recipient, most often a patient with some medical or surgical condition. Certain technics have been devised to determine the relative safety of such a procedure and to prevent a blood transfusion reaction. The first step is called the *major cross match,* and in this the red blood cells of the donor are mixed with the serum of the person to receive the blood. The mixture is carefully observed for any sign of clumping of the red blood cells, and any agglutination means that the donor blood is incompatible with the

---

*Synonyms are hepatitis B, serum hepatitis, incubation hepatitis, tattoo hepatitis, postvaccinal hepatitis, HAA-positive hepatitis, hemologous serum jaundice, syringe hepatitis.

*Trade name: RhoGAM.

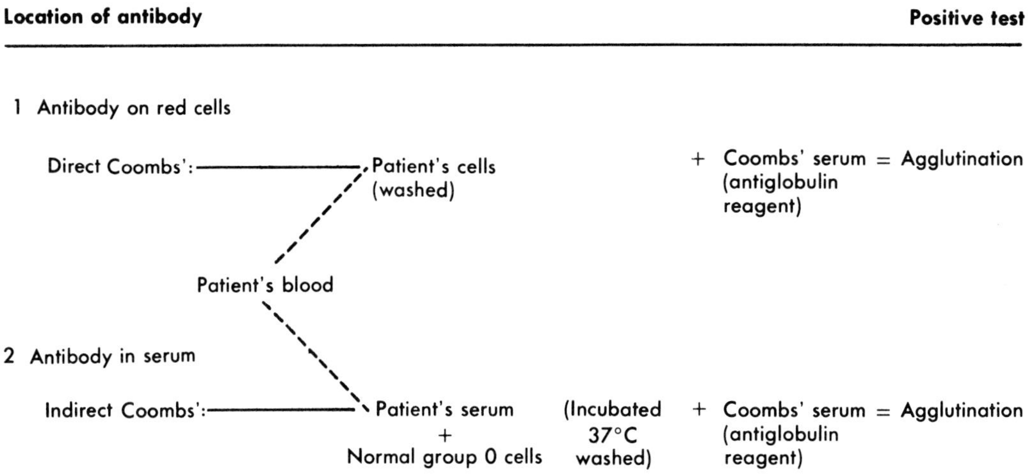

Location of antibody                                                         Positive test

1 Antibody on red cells

Direct Coombs': ——————————→ Patient's cells          + Coombs' serum = Agglutination
                                      (washed)                    (antiglobulin
                                                                  reagent)

                          Patient's blood

2 Antibody in serum

Indirect Coombs': ——————————→ Patient's serum    (Incubated   + Coombs' serum = Agglutination
                                   +                  37°C          (antiglobulin
                              Normal group O cells   washed)        reagent)

**Fig. 12-7.** Coombs' antiglobulin test (direct and indirect). The antiglobulin test (patient's cells plus Coombs' serum) indicating presence of antibodies on red blood cells is *direct* Coombs' test. The indirect Coombs' test (patient's serum plus O cells plus Coombs' serum) identifies presence of antibodies in patient's serum. No agglutination is a negative test. (Modified from Bove, J. R.: J.A.M.A. **200:**459, 1967.)

blood of the recipient. If the recipient were to receive this blood even in small quantities, a transfusion reaction could easily occur.

The second step is the *minor cross match,* in which red blood cells, this time from the recipient, are admixed with serum from the donor. Again the mixture is carefully observed for any sign of clumping of the red blood cells, which would mean an incompatibility of the two bloods. Agglutination at this step indicates the possibility of a transfusion reaction should the donor blood be transfused into the recipient, but the reaction would probably not be so severe as an incompatibility picked up in the major cross match.

A third step is further indicated to detect unusual or uncommon antibodies that for some reason are not demonstrated in the major or minor cross match. In many blood bank laboratories this is accomplished by the use of the *Coombs' test* (also known as the antiglobulin test). If we remember that antibodies are primarily related to the globulin fraction of the plasma proteins and if we know that the protein globulin itself can function as an antigen to stimulate the production of antibodies, then it should be easy to understand that an antihuman globulin serum (Coombs' serum) can be prepared by successively injecting human serum into a suitable animal such as a rabbit or goat. The serum of this immunized animal will then contain an antibody against the globulin of human serum. Since the globulin fraction contains the antibodies, it means that this Coombs'

serum will also have an action against antibodies, an action, as one can see, of a general or nonspecific nature. The Coombs' test does not in any way identify antibodies; its chief use lies in the fact that it can detect antibodies or indicate that they are present and attached to red blood cells. (See Fig. 12-7.) It helps to indicate the presence of antibodies even when an antigen-antibody combination has not resulted in an observable reaction. Such a test is of immeasurable value in blood typing and, on the whole is easily carried out. If this test is negative when donor red blood cells and recipient serum are used in the procedure and if the major and minor cross matches show no incompatibility, it is then considered safe for the donor blood to be given as a transfusion to the recipient in question.

## Questions for review

1 Fill out the table on p. 115, indicating whether each example of acquired immunity (a) is obtained naturally or artificially and (b) is active or passive.
2 Classify immunity. Give an example of each kind.
3 What type of immunity is of the longest duration? The shortest? Explain.
4 What are the immunoglobulins? How may they be classified?
5 Compare humoral immunity with cellular immunity.
6 What is the role of the lymphoid system in immunity? Role of the thymus gland?
7 Comment on the immunologically competent cell.
8 Categorize in general terms the disturbances in immunity.

| CAUSE OF IMMUNITY | ACQUIRED | | | |
| --- | --- | --- | --- | --- |
| | NATURALLY | ARTIFICIALLY | ACTIVE | PASSIVE |
| Attack of measles | | | | |
| Attack of smallpox | | | | |
| Vaccination against poliomyelitis | | | | |
| Vaccination against smallpox | | | | |
| Pasteur treatment | | | | |
| Diphtheria antitoxin | | | | |
| Diphtheria toxoid | | | | |
| Tetanus antitoxin | | | | |
| Tetanus toxoid | | | | |
| Immune globulin | | | | |
| Bacterial vaccine | | | | |
| Placental transmission of antibodies | | | | |

9 In the following diagram, place arrows pointing from the serum of each blood group to the cells agglutinated by that serum.

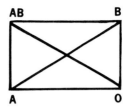

10 Why is a transfusion reaction more likely to occur when the donor's cells are agglutinated by the recipient's serum than when the recipient's cells are agglutinated by the donor's serum?

11 List the different kinds of transfusion reactions. Briefly explain.

12 Cite examples of immunosuppressive therapy.

13 What is meant by graft versus host reaction? How is it thought to come about?

14 State the importance of the transplantation antigens.

15 Explain the difference between autograft and heterograft; between isograft and homostatic graft.

16 Define or briefly explain: immunity, immunology, immunopathology, immunoglobulin, immunochemistry, immunobiology, immunosuppression, agglutination, antigenic determinant, isoantigen, adjuvant, immune system, and susceptibility.

17 What practical application is made of the Coombs' test?

**References on pp. 135 to 138.**

# CHAPTER 13

# Immunologic reactions

## Reactions for humoral immunity

Because of the specificity of the antigen-antibody reaction, if either the antigen or antibody is known, it is possible to identify the other. In many instances, by diluting the one known it is possible to obtain reliable information as to how much of the other is present. Since antigen-antibody reactions are usually measured in serum,* they are called *serologic reactions*. In the clinical laboratory, *serology* is the study of antigen-antibody reactions in a specimen of serum. With a positive serologic test, the unit that measures the number of antibodies present is the *titer*. There are a variety of technics available. Some of the important ones will be discussed here.

### DETECTION OF ANTIBODIES

The type of antigen-antibody reaction that applies in any given situation depends largely on the physical state of available antigen. Practically speaking, antibodies (immunoglobulins) are detected by what they do to produce a *visible* reaction with a specific antigen under specified conditions (Table 13-1). In the hospital and clinical laboratory antibodies are ordinarily classified as (1) complement-fixing antibodies, (2) antitoxins (neutralizing), (3) precipitins, (4) cytolysins, (5) agglutinins, (6) opsonins, (7) virus-neutralizing antibodies, and (8) fluorescent antibodies. In Table 13-1 this list of antibodies is tied in with antigens involved, and the nature of the antigen-antibody reaction is briefly indicated.

### KINDS OF REACTIONS

**Complement fixation.** The complement fixation test is designed to detect complement-fixing antibodies and is based on this fact: When serum containing the complement-fixing antibodies against the etiologic agent of a disease, the microbe itself, and complement are mixed in suitable proportions and in-

cubated, the three enter into a kind of combination whereby the complement is destroyed or inactivated (fixed). Since this combination is not accompanied by any visible change, some kind of indicator system must be used to detect it. Because hemolysis is dramatic, a hemolytic system is a good indicator. In this system the combination of *hemolysin (amboceptor),* complement, and sensitized red cells of the species of animal against which hemolysin was prepared effects *hemolysis* or dissolution of the red cells.

If a sample of serum from a patient is mixed with complement and a bacterial suspension and incubated, complement will be fixed when complement-fixing antibodies to the given bacteria are present in that serum. If suitable proportions of hemolysin and red blood cells are then added and the mixture incubated a second time, hemolysis *cannot* occur. This is a positive test. If, on the other hand, the patient's serum does not contain the specific antibodies, the complement is *not* fixed during the first incubation, and hemolysis occurs when hemolysin and red blood cells are combined with complement. This is a negative test, graphically illustrated in Schema 4.

*Wassermann test.* The Wassermann test for syphilis depends on the principle of complement fixation. It has always been impossible to grow the causative organisms of syphilis by artificial methods. When the Wassermann test first came into use, extracts of the livers of syphilitic fetuses were used as antigens. These extracts were used because the liver of a syphilitic fetus was known to contain myriads of the spirochetes of syphilis and as such were the nearest approach to extracts of the organisms themselves. Today certain lipid extracts of normal organs are efficient antigens. A lipid extract of beef heart gives clinically reliable and consistent results. Of course, the term *antigen* applied to extracts of normal tissue used in the Wassermann test is scientifically incorrect. In other diseases the antigens used in complement fixation tests are derived directly from the organisms themselves.

*Assay of complement.* The complement system itself can be measured by the pattern of complement

---

*To collect serum: Allow a sample of blood to clot. The fibrin formed in the process entraps the blood cells. When the clot shrinks, the fluid expressed is the serum, an important source of antibodies.

**Table 13-1**
Detection of important antigen-antibody combinations

| REACTION | ANTIGEN | ANTIBODY (IN SERUM) | NATURE OF REACTION |
|---|---|---|---|
| Complement fixation | Microbes | Complement-fixing antibodies | Inactivation of complement detected by hemolytic indicator system; *absence* of hemolysis a positive test |
| Flocculation | Exotoxins | Antitoxins | Flocculent precipitate |
| Precipitation | Microbes | Precipitins | Fine precipitate from clear solution |
| | Animal proteins | | |
| Cytolysis | Intact cells | Cytolysins | Cells dissolved |
| Bacteriolysis | Bacteria | Bacteriolysins | |
| Hemolysis | Red blood cells | Hemolysins | |
| Agglutination | Agglutinogens | Agglutinins | Gross clumping of cells |
| | Bacteria | | |
| | *Proteus* bacilli | Heterophil antibodies | |
| | Human red blood cells | Isoantibodies | |
| | Sheep red blood cells | Heterophil antibodies | |
| Inhibition of viral hemagglutination | Human type O red cells coated with viral antigen | Inhibiting antibodies | Clumping of red cells blocked |
| Opsonization | Bacteria | Opsonins | Bacteria phagocytosed in greater numbers by leukocytes |
| Neutralization or protection | Viruses | Virus-neutralizing antibodies | Protection of animal or tissue culture from harmful effects of agent |
| | Toxins | Antitoxins | |
| Fluorescence under ultraviolet light | Microbes | Fluorescein-tagged antibodies | Reaction tagged with marker |

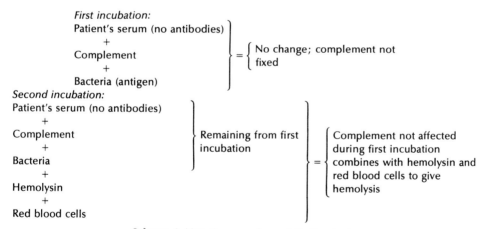

**Schema 4.** Negative complement fixation test.

fixation outlined above. The level of complement is altered in many disease states. Beta-1-complement (C3) is down in important diseases. Assay of complement with a hemolytic system can indicate both amount of complement (quantity) and its functional activity (quality).

**Toxin-antitoxin flocculation.** Antitoxins are antibodies that neutralize toxins, a combination demonstrable by flocculation. Flocculation refers to the presence of aggregates visible microscopically or macroscopically with certain antigen-antibody reactions. Toxin-antitoxin flocculations are similar to pre-

**117**

cipitin reactions (see below) but show a very sharp end point, the reaction being blocked by either too much antigen or too much antibody.

**Precipitation.** When a suitable animal is immunized with certain bacteria, the animal's serum acquires the ability to cause a fine powdery precipitate from the clear filtrate of the bacterial growth (*soluble* antigen of the bacterial extract is present). The antibodies formed are *precipitins*. The same phenomenon is noted when animals are immunized with the soluble antigens of certain animal and vegetable proteins. Precipitins are specific; bacterial precipitins react only with the filtrates of the bacteria that produced them, and precipitins formed by immunizing an animal with the serum of an animal of a different species react only with the proteins of the species used for immunization. Precipitins do not form regularly in infectious disease, but where they are present, they are nicely demonstrated by technics of immunodiffusion (see below).

The precipitin reaction has a wide medicolegal application in determining whether bloodstains are of human origin and in detecting the adulteration of one kind of meat with another. It is the test on which Lancefield's classification of streptococci is based. Flocculation tests for syphilis, such as the Kline, Kahn, and VDRL, are modified precipitation tests.

*C-reactive protein.* A biologic coincidence occurs in a number of inflammatory conditions of either infectious or noninfectious nature. A peculiar protein (a globulin) that can form a precipitate when in contact with the somatic C-polysaccharide of pneumococci appears in the blood of the affected person. For this reason the protein is spoken of as C-reactive protein; it is *not* an antibody. The serum of an animal immunized to this protein is used in a precipitation test to detect C-reactive protein in serum of persons suspected of having one of the diseases in which the protein appears. Among such diseases, both infectious and noninfectious, are acute rheumatic fever, subacute bacterial endocarditis, staphylococcal infections, infections with enteric bacteria, and neoplasms.

**Cytolysis.** Antibodies that dissolve or lyse cells are known as cytolysins or *amboceptors*. *Bacteriolysins,* cytolysins that lyse bacteria, are produced or at least increased by bacterial infection. Cytolysis is dependent on the presence of both cytolytic antibodies and complement; if only one is present, cytolysis will not occur. A cytolysin of great importance in immunologic procedures is *hemolysin,* which effects dissolution of red blood cells. It is prepared by giving an animal (most often a rabbit) a series of injections of the washed red blood cells from an animal of another species (most often man or sheep). Hemolysin develops in the serum of the recipient animal. It is spe-cific for the red blood cells of the species used; it does *not* affect the red blood cells of other species.

**Agglutination.** If the serum of a person who has had a disease such as salmonellosis is mixed with a suspension of the bacteria that cause the disease, the bacteria will adhere to one another and in the test tube will form easily visible clumps that sink to the bottom of the tube. Likewise, if an animal receives several injections of a given microbe, its serum will acquire the ability to clump or *agglutinate* the microorganisms used. This kind of clumping is *agglutination* (Figs. 13-1 and 13-2), and the antibodies that bring it about are called *agglutinins.* Particulate substances (antigens) that when injected into an animal induce the formation of agglutinins are known as *agglutinogens.* Agglutinogens may be microorganisms, red blood cells, or latex spheres coated with absorbed antigen. In each instance there must be particles for the characteristic clumping to occur.

Motile bacteria lose their motility before agglutination occurs. Bacteria are not necessarily killed by agglutination, and dead bacteria are agglutinated as easily as live ones. Agglutinated microorganisms are more easily taken up by phagocytic cells.

*Kinds of agglutinins.* Normally occurring agglutinins exist in the blood of certain persons. For instance, the human serum sometimes shows a weak agglutinin content against typhoid bacilli although the person has never been knowingly infected with the organisms. The agglutinin content is so low, however, that when the serum is diluted 20 or 40 times and then mixed with a suspension of the organisms, agglutination does not occur.

*Immune agglutinins* are agglutinins brought about by infection or artificial immunization. Such agglutinins can occur plentifully in serum, and such serum will cause agglutination though diluted 500 to 1000 times. Agglutinin formation is usually specific; that is, when an organism is introduced into the body, the body forms agglutinins against that organism only or, in some cases, against very closely related organisms. Agglutinins for closely related organisms are known as *group agglutinins.* However, the agglutinin content of the serum is much higher for the organism directly inducing the production of the agglutinins than it is for the closely related organisms. Usually in an infection the human (or animal) body has not manufactured enough agglutinins for positive identification until infection has lasted 7 to 10 days.

Comparatively few organisms induce appreciable agglutinin formation with infection or artificial immunization. Most important of these are *Salmonella typhi,* other *Salmonella* species, *Brucella* species, and *Francisella tularensis.* In infections with these (salmonellosis, undulant fever, and tularemia) the agglu-

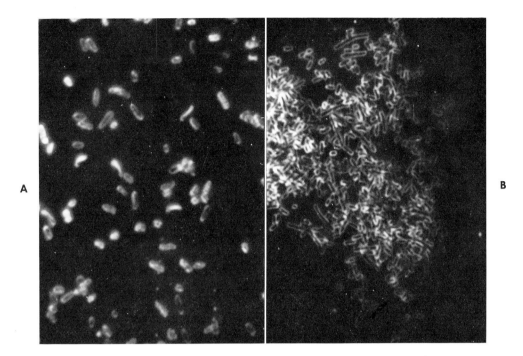

**Fig. 13-1.** Bacterial agglutination, dark-field illumination. **A,** Saline suspension of killed *Salmonella,* bacteria evenly spread with no clumping. **B,** Addition of positive antiserum. Note large clump of organisms. (Courtesy Gwyn Hopkins and Dr. Gerard Noteboom, Dallas.)   *WIADL REACTION*

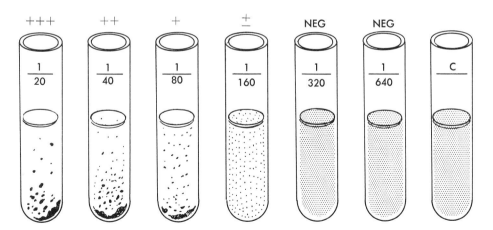

**Fig. 13-2.** Bacterial agglutination, test tube method. Dilute 0.2 ml. of patient's serum serially in iso-tonic saline through first *six* tubes (left to right). Add 1 ml. of suspension of bacteria to each tube through all seven. Final dilutions indicated by numbers on each tube (as 1 part serum in 20 parts, etc., suspension). Control tube on far right contains only bacterial suspension and saline. Note maximal agglutination of bacteria (large masses) in first three tubes on left, some in fourth, and none in fifth and sixth. *Agglutination test positive; titer of serum 1:160.*

tination test becomes an important diagnostic tool. For example, serum from a patient is mixed with a suspension of *Salmonella typhi* in the *Widal test* for typhoid fever; if agglutination occurs when the serum is diluted to exclude the action of natural and group agglutinins, we know that the patient's serum contains immune agglutinins against *Salmonella typhi*. We may not know, however, whether the agglutinins result from a current attack of typhoid fever, a previous attack, or the recent administration of vaccine. (The diagnosis of typhoid is usually resolved with the case history and clinical manifestations.) In lower animals the agglutination test is used to detect Bang's disease (contagious abortion of cattle) and bacillary white dysentery in chickens caused by *Salmonella gallinarum*.

Sometimes *nonspecific agglutinins* are produced against organisms with apparently no relation to the disease. Nonspecific agglutination is of special diagnostic value in typhus fever and other rickettsial diseases. In typhus fever nonspecific agglutinins develop against certain members of the *Proteus* genus of bacteria; typhus fever is caused by rickettsias, not by *Proteus*. It is thought that many such agglutinins are formed as the result of the introduction into the body of *heterophil* antigens* (*hetero,* from an individual of a *different* species). Heterophil antigens cause heterophil antibodies to be formed not only against themselves but against other antigens as well. Such antigens are common in the lower orders of life. In typhus fever the causative agent of the disease, a rickettsia, seems to act as a heterophil antigen, and the antibodies formed react not only to the rickettsias but to certain types of *Proteus* bacilli as well. The agglutination of certain *Proteus* organisms by the serum of a patient with typhus fever constitutes the *Weil-Felix reaction*.

The serum of human patients with infectious mononucleosis agglutinates the red blood cells of the sheep. The antibody that agglutinates the red cells is a *heterophil antibody* since it agglutinates an antigen (in the red cells) of a different species. This important diagnostic test is the *heterophil antibody test* or the *Paul-Bunnell test*.

Agglutination tests are utilized in the laboratory for the identification of bacteria. Agglutinating serums are prepared by artificially immunizing separately several individual animals of the same species with known species or types of bacteria so that a battery of typing serums is available. After an immunized animal is bled, its serum is separated and preserved for use. Such typing serums retain their potency for

months. A suspension of unknown bacteria may be mixed with the battery of typing serums. If one of the serums shows agglutination, the unknown bacteria must be the same as those against which the serum was prepared.

In the application of the agglutination test to the identification of bacteria, the antibody is known and the antigen is unknown; in its application to the diagnosis of disease, the antigen is known and the antibody (in serum from a patient) is unknown.

Agglutination forms the basis of many useful laboratory tests and is thought to represent a body mechanism for clearing the blood stream of would be invaders.

*Hemagglutination.* Many types of antigens can be absorbed onto the surface of a red blood cell. A red cell properly prepared with a test antigen can serve as a reagent for the detection of antibodies in the serum of a patient. This technic is *hemagglutination*. The *titer* of antibody is the dilution of serum in which no further agglutination of red cells occurs.

*Hemagglutination-inhibition.* Red cell agglutination is used to identify certain viruses (p. 289). The action of a virus to clump red cells (viral hemagglutination) can be blocked by specific antibody to the virus. This is *hemagglutination-inhibition,* and is a very important diagnostic test in a number of viral infections.

**Opsonization.** Opsonins are substances that act on bacteria or other cells in such a manner (opsonization) as to render them more easily ingested by phagocytes and to favor their breakdown within the cytoplasm of the phagocyte. When the white blood cells of a person or animal suspected of having a disease are mixed with a suspension of the bacteria causing the disease, the degree of phagocytosis taking place is of diagnostic significance and can be evaluated in the *opsonocytophagic* test. This test has been used in the diagnosis of undulant fever and tularemia.

Phagocytosis (p. 94) is not an activity of the phagocytes alone but is dependent on the action of opsonins in the serum. Opsonins are to some degree present in normal serum but are present in an increased amount in immune serum, and their action is enhanced by complement. This is not a test in wide use today.

*Nitroblue tetrazolium (NBT) test.* When normal neutrophils (microphages) in an individual with a normally functioning immune system are confronted by bacterial pathogens, certain metabolic changes consequent to their phagocytic activity take place within them. These changes probably relate to the cell membrane; opsonins are not pinpointed. Because of these the neutrophils can be shown to reduce appre-

---

*The heterophil antigen is an exception to the tenet of antigen specificity.

ciably a supravital dye, pale yellow nitroblue tetrazolium to blue-black formazan crystals. An in vitro test, the nitroblue tetrazolium (NBT) test, has been devised to display in human blood the ability of the neutrophils to do so. This test helps to separate certain bacterial infections from nonbacterial illness in patients where clinical manifestations are confusing and to monitor patients with increased vulnerability to infection (because of tissue transplant, immunosuppressive therapy, and the like).

**Neutralization or protection tests.** Neutralization tests are important in a number of infections caused by viruses and a few caused by bacteria. Antibodies that give immunity to viruses are known as *virus-neutralizing antibodies.* They can block the infectivity of a given viral agent under test conditions in a susceptible host. (See p. 289.)

**Immunofluorescence.** In recent years it has been demonstrated that antibodies can be chemically tied to the fluorescent dye fluorescein without changing their basic properties as antibodies. Such tagged antibodies (*fluorescent antibodies*) react with their specific antigens in the usual way. When fluorescent antibodies are allowed to react with their specific antigens in cultures or smears containing certain microorganisms or in the tissue cells of the human or animal body (*the direct test*), the result is a precipitate formed from the combination of antigen and antibody that, because of the accompanying fluorescein, can be seen as a luminous area when viewed under ultraviolet light. A special type of microscope has been devised with which one can do just this. Specimens for testing with fluorescent antiserums may be taken from the various body fluids and sites of disease.

The direct test is applicable to infections with the following agents:

*Actinomyces*
*Blastomyces dermatitidis*
*Bordetella pertussis*
*Brucella*
*Candida albicans*
*Cryptococcus neoformans*
Enteropathogenic *Escherichia coli*
Enteroviruses
Group A streptococci
*Haemophilus influenzae*
Herpesvirus
*Histoplasma capsulatum*
Influenza virus
*Listeria monocytogenes*
*Neisseria gonorrhoeae*
*Neisseria meningitidis*
Parainfluenza viruses
Rabies virus
*Shigella*

*Staphylococcus aureus*
*Streptococcus (Diplococcus) pneumoniae*

In the *indirect test,* nonfluorescent antibody is bound to its antigen. The combination is made visible after application of a second antibody (antihuman serum), this time a fluorescent one. The test is set up so that the unconjugated serum acts as antibody in the first part and as antigen when exposed to fluorescent serum in the second part. The indirect test has been used with infections caused by the following:

*Brucella*
*Chlamydia trachomatis*
*Cryptococcus neoformans*
Cytomegalovirus
Epstein-Barr virus
*Haemophilus influenzae*
Herpesvirus
*Leptospira*
*Mycoplasma pneumoniae*
*Plasmodium* of malaria
*Rickettsia prowazekii*
Rubella virus
*Toxoplasma gondii*
*Treponema pallidum*

Because of the rapid results with this technic, there is a wide variety of applications in identification of antigens related to bacteria, rickettsias, viruses, fungi, and protozoa. Pathogenic amebas can be quickly distinguished from nonpathogenic ones, streptococci may be detected quickly in throat swabs, and rabies virus can be tagged in animals. In tissues fluorescent staining helps to localize the precise anatomic sites of antigen-antibody combination in diseases such as lupus erythematosus, rheumatoid arthritis, and certain hypersensitivity reactions.

**Special technics.** There are several other laboratory tests important to the study of the structure and nature of antibodies (immunoglobulins) and to the elucidation of the immunologic disorders.

*Electrophoresis.* When proteins are placed in an electrical field at a given pH, they will move in a distinctive path according to their own specific electrical charges. The pattern of migration of different proteins can be visualized under prescribed test conditions on a suitable strip, such as paper, stained with dye. (See Figs. 13-3 and 13-4.) *Zone electrophoresis* refers to the technic of using a stabilizing medium to trap migrating proteins into more or less separate areas of zones that can then be stained and identified later. Routinely used solid support media include paper, starch, agar, and cellulose acetate. Antibodies with zone electrophoresis tend to show up as an undifferentiated group. They can be sorted, however, by technics indicated below.

*Radial diffusion immunoassay.* Under the appro-

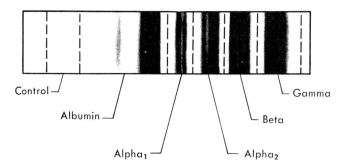

**Fig. 13-3.** Electrophoresis of normal human serum. Serum sample is placed near one end of cellulose acetate strip moistened with buffer. An electric potential is applied. Serum proteins migrate along strip at different speeds. Afterward strip is dried, and proteins fixed and stained (bromphenol blue). Black bands correspond to separated and stained proteins, depth of color in each band proportional to amount of that protein present. Strip may be cut crosswise as indicated, and protein fractions analyzed further. (From Bauer, J. D., and others: Clinical laboratory methods, ed. 8, St. Louis, 1974, The C. V. Mosby Co.)

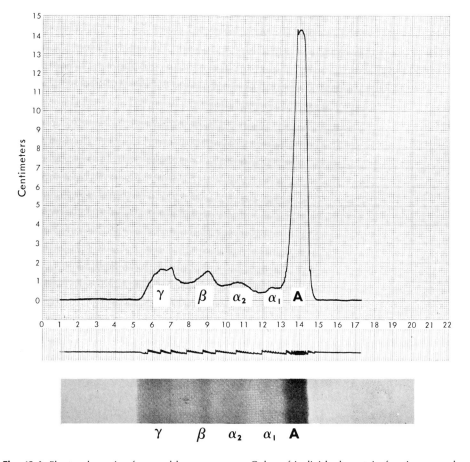

**Fig. 13-4.** Electrophoresis of normal human serum. Color of individual protein fractions may be measured directly on cellulose acetate strip with a recording densitometer and a curve obtained as above. (From Bauer, J. D., and others: Clinical laboratory methods, ed. 8, St. Louis, 1974, The C. V. Mosby Co.)

priate conditions antigen-antibody combinations form a visible precipitate. *Gel diffusion* is a term used for the antigen-antibody precipitin reaction detected in semisolid media. If protein (or antigen) is placed in a specially designed hole or well in an agar gel medium (no electrical charge), the protein diffuses concentrically out of the well. Just as specific antibody precipitates antigen in gels, this radial diffusion can be shown nicely in the clear gel if specific antibody has been impregnated into it. As antigen diffuses out of the well, it forms a ring of precipitate at the points of contact with specific antibody. This reaction can be quantitated easily for amounts of protein (or antigen). Known also as *single gel diffusion*, this is an important method for analysis of immunoglobulins.

*Electroimmunodiffusion* is single gel diffusion in an electric field.

*Double gel diffusion.* In this method antibody is not incorporated throughout the agar as in single gel diffusion but is placed in a trench (or other reservoir) cut in the medium. The arrangement is such that soluble protein (antigen) and antibody diffuse out into the agar to form a band or line of precipitate at points of contact. If a mixture of proteins (or antigens) is analyzed, each specific antigen-antibody combination tends to present as a separate band at a definite position in the medium between the reservoir for the antigen and that for the antibody. This reaction is also a quantitative one.

In the Ouchterlony technic, microslides are covered with suitable diffusion medium, the center well is filled with serum (human or animal) containing known antibodies, test serums are placed in wells opposite the center one, and the microslide is incubated in a moist chamber for 24 to 48 hours. The combination of specific antibody with antigen from a test serum is read from the precipitation line. This particular precipitin-in-agar technic may be used at times as a simple, fairly rapid screening technic for the identification of various microorganisms.

*Immunoelectrophoresis.* If the technics of electrophoresis and double gel diffusion are combined, we have the process of *immunoelectrophoresis*, a valuable method for separating complex mixtures of proteins (antigens). In the test specimen in an electrical field, the unknown proteins are spread out in a series of differently charged masses. Specific antibody is placed in a trough parallel to the line of migration of the proteins in the gel. After electrophoresis proteins diffuse outward; antibody diffuses inward in an incoming wave. As specific antibody meets antigen, precipitation occurs in a series of arcs. (See Fig. 13-5.) The immunoprecipitin bands are readily seen, and the position and shape are consistent and stable for known proteins. Deviations represent abnormal constituents. (See Fig. 13-6.)

## Procedures for cellular immunity

Cellular immunity may be measured by immunologic yardsticks although the technics are not so well established as those with which we evaluate humoral immunity.

**Lymphocytes in peripheral blood.** The presence, number, and kind of lymphocytes circulating in the peripheral blood can be determined. This is informa-

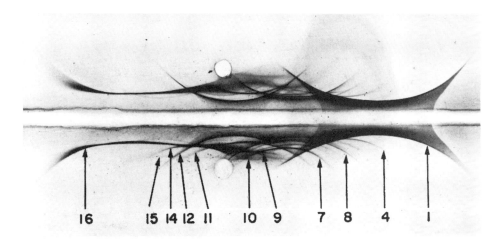

**Fig. 13-5.** Immunoelectrophoresis. Demonstration of normal serum proteins when tested against polyvalent antiserum. Note pattern of arcs: *1*, albumin; *4*, antitrypsin; *10*, beta lipoprotein; *14*, IgA globulin; *15*, IgM globulin; *16*, IgG globulin; *7* to *9*, *11*, and *12*, other proteins. (From Miale, J. B.: Laboratory medicine: hematology, ed. 4, St. Louis, 1972, The C. V. Mosby Co.)

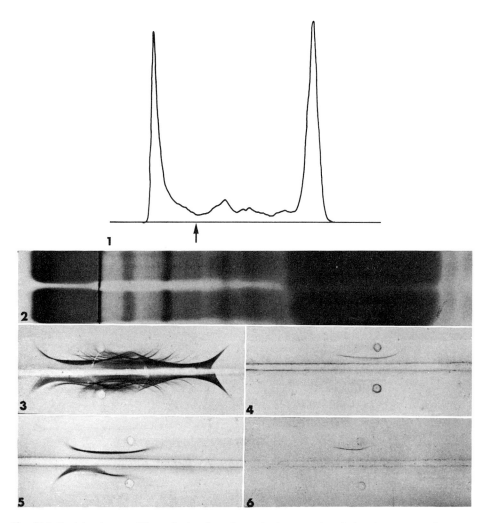

**Fig. 13-6.** Protein abnormalities, electrophoretic study. In several technics demonstrated, an example of a malignant proliferation of lymphoid system—multiple myeloma—is used, a disease associated with large quantities of abnormal globulins. **1,** Paper electrophoresis showing abnormal peak (arrow). **2,** Starch gel electrophoresis showing abnormal gamma globulin component. **3 to 6,** Immunoelectrophoresis (in each instance normal control sample is at top, patient specimen at bottom). **3,** Testing with polyvalent antiserum. **4,** Testing with anti-IgA. **5,** With anti-IgG (which picks up, identifies, and locates the IgG) there is an increase of IgG. **6,** With anti-IgM there is a decrease of IgM. (From Miale, J. B.: Laboratory medicine: hematology, ed. 4, St. Louis, 1972, The C. V. Mosby Co.)

tion of a general nature, but it can nonetheless be useful. If the total number of lymphocytes is decreased (lymphopenia), a significant finding, this is reflected in the total lymphocyte count (sometimes done sequentially). The critical level for lymphocytes is 1200 per cubic millimeter. The morphology of the lymphocytes may be studied in peripheral blood smears, and differential counts made. Thymus derived T cells are easily recognized: they are small, mostly nucleus with little cytoplasm about it. Approxi-

mately 70% of peripheral blood lymphocytes are T cells; some 25% are B cells.

**Battery of skin tests.** Skin testing is fairly straightforward for the presence or absence of cellular immunity. A battery of antigens is selected with the idea that most normal adults should have a positive skin test to at least one of them. The antigens used routinely include one for *Candida,* a mumps antigen, streptokinase-streptodornase, trichophytin, and purified protein derivative (PPD, tuberculin). Children, however, even under normal circumstances may show negative skin test results with all of these. In a child, sensitivity may be artificially induced with dinitrochlorobenzene, and challenge made 2 weeks later.

**Immunologic competency in vitro.** There are tests based on the premise that cell-mediated immunity requires for its expression a direct interaction between the host lymphoid cell and the agent (microbe, foreign cell, and the like) that carries the antigen into the arena of contact. When the natural situation is simulated, the immunologic behavior of the lymphocytes can be observed. Rather precise assays are being developed along these lines. One such starts with peripheral lymphocytes isolated in cell culture. A mitogen such as phytohemagglutinin (PHA) is added

to stimulate increased DNA and RNA synthesis, a response of the lymphocytes measurable in two ways. One method quantitates the uptake of radioactive thymidine. A second method is differential counting of the cells. Small lymphocytes exposed to PHA become larger cells. After suitable staining, one can record the number of the enlarged blast cells.

Another assay starts with a mixed white cell culture, one in which test lymphocytes from a given person are cultured with lymphocytes from an unrelated donor. Competent lymphocytes can recognize the cells that do not belong, the nonself. This they do because of the histocompatibility HL-A antigens foreign to them on the donor cells. In severe immunologic deficiency disorders involving cell-mediated immun-

**Table 13-2**
Immunologic approach to disease

| TEST(S) | APPLICATION |
|---|---|
| *Serologic* | |
| 1. Complement fixation | Diagnosis of syphilis, viral infections, and certain bacterial infections |
| 2. Flocculation | Diagnosis of syphilis |
| 3. Precipitation | Diagnosis of syphilis |
| Protein precipitation | Detection of origin of blood stains; detection of meat adulteration |
| 4. Agglutination | Identification (serologic typing) of bacteria; diagnosis of undulant fever, tularemia, and salmonellosis |
| a. Widal | Diagnosis of typhoid fever |
| b. Weil-Felix | Diagnosis of typhus fever and Rocky Mountain spotted fever |
| c. Paul-Bunnell (heterophil antibody) | Diagnosis of infectious mononucleosis |
| d. Viral hemagglutination | Diagnosis of viral infections—rubella, rubeola, influenza, parainfluenzal infection |
| 5. Virus neutralization | Diagnosis of viral infections |
| 6. Fluorescent antibody | Identification of protozoa, fungi, bacteria, rickettsias, chlamydiae, and viruses; diagnosis of rabies, syphilis, amebiasis |
| *Intradermal* (skin) | Diagnosis of infection, past or present, caused by microorganisms of: |
| 1. Cell-mediated immunity to infection with: | |
| a. Bacteria | |
| Brucellergen | Brucellosis |
| Lepromin | Leprosy |
| Mallein | Glanders |
| Tuberculin | Tuberculosis |
| b. Fungi | |
| Blastomycin | Blastomycosis |
| Coccidioidin | Coccidioidomycosis |
| Trichophytin | Epidermophytosis |
| Oidiomycin | Candidiasis |
| Histoplasmin | Histoplasmosis |
| Sporotrichin | Sporotrichosis |
| c. Chlamydiae | |
| Frei | Lymphopathia venereum |
| d. Viruses | |
| Mumps | Mumps |
| 2. Susceptibility | |
| Schick | Susceptibility to diphtheria |
| Dick | Susceptibility to scarlet fever |

ity the ability to recognize and respond to HL-A antigens is lost.

**Migration inhibitory factor assay.** Several methods have been devised to assay factors released after the interaction of the sensitized lymphocytes with specific antigen. One such is the assay of the migration inhibitory factor (MIF). For this test, cellular suspensions are prepared from the peritoneal exudates of guinea pigs sensitized to antigen(s). In this material there are macrophages (70%), polymorphonuclear leukocytes (only a few), and lymphocytes, specifically sensitized. The exudative material is placed into capillary tubes, and the macrophages observed as they migrate out of the tubes onto glass coverslips in culture chambers *in the absence of antigen*. When the antigen is added, the migration is stopped. It takes only 1 sensitized lymphocyte to block movement of 99 macrophages. This reaction can also be quantitated. First, the patient is studied to determine whether sensitized lymphocytes are circulating and then as to what sensitivities are present to a given variety of tissue antigens.

**Rosettes.** When T cells and sheep red blood cells are incubated together for a short time, about 25% of the T lymphocytes form rosettes with the sheep red cells. B cells can be identified with fluorescent anti-immunoglobulin serum designed to indicate surface receptors. When red cells coated with anti–red cell antibody and complement are added to red cells to demonstrate the receptors for complement on the B cell surface, the red cells cluster about the B cells forming rosettes.

## Application of immunologic methods

Some of the more frequently used immunologic methods for identifying and studying microbes and for defining their role in disease production are given in Table 13-2.

## Questions for review

1 What is an agglutination test? Name diseases in which it is used as a diagnostic procedure.
2 Briefly define antitoxin, cytolysin, agglutinin, precipitin, precipitation, serology, heterophil antibody, opsonin, hemolysis, hemolysin, amboceptor, serum, hemagglutination, virus-neutralization, flocculation, migration inhibitory factor, lymphopenia.
3 How may antibodies be detected?
4 What is meant by the titer of a serum?
5 What are the advantages of the immunofluorescent technics?
6 Explain the difference between the direct and the indirect fluorescent antibody test.
7 Briefly discuss immunoelectrophoresis and its applications.
8 Diagram a positive complement fixation test.
9 State ways in which cell-mediated immunity may be evaluated.

**References on pp. 135 to 138.**

# CHAPTER 14

# Allergy

## Allergic disorders

**General characteristics.** Some persons exhibit unusual and heightened manifestations on contact with certain substances that are often, but not necessarily, protein, and that do not affect the average or another person. For example, an individual may have asthma on contact with horse dander,* and many persons have hay fever on contact with plant pollens.

We have learned that immunity is a state wherein by prior contact a person obtains protection against an agent that would otherwise harm him. The reaction is specific for the particular agent, and a benefit comes from the immune setup. If we think of another situation, comparable immunologically but one in which the immune mechanisms injure or damage instead of protect, then we are referring to the state of *allergy* or *hypersensitivity*.† Allergy or hypersensitivity is a state of altered reactivity directly related to the operation of the immune system. The study of the effects in body tissues of the allergic reaction is included in *immunopathology*. (See also p. 501.)

An antigenic substance that can trigger the allergic state is an *allergen*. It may be a protein or frequently a nonprotein of low molecular weight. Allergens may reach the body by way of the respiratory tract or the digestive tract, by direct contact with skin or mucous membranes, and by mechanical injection. Of these routes, the respiratory pathway is most regular. It is thought that unchanged protein must pass through the intestinal wall to the bloodstream for sensitization via the intestinal tract to occur. This can occur in children and adults with digestive disturbances. A passive sensitization may be transmitted from the mother to her child in utero via the placenta.

---

*Dander is animal dandruff—the composite of cast-off epithelial cells of the skin, sebum, and other body oils.
†Both terms are commonly used to mean conditions such as emotional upsets, nonallergic food reactions, toxic responses to drugs, and others that are nonimmunogenic. Since *hypersensitivity* is more often so used than *allergy*, some authorities believe that the term *allergy* has priority.

This type of sensitization is short lived, as is true of passive immunity in the newborn infant.

An allergic person is often sensitive to several different allergens. At least 10% to 20% of persons in the United States develop allergic disorders under the natural conditions of life.

**Kinds.** As would be expected from our discussion of immunity, the reactions of allergy are separated into two main divisions (Table 14-1): (1) those in which the allergic responses result from the presence of humoral antibody, reactions of the *immediate* type, and (2) those in which the responses are not mediated by circulating antibodies but by specifically sensitized cells (that is, they are cell-mediated), reactions of the *delayed* type.

**Mechanisms.** The mechanisms of allergy are enormously complex and poorly understood. Only a sketch (Fig. 14-1) is given of some of the background factors.

In the immediate type of allergy, it is postulated that as a consequence of injury to a certain kind of cell, allergen combining with humoral antibody triggers a release of a number of highly active substances. The cell believed to be sensitized by circulating antibody and vulnerable is the mast cell, a cell widely distributed in the connective tissues of the body. The substances released include histamine, bradykinin, heparin, and slow-reacting substance, Each of these has the chemical potential to induce responses associated with immediate-type allergy. The spectrum of effects in immediate-type allergy includes contraction of smooth muscle, increase of gastric secretion, increase of nasal and lacrimal secretions, increase of vascular permeability, and vascular changes that can lead to circulatory collapse (shock). Of the chemical mediators of allergy, histamine has been the most extensively studied, and the allergic reaction has even been said to constitute a response to too much histamine.

The mast cell (the basophil of peripheral blood) is a cell about 15 $\mu$m. ($\mu$) wide and is known for its distinctive appearance (Fig. 14-2). Large, densely placed, metachromatically staining granules found in

**Table 14-1**

Kinds of allergic disorders

|  | IMMEDIATE-TYPE REACTIONS (ANAPHYLACTIC TYPE) | DELAYED-TYPE REACTIONS (BACTERIAL OR TUBERCULIN TYPE) |
|---|---|---|
| Clinical state | Hay fever | Drug allergies |
|  | Asthma | Infectious allergies |
|  | Urticaria | Tuberculosis |
|  | Allergic skin conditions | Tularemia |
|  | Serum sickness | Brucellosis |
|  | Anaphylactic shock | Rheumatic fever |
|  |  | Smallpox |
|  |  | Histoplasmosis |
|  |  | Coccidioidomycosis |
|  |  | Blastomycosis |
|  |  | Trichinosis |
|  |  | Contact dermatitis |
| Onset | Immediate | Delayed |
| Duration | Short—hours | Prolonged—days or longer |
| Allergens | Pollen | Drugs |
|  | Molds | Antibiotics |
|  | House dust | Microbes—bacteria, viruses, fungi, animal parasites |
|  | Danders | Poison ivy and plant oils |
|  | Drugs | Plastics and other chemicals |
|  | Antibotics | Fabrics, furs |
|  | Horse serum | Cosmetics |
|  | Soluble proteins and carbohydrates |  |
|  | Foods |  |
| Passive transfer of sensitivity | With serum | With cells or cell fractions of lymphoid series |

its cytoplasm are notable for their high concentration of pharmacologically potent compounds such as histamine, heparin, and proteolytic enzymes, Injury to the cell means degranulation. As the cell loses its unique granules, the substances contained therein are released into tissue fluids. Nonimmune as well as immune factors can cause degranulation.

Of 5000 different immunoglobulin molecules found in normal persons, only one seems to be an immunoglobulin E (IgE). However, allergic individuals seem to produce considerably more of their antibodies from this class. IgE is formed mainly by plasma cells in the mucosa and submucosa of the respiratory, alimentary, and genitourinary tracts and their regional nodes. Only small amounts come from the spleen. IgE is thought to be secreted directly from these surfaces along with immunoglobulin A. IgE selectively attaches to the mast cells (basophils), whereon it has been identified. It is involved with the release of histamine and other substances and is thought to play an important role in governing the allergic response.

In immediate-type allergy the consequences of the antigen-antibody combination follow shortly thereafter, even within minutes, and the reaction reaches a maximum within a few hours. The responses occur in vascularized tissues and relate primarily to smooth muscle, blood vessels, and connective tissues. A specific shock tissue is important, that is, a target tissue or organ that, because of its anatomic makeup, shows maximal effects. Manifestations are acute and short-lived. Epinephrine, antihistaminic drugs, and related compounds are of benefit. This type of reactivity can be transferred passively to a nonsensitized person by antibody-containing serum.

In delayed-type allergy, by contrast, there is no relation to conventional antibody. The phenomenon is closely associated with cells. The responses are set in motion by lymphocytes specifically modified so that they can respond to the specific allergen deposited at a given site. The main feature of the reaction is the direct destruction of target tissue containing the antigen. The condition may be passively transferred to a nonsensitized person if immunologically competent cells (lymphoid cells) are used.

In allergic reactions of this type a much longer

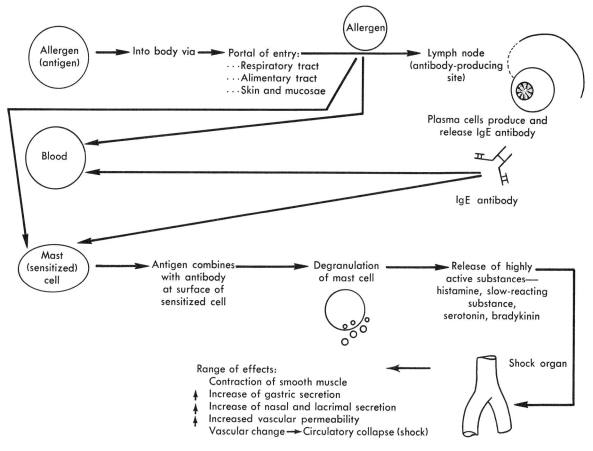

**Fig. 14-1.** Simplified schema of immediate-type allergy.

period of time elapses between the presentation of the antigen and the manifestations of the disorder. The period of incubation ranges from 1 to several days. Reactions do not favor any particular tissue but may occur anywhere. There is no specific shock organ or tissue as with immediate-type allergy. Many cells in the body are vulnerable. Manifestations tend to be slow in onset and prolonged. No histamine effect is demonstrated as in the immediate-type reactions, and antihistamines are without effect. The steroid hormones seem to help in the treatment of some allergic disorders of this kind and in some of these of the immediate type as well. The exact mode of their action is not known.

## IMMEDIATE-TYPE ALLERGIC REACTIONS

**Anaphylaxis.** In immediate-type allergy, if there is sudden release of the chemical mediators, the response is acute. The acute reaction is *anaphylaxis,* the prototype of immediate-type hypersensitivity. If a small amount of foreign protein (such as serum or egg white), within itself nonpoisonous, is injected into a suitable animal, the first dose will be without noticeable effect; but if a second injection is given after an interval of 10 to 14 days, severe manifestations promptly appear within *minutes,* and even death may occur. This condition is known as anaphylaxis. The first dose is known as the *sensitizing dose;* the second, the *provocative dose.*

Systemic anaphylaxis, or anaphylactic shock, is a generalized reaction brought about in a sensitized animal on contact with adequate amounts of antigen administered so that rapid dissemination occurs (as intravascularly).

Anaphylaxis or *systemic shock* may best be demonstrated in a guinea pig. A small sensitizing injection of horse serum is followed at the end of 10 to 14 days by a second but larger injection of horse serum. Within *1 or 2 minutes* after the provocative dose, the pig becomes restless and breathes with difficulty. Frantic activity with extreme breathlessness is followed by the pig's death in respiratory failure.

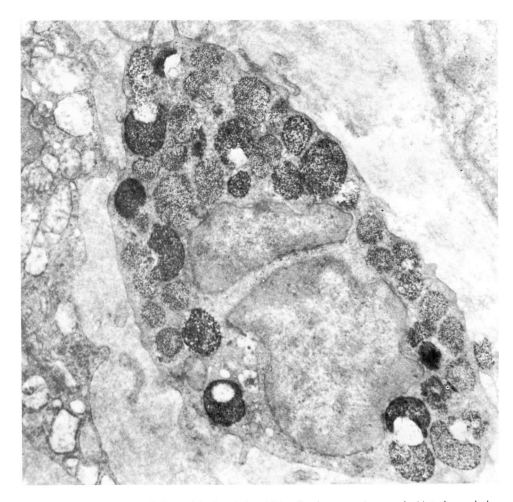

**Fig. 14-2.** Human mast cell (basophil of peripheral blood), electron micrograph. Note large dark granular masses (large, dark blue cytoplasmic granules of Wright-stained blood smears). They store histamine and heparin. (From Barrett, J. T.: Textbook of immunology, ed. 2, St. Louis, 1974, The C. V. Mosby Co.)

Anaphylaxis is specific; that is, for anaphylaxis to occur, the sensitizing and provocative doses must be of the same substance. If the serum of a sensitized animal is injected into a normal animal and if after an interval of 6 to 8 hours the normal animal is injected with some of the material to which the first animal is sensitive, signs of anaphylaxis appear in the normal animal. This is *passive anaphylaxis*. The passive transfer of the hypersensitive state assumes considerable importance when it is realized that the use of an allergic donor for blood transfusion may render the recipient hypersensitive. One interesting case is reported in which, after receiving blood from a donor sensitive to horse dander, the recipient had an attack of asthma on contact with a horse. If an actively sensitized animal survives an anaphylactic attack, it is

desensitized for a few days, but it eventually becomes sensitive again.

*Role of smooth muscle.* The dramatic manifestations of anaphylaxis result from the contraction of smooth muscle fibers, and the part of the body primarily attacked in a given animal depends on the distribution of smooth muscle fibers in the species. In the guinea pig, smooth muscle fibers are plentiful in the lungs; contraction of these closes bronchioles and bronchi and leads to death from respiratory tract obstruction. In the rabbit, smooth muscle is plentiful in the pulmonary arteries. If the rabbit is used as a test animal, these arteries contract, and a burden that leads to failure is thrown on the right side of the heart.

That anaphylactic shock causes contraction of smooth muscle may be proved in the following man-

**Table 14-2**

Makeup of the anaphylactic set*

| ITEM | NUMBER NEEDED | ITEM | NUMBER NEEDED |
|---|---|---|---|
| Ampules of 1:1000 solution of epinephrine (1 ml.) | 2 | Syringes, 2 ml. | 2 |
| Hypodermic needles | 2 | Needles (1 and 4 in. long) | 2 |
| Ampules of aminophylline (0.24 gm. each) | 2 | Bottles of 5% solution dextrose in distilled water, 1000 ml. | 1 |
| Intravenous set | 1 | Ampule of diphenhydramine hydrochloride, 10 ml. (10 mg./ml.) | 1 |
| Bottle of hydrocortisone (dilution to 2 ml. gives 50 mg./ml.) | 1 | Ampule of sterile water | 1 |
| Scalpel | 1 | Hemostat | 1 |
| Ampule of absorbable surgical suture (catgut) with needle | 1 | Syringe, 20 ml. | 1 |
| Tongue depressors | | Alcohol, 70% (disinfectant) | |
| Gauze sponges | | | |

*This kind of emergency must be anticipated. At the Mayo Clinic, Rochester, Minn., "anaphylactic sets" are placed in strategic areas. They contain the above items, quickly available, to be used in the event of such a reaction.

ner. Take a strip of fresh tissue containing an abundance of smooth muscle (for instance, the uterine muscle of the guinea pig) from an animal that has been sensitized and place it in a bath of Ringer's solution. Make one end of the strip stationary and attach the other end to a recording instrument (kymograph). When only a small amount of the sensitizing substance is added to the solution, vigorous contraction of the smooth muscle will occur and be registered on the kymograph. This is the *Schultz-Dale reaction.*

*Anaphylaxis in man.* In man anaphylaxis can be an immediate, severe, and fatal reaction, running its course within seconds or minutes. (See Table 14-2.) If the person is sensitive to the given allergen, a very small amount can precipitate the reaction.

When anaphylaxis was first described at the turn of the century, one of the chief causes then was a sting by a member of the insect Order Hymenoptera. Included in this order are bees, yellow jackets, wasps, and hornets. This is still true. It is said today that far more deaths occur from insect stings than from snakebites.*

In all areas of our complex society the number of different substances to which man may become sensitized is astonishing. This is especially true in the field of medicine where a variety of chemicals is used for

many reasons, so that most of the anaphylactic reactions today are the result of sensitivity to drugs that have been used in one way or another for diagnosis and treatment of disease. Reactions of this type are referred to as *iatrogenic* reactions. Table 14-3 lists chemical agents known to have caused systemic anaphylaxis in man.

**Atopic allergy.** Atopic allergy is the designation for a group of well-known human allergies to naturally occurring antigens, chronic manifestations of immediate-type allergy. Here are found hay fever and asthma. By contrast with systemic anaphylaxis, where large doses of antigen are given intravenously, low doses of antigen repeatedly contact mucous membranes.

Allergic diseases are not inherited, but the special tendency for the individual to develop the state of altered reactivity in tissues is. Atopic allergy seems to be present more in some families than in others; however, all the members of an affected family do not have the same condition. One may have hayfever; another, asthma; and still another member, some type of skin eruption. Seldom will all the members of a family manifest the hypersensitive state.

Atopic allergy is associated with the type of antibody called *reagin*, with a special ability to bind to skin or other tissues. Recent observations indicate that reaginic antibody mostly belongs in immunoglobulin class IgE.

*Asthma.* Asthma is a recurrent type of breathlessness coming in acute episodes and described by certain types of respiratory movements and wheezing. It is an allergic condition most often caused by animal

---

*A person with no history of allergy can have a fatal reaction to an insect bite. If one has had a reaction, he should take every precaution in areas of contact, wear the necessary protective clothing, and if need be, carry an emergency kit of appropriate medication. Insect-sting kits are available commercially.

**Table 14-3**

Systemic anaphylaxis in man—documented agents*

| CHEMICAL CLASS | TRADE NAME OF CLINICAL DRUG | ROUTE OF INOCULATION | DEATH |
|---|---|---|---|
| *Proteins* | | | |
| Antiserum of horse (in passive immunization) | | Parenteral | Yes |
| Antirabies serium | | | |
| Tetanus antitoxin | | | |
| Bivalent botulism antitoxin | | | |
| Hormones | | | |
| Insulin | | Subcutaneous | |
| Corticotropin | Acthar Corticotropin | Intravenous | |
| Enzymes | | | |
| Chymotrypsin | | Intramuscular | |
| Trypsin | Parenzyme | Intramuscular | |
| Penicillinase | Neutrapen | Intramuscular | |
| Sting of Hymenoptera (bees, wasps, hornets, and yellow jackets) | | Subcutaneous (insect bite) | Yes |
| Pollen | | | |
| Bermuda grass | | Intradermal | Yes |
| Ragweed | | Intradermal | Yes |
| Food | | | |
| Egg white | | Intradermal | Yes |
| Buckwheat | | Intradermal | Yes |
| Cotton seed | | Intradermal | Yes |
| Glue | | Intradermal | Yes |
| *Polysaccharides* | | | |
| Acacia (emulsifier) | | Intravenous | |
| Dextran (plasma expander) | Expandex, Gentran | Intravenous | |
| *Others: action as haptens* | | | |
| Antibiotics | | | |
| Penicillin | | Oral and parenteral | Yes |
| Demethylchlortetracycline hydrochloride | Declomycin | Oral | |
| Nitrofurantoin | Furadantin | Oral | |
| Streptomycin | | Intramuscular | |
| Other medications | | | |
| Sodium dehydrocholate | Decholin | Intravenous | Yes |
| Thiamine | | Subcutaneous and intravenous | Yes |
| Salicylates (aspirin) | | Oral | |
| Procaine | Novocaine | Parenteral | Yes |
| Diagnostic agents | | | |
| Sulfobromophthalein | Bromsulphalein (BSP) | Intravenous | Yes |
| Iodinated organic contrast agents | | Oral and intravenous | Yes |

*Data from Austen, K. F.: Systemic anaphylaxis in man, J.A.M.A. **192:**108, 1965.

hair, feathers or dander, house dust, foods, microbes, and certain cosmetics. Important asthma-producing foods are milk, milk products, eggs, meat, fish, and cereals. A person may become sensitive to the bacteria normally inhabiting the upper respiratory tract and thereby become a victim of asthmatic attacks. This type of asthma is spoken of as *endogenous* asthma. An estimated 4% of the population has asthma.

*Hay fever.* Hay fever, with its well-known nasal symptoms, results from sensitivity to pollens, and the period of attack corresponds to the time of pollination of the offending plant or plants. To be important as a cause of hay fever, a plant must produce a light dry pollen that is easily carried a long distance by the wind. This excuses both goldenrod and roses, long accorded an unearned distinction as causes of hay fever. Early spring hay fever is usually caused by the pollen of trees. Late spring and early summer hay fever is most often from grass pollens, and more than 80% of the cases of fall hay fever results from ragweed pollen. Ragweed is found only in the United States, parts of Canada, and Mexico. The importance of individual trees, grasses, or other plants depends on geographic location. Ten percent of the population has hay fever.

**Urticaria and allergic skin eruptions.** Allergic skin conditions may come from foods, drugs, chemicals, and a wide variety of other allergens. Urticaria, known sometimes as nettle rash, is an allergic disorder of the skin depicted by the presence of wheals (whitish swellings) or hives (lesions of a strikingly transitory nature at times).

**Serum sickness.** After the administration of an immune serum a reaction known as serum sickness may appear in persons who have never had a previous injection of horse serum and, so far as is known, are not sensitive to horse proteins.

Serum sickness is common, and its manifestations are unpleasant but seldom life-threatening. It usually begins 8 to 12 days after the injection of an immune serum and is typified by skin eruption, swollen, painful, and stiff joints, enlargement of the lymph nodes, leukopenia, and decreased coagulability of the blood. A reaction may occur only around the site of injection (local serum disease). Serum sickness is thought to be caused by the combination of antibodies formed right after the injection with an excess of the serum. (Serum sickness is here classified as an immediate-type response, although it is a disorder combining features of the two major categories of hypersensitivity.)

An immune serum should be administered with extreme caution to asthmatic patients and to those who have had a previous injection of horse serum. Before an immune serum is given, tests to detect sensitivity to horse serum should always be done because the factor responsible for untoward reactions is the horse protein, the medium for some antitoxins and immune serums. The fall in blood pressure, drop in body temperature, and respiratory difficulty resulting from the injection of an immune serum are most likely to appear when the second injection is given 2 or 3 weeks after the first, but severe reactions may occur when a second injection is given months or even years after the first. Anaphylaxis is most likely to occur in man after intravenous injection. Rarely, manifestations may lead to immediate collapse and death.

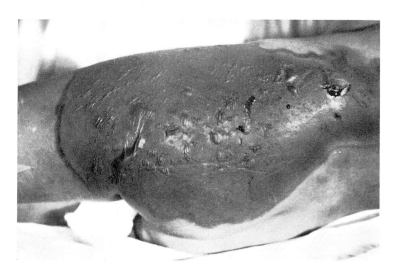

**Fig. 14-3.** Arthus phenomenon in sharply set-off area in skin of hip and thigh. Note discoloration associated with hemorrhage and death of tissue. (From Top, F. H., Sr.: Communicable and infectious diseases, ed. 6, St. Louis, 1968, The C. V. Mosby Co.)

*Arthus phenomenon.* The Arthus (toxic complex) phenomenon (Fig. 14-3) shows us how immunologic mechanisms may damage tissues. When material (an antigen) to which an individual is sensitized is *re*introduced into his body, the Arthus phenomenon may develop in a localized area of skin about the injection site. Although considered an immediate type of allergy, this reaction appears after a delay of several hours at least. Skin involvement results from an intricate sequence of events set in motion when the injected antigen combines with antibody present and precipitates as a complex in the subendothelial layer of blood vessels. The complex fixes complement and, in so doing, triggers an inflammatory response. The net effect is injury to tissues and primarily to small blood vessels. The area of skin becomes swollen, reddened, hemorrhagic, and may even be necrotic (dead).

## Delayed-type allergic reactions

**Sensitivity to drugs.**\* It is not hard to find persons who exhibit drug allergy, that is, an untoward reaction, to a certain drug or drugs. It is believed that when drugs are regularly taken into the body, a chemical combination may occur between the drug and certain body proteins, forming a complete antigen in a protein compound foreign to the body and one against which the mechanisms responsible for allergic manifestations are directed. True allergic drug reactions may be associated either with humoral antibodies or cell-mediated responses.

It has been estimated that about 500 drugs are capable of bringing about the allergic state. The ones most commonly responsible for a hypersensitive state in the person using them are the opiates (morphine, codeine), salicylates (aspirin), barbiturates, iodides, bromides, arsenicals, sulfonamides, and antibiotics. Among the drugs inducing allergy, penicillin is the worst offender; an allergy to the drug occurs in 10% to 15% of the instances where it is given. For other drugs, fortunately, the incidence is much lower.

Sensitivity to the sulfonamide drugs is most likely when the drugs are used in the form of topical ointments. Because of the likelihood that sensitivity might occur after the local use of the sulfonamide drugs and penicillin as well, this type of therapy has almost completely disappeared. Sensitivity to the antibiotics regularly appears as a skin eruption. In a gen-

eral way a reaction to penicillin and certain other antibiotics often closely resembles serum sickness. The same is true of reactions to insulin and liver extract. If a previous reaction to penicillin has taken place or if there is reason to think that the patient is hypersensitive to the drug, it should *not* be given. Penicillin is said to have caused more deaths than has any other drug.\* No reliance should be placed on desensitization.

**Infectious allergies (hypersensitivity to infection).** Repeated or chronic infections may sensitize a patient to the microbes causing the infection. This is well illustrated in the allergy to *Mycobacterium tuberculosis* and its products. When an extract of *Mycobacterium tuberculosis* is applied to the skin of the person who has or has had tuberculosis, there is a reaction, and the tuberculin test is said to be positive. Patients may likewise be hypersensitive to other organisms such as *Brucella* (the causative agents of undulant fever). In fact, the manifestations of acute rheumatic fever are considered as an allergic reaction to streptococci.

Other infections in which hypersensitivity to causative agent are measured are leprosy, chancroid, lymphopathia venereum, coccidioidomycosis, blastomycosis, and histoplasmosis. In veterinary medicine hypersensitivity of infection is seen in glanders, Bang's disease (undulant fever), and Johne's disease. In some of these, diagnostic skin tests are used to detect sensitivity. (See Table 13-2.)

**Contact dermatitis.** Contact dermatitis localizes in the skin, especially in areas exposed to direct physical contact with irritant substances of many different kinds. As would be expected, this inflammatory condition is often seen on the hands. The first time that the skin contacts the offending substance there is no visible effect, but sensitization means that subsequent contacts will result in skin changes. Contact dermatitis is sometimes referred to as eczema or eczematous dermatitis. The list of offenders is a long one. It includes the well-known poisons of poison ivy and poison oak† and a vast host of substances related to trade and industry, such as dyes, soaps, lacquers, plastics, woods, fabrics, furs, formalin, cosmetics, drugs, chemicals, metals, and explosives. (See Fig. 14-4.)

**Autoallergies.** See p. 501.

---

\**Drug intolerance* is the state in which a person receiving the drug reacts in a characteristic way to unusually small doses of the drug, doses that have no physiologic effect.

*Drug idiosyncrasy* refers to the situation in which the recipient of the drug reacts in an unusual way, as for example when a dose of a barbiturate (a sedative) produces excitement.

---

\*Penicillin as such does not induce hypersensitivity; it is the degradation products that can become haptens. A skin test can be done with one of these, penicilloyl-polylysine, to indicate the probable risk of an allergic reaction.

†Poison ivy, oak, and sumac belong to the *Rhus* genus of trees and shrubs; the skin lesions may be called rhus dermatitis. The *Rhus* plants are responsible for more allergic contact dermatitis than all other allergens combined.

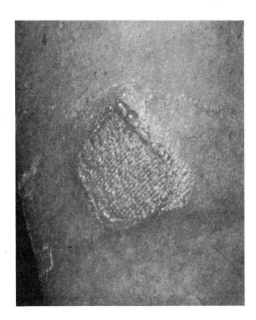

**Fig. 14-4.** Contact dermatitis—positive patch test to rubber from bathing cap. Note blisters and texture of skin. Similar reaction occurs with formalin, mercury, or other simple chemicals used as test antigens in a sensitized person. (From Leider, M.: Practical pediatric dermatology, ed. 2, St. Louis, 1961, The C. V. Mosby Co.)

## Laboratory tests to detect allergy*

If some of the antigen to which a person is sensitive is rubbed in a scratch on the skin or if some of the dilute antigen is injected between the layers of the skin, a wheal and flare of 0.5 to 2 cm. in diameter will occur at the site of contact within 20 to 30 minutes (cutaneous anaphylaxis). If the person is not sensitive to the antigen, no reaction will occur. This is the *skin test*.

The *ophthalmic test* helps to detect sensitization to serum. A drop of the *diluted* serum is instilled into the conjunctival sac; if the patient is sensitive to horse serum, redness of the conjunctiva and a watery discharge will appear within 10 to 20 minutes. The reaction may be controlled by epinephrine.

The *patch test* is useful in detecting the cause of contact dermatitis. In this test the suspect material is applied directly to the skin and held in place by means of adhesive tape for 1 to 4 days. A positive reaction reproduces the lesion from which the patient is suffering, with blister and papule formation.

## Desensitization

In some cases desensitization may be accomplished by giving repeated injections of very small

---

* See also p. 407.

amounts of the antigen to which the patient is sensitive. A patient hypersensitive to horse serum may sometimes be given an immune serum if the administration is preceded by several injections of very small amounts at 30-minute intervals. The desensitizing doses are graded by the reaction of the patient, and the administration of an immune serum to a hypersensitive person should be undertaken only by those with experience in immune therapy. A similar but much prolonged method of desensitization is used in the treatment of hay fever and selected cases of asthma and urticaria. Desensitization, unlike sensitization, is of relatively short duration. In some forms of allergy it is accomplished with great difficulty.

## Questions for review

1 Compare the two major categories of allergic disorders.
2 Briefly discuss anaphylaxis.
3 Describe briefly the most important allergic diseases.
4 What is serum sickness? Why is it less common than previously?
5 What effect has the development of sensitivity to the sulfonamides and antibiotics had on the topical use of these drugs?
6 Outline the laboratory diagnosis of allergy.
7 Explain the role in allergy postulated for immunoglobulin E.
8 Explain the relation of the basophil to allergic disorders.
9 How is desensitization accomplished?
10 List five agents known to have caused anaphylaxis in man.
11 What are the infectious allergies? How can they be detected?
12 Define or briefly explain: hypersensitivity, allergy, sensitizing dose, provocative dose, allergen, immunopathology, Arthus phenomenon, Schultz-Dale reaction, reagin, iatrogenic, endogenous, insect sting kit, drug intolerance, drug idiosyncrasy, cutaneous anaphylaxis.

**REFERENCES** (Chapters 10 to 14)

Abrams, B. L., and Waterman, N. G.: Dirty money, J.A.M.A. **219:**1202, 1972.

Anderson, C. L.: Community health, ed. 2, St. Louis, 1973, The C. V. Mosby Co.

Bahn, A. K.: Epidemiology as a field of practice, J. Am. Med. Wom. Assoc. **29:**387, 1974.

Barnako, D.: The environment: rats, J.A.M.A. **218:**663, 1971.

Barnett, S. A.: Rats, Sci. Am. **216:**78, Jan., 1967.

Barr, S. E: Allergy to Hymenoptera stings, J.A.M.A. **228:** 718, 1974.

Barrett, J. T.: Textbook of immunology, ed. 2, St. Louis, 1974, The C. V. Mosby Co.

Bazaral, M., and others: IgE levels in normal infants and mothers and an inheritance hypothesis, J. Immunol. **107:** 794, 1971.

Bellanti, J.: Immunology, Philadelphia, 1971, W. B. Saunders Co.

Benenson, A. S., editor: Control of communicable diseases in man, New York, 1970, American Public Health Association.

Bergman, N., and others: Antibacterial activity of human amniotic fluid, Am. J. Obstet. Gynecol. **114:**520, 1972.

Berland, T.: Mrs. Berland, your son is just plain lousy, Today's Health **52:**39, June, 1974.

Bernton, H. S., and Brown, H.: Insect allergy: allergenicity of excrement of the cockroach, Ann. Allergy **28:**543, 1970.

Billingham, R., and Silvers, W.: The immunobiology of transplantation, Englewood Cliffs, N.J., 1971, Prentice-Hall, Inc.

Black, F. L.: Infectious diseases in primitive societies, Science **187:**515, 1975.

Block, V.: Wild pets could turn them off, Today's Health **46:**56, Dec., 1968.

Booth, B., and others: Modern concepts in clinical allergy, New York, 1973, Medcom Books, Inc.

Bruninga, G. L.: Complement—a review of the chemistry and reaction mechanisms, Am. J. Clin. Pathol. **55:**273, 1971.

Buckley, C. E., III: Immunologic evaluation of older patients, Postgrad. Med. **51:**235, 1972.

Burnet, F. M.: Immunological surveillance, New York, 1970, Pergamon Press, Inc.

Burnet, F. M.: Auto-immunity and auto-immune disease, Philadelphia, 1972, F. A. Davis Co.

Cancer antigens (editorial), J.A.M.A. **221:**66, 1972.

Cartwright, R. Y.: Commensal bacteria of the human respiratory tract, Nurs. Times **70:**418, March 21, 1974.

Castillo, P.: Methods of warming blood, AORN Journal **14:**82, Aug., 1971.

Cawley, L. P.: Electrophoresis and immunoelectrophoresis, Boston, 1969, Little, Brown & Co.

Chandor, S. B.: Serum immunoglobulin levels in older individuals, Lab. Med. **4:**25, June, 1973.

Chapman, J. S.: The environment: animal to human infection, J.A.M.A. **213:**1559, 1970.

Civantos, F., and others: Protein immunoelectrophoresis, Lab. Med. **4:**37, March, 1973.

Cline, M. J., and others: UCLA Conference, Granulocytes in human disease, Ann. Intern. Med. **81:**801, 1974.

Cohen, E. P.: Must you have shots for hay fever? Today's Health **52:**54, July, 1974.

Craven, R. F.: Anaphylactic shock, Am. J. Nurs. **72:**718, 1972.

Culliton, B. J.: Immunology: two immune systems capture attention, Science **180:**45, 1973.

Culliton, B. J.: Restoring immunity: marrow and thymus transplants may do it, Science **180:**168, 1973.

Danilevicius, Z.: HL-A system and rheumatic disease, J.A.M.A. **231:**283, 1975.

Diamond, L. K.: The Rh problem through a retrospectroscope, Am. J. Clin. Pathol. **62:**311, 1974.

Dixon, F. J., and Kunkel, H. G., editors: Advances in immunology, vol. 19, New York, 1974, Academic Press, Inc.

Dodd, R. Y.: Transmissible disease and blood transfusion Science **186:**1138, 1974.

Dong, E., Jr., and Shumway, N. E.: The current status of heart transplantation (editorial), South. Med. J. **67:**255, 1974.

Edelman, G. M.: Antibody structure and molecular immunology, Science **180:**830, 1973.

Ellis, F. R., and others: Application of Gm typing in cases of disputed paternity, J. Forensic Sci. **18:**290, 1973.

Erskine, A. G., and Wiener, A. S.: The principles and practices of blood grouping, St. Louis, 1973, The C. V. Mosby Co.

Evans, H. E., and others: Factors influencing the establishment of neonatal bacterial flora. Part II, Arch. Environ. Health **21:**643, 1970.

Evans, H. E., and others: Flora in newborn infants, Arch. Environ. Health **26:**275, 1973.

Fahey, J. L.: Cancer in the immunosuppressed patient (editorial), Ann. Intern. Med. **75:**310, 1971.

Federman, S.: Underwater weapon in war on mosquitoes, Today's Health **46:**14, June, 1968.

Fenner, F.: Infectious disease and social change. Part 2, Med. J. Aust. **1:**1099, 1971.

Finkel, A., and others: Intrauterine infection and cord immunoglobulin M, Can. Med. Assoc. J. **110:**38, 1974.

Fisher, A. A.: Tracking the mystery rash, Today's Health **47:**66, Jan., 1969.

Fite, G. L.: Canine zoonoses (editorial), J.A.M.A. **231:**497, 1975.

Force, D. C.: Ecology of insect host-parasitoid communities, Science **184:**624, 1974.

Forrester, R. H.: Army research in military blood blanking, South. Med. Bull. **57:**17, June, 1969.

Fort, A. T., and Walker, R. H.: Passive transfer of maternal antibody to the fetus, Lab. Med. **1:**40, June, 1970.

Fotino, M.: Tissue typing for organ transplantation, Bull. S. Cent. Assoc. Blood Banks **14:**4, Nov.-Dec., 1970.

Frazier, C. A.: Coping with food allergy, New York, 1974, Quadrangle/The New York Times Book Co.

Frazier, C. A.: Those deadly insects, RN **34:**49, April, 1971.

Freedman, S. O.: Clinical immunology, New York, 1971, Harper & Row, Publishers.

Fudenberg, H. H., and others: Basic immunogenetics, New York, 1972, Oxford University Press.

Fudenberg, H. H., and others: The therapeutic uses of transfer factor, Hosp. Pract. **9:**95, Jan., 1974.

Giannella, R. A., and others: Influence of gastric acidity of bacterial and parasitic enteric infections, Ann. Intern. Med. **78:**271, 1973.

Gillett, J. D.: The mosquito, its life, activities, and impact on human affairs, New York, 1972, Doubleday & Co., Inc.

Glenn, G. C.: Primary immunologic deficiency diseases, Lab. Med. Bull. Pathol. **10:**293, Sept., 1969.

Goldman, L.: Prevention and treatment of eczema, Am. J. Nurs. **64:**114, March, 1964.

Good, R. A.: On threshold of biologic engineering, Am. J. Med. Technol. **38:**153, May, 1972.

Good, R. A., and Fisher, D. W., editors: Immunobiology, Stamford, Conn., 1971, Sinauer Associates, Inc.

Gotoff, S. P.: Cell-mediated immune deficiency (editorial), J. Pediatr. **78:**379, 1971.

Grothaus, R. H., and Adams, J. F.: An innovation in mosquito-borne disease protection, Milit. Med. **137:**181, 1972.

Grzybowski, S., and others: Tuberculosis in Eskimos, Arch. Environ. Health **25**:329, 1972.

Gunther, M.: Don't feed the rats, Today's Health **53**:48, Jan., 1975.

Guttman, R. D., and others, guest editors: Scope monograph on immunology, Kalamazoo, Mich., 1972, The Upjohn Co.

Haesler, W. E., Jr.: Immunohematology, Medical Technology Series, Philadelphia, 1972, Lea & Febiger.

Halliday, W. J.: Glossary of immunological terms, London, 1971, Butterworth & Co. (Publishers) Ltd.

Headington, J. T.: Applied microbiology in skin diseases, Lab. Med. **1**:45, Sept., 1970.

Heinz, W. C.: The man who said, "They don't have to die," Today's Health **49**:26, Jan., 1971.

Henderson, L. L.: Acute reaction to insect sting, Postgrad. Med. **49**:191, May, 1971.

Herbert, W. J., and Wilkinson, P. C., editors: A dictionary of immunology, Philadelphia, 1971, F. A. Davis Co.

Higdon, R. S.: Common insect, mite, and parasite problems in the United States, GP **37**:84, May, 1968.

Holborow, E. J.: An ABC of modern immunology, ed. 2, Boston, 1973, Little, Brown & Co.

Immunological power of the lymphocyte (editorial), J.A.M.A. **206**:2514, 1968.

Irwin, T.: Fever: how to play it cool, Today's Health **46**:52, Dec., 1968.

Isler, C.: Blood, the age of components, RN **36**:31, June, 1973.

Kelly, J. F., and Patterson, R.: Anaphylaxis, course, mechanisms, and treatment, J.A.M.A. **227**:1431, 1974.

Klebanoff, S. J.: Neutrophils and host defense (editorial) Calif. Med. **114**:47, June, 1971.

Kolata, G. B.: Antibody diversity: how many antibody genes? Science **186**:432, 1974.

Kountz, S. L.: Current status of kidney transplantation, New Physician **22**:550, Sept., 1973.

Kountz, S. L., and Pindyck, J. L.: Tissue typing for clinical transplantation, New Physician **23**:56, Sept., 1974.

Laskin, A. I., and Lechevalier, H., editors: Macrophages and cellular immunity, Cleveland, 1972, CRC Press.

Lehrer, R. I.: The role of phagocyte function in resistance to infection, Calif. Med. **114**:17, June, 1971.

Levine, P.: Suppression of Rh sensitization by Rh immunoglobulin, Bull. Pathol. **9**:46, 1968.

Limax, A.: What immunity to disease means to you, Today's Health **43**:54, Nov., 1965.

Lockey, R. F.: Systemic reactions to stinging ants, J. Allergy Clin. Immunol. **54**:132, Sept., 1974.

Marples, M. J.: Life on the human skin, Sci. Am. **220**:108, Jan., 1969.

Maugh, T. H., II: Tissue cultures: transplantation without immune suppression, Science **181**:929, 1973.

McAllen, M. K.: Hay fever, Nurs. Mirror **138**:63, May 24, 1974.

McCluskey, R. T., and Cohen, S., editors: Mechanisms of cell-mediated immunity, New York, 1974, John Wiley & Sons, Inc.

McDevitt, H. O.: Genetic control of the antibody response, Hosp. Pract. **8**:61, April, 1973.

McDonald, J. C., and Wallace, J.: I. Transplantation immunology. II. Histocompatibility testing. III. Renal transplantation. IV. Transplantation of organs other than kidney. V. Providing transplantation to the population, South. Med. Bull. **58**:9, Feb., 1970.

McKelvey, J. H., Jr.: Man against Tsetse, struggle for Africa, Ithaca, N.Y., 1973, Cornell University Press.

Medawar, P. B.: The new immunology, Hosp. Pract. **9**:48, Sept., 1974.

Milam, J. D.: Clinical use and risks of certain blood derivatives. J. S. Cent. Assoc. Blood Banks **17**:9, July-Aug., 1974.

Miller, M. E.: WHO's immunodeficiencies (editorial), Ann. Intern. Med. **77**:149, 1972.

Minkin, W., and Lynch, P. J.: Incidence of immediate systemic penicillin reactions, Milit. Med. **133**:557, 1968.

Mollison, P. L.: Blood transfusions in clinical medicine, Philadelphia, 1973, F. A. Davis Co

Montes, L. F., and others: Microbial flora of infant's skin, Arch. Dermatol. **103**:400, 1971.

Moody, L.: Asthma: physiology and patient care, Am. J. Nurs. **73**:1212, 1973.

Moore, F. D.: Transplant, the give and take of tissue transplantation, New York, 1972, Simon & Schuster, Inc.

Movat, H. Z., editor: Inflammation, immunity and hypersensitivity, New York, 1971, Harper & Row, Publishers.

Murillo, G. J.: Synthesis of secretory IgA by human colostral cells, South. Med. J. **64**:1333, 1971.

Murray, J. E., and Barnes, B. A.: Organ transplant registry (editorial), J.A.M.A. **217**:1546, 1971.

Ness, P. M.: Plasma fractionation in the United States; a review for clinicians, J.A.M.A. **230**:247, 1974.

Nichols, G. A., and Kucha, D. H.: Taking adult temperatures: oral measurements, Am. J. Nurs. **72**:1090, 1972.

Notkins, A. L.: Viral infections: mechanisms of immunologic defense and injury, Hosp. Pract. **9**:65, Sept., 1974.

Organ transplantation (editorial), J.A.M.A. **223**:320, 1973.

Oxborrow, G. S., and Puleo, J. R.: Microbiological studies of spacecraft, Lab. Med. **1**:17, Oct., 1970.

Paine, R. T., and Zaret, T. M.: Ecological gambling, the high risks and rewards of species introductions, J.A.M.A. **231**:471, 1975.

Palmer, R. L.: Diagnostic aids for immunological disorders, Tex. Med. **67**:79, March, 1971.

Patterson, R., and others: Mast cells from human respiratory tissue and their in vitro reactivity, Science **175**:1012, 1972.

Petersdorf, R. G.: The physiology, pathogenesis and diagnosis of fever, Resident Physician **14**:67, March, 1968.

Petersdorf, R. G.: Penicillin (editorial), J.A.M.A. **209**:1520, 1969.

Pierce, J. C., and others: Lymphoma, a complication of renal allotransplantation in man, J.A.M.A. **219**:1593, 1972.

Porter, R. R.: The structure of antibodies, Sci. Am. **217**:81, Oct., 1967.

Porter, R. R.: Structural studies of immunoglobins, Science **180**:713, 1973.

Potter, H., and others: Transfer factor, Ann. Intern. Med. **81**:838, 1974.

Race, R. R., and Sanger, R.: Blood groups in man, Philadelphia, 1968, F. A. Davis Co.

Reeves, W. C.: Can the war to contain infectious diseases be lost? Am. J. Trop. Med. Hyg. **21:**251, 1972.

Reisfeld, R. A., and Kahan, B. D.: Makers of biological individuality, Sci. Am. **226:**28, June, 1972.

Remington, J. S.: The compromised host, Hosp. Pract. **7:**59, April, 1972.

Richards, F. F., and others: On the specificity of antibodies, Science **187:**130, 1975.

Ritzmann, S. E., and Daniels, J. C.: Immunology of transplantation, Tex. Med. **66:**48, May, 1970.

Rogers, R. S., III, and Callaway, J. L.: Contact dermatitis. Part I. Plants (Rhus) and chemicals as causative agents, Hosp. Med. **7:**6, 1971.

Rose, N. R., and others, editors: Methods in immuno-diagnosis, New York, 1973, John Wiley & Sons, Inc.

Rosenstein, D. L.: Transfusion therapy, Bull. S. Cent. Assoc. Blood Banks, **15:**11, May-June, 1971.

Roueché, B.: Poison ivy: "its purpose has yet to be established," Today's Health **49:**38, May, 1971.

Safran, C.: Those summer allergies, Today's Health **51:**18, July, 1973.

Schwartz, L. M., and Schwartz, P.: An exercise manual in immunology, Medcom Workbook/Manual Series, New York, 1975, Medcom Books, Inc.

Scott, B.: Asthma—the demon that thrives on myths, Today's Health **48:**42, June, 1970.

Segal, A. W., and others: Reevaluation of nitroblue tetrazolium test, Lancet **2:**879,1973.

Sell, S.: Immunopathologic mechanisms. Part I. Allergic phenomena mediated by antibody. Part II. Allergic phenomena mediated by cells, Bull. Rheum. Dis. **19:**546, 1969.

Sell, S.: Immunology, immunopathology and immunity, New York, 1972, Harper & Row, Publishers.

Shaffer, J. H., and Sweet, L. C.: Allergic reactions to drugs, Am. J. Nurs. **65:**100, Oct., 1965.

Sindermann, C. J.: Diseases of marine animals transmissible to man, Lab. Med. **1:**50, Jan., 1970.

Smith, G. P.: The variation and adaptive expression of antibodies, Cambridge, Mass., 1973, Harvard University Press.

Sokol, A. B., and Houser, R. G.: Dog bites: prevention and treatment, Clin. Pediatr. **10:**336, 1971.

Stastny, P.: HL-A antigens in mummified pre-Columbian tissues, Science **183:**864, 1974.

Steele, J. H.: What is the current state of the zoonoses? Lab. Med. **1:**28, Dec., 1970.

Stiehm, E. R., moderator: UCLA Conference—Diseases of cellular immunity, Ann. Intern. Med. **77:**101, 1972.

Stiehm, E. R., and Fulginiti, V. A.: Immunologic disorders in infants and children, Philadelphia, 1973, W. B. Saunders Co.

Sumida, S.: Transfusion of blood preserved by freezing, Philadelphia, 1973, J. B. Lippincott Co.

Sussman, L. N.: Au antigen test—a simplified technique, Lab. Med. **2:**11, Nov., 1971.

The control of lice and louse-borne diseases. Proceedings of a symposium, Washington, D.C., Dec., 1972, Washington, D.C., 1973, Pan American Health Organization, Sci. Pub. No. 263.

Thompson, E., and others: Changes in antigenic nature of lymphocytes caused by common viruses, Br. Med. J. **4:**709, Dec. 22, 1973.

Valentry, D.: The fantastic fly, Today's Health **47:**56, Aug., 1969.

Van Boxel, J. A., and others: IgD-bearing human lymphocytes, J. Immunol. **109:**648, 1972.

Van Furth, R., editor: Mononuclear phagocytes, Philadelphia, 1970, J. B. Lippincott Co.

Walls, K. W., and Hall, L. S.: New concepts in automated diagnostic complement fixation techniques in microbiology, Lab. Med. **4:**31, April, 1973.

Ward, F. A.: A primer of immunology, New York, 1970, Appleton-Century-Crofts.

Weiser, R. S., and others: Fundamentals of immunology, Philadelphia, 1969, Lea & Febiger.

Weiss, H. J.: Aspirin—a dangerous drug? J.A.M.A. **229:**1221, 1974.

Weiss, L.: The cells and tissues of the immune system; structure, functions, interactions, Englewood Cliffs, N.J., 1972, Prentice-Hall, Inc.

Wilson, D.: Body and antibody; a report on the new immunology, New York, 1972, Alfred A. Knopf, Inc.

Wolkomir, R.: Stinging insects—armed and dangerous, Today's Health **47:**48, June, 1969.

Wright, D. N., and Alexander, J. M.: Effect of water on bacterial flora of swimmer's ears, Arch. Otolaryngol. **99:**15, 1974.

Wybran, J., and Fudenberg, H.: How clinically useful is T and B cell quantitation? (editorial), Ann. Intern. Med. **80:**765, 1974.

Yates, U. M.: Transplantation: today and tomorrow, Today's Health **46:**33, April, 1968.

Zmijewski, C. A., and Fletcher, J. L.: Immunohematology, ed. 2, Englewood Cliffs, N.J., 1972, Prentice-Hall, Inc.

CHAPTER 15

# Physical agents in sterilization

*Sterilization* is the process of killing or removing all forms of life, especially microorganisms, associated with a given object or present in a given area. This includes bacteria and their spores, fungi (molds, yeasts), and viruses (which must be either destroyed or inactivated). An object on and within which all microbes are killed or removed is said to be *sterile*. The length of time that an object remains sterile depends on how well it is protected from microorganisms after it is sterilized. For instance, the outside of a tube of culture medium soon becomes contaminated because it is in direct contact with the microorganisms of the air, whereas inside the tube the culture medium, protected from microorganisms by the cotton plug, remains sterile indefinitely. Bacteria that have been killed are unable to multiply, but their bodies are not necessarily completely destroyed. The dead bodies of certain bacteria may retain their shape and staining qualities and even promote the production of antibodies when introduced into the bodies of man or lower animals.

Sterilization may be accomplished by mechanical means, by heat, or by chemicals.

## Removal of microbes by mechanical means

There are three chief mechanical methods of removing microbes: (1) scrubbing, (2) filtration, and (3) sedimentation.

**Scrubbing.** Scrubbing is usually done with water to which some chemical agent such as soap, detergent, or sodium carbonate has been added. The process is both mechanical and chemical. Scrubbing, by itself, removes many microorganisms mechanically while the incorporated chemical acts on them chemically. Scrubbing with soap (or detergent) and water is a very important process basic to any discussion of sterilization, since the removal of dirt, debris, and extraneous matter from an area or object is a preliminary step to the effective removal of microbes therefrom by any method. Hands and person, floors, walls, woodwork, furniture, utensils of all kinds, glassware, linens, clothing, instruments, thermometers—all must be clean.

**Filtration.** Bacterial filtration is the process of passing a liquid containing bacteria through a material whose pores are so small that the bacteria are held back. The mechanical removal or separation of the bacteria from the fluid renders it sterile. In the laboratory this process is used for sterilizing liquids and culture media that cannot be heated and for separating toxins, enzymes, and proteins from the bacteria that produced them. Certain pharmaceutical preparations are sterilized in this way. The materials most often used for bacterial filtration are unglazed porcelain, diatomaceous earth, asbestos, sintered glass, and cellulose membranes. (The finest-mesh filter paper of the best quality will not hold back bacteria, but the pore size of a cellulose membrane filter may be reduced so that even certain viruses are retained.) Bacterial filters are constructed so that the material to be filtered is made to pass through a disk or the wall of a hollow tube made of the filtering material. Viruses passing through bacteria-retaining filters are said to be *filtrable*.

Filtration is an important step in the purification process of a city water supply (p. 382). Bacterial filtration by a plastic membrane technic is widely used as a laboratory procedure in sanitary microbiology (p. 381).

**Sedimentation.** The process by which suspended particles settle to the bottom of a liquid is sedimentation. It finds practical application in the purification of water by natural or artificial means. In nature large particles and suspended bacteria sink to the bottom of lakes, ponds, and flowing streams. Sedimentation plays a significant role in the artificial purification of water (p. 381).

## Sterilization by moist heat

The most widely applicable and effective sterilizing agent is heat. It also is the most economical and easily controlled. The temperature that kills a 24-hour liquid culture of a certain species of bacteria at a pH of 7 (neutral reaction) in 10 minutes is known as the *thermal death point* of that species. Since this represents the temperature at which all bacteria are killed, it is obvious that many are destroyed before this temperature is reached. In fact, most are destroyed within the first few minutes. For purposes of standardization bacteria must be in a neutral medium when their thermal death point is determined because in either a highly acid or a highly alkaline medium they are more susceptible to heat. The *thermal death time* is the time required to kill all bacteria in a given suspension at a given temperature.

Aside from burning (really a chemical process) heat may be applied in the form of *moist heat* or *dry heat*. Moist heat may be applied as hot water or as steam and is the method of choice in sterilization except for those objects altered or damaged by it. See Table 15-1 for applications of heat sterilization.

**Boiling.** A commonly employed, although incompletely effective, method of sterilizing by moist heat is boiling. Boiling kills vegetative forms of pathogenic bacteria, fungi, and viruses in a matter of a few minutes. Hepatitis viruses are destroyed at the end of 30 minutes. For practical elimination of hepatitis viruses, however, boiling is *not* recommended. Spores are less readily destroyed. Although most of the spores of pathogenic bacteria can be destroyed in a boiling time of 30 minutes, boiling is not a reliable method when materials are likely to contain spores. Certain heat-loving saprophytes can survive at high temperatures, and their spores resist *prolonged* boiling for many hours.

The addition of sodium carbonate to make a 2% solution in boiling water hastens the destruction of spores and helps to prevent rusting of instruments. Surgical instruments, needles, and syringes that are boiled must be clean and free of organic material. Remember that microbes will not be eliminated in the interior of the materials boiled until heat has penetrated there. Boiling must be continued long enough to ensure even distribution of heat through the object being sterilized. Such objects must be completely immersed in the boiling water. Boiling time should be prolonged 5 minutes for each 1000 feet above sea level.

**Sterilization by steam.** Steam gives up heat by condensing back into water. For instance, when a bundle containing fabrics such as pads or sponges is sterilized by steam, the steam contacts the outer layer, where a portion of it condenses into water and gives up heat. The steam then penetrates to a second layer, where another portion condenses into water and gives up heat. The steam thus approaches the center of the package, layer after layer, until the whole package is sterilized.

Steam may be applied as free-flowing steam or as steam under pressure. Free-flowing steam has about the same sterilizing action as boiling water. Steam under pressure is the most powerful method

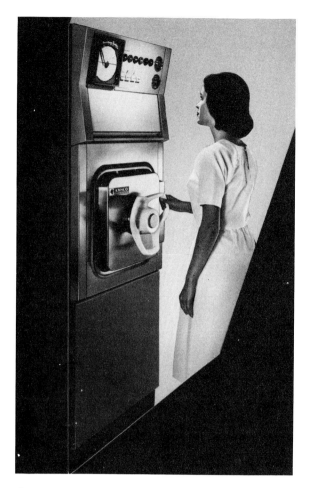

**Fig. 15-1.** Pressure steam sterilizer or autoclave, cabinet model. (Courtesy American Sterilizer Co., Erie, Pa.)

of sterilizing that we possess and is the preferred method unless the material being sterilized is injured by heat or moisture. The process is carried out in the *pressure steam sterilizer*, familiarly known as the *autoclave* (Figs. 15-1 and 15-2). It consists of a square sterilizing chamber surrounded by a steam jacket. The outside of the steam jacket is insulated and covered. The chamber is loaded with supplies to be sterilized (the load) through a door that closes the front end of the sterilizing chamber. This is a safety steam-locked door made tight against a flexible heat-resistant gasket. The design is such that steam can be admitted to the closed chamber under pressure. The source of the steam varies; it may come from the central boiler supply of a large hospital or from an electrically heated boiler on the instrument itself. Valves on the autoclave control the flow and exhaust of steam. On some of the pressure steam sterilizers, these valves are operated by hand, but in the modern ver-

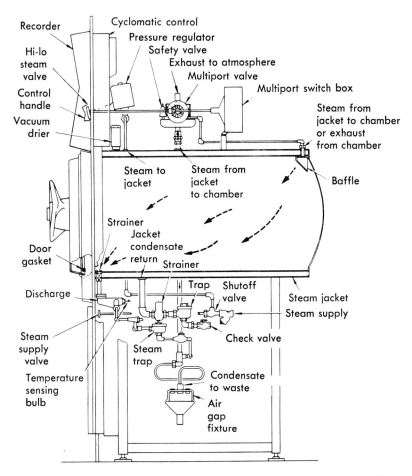

**Fig. 15-2.** Autoclave (pressure steam sterilizer), gravity air removal type. Diagram of longitudinal cross section. (Courtesy American Sterilizer Co., Erie, Pa.)

sions the entire operation of the instrument is automatically designed.

*Steam under pressure* is hotter than free-flowing steam, and the higher the pressure, the higher the temperature. The temperature of free-flowing steam is 100° C. At 15 pounds' pressure (atmospheric pressure at sea level) the temperature of steam is 121° C., and at 20 pounds' pressure it is 126° C. *Sterilization by steam under pressure is the result of the heat of the moist steam under pressure and not of the pressure itself.* Steam under a pressure of 15 or 20 pounds will kill all organisms and spores in 15 to 45 minutes (depending on the materials involved). To maintain these temperatures at higher altitudes, the pressure must be increased 1 pound for each 2000-foot increase in altitude.

*Operation of an autoclave.* In the method of steam sterilization carried out in an autoclave (see Fig. 15-2) the long-used principle has been the "down-ward displacement gravity system." (Steam is admitted to the sterilizing chamber in such a way as to drive air down and out. Steam being lighter than air displaces air downward.) In the operation of an autoclave, pressure is first generated in the steam jacket. The connection to the sterilizing chamber is kept closed until jacket pressure is constant at 15 to 17 pounds. (The pressure within the steam jacket is kept constant during the procedure to keep the walls of the chamber heated and dry.) The load is placed in the chamber, and the door secured. Then steam is admitted to the sterilizing chamber, and the load is heated to the temperature of the steam in the chamber. At the time steam enters the chamber, the load and the chamber are both filled with air, which, if not evacuated, would reduce the moisture content of the autoclave and lessen its sterilizing capacity. Pressure steam sterilizers are provided with a vent arrangement whereby the air can escape to the atmosphere as the temperature is raised. When all the air has been evacuated, steam will contact the thermostatic valve, and it closes. The moisture that condenses on the door or back part of the sterilizing chamber drains downward from behind a steam deflector plate to the bottom part of the chamber and is then discharged to the waste line. After the end of the sterilizing cycle, the steam is exhausted from the chamber but not from the jacket. At this point, a drying cycle is effected before the door is opened. This is done by creating a partial vacuum in the chamber with steam from the jacket through an ejector tube on the autoclave and at the same time admitting air through a presterilized filter.

Since sterilization by steam under pressure is primarily a matter of temperature and the increase in pressure plays its part in the sterilizing process by increasing the temperature, the height to which the thermometer rises, rather than the reading on the pressure gauge, should be the guiding factor in the operation of the autoclave. This is particularly true because many pressure gauges are inaccurate. (Autoclaves usually have two pressure gauges, one to indicate the pressure in the steam jacket and the other to indicate the pressure in the sterilizing chamber.) As a whole, inaccurate pressure gauges read too high. A thermometer or the sensing element of a thermometer placed at the bottom of the sterilizer is a better indicator of the efficiency of the sterilizing process than one placed at the top, since if any part of the autoclave fails to receive the full benefit of the steam, it is the bottom part. If the thermometer is placed in the discharge path of air and moisture coming from the sterilizing chamber, it can never indicate less than the lowest temperature in the system.

Modern autoclaves are equipped with a number of controls to increase the efficiency of sterilization and to remove insofar as possible the human factor. The *recording thermometer* is a clock-thermometer mechanism that indicates (1) the time at which the material being sterilized reaches the desired temperature, (2) whether the temperature remains stable, (3) how long the exposure lasts, and (4) how many times the autoclave is in operation during the day. The *indicating potentiometer* is an instrument for actually measuring the temperature of material in the autoclave. The *automatic time-temperature control* (1) operates the autoclave at the time and temperature for which it is set, (2) exhausts the steam from the chamber, (3) governs the process of drying, and (4) sounds an alarm indicating that the operation is complete.

*Indicators* are placed in with the load to be sterilized. An indicator changes in a predictable way

its physiochemical properties or biologic nature when the prescribed temperature for sterilization has been reached. Indicators used are strips of paper impregnated with biologic material such as the dried spores of *Bacillus stearothermophilus*, the thermal death time of which is known. For steam sterilizers, *Bacillus stearothermophilus* is the indicator or challenge microorganism of choice; it grows readily and is more resistant to heat than the microbes usually found on the material being sterilized. For dry heat and ethylene oxide sterilizers (p. 164) *Bacillus subtilis* (var. *globigii* or *niger*) is preferred.

*High-prevacuum sterilizer.** An improved pressure

---

*Basic principles for sterilization are the same in both the gravity air-removal type of sterilizer (just described) and the high-prevacuum one.

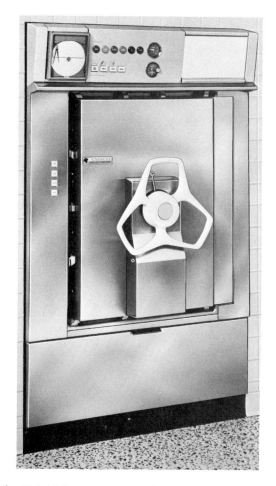

**Fig. 15-3.** High-prevacuum sterilizer (Medium Rectangular Vacamatic). Panel of controls for manual operation behind white panel in upper right of instrument. (Courtesy American Sterilizer Co., Erie, Pa.)

steam sterilizer, the high-prevacuum sterilizer, is in wide use (Fig. 15-3). With a vacuum system incorporated into the sterilizer unit, a precisely controlled vacuum is pulled at the beginning and the end of the sterilizing cycle. Saturated steam at a temperature of 275° F. (under a pressure of 28 to 30 pounds) enters the preevacuated chamber and instantly penetrates the load to be sterilized. Microbes present are killed within a few minutes. Under these high temperature–high pressure conditions of steam sterilization there is a considerable shortening of the sterilizing (exposure) time (sometimes only 3 minutes). The vacuum pulled at the end of the sterilizing cycle dries the load. There is less damage to fabrics and to such items as rubber gloves because of reduced exposure.

**Fractional sterilization (intermittent sterilization).** When something that cannot withstand the temperature of an autoclave has to be sterilized, the procedure known as fractional or intermittent sterilization is used. This consists in exposing the material to free-flowing steam at atmospheric pressure for 30 minutes on 3 successive days; between times it is stored under conditions suitable for bacterial growth. With the first application of heat, all vegetative bacteria are killed, but the spores are not affected. Under conditions suitable for bacterial growth the spores develop into vegetative bacteria, and the second application of heat kills them. The second incubation and third application of heat are added to ensure complete sterilization. This method is of no value unless the material being sterilized is of such a nature as to promote the germination of spores. Therefore it would be most applicable to the sterilization of culture media. Sometimes referred to as *tyndallization*, it is infrequently used.

The low-temperature method of sterilizing vaccines (p. 173) may be applied in a fractional manner to materials such as serums that cannot withstand a temperature of 100° C. Such materials may be sterilized by being heated to a temperature of 55° to 60° C. for 1 hour on 5 or 6 successive days.

**Pasteurization.** All nonsporebearing disease-producing bacteria and most nonsporebearing nonpathogenic bacteria are killed when exposed in a watery liquid to a temperature of 60° C. for 30 minutes. This is the basis of pasteurization (p. 387), a special method of heating milk or other liquids for a short time to destroy undesirable microorganisms without changing composition and food value of the material itself.

## Sterilization by dry heat

Dry heat (hot air) sterilization consists of baking the material to be sterilized in a suitable oven. Dry heat at a given temperature is not nearly so effective a sterilizing agent as moist heat of the same temperature. Under controlled conditions a dry temperature of 120° to 130° C. kills all vegetative bacteria within 1½ hours, and a dry temperature of 160° C. kills all spores within 1 hour; but a moist temperature of 120° C. kills all vegetative bacteria and most spores within 15 to 20 minutes. Whereas moist heat sterilization is primarily a process of protein coagulation, dry heat sterilization is a process of protein oxidation; and that oxidation goes on more slowly than coagulation. Moist heat also has greater penetrating power than dry heat.

**Table 15-1**

Heat (physical) sterilization of reusable instruments and supplies

| METHOD | ADMINISTRATION | | APPLICATION |
| --- | --- | --- | --- |
| | TEMPERATURE | TIME* | |
| Autoclave | 121°-123° C. (250°-254° F.), 15-17 lb. pressure | 30 min. | Gloves, drapes, towels, gauze pads, instruments, glassware, and metalware |
| Dry heat | 170° C. (340° F.) | 1 hr. | Glassware, metalware, and dull instruments (any temperature listed) |
| | 160° C. | 2 hr. | Small quantities of powders, petrolatum (Vaseline), oils, and petrolatum gauze |
| | 150° C. | 3 hr. | Sharp instruments and metal-tip syringes |
| | 121° C. (250° F.) | 6 hr. or longer | |
| Boiling | 100° C. (212° F.) | 30 min.† | Method not recommended when dry heat and autoclave sterilization available |

*With a high pre-vacuum sterilizer, sterilizing (exposure) times are shorter; at a temperature of 132.8° to 135.5° C. (271° to 276° F.), sterilizing time is 4 minutes.
†Atmospheric pressure, sea level.

For temperatures and times in practical dry heat sterilization, see Table 15-1. A temperature of more than 200° C. causes cotton and cloth to turn brown. Even a moderate degree of dry heat is injurious to most fabrics. Hot air is used mostly to sterilize glassware, metal objects, and articles injured by moisture or items such as petrolatum (Vaseline), oils, and fats that resist penetration by steam or water. An advantage is that dry heat does not dull cutting edges. In this form of sterilization the temperature should be slowly raised, and after sterilization is complete, the oven should be allowed to cool slowly to prevent breakage of glassware.

There are two causes of ineffective dry heat sterilization: (1) the materials to be sterilized are too closely packed and (2) the temperature is not uniform within the sterilizing oven. An attempt to overcome the uneven distribution of heat has been made in sterilizers and sterilizing ovens constructed in such a manner that either gravity aids in the circulation of hot air through the sterilizer (gravity convection) or circulation is carried on by means of blowers (mechanical convection). Mechanical convection is more satisfactory than gravity convection. *Instruments to be sterilized must be clean and free of oil or grease films.*

**Burning (incineration).** Burning is a form of intense dry heat very effective in removing infectious materials of various kinds. The platinum wire loop used to inoculate cultures is repeatedly and quickly sterilized by *flaming*—heating the wire in an open flame until it glows. This form of sterilization is most important when materials and supplies are disposable or expendable.

*All contaminated objects that are of no value or that cannot be used again are best burned.*

## Sterilization by other physical means

**Natural methods of removing or eliminating microbes.** If a culture of bacteria is dried, the majority of the bacteria are quickly killed, but some may live for quite a while. Spores and encysted protozoa resist drying for a long time. Although drying is an important natural method of removing or destroying microbes, it has little practical application to "artificial" sterilization except that sterile dressings and similar objects should be kept dry.

Sunlight has a marked inhibitory and destructive action on microbes. It will kill *Mycobacterium tuberculosis* within a few hours and will kill many other bacteria in a shorter time. Sunlight is nature's great sterilizing agent but so irregular in its presence that one cannot depend on its action. The antimicrobial action of both drying and sunlight is advantageous in home-drying of food.

**Ultraviolet radiation.** The purity of the air in the wide open spaces has long been recognized, and it is well known that the sterilizing effect of sunlight there comes from the ultraviolet rays present. This fact has been applied to the construction of ultraviolet lamps in wide use to prevent the airborne spread of disease-producing agents, especially in public places, in hospitals (operating rooms, treatment rooms, nurseries), in microbiologic laboratories, and in quarters used to house animals.

Ultraviolet radiation is especially effective in killing organisms contained in the minute dried respiratory droplets tending to disperse rapidly through the atmosphere of a building or hospital. It is not so active against dust-borne agents and microorganisms on surfaces. It inactivates certain viruses. Its bactericidal effect drops sharply when the humidity of the area exceeds 55% to 60%. In appropriate amounts it damages skin and conjunctivae.

**X rays and other ionizing radiations.** X rays and other ionizing radiations are known to be lethal to microbes and to living cells as well, but there is no practical application for their use in routine sterilization. In industry beta rays or electrons sterilize prepackaged materials such as sutures and plastic tubing. High-energy electrons have been proposed for the treatment of sewage and wastewater.

One interesting application is the combination of heat and gamma radiation for the sterilization of spacecraft. If heat alone is used, the spaceship is subjected to a temperature of 125° C. (257° F.) for 60 hours. The temperature has to be controlled carefully to prevent heat damage to, and failure of components in, such items as silver-zinc batteries and tantalum capacitors. If the spaceship with its equipment is sprayed with 150,000 rads of gamma radiation, the time at the temperature of 125° C. can be cut down to 2 hours.

**Lasers.** Recent investigation suggests the use of a laser to sterilize medical instruments, clear the air in operating rooms, and pick organisms off a wound surface. The technical problem is that the laser beam must reach all parts of the item to be sterilized. If feasible, laser sterilization would be split-second, and heat-resistant spores could easily be eliminated.

**Ultrasonics.** Sound waves are mechanical vibrations. In the range of vibration (18,000 or more cycles per second) where they are no longer heard as sound (supersonic or ultrasonic), these waves have been demonstrated to coagulate protein solutions and to destroy bacteria. Cold boiling results from the passage of ultrasonic pressure waves through a cleaning solution. Very tiny empty spaces in the liquid form and collapse thousands of times a second. This type of scrubbing action can blast material from the surface of objects made of metal, glass, or plastic. The use of such vibrations (pitched too high to be heard) is not widely practical, but the principle has been incorporated into a commercially available dishwasher. Cleaning medical instruments is a common application. The use of ultrasonics (noiseless sound) is being applied experimentally to treatment of sewage water to effect disintegration of viruses, bacteria, and certain chemical substances such as phosphates and nitrogen-containing compounds.

**Action of fluorescent dyes.** Certain dyes with the property of fluorescence, such as methylene blue, rose bengal, and eosin, are lethal to bacteria and viruses if in contact with these microbes in strong visible light.

## Questions for review

1 Name three ways in which sterilization may be accomplished.
2 Define sterilization, bacterial filtration, sedimentation, thermal death point, pasteurization.
3 Name and describe briefly three mechanical methods of removing or destroying microbes.
4 Why is moist heat more effective than dry heat as a sterilizing agent?
5 What is the effect of pressure on steam sterilization?
6 Explain intermittent or fractional sterilization.
7 What is an autoclave? Indicate the basic principles of its operation.
8 Briefly describe the high-prevacuum sterilizer. State its advantage.
9 How is dry heat applied for sterilization? Cite items that must be sterilized in this way.
10 Tabulate all physical agents used for sterilization.

**References on pp. 173 to 175.**

## CHAPTER 16

# Chemical agents

## Effects of chemical agents on microbes

**Definitions.** Certain definitions are important for material to follow. As we have learned, "sterilization" is an absolute term referring to the destruction or removal of all microorganisms present under given conditions. *Disinfection,* on the other hand, means death to disease-producing organisms and the destruction of their products. (A more practical definition of the process might indicate that disinfection halts the spread of undesirable microorganisms by inducing structural or metabolic derangements in them.) Disinfection does not consider directly the saprophytic organisms present in a given area that may or may not be killed. Disinfection is usually accomplished with chemical agents known as *disinfectants. Antiseptics* are agents that prevent the multiplication of bacteria but do not necessarily kill them. The terms *disinfection* and *disinfectant* are applied to procedures and chemical agents used to destroy microorganisms associated with inanimate objects. The term *antiseptic* is usually applied to an agent that acts on microorganisms associated with the living body. For instance, we disinfect the excretions from a sick person but apply an antiseptic to his wounds. True, the terms are often interchanged.

*Germicides* are chemicals that kill microbes (not necessarily their spores). *Bactericides* are chemicals that kill bacteria. *Viricides* are agents that destroy or inactivate viruses. *Fungicides* destroy fungi. *Amebicides* destroy amebas, especially the protozoan *Entamoeba histolytica. Asepsis* means the absence of pathogenic microorganisms from a given object or a given area. In aseptic surgery the field of operation, the instruments, and the dressings are rendered free of microorganisms by sterilization. The operation is conducted in such a manner that the field is kept as free of microbes as possible. The purpose of all of this is to avoid infection of the patient. *Fumigation* is the liberation of fumes or gases to destroy insects or small animals. *Deodorants* are substances that destroy or mask offensive odors. They may have neither disinfectant nor antiseptic action and may generally tend to obscure infectious material rather than destroy it.

*Bacteriostasis* is that condition in which bacteria are prevented from multiplying (but in no other manner affected) by such agents as low temperature, weak antiseptics, and dyes. *Agents causing bacteriostasis are known as bacteriostatic agents. Antiseptics* and *chemical bacteriostatic agents* are synonymous terms. *Preservatives* are antiseptics or bacteriostatic agents used to prevent the deterioration of foods, serums, and vaccines.

Two terms with increasing applications are *degerm* and *sanitize.* To degerm is to remove bacteria from the skin by mechanical cleaning or application of antiseptic. To sanitize means to reduce the number of bacteria to a safe level as judged by public health requirements. It refers to the day-by-day control of the microbial population of utensils and equipment used in dairies and establishments where food and drink are served. In short, sanitization refers to a "good cleaning" and is basic to technics of sterilization. As used, the term *sterilization* implies a mechanically clean item. The word *decontamination* applies to the process of killing all microbes from an item known to be mechanically dirty and containing a heavy growth of microorganisms.

**Qualities of a good disinfectant.** There are certain qualities that a chemical should have in order to be an ideal disinfectant for general use. Unfortunately, at the present time none possesses all of them, and the selection of a disinfectant must depend on the conditions under which it is to be used. The more of the following qualities that a chemical has, the more nearly it qualifies as an ideal general disinfectant. It should

1. Attack all types of microorganisms
2. Be rapid in its action
3. Not destroy body tissues or act as a poison if taken internally
4. Not be retarded in its action by organic matter
5. Penetrate material being disinfected
6. Dissolve easily in or mix with water to form a stable solution or emulsion
7. Not decompose when exposed to heat, light rays, or unfavorable weather conditions

8. Not have a deleterious effect on materials being disinfected, such as instruments or fabrics
9. Not have an unpleasant odor or discolor the material being disinfected
10. Be easily obtained at a comparatively low cost and readily transported

The most important feature of a disinfectant is its ability to form lethal combinations with microbial cells. *Remember that different species of microbes, especially bacteria, show much greater variation in their susceptibility to disinfectants than they do to sterilization by physical agents.*

**Action of antiseptics and disinfectants.** Antiseptics and disinfectants act by (1) oxidation of the microbial cell, (2) hydrolysis, (3) combination with microbial proteins to form salts, (4) coagulation of proteins, (5) modification of the permeability of the microbial plasma membrane, (6) inactivation of vital enzymes of microorganisms, and (7) disruption of the cell.

*Factors influencing the action of disinfectants.* The factors influencing the action of disinfectants may be classified as to (1) the qualities of the disinfectant, (2) nature of the material to be disinfected, (3) concentration of the disinfectant, and (4) manner of application. A chemical in a solution of one strength may be a disinfectant, whereas in a weaker solution it may act only as an antiseptic, and in certain very weak solutions it may actually stimulate microbial growth. The relative germicidal properties of the salts of a heavy metal are proportional to their ionization.

The item for disinfection is evaluated as to (1) kind and number of microbes present, (2) presence of vegetative forms or spores, (3) distribution of microbes in clumps or in an even suspension, and (4) presence of organic compounds or other chemicals that inactivate the disinfectant.

Most chemical agents in common use as disinfectants are *germicidal but are not absolutely sporicidal;* that is, they do not kill all spores present. As a rule, the process of disinfection is a gradual one, and a few microbes survive longer the majority. To be effective, the disinfectant must be applied for a length of time sufficient to destroy all microorganisms. Many chemical disinfectants must be used for a long time to obtain the maximal effect; this often means 18 to 24 hours. An important factor relating to the disinfectant is the temperature at which it is applied. The higher the temperature, the more active it is. Remember that a disinfectant must penetrate all parts of the material being disinfected because it must contact microbes to destroy them. An article being disinfected must be *completely covered* by the disinfectant solution. Also, a disinfectant should be properly chosen in

accordance with the physiochemical nature of the material to be disinfected.

*Surface tension in disinfection.* The molecules lying below the surface of a liquid are acted on in all directions by the cohesive forces of neighboring molecules. Those at the surface are pulled downward and sideways by adjacent molecules but are not pulled upward because there are no molecules above the surface to attract them. This phenomenon is known as surface tension. Surface tension may be nontechnically defined as *that property resulting from molecular forces by which the surface film of all liquids tends to bring the contained volume into a shape having the least superficial area.* Since a sphere has the least area for a given volume, surface tension causes drops of liquid to become spherical.

If a drop of mercury is placed on a flat surface of metal or glass, it remains a distinct globule, rolling from place to place. If, on the other hand, a drop of alcohol is placed on a surface, it does not form a globule but spreads out into a very thin layer over a large area. The surface tension of mercury is high; that of alcohol, low.

Surface tension is important in disinfection because liquids of low surface tension spread over a greater area and contact cells more intimately than do liquids of high surface tension. Such low surface tension liquids are often spoken of as *wetting agents*. A good wetting agent spreads over a surface rapidly and remains in a thin film. Chemicals that reduce the surface tension of water when dissolved in it accumulate on the surface of cells in a more concentrated form than that in which they exist throughout the solution. Some wetting agents are also effective antiseptics. Wetting agents thought of primarily as surface-cleaning agents are *detergents*. Many detergents act as both cleaning agents and inhibitors of bacterial growth. The classic example of a wetting agent or detergent is soap. However, soap does not have the antiseptic action of certain other detergents. Many new synthetic organic detergents (liquids, granules, and such) that have been placed on the market are sometimes spoken of as soapless soaps or as nonsoap cleaners. Some detergents such as Tween 80 do not have an antiseptic action but promote bacterial growth.

**Standardization.** Many types of procedures have been designed to evaluate the antimicrobial activity of a given chemical agent as well as indicate its toxicity for tissues. Rideal and Walker in 1903 devised the original phenol coefficient test, which compared the disinfectant or antiseptic activity of a given compound with that of phenol under identical conditions. In this test a phenol coefficient of greater than 1 indicated a stronger agent than phenol; a coefficient less than 1 indicated a weaker one. Despite the variety and number of methods existing today, inadequacies still remain, and the tests fail to give all the information needed.

## Common disinfectants and antiseptics

Myriads of cleaning and disinfecting chemicals and combinations exist. With a few exceptions, there seems to be no general uniformity of opinion today as to which of these is best for application in any given situation, and the use of such chemical agents varies considerably, even in the same community. Only a few of the better known ones are considered in this chapter. At the end of the listing of chemical agents is placed Table 16-1, a summary statement and comparison of the antimicrobial activity of some of the more important ones discussed. It does reflect, as indicated, material from a given source.

### SURFACE-ACTIVE COMPOUNDS

*Soap* is our most important cleaning agent. Although its utility as a disinfectant is limited, it is generally used before one is applied. The major action of soap is to aid the mechanical removal of microbes, primarily through scrubbing. In cleaning, soap and water separate particulate contamination of whatever kind from a given area, for example, the skin surface of the human body. This is an area constantly collecting dead cells, oily secretions, dust, dried sweat, dirt, soot, and varied microorganisms. Soap breaks up the grease film into tiny droplets; water and soap acting together lift up the emulsified oily materials and dirt particles, floating them away as the lather is washed off.

Although the term *detergent* means any cleaning agent, even water, it is used to distinguish the synthetic compounds from soap, both of which lower the surface tension of water. Soap is made from fats and lye; detergents are made from fats and oils by complicated chemical processes, and most contain a biodegradable linear sulfonate derivative of petroleum. Soaps depend for their cleaning action on their content of alkali, which suspends the grime from the surface of an object in the water to be washed off. The detergent ionizes in water; its electrically charged ions attach themselves to the dirt. The washing action releases the ions, which carry the dirt away. Detergents dissolve readily in cold water and completely in even the hardest water. Soap combines with the calcium and magnesium salts in hard water to form an insoluble scum.

*Enzyme detergent* refers to laundry presoak products in which certain proteolytic enzymes from bacteria are incorporated (in amounts up to 1.0% active enzyme). Enzymes are obtained through a fermentation process from the widely distributed nonpathogenic soil organism, *Bacillus subtilis.* Enzyme detergent dissolves organic (protein) stains such as blood, feces, and meat juices without harming fabric or user. Enzyme activity is quickly dissipated during the washing process and is inactivated by chlorine bleach.

Soap is mildly antiseptic because of its sodium an alkali content, but to remove most bacteria effectively, scrubbing must be followed by the application of a suitable disinfectant. Organisms susceptible to the germicidal action of soap are pneumococci, streptococci, gonococci, meningococci, *Treponema pallidum,* and influenza viruses.[*]

*If soap is to be followed by some germicide, it should be thoroughly washed off with 70% alcohol before the germicide is applied, because soap and germicide might combine to form an inert compound.* The so-called germicidal soaps generally have little or no advantage over ordinary soaps. If soap is not properly handled and dispensed, it may become a source of infection by itself.

*Benzalkonium chloride (Zephiran Chloride)* is a mixture of high molecular weight alkyl dimethyl-benzylammonium chlorides and one of the most important members of the surface-active chemical disinfectants known as quaternary ammonium disinfectants, or quats.[†] It is widely used in hospitals for the disinfection of hands and preparation of the field of operation. A 1:1000 aqueous solution may be used for the disinfection of instruments, especially endoscopes and sharp-edged cutting instruments, the blades of which would be dulled by autoclaving. Such a solution kills vegetative bacteria (except tubercle bacilli) in 30 minutes. *It has no effect on tubercle bacilli. It is not effective against spores or viruses.* The presence of serum or alkali retards its action. The same is true of soap; when Zephiran Chloride is used as a skin antiseptic, soap should be removed by thorough rinsing with 70% alcohol for 1 minute or more before the Zephiran Chloride solution is applied. (Water usually does not remove all soap,

---

[*] Most pathogenic bacteria and viruses are removed or chemically killed by the soaps and detergents ordinarily used in the commercial self-service laundry machine. The temperature of the dryer usually is high enough to eliminate any remaining bacteria. If the clothes are then ironed, the heat of the hot iron destroys any microbes that possibly could have survived.

[†] A quaternary ammonium compound is built around a nitrogen atom of five valence bonds. Four of these bonds are attached to adjacent carbon atoms of organic radicals, and one is attached to an inorganic or organic radical. Soap reduces the germicidal action of the quats, as would hard water were it used to dilute a stock solution to make an aqueous preparation.

since soap and water constitute a colloidal solution.) Soap is completely soluble in 70% alcohol. When metal instruments are to be stored in a solution of Zephiran Chloride for a period of time, it is well to add an antirust agent or antirust tablets. One antirust tablet available commercially is a combination of sodium carbonate and sodium nitrite.

*Diaparene Chloride* is a quaternary ammonium compound particularly bacteriostatic toward *Brevibacterium ammoniagenes*, the intestinal saprophyte chiefly responsible for the production of ammonia in decomposed urine. It therefore is useful in the prevention of ammonium dermatitis in infants when used for the disinfection of diapers.

*Ceepryn Chloride* bears a close resemblance to the quaternary ammonium compounds just described. A commercially available 1:1000 solution is recommended as a mouthwash or gargle. It combines a foaming detergent cleaning action with an antibacterial activity against certain pathogenic organisms found in the mouth and throat.

## HEAVY METAL COMPOUNDS

*Merbromin (Mercurochrome)*[*] is a combination of mercury and a derivative of fluorescein. A 2% solution is used as a disinfectant of wounds. Stronger solutions are used as skin antiseptics. A 1% solution is tolerated by the bladder and kidney pelvis. A 2% solution in water (35%), alcohol (55%), and acetone (10%) is known as *surgical merbromin solution*. This antiseptic has probably received more publicity than its effectiveness warrants.

*Nitromersol (Metaphen)* is an organic mercury compound for the sterilization of instruments, for skin antisepsis, and for irrigation of the urethra. It is used in strengths ranging from 1:10,000 to 1:1000. It is said to be comparatively nontoxic, nonirritating, and nondestructive to metallic instruments and rubber goods. It kills pathogenic bacteria that do not form spores, other than tubercle bacilli. *Organic mercurials have no action against spores.*

*Thimerosal (Merthiolate)* is another organic mercury preparation with the advantages of ready solubility in water and body fluids and low toxicity for tissues. It is used for disinfecting instruments, skin, and mucous membranes and as a biologic preservative for vaccines, serums, and blood cells. This agent in aqueous solutions is considered to be fungistatic and bacteriostatic for nonsporeforming bacteria. The

tincture or alcoholic solution is rather rapidly germicidal.

*Mercresin* combines the germicidal action of the mercurials with that of the phenolic derivatives, giving a maximum disinfectant action with a minimum of tissue injury. Its action is not inhibited by the presence of serum. It is widely used for local antisepsis of the skin.

*Silver nitrate* pencils are used to cauterize wounds. A 1:10,000 solution inhibits the growth of bacteria, and increasing the strength of solution, even up to 10% in certain instances, enhances germicidal activity. Silver nitrate has a selective action for gonococci. A 1% solution is instilled into the eyes of newborn babies to prevent ophthalmia neonatorum. Silver nitrate 0.5% solution is used in the continuously soaked dressings applied to burns. It reduces infection, but *Pseudomonas* can still grow beneath the dry black eschar that results. The action of silver nitrate is retarded by chlorides, iodides, bromides, sulfates, and organic matter. It is reduced on exposure to light and because of its many incompatibilities should be used only with distilled water.

There are various unofficial salts of silver on the market, such as colloidal iodides, albuminates, and proteins, with fewer incompatibilities than silver nitrate. They have been used in various strengths, with varying results.

*Protargol, Argyrol, Silvol,* and *Neo-Silvol* are colloidal solutions of silver salts used because of their nonirritating qualities.

Zinc salts are mild antiseptics and also astringents. *Medicinal Zinc Peroxide* is a mixture of zinc peroxide, zinc carbonate, and zinc hydroxide. The commercial powder should be sterilized at 140° C. dry heat for 4 hours. It is used in watery suspensions and ointments and is of special value in controlling infections caused by anaerobic and microaerophilic organisms in injuries such as gunshot wounds, bites, and deep puncture wounds.

*Calamine Lotion* is mostly zinc oxide with some ferric oxide.

*Copper sulfate* is valuable chiefly for its destructive action on the green algae that often grow in reservoirs and that render water obnoxious. A copper sulfate concentration of 1 part per million (p.p.m.)[*] parts of water kills algae if the water does not contain an excess of organic matter. One part of copper sulfate added to 400,000 parts of water destroys typhoid

---

[*] To avoid the toxicity of the inorganic mercurials and still retain the disinfecting qualities of mercury, a number of organic mercury compounds have been developed. Among these are Mercurochrome, Metaphen, Merthiolate, and Mercresin (a mixture instead of a definite compound).

[*] 1 p.p.m. = 1 inch in 16 miles; 1 minute in 2 years; a 1-gram needle in a ton of hay; 1 penny in $10,000; 1 large mouthful of food when compared with the food a person will eat in a lifetime.

bacilli in 24 hours. For a short time it is not harmful to drink water that contains this amount of copper sulfate. Copper sulfate is an important ingredient of sprays used to combat fungous diseases of plants.

## ALCOHOLS AND ALDEHYDES

*Ethyl alcohol* is one of the most widely used disinfectants and one of the best. For alcohol to coagulate proteins (its disinfectant action), water must be present. Because of this fact, 70% has long been considered the critical dilution of ethyl alcohol. However, there is good reason to think that against microorganisms in a moist environment alcohol acts over a range including 70% and up to 95%. Alcohol in a 70% dilution may be used for the disinfection of certain delicate surgical instruments, although it tends to rust instruments and dissolves the cement from around the lights of endoscopes. It does not kill spores. Alcohol kills tubercle bacilli rapidly and is a tuberculocidal disinfectant of choice.

*Isopropyl alcohol* is slightly superior to ethyl alcohol as a disinfectant. It is also cheaper, and its sale is not subject to legal regulations. Like ethyl alcohol, its acts against vegetative bacilli (not spores) and tubercle bacilli. Recent evidence indicates that this agent is an effective disinfectant in dilutions stronger than the conventional 70% and that the most effective one may well be full strength (99%).

*Formaldehyde,* a gas, occurs in commerce in a watery 37% solution known as *formalin.* In addition to disinfecting properties, formaldehyde serves as a deodorizer and as a preservative of tissues. It is used to convert toxins into toxoids. Its action depends on the presence of moisture, the concentraton of the gas, temperature, and condition of the object to be sterilized. The presence of 1% of the gas in a room or chamber destroys all nonsporulating pathogenic bacteria. Cystoscopes and certain specialized instruments that would be damaged by heat are sometimes disinfected in airtight sterilizing cabinets equipped with electric terminals so that formaldehyde pastils can be vaporized in them. The instruments are left in the cabinet exposed to the formaldehyde fumes for 24 hours.

Mixtures of alcohol, formalin, and hexachlorophene are frequently used for sterilizing surgical instruments. This combination makes one of the most active germicidal solutions commercially available; bacteria, spores, tubercle bacilli, and most viruses are speedily killed thereby. An example of such a mixture is *Bard-Parker Germicide,* a commercial mixture of formaldehyde, isopropanol, methanol, and hexachlorophene. It is especially useful in the sterilization of knife blades and suture needles.

*Glutaraldehyde* (Cidex) is one of the latest additions to any list and one of the best. *Activated glutaraldehyde solution* is bactericidal, viricidal, and sporicidal in short exposure times. It does however corrode rubber tubing and materials, etches plastic with repeated exposure, and irritates the skin. It is useful for sterilization of anesthetic equipment and the intermittent positive-pressure breathing apparatus and is recommended for use with instruments containing optical lenses.

## PHENOLS AND DERIVATIVES

*Phenol* (carbolic acid) is a corrosive poison. A 1:500 solution inhibits the growth of bacteria. A 5% solution kills all vegetative bacteria and the less resistant spores in a short time. Contact with alcohol or ether decreases its action, which is also inhibited by soap. The addition of 5% to 10% hydrochloric acid increases its efficiency. Since the action of phenol is not greatly retarded by the presence of organic matter, it is an excellent disinfectant for feces, blood, pus, sputum, and proteinaceous materials. It does not injure metals, fabrics, or painted surfaces. The crude acid may be used for woodwork because it is cheaper and more effective than the pure substance. The crystals or strong solutions should not be allowed to touch the skin. If this happens, alcohol should be applied at once. Dilute solutions should not be left in contact with the skin or mucous membrane for more than 30 minutes or 1 hour because they injure tissues.

*Cresol* has a higher germicidal power than does phenol and is less poisonous. *Saponated cresol solution* is an alkaline solution of cresol in soap. (Similar but generally more expensive proprietary preparations are on the market.) A 2.5% solution of saponated cresol makes a good disinfectant for feces and sputum.

*Lysol,* a widely used and popular disinfectant, is essentially a solution of cresol with soap, sold under a trade name. In recent years improvements have been made in the mixture. Lysol is most important in the disinfection of inanimate objects, including instruments, furniture, table surfaces, floors, walls, rubber goods, rectal thermometers, and contaminated objects of varied description, especially when these have been contaminated by *Mycobacterium tuberculosis.*

In general, phenol derivatives such as cresol and Lysol can be used to disinfect excreta or contaminated secretions from patients with infectious diseases but have special value in the disinfection of tuberculosis. They are of little value in antisepsis of the skin because in concentrations that would not injure the skin they possess little bactericidal activity. They do not destroy all spores present.

*Amphyl* is one of the modern and greatly improved phenolic disinfectants with wide and varied applications as a germicide. (Chemically it is a mixture of ortho-phenylphenol and paratertiary amylphenol with potassium ricinoleate in propylene glycol and alcohol.) Nontoxic, noncorrosive to metals, and nonirritating to skin and mucous membranes, Amphyl can be mixed with soap and certain other antiseptics. Because it is an agent with low surface tension, it spreads and penetrates materials. Surfaces treated with it tend to retain an antimicrobial action for several days. It is effective in dilutions of 0.25% to 3% for a range of routine disinfecting procedures involving skin, mucous membranes, floors, walls, furniture, dishes, utensils, and surgical instruments. Fungi, bacteria (including the tubercle bacillus), and viruses, but *not* spores, are destroyed by its action; heating increases its germicidal properties.

*Staphene* is a phenolic disinfectant related to Amphyl. It is a mixture of four synthetic phenols* (paratertiary amylphenol, ortho-benzyl-para-cholorophenol, orthophenylphenol, and 2, 2'-methylene-bis[3, 4, 6-trichlorophenol]).

*O-syl,* an antiseptic, germicide, and fungicide, is considered to be especially effective against the causative agent of tuberculosis. Chemically it is one synthetic phenol (orthophenylphenol).

*Hexachlorophene (G-11),* a diphenol, is one of the few antiseptics and disinfectants not affected by soap. Therefore in concentrations from 1% to 3% it has been incorporated into soaps and combined with detergents that have been used for the preoperative hand scrubs of the surgical team and for the preoperative and postoperative preparation of the skin of the patient. Hexachlorophene is long retained on the skin, from where it can be recovered more than 48 hours after use. Its benefit is attributed to the bactericidal film left on the skin after repeated application; the concentration on the skin is cumulative up to 2 or 4 days. (The skin cannot be completely sterilized.) Mechanical cleaning plus the use of germicidal agents removes the superficial growth of bacteria from the skin surface, which fortunately includes most of the pathogens. Hexachlorophene has been so widely used because of its bacteriostatic action against gram-positive microbes, notably the staphylococcus. Bathing of infants with a detergent containing hexachlorophene has been shown to reduce considerably the incidence of staphylococcal infection in a population of newborns.

Generally hexachlorophene is not irritating to the skin although it is sometimes associated with allergic

---

*Some of the phenolic detergent germicides widely used in cleaning solutions can cause depigmentation of the skin of the user.

manifestations. However, it is readily absorbed through normal skin, more easily so through abraded or burned skin. Its use has been blamed for brain seizures developing in young burn victims who had been washed with it. Animal experiments relate the uptake through the skin over a period of days to subsequent brain damage and even paralysis.

The United States Food and Drug Administration warns against total body bathing of infants and adults with products containing 2% and 3% concentrations of hexachlorophene and bans the over-the-counter sale of most products containing it.* Although available only by prescription, it is still used in hospitals and similar institutions because of its effective antibacterial action.

Recently the Committee on Fetus and Newborn of the American Academy of Pediatrics has recommended that only with a serious outbreak of staphylococcal infection may one resort to total body bathing of newborns with hexachlorophene, and then, only if (1) a solution of not more than 3% is used, (2) it is applied to full-term infants only, (3) it is washed off thoroughly after each application, and (4) it is applied no more than two times to a given infant.

*pHisoderm,* a detergent cream, is not a single compound but a proprietary mixture of wool fat, cholesterol, lactic acid, and sulfonated petrolatum. It cleans faster and more effectively than soap and is used for degerming the hands and other skin areas. It may be used alone but is most often combined with hexachlorophene.

*pHisoHex* is the name given to the mixture of the detergent base pHisoderm and 3% hexachlorophene. It is still popular for surgical hand scrubs because regular use gives maximal bactericidal effect. It is nonirritating, only small amounts need be used, and the time required for surgical scrubbing of hands is much shorter than with soap preparations. Its emulsifying action on oily material and its ability to form suds are desirable characteristics.

*Hexagerm* is another antiseptic skin detergent containing 3% hexachlorophene.

## HALOGEN COMPOUNDS

*Iodine* is one of the best known and most widely used disinfectants. It is a potent amebicide, a bactericide in a wide spectrum, a good tuberculocide, a fun-

---

*Hexachlorophene has been perhaps the most universal of the antibacterial agents, having been incorporated into a wide variety of consumer products—soaps, shampoos, toothpastes, deodorants, lotions, powders, ointments, cosmetics, and medicinal cleaners. According to the FDA the ingredient replacing hexachlorophene in many antibacterial products—tribromsalan—should also be eliminated.

gicide, and a viricide. The ubiquitous *tincture of iodine* containing 2% iodine in alcohol is one of the best disinfectants for small areas of skin, minor cuts, abrasions, and wounds. The strong tincture of iodine (7% in alcohol) is too toxic for most purposes. Iodine becomes freely soluble in water in the presence of soluble iodides such as those of sodium and potassium. *Iodine solution* (aqueous) containing 2% iodine is as effective as the alcoholic solutions (tinctures), but higher concentrations are sometimes used. Very strong and very old solutions of iodine burn the skin. It should not be applied under a bandage. Although in some persons iodine compounds produce allergic skin rashes, iodine is less toxic than other routinely used germicides. Within the last few years iodine has been used for disinfection of water in swimming pools.

*Iodophors* are compounds in which iodine is carried by a surface-active solvent. The germ-killing action results from release of free iodine when the compound is diluted with water; only the free iodine has any appreciable disinfectant action. An iodophor enhances the bactericidal action of iodine and reduces odor. It does not stain the skin or materials on which it is placed as does the tincture. One such is the proprietary preparation *Wescodyne*, an iodine detergent germicide (also a good tuberculocide). Other examples are *Hi-Sine, Iosan,* and *Betadine* (povidone-iodine complex).

*Chlorine* is one of the most effective and widely used of all chemical disinfectants. It is used in the disinfection of drinking water, purification of swimming pools, and treatment of sewage. It is applied by releasing the gas from cylinders or by the use of compounds that liberate free chlorine. The chlorine from chlorine-liberating compounds is spoken of as "available" chlorine. For effective disinfection, the chlorine content of water must reach a concentration of 0.5 to 1 p.p.m. If no organic material is present, 0.1 p.p.m. destroys the poliovirus, but in a strength of 1 p.p.m., chlorine has no effect on the cercariae that represent one stage in the development of flukes (p. 356). (Nor are these minute worms removed by sand filtration or aluminum sulfate clarification of the water.) Cysts of *Entamoeba histolytica* (p. 342), the cause of amebic dysentery, can live as long as 1 month in water. The usual chlorination treatment for drinking water does not kill them; water containing an adequate amount of chlorine to destroy them would not be fit to drink. The World Health Organization recommends that commercial airlines filter their water supply and overchlorinate it, 8 to 10 p.p.m. of free available chlorine, in order to kill cysts of *Entamoeba histolytica* and viruses of infectious hepatitis. The water must then stand for at least 30 minutes. It is dechlorinated to eliminate the disagreeable taste and smell.

*Sodium hypochlorite* (NaOCl), made by reaction of chlorine on sodium hydroxide, is a powerful oxidizing agent. It cannot be prepared in the form of a powder but is manufactured in solutions of varying strength. The stronger solutions are used as bleaches by laundries and other establishments. The weaker solutions (example: Clorox) are used as household bleaches and for the bactericidal treatment of food-handling equipment. Hypochlorite solutions prepared fresh daily are active against viruses if they contain 5000 to 10,000 p.p.m. of available free chlorine (0.5% to 1.0% solutions) and may be used in hemodialysis units, laboratories, and blood banks for disinfection of nonmetal equipment and surfaces likely to contain hepatitis viruses.

*Dakin's solution* and modifications are weak neutral solutions of sodium hypochlorite, liberating from 0.5% to 5% available chlorine.

*Chloramines* are organic chlorine compounds that decompose slowly and liberate chlorine. They are used to sanitize glassware and eating utensils and to treat dairy and food-manufacturing equipment. They are inferior when rapid action is required. Their value lies in their prolonged action. The ones in most common use are chloramine-T, chloroazodin, and halazone. Halazone is used for the sterilization of relatively small amounts of drinking water.

## ACIDS

*Boric acid* is a weak antiseptic most often used as an eyewash. However, when taken internally, boric acid is highly toxic. Because of the risk of accidental poisoning, its use in hospitals has been condemned. It has no place in the pediatric division or in any nursery. If even a dilute solution of boric acid mistaken for distilled water should be used in an infant formula or in a parenteral fluid, the results could be disastrous. Dusting the powder repeatedly over the diaper area of a baby to remedy diaper rash can cause death. A so-called bland ointment applied to abraded areas of the skin can produce an unfavorable reaction.

*Fuming nitric acid* is the best agent for cauterizing the wounds inflicted by rabid animals.

*Benzoic acid* and *salicylic acid* are fungistatic agents. A mixture of benzoic acid 6% and salicylic acid 3% (*Whitfield's ointment*) is used to treat fungous infections of the feet.

*Undecylenic acid (Desenex)* is used for athlete's foot and other fungous infections of the skin.

## OXIDIZING AGENTS

*Hydrogen peroxide* owes its disinfecting qualities to the free oxygen that it liberates. It is a spectacular but not overly reliable antiseptic that deteriorates rapidly.

*Sodium perborate* is an oxidizing agent used in the treatment of trench mouth (p. 239). It is a common ingredient of tooth powders.

*Potassium permanganate* owes its effectiveness to strong oxidizing qualities. However, its action is weakened by the presence of organic matter. It was once used extensively in the treatment of infections of the genitourinary tract.

## DYES

Dyes such as gentian violet and crystal violet in high dilutions inhibit the growth of gram-positive bacteria but have little effect on gram-negative bacteria, whereas dyes such as acriflavine and proflavine inhibit the action of gram-negative bacteria but have little effect on gram-positive bacteria. Dyes are used to obtain pure cultures and to treat certain infectious processes. If it had not been for the advent of the sulfonamide drugs, the use of dyes as therapeutic agents would be presently more advanced.

## MISCELLANEOUS AGENTS

*Ethylene oxide* is a gas with a broad range of antimicrobial activity that has been used in industry for years for such purposes as the disinfection of the furnishings of railway cars. It is an odorless, poisonous, and explosive gas that can be easily kept as a liquid. Since its vapor is highly inflammable in air, it is transported commercially in a noninflammable mixture with carbon dioxide. This gas is used especially to treat items that are damaged by heat, water, or chemical solutions and is a potent agent if properly used. The article to be disinfected must be exposed to the gas in an appropriately designed sterilizing chamber in which the temperature can be raised and from which the air must be evacuated. Polyethylene and paper are suitable for packaging. A prolonged period of exposure is required—in one large model, at least 8 hours. Bacteria (including tubercule bacilli and staphylococci) and spores are killed. The hepatitis viruses are destroyed. Ethylene oxide properly used has an irreversible chemical reaction with all organisms including their spores. The reaction is speeded by heat. Ethylene oxide sterilization is safe and effective provided adequate aeration time is allowed for the gas to elude from items so sterilized. This is important because the gas and its by-products are highly irritating to skin and mucous membranes (including those of the eye). This form of *cold* sterilization is being widely used for delicate surgical instruments with optical lenses and for the tubing and heat-susceptible plastic parts of the heart-lung machine. Many prepackaged commercial items such as rubber goods and plastic tubes are sterilized with ethylene oxide. Because of the penetration of the gas, this form of sterilization is effective for blankets, pillows, mattresses, and bulky objects.

*Lime* is one of the most common and, when properly used, one of the most effective germicidal agents. Limestone (calcium carbonate), which occurs plenti-

## Table 16-1
Antimicrobial activity of commonly used cold "sterilants"*

| AGENT | DESTRUCTIVE ACTION AGAINST | | | | |
| --- | --- | --- | --- | --- | --- |
| | BACTERIA | TUBERCLE BACILLI | SPORES | FUNGI | VIRUSES |
| Alcohol—ethyl (70% to 90%) | + | + | 0 | + | ± |
| Alcohol—isopropyl (70% to 90%) | + + | + | 0 | + | ± |
| Alcohol-formaldehyde (Bard-Parker Germicide) | + + | + | + | + | + |
| Alcohol-iodine (2%) | + + | + | ± | + | + |
| Formalin (37%) | + | + | + | + | + |
| Glutaraldehyde (buffered, 2%) (Cidex) | + + | + | + + | + | + |
| Iodine (2% to 5% aqueous) | + + | + | ± | + | + |
| Iodophors (1%) (povidone-iodine complex) | + | + | ± | ± | + |
| Mercurials (Merthiolate) | ± | 0 | 0 | + | ± |
| Phenolic derivatives (0-syl 1% to 3%) | + | + | 0 | + | ± |
| Quats (benzalkonium chloride 1:750 to 1:1000) | + + | 0 | 0 | + | 0 |

*Based on data from DiPalma, J. R., editor: Drill's pharmacology in medicine, ed. 4, New York, 1971, McGraw-Hill Book Co.
+ +, Very good; +, good; ±, fair (greater concentration or more time needed); 0, no activity.

fully in nature, is converted by heating into *quicklime* (calcium oxide), with release of carbon dioxide. When quicklime is treated with one-half its weight of water. *slaked lime* (calcium hydroxide) is formed. Slaked lime, a powerful disinfectant, is used in the form of *milk of lime,* prepared by mixing 1 part of freshly slaked lime with 4 parts of water. Milk of lime is especially useful as a disinfectant for feces. A more dilute suspension of slaked lime is *whitewash.* Lime preparations must not be exposed to the air because they combine with the carbon dioxide of the air to form calcium carbonate without any antiseptic action.

*Chlorinated lime* (chloride of lime, bleaching powder, calcium hypochlorite), made by passing chlorine through freshly slaked lime, is one of the most important of the chlorine-liberating compounds used as disinfectants. An unstable compound, its antiseptic action results from its release of hypochlorous acid toxic to the bacterial cell. A 0.5% to 1% solution kills most bacteria in from 1 to 5 minutes. A 1:100,000 solution destroys typhoid bacilli in 24 hours. Chlorinated lime bleaches and destroys fabrics and decomposes when exposed to the air. As a means of disinfecting excreta, chlorinated lime is probably without rival.

*Sulfur dioxide* is a gas formed by burning sulfur. It was formerly used extensively for house and room fumigation. Its germicidal action depends on the presence of moisture because it combines with water to form sulfurous acid, the destructive agent. It damages fabrics and metals.

*Ferrous sulfate* (copperas) is used in the form of the impure commercial salt. Besides being a good disinfectant, it is a good deodorant because it combines with both ammonia and hydrogen sulfide. It is an ideal disinfectant for use in damp musty places and around houses.

*Chlorophyl* in the form of its water-soluble components has been used in the local treatment of wounds. It cleans the wound, stops pus formation, destroys odors, and promotes healing.

## Therapeutic chemicals for microbial diseases

### CHEMOTHERAPEUTIC AGENTS

Although it is possible to treat many local infections with chemicals, the finding of a chemical that, taken orally or parenterally, destroys microorganisms without injuring the body cells is not easy. Examples of such chemicals are quinine, against the parasites of malaria, and emetine (the active principle of ipecac), against *Entamoeba histolytica,* the organism causing amebic dysentery. These agents are known as *chemotherapeutic agents.* The treatment of disease with chemotherapeutic agents is *chemotherapy.* The *chemotherapeutic index* compares the toxicity of a drug for the body with its toxicity for a disease-producing agent. It is obtained by dividing the maximal tolerated dose per kilogram of body weight by the minimal curative dose per kilogram of body weight.

Within recent years there have been phenomenal developments in the field of chemotherapy, beginning with the discovery of the sulfonamide compounds. A brief discussion of these and certain specifically acting chemotherapeutic drugs follows.

*Sulfonamide compounds* contain the group $-SO_2N<$. Many of them are derived from the compound known as sulfanilamide, which was among the first of the sulfonamides to be developed as a chemotherapeutic agent. Sulfanilamide was derived from a dye known by the trade name of Prontosil, that had been found effective in treating streptococcal infections. Prontosil was used for only a short time, and sulfanilamide itself was soon replaced by less toxic drugs.

The sulfonamide compounds are bacteriostatic in their mode of action; they interfere with certain enzymes in the affected bacterial cells. The sulfonamide compounds are not self-sterilizing, and their action is inhibited by pus. Sulfonamides are effective against gram-positive bacteria, some gram-negative diplococci and bacilli, chlamydiae, and *Actinomyces.* Generally the sulfonamides have been replaced by antibiotics that are not so toxic and that are more certain and rapid in their action. Where an antibiotic and a sulfonamide are of equal value, it is customary to give the antibiotic. The sulfonamides have been used for treatment of epidemic meningitis because the sulfonamides pass into the cerebrospinal fluid more easily than do the antibiotics. The highly soluble sulfonamides are important in the treatment of some infections of the urinary tract as well. Certain sulfonamides for intestinal use suppress the growth of the intestinal flora, an important measure in the preparation of the patient for surgery of the large bowel.

A patient receiving sulfonamide therapy should be continuously observed for early toxic symptoms. If such appear, the drug must be discontinued.

Today there are many sulfonamide compounds with varying actions on bacteria and varying toxic effects on the body. The ones most readily available are sulfadiazine, sulfamerazine, sulfamethazine, sulfacetamide (Sulamyd), sulfadimethoxine (Madribon), sulfisoxazole (Gantrisin), sulfamethoxypyridazine (Kynex), sulfachloropyridazine (Sonilyn), sulfisomidine (Elkosin), sulfamethizole (Thiosulfil), and sulfaethidole, all for systemic use. Other compounds include sulfaguanidine, succinylsulfathiazole (Sulfasuxidine), and phthalylsulfathiazole (Sulfathalidine) for intestinal use.

*Isoniazid* (isonicotinylhydrazine) (INH) is a remarkably potent bacteriostatic agent against *Mycobacterium tuberculosis*, but it has little effect on most other microbes. Its mode of action is not known at the present time. Isoniazid is an effective drug not only in treating tuberculosis but also in preventing tuberculous infection from becoming active disease. The American Thoracic Society recommends ideally that all tuberculin-positive individuals should receive a year of isoniazid prophylaxis. (See also p. 253.) Generally there have been few untoward reactions, but recently instances of drug toxicity have appeared. Some 10 out of 1000 individuals receiving isoniazid prophylacti-

**Table 16-2**
Microbial sources of antibiotics

| MICROBE | ANTIBIOTIC | MICROBE | ANTIBIOTIC |
|---|---|---|---|
| *Arachniotus aureus* | Aranotin (antiviral) | *Streptomyces fradiae* | Neomycin |
| **Bacteria** | | *Streptomyces spheroides* | Novobiocin |
| *Bacillus subtilis* group | Bacitracin | *Streptomyces noursei* | Nystatin (Mycostatin) |
| *licheniformis* | | *Streptomyces antibioticus* | Oleandomycin |
| *Bacillus polymyxa* var. | Colistin | *Streptomyces rimosus* | Oxytetracycline (Terramycin) |
| *colistinus* | | *Streptomyces rimosus* | Paromomycin (Humatin) |
| *Bacillus polymyxa* | Polymyxin | | |
| *Bacillus brevis* | Tyrothricin | *Streptomyces lincolnensis* | Ranimycin (antibiotic) |
| **Streptomycetes** | | *Streptomyces* | Rifampin (Rimactane) |
| *Streptomyces parvullus* | Actinomycin D (Dactinomycin) (antineoplastic) | *mediterranei* | |
| *Streptomyces nodosus* | Amphotericin B (Fungizone) (antifungal) | *Streptomyces spectabilis* (variant) | Spectinomycin (Trobicin) |
| *Streptomyces tenebrarius* | Apramycin (Ambylan) | *Streptomyces griseus* | Streptomycin |
| *Streptomyces fragilis* | Azaserine (antineoplastic) | *Streptomyces lavendulae* | Streptothricin |
| *Streptomyces verticillus* | Bleomycin (antineoplastic) | *Streptomyces* | Streptozotocin |
| *Streptomyces griseus* | Candicidin (antifungal) | *achromogenes* | |
| *Streptomyces capreolus* | Capreomycin (Capastat) | *Streptomyces aureofaciens* (mutant) | Tetracycline |
| *Streptomyces venezuelae* | Chloramphenicol (Chloromycetin) | *Streptomyces orientalis* | Vancomycin |
| *Streptomyces aureofaciens* | Chlortetracycline (Aureomycin) | *Streptomyces antibioticus* | Vidarabine (adenine arabinoside, ara-A) (antiviral) |
| *Streptomyces bellus* var. *cirolerosis*, var. *nova* | Cirolemycin (antineoplastic) | *Streptomyces puniceus* | Viomycin |
| *Streptomyces noursei* | Cycloheximide (Actidione) | *Streptomyces bikiniensis* (variant) | Zorbamycin |
| *Streptomyces peucetius* | Daunomycin (antineoplastic) | **Actinomycetes** | |
| *Streptomyces aureofaciens* (mutant) | Demeclocycline (Declomycin) | *Micromonospora purpurea* | Gentamicin |
| *Streptomyces peucetius* var. *caesius* | Doxorubicin (Adriamycin) (antineoplastic) | *Nocardia lurida* | Ristocetin (Spontin) |
| *Streptomyces erythraeus* | Erythromycin (Ilotycin) | *Micromonospora inyoensis* | Sisomicin |
| *Streptomyces fradiae* | Fosfomycin (antibiotic) | **Fungi** | |
| *Streptomyces fradiae* | Fradicin (antifungal) | *Cephalosporium acremonium* | Cephaloridine (Loridine) |
| *Streptomyces tanashiensis* | Kalafungin (antibiotic) | *Cephalosporium* | Cephalothin (Keflin) |
| *Streptomyces kanamyceticus* | Kanamycin (Kantrex) | *Aspergillus fumigatus* | Fumagillin |
| *Streptomyces lincolnensis* | Lincomycin (Lincocin) | *Penicillium griseofulvum dierckx* and *Penicillium janczewski* | Griseofulvin (Fulvicin) |
| *Streptomyces melanogenes* | Melanomycin | | |
| *Streptomyces plicatus* | Mithramycin (antineoplastic) | *Aspergillus giganteus* | Nifungin (antifungal) |
| *Streptomyces caespitosus* | Mitomycin | *Penicillium notatum* and *chrysogenum* | Penicillin |
| *Streptomyces carzinostaticus* (variant) | Neocarzinostatin (antineoplastic) | *Penicillium stoloniferum* | Statolon (antiviral in animals) |

cally develop evidence of liver dysfunction, rarely severe hepatitis. Most authorities believe this is no reason to discontinue the regimen but rather an indication to screen the recipients initially and, once on the drug, to check them at monthly intervals for any sign of liver disorder.

*Para-aminosalicylic acid* (PAS) is another chemotherapeutic agent effective against the tubercle bacillus; it is often used in combination with isoniazid and streptomycin in the treatment of tuberculosis.

*Ethambutol* (2,2'-[ethylenediimino]-di-1-butanol dihydrochloride) is often used in combination with isoniazid for the treatment of tuberculosis. It is valuable in the treatment of disease caused by tubercle bacilli resistant to other tuberculostatic drugs and is effective against certain atypical mycobacteria.

*Nitrofurans* are a group of synthetic antimicrobial drugs with activity against gram-positive and gram-negative bacteria, fungi, and protozoa but little toxicity for tissues. Their mode of action is to interfere with basic enzyme systems within the microbial cell. An important one is *nitrofurazone* (Furacin), applied topically to prevent infections of wounds, burns, ulcers, and skin grafts. *Nitrofurantoin* (Furadantin) is used in bacterial infections of the urinary tract. *Furazolidone* (Furoxone) is effective against *Giardia lamblia* in intestinal infections; in a mixture with *nifuroxime* (Micofur) it is used in the treatment of vaginitis caused by bacteria, by *Trichomonas vaginalis,* and by *Candida albicans.*

## ANTIBIOTICS

Experiments and observations carried on during the last three decades have proved that numerous organisms can produce substances with the power to inhibit the multiplication of other organisms or even to kill them. Such substances are known as antibiotics.*

---

*This information is not so new as it might seem, because Pasteur in 1877 demonstrated that the growth of anthrax bacilli was retarded by the presence of common soil organisms, and several antibiotic-like substances (for example, pyocyanase) were prepared before 1900. The term *antibiosis* was introduced in 1889 by Vuillemin, who said: "No one considers the lion which leaps on its prey to be a parasite nor the snake which injects venom into the wounds of its victim before eating it. Here there is nothing equivocal; one creature destroys the life of another to preserve its own; the first is completely active, the second completely passive. The one is in absolute opposition to the life of the other. The conception is so simple that no one has ever thought of giving it a name. This condition, instead of being examined in isolation, can appear as a factor in more complex phenomena. In order to simplify words we will call it antibiosis. . . ." (Florey, H.: Antibiotics, Fifty-second Robert Boyle Lecture presented to the Oxford University Scientific Club, Springfield, Ill., 1951, Charles C Thomas, Publisher, p. 1.)

**Table 16-3**
Antibiotics—range of activity

| NARROW-SPECTRUM ANTIBIOTICS | BROAD-SPECTRUM ANTIBIOTICS |
| --- | --- |
| Penicillin | Chloramphenicol |
| Streptomycin | Chlortetracycline |
| Dihydrostreptomycin | Demeclocycline |
| Erythromycin | Oxytetracycline |
| Lincomycin | Tetracycline and derivatives |
| Polymyxin B | Kanamycin |
| Colistin | Ampicillin |
| Oleandomycin | Cephalothin |
| Vancomycin | Rifampin |
| Nystatin | Gentamicin |
| Spectinomycin | Paromomycin |

In 1941 the term *antibiotic* was defined by Waksman as follows: "An antibiotic is a chemical substance produced by microorganisms which has the capacity to inhibit the growth of bacteria and even destroy bacteria and other microorganisms in dilute solution."*

Antibiotics are elaborated by bacteria, fungi, actinomycetes, streptomycetes, and plants including certain flowering ones. Some organisms produce more than one, and certain antibiotics are produced by more than one organism. Table 16-2 gives such sources. Although thousands of species of microorganisms biosynthesize antibiotics and hundreds of them are known, only a few are practically useful in the treatment of disease. We consider them collectively, yet their physical, chemical, and pharmacologic properties are widely divergent.

**Spectrum of activity.** Some antibiotics affect mainly gram-positive bacteria, with little or no effect on gram-negative bacteria. Others seem to affect only certain species of bacteria regardless of whether they are gram-negative or gram-positive. A few attack fungi. A few are active against the rickettsias and the chlamydiae (bedsoniae).

The susceptibility (or resistance) of bacteria to different antibiotics may be determined by suitable laboratory tests, designated susceptibility tests (p. 68), and there are also satisfactory tests for determining the amount of certain antibiotics in the blood.

The *spectrum* of a compound is its range of antimicrobial activity. A *broad spectrum* indicates a wide variety of microorganisms affected, including usually both gram-positive and gram-negative bacteria. A *narrow-spectrum* antibiotic limits only a few. Table 16-3 lists some antibiotics of both categories.

---

*Waksman, S. A.: Bull. N.Y. Acad. Med. **42:**623, 1966.

**Table 16-4**
Cellular disturbances (mode of action) related to antimicrobial agents

| INHIBITORY EFFECT ON | | | | | METABOLISM ANTAGONISM—COMPETITIVE INTERFERENCE IN CELL METABOLISM |
|---|---|---|---|---|---|
| CELL WALL SYNTHESIS | NUCLEIC ACID SYNTHESIS | PROTEIN SYNTHESIS | | CELL MEMBRANE FUNCTION | |
| | | RIBOSOME FUNCTION | OTHER | | |
| Bacitracin | Actinomycin D | Chloramphenicol | Chlortetracycline | Amphotericin B | Isoniazid |
| Cephalosporins | Griseofulvin | Dihydrostreptomycin | Erythromycin | Benzalkonium | Nitrofurans |
| Penicillins | Idoxuridine | Gentamicin | Lincomycin | chloride | Para-aminosalicylic |
| Vancomycin | Rifampin | Kanamycin | Methacycline | Colistin | acid |
| | | Neomycin | Oleandomycin | Nystatin | Sulfonamides |
| | | Paromomycin | Oxytetracycline | Polymyxins | |
| | | Streptomycin | Tetracycline | | |

**Mode of action of antimicrobial drugs.** Several mechanisms explain in part the harmful or lethal effects that antimicrobial drugs have for microbes. Most of the time the mechanisms of injury are subtle ones, usually reflecting an inhibitory effect on some aspect of microbial physiology. The first mechanism studied was the role of the sulfonamides in competition for a place in the metabolic activities of the cell (*metabolic antagonism*). A drug utilized by mistake because of a close chemical resemblance to a vital cytoplasmic substance could halt growth and function. The physiologic integrity of the microbial cell depends on key macromolecules and the processes in which they are involved. Certain ones known to be vulnerable to commonly used antimicrobials include (1) bacterial cell wall synthesis, (2) nucleic acid synthesis, (3) protein synthesis, and (4) cell membrane function. Table 16-4 lists antimicrobial compounds as to category of action.

The rigid cell wall jackets bacterial cell cytoplasm with its characteristically high osmotic pressure. If the cell wall is faulty in its construction and weakened because of the action of penicillin, the cytoplasmic membrane cannot withstand the internal pressure. In a medium of ordinary tonicity the bacterial cell explodes.

Antibiotics can interfere with the synthesis of the nucleic acids within the cell. Some complex with DNA and block the formation of the messenger RNA. Other antibiotics inhibit the ribosomes (RNA) directly, thereby materially affecting the elaboration of proteins within the cell. As a result so-called "nonsense" proteins appear, indicating a chemical mixup. Since the biochemical activities relating to nucleic acid and protein synthesis are complicated, the possibilities for injury to the cell are many.

One of the antifungal antibiotics combines with sterols in the cell membrane of the susceptible fungus, destroying membrane function. Cell contents leak out, and the cell dies. Some antibiotics alter the permeability of the plasma membrane. Benzalkonium chloride can disrupt a bacterial cell membrane by its detergent action.

An important factor in any consideration of the mode of action of antimicrobial compounds is that of *selective toxicity:* The agent, to be useful, must kill the microbial cells without damaging the cells of the animal host. Agents such as disinfectants that coagulate proteins in *all* living cells are *nonselective*.

**Side effects.** There are four serious complications of antibiotic therapy: (1) hypersensitivity or allergy, (2) toxicity, (3) effects of the replacement flora, and (4) induction of bacterial resistance.

The turnover of drugs by the human body involves a series of complex, enzymatically mediated reactions. It is increasingly apparent that there can be vast individual differences. Signs of hypersensitivity to the antibiotics are variable in different persons but include skin rashes, joint paints, lymph node enlargement, lowered white blood cell count, and sometimes hemorrhages (p. 546). Examples of toxicity* to antibiotic therapy include the aplastic anemia induced by chloramphenicol and the deafness sometimes produced by streptomycin. Table 16-5 gives additional examples indicating the background and the lesion.

*Replacement flora.* The appearance of a replacement microbial flora is quite troublesome at times. Not

*Some antibiotics in the doses ordinarily given are associated with psychiatric disturbances. Depression and hallucinations have been related to certain long-acting sulfonamides. Psychosis, especially in the elderly, can be precipitated with the antiviral amantadine. A buoyant state of well-being and elation has been noticed in isoniazid-treated patients with tuberculosis.

**Table 16-5**

Some examples of pathologic complications to antibiotic therapy

| ANTIBIOTIC | THERAPEUTIC BACKGROUND | PHYSIOLOGIC DERANGEMENT | PATHOLOGIC LESION |
|---|---|---|---|
| Neomycin | Prolonged administration | Changes in lining of small intestine (jejunum) with interference in absorption of glucose, iron, vitamin $B_{12}$ | Malabsorption syndrome* |
| Tetracycline | Administration during pregnancy or to infants | Deposition of antibiotic in tooth enamel | Dental defects—pigmentation |
| Tetracycline | Large doses given intravenously | Toxic effect on liver | Liver disease (injury from hepatotoxin) |

*See p. 570.

being affected by the drug themselves, such organisms tend to increase during the period of therapy, being no longer held back by the organisms that succumb to the antibiotic. They can multiply in an uncontrolled way, and if potential or opportunist pathogens, they may start a disease process difficult to treat. The replacement flora can be quite resistant to standard antibiotics. Such secondary infections are often caused by *Proteus* or *Pseudomonas* species, and infections with *Candida albicans* easily follow prolonged and extensive antibiotic therapy, especially with broad-spectrum preparations. *Superinfection* as a complication is more likely with the broad-spectrum antibiotics than with the narrow-spectrum ones.

*Drug resistance.* Bacteria vary in their capability to develop resistance to a given drug. Resistance means that the drug is no longer effective in suppressing their growth and multiplication. Remember that resistance is always a possibility whenever a bacteriostatic drug is given, since such a drug merely limits the activities of given microbes—body mechanisms dispose of them! Many antibiotics are bacteriostatic within the human body. If only *bactericidal* (lethal) antibiotics were given, resistance would cause less concern.

In food processing, antibiotics are used to control bacterial spoilage of foods. Farmers use antibiotics freely in treating mastitis in cows producing market milk. Some 16 antibiotics are used as additives in livestock feed. All these factors are believed to contribute significantly to the problem of bacterial resistance.

The best known mechanism of drug resistance by disease-producing staphylococci and coliform bacteria is the production of the adaptive enzyme *penicillinase*, which inactivates penicillin G.

One of the most interesting mechanisms yet described concerns the *R*, or *resistance*, factors (also called resistance transfer factors, RTF). First detected in Japan in 1959, they were later identified in the United States as circular molecules of double-stranded DNA separate from the bacterial chromosome that could be passed by bacterial conjugation from one microorganism to another within a species or even from one member of a genus to another (Fig. 3-9). The particles replicate independently of the main genetic material, and the resistance is passed to successive generations. R factors are an example of bacterial *plasmids*, extrachromosomal genetic elements carrying information not normally necessary for the survival of the bacterial host. This genetic material, free-floating in the cytoplasm, endows its possessor with an all-inclusive type of resistance to diverse antibacterial agents—sulfonamides, streptomycin, tetracyclines, chloramphenicol, penicillin, neomycin, even experimental antibiotics—with obviously different modes of antibacterial activity. About two dozen gram-negative bacteria transfer the R factors. From Bergey's Family Enterobacteriaceae they include members of the genera *Enterobacter, Escherichia, Klebsiella, Salmonella, Shigella, Serratia, Proteus, Citrobacter;* from Bergey's Family Pseudomonadaceae, *Pseudomonas;* and from Bergey's Family Vibrionaceae, *Vibrio.*

**The roster**

Short discussions of well-known antibiotics follow.

*Tyrothricin,* one of the first antibiotics to be studied carefully, was isolated from an aerobic, motile, nonpathogenic bacillus (*Bacillus brevis*) growing in the soil. From tyrothricin were obtained two polypeptide products—*gramicidin* (named in honor of the bacteriologist Gram) and *tyrocidine,* both highly antagonistic to gram-positive cocci and very toxic. Tyrothricin is without effect when given orally and very dangerous when given parenterally. It therefore must be used locally. It prevents bacterial growth and causes bacteria to lyse.

*Penicillin* is an organic acid and a beta-lactam antibiotic. Accidentally discovered, this important antibiotic is isolated from certain molds, the most impor-

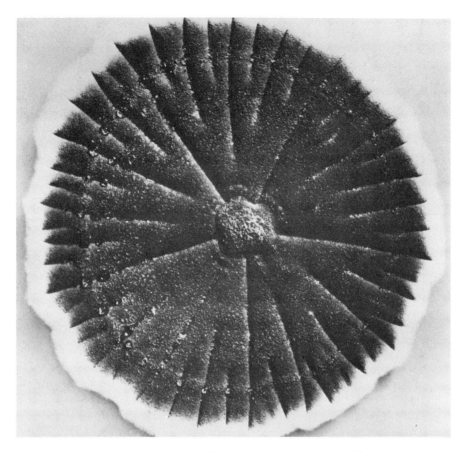

**Fig. 16-1.** *Penicillium chrysogenum,* giant colony. From this mutant form of the green mold, almost all of the world's supply of penicillin is obtained. (Courtesy Pfizer Inc., New York.)

tant of which are *Penicillium notatum* and *Penicillium chrysogenum* (Fig. 16-1). The first antibiotic to come into general use, it is still in many ways the best.* It may be administered intravenously, subcutaneously, into body cavities, orally, and locally, and in contrast to many antibiotics that are bacteriostatic, it is also bactericidal. It is one of the most important anti-infectives because it is bactericidal! Penicillin acts by interfering with synthesis of the bacterial cell wall and therefore affects actively growing bacteria. In the individual not allergic to penicillin its toxicity for human tissue is almost nonexistent. It is an effective agent, with some exceptions, against staphylococci, streptococci (Group A), pneumococci, meningococci, and other organisms, and its use revolutionized the treatment of syphilis. It does not have an effect on most gram-negative bacilli with the usual doses given. Most of the microorganisms originally

sensitive to penicillin still are, with the notable exceptions coming from the penicillinase-producing staphylococci and gonococci. The enzyme penicillinase accounting for penicillin resistance in both gram-positive and gram-negative microorganisms inactivates penicillin by opening the beta-lactam ring. Its formation has been directed by the bacterial plasmid.

Penicillin has been isolated in six closely related forms called F, G, X, K, O, and V. Penicillin G is the most satisfactory type to manufacture and use. Therefore about 90% of commercial penicillin is of this type. The sodium, potassium, and procaine salts are the common ones. Penicillin G is the agent of choice in the nonallergic individual for the treatment of infections caused by group A hemolytic streptococci.

The strength of penicillin is designated in *units*. A unit (International) corresponds to the activity of 0.6 $\mu$g. (0.000006 gm.) of pure sodium penicillin G.

The generic name *penicillin* includes all antibacterials isolated from the genus *Penicillium*. The natural penicillins are extracted from cultures.

*Semisynthetic penicillins* are the sequel to a basic

---

*Penicillin is an inexpensive drug. The chances are that a course of penicillin will cost only a fraction of that with another antibiotic.

observation on the chemical structure of penicillin made in Great Britain in 1959. When the chemist learns how the molecule can be modified, he can change it to give the new product more desirable properties than those of the natural substance. Consequently, more than 500 semisynthetic penicillins have been made. Phenethicillin potassium (Syncillin), an oral preparation, was the first one to be dispensed by prescription.

Penicillin resistance is most important from a pathogenic staphylococcus. In a general way the newer penicillins are indicated for pathogenic staphylococci resistant to penicillin G; otherwise, the potency of these new drugs is less than that of the original penicillin. Compounds designed to counteract staphylococcal penicillinase are methicillin sodium (Staphcillin), oxacillin sodium (Prostaphlin), nafcillin sodium (Unipen), cloxacillin (Tegopen), and sodium dicloxacillin monohydrate (Pathocil).

*Ampicillin* (Polycillin) is a broad-spectrum semisynthetic penicillin with activity against a number of gram-positive and gram-negative bacteria, including *Salmonella, Shigella, Escherichia coli,* and *Proteus.* If disease of the biliary tract is not present, ampicillin can be used to treat the typhoid carrier, and it has value in the treatment of intestinal amebiasis. It is ineffective in the presence of penicillinase.

*Carbenicillin* (Pyopen) is a British semisynthetic penicillin with reported activity against *Pseudomonas. Disodium carbenicillin* (Geopen) is active against the gram-negative *Pseudomonas* and *Proteus.*

*Cross allergenicity* exists among the penicillins; that is, a person sensitive to penicillin G will be found sensitive to one of the semisynthetic penicillins. It is estimated that 5% to 6% of the population are allergic to penicillin.

*Cephalothin, cephaloridine, cephaloglycin,* and *cephalexin* are cephalosporins, a group of antibiotics of an entirely new class, though closely related chemically to penicillin (also beta-lactam antibiotics). They are semisynthetic derivatives from the fermentation products of the fungus *Cephalosporium* (Fig. 16-2), whose natural habitat is the seacoast of Sardinia in Italy. Sodium cephalothin (Keflin) is a broad-spectrum antibiotic bactericidal against gram-positive and gram-negative bacteria. It must be given parenterally; it is unaffected by penicillinase and is of low toxicity. Cephaloridine (Loridine) is similar to cephalothin. Cephaloglycin (Kafocin) and cephalexin (Keflex) can be given orally. An advantage to the cephalosporins is the general lack of cross allergenicity with penicillin.

*Streptomycin,* an organic base, was isolated from *Streptomyces griseus,* an organism growing in the soil, and is one of a large group of chemically related

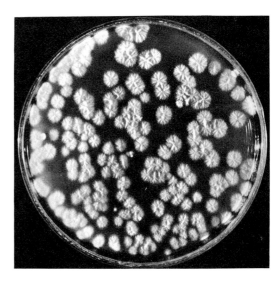

**Fig. 16-2.** *Cephalosporium* colonies on agar plate. Important antibiotics are derived from this fungus. (From Profile of an antibiotic, Indianapolis, 1966, Eli Lilly & Co.)

antibiotics, the aminoglycoside antibiotics, whose discovery came as a result of a deliberate search. Its action in a general way is bactericidal, like that of penicillin. It is active against gram-negative and acid-fast bacilli. Although seldom given intravenously, it may be administered by many routes. There are three disadvantages to streptomycin: (1) toxicity—its use may induce injury to the auditory portion of the eighth cranial nerve, with deafness; (2) drug resistance—bacteria sensitive to it can quickly become resistant during the course of therapy; and (3) poor oral absorption—if the drug is given by mouth, it is not significantly absorbed. A unit of streptomycin corresponds to the activity of 1 $\mu$g. of pure crystalline streptomycin base.

*Dihydrostreptomycin* is a derivative of streptomycin and much like it. Its use also may be followed by neurotoxic symptoms, but as a rule, it is less toxic than streptomycin.

*Neomycin* and *viomycin,* also aminoglycosides, are similar to streptomycin. Neomycin is derived from *Streptomyces fradiae.* Viomycin is derived from *Streptomyces puniceus.* Neomycin can damage the kidney. Viomycin is sometimes used in the treatment of tuberculosis, although it also is nephrotoxic.

*Kanamycin* (Kantrex), a broad-spectrum aminoglycoside antibiotic obtained from *Streptomyces kanamyceticus,* must be given parenterally. Its activity is directed against many aerobic gram-positive and gram-negative bacteria, including most strains of staphylococci and many strains of *Proteus.* The major toxic manifestation of this drug is partial or complete deafness resulting from its action on the auditory portion of the eighth cranial nerve. It is also nephrotoxic.

*Gentamicin sulfate* (Garamycin), an aminoglycoside, is a broad-spectrum antibiotic, chemically related to neomycin and kanamycin, which can be given parenterally. It is becoming a drug of choice for serious systemic infections caused by gram-negative bacteria. Like the other aminoglycoside antibiotics, it is nephrotoxic and ototoxic. Loss of hair including that of the eyebrows has been reported with its use.

*Spectinomycin* (Trobicin), a new member of the streptomycin-kanamycin family, is designed for the one-dose intramuscular treatment of gonorrhea. Although an aminoglycoside antibiotic, it is not thought to be nephrotoxic or ototoxic.

*Erythromycin* (Ilotycin), a macrolide, is derived from *Streptomyces erythraeus*. A valuable antibiotic, it is effective when given orally against gram-positive bacteria and some of the gram-negative bacteria. It is especially recommended for the treatment of infections caused by organisms that have become resistant to penicillin. Its use is seldom followed by toxic manifestations.

*Lincomycin* (Lincocin), is a medium-spectrum antibiotic that can be administered orally or by injection. It inhibits the growth of gram-positive cocci, including staphylococci, which produce penicillinase. Although its action is similar to that of erythromycin, erythromycin is antagonistic to it (as are the cyclamate artificial sweeteners formerly used in various low-calorie preparations). Lincomycin is a parent drug to *clindamycin* (Cleocin), which may be the first antibiotic that is also an antimalarial drug. Clindamycin, an oral agent, is particularly useful in treatment of anaerobic infections, especially those of *Bacteroides*.

*Polymyxin* is a general name for a number of polypeptide antibiotics derived from different strains of *Bacillus polymyxa*, known as polymyxin A, B, C, and D. Polymyxin is toxic, especially to the kidney* and brain. It is used locally and as an intestinal antiseptic. It is important in topical preparations, but its systemic use is hazardous. Polymyxin B is usually effective against infections with *Pseudomonas aeruginosa*. However, *Proteus* resists it.

*Colistin* (Coly-Mycin), a polypeptide antibiotic isolated in Japan from *Bacillus polymyxa* var. *colistinus*, is chemically similar to polymyxin. It is effective against gram-negative bacteria in general and, like polymyxin B, against *Pseudomonas aeruginosa* in particular. Less toxic than polymyxin B and with fewer side reactions in the central nervous system and kidney, it is of special value in urinary tract infections. It is given intramuscularly.

*Bacitracin* is a polypeptide antibiotic produced by *Bacillus subtilis* group *licheniformis*. It inhibits the growth of many gram-positive organisms including penicillin-resistant staphylococci and of the gram-negative gonococci and meningococci, but can only be used locally.

*Capreomycin*, a new polypeptide antibiotic, is derived from *Streptomyces capreolus* and is related to viomycin. It is mentioned because of its activity against atypical mycobacteria and in combination with other drugs against tubercle bacilli resistant to standard antituberculosis drugs.

*Vancomycin* (Vanocin) must be given intravenously. It is a bactericidal drug isolated from *Streptomyces orientalis*, promoted for the therapy of infections caused by antibiotic-resistant gram-positive bacteria, especially staphylococci.

*Oleandomycin*, isolated from *Streptomyces antibioticus*, is similar to erythromycin but less active. It can be given orally but is hepatotoxic.

*Rifampin* (Rifadin, Rimactane), one of the rifamycins, is a semisynthetic broad-spectrum antibiotic taken by mouth, with bactericidal activity notable against the tubercle bacillus. It is effective in the treatment of carriers of the meningococcus and has been used in the treatment of leprosy. It has an effect against the causative chlamydiae (bedsoniae) of trachoma and inhibits replication of poxvirus by blocking synthesis of viral protein. Adverse reactions are infrequent. The urine, feces, saliva, sputum, tears, and sweat may take on an orange color because of therapy with the drug.

*Tetracycline* is one of a group of broad-spectrum antibiotics and represents the chemical moiety common to the group. It is produced chemically from oxytetracycline and has been isolated from a streptomycete found in Texas. As a group tetracyclines sometimes irritate the alimentary tract. They are given orally to treat intestinal amebiasis. Tetracyclines sometimes pigment the teeth. If tetracycline gains access to the circulation of an unborn baby because the drug is given to the mother, it is deposited in areas of developing bones and teeth. The damage results in staining of tooth enamel (Fig. 16-3).

*Chlortetracycline* (Aureomycin), a broad-spectrum antibiotic isolated from *Streptomyces aureofaciens*, is effective against a wider range of organisms than are such antibiotics as penicillin and streptomycin. It affects gram-positive bacteria, certain gram-negative bacteria, rickettsias, and chlamydiae. It may be given orally or intravenously.

*Oxytetracycline* (Terramycin) is derived from *Streptomyces rimosus*. Like chlortetracycline, it has a

---

*The polypeptide antibiotics, polymyxin, colistin, and bacitracin, are all nephrotoxic.

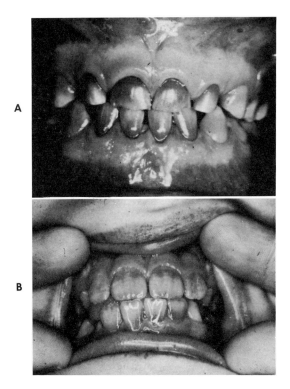

**Fig. 16-3.** Discoloration of teeth caused by tetracycline. **A,** Deciduous teeth, brownish gray. **B,** Permanent teeth, yellowish gray. (From Gorlin, R. J., and Goldman, H. M.: Thoma's oral pathology, ed. 6, St. Louis, 1970, The C. V. Mosby Co.)

wide range of antibacterial activity. It is given orally and is comparatively nontoxic.

*Demeclocycline** (Declomycin) another member of the group of tetracyclines, was first prepared chemically. It was later found in a mutant strain of *Streptomyces aureofaciens*. In general, its antibacterial activity is similar to that of the other tetracyclines, perhaps somewhat prolonged. Cases of photosensitization (sensitivity to light) have followed its use. Other derivatives of tetracycline and comparable to it pharmacologically are *methacycline* (Rondomycin), *minocycline* (Minocin), *rolitetracycline* (Syntetrin), and *doxycycline* (Vibramycin).

*Chloramphenicol* (Chloromycetin), the first of the broad-spectrum antibiotics, was isolated from *Streptomyces venezuelae* (found in the soil of Venezuela) but has now been crystallized. It is effective against certain bacteria, rickettsias, and the chlamydiae (bedsoniae). It is the best antibiotic for the treatment of typhoid fever. It is usually given orally, but it may be given intramuscularly or intravenously. Two peculiar

---

*Demethylchlortetracycline.

toxic disturbances occasionally complicate chloramphenicol therapy. One is hematologic; an aplastic anemia develops, with cessation of blood cell formation. The other is cardiovascular collapse seen in babies 2 months of age and younger. This is *gray syndrome*. Since chloramphenicol is toxic, it should not be used in those cases where tetracyclines are effective.

*Nystatin* (Mycostatin), an antifungous, polyene antibiotic produced by *Streptomyces noursei*, is used with favorable results in infections caused by *Candida albicans*. It is often given with a broad-spectrum antibiotic to suppress the growth of the resistant intestinal fungi (replacement flora), which might produce lesions in the bowel after prolonged antibiotic therapy.

*Amphotericin B* (Fungizone), a broad-spectrum antifungal drug and another polyene obtained from *Streptomyces nodosus*, should be given intravenously. It is said to be effective in the treatment of deep-seated fungous infections, those involving the internal organs and widely spread within the body, but it has no effect on bacteria. The initial infusion of this drug is regularly accompanied by a chill-fever reaction.

*Fumagillin* is produced during the growth of *Aspergillus fumigatus*. It is inactive against most bacteria, fungi, and viruses but is destructive to *Entamoeba histolytica* (the cause of amebic dysentery).

*Griseofulvin* (Fulvicin) is an oral antibiotic obtained from at least four species of *Penicillium*. A *fungistatic* drug, not a fungicidal one, it has a wide range of antifungal activity against practically all the dermatophytic fungi (*Microsporum*, *Epidermophyton*, and *Trichophyton*). Although systemically administered, it does not act on *Candida albicans*, the deep systemic fungi, or bacteria. The drug can be demonstrated to attack the advancing hyphal threads of invading fungi in skin, nails, and hair, causing these segments to shrivel and curl. Toxicity seems to be low; in anticipation of an effect on the blood-forming organs, periodic white blood cell counts are advised.

*Paromomycin* (Humatin), an amebicide, is a broad-spectrum antibiotic obtained from *Streptomyces rimosus*. Because of its nephrotoxicity it is given not by injection but orally, although it is poorly absorbed from the gastrointestinal tract. It is effective against *Entamoeba histolytica* and holds back the secondary infection of the bowel that complicates amebiasis. In addition to paromomycin, the antibiotics with amebicidal activity are neomycin, kanamycin, and the tetracyclines.

## ANTIVIRALS

Although antiviral agents are still largely under investigation, there is a great deal of interest in them; many compounds are being studied, some released;

and several major developments have occurred in the last few years. Currently three important categories have emerged: (1) thiosemicarbazone, (2) a group of pyrimidine nucleosides, and (3) amantadine.

*Methisazone* (N-methylisatin-β-thiosemicarbazone) has been shown to prevent smallpox in susceptible persons exposed in the epidemics studied in India.

*Idoxuridine* (5-iodo-2'-deoxyuridine, or *IDU*), an antimetabolite and pyrimidine analog that inhibits normal cellular DNA synthesis, has been found effective against eye infection caused by the herpes simplex virus. Idoxuridine represents an achievement—the results of treatment with it in herpetic keratitis have been spectacular.

From *Streptomyces antibioticus* comes the purine nucleoside *vidarabine*, also known as adenine arabinoside or ara-A. It is a nonspecific inhibitor of viral replication, with a wide range of activity and almost no acute toxicity.

*Cytarabine* (Cytosar), also known as cytosine arabinoside or ara-C, is also a purine analog. It was studied as an antileukemic agent in the laboratory and found to be an antagonist of DNA synthesis with potent antiviral properties in vitro. Both ara-C and idoxuridine are rapidly inactivated in vivo, and both can suppress bone marrow function.

*Ribavirin* (Virazole), a synthetic nucleoside, is active in tissue culture against a number of DNA and RNA viruses. Its action is to prevent replication, not to destroy viruses.

*Amantadine hydrochloride* (Symmetrel) is a synthetic compound with a selective antiviral action. It has been used for the prevention of influenza due to $A_2$ strains of the virus only. It also has been used against rubella virus. Amantadine blocks penetration of the virus into the host cell. It stimulates the central nervous system and can cause convulsions in large doses.

*Interferon,* a naturally occurring nonimmune protein, was the first substance to be associated with an antiviral action. An integral part of the host defense, it is a diffusible substance produced by a living cell infected with virus that blocks further viral infection of that cell (p. 291). It can also be induced by bacteria, bacterial products, chlamydiae, and protozoa. Certain chemicals such as double-stranded RNA from a synthetic source can act as *interferon inducers*. Their use in enhancing resistance to viral infection is still experimental.

## Questions for review

1 Define disinfection, germicide, bactericide, antiseptic, asepsis, fumigation, bacteriostasis, preservative, antibiotic, iodophor, R transfer factors, penicillinase, interferon, detergent, cross allergenicity, enzyme detergent.
2 How do chemical disinfectants act?
3 Broadly classify antiseptics and disinfectants.
4 What is the current status of the antivirals?
5 Name 5 sulfonamide compounds used in medicine.
6 What is meant by chemotherapy and chemotherapeutic agent?
7 Discuss ethylene oxide as a sterilizing agent.
8 Explain *cold* sterilization.
9 What are broad-spectrum antibiotics? Name five.
10 What agents are most effective in the disinfection of articles contaminated with *Mycobacterium tuberculosis*?
11 List chemotherapeutic drugs used in the treatment of pulmonary tuberculosis.
12 Briefly discuss harmful side effects of antibiotic therapy. What is meant by a replacement flora?
13 What is a narrow-spectrum antibiotic? Name three.
14 Briefly describe one antifungous agent and one amebicide.
15 Briefly indicate the mode of action of antibiotics.

**References on pp. 173 to 175.**

# CHAPTER 17

# Practical technics

## Surgical disinfection and sterilization

Many different methods of sterilizing surgical instruments and supplies and of disinfecting wounds, the field of operation, and the hands of persons taking part in surgical operations are used in different hospitals and related medical or health field settings. An overview of the standard methods as evaluated in an experimental and testing laboratory is presented in Table 17-1. In the following paragraphs some of the ones commonly used are presented.

*The method of choice wherever applicable is sterilization by steam under pressure as usually carried out in a pressure steam sterilizer* (preferably the modern high-prevacuum steam autoclave) (Figs. 15-1, 15-3, and 17-1). There are exceptional circumstances in which chemical disinfection, including sterilization with ethylene oxide gas, has to be substituted for autoclave sterilization. Certain items are damaged by the environment of the pressure steam sterilizer, such as surgical instruments with optical lenses, instruments or materials made of heat-susceptible plastics, articles made of rubber, certain delicately constructed surgical instruments, and nonboilable gut sutures.

Generally, the pressure steam sterilizer (gravity air removal type) for most routine purposes of sterilization is maintained at 121° to 123° C. (250° to 254° F.), 15 to 17 pounds of pressure, for 30 minutes (Table 15-1). For certain items of rubber subjected to steam sterilization the time is shorter, 15 to 20 minutes. (Note the shorter time with the higher temperatures in the high-prevacuum sterilizer.)

**Gas sterilization.** Ethylene oxide is widely applied today to the sterilization of many items that cannot be steam sterilized. Gas sterilization is carried out in a specially devised chamber (Fig. 17-2). Table 17-2 compares this form with that of steam under pressure.

### SURGICAL INSTRUMENTS AND SUPPLIES

In Table 17-3 practical suggestions are given for the sterilization or chemical disinfection of specific instruments and supplies. (See also Table 17-4.)

Syringes and needles contaminated by even minute traces of serum or plasma may be sterilized by one of the methods recommended in Table 17-4. Disposable needles, blood lancets, and syringes are available commercially, and their use is strongly recommended wherever feasible, since one important method of spreading the hepatitis viruses is thereby blocked. (Disposable items are designed to be used once only and should never be sterilized and reused.)

The proper disposition of disposables must be stressed! Disposable syringes and needles must be kept away from children and drug addicts and must not wound the hand of the garbage collector. Once used, they can be incinerated, deformed in boiling water, or crushed in a machine.

One method for safe discard of disposable syringes and needles is as follows. The needle is placed inside the syringe, needle point upward toward the piston. The piston is inserted into the syringe and jammed down, locking the needle tightly between the barrel of the syringe and the plunger. The unit may then be thrown into the trash.

It is hard to render instruments with optical lenses completely free of microbes. To kill completely all microbes present might well loosen the cement of the lens system in the process or corrode the metal in some of the instruments. A recently developed, heat-resistant cement makes it possible to carry out a type of pasteurization wherein endoscopes are submerged in hot (not boiling) water at a temperature of 85° C. for 1 hour. This method kills most of the ordinary bacterial contaminants. Telescopic instruments with the modern improved cements in the lens systems can also be sterilized with ethylene oxide.

Formerly the preparation and care of rubber tubing used for intravenous medication was a difficult and time-consuming task. The use of plastic disposable units *should completely eliminate* the need for rubber tubing for intravenous medication and blood transfusion.

**Dressings and linens.** Towels, gowns, and other articles of cloth may be sterilized by autoclaving at

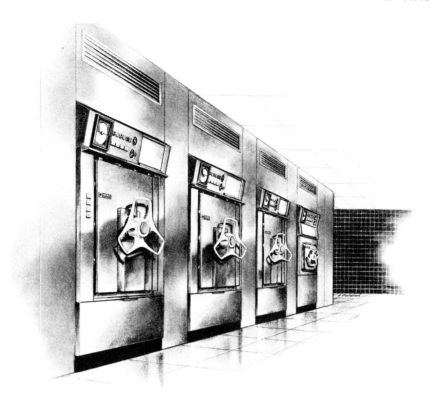

**Fig. 17-1.** Bank of recessed autoclaves in modern hospital. (Courtesy American Sterilizer Co., Erie, Pa.)

## Table 17-1
Comparison of methods for controlling microbial life*

| METHOD | TEMPERATURE REQUIRED | MINIMUM EXPOSURE TIME IN MINUTES |
|---|---|---|
| | | 0'  2'  10'  12'  15'  20'  90'  120'  150'  180' |
| *Sterilization*† | | |
| Saturated steam under pressure | 285° F. (140° C.) | (Instantaneous) |
| | 270° F. (132° C.) | |
| | 250° F. (121° C.) | |
| Ethylene oxide gas (12% ETO, 88% Freon-12) | 130° F. (54° C.) | |
| | 105° F. (40° C.) | |
| Hot air | 320° F. (160° C.) | or more |
| Chemical sporicide (solution) | Room temperature | or more |
| *Disinfection* | | |
| Steam—free flowing or boiling water | 212° F. (100° C.) | |
| Chemical germicide (solution) | Room temperature | |
| *Sanitization* | | |
| Water, detergents, or chemicals aided by physical means for soil removal | Maximum 200° F. (93° C.) | |

*Modified from chart copyrighted 1967, Research and Development Section, American Sterilizer Co., Erie, Pa.
†See pp. 139 and 146 for definitions.

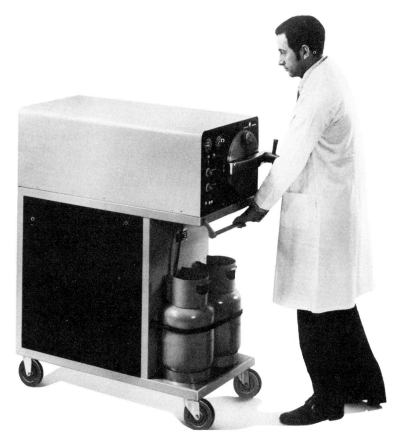

**Fig. 17-2.** Gas sterilizer, mobile unit. (Courtesy American Sterilizer Co., Erie, Pa.)

## Table 17-2
Comparison of steam sterilization with gas sterilization*

| | STEAM | GAS |
|---|---|---|
| Medical indications | Syringes, instruments, drapes, gowns, some plastics, rubber | Heat-sensitive plastics, rubber, bulky equipment (ventilators, telescopic instruments†) |
| Equipment | Automatic chamber (large and bulky) | Automatic chamber (large and bulky); also portable model |
| Penetration of material to be sterilized | Rapid | Very rapid |
| Time required | Minutes (15 minutes or less in some models) | Hours (4 to 12) |
| Efficiency | Excellent | 100% |
| Technical snags | Removal of air | Prevacuum; correct humidification; temperature over 70° C. |
| Danger | None | Undiluted ethylene oxide, explosive‡ |
| Hazard | Sterilization inadequate if air not completely removed | Toxic residues if aeration inadequate |
| Contraindications | Many plastics; sharp instruments; rubber deteriorates | Previously irradiated plastics such as polyvinyl chloride |

*Modified from Rendell-Baker, L., and Roberts, R. B.: Gas versus steam sterilization: when to use which, Med. Surg. Rev. **5:**10 (Fourth quarter), 1969.
†Modern day cements used on the optical lenses of such instruments have been sufficiently improved to permit sterilization with ethylene oxide gas.
‡The mixture of 12% ethylene oxide (ETO) and 88% Freon-12, which is generally used, is a safe one.

## Table 17-3
Technics of sterilization (or disinfection) of commonly used items in the clinical setting

| ITEM TO BE STERILIZED | AUTOCLAVE (METHOD OF CHOICE) | CHEMICAL DISINFECTION (CHOICE INDICATED)* | OTHER TECHNICS APPLICABLE |
|---|---|---|---|
| Surgical instruments and supplies, mechanically clean | | | |
| Noncutting instruments | Yes | 1. Amphyl 2%, 20 min.<br>2. Bard-Parker Germicide, 10 min. to 2 hr.<br>3. Ethylene oxide gas, 2 to 12 hr. | Boil completely submerged 30 minutes |
| Sharp instruments | Yes, in certain instances | 1. Amphyl 2%, 20 min.<br>2. Bard-Parker Germicide, 10 min. to 2 hr.<br>3. Ethylene oxide gas, 2 to 12 hr. | 1. Bake in hot-air sterilizer, 150° C., 3 hr.<br>2. Boil 30 min. (the cutting part wrapped with cotton and the instrument kept from tossing about; water should be boiling before instruments are placed in it† |
| Surgical needles | Yes, in packages | 1. Amphyl 2%, 20 min.<br>2. Isopropyl alcohol 70% to 90%, 20 min.<br>3. Ethylene oxide gas, 2 to 12 hr.<br>Wash needles in sterile water | Hot air at 160° C., 2 hr. |
| Hypodermic syringes and needles | Yes | Cold sterilization inadequate to remove viruses of hepatitis | 1. Dry heat, 160° C., 2 hr.<br>2. Boil 30 min. |
| Hinged instruments | Yes, in certain instances | 1. Isopropyl alcohol 70% to 90%, 20 min.<br>2. Activated glutaraldehyde (2% aqueous), 20 min. to 10 hr.<br>3. Ethylene oxide gas, 2 to 12 hr. | — |
| Transfer forceps | Yes, for the container | Bard-Parker Germicide (change solution once a week) | — |
| Endoscopes and instruments with optical lenses (cystoscopes and others) | — | 1. Ethylene oxide gas, 2 to 12 hr. (method of choice)<br>2. Aqueous formalin 20%, 12 hr.<br>3. Activated glutaraldehyde (2% aqueous), 10 hr.‡ | — |
| Polyethylene tubing | — | Immerse tubing carefully filled with disinfectant:<br>1. Bard-Parker Germicide, 12 hr.<br>2. Ethylene oxide gas 2 to 12 hr.<br>3. Aqueous formalin 20%, 12 hr. | — |
| Rubber tubing, silk catheters, and bougies | — | 1. Ethylene oxide gas, 2 to 12 hr. (method of choice)<br>2. Iodophor, 500 p.p.m. available iodine, 20 min.§ | — |

*Sodium nitrite should be added to alcohols, formalin, formaldehyde-alcohol, quaternary ammonium, and iodophor solutions to prevent rusting. Sodium bicarbonate should be added to phenolic solutions to prevent corrosion. Antirust tablets are available commercially.
†Boiling dulls knives and other sharp instruments because iron tends to enter solution in the ferrous state when heated. The site of corrosion—that part that is electropositive—is the sharp edge of the instrument. A "cathodic" sterilizer is so equipped electrically that such instruments are connected with the negative pole of a battery and corrosion prevented. This permits long-continued boiling without dulling.
‡Exposure to Nos. 2 or 3 for 15 min. eliminates tubercle bacilli and enteroviruses.
§To eliminate tubercle bacilli and enteroviruses, tubing must be filled.

*Continued.*

**Table 17-3**

Technics of sterilization (or disinfection) of commonly used items in the clinical setting—cont'd

| ITEM TO BE STERILIZED | AUTOCLAVE (METHOD OF CHOICE) | CHEMICAL DISINFECTION (CHOICE INDICATED) | OTHER TECHNICS APPLICABLE |
|---|---|---|---|
| | | 3. Amphyl 2%, 20 min.§ | |
| | | 4. Activated glutaraldehyde (2% aqueous), 15 min.§ | |
| Inhalation and equipment for anesthesia | — | 1. Ethylene oxide gas, 2 to 12 hr. | — |
| | | 2. Activated glutaraldehyde (2% aqueous), 10 hr. | |
| Thermometers | — | 1. Bard-Parker Germicide, 12 hr. | — |
| | | 2. Ethylene oxide gas, 2 to 12 hr. (cold cycle only) | |
| | | 3. Isopropyl alcohol 70% to 90% plus iodine 0.2%, 15 min. (to eliminate tubercle bacilli and enteroviruses) | |
| Surgical instruments and supplies, contaminated | Yes, wherever possible | Ethylene oxide gas, 2 to 12 hr. | — |

15 pounds of pressure for 30 minutes. They may be arranged in packs $12 \times 12 \times 20$ inches in size and wrapped in two layers of muslin or one layer of muslin and one or two layers of heavy paper.

**Reusable gloves.** When an operation is finished, the surgeon and his assistants should wash their gloves in cold water before removing them. After removal the gloves are washed outside and inside with tincture of green soap, thoroughly rinsed, and dried. They are then powdered, placed in glove envelopes, and wrapped. They are sterilized as follows: (1) autoclave at 15 pounds of pressure for 20 minutes, (2) follow with a vacuum for 5 to 10 minutes, (3) open the door of the sterilizer slightly and allow the gloves to dry in the sterilizer for about 5 minutes, and (4) re-move and separate the packages to allow rapid cooling (this prevents sticking). *Caution:* Gloves are often ruined by being allowed to remain in the sterilizer too long.

*Note:* In some of the modern sterilizer models all these steps will not be necessary.

By putting an iodine solution in the water used to wash off glove powder and by taking advantage of a well-known color change, one can detect holes in gloves. If there is even a very tiny hole, a brownish discoloration of the hand is seen after the glove is removed.

**Hand brushes.** To sterilize hand brushes, (1) clean thoroughly, rinse free of soap under running water, and submerge in 1:1000 aqueous benzalkonium chloride (Zephiran Chloride)* for 30 minutes (leave in the disinfectant until needed) or (2) autoclave and store in a sterile dry container. (Note the availability and practicality of prepackaged, sterile, disposable hand brushes.)

**Materials of fat or wax, oils, and petrolatum gauze.** To sterilize these heat-susceptible objects, place them in the sterilizing oven at 160° C. for 2 to 2½ hours.

**Sutures and ligatures.** To sterilize sutures and

**Table 17-4**

Methods of physical sterilization to eliminate hepatitis viruses*

| METHOD | TIME | TEMPERATURE |
|---|---|---|
| Autoclave† | 30 min. | 121.5° C. (15 lb. pressure) |
| Dry heat | 2 hr. | 170° C. |
| Boiling (active) | 30 min. | 100° C. |

*Most human viruses are destroyed at 60° C. for 30 minutes, with the exception of the hepatitis viruses. At this temperature a 10-hour period is required for inactivation.

†The autoclave is definitely the preferred method and strongly advised over the other two.

*Although only one disinfectant, such as benzalkonium chloride (Zephiran Chloride), may be mentioned for various purposes in the pages of this chapter, it does not follow that the one cited is necessarily the best. There are certainly many other good ones.

ligatures, (1) scrub the glass tubes with soap and water to remove greasy film, (2) rinse well with water to remove soap, (3) submerge in alcohol-formalin solution of the Bard-Parker type for 1 hour, (4) place in a sterile suture jar containing the foregoing antiseptic, and (5) remove with sterile forceps and rinse in sterile water before using.

Silkworm-gut, silk, horsehair, and metal ligatures may be sterilized by boiling. Surgical gut sutures in sealed tubes are available commercially. The tubing fluid is usually a mixture; one is isopropyl alcohol 90%, phenyl mercuric benzoate 0.025%, and water sufficient to make 100%. The tubes are handled and shipped in jars that contain a storage disinfectant. Such solutions are usually mixtures of isopropyl alcohol, formaldehyde, sodium nitrite, sodium bicarbonate, and distilled water and are of such a density that the tubes remain completely submerged and covered by the solution. (If hexachlorophene is added to this storage solution, the spore-killing time is reduced from 18 to 3 hours.)

**Water and saline solutions.** Water and saline solutions are placed in suitable containers and autoclaved at 15 pounds of pressure for 30 minutes. Great care should be exercised to prevent fibers of lint or other particles from getting into solutions that are to be given intravenously.

## SURGICAL SUITE

The operative field is exposed to pathogenic bacteria floating in the air. These arise from the noses and throats of the occupants of the surgical suite and may be destroyed by ultraviolet radiation.

Terminal disinfection of the operating room is done at the end of an operative procedure, after the patient has been removed. One of the phenol derivatives is usually used for this.

## BODY SITES

**Hands.** There are many methods of disinfecting the hands. The following method gives good results.
1. Wash the hands and arms well with soap and water.
2. With soap and sterile brush, scrub the nails and knuckles of both hands.
3. Scrub the hands, beginning with the thumbs and in succession scrubbing the inner and outer surfaces of the thumbs and fingers, giving several strokes to each area.
4. Scrub the palms and the backs of the hands and then the forearms to 3 inches above the elbow for 3 minutes; rinse well with running water.
5. With a sterile orange stick, clean under each nail thoroughly.
6. With a second sterile brush, scrub the hands and arms for 7 minutes in the same manner as with the first brush.
7. Thoroughly rinse off all soap with water and then rinse the hands in 70% alcohol.
8. With one end of a sterile towel, dry one hand and, with a circular motion, dry the forearm to the elbow. With the other end of the towel, dry the other hand and forearm in the same manner.

When one is scrubbing the hands for a surgical operation, plenty of soap should be used, and the scrubbing should be done with running water. When one is using cake soap, the soap is held between the brush and the palm until the scrubbing is complete. During the entire procedure the hands should be held higher than the elbows in order to prevent contamination.

At the present time the methods of disinfection of the hands are shortened by the habitual use of detergent soaps containing germicidal substances. The following method, known as the Betadine (p. 152) Surgical Scrub regimen, is widely used today. Because some members of the surgical team as well as some patients are allergic to iodine, pHisoHex (p. 151) can still be found in the health field setting.
1. Clean under the nails. Keep the fingernails short and clean.
2. Wet the hands and forearms.
3. Apply to the hands two portions, about 5 ml., of Betadine Surgical Scrub from a dispenser. (Depress Betadine dispenser foot pedal twice.)
4. Without adding water, wash the hands and forearms thoroughly for 5 minutes. Use a brush if desired.
5. With a sterile orange stick, clean under the nails. Add a little water for copious suds. Rinse thoroughly with running water.
6. Apply 5 ml. from the dispenser to the hands. Repeat steps just given. Rinse with running water.

Actual sterilization of the hands is not possible. Microbes live not only on the surface of the skin but also in its deeper layers, in the ducts of sweat glands, and around the hair follicles. These resident microbes are chiefly nonpathogenic staphylococci and diphtheroid bacilli and are plentiful about the nails.

**Site of operation.** Although the deeper portions of the skin cannot be absolutely sterilized, enough bacteria can be removed to make infection unlikely. The selection of an antiseptic for preoperative skin preparation has had the attention of surgeons since the earliest times, and many different ones have been used. The following outline represents a satisfactory method of skin preparation.

*Preliminary preparation.* This is carried out several hours before the operation.

1. Wash the part thoroughly with tincture of green soap; detergent soaps containing hexachlorophene may be used.
2. Shave the part.

There is no need to scrub the part with ether or alcohol during the preliminary preparation or to cover the area with sterile towels, as was once the custom, since this may increase the apprehension of the patient and is not necessary from the surgical standpoint.

Some authorities object to the skin shave being done ahead of the time the patient is taken to the operating room. They feel the best time is right before the surgical operation, in the operating room, after the patient has been put to sleep and positioned. If lather from a dispenser can and a new razor blade are used, there is no danger of cross infection, and the lather traps the hair. When the skin shave is done many hours before surgery, there is a good chance bacteria will grow in the inflammatory reaction about small razor nicks. The incision the surgeon makes is then likely to go through minute abscesses.

*Preparation at operation*

1. Clean the umbilicus with an applicator stick containing soap or detergent if the skin of the abdomen is being scrubbed.
2. Scrub the skin with detergent or soap, beginning with the imaginary line of incision and working laterally to the bed line.
3. Apply benzalkonium chloride 1:1000 to the umbilicus of abdomen with the applicator.
4. Paint the skin with benzalkonium chloride 1:1000 on a sponge. Begin at the imaginary line of incision and proceed as in step 2. (Tint a colorless solution so that the area of skin prepared will be outlined for the surgeon.)

*Note I.* Tincture of iodine mixed with 70% to 90% isopropyl alcohol, tincture of Merthiolate 1:1000, tincture of Mercresin, tincture of iodine, and other disinfectants may be used instead of benzalkonium chloride. If tincture of iodine is used, the iodine must be removed from around the edges of the field with an alcohol sponge.

*Note II.* When any skin area is prepared for operation, the imaginary line of incision is never painted with the same sponge more than once.

The following method utilizes Betadine Surgical Scrub and can be modified as indicated.

1. Shave the field of operation. Wet with water.
2. Apply Betadine on a sponge to the umbilicus, if the skin of the abdomen is being scrubbed, and discard sponge.
3. Scrub the imaginary line of incision with Betadine on a sponge for 1 minute, using a rotating motion.
4. Carry the same sponge out from the line of incision and scrub the outer portions of the surgical area for 1 minute; again, use a circular motion and discard the sponge.
5. Repeat this entire maneuver for five separate instances.
6. Use a little water to make suds. Use wet sterile gauze to rinse surgical area.
7. Pat dry with sterile towel.
8. Paint area with Betadine Solution. Allow to dry. The surgical area is now ready for the drapes.

The operating room personnel and those who prepare patients for operations should not let the fact that many surgical infections may be controlled by antibiotics lull them into satisfaction with careless antiseptic or aseptic technic.

**Other areas of skin.** For the rapid sterilization preceding routine hypodermic injections and venipunctures for intravenous medication, 70% to 90% ethyl or isopropyl alcohol or 2% iodine in 70% alcohol is effective when applied to a clean area of skin for 30 to 60 seconds. When lumbar puncture is to be done, the overlying skin should be cleansed with soap or detergent, rinsed, dried, and disinfected with a suitable preparation.

**Mucous membranes.** Absolute disinfection of mucous membranes is impossible. The mouth and throat may be cleansed with Dobell's solution, hydrogen peroxide, hexylresorcinol, or Ceepryn Chloride 1:10,000 to 1:5000. The vagina may be irrigated with benzalkonium chloride 1:5000 to 1:2000.

**Wound disinfection.*** Antiseptics that may be used for disinfection of wounds are Ceepryn Chloride 1:1000, hexachlorophene, soap, and Furacin 1:500. In some parts of the United States Furacin seems to be the most generally used wound antiseptic. Bacitracin in the form of an ointment and water-soluble chlorophyl derivatives such as Chloresium ointment (0.5%) are often applied to wounds. Chloresium acts as a deodorizer and, according to some observers, promotes the formation of granulation tissue, the tissue of repair. The chloramines (which slowly liberate chlorine) are sometimes used, as are such dyes as gentian violet, crystal violet, brilliant green, and malachite green, since these dyes are effective against the gram-positive bacteria so often responsible for wound infections. The dyes have a moderately destructive action on tissue cells. Favorable reports have been given the efficacy of Medicinal Zinc Peroxide

---

*Remember that local treatment of a wound with sulfonamides or penicillin can result in the patient's developing a sensitivity of these antibacterial agents (p. 157).

in the treatment of certain wounds (p. 149). *The use of antiseptic solutions should never be substituted for indicated surgical cleaning of infected wounds.*

## Disinfection of excreta and contaminated materials from infectious diseases

A patient with a communicable disease is not properly supervised until every avenue by which the infectious agent may be spread from the patient to others has been closed. These avenues are not closed until all excreta and all objects that may convey the infection have been properly disinfected. A patient who is being cared for in such a manner that all avenues by which the infection may spread to others are closed is said to be *isolated.* A ward patient with a conscientious and capable nurse is more strictly isolated from the microbiologic point of view than is the patient in a room with plastered walls and airtight doors who has a careless or incompetent nurse. Isolation refers to avenues of infection, not to walls and doors. *Remember that pathogenic microbes are most virulent when first thrown off from the body.*

Disinfection in infectious diseases is of two types: concurrent and terminal. *Concurrent disinfection* means the immediate disinfection of the patient's excreta or objects that have become contaminated by the patient or his excreta. *Terminal disinfection* means the final disinfection of the room, its contents, and environs after it has been vacated by the patient. The final chapter is written when it has been proved that patient and attendants are free of the agent that caused the disease—that is, they have not become carriers. In the following paragraphs are given methods of disinfecting excreta, materials, and objects by which infection is most often spread from the sick to the well.

**Hands of the nurse.** Unless properly disinfected, the hands of nurses, doctors, or other persons in contact with the patient are almost certain to transfer the infectious agent to themselves or to others. Although disinfection of the hands to prevent the spread of communicable diseases is not so time-consuming as for a surgical operation, it should be just as conscientiously done. The hands and lower arms should be submerged in a basin of 1:1000 aqueous benzalkonium chloride and rubbed vigorously for 2 minutes. It is good to follow this by washing the hands with soap and running water. It is not necessary to use a brush for scrubbing the hands and arms, although in some institutions this is required. The cleaned hands should be dried thoroughly. Hand lotion keeps the skin in good condition. The nails should be kept clean at all times. The hands should be cleaned in this way every time that they contact the patient for

any purpose whatsoever. To allow one's hands to contact a person suffering from a communicable disease and then, without disinfection, allow them to contact another person is little short of criminal neglect.

**Soiled linens and clothing.** All linens and clothing that have come in contact with the patient should be considered contaminated and should be kept in the patient's room until ready for final disposal. In the hospital they may be wrapped in sheets or placed in pillow cases and put in a special bag, care being taken that the outside of the bag does not become contaminated. Before the bag is full, it is closed tightly, marked to indicate that it contains infectious material, and sent to the laundry. On reaching the laundry, the bag itself is put in the washer. The washer is then closed and live steam introduced for 15 to 20 minutes. After this the regular procedure of the laundry is carried out. In the home the linen or bedclothes are bundled and carried to the kitchen or home laundry to be placed in a boiler containing warm water and soapsuds and boiled for from 10 to 15 minutes. After boiling, the process of laundering may be completed in the home or by a commercial laundry. On occasion, the boiler is carried to the patient's room to receive the soiled linen.

Mattresses, pillows, and blankets may be sterilized by heat in special sterilizing chambers, or they may be sterilized in a formaldehyde chamber. They also may be dried in the sunlight for an exposure period of 24 hours. Mattresses may be encased in plastic covers that have been cleaned with antiseptic solutions.

**Shoes.** Disinfection of shoes is best accomplished by placing a pledget of cotton saturated with formalin in each shoe and allowing the shoes to stay in a closed box for 24 hours. Shoes may also be disinfected by being sprayed with formalin from an atomizer for three successive evenings.

**Feces and urine.** Where connections exist to modern sewage disposal systems, feces and urine are disposed of in the commode without disinfection. Otherwise, feces and urine, especially from patients with typhoid fever, infectious hepatitis, and similar disorders, should be mixed with either 5% phenol (carbolic acid) or preferably chlorinated lime. The volume of disinfectant should be three times that of the material to be disinfected. Feces should be thoroughly broken up in order to ensure penetration. After the urine and feces are thoroughly mixed with the disinfecting solution, the mixture is allowed to stand for at least 2 hours before disposal of it is made. Contaminated colon tubes and such may be disinfected in Amphyl 2% solution for 20 minutes.

**Discharges from the mouth and nose.** Discharges from the mouth and nose are received on squares of tissue and placed in a paper bag pinned to the side of the bed. After the bag is wrapped in several layers of clean newspaper it is burned in the incinerator.

**Sputum.** Sputum should not be allowed to dry so as to permit particles to float off in the air. It should be received in a paper cup held in a special metal holder. The paper cup is discarded and the metal holder sterilized at least twice daily (more often if necessary). To discard a paper cup, remove the cup from the holder with forceps and set it on several thicknesses of newspaper. The cup is then filled with sawdust to decrease the amount of moisture and to make the cup burn more easily. The paper is wrapped around the cup and tied securely; next the packet is placed in the incinerator or in a special receptacle to be carried to the incinerator later. After this has been done, the metal holder is autoclaved or boiled for 30 minutes. Ambulatory patients often use collapsible cups.

Sputum can be received into a waxed paper cup with a tight-fitting lid that can be secured before the cup is discarded.

**Clinical thermometers.** A clinical thermometer must be sterile each time it is used. After a thermometer is used and the temperature recorded, the thermometer must be washed with soap or detergent and water (with friction applied). It may be disinfected as indicated in Table 17-3.

After sterilization a thermometer is wiped with sterile cotton and placed in a sterile container for later use. Preferably it is stored in alcohol or in fresh-daily solutions of tincture of iodine 0.5% or 150 p.p.m. of an aqueous iodophor. Alcoholic solutions of the quats must be used, since the aqueous solutions do *not* kill tubercle bacilli. Thermometers are rinsed in cold water before use.

A patient with hepatitis should have his own thermometer, which is destroyed when he leaves the hospital.

**Eating utensils.** A special covered container is placed in the sickroom, and the dishes are placed therein, preferably by the patient himself. Care to prevent contamination of the outside of the container must be exercised. After the dishes, knives, and forks are placed in the container, it is carried to the kitchen and boiled in soapy water for 5 minutes. Sometimes the eating utensils are carried to the kitchen before they are placed in the container. Left-over bits of food may be placed in a paper sack, wrapped well with newspaper, and burned in the incinerator. If this is not practical, the food remains are placed in chlorinated lime or phenol solution and left for 1 hour.

**Terminal disinfection of hospital room.** When a patient is removed from a room, the floors, walls,

woodwork, and furniture should be scrubbed with soapsuds and thoroughly aired. The phenol derivatives are valuable and widely used in terminal disinfection. Other good housekeeping disinfectants are 1% sodium hypochlorite and Wescodyne or other iodophor, 500 p.p.m. available iodine.

## Disinfection of articles for public use

**Rest rooms and bathroom fixtures.** The woodwork, floors, sinks, basins, and toilets of public rest rooms should be washed frequently with hot soapsuds or detergent and rinsed thoroughly. Phenolic disinfectants or one of the iodophors such as Wescodyne are suitable for disinfection.

**Woodwork.** The woodwork of schoolhouses, churches, theaters, or other places of public assembly should be washed frequently with a detergent-germicide solution.

**Public conveyances.** All parts touched by the hands of passengers should be frequently washed with a detergent-germicide solution.

## Fumigation of rooms and disinfection of air

**Fumigation.** In former years it was an almost universal procedure to put a sickroom "into fumigation" as soon as the room was vacated. Fumigation at that time meant terminal gaseous disinfection with formaldehyde, the gas of choice. This gaseous method of disinfection has been abandoned because the formaldehyde does not kill insects, small animals, or pathogenic microbes. The scrubbing of walls and floors to clean them thoroughly has replaced fumigation in the control of communicable disease; natural drying of surfaces effects the destruction of bacteria.

The term *fumigation* now denotes the destruction of disease-carrying animals, insects, or vermin. The fumigant of choice is hydrocyanic acid, a deadly poison that must be handled with extreme care. Sulfur dioxide is a splendid insecticide, but because of its destructive action on metals and household goods, it is seldom used in homes, public buildings, or hospitals.

**Air disinfection.** Two methods of destroying bacteria and other disease-producing agents as they are dispersed through the air are ultraviolet radiation and chemical disinfection by means of aerosols.

Aerosols are chemical vapors liberated into the air for disinfection. Two of the most potent are propylene glycol, effective in a dilution of 1 part in 100 million parts of air, and triethylene glycol, effective when diluted to 1 part in 400 million parts of air. The vapors may be introduced into rooms through ventilating systems, bombs, or special equipment. The importance of thorough cleaning and disinfection of air conditioning units must be kept in mind.

## Sterilization of biologic products

In the preparation of bacterial vaccines it is necessary to kill the bacteria at as low a temperature as possible because a temperature of more than 62° C. coagulates the bacterial protein and renders the vaccine worthless. It has been found that an exposure for 1 hour to a water bath temperature of 60° C. kills any of the ordinary bacteria used in making vaccines. Bacterial vaccines are sometimes sterilized by the addition of chemicals such as phenol or cresol. Mercury-vapor lamps as a source of ultraviolet radiation are used in the preparation of bacterial as well as viral vaccines, but ultraviolet radiation, ideal in theory, is practically ineffective at times. Ethylene oxide gas is also used for this purpose.

Hepatitis viruses may be eliminated in pooled plasma or serum by exposure to ultraviolet light followed by the use of beta-propiolactone, 1.5 gm./liter of material.

## Questions for review

1  How may knives be sterilized?
2  What is the preferred method of sterilization for endoscopes? What is meant by pasteurization of endoscopes?
3  List three surgical items easily damaged by heat.
4  Give a method of preparing the skin for operation.
5  How may the air be kept free of pathogenic bacteria during the time of operation?
6  What is the difference between physical and microbiologic isolation?
7  How would you dispose of the feces and urine of a patient with typhoid fever?
8  Discuss the drugs used in wound disinfection.
9  Explain what is meant by concurrent disinfection. Terminal disinfection.
10  What precaution should be taken in handling sputum from a patient with tuberculosis? How is sputum sterilized?
11  How are clinical thermometers sterilized?
12  Briefly discuss the use of hydrocyanic acid as a fumigant.
13  How may hepatitis viruses be eliminated?
14  How are biologic products sterilized?
15  Compare steam sterilization with gas sterilization.

**REFERENCES** (Chapters 15 to 17)

AMA Council on Drugs: Evaluation of a new antituberculous agent, Rifampin (Rifadin, Rimactane), J.A.M.A. **220:**414, 1972.

AMA drug evaluations, ed. 2, Acton, Mass., 1973, Publishing Sciences Group, Inc.

American Academy of Pediatrics, Committee on Fetus and Newborn: Skin care of newborns, Pediatrics **54:**682, 1974.

Ballinger, W. F., II, and others: Alexander's care of the patient in surgery, ed. 5, St. Louis, 1972, The C. V. Mosby Co.

Bauer, D. J.: Antiviral chemotherapy: first decade, Br. Med. J. **3:**275, Aug. 4, 1973.

Bell, A. N.: Personal communication, 1976.

Bickel, L.: Rise up to life; a biography of Howard Walter Florey who gave penicillin to the world, New York, 1973, Charles Scribner's Sons.

Blumberg, P. M., and Strominger, J. L.: Interaction of penicillin with the bacterial cell: penicillin-binding proteins and penicillin-sensitive enzymes, Bacteriol. Rev. **38:**291, 1974.

Borick, P. M., editor: Chemical sterilization, Stroudsburg, Pa., 1973, Dowden, Hutchinson & Ross, Inc.

Brunn, J. N., and Solbert, C. O.: Hand carriage of gram-negative bacilli and *Staphylococcus aureus*, Br. Med. J. **2:**580, June 9, 1973.

Byrd, C. B., and others: Isoniazid toxicity, J.A.M.A. **220:**1471, 1972.

Caldwell, J. R., and Cluff, L. E.: Adverse reactions to antimicrobial agents, J.A.M.A. **230:**77, 1974.

Carter, W. A., editor: Selective inhibitors of viral functions, Cleveland, 1973, CRC Press.

Chloramphenicol-induced bone marrow suppression (editorial), J.A.M.A. **213:**1183, 1970.

Cohen, S.: A decade of R factors (editorial), J. Infect. Dis. **119:**104, 1969.

Copeland, E. M., and others: Prevention of microbial catheter contamination in patients receiving parenteral hyperalimentation, South. Med. J. **67:**303, 1974.

Coriell, L. L., and others: Medical applications of dust-free rooms, J.A.M.A. **203:**1038, 1968.

Culliford, A. T., and others: Sudden death and hexachlorophene, Arch. Surg. **109:**434, 1974.

Dineen, P.: Duration of shelf life—an evaluation, AORN J. **13:**63, March, 1971.

Dineen, P.: Personnel, discipline, and infection, Arch. Surg. **107:**603, 1973.

Duncalf, D.: Care of anesthetic equipment and other devices, Arch. Surg. **107:**600, 1973.

Easley, J. R.: Personal communication, 1976.

Evans, M. J.: Some contributions to prevention of infections, Nurs. Clin. North Am. **3:**641, 1968.

Fason, M. F.: Controlling bacterial growth in tube feedings, Am. J. Nurs. **67:**1246, 1967.

Finland, M., and Kass, E. H., editors: Trimethoprim-sulfamethoxazole: microbiological, pharmacological, and clinical considerations, Chicago, 1974, The University of Chicago Press.

Fox, F.: A review of the types and problems of sterilization, Hosp. Man. **103:**135, March, 1967.

Fox, M. K., and others: How good are hand washing practices? Am. J. Nurs. **74:**1676, 1974.

Friedman, R. M.: Interferons and virus infections, Am. J. Nurs. **68:**542, 1968.

Garner, J. S., and Kaiser, A. B.: How often is isolation needed? Am. J. Nurs. **72:**733, 1972.

Ginsberg, F.: Sterilizing anesthesia equipment is difficult but it is necessary, Mod. Hosp. **109:**108, July, 1967.

Ginsberg, F.: Gas sterilizers: handle with care, Mod. Hosp. **111:**84, Aug., 1968.

Ginsberg, F.: Hair, long or short, must be covered in O.R., Mod. Hosp. **117:**106, July, 1971.

Goth, A.: Medical pharmacology: principles and concepts, ed. 7, St. Louis, 1974, The C. V. Mosby Co.

Gröschel, D.: Fact and fiction in hospital disinfection, ASM News **38:**479, 1972.

Grove, V. E., Jr.: Common drugs cause psychiatric illness, Tex. Med. **67:**30, March, 1971.

Hall, E. D.: The cleanup is as important as the setup, Hosp. Man. **99:**105, March, 1965.

Heller, W. M.: The United States Pharmacopeia, its value to the professions, J.A.M.A. **213:**576, 1970.

Hiel, R. M.: Will this drug harm the unborn infant? The doctor's dilemma, South. Med. J. **67:**1476, 1974.

Hitchings, G. H.: A quarter century of chemotherapy, J.A.M.A. **209:**1339, 1969.

Hobby, G. L., editor: Antimicrobial agents and chemotherapy, Ann Arbor, Mich., 1967, American Society for Microbiology.

Irey, N. S.: Adverse reactions to drugs and chemicals, a resumé and progress report, J.A.M.A. **230:**596, 1974.

Isoniazid-associated hepatitis (current trends), summary of report of Tuberculosis Advisory Committee and special consultants to the director, Center for Disease Control, Morbid. Mortal. Wk. Rep. **23:**97, 1974.

Jackson, G. G.: Influenza; the present status of chemotherapy, Hosp. Pract. **6:**75, Nov., 1971.

Jackson, G. G.: Perspective from a quarter century of antibiotic usage, J.A.M.A. **227:**634, 1974.

Jeanes, C. W. L., and others: Inactivation of isoniazid by Canadian Eskimos and Indians, Can. Med. Assoc. J. **106:**331, 1972.

Kagan, B. M., and others: Spotlight on antimicrobial agents—1973, J.A.M.A. **226:**306, 1973.

Keitel, H. G., and Soentgen, M. L.: Dental staining, tetracycline induced, Med. Sci. **17:**57, Jan., 1966.

Keitel, H. G., and Soentgen, M. L.: Hazards and benefits of tetracycline administration in children, Med. Sci. **17:**80, Nov., 1966.

Kundsin, R. B., and Walter, C. W.: The surgical scrub—practical consideration, Arch. Surg. **107:**75, 1973.

Kunin, C. M.: Nephrotoxicity of antibiotics, J.A.M.A. **202:**204, 1967.

Laufman, H., editor: Symposium on operating room hazard control, surgical hazard control, Arch. Surg. **107:**552, 1973.

Lal, S., and others: Effect of rifampicin and isoniazid on liver function, Br. Med. J. **1:**148, Jan. 15, 1972.

Lee, S., and others: Comparison of use of alcohol with that of iodine for skin antisepsis in obtaining blood cultures, Am. J. Clin. Pathol. **47:**646, 1967.

Litsky, B. M. Y.: Are pathogenic spores a hospital threat? Hosp. Man. **101:**74, May, 1966.

Litsky, B. M. Y.: How do you know how well you are doing—in getting rid of the pathogens? Hosp. Man. **103:**94, March, 1967.

Litsky, B. M. Y.: Environmental control: the operating room, AORN J. **14:**39, July, 1971.

MacKenzie, A. R.: Effectiveness of antibacterial soaps in a healthy population, J.A.M.A. **211:**973, 1970.

Maddrey, W. C., and Boitnott, J. K.: Isoniazid hepatitis, Ann. Intern. Med. **79:**1, 1973.

Mathews, R.: TLC with the penicillin, Am. J. Nurs. **71:**720, 1971.

McArthur, B. J., and others: Stopcock contamination in an ICU, Am. J. Nurs. **75:**96, 1975.

McInnes, B.: Essentials of communicable disease, ed. 2, St. Louis, 1975, The C. V. Mosby Co.

Meeks, C. H., and others: Sterilization of anesthesia apparatus, J.A.M.A. **199:**276, 1967.

Merigan, T. C., Jr.: Interferon and interferon inducers: the clinical outlook, Hosp. Pract. **4:**42, March, 1969.

Meyer, C.: Don't wash labware: "incinerate" it, Lab. Man. **13:**40, Jan., 1975.

Modell, W., editor: Drugs of choice 1976-1977, St. Louis, 1976, The C. V. Mosby Co.

Moravec, D. F.: All drugs should be respected but not feared, Hosp. Man. **106:**62, Oct., 1968.

Morse, R. A.: Environmental control in beehive, Sci. Am. **226:**92, April, 1972.

Nelson, J. P.: OR clean rooms, AORN J. **15:**71, May, 1972.

Nichols, G. A., and Dobek, A. S.: Sterility of items sealed in plastic, Hosp. Top. **49:**84, Dec., 1971.

Notes on the package insert (editorial), J.A.M.A. **207:**1335, 1969.

Osol, A., and others, editors: United States dispensatory, Philadelphia, 1973, J. B. Lippincott Co.

Oviatt, V. R.: How to dispose of disposables, Med. Surg. Rev. **5:**57, Second quarter, 1969.

Peers, J. G.: Cleanup techniques in the operating room, Arch. Surg. **107:**596, 1973.

Perkins, J. J.: Principles and methods of sterilization in health sciences, Springfield, Ill., 1970, Charles C Thomas, Publisher.

Perlman, D.: Evolution of the antibiotics industry, 1940-1975, ASM News **40:**910, 1974.

Petersdorf, R. G.: Penicillin (editorial), J.A.M.A. **209:**1520, 1969.

Physicians' desk reference to pharmaceutical specialties and biologicals, Oradell, N.J., 1976, Medical Economics, Inc.

Poupard, J. A., and others: A general reference chart for common bacterial agents, Lab. Med. **2:**26, April, 1971.

Prioleau, W. H.: Fashion hides its head in the OR, Hospitals **46:**107, May 1, 1972.

Quintiliani, R.: Current concepts in therapy: general concepts in the use of antibiotics in adults, South. Med. J. **66:**940, 1973.

Rees, R. B.: Cutaneous drug reactions, Tex. Med. **66:**92, Feb., 1970.

Regamey, C., and others: Cefazolin vs. cephalothin and cephaloridine, Arch. Intern. Med. **133:**407, 1974.

Resistance to antibiotics (editorial), J.A.M.A. **203:**1132, 1968.

Riley, H. D., Jr.: Current concepts in therapy: rifampin, South. Med. J. **66:**273, 1973.

Roberts, R. B., and Rendell-Baker, L.: Ethylene-oxide sterilization, Hosp. Top. **50:**60, May, 1972.

Roberts, R. B., and Stark, D. C. C.: Sterile procedures in the doctor's office, Med. Surg. Rev. **6:**24, June-July, 1970.

Rudolph, A. H., and Price, E. V.: Penicillin reactions among patients in venereal disease clinics, a national survey, J.A.M.A. **223:**499, 1973.

Schwabe, C. W.: Veterinary medicine and human health, Baltimore, 1969, The Williams & Wilkins Co.

Scott, A. J., and others: Lincomycin as cause of pseudo-membranous colitis, Lancet **2:**1232, Dec. 1, 1973.

Selwyn, S., and Ellis, H.: Skin bacteria and skin disinfection reconsidered, Br. Med. J. **1:**136, Jan. 15, 1972.

Sheely, L. L., and Volpitto, P. P.: An inexpensive and satisfactory method for gas sterilization of anesthetic equipment, Anesthesiology **27:**95, 1966.

Shirkey, H. C.: The package insert dilemma, J. Pediatr. **79:**691, 1971.

Shuman, R. M., and others: Neurotoxicity of hexachlorophene in the human. 1. A clinicopathologic study of 248 children, Pediatrics **54:**689, 1974.

Slepecky, R. A.: Sonication—germicide treatment in surgical instrument cleaning, Hosp. Top. **44:**133, April, 1966.

Smylie, H. G., and others: From Phisohex to Hibiscrub, Br. Med. J. **4:**586, Dec. 8, 1973.

Spaulding, E. H.: Principles and application of chemical disinfection, AORN J. **1:**36, May-June, 1963.

Stead, W. W., and Texter, E. C., Jr.: Isoniazid hepatitis: backlash of progress (editorial), Ann. Intern. Med. **79:**125, 1973.

Strominger, J. L.: The bactericidal mechanisms of antibiotic drugs, Hosp. Pract. **2:**54, July, 1967.

Summary of the report of the Ad Hoc Advisory Committee on Isoniazid and Liver Disease (current trends), Morbid. Mortal. Wk. Rep. **20:**231, 1971.

Sutherland, R., and others: Amoxycillin: new semi-synthetic penicillin, Br. Med. J. **3:**13, July 1, 1972.

Swenson, O., and Grana, L.: A new, improved sterilization set-up for the operating room, AORN J. **13:**80, Jan., 1971.

Taylor, J. W., and others: For effective thermometer disinfection, Nurs. Outlook **14:**56, Feb., 1966.

The cost of disposables (editorial), J.A.M.A. **217:**1859, 1971.

The package insert (editorial), J.A.M.A. **207:**1342, 1969.

Walter, C. W.: Disinfection of hands, Am. J. Surg. **109:**691, 1965.

Walter, C. W., and Kundsin, R. B.: The airborne component of wound contamination and infection, Arch. Surg. **107:**588, 1973.

Weinstein, L.: The present status of antimicrobial therapy, Resident Staff Physician **15:**63, Feb., 1969.

Weinstein, L., and Chang, T. W.: Interferon: nonviral infections and nonviral inducers (editorial), Ann. Intern. Med. **69:**1315, 1968.

Winner, H. I.: A bacteriologist looks at hospital bedding, Nurs. Times **62:**529, 1966.

Winters, R. E., and others: Combined use of gentamicin and carbenicillin, Ann. Intern. Med. **75:**925, 1971.

## CHAPTER 18

# Gram-positive pyogenic cocci

The pathogenic cocci are often called the *pyogenic* cocci because of their ability to cause pus formation. The important gram-positive cocci are the staphylococci, the streptococci, and the pneumococci (genera *Staphylococcus* and *Streptococcus.*)

The pneumococcus has long been considered as a streptococcus by many authorities who have even classified it in the same genus. Recognizing the biologic similarity of the two, the eighth edition of *Bergey's Manual* reclassifies the pneumococcus. Formerly *Diplococcus pneumoniae,* it is now *Streptococcus pneumoniae*. In this chapter, because of certain properties peculiar to it and because of its relation to an important disease, it is discussed separately.

### Staphylococcus species (the staphylococci)

**General characteristics.** Staphylococci occur typically in grapelike clusters (Fig. 18-1). Under special conditions they may occur singly (Fig. 18-2), in pairs, or in short chains. They are gram-positive, nonmotile, and nonsporeforming and grow luxuriantly on all culture media. Most of them grow best in the presence of oxygen, but they easily grow in its absence. A few are strictly anaerobic. They grow best between 25° and 35° C. but may grow at a temperature as low as 8° or as high as 48° C.

When staphylococci are grown on blood agar, there is characteristic pigment production, the colors ranging from a deep gold to lemon yellow to white. The deep golden color observed with growth was originally responsible for the species name *aureus.* We now know that there are white variants of the golden staphylococci.

Staphylococci are most resistant to the action of heat, drying, and chemicals. Although most vegetative bacteria are destroyed by a temperature of 60° C. for 30 minutes, staphylococci frequently resist a temperature of 60° C. for 1 hour, and some strains may resist a temperature of 80° C. for 30 min-

utes. In dried pus they live for weeks or months. Another mechanism for survival of the staphylococcus is its tolerance to salt or a salty medium, as would be found in preserved foods. Staphylococci also tend to become resistant to the sulfonamides and antibiotics. They adapt quickly and easily to such agents. Many (about 80%) are penicillin resistant.

There are two species of note for the genus *Staphylococcus: Staphylococcus aureus (Staph. aureus)* and *Staphylococcus epidermidis (Staph. epidermidis),* two organisms separated by a biochemical reaction and the presence of an enzyme. *Staph. aureus* ferments mannitol, which the other staphylococcus does not, and *Staph. aureus* is coagulase-positive. *Staph. epidermidis* is coagulase-negative.

**Toxic products.** Several important metabolic products are elaborated by staphylococci. Among the ones with toxic properties are those that (1) destroy red blood cells (hemolysins, staphylolysins), (2) destroy leukocytes (leukocidin), (3) cause necrosis of tissue (necrotizing exotoxin), (4) produce death

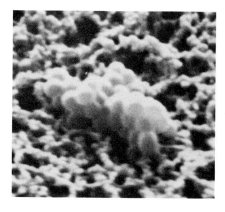

**Fig. 18-1.** Staphylococci, scanning electron micrograph. Note typical grapelike cluster. (Courtesy Millipore Corp., Bedford, Mass.)

(the lethal factor), and (5) cause gastroenteric symptoms (enterotoxin). Probably no single strain produces all of these poisons, and many produce none of them.

In addition, some staphylococci produce the enzyme *coagulase*, by means of which they cause the plasma of blood to clot. The *coagulase test* indicates the presence of coagulase, which is generally considered the best single bit of evidence that a given staphylococcus is pathogenic. Because of coagulase activity a surface layer of fibrin accumulates on an individual staphylococcus and protects it from phagocytic attack. The production of coagulase correlates with the production of other toxic products. Staphylococci also produce staphylokinase, which dissolves fibrin, and hyaluronidase.

**Pathogenicity.** Some staphylococci are nonpathogenic; others can cause severe infections. Severe infections are caused by *Staph. aureus. Staph. epidermidis*, though sometimes responsible for very mild, limited infections, is generally considered nonpathogenic except under unusual medical circumstances.

The best known staphylococcal infections are those of the skin and superficial tissues of the body, the features of which are greatly influenced by the age of the patient. The scalded-skin syndrome (Fig. 18-3) is an example of staphylococcal disease produced by certain strains with a predilection for the newborn and very young. Its manifestations are clearly depicted by the name. Staphylococci cause boils, pustules, pimples, furuncles, abscesses, carbuncles, paronychias, and infections of accidental or surgical wounds.

Staphylococci also produce systemic disease, and all organ systems in the body may be affected. They are one cause of pneumonia, empyema, endocarditis, meningitis, brain abscess, puerperal fever, parotitis, phlebitis, cystitis, and pyelonephritis. Staphylococci can infect a valve prosthesis in the heart. Staphylococcal pneumonia was a fatal complication to cases of influenza in recent epidemics. Staphylococci are the commonest cause of osteomyelitis and impetigo contagiosa (Fig. 18-4). Systemic staphylococcal disease is often acquired in the hospital, especially in

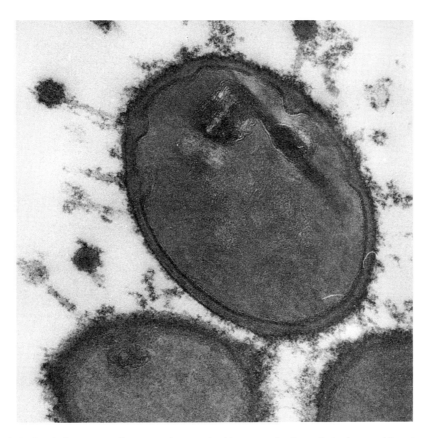

**Fig. 18-2.** *Staphylococcus,* electron micrograph. Note attached staphylophages. (Courtesy S. Tyrone, Dallas.)

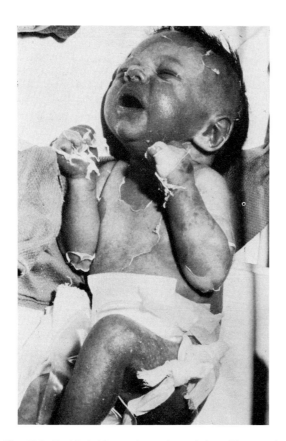

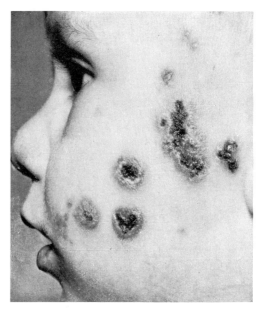

**Fig. 18-4.** Impetigo contagiosa, highly communicable skin disease. Note various sized lesions, some of which are dark and encrusted. (From Top, F. H., Sr., and Wehrle, P. F., editors: Communicable and infectious diseases, ed. 7, St. Louis, 1972, The C. V. Mosby Co.)

**Fig. 18-3.** Scalded-skin syndrome in an infant. Note peeling of superficial skin layer. (From Melish, M. E., and Glasgow, L. A.: N. Engl. J. Med. **282:**1114, 1970.)

patients already ill with a serious disease, and staphylococcal pneumonia as a superinfection is a threat after large doses of antibiotics have been given.

Staphylococcal septicemia assumes two forms. The first is a fulminating, profound toxemia with death a few days later. The second and more frequent is of longer duration and characterized by severe clinical disease, formation of metastatic abscesses in different parts of the body, and slightly reduced mortality. Staphylococcal septicemia may be a primary condition, but mostly it results from secondary invasion of the bloodstream by organisms from a localized site of infection in the skin (often a trivial one). It can come from an infected wound, a dental abscess, a pneumonia, or an infected intravenous catheter site. An indwelling intravenous catheter should not remain in place longer than 3 to 4 days because of the likelihood of serious infection. Boils about the nose and lip are likely to be so complicated and for this reason should not be traumatized.

There is an area of the face, triangular in shape, lying with its base along the opening of the mouth and its apex placed in the region above the upper part of the nose. It is called the "dangerous triangle" (Fig. 18-5) because of the threat to a person's life if infection originating there spreads backward into the cranial vault. It is a peculiar area in that anatomic factors operate there to favor just such a disaster. (A comparable lesion in another part of the body would be inconsequential.) These factors include poor connective tissue supports that provide no mechanical barriers, veins without valves connecting with veins that drain backward, and muscles of the face that are more or less constantly in motion.

If piercing of the ears (for cosmetic reasons) is done in an unsanitary setting, there is the danger of secondary infection with potentially deadly staphylococci. They can easily enter such a wound that is kept open for several days, and in rare instances the spread of infection to the bloodstream has been tragic.

On occasion, implantation of staphylococci in the intestinal tract after antibiotic therapy results in enteritis or enterocolitis causing dysentery. Staphylococcal food poisoning is the most frequent type of food poisoning from ingestion of a bacterial toxin.

Staphylococci are an important cause of suppurative conditions in cattle and horses. Mastitis of staphylococcal origin in cows can be transmitted to other

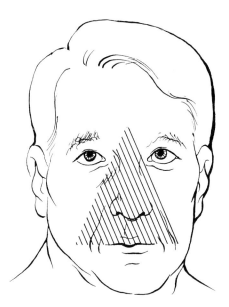

**Fig. 18-5.** Triangular area of the face where staphylococcal infection is very dangerous.

cows by the hands of the milker. Staphylococcal bacteremia may follow tick bites in lambs.

**Pathology.** The hallmark of staphylococcal infection is the *abscess,* the type lesion. It reflects the excellent pus-forming ability of staphylococci and their limited capacity for spread. Since the microbes occur on the skin, this is the area most frequently involved. A boil is a skin abscess. The type lesion is modified by anatomic location and degree of involvement. Staphylococcal pneumonia means multiple abscesses in the lungs. Pyelonephritis means multiple abscesses extending down the tubular system of the kidney. Staphylococcal septicemia is the development of multiple abscesses over the body; the word *pyemia,* literally meaning "pus in the blood," is more appropriate. Staphylococci, as an important cause of wound infections, are responsible for pus formation therein.

**Hospital-acquired (nosocomial) staphylococcal infection.** Because of man's intimate contact with this microbe and because of its ubiquity, there are unique features to its infections at any time. For a number of years, staphylococcal infections have been especially troublesome in hospitals all over the world. To begin with, there are several background factors. In one regard, the problem is a complication to modern antibiotic therapy. Important antimicrobial agents have been freely given. Antibiotics generally are bacteriostatic, *not* bactericidal. Staphylococci are well endowed for survival, and consequently antibiotic-resistant strains have developed. Moreover, with prepaid medical plans and medical advances favoring

early detection of disease, more persons now are treated in hospitals. Modern surgery is expanded. Complicated surgical technics can be done with a greater exposure of tissue at operation for a longer period of time than ever before. In certain instances drugs such as the corticosteroids that depress the patient's resistance to infection are indicated.

The hospital population is already large and complex, but it is growing with the increased demand for persons with specialized technical skills. Here, then, is a patient, sometimes seriously ill, confined within a large institution where the contacts with all kinds of persons are many and varied. Consider these factors in light of the fact that staphylococci are everywhere. Is it any wonder that in this kind of setting the staphylococcus can be a troublemaker!

Four major categories of disease caused by antibiotic-resistant staphylococci related to hospital-acquired infection are stressed:

1. Skin abscesses (impetigo and pyoderma) in newborn infants. Many of these infants develop breast abscess. Fatal staphylococcal pneumonia or septicemia is prevalent. The nursing mother can pick up a virulent organism from her baby. Abscess formation in her breast may result.
2. Wound infections, especially of surgical wounds.
3. Secondary staphylococcal infections in hospitalized elderly and debilitated persons.
4. Gastroenteritis, as a result of a change in the bacterial flora of the intestinal tract.

**Sources and modes of infection.** Staphylococci are normal inhabitants of the skin, mouth, throat, and nose of man. They live in these areas without effect, but once past the barrier of the skin and mucous membrane, they can cause extensive disease. They may pass through the unbroken skin via the hair follicles and ducts of the sweat glands under certain conditions. The natural invasive characteristics of staphylococci and the resistance of the body are so well balanced that infection probably never occurs unless a highly virulent organism is encountered or body resistance is lowered. As a rule, a localized process such as an abscess or a boil is first formed. Healing without widespread dissemination of infection usually takes place, but in some cases organisms do escape from the localized process, invade the bloodstream, and affect distant parts of the body.

Important to the spread of staphylococcal infections are direct, person-to-person contacts. For example, in the hospital the hands of the doctor or nurse or attendant may carry the infection from one patient to another. The hospital staff generally has a higher carrier rate, and cross infection is significant. Staphylococci are abundant in hospitals. Nasal carriers are an important source. Virulent organisms may also be passed to man from livestock and household pets.

**Bacteriologic diagnosis.** A bacteriologic diagnosis of a staphylococcal infection is made easily by smears and cultures. When blood cultures for staphylococci are made, special pains must be taken to exclude those inhabiting the skin. The coagulase test (slide and test tube methods) is performed to differentiate nonpathogenic from pathogenic staphylococci. A freshly isolated staphylococcus is most likely to be a virulent pathogen if it produces a yellow pigment, hemolyzes blood, ferments mannitol, elaborates deoxyribonuclease, and is coagulase-positive.

The bacteriophage typing of staphylococci deserves special mention. Bacteriophages (p. 292) are viruses that attack bacteria and in certain instances dissolve the bacterial cell parasitized. The action of phages is specific; that is, only a certain phage or group of phages affects the given strain of bacteria. It has been found that specific bacteriophages (staphylophages) react with about 60% of coagulase-positive staphylococci. Coagulase-negative strains of staphylococci are not so susceptible. Because of this specificity, phage typing of staphylococci can be done. For convenience, bacteriophages have been given identifying numbers, and the strains of staphylococci related to these particular phages are designated by the number of the bacteriophage or phages dissolving them. On this basis, *Staph. aureus* can be classified into phage lytic groups as follows:

| | |
|---|---|
| Group I | 29, 52, 52A, 79, and 80 |
| Group II | 3A, 3B, 3C, 55, and 71 |
| Group III | 6, 7, 42E, 47, 53, 54, 75, 77, and 83A |
| Group IV | 42D |
| Not allotted | 81 and 187 |

**Immunity.** Man possesses considerable natural immunity to staphylococci. Specific serum antibodies to staphylococci can be demonstrated in most human beings to suggest that almost everyone has had a staphylococcal infection at some time and that acquired immunity of a protective nature may exist. However there is little reason to think that acquired immunity is a practical mechanism against serious infection. Patients with debilitating diseases, especially diabetes, are especially vulnerable.

**Prevention and control of staphylococcal infection.** The crucial measures in control of staphylococcal infections are maintenance of good housekeeping standards* and adherence to strict aseptic

*As Welton Taylor has said: "Perhaps the most important ally in the hospital's campaign against hospital-borne infection is the housekeeper, who merely has to employ the common-sense sanitation that any good housewife knows." (From Hosp. Trib. **7:**3, Oct. 9, 1967.)

technics. There is strong evidence that the currently pathogenic strains of staphylococci are as susceptible to the action of chemical germicides as are the ordinary nonpathogenic strains. The detection of nasal carriers, especially in the nurseries for newborn infants, is important.

Phage typing of coagulase-positive staphylococci has proved valuable in the epidemiologic study of hospital-acquired infections to track down the sources to carriers or other foci of staphylococcal disease. Bacteriophage types 52, 52A, 80, and 81 are the prevalent ones in the hospital environment today. For many years the 80/81 phage type has been an epidemic strain largely instrumental in producing infections in hospitals over wide geographic areas. It is known to be resistant to penicillin, streptomycin, and the tetracyclines. In some cases it may be sensitive to other antibiotics. Vaccine therapy has not proved effective in dealing with this organism because of certain of its immunochemical peculiarities. A staphylococcal phage lysate designed to call forth cell-mediated immunity is more promising.

If one strain of coagulase-positive staphylococcus is biologically anchored to a given site in the human body, another coagulase-positive strain cannot implant there. The colonization of the second strain is blocked. There is *bacterial interference* between the two. Today in newborn nurseries of hospitals practical application of this phenomenon is made to protect newborn infants against current epidemic strains of staphylococci.

## Streptococcus species (the streptococci)
### GENERAL CONSIDERATIONS

The term *streptococcus* has a morphologic meaning and includes cocci that occur in pairs and chains. A biochemical feature distinguishing the genus *Streptococcus* is the fermentation of glucose by the hexose diphosphate pathway to yield mainly dextrorotatory lactic acid. Within this genus of organisms are found significant variations in cultural characteristics and disease-producing properties. Some produce deadly disease, others do so only under special conditions, and still others are nonpathogenic. As a whole, streptococci are probably responsible for more illness and can cause more different kinds of disease than any other group of organisms. They attack any part of the body and can cause primary as easily as secondary disease. They attack both man and lower animals. Some occur as saprophytes in milk and other dairy products.

A great deal of research is carried out on the biology of the streptococcus. The individual streptococci are being studied in great detail as are the reactions they induce on contact with a given host.

**Characteristics.** Typical streptococci occur in varying sizes arranged in long or short chains. Long chains contain fifty or more organisms; short chains contain as few as four or six, the bacteria arranged in pairs within the chains. Chains form when bacteria divide in one plane and cling together after division. Streptococci are nonmotile, gram-positive organisms that do not form spores. Capsule formation is variable. Some species form distinct capsules; most do not.

The majority of streptococci grow best in the presence of oxygen, but they may grow in its absence. A few species are strict anaerobes. They grow well on all fairly rich media, and visible growth usually appears within 24 to 28 hours. Growth is especially luxuriant on hormone media or media containing unheated serum, whole blood, or serous fluid. Streptococci multiply in milk. They grow best at body temperature but may grow through a temperature range of 15° to 45° C. Most are not soluble in bile and do not ferment inulin.

Streptococci may remain alive in sputum or other excreta for several weeks and may live in dried blood or pus for several months. They are destroyed at a temperature of 60° C. within 30 to 60 minutes. They are killed in 15 minutes by 1:200 phenol solution, tincture of iodine, or 70% isopropyl alcohol. Penicillin is the most effective antibiotic against most types, except the enterococci.* Streptococci readily acquire a resistance to the other antimicrobial drugs.

**Classification.** Streptococci may be classified on the basis of their action on blood agar, their biochemical properties, or their serologic behavior (agglutination and precipitation).

To determine their action on blood agar, plates of blood agar are prepared. Nutrient agar is melted and cooled to 45° C.; sterile defibrinated blood is added: 5 to 10 parts of blood to 100 parts of nutrient agar. The mixture is poured into Petri dishes and allowed to cool. The plates are streaked with the material containing the streptococci and incubated at 37° C. for 24 hours or longer. Corresponding to their action on the blood agar plates, streptococci may be classified broadly as

1. Alpha hemolytic or viridans—colony surrounded by a green halo; hemolysis slight or incomplete

---

*Against beta hemolytic streptococci, penicillin is still the drug of choice.

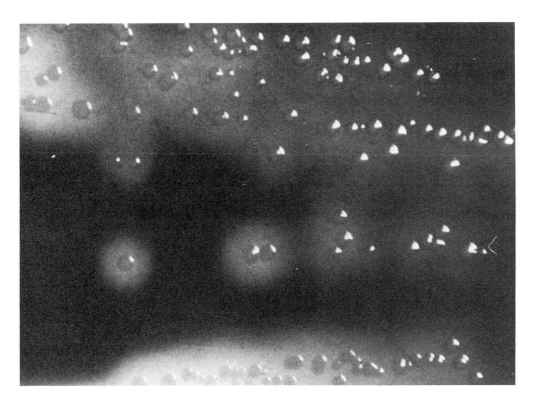

**Fig. 18-6.** Beta hemolytic streptococci, routine blood agar plate. Note wide clear zones about small gray colonies.

2. Beta hemolytic—colony surrounded by a clear, wide, colorless zone of hemolysis (Fig. 18-6)
3. Gamma—colonies showing neither hemolysis nor color change (Fig. 18-7)

As a general rule, the beta hemolytic streptococcus is the most virulent and is usually associated with acute fulminating infections; the viridans type is most often associated with chronic low-grade infections in man. However, infections caused by the viridans type (example: subacute bacterial endocarditis) may be as serious as infections with beta hemolytic streptococci. Alpha hemolytic streptococci are also responsible for such nonlethal infections as tooth abscesses and sinus infections. Many, but not

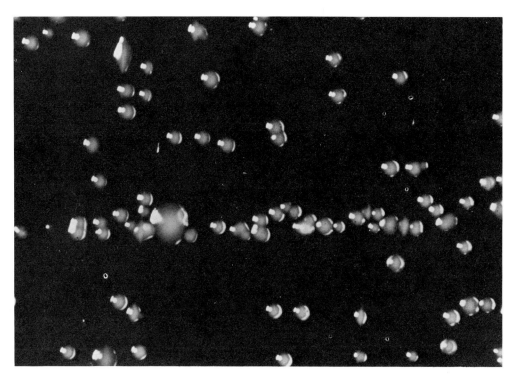

**Fig. 18-7.** Gamma hemolytic streptococci. No hemolysis indicated about these colonies.

## Table 18-1
Biologic properties of streptococci

| DIVISION | HEMOLYTIC STREPTOCOCCUS | VIRIDANS STREPTOCOCCUS | ENTEROCOCCUS | LACTIC STREPTOCOCCUS |
|---|---|---|---|---|
| Serologic group | A, B, C, E, F, G, H, K, L, M, O | None | D | N |
| Hemolysis on blood agar | Usually beta | Usually alpha | Alpha, beta, or gamma | Alpha or gamma |
| Growth in 0.1% methylene blue milk | − | − | + | + |
| Growth in 6.5% salt broth | − | − | + | − |
| Growth on 40% bile blood sugar | − | ± | + | + |
| Antibiotic susceptibility (bacitracin) | Usually sensitive | May be resistant | May be resistant | (Nonpathogenic) |

all, strains of streptococci of the gamma type are nonpathogenic.

Another classification divides the streptococci into (1) the pyogenic group, (2) the viridans group, (3) the lactic group, and (4) the enterococcus group. (See Table 18-1.) Enterococci, of which *Streptococcus faecalis* is an important species, are frequently responsible for infections of the genitourinary tract and occasionally for respiratory infections; they are rare causes of subacute bacterial endocarditis. The lactic group, found in sour milk, includes *Streptococcus lactis* and *Streptococcus cremoris*. It is not pathogenic but is important in the dairy industry and in certain types of biologic assay. The important member of the viridans group is *Streptococcus mitis,* often referred to as *Streptococcus viridans*. It is responsible for 90% of the cases of subacute bacterial endocarditis. The type organism of the pyogenic group is *Streptococcus pyogenes (Strep. pyogenes),* one of the most important of pathogenic bacteria.

By serologic (precipitin) methods streptococci fall into thirteen groups (the classification of Lancefield and others), which correspond in a general way to their pathologic action (Table 18-2). These groups

may be further subdivided into types given Arabic numbers. For over 50 types in group A, the antigenic substance determining type specificity is the *M protein*. Superficially attached to the cell wall, it protects the virulent streptococci of this group from the phagocytes of the host. Most human infections are caused by group A streptococci *(Strep. pyogenes)*. Streptococci of all other groups except those of N are indigenous to man and therefore potential pathogens. Certain members of groups B, C, D, H, K, and O and all members of group N are nonhemolytic. Although not listed in Table 18-2, groups P, Q, R, S, and T have been described.

**Toxic products.** Streptococci elaborate certain extracellular poisons, some of which can be called exotoxins. Among these are (1) hemolysins, (2) leukocidin, (3) streptokinase, (4) streptodornase, (5) hyaluronidase, and (6) erythrogenic toxin.

The hemolysins or *streptolysins* produced by streptococci are of two types, S and O. Streptolysin S is produced primarily by members of group A; streptolysin O is elaborated by most members of group A, by the "human" members of group C, and by certain members of group G. Most workers be-

**Table 18-2**

Serologic groups of streptococci

| GROUP | SPECIES | SIGNIFICANCE |
|-------|---------|--------------|
| A | *Streptococcus pyogenes* | Important human diseases (infection by beta hemolytic streptococci initiates acute rheumatic fever); group sensitive to penicillin |
| B | *Streptococcus agalactiae* | Bovine mastitis |
| C | *Streptococcus equi* | Animal diseases; mild respiratory infections in man |
| | *Streptococcus zooepidemicus* | |
| | *Streptococcus equisimilis* | |
| | *Streptococcus dysgalactiae* | |
| D | *Streptococcus faecalis* | Enterococci; genitourinary tract infections, endocarditis, wound infections in man; found in dairy products |
| | *Streptococcus faecalis,* subsp. *liquefaciens* | |
| | *Streptococcus faecalis,* subsp. *zymogenes* | |
| | *Streptococcus faecium* | |
| E | | Disease of swine; found in normal milk |
| F | *Streptococcus minutus* | Found in respiratory tract of man |
| G | *Streptococcus anginosus* | Mild respiratory infections in man; genital infections in dogs |
| H | *Streptococcus sanguis* | Found in respiratory tract of man |
| K | *Streptococcus salivarius* | Found in respiratory tract of man |
| L | | Genital tract infections in dogs |
| M | | Genital tract infections in dogs |
| N | *Streptococcus lactis* | Lactic group; found in dairy products |
| | *Streptococcus cremoris* | |
| O | | Viridans group; subacute bacterial endocarditis; found in upper respiratory tract in man |
| | | Microaerophilic streptococci |
| | | Anaerobic streptococci—13 species |

lieve that the leukocidin of streptococci and strepto-lysin O are identical. *Streptokinase* or *fibrinolysin* is important in that it activates an enzyme that destroys fibrin (the component that forms the framework of blood clots). Blood clots play an important part in wound healing and in blocking the spread of local infections.

*Streptodornase (streptococcal deoxyribonuclease)* acts to liquefy the thick, tenacious exudates such as are seen in pneumonia. The enzymatic activity of the deoxyribonuclease is directed against the de-oxyribonucleoprotein content of the exudate, the factor responsible for its viscosity. *Hyaluronidase* (the spreading factor, *invasin*) is a factor increasing the permeability of the tissues to bacteria and toxins by breaking down hyaluronic acid, one of the sub-stances that cement tissue cells together. The *erythro-genic toxin* produces erythema or redness when injected into the superficial layers of the skin, and with a large enough dose, a generalized rash. The scarlet fever toxin of Dick, it occurs in two immuno-logic types, A and B.

**Pathogenicity.*** Streptococci may be responsible for a localized inflammatory reaction, such as abscess, or a generalized reaction, such as septicemia. The nature of the lesion depends on the virulence of the streptococci, the number introduced into the body, the mode of introduction, the tissue invaded, and the resistance of the host.

**Pathology.** Pathologically, the type lesion of hemolytic streptococci is the diffuse, ill-defined, spreading lesion of *cellulitis*. The exudate contains few cells and consists largely of fluid with little fibrin. The toxic products of the microbes greatly aid their extension through both natural tissue and inflam-matory barriers, and they tend to infect the lymphatic vessels at the site of invasion. Many well-known forms of streptococcal infection can be designated as an expression of cellulitis. Erysipelas is cellulitis with a specific anatomic pattern; septic sore throat is cel-lulitis of the throat. Streptococcal bronchopneumonia is an inflammatory process comparable to cellulitis in the lung. Streptococci are also important in wound infections.

Allergic manifestations follow certain streptococcal infections. For instance, acute rheumatic fever and one form of kidney disease (glomerulonephritis) are considered to be allergic reactions to streptococcal infection, usually in the upper respiratory tract.

As a rule, the more virulent an infection, the more virulent are the streptococci isolated from the lesions for animals of the same species. Usually their viru-lence is lowered when they are introduced into ani-

mals of another species. When transferred from one animal to another, streptococci tend to produce the same type of lesion in the new host as in the original one. Rabbits and white mice are more susceptible to streptococci of human origin than other laboratory animals.

*Streptococci in human diseases.* In addition to being the cause of erysipelas and of two epidemic diseases, scarlet fever and epidemic sore throat, streptococci belonging to group A *(Strep. pyogenes)* are the commonest cause of acute endocarditis, sep-ticemia, and puerperal sepsis. They may cause pneu-monia, boils, abscesses, cellulitis, peritonitis, tonsil-litis, lymphangitis, infection of surgical wounds, osteomyelitis, and empyema. From an infection of the middle ear (otitis media) streptococci may spread to the mastoid cells and cause mastoiditis. From either the middle ear or the mastoid cells, spread of infection to the meninges means streptococcal meningitis.

*Strep. pyogenes* is responsible for the majority of bronchopneumonias complicating whooping cough, measles, and influenza. Such bronchopneumonias are often fatal and may reach epidemic proportions when outbreaks of whooping cough, measles, or influenza occur in communities containing numerous carriers of *Strep. pyogenes*. Streptococcal pneumonia is often the terminal phase of chronic diseases such as tuberculosis and cancer. Streptococci as well as staphylococci (often acting together) are responsible for the highly communicable skin disease known as *impetigo contagiosa*.

*Streptococcal infections in lower animals.* The majority of streptococcal infections in lower animals are caused by streptococci in Lancefield's groups B and C. Strangles, an acute communicable disease of the upper respiratory passages of horses, is caused by *Streptococcus equi*. Streptococcal mastitis, a serious disease of cows that renders milk unfit for use, is caused by *Streptococcus agalactiae* and is most likely spread from cow to cow by the hands of the milker. *Streptococcus agalactiae* does not affect man.

**Sources and modes of infection.** Streptococci are normal inhabitants of the mouth, nose, throat, and respiratory tract. They may be conveyed from person to person by direct contact or by contami-nated objects, hands, and surgical instruments. The hands are important conveyors of infection in puer-peral sepsis and wound infections. Milk can be an important source. Streptococcal diseases, especially scarlet fever and septic sore throat, may be spread by milk that has been contaminated with the mouth and nose secretions of a carrier or by milk from a cow with mastitis caused by *Strep. pyogenes*.

Streptococci usually enter the body by the respi-ratory tract or through wounds of the skin. Only a

---

*See also p. 489.

minute abrasion is necessary, and streptococcal infections in such abrasions have many times led to fatal septicemias in physicians and nurses. Streptococci leave the body by way of the mouth and nose and in the exudates from areas of infection. The nasal carrier is an important source of infection. The enterococci are normal inhabitants of the intestinal canal and are excreted in the feces.

**Laboratory diagnosis.** Streptococci are detected by smears and cultures from the site of disease. In septicemias caused by beta hemolytic streptococci, the organisms can usually be detected by blood cultures. In subacute bacterial endocarditis, since the viridans organisms escape into the blood intermittently, repeated cultures may have to be made.

A presumptive test of value in the identification of streptococci is the *bacitracin disk test*. Even in low concentrations this antibiotic appears to be specifically active against members of Lancefield group A streptococci; it is without effect on other groups. A paper disk containing a known unit of bacitracin is placed on a blood agar plate previously streaked with the streptococci in question. A zone of inhibition of growth found around the streptococci identifies them in group A. This method is practical and is as accurate as precipitin tests to catch group A.

When an infection with streptococci that produce streptolysin O takes place, antibodies against the streptolysin O appear in the blood of the patient. The detection and quantitation of these antibodies form an important diagnostic procedure in streptococcal infections of a chronic and persistent nature. This is the *antistreptolysin O titer* (ASTO), useful in the diagnosis and management of acute rheumatic fever and acute hemorrhagic glomerulonephritis (allergic reactions to beta hemolytic streptococci). The course of these diseases relates to the titer. The test helps to differentiate certain diseases similar to rheumatic fever where the streptococcus is not comparably implicated. The titer in these diseases is not significant.

**Immunity.** With the exception of scarlet fever, streptococcal infections are not followed by an immunity to subsequent attacks, and in scarlet fever the immunity is established only against scarlet fever toxin, not against the organisms.

**Prevention.** When caring for a patient with a streptococcal infection, nurses should remember that they are dealing with an infection that may be most virulent and easily spread. Physicians and nurses attending such infections, especially scarlet fever and erysipelas, should not attend an obstetric case or surgical operation until they are incapable of spreading the infection. Obstetric cases should be handled with strictest aseptic care because the recently emptied uterus is extremely vulnerable.

The buccal and nasal secretions from a patient with streptococcal bronchopneumonia should be handled in the same manner as those from a patient with diphtheria. A patient with streptococcal bronchopneumonia should be isolated from patients with measles or influenza. Conditions favoring contact infection should be avoided, and all wounds and abrasions on the body should be thoroughly disinfected.

The fact that more than 50 types exist among group A streptococci, all immunologically specific, explains the delay in the development of a clinically feasible vaccine. Vaccine production centers around the highly antigenic M protein in the streptococcal cell membrane that is significantly related to virulence.

## SCARLET FEVER

Scarlet fever (scarlatina) is an acute infection of childhood characterized by sore throat, severe constitutional symptoms, and a distinct skin eruption with massive exfoliation. The rash results from an acute hyperemia of the skin with petechial hemorrhages. The nasopharynx and tonsils may be covered with a membrane. The lymph nodes, especially those of the neck, are swollen and inflamed. The white blood count ranges from 15,000 to 30,000 cells per cubic millimeter, of which 85% to 95% are neutrophils.* Scarlet fever is caused by streptococci that produce erythrogenic toxin. In almost all cases streptococci are of Lancefield's group A, and only on the rarest occasion is scarlet fever produced by streptococci belonging in groups C and D.

The present opinion is that scarlet fever and streptococcal sore throat are different manifestations of the same basic disease. If the streptococci causing the sore throat produce erythrogenic toxin and the recipient of the infection is not immune to the toxin, scarlet fever results. If the streptococci do not produce erythrogenic toxin or if the recipient is immune to the toxin, then only the sore throat is present. There is a close relation between the streptococci causing scarlet fever, erysipelas, and puerperal sepsis.

In the past, scarlet fever was a disease of great severity, often fatal. Now it is relatively benign but may be complicated by suppurative otitis media and peritonsillar abscess or be followed by rheumatic fever and acute nephritis. It is more prevalent in Europe than in North America.

**Sources and modes of infection.** The sources of scarlet fever are the nose and throat secretions of patients or carriers and pus from infected lymph

---

*Normal white count is 5000 to 9000 cells per cubic millimeter, with 55% to 65% neutrophils.

nodes, ears, and other lesions. The organisms are present throughout the course of the illness and may persist in the nose and throat or in the exudates for weeks or months thereafter. As long as a person harbors the organism, he is a dangerous source of infection. The desquamated scales are not infectious.

The organisms usually enter the body through the mouth and nose, less often through wounds, burns, and the parturient uterus. Infection may be transmitted by direct contact or by contaminated objects such as handkerchiefs, towels, pencils, toys, and dishes.

**Erythrogenic toxin.** The erythrogenic toxin of scarlet fever streptococci is released by the organisms at the primary site, is absorbed into the body, and brings about the rash and other constitutional effects of the disease. It may be found in the blood in a concentration as high as 300 units per milliliter and also in the urine. It is prepared artificially by growing scarlet fever streptococci for 5 days in broth and then filtering the bacteria from the broth. The filtrate contains the toxin. Toxin prepared in this manner causes scarlet fever when given in large doses. When injected in very small amounts into the skin of persons susceptible to scarlet fever, it gives rise to an inflammatory reaction, the basis of the *Dick test*. It can induce an active immunity and the formation of antitoxin when injected into the animal body. The unit of measurement of scarlet fever toxin is known as the skin test dose (STD), the smallest amount of toxin causing an inflammatory reaction in the skin of a susceptible person. It is necessary to use susceptible persons for the test, since the majority of laboratory animals do not react.

**Immunity.** Immunity to scarlet fever relates to scarlet fever antitoxin in the blood. Infants inherit an immunity from their mothers that is lost within 1 year, and susceptibility increases until the sixth year. After the sixth year susceptibility decreases until adult life, at which time the majority of people are immune. An attack of scarlet fever is usually followed by permanent immunity. Remember that although an immune person will not be harmed by scarlet fever toxin, the streptococci themselves may invade his body and cause tonsillitis, abscesses, or otitis media. Immune persons may harbor the organisms for a long time and spread the infection widely.

*Dick test.* The Dick test is performed by injecting between the layers of the skin of the forearm 0.1 ml. of scarlet fever toxin so diluted that 1 STD is given. In immune persons the antitoxin in the blood neutralizes the injected toxin, and no reaction occurs. In susceptible persons without antitoxin the toxin injures the cells around the injection site, producing within 24 hours an area of inflammation and redness

at least 1 cm. in diameter. The test is positive at the beginning but becomes negative during the course of scarlet fever.

*Schultz-Charlton phenomenon.* If a small amount of the serum of a person convalescent from scarlet fever or of an animal immunized against scarlet fever is injected intradermally into an area of scarlet fever rash, the skin blanches at the injection site because the toxin in the area is neutralized by the injected antitoxin. This test differentiates scarlet fever from measles, German measles, and other skin diseases.

**Prevention.** The patient with scarlet fever should be isolated, and the discharges from the mouth and nose as well as all contaminated articles should be disinfected. The disinfecting procedures are the same as those for diphtheria (p. 244). Persons attending a patient should exercise every precaution to prevent the spread of infection to others, especially to obstetric or surgical cases. The patient should remain isolated until the discharges from the mouth and nose are free of scarlet fever streptococci and all complications have healed. Remember that during epidemics of scarlet fever persons with rhinitis and sinusitis may just as effectively spread the disease as those with a skin eruption. Pasteurization prevents milk-borne epidemics.

### ERYSIPELAS

Erysipelas (St. Anthony's fire)* is an acute inflammation of the skin caused by hemolytic streptococci of Lancefield's group A or, infrequently, of group C or D. The organisms grow at the site of infection and elaborate toxic substances responsible for the constitutional state. They are present not in the central portion of the inflamed area but at the periphery.

**Mode of infection.** The portal of entry for the streptococci is a wound, fissure, or abrasion. The lesion begins at the site of infection and extends peripherally as a hard red thickening of the skin. The streptococci grow almost exclusively in the lymph channels of the inflamed area, and as the disease progresses, they spread peripherally several centimeters beyond the line limiting the area of obvious inflammation. When streptococci enter the blood, the prognosis is bad. Erysipelas may be complicated by abscesses, pericarditis, arthritis, endocarditis, septicemia, and pneumonia. Patients with uncom-

---

*Erysipelas should not be confused with erysipeloid, a localized infection of the skin caused by *Erysipelothrix rhusiopathiae* (gram-positive rod with a tendency to form long filaments) and occurring in those who handle fish or meats.

plicated disease without open wounds or superficial discharges will not transmit the infection to others. Erysipelas may occur in association with other group A streptococcal infections.

**Immunity.** Instead of inducing immunity, an attack of erysipelas seems to render the patient more vulnerable to future attacks. Penicillin is the drug of choice in the treatment of erysipelas.

## STREPTOCOCCAL SORE THROAT (SEPTIC SORE THROAT)

Septic sore throat is an ulcerative inflammation of the throat accompanied by severe symptoms and a high mortality. This is the disease referred to as "strep throat." It is caused by hemolytic streptococci belonging to Lancefield's group A or, in a small proportion of cases, group C. It may be transferred by direct contact or droplet infection. However, direct transfer from person to person is not frequent.

Streptococcal sore throat may extend to the lungs to produce streptococcal pneumonia. Like scarlet fever, it may be followed by nephritis or rheumatic fever. Penicillin is the drug of choice in treatment.

## PUERPERAL SEPSIS

Puerperal sepsis (puerperal septicemia) is usually caused by a hemolytic streptococcus that reaches the uterus via hands or instruments contaminated from the nose and throat of the patient herself or from those in close association with her. Most of such streptococci belong to Lancefield's group A of organisms exogenous to the generative tract, but 20% to 25% of the cases come from anaerobic streptococci that are normal inhabitants of the vagina.

## STREPTOCOCCUS (DIPLOCOCCUS) PNEUMONIAE (THE PNEUMOCOCCUS)

**General characteristics.** The organism *Streptococcus (Diplococcus) pneumoniae*, best known in relation to pneumonia, occurs typically in pairs of lancet-shaped diplococci with their broad ends in apposition. Within the animal body or in excretions each pair is enclosed within a capsule. They are gram-positive, nonmotile, and nonsporeforming.

Pneumococci grow equally well in the presence or absence of oxygen. Their optimum temperature is 37° C., and they grow best in a slightly alkaline medium. Growth is most abundant on such enriched media as hormone agar and blood agar (Fig. 18-8). On the latter medium the green zone of slight hemolysis surrounding the colony is an important diagnostic feature. The power to form capsules is lost when pneumococci are cultivated for a long time on artificial media.

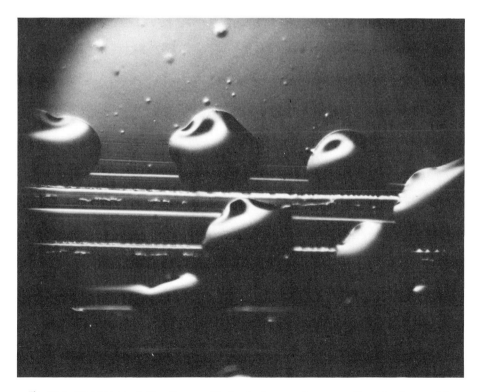

**Fig. 18-8.** Pneumococci. Greatly magnified colonies growing on routine blood agar plate.

*[handwritten margin note: organisms responsible for disease destroyed by Pasteurization]*

The pneumococcus is not a very hardy organism and has no natural existence outside the animal body. In the finely divided spray thrown off from the nose and mouth pneumococci live about 1½ hours in sunlight. In large masses of sputum they live for 1 month or more in the dark and about 2 weeks in sunlight. They are more susceptible to ordinary germicides than are most other bacteria and are destroyed in 10 minutes by a temperature of 52° C.

**Types.** Although all pneumococci are very much alike microscopically and culturally, they show distinct differences immunologically. This was discovered in 1910, when different cultures of pneumococci were used to immunize animals, and the serum of these animals was used to agglutinate pneumococci from various other sources. It was found that the majority of pneumococci fell into one of three rather distinct types (types I, II, and III) and that an antiserum prepared by immunizing an animal against pneumococci of one type agglutinated pneumococci of that type only. Pneumococci that did not fall into any of the three types were placed in group IV, which later was divided into 29 types. Other types were described in rapid succession, until at the present time there are at least 82 types or subtypes. All can cause pneumonia, but 50% to 80% of adult cases are due to types I, II, and III. Type III pneumonias menace the aged. In the pneumonias of children the primary types of pneumococci are XIV, I, VI, V, VII, and XIX (in order of frequency).

Formerly, therapeutic serums made from rabbits were available for the treatment of pneumonia caused by at least 30 of the types known at that time, and the determination of the type of pneumococcus causing the infection was necessary before serum therapy could be instituted. Today serum therapy for pneumonia has been replaced by antimicrobial therapy.

Pneumococcus type III differs somewhat from other pneumococci, with its wide capsule and slimy growth on culture media. It is not lancet-shaped. There seems to be a direct relation between capsule development and virulence of pneumococci, thus explaining why type III infections have such a high mortality.

The soluble carbohydrates that give pneumococci their type characteristics are polysaccharides in the capsules, spoken of as *specific soluble substances* (SSS). They can be detected by the precipitin reaction in broth cultures of pneumococci and in the blood and urine of patients with pneumonia. In addition to these, a somatic antigen is common to pneumococci.

**Toxic products.** The clinical features of pneumococcal disease indicate that the disease is a toxemia, but a toxin similar to that elaborated by the diphtheria bacillus has never been found. Pneumococci do, however, produce hemolysins, leukocidins, and necrotizing substances. Many strains produce hyaluronidase.

**Pathology.** The hallmark of pneumococcal infections is the presence of an abundance of fibrin in the areas of inflammation. In lobar pneumonia there is much fibrin in the lungs; in pneumococcal meningitis, much fibrin deposited in the subarachnoid space.

*Pneumonia* is an inflammatory condition of the air sacs (alveoli), bronchioles, and smaller bronchi of the lungs, in which these structures are filled with fibrinous exudate (Fig. 18-9). The pneumococcus is the most important cause of two kinds: lobar pneumonia and bronchopneumonia.

*Lobar pneumonia* is an acute disease characterized by a severe toxemia and a massive inflammatory exudation that fills the air spaces of one or more lobes of the lungs (*consolidation*). Rapid, shallow breathing, increased pulse rate (tachycardia), cyanosis, nausea, and vomiting are signs and symptoms related to the interference with respiration. With recovery and resolution the exudate in the lungs liquefies and is removed partly by absorption and partly by expectoration. Air reenters the affected lobe or lobes, and the lung completely returns to its former efficiency. Occasionally, delayed resolution leads to abscess formation or a chronic organizing pneumonia. Pleurisy (inflammation of the pleura) is a part of the disease. This disease has yielded so dramatically to the use of sulfonamides and antibiotics that the pathologic stages described years ago are rarely seen today.

Lobar pneumonia is a primary disease, and 95% of cases are pneumococcal. However, it may also be caused by the Friedländer bacillus, the influenza bacillus, or other streptococci. (See Fig. 26-3, p. 260.)

*Bronchopneumonia* is usually pneumococcal, but it may be caused by any one of a number of microbes, including other streptococci, staphylococci, and influenza bacilli, operating singly or in variable combinations.

Bronchopneumonia, more often secondary than primary, is a serious complication to measles, influenza, whooping cough, and chronic diseases of the heart, blood vessels, lungs, and kidneys. It peaks in the early and late years of life and frequently is the terminal event in debilitating diseases of the very young and extremely old. (It has long been called the "old man's friend.") Bronchopneumonia may follow the administration of an anesthetic or the aspiration of infectious material into the lungs during an operation. In newborn infants it is often caused by aspiration of infected amniotic fluid.

Unlike lobar pneumonia, bronchopneumonia

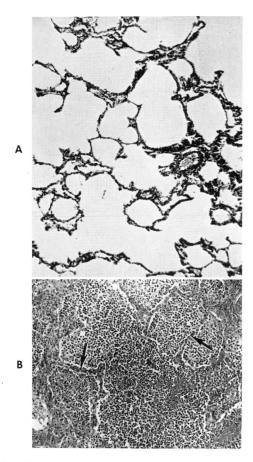

**A**

**B**

**Fig. 18-9.** Lobar pneumonia, microscopic section. (See also Fig. 50-3, p. 556.) **A,** Normal lung for comparison. Note air spaces with thin walls. **B,** Pneumonia–air sacs plugged solidly with exudate of fibrin and neutrophils (many small irregular, closely packed, dark nuclei). Arrows point to alveolar walls about consolidated air spaces. (×800.)

*TYPICAL PNEUMONIA*

consists of scattered small inflammatory foci, usually more numerous at the lung bases. The exudate consists of leukocytes, fluid, and bacteria but little or no fibrin or red blood cells. Pleurisy and empyema are complications. This kind of pneumonia does not always resolve readily, and chronic pneumonia often persists. *Hypostatic* pneumonia is bronchopneumonia complicating the hypostatic congestion of heart failure.

Pneumococci cause other diseases such as empyema, endocarditis, meningitis, arthritis, otitis media, peritonitis, and corneal ulcers. Some complicate pneumonia; others occur as primary conditions. Pneumococcal peritonitis is primary in children. Pneumococcal otitis media tends to spread to the meninges, with resultant pneumococcal meningitis.

*ANY OTHER IS ATYPICAL*

**Sources and modes of infection.** Lobar pneumonia is endemic in all centers of population. Epidemics seldom occur but can if conditions enhance exposure to infection with a concomitant lowering of host resistance. The sources of infection are active cases and carriers.

Pneumococci enter and leave the body by the same route, the mouth and nose. Infection is usually transferred directly, most often by droplets from the mouth and nose, but indirect transmission by contaminated objects is possible.

Practically everyone becomes a carrier of pneumococci for a short time during the year. Those who have contacted a patient may carry the organisms in their throats for a few days or weeks. Most carriers not in contact with pneumonia harbor comparatively avirulent pneumococci and are of little danger, although type III pneumococci may be found in such carriers. That carriers of type III pneumococci are common while type III infections are comparatively rare is difficult to explain.

**Laboratory diagnosis.** Pneumococci may be detected in sputum and other body fluids with some degree of certainty by direct microscopic examination of smears stained for capsules and by Gram's method. Confirmatory methods are cultures and the inoculation of white mice. (Rabbits and mice are very susceptible to pneumococci.) One milliliter of the emulsified sputum is injected into the peritoneal cavity of the mouse, wherein the pneumococci outstrip all other organisms. The mouse becomes ill after 5 to 8 hours, at which time it is killed. The peritoneal cavity contains many pneumococci to be identified by microscopic, cultural, and typing methods. Animal inoculation demonstrates pneumococci when direct smears fail to do so, and it always demonstrates them more quickly than do cultures.

Since serum therapy of pneumonia has yielded to antimicrobial drugs, typing is done primarily to determine whether a highly virulent type of the organism is present. There are several methods. All depend on the action of agglutinating and precipitating serums (typing serums) prepared by immunizing animals against the different types of pneumococci. In the method devised by Neufeld, flecks of sputum or other pneumococcus-containing material are mixed with the battery of type-specific serums. Where the type of pneumococcus matches that of the serum, the capsules of the pneumococci swell (Fig. 18-10). If the sputum contains too few pneumococci or if the typing is otherwise unsatisfactory, some of the sputum may be injected into a white mouse, as previously described, and in the course of a few hours typing may be carried out on the pneumococci from the peritoneal exudate.

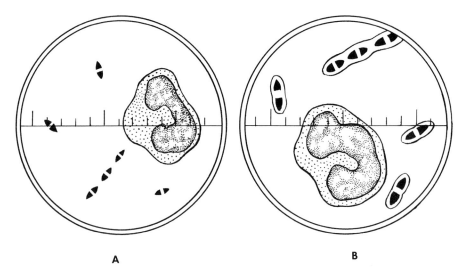

**Fig. 18-10.** Neufeld reaction (capsular swelling), sketch. **A,** No detectable change in capsule of lancet-shaped diplococci. **B,** Swelling of pneumococcal capsule in presence of type-specific serum.

*Differentiation of pneumococci from other strepto-cocci.* Pneumococci and the other streptococci bear such a close microscopic resemblance to each other that their differentiation is always an important laboratory problem. In fact, they are so closely related that in the eighth edition of *Bergey's Manual*, pneumococci are classified as a species of the genus *Streptococcus* and given a name long used for them in some parts of the world—*Streptococcus pneumoniae*.

Distinguishing points are that (1) on blood agar the colonies differ; (2) in animal tissues pneumococci have capsules whereas so-called streptococci seldom do; (3) when 1 part of bile is added to 3 parts of a liquid culture, pneumococci are dissolved whereas streptococci are not; (4) pneumococci ferment inulin, streptococci do not; (5) pneumococci are inhibited by optochin (ethylhydrocupreine hydrochloride) whereas streptococci are not; and (6) pneumococci are more pathogenic for mice than are streptococci. Other differential aids are agglutination and precipitation tests with specific antiserums.

**Immunity.** Recovery from a pneumococcal infection confers 6- to 12-month immunity to the type of pneumococcus causing the infection but none to other types. (Instances have been reported in which a person has had pneumonia more than a dozen times.) The natural resistance of man against the pneumococcus is comparatively high, and a person probably never contracts the disease unless his resistance is lowered. Blacks are more susceptible than whites, and men more so than women.

**Prevention.** The number of persons contacting a patient with pneumonia should be restricted. The discharges from the mouth and nose of the patient should be burned or disinfected. The hands and all objects, such as spoons, cups, and other utensils, possibly contaminated by the discharges of the patient should be disinfected. Measures should be taken to minimize droplet infection in the spray leaving the mouth of the patient when he talks or coughs.

Because of the antibiotic resistance encountered in pneumococci, vaccine therapy is coming back. The model is new. In process is the design of a polyvalent vaccine given in a single injection. It incorporates the purified capsular polysaccharides from the 12 or 14 types of pneumococci most likely to cause disease. Vaccines under investigation comprise types I to IX, XII, XIV, XVIII, XIX, and XXIII.

## Questions for review

1 Name important gram-positive cocci. Why are pyogenic cocci so called?
2 Characterize staphylococci.
3 List diseases caused by staphylococci.
4 Describe the localization and invasion of the body by staphylococci.
5 How is pathogenicity of a staphylococcus established?
6 Comment on the background factors in hospital-acquired infections. How are they studied epidemiologically?
7 Outline the streptococci according to the following categories: morphology, general features, classification, pathogenicity.
8 Name 10 diseases of man caused by streptococci. Name 2 diseases of animals. State the Lancefield groups responsible.
9 How are streptococci and pneumococci transmitted from person to person?

10 What is the Dick test? Neufeld reaction? Bacitracin disk test? Coagulase test? Schultz-Charlton phenomenon? Optochin test?

11 How is the antistreptolysin O titer used clinically?

12 Briefly discuss septic sore throat, puerperal sepsis, and erysipelas.

13 What is the relation between streptococcal disease and rheumatic fever?

14 Compare lobar pneumonia with bronchopneumonia.

15 Contrast the type lesion of staphylococcal and streptococcal infections. State the notable feature of pneumococcal injury.

16 What is the current status of vaccines against pyogenic cocci?

**References on pp. 276 to 280.**

# CHAPTER 19

# Gram-negative neisseriae

Distinctive gram-negative cocci or plump cocco-bacilli, sometimes called neisseriae, are found in the family Neisseriaceae, which includes three parasitic genera—*Neisseria, Branhamella,* and *Moraxella.* The most important ones are the gonococcus (*Neisseria gonorrhoeae*) and the meningococcus (*Neisseria meningitidis*), two pathogenic neisseriae of genus *Neisseria,* whose members are aerobic or faculta-tively anaerobic, oxidase-positive, and parasites of the mucous membranes of man. Members of the genera *Branhamella* and *Moraxella* and certain minor *Neisseria* species are important, not because of their pathogenicity but because of their habitat in the mouth and upper respiratory passages.

## NEISSERIA GONORRHOEAE (THE GONOCOCCUS)

*Neisseria gonorrhoeae* is the cause of gonorrhea, one of the most prevalent diseases affecting man, the most common of the venereal diseases, and the num-ber one communicable disease problem today in the United States. A disease known to the ancient Chi-nese and Hebrews, it was termed *gonorrhea* by Galen around 130 A.D. The gonococcus is sometimes called the diplococcus of Neisser after its discoverer, and its infections are referred to as neisserian infections.

**General characteristics.** The gonococcus is a gram-negative, nonmotile, nonencapsulated, non-sporeforming diplococcus (Fig. 19-1). In smears the cocci are placed like two coffee beans lying with their flat sides together.

Gonorrhea is a disease accompanied by a discharge from the genital tract that is at first thin and watery, then later purulent. The incubation period is 3 to 5 days. During the early stages the gonococci are found free in the serous exudate or attached to epithelial cells; but when the exudate becomes purulent, phago-cytosis takes place, and the gonococci are found char-acteristically within the cytoplasm of pus cells (poly-morphonuclear neutrophilic leukocytes). A single white blood cell may contain from 20 to 100 micro-organisms. These gonococci are not dead and are still infectious. In later stages of the disease they may be found outside the white blood cells, and when the dis-ease becomes chronic, they often cannot be found at all.

This fastidious organism will not grow on ordinary culture media and is somewhat difficult to cultivate even on media prepared especially for it. Gonococci grow best at or slightly below body temperature (35° to 37° C.) and in an atmosphere containing oxygen and carbon dioxide (3% to 10%). The appearance of colonies of gonococci is variable, and four types refer-able to the differences are described and related to virulence. Colony types 1 and 2 come from infective organisms; colony types 3 and 4 from gonococci, prob-ably noninfective. The cocci of types 1 and 2 possess pili, which may help the bacteria to attach themselves to epithelial cells and so resist phagocytosis. Gono-cocci produce the enzyme *oxidase,* as do other mem-bers of the genus *Neisseria.* The *oxidase reaction* is used to identify colonies of neisserian species in cultures.

Although gonococci are difficult to destroy within the body, they possess little resistance outside it. They are killed in a very short time by sunlight and drying. In pus or on clothing in moist, dark surroundings they may live from 18 to 24 hours. They are very suscep-tible to disinfectants, especially silver salts, and are killed by a temperature of 60° C. within 10 minutes. Although gonococci are susceptible to the action of the modern antibiotics, drug resistance is an ever-present problem, especially with the number of drug-resistant strains coming in from southeast Asia and the Philippine Islands. Gonococci are not exactly alike immunologically but cannot be typed. There is only one defined strain.

**Pathogenicity.** The gonococcus is parasitic spe-cifically for man. Spontaneous infection does not occur. Nothing comparable to any of the clinical forms of gonorrhea had been produced artificially in lower animals until recently, when gonococcal urethritis was produced experimentally in the chimpanzee and the male-to-female animal transmission demonstrated.

In typical cases of gonorrhea the sites of primary infection in the female are the urethra and cervix; in

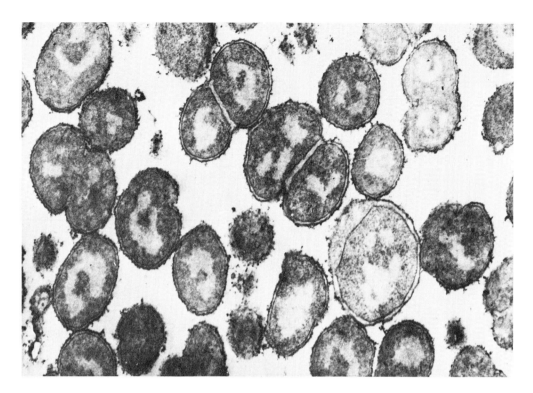

**Fig. 19-1.** *Neisseria gonorrhoeae* in cross section, electron micrograph. (×100,000.) (Courtesy Technical Information Services, State and Community Services Division, Center for Disease Control, Health Services and Mental Health Administration, Department of Health, Education and Welfare, Atlanta.)

the male the site is the urethra. Gonococci injure columnar epithelium like that lining the cervix uteri and the rectum and the transitional (urothelial) epithelium lining the urinary tract. Vaginal infection is not seen because the epithelium lining the vagina of adult women is a cornified stratified squamous type resistant to gonococci. Before the age of puberty the vagina is lined with a softer, extremely susceptible epithelium. Gonorrheal vulvovaginitis in prepubertal girls may be epidemic and difficult to eradicate. The change in the epithelium with the onset of puberty usually eliminates a childhood infection completely.

An important site of primary infection seen more and more today is the conjunctiva of the eye (gonorrheal conjunctivitis and keratitis), and the process is one that actively damages the tissues of the eye (Fig. 19-2). *Ophthalmia neonatorum*, gonorrheal conjunctivitis in newborn infants, results when the eyes are infected during the birth passage. A profuse purulent discharge in the eyes of a neonate can build up a considerable pressure behind the lids. If the lids are forced apart, pus spurts out. The physician and attendants of these babies must be careful to protect

their own eyes. In babies or adults the infection may easily result in blindness or serious sight impairment because of the inflammatory distortion of the structures in the eye. Ophthalmia neonatorum can be prevented by the Credé method, as is required by law for all babies.

From the urethra of the male, gonococcal infection may spread by direct extension to the other parts of the male reproductive system. In the female it may likewise spread to other parts of the tract, especially to Bartholin's glands and the fallopian tubes. The lining of the uterus seems to resist the action of gonococci. Invasion of the fallopian tubes usually occurs with the first or second menstrual period after infection; however, in some cases it may not occur until later. Involvement of the fallopian tubes is associated with considerable distortion and scarring if the disease becomes chronic. Scarring of the urethra in the male may lead to stricture or closure of the urethral lumen at one or more focal points.

Gonococci sometimes pass from the genitourinary tract via the lymphatics or the bloodstream to set up distant sites of infection. Serious consequences

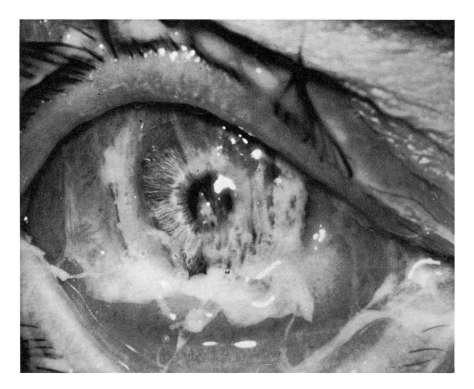

**Fig. 19-2.** Acute gonococcal conjunctivitis (gonorrheal ophthalmia of adults). Note marked inflammation, redness and irritation of conjunctivae, and copious amounts of pus. Smear of exudate showed pus cells with intracellular diplococci. Culture grew out gonococci. Patient also had gonococcal pelvic inflammatory disease. (From Donaldson, D. D.: Atlas of external diseases of the eye, vol. 1, St. Louis, 1966, The C. V. Mosby Co.)

would be an endocarditis or meningitis. Gonococcemia is associated with varied skin lesions from which organisms may be identified. An important manifestation of extragenital gonococcal infection is a purulent, destructive arthritis. As the overall incidence of gonorrhea increases, extragenital lesions become more prominent.

**Sources and modes of infection.** Gonococci are never found outside the human body unless they are on objects very recently contaminated with gonorrheal discharges, and here they live only for a short time. Therefore gonorrheal infections are practically always spread by direct contact, and mostly the mode of contact is sexual intercourse. It is not to be denied that gonorrhea is sometimes transmitted indirectly by contaminated objects, but this is very rare.

Gonorrheal ophthalmia of adults is usually accidental. Infection from the genitourinary tract is inadvertently transferred to the eyes by the hands of the same or a different person. Vulvovaginitis in children is spread by the use of common bed linen, bathtubs, toilets, and such. It has been known to result from the use of contaminated rectal thermometers. It usually occurs where children live in closely crowded quarters.

Untreated gonococcal infections tend to become chronic. Females, especially, who are untreated or inadequately treated become infectious carriers for years after manifestations of disease have disappeared. An estimated 60% to 80% of females with the infection are asymptomatic.

**Laboratory diagnosis of gonorrhea.** The microbiologist has at his command several procedures applicable to the diagnosis of gonorrhea. Smears, cultures, and the oxidase reaction are the *presumptive* tests. To confirm the results of these and to establish the diagnosis of gonorrhea he uses fluorescent antibody technics and carbohydrate fermentation reactions.

Direct smears of genital discharges may be stained with the Gram stain. There are rare exceptions to the rule that for all practical purposes the finding of gram-negative diplococci within the pus cells of an exudate from a genital infection strongly *suggests* that they are gonococci. This is especially true if the exudate is from the male urethra. In the male with typical acute purulent urethritis, the gram-stained smear of the

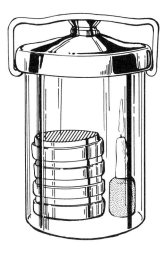

**Fig. 19-3.** Culture under increased carbon dioxide tension, a simple method for partially anaerobic conditions. Cultures and lighted candle are placed in container, and container is made airtight. Candle burns until oxygen is almost completely exhausted, then goes out.

exudate containing the distinctive intracellular diplococci ordinarily makes the diagnosis. In the female, early in the disease, typical diplococci may be seen in smears of material from Skene's and Bartholin's glands, but even a working diagnosis cannot be made on this basis alone. The reasons for this are several—gram-negative diplococci other than gonococci occur outside cells. Gonococci occur outside cells, singly or in pairs, and gram-positive organisms having the morphology of gonococci occur within cells. All that can be said about gram-negative diplococci found outside cells is that they *may be* gonococci. Very infrequently are gram-negative diplococci other than gonococci found within the pus cells of a genital exudate, but it is possible. The smear prepared from gonorrheal exudates should be very thin because gonococci react to the Gram stain in an erratic way if the smear is thick and uneven. The microbes usually are not found in the exudate of chronic gonorrhea.

Cultural methods are of special value in the diagnosis of chronic gonorrhea and in the determination of a cure. Cultures are incubated under increased carbon dioxide tension (Fig. 19-3). Enriched media such as chocolate agar, Hirschberg's egg medium, and, currently, the Thayer-Martin medium are used to cultivate the delicate gonococcus. Thayer-Martin (T-M)

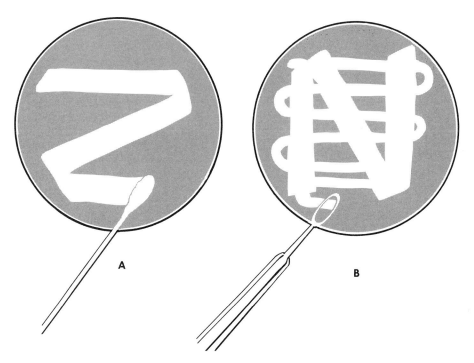

**Fig. 19-4.** Two-step method of streaking plate for culture of gonococci. **A,** Cervical (or rectal) secretions on swab rolled gently onto plate in Z pattern. **B,** Cross streaking of inoculum in **A** done with platinum loop.

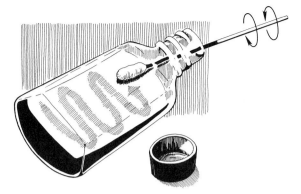

**Fig. 19-5.** Inoculation of Transgrow medium. Note neck of bottle elevated. (From Criteria and techniques for the diagnosis of gonorrhea, Atlanta, 1972, Center for Disease Control.)

medium* contains hemoglobin, certain chemicals to enhance gonococcal growth, and antimicrobial agents to inhibit selectively fungi, gram-positive organisms, and many gram-negative ones. The plates of T-M medium to be inoculated must be streaked in a specified way so as to spread the organisms out of the associated mucus, which tends to lyse them (Fig. 19-4). A modification of Thayer-Martin medium, Transgrow, has been developed so that suspect cultures can be sent into central laboratories. Transgrow comes in a screw-cap bottle containing a mixture of air and carbon dioxide. To inoculate Transgrow, one holds the bottle upright to prevent carbon dioxide from escaping and unscrews the cap (Fig. 19-5). The swab with the test material on it is rolled over the medium. The cap is returned, and the bottle is ready for shipping. The unopened bottle can be incubated directly at the receiving laboratory. Gonococci survive and grow 48 to 96 hours in this medium.

Public health authorities today recommend that suspect material for culture be obtained from the anorectal area and pharynx as well as from the urogenital tract (anterior urethra, endocervical canal). Rectal gonorrhea is easily overlooked. Carefully taken swabs are important in male homosexuals, and in females both cervical and rectal swabs are needed because half the women infected harbor the gonococcus in the rectum. Infection may persist there after it has been eliminated in the cervix.

Gonococci can be recovered in urine from the male if the first 10 ml. of voided urine is centrifuged and the sediment cultured. In a simpler screening method,

---

*Also called VCN medium for the three antibiotics it contains —vancomycin hydrochloride, colistimethate sodium, and nystatin.

the first few drops of urine caught on a dry swab are immediately passed across Thayer-Martin medium. Cultures of urine in screening programs have helped to define a reservoir existing in the asymptomatic male as well as female.

The next steps in the bacteriologic study of the gonococcus are the determination of the biochemical reactions and identification of the organisms with fluorescein-labeled antiserums. The biochemical reactions of *Neisseria* species discussed in this chapter are given in Table 19-1. The fact that the gonococcus possesses a specific K-type antigen is the basis for the fluorescent antibody test to detect gonococci in direct smears of exudate or in smears made from cultures.

Several serologic tests under study are still in pilot stages, but results are discouraging. A serologic test to catch the large number of women in the silent, communicable reservoir, although highly desirable, is associated with problems. One of these is that the gonococcus seems to share its antigens with other, harmless neisseriae.

It is never within the province of the laboratory alone to say that a person is cured of gonorrhea, and in many cases the efforts of both laboratory and clinician do not determine whether the disease is completely eradicated. In dealing with a case of gonorrhea, physicians and nurses should consider its medicolegal potential.

**Social importance of gonorrhea.** In the United States today gonorrhea, the single most prevalent bacterial infection, is increasing in frequency to epidemic and pandemic proportions. It is estimated that there are 3 million new cases annually, about 1, it is said, every 15 seconds. More than half of the cases occur in teenagers and young adults under 25 years of age.

Generally three males are treated and reported for each female, since in males the manifestations of disease are usually sufficiently disagreeable to motivate them to seek medical attention. Since females are often asymptomatic or relatively so, many of them are reported and diagnosed only because of information from male consorts. The silent reservoir of asymptomatic females constitutes a primary obstacle to control of disease, and if widespread screening of the female population is not done, it may remain so. Some health authorities recommend that a culture for *Neisseria gonorrhoeae* be considered an essential part of prenatal care and that a routine culture be taken more often at the time a pelvic examination is done in any woman.

The most destructive piece of misinformation that has been handed down from generation to generation is that gonorrhea is no worse than a cold. Such a fallacy both underestimates the danger of gonorrhea and creates the impression that colds are of no conse-

**Table 19-1**

Characteristics of the neisseriae

| ORGANISM | GROWTH ON THAYER-MARTIN MEDIUM | GROWTH ON NUTRIENT AGAR AT 22° C. | OXI-DASE | FERMENTATION OF SUGARS WITH ACID ONLY | | | | | PIGMENT PRO-DUCTION | HABITAT |
|---|---|---|---|---|---|---|---|---|---|---|
| | | | | GLU-COSE | MAL-TOSE | SU-CROSE | FRUC-TOSE | MAN-NITOL | | |
| *Neisseria gonorrhoeae* | + | − | + | + | − | − | − | − | − | Found only in genital infections of man |
| *Neisseria meningitidis* | + | − | + | + | + | − | − | − | − | Nasopharynx of man |
| *Neisseria sicca* | −* | + | + | + | + | + | + | − | Variable | Nasopharynx of man |
| *Neisseria flavescens* | −* | + | + | − | − | − | − | − | Golden yellow | Nasopharynx of man |
| *Neisseria subflava* | −* | + | + | + | + | − | + | − | Greenish yellow | Nasopharynx of man |

*Growth with heavy inoculum.

quence. The medical, social, psychologic, and even medicolegal implications of gonorrhea are sizable.

Gonorrhea is said to be the most common cause of sterility in both sexes. In women, sterility results from occlusion of the fallopian tubes by scar tissue formed during the healing of gonorrheal salpingitis. In men it results from occlusion of the vasa deferentia by a similar process of gonorrheal inflammation and healing, with scarring.

**Immunity.** An attack of gonorrhea confers little if any immunity to subsequent attacks.

**Prevention.** The general public should be warned of the dangers of gonorrhea and the difficulty of its cure. It is unfortunate that use of the wonder drugs has engendered an attitude that the disease is unimportant. The dangers of quack doctors and folk remedies should be stressed. The patient must not allow his discharges to soil toilets or articles used by others. He must be warned of the danger of transferring the infectious material to his eyes by means of his hands.

Prophylactic treatment in newborn babies is as follows. Immediately after birth, the eyelids of the baby are cleaned with sterile water. A different piece of cotton is used for each eye, and the lids are stroked (or irrigated) from the nose outward. Next, the lids are opened, and one or two drops of 1% silver nitrate solution is instilled into each eye, care being taken that the conjunctival sac is completely covered with the solution. After 2 minutes the eyes are irrigated with isotonic saline solution. (A mild irritation of the lining membranes of the eye may be produced but is short lived.) This is known as *Credé's method,* a procedure so important that it is required by law in most of the fifty states. It appears that penicillin and other antibiotics are as effective as silver nitrate in the preven-

tion of ophthalmia neonatorum, but where the law requires silver nitrate, such antibiotics are not used. A few states have passed laws allowing a suitable antibiotic to be used instead of silver nitrate. However, the National Society for the Prevention of Blindness (New York) is currently recommending that the silver nitrate method be continued as the standard and preferred procedure.

Vulvovaginitis in children may be prevented by proper care of bed linen, bathtubs, night clothes, and wash water. All children should be examined for gonorrhea before admission to children's institutions or to hospital wards with other children. It has been noted that vulvovaginitis in children spontaneously regresses within a few weeks in more than 85% of the cases.

The U. S. Public Health Service, although presently concerned with the development of a vaccine for gonorrhea, is not optimistic. Because of the nature of the disease and the mode of transfer, every person who has gonorrhea should be serologically tested for syphilis.

**The VD pandemic.** Every 2 minutes somewhere in the United States a teenager contracts a venereal disease. Because of changing factors in our society, forms of disease contracted primarily through intimate sexual contact and some that may be contracted this way are on the rise. This is a matter of great concern to public health officials and agencies. Table 19-2 gives a list of diseases so transmitted with causative agents.*

Venereal disease treatment information is available

---

*With the exception of gonorrhea, these diseases are discussed in subsequent chapters.

**Table 19-2**

The venereal diseases

| DISEASE | AGENT |
|---|---|
| The "classic five" | |
| 1 Gonorrhea | Bacterium |
| | *Neisseria gonorrhoeae* |
| 2 Syphilis | Spirochete |
| | *Treponema pallidum* |
| 3 Chancroid | Bacterium |
| | *Haemophilus ducreyi* |
| 4 Granuloma | Bacterium (Donovan bodies) |
| inguinale | *Calymmatobacterium granulomatis* |
| Lymphopathia | Chlamydia |
| venereum* | *Chlamydia trachomatis* |
| Newcomers | |
| Herpes | Virus |
| progenitalis | *Herpesvirus hominis* type II |
| Molluscum | Virus (Molluscum bodies) |
| contagiosum | Poxvirus group |
| Mycoplasmosis | Mycoplasma—T strains |
| Candidiasis | Fungus |
| | *Candida albicans* |
| Trichomoniasis | Protozoan |
| | *Trichomonas vaginalis* |
| Condyloma | Virus |
| acuminatum | |

*Lymphogranuloma venereum.

from a toll-free, nationwide "hot line," Operation Venus, financed by a volunteer organization, the United States Alliance for Eradication of Venereal Disease. The number is 800-462-4966 in Pennsylvania and 800-523-1885 for the rest of the nation.

## NEISSERIA MENINGITIDIS (THE MENINGOCOCCUS)

The meningococcus *Neisseria meningitidis* is the cause of meningococcal septicemia with or without localization in the leptomeninges to produce epidemic cerebrospinal meningitis. Epidemic cerebrospinal meningitis is known also as cerebrospinal fever, spotted fever, and meningococcal meningitis and is one form of acute bacterial meningitis.* During World War II more soldiers in the Army of the United States died as a result of meningococcal infection than of any other infectious disease.

**General characteristics.** Meningococci are gram-negative diplococci with a striking resemblance to gonococci but with more irregularity in size and shape. They are nonmotile and do not form spores. Capsules are usually not seen in ordinary smears but may be demonstrated by special methods. Meningococci produce endotoxins liberated when the cocci

*Nonepidemic forms of meningitis are discussed on p. 622.

disintegrate; these toxins are partly responsible for the manifestations of meningitis. In the cerebrospinal fluid meningococci appear both within and without the polymorphonuclear neutrophilic leukocytes. (One must know the source of the specimen to determine whether gram-negative intracellular diplococci found in a smear are meningococci or gonococci.)

Meningococci grow best at body temperature in an atmosphere containing 10% carbon dioxide (Fig. 19-3). They do not grow at room temperature. Growth requires special media containing enriching substances such as whole blood, serum, or ascitic fluid. Agar containing laked rabbit blood and dextrose supports the growth of meningococci especially well, as does enriched hormone agar. Different strains of meningococci may vary considerably in the ease with which they grow on artificial culture media. Salt has a toxic effect on meningococci and should be left out of media on which they are to be grown. Like gonococci, they are oxidase-positive.

Meningococci are such frail organisms that they survive only a short time outside the body. Sunlight and drying kill them within 24 hours. Away from the body, they are easily killed by ordinary disinfectants, but in the nasopharynx they are very resistant. They are quite susceptible to heat and cold. Meningococci quickly lyse in cerebrospinal fluid removed from the body. Therefore, specimens of suspect fluid should be examined as quickly as possible.

**Meningococci and gonococci compared.** Meningococci and gonococci are alike in that (1) both are strict parasites and cause disease only in man, (2) they show little difference in resistance to injurious agents, (3) their distribution in the inflammatory exudate is the same, (4) they grow on artificial media with difficulty, and (5) their disease-producing properties are comparable. Skin lesions of gonococcemia may be similar to those of meningococcemia, and gonococci have caused the Waterhouse-Friderichsen syndrome (see below). It may be said that they are morphologically, physiologically, and pathogenetically much alike.

**Groups of meningococci.** By serologic reactions, including a capsular swelling test similar to that used in typing pneumococci, meningococci are classified into four main groups—A, B, C, and D.* (The U. S. Public Health Service Center for Disease Control in Atlanta, Ga., recognizes at least seven different types of meningococci with specific antigenic and epidemiologic differences—A, B, C, D, X, Y, and Z.)

Groups A and C are encapsulated and possess a specific capsular polysaccharide. There is a polysac-

*Groups A, B, C, and D correspond respectively to groups I, II, II alpha, and IV in the formerly used classification.

charide-polypeptide component in group B, but usually no capsule. In the past, group A meningococci have been responsible for 95% of cases of epidemic meningitis; group A was especially troublesome during World War II. Groups B and C have been the endemic organisms figuring in sporadic outbreaks between major epidemics. Until the mid-1960s, group B was the prevalent one. Since then group C is causing an increasing number of epidemics at military bases. There are few meningococci of group D in this country.

**Pathology.** The meningococcus is not very pathogenic for the lower animals, and typical epidemic cerebrospinal meningitis occurs only in man. Invasion of the body by meningococci occurs in three steps: (1) implantation in the nasopharynx, (2) entrance into the bloodstream, with the production of a septicemia, and (3) localization in the meninges (cerebrospinal meningitis). For most patients the invasion ends with implantation in the nasopharynx (the carrier state).

About one third of meningococcal infections are septicemias of such severity that without treatment the patient dies before meningeal infection can occur. Meningococci proliferate as massively in blood and tissues as though growing in laboratory broth culture. The events of meningococcal septicemia come together under the designation *Waterhouse-Friderichsen syndrome,* an acute fulminating condition characterized by many small areas of hemorrhage in the skin (Fig. 19-6) and, within a few hours, death in peripheral circulatory failure.* At autopsy large areas of hemorrhage are seen in the adrenal glands. (See Fig. 19-7.)

In only a few patients do bacteria in the bloodstream infect the meninges or other body tissues.

---

*The rapid course of events possible with meningococcal disease—collapse and death within an hour or so—is terrifying to the social group. The disease upsets people to the point of mass hysteria.

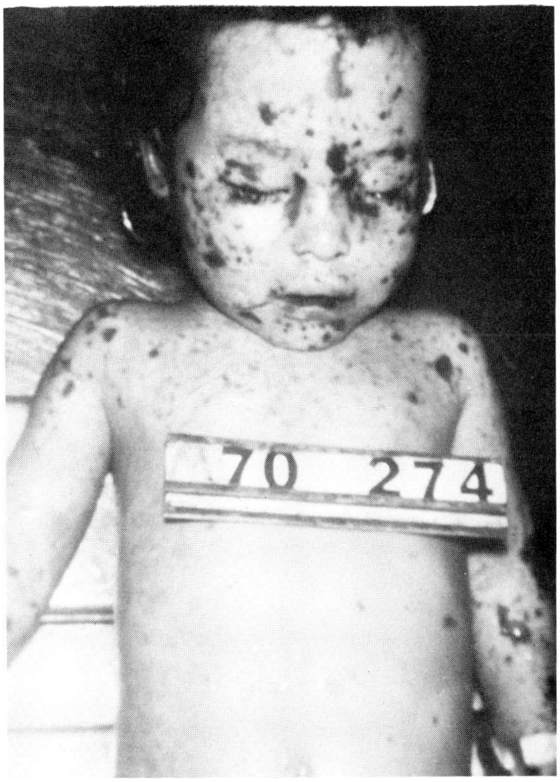

**Fig. 19-6.** Acute fatal meningococcemia in small child (Waterhouse-Friderichsen syndrome). Note hemorrhages over face and upper trunk.

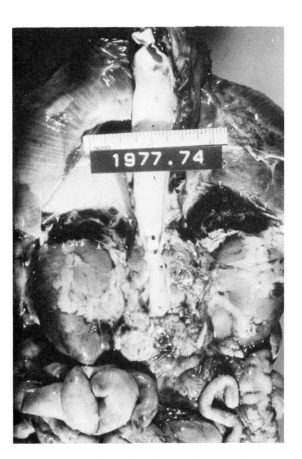

**Fig. 19-7.** Hemorrhagic adrenal glands in normal position overlying kidneys at autopsy of patient in Fig. 19-6 (Waterhouse-Friderichsen syndrome). You are looking at retroperitoneal area of abdomen. The aorta has been opened (in center). Note its smooth inner surface.

When meningococci do infect the meninges of the brain, purulent inflammation results. An exudate composed of leukocytes, fibrin, and meningococci forms in the subarachnoid space, the area between the two meningeal coverings, the arachnoid and the pia mater. Most prominent along the base of the brain, the exudate extends into the cerebral ventricles and down the spinal subarachnoid space. The cerebrospinal fluid may be so purulent that it scarcely flows through the lumen of the lumbar puncture needle.

Among the complications of epidemic meningitis are arthritis, hydrocephalus, otitis media, retinitis, deafness from involvement of the eighth nerve, pericarditis, endocarditis, conjunctivitis, pneumonia, and blindness.

**Sources and modes of infection.** Since meningococci are such frail organisms and seldom found outside the body, the source of infection must be a patient or a carrier. The organisms reside in the nasopharynx of both patients and carriers and leave the body in the nasal and buccal secretions. The mode of transfer is by close contact, and the organisms enter the body by the nose and mouth. Venereal transmission is reported. When meningococci reach a new host, they localize in the nasopharynx and multiply. Infection traced to articles recently contaminated by infected nasal and buccal secretions seldom occurs.

Meningococcal infections are not highly communicable, and there seems to be a high degree of natural immunity to them. Many persons exposed become carriers, but few develop disease. It is estimated that about 1 carrier in 1000 develops meningococcemia or meningitis. In the absence of immunity, the great numbers of carriers in the general population would maintain an epidemic at all times. Since meningococcal infection is endemic in all densely populated centers, it may become epidemic under overcrowded conditions, as in army camps. Overcrowding concentrates the carriers and promotes factors that lower individual resistance. When troops are mobilized it is one serious disease to which the men seem to be exceedingly vulnerable.

Under ordinary conditions probably 2% to 5% of the general population are carriers. When epidemics occur, the number of carriers, especially of group A meningococci, increases. In military establishments, 50% of the personnel may become carriers. About two thirds of those who contract meningitis harbor the organisms for a variable time after convalescence. The carrier state lasts about 6 months. However, healthy persons who have never had meningitis but nevertheless harbor meningococci in their nasopharynx play a more important part in the spread of meningitis than do those who harbor the organisms after recovery from the disease.

At times the meningococcus has been recovered from the vagina and cervix in situations where its relation to disease was not clear. This finding emphasizes the importance of adequately identifying organisms from the female genital tract. Meningococci, although thought of as respiratory pathogens, may invade on occasion other parts of the body.

**Laboratory diagnosis.** To give the patient the advantage of early treatment, which means so much in meningococcal infections, meningococcal septicemia should be diagnosed clinically. The diagnosis is confirmed by blood cultures. A valuable diagnostic adjunct is the demonstration of meningococci by smears or cultures in the hemorrhagic skin lesions associated with septicemia (Fig. 19-6). When cultures for meningococci are made, the specimen must not cool before inoculation onto media warmed to room temperature. The inoculated cultures are promptly incubated.

In epidemic meningitis the cerebrospinal fluid is first turbid and then purulent. In smears of cerebrospinal fluid the typical arrangement of gram-negative diplococci within the pus cells is sufficient for practical purposes to make a working diagnosis of epidemic meningitis. However, cultures must confirm the diagnosis. Because of the tendency of the organisms to undergo autolysis, the specimen must be examined as quickly as possible after it is withdrawn.

Fluorescent antibody technics detect the organisms, and immunoelectrophoresis can be used to test for the presence of meningococcal antigen in cerebrospinal fluid and serum. Group typing is also done by immunoelectrophoresis.

**Immunity.** That epidemics of meningeal infection are not more common stems from the fact that whereas nasopharyngeal infection is prevalent (low immunity of localization), resistance to invasion of the bloodstream or body tissues is high. Some observers believe that a moderate degree of immunity results from an attack of meningitis. Others believe that no protection is acquired. Immunity seems to increase with age, since the disease is more prevalent in children than in adults.

Before the advent of the antimicrobial compounds the mainstay in the treatment of epidemic meningitis was antimeningococcal serum of two types, bactericidal and antitoxic. Although serum therapy reduced the mortality, its results did not equal those now obtained with the antimicrobial drugs. The death rate was 40% to 50%; it is now 5% to 10%.

**Prevention.** The patient with a meningococcal infection should be isolated until cultures fail to show meningococci in his nasopharynx. All discharges from the mouth and nose and articles soiled therewith should be disinfected. The urine occasionally contains the organisms and therefore should be disinfected.

The physician and nurse should use every precaution to avoid infection or the carrier state. Nurses should exercise care lest their hands convey the infection. Dishes used by the patient should be properly sterilized. Persons who have been in close contact with a patient should not mingle with others until bacteriologic examination has proved them to be free of meningococci.

General preventive measures include the proper supervision of carriers. The wholesale isolation of carriers does not eliminate infection, and the trend presently is to isolate only those in immediate contact with a patient. Nose sprays are probably of little value. The antibiotic rifampin is used to eliminate the carrier state.

The control of epidemic meningitis is yet to be accomplished. For reasons that we do not understand, it suddenly becomes virulent in a community, attains epidemic form, persists for a time, and then disappears.

Field testing continues, with the expectation of a polyvalent vaccine against groups A, B, and C. Polysaccharide antigens are used, and results are good. A polysaccharide vaccine has been shown effective in preventing group C meningococcal disease and also the carrier state.

## OTHER GRAM-NEGATIVE COCCI (AND COCCOBACILLI)

**Branhamella (Neisseria) catarrhalis.** The organism *Branhamella (Neisseria) catarrhalis* is a normal inhabitant of the mucous membranes, especially those of the respiratory tract. It is important to the microbiologist because it may be confused with the meningococcus or the gonococcus. Like these organisms it is a gram-negative, biscuit-shaped diplococcus that on rare occasions may assume the intracellular position. Differentiation depends on agglutination tests and the ability of *Branhamella (Neisseria) catarrhalis* to grow on ordinary culture media at room temperature.

**Other neisseriae.** Other gram-negative diplococci that may lead to errors in microbiologic diagnosis are *Neisseria subflava* and *Neisseria sicca,* both of which are normal inhabitants of the pharynx and nasopharynx (Table 19-1). *Neisseria flavescens* has been recovered from the cerebrospinal fluid of patients with meningitis, and its colonies look like those of *Neisseria meningitidis,* but it does produce a golden yellow pigment when first isolated.

**Moraxella lacunata (the Morax-Axenfeld bacillus).** The oxidase-positive, gram-negative, strictly aerobic coccobacilli of the genus *Moraxella* are very similar to members of the genus *Branhamella* and, like *Branhamella,* are parasitic on mucous membranes of man and animals. *Moraxella lacunata* causes a subacute or chronic inflammation of the conjunctiva, eyelid, and cornea.

## Questions for review

1 Name and describe the microbe causing gonorrhea.
2 What is the social importance of gonorrhea?
3 Briefly discuss the venereal disease pandemic.
4 List 10 diseases venereally transmitted. Give the causative organism for each.
5 Outline the laboratory diagnosis of gonorrhea.
6 What are the sources and modes of infection in gonorrhea?
7 How is gonorrheal ophthalmia contracted in adults? In infants?
8 What is Credé's method?
9 Compare gonococci with meningococci.
10 Name and describe the microbe causing epidemic meningitis.
11 What are the sources and modes of infection in epidemic cerebrospinal meningitis?
12 State the importance of the carrier in meningococcal infections.
13 Give the nursing precautions in epidemic meningitis.
14 How is the diagnosis of meningococcal infection made in the laboratory?
15 List 10 microorganisms causing meningitis. See p. 622.
16 Explain what is meant by the Waterhouse-Friderichsen syndrome.

**References on pp. 276 to 280.**

# CHAPTER 20

# Gram-negative enteric bacilli

The *enteric bacilli*, a large, heterogeneous group in the family Enterobacteriaceae, include several closely related genera of short, nonsporeforming, gram-negative rods, facultatively anaerobic, that inhabit or produce disease in the alimentary tract of man and warm-blooded animals. Here are the nonpathogenic bacteria that normally inhabit the intestinal canal and the highly pathogenic bacteria that invade and injure it. Heading any list of enteric pathogens are the consistent troublemakers, the *Salmonella* and *Shigella* species. Normal residents include many species in a number of genera, and if given the right opportunity, many of these supposedly benign bacteria can be awesome in their behavior. Not all members of Enterobacteriaceae are intestinal parasites; they have been placed here because of other similarities.

Today, members of this family of bacteria are notorious as causes of urinary tract infection and are recovered from a variety of clinical specimens taken from diseased foci other than in the gastrointestinal tract. The Enterobacteriaceae are probably responsible for more human misery than any other group.

Enteric microorganisms of this chapter are defined in the classification most widely used in microbiologic laboratories. The starting point is Bergey's Family I of Part 8, Enterobacteriaceae. The breakdown as proposed by W. H. Ewing and approved by the subcommittee of the American Society for Microbiology is shown in Schema 5.*

---

*Note departure from Bergey's classification in Schema 5.

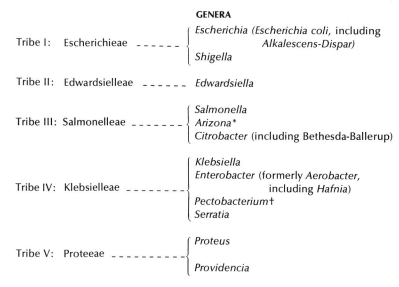

**Schema 5.** Ewing's classification of enteric microorganisms.
*The term *paracolon bacilli* was formerly used for enteric bacilli resembling *Escherichia coli* but fermenting lactose much more slowly. They were placed in the genus *Paracolobactrum* and separated into the Bethesda-Ballerup group, the Arizona group, the Providence group, and the Hafnia group. In the above schema, paracolon bacilli are regrouped, and the term *paracolon* discarded.
†A genus of plant pathogens (soft rot coliforms), it is not implicated in human infection. As might be expected, it is the only genus in the family liquefying sodium pectate.

Enteric bacilli may be studied as to disease production, physiologic behavior, and immunologic reactions. The practical identification of the enteric gram-negative bacilli, however, involves the use of an elaborate array of biochemical reactions. To demonstrate biologic activities of test organisms is usually a complex maneuver in the clinical laboratory. In a greatly simplified scheme, Table 20-1 presents key reactions for the bacteriologic separation of some of the enteric organisms to be discussed.

## Salmonella species*

**General characteristics.** The genus *Salmonella* comprises the causative organisms of the salmonelloses, some 250 species in 4 subgenera† of motile enteric bacilli, which are found everywhere that there are animals and man. Of the numerous strains, all can produce disease in their natural hosts.

Although the members of the different species are similar in morphology, staining reactions, and cultural characteristics, they can be separated by fermentation

---

*The *Salmonella* genus was named for Daniel Elmer Salmon (1850-1914), American veterinary pathologist who first isolated the organisms in 1885.

†In sharp contrast to the complexity of the breakdown of the genus *Salmonella* found in the eighth edition of *Bergey's Manual* (Table 1-1, p. 7), Dr. Ewing recognizes only three species in genus *Salmonella*—*Salmonella cholerae-suis* as type species, *Salmonella typhi* as unique pathogen of man, and *Salmonella enteritidis* to comprise all other serotypes and serobiotypes. By this schema, *Salmonella enteritidis* would now be *Salmonella enteritidis* ser. *enteritidis*, and *Salmonella typhimurium* would be *Salmonella enteritidis* ser. *typhimurium*. Since this approach is not yet widely accepted, we shall continue with traditional species names.

## Table 20-1
Simplified scheme for the separation of some gram-negative enteric bacilli

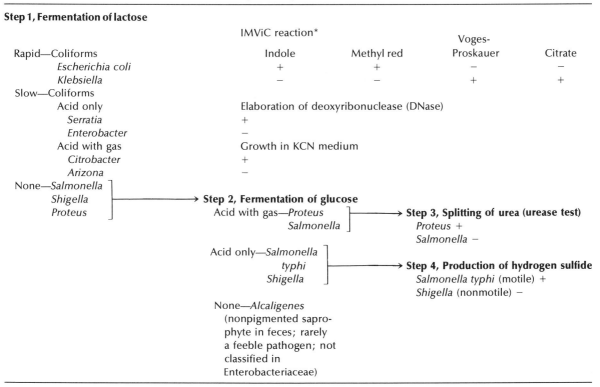

**Step 1, Fermentation of lactose**

| | IMViC reaction* | | Voges- | |
| | Indole | Methyl red | Proskauer | Citrate |
|---|---|---|---|---|
| Rapid—Coliforms | | | | |
|   *Escherichia coli* | + | + | − | − |
|   *Klebsiella* | − | − | + | + |
| Slow—Coliforms | | | | |
|   Acid only | Elaboration of deoxyribonuclease (DNase) | | | |
|    *Serratia* | + | | | |
|    *Enterobacter* | − | | | |
|   Acid with gas | Growth in KCN medium | | | |
|    *Citrobacter* | + | | | |
|    *Arizona* | − | | | |

None—*Salmonella*
 *Shigella* → **Step 2, Fermentation of glucose**
 *Proteus*

  Acid with gas—*Proteus* → **Step 3, Splitting of urea (urease test)**
      *Salmonella*   *Proteus* +
               *Salmonella* −

  Acid only—*Salmonella*
       *typhi* → **Step 4, Production of hydrogen sulfide**
     *Shigella*   *Salmonella typhi* (motile) +
              *Shigella* (nonmotile) −

  None—*Alcaligenes*
    (nonpigmented sapro-
    phyte in feces; rarely
    a feeble pathogen; not
    classified in
    Enterobacteriaceae)

---

*The pattern of the IMViC reaction is important to the differentiation of the coliform bacilli (normal residents of the enteron). It refers to four biochemical color reactions. The first reaction, "I," is the production of indole from tryptophan (pink or red color). The next two, the methyl red reaction, "M," and the Voges-Proskauer reaction, "Vi," indicate a difference in the fermentation of glucose in a special test medium after 2 to 4 days' incubation. If the test organism ferments glucose with the accumulation of acid end products, the methyl red indicator gives a red color (pH below 4.5), a positive test. If glucose has been fermented with the accumulation of neutral end products, the Voges-Proskauer test is positive, a red-orange color showing the presence of acetylmethylcarbinol. The fourth reaction, "C," refers to the utilization of Simmons citrate agar and indicates that the test organism can use the citrate as its sole source of carbon.

**Table 20-2**
Biochemical patterns for *Salmonella* species

| ORGANISM | PRODUCTION OF HYDROGEN SULFIDE | REDUCTION OF NITRATES | PRODUCTION OF INDOLE | LIQUEFACTION OF GELATIN | FERMENTATION OF CARBOHYDRATES | | | | | |
|---|---|---|---|---|---|---|---|---|---|---|
| | | | | | GLUCOSE | LACTOSE | MALTOSE | SUCROSE | MANNITOL | DULCITOL |
| *Salmonella typhi* | + | + | – | – | Acid | – | Acid | – | Acid | – |
| *Salmonella paratyphi-A* | – | + | – | – | Acid, gas | – | Acid, gas | – | Acid, gas | Variable |
| *Salmonella schottmuelleri* | + | + | – | – | Acid, gas | – | Acid, gas | – | Acid, gas | Variable |
| *Salmonella hirschfeldii* | + | + | – | – | Acid, gas | – | Acid, gas | – | Acid, gas | Acid, gas |
| *Salmonella typhimurium* | + | + | – | – | Acid, gas | – | Acid, gas | – | Acid, gas | Variable |
| *Salmonella cholerae-suis* | Variable | + | – | – | Acid, gas | – | Acid, gas | – | Acid, gas | Variable |
| *Salmonella enteritidis* | + | + | – | – | Acid, gas | – | Acid, gas | – | Acid, gas | Variable |
| *Salmonella gallinarum* | Variable | + | – | – | Acid | – | Acid | – | Acid | Acid |

reactions* (Table 20-2) and agglutination tests. Serologic typing is the important last step in their bacteriologic identification. More than 1600 serotypes have been identified. The immunologic classification of *Salmonella* is complex but important in tracing epidemiologic patterns of disease. Salmonellae are susceptible to the action of heat, disinfectants, and radiation. At the temperature of the refrigerator, they do not multiply but remain viable.

**Sources and modes of infection.** Since only a few species, such as *Salmonella typhi* (*S. typhi*), are indigenous to man, most infections come from species in lower animals. In nature, salmonellae occur in the intestinal tract of man and animals. Therefore they must be spread by feces either directly or indirectly from one host to another. Excreta contain bacilli because the infected host has obvious disease or inapparent infection or is a carrier. The principal vehicle is water, milk, or food contaminated by feces. The most dangerous link in a chain of infection is the food handler who is a carrier.

If the food ingested contains only a small number of salmonellae, the acid in the stomach of the host destroys them readily. If the food is heavily contaminated, some of the bacilli escape the effects of the gastric acid to enter and injure the small bowel.

**Pathogenicity.** Infection with *Salmonella* is salmonellosis, the major site of which is the lining of the intestinal tract. Because of their toxic properties, every known strain of *Salmonella* can cause any one of three types of salmonellosis: (1) acute gastroenteritis of the food infection type, (2) septicemia or acute sepsis similar to pyogenic infections, and (3) enteric fever such as typhoid or paratyphoid fevers.

Most of the time, however, *Salmonella* infection is acute gastroenteritis, a condition characterized by fever, nausea, vomiting, diarrhea, and abdominal cramps. Sometimes gastroenteritis is the forerunner of septicemia. Once the bacilli have spread, they can cause a wide range of lesions in different parts of the body. Examples are abscesses of various organs, arthritis, endocarditis, meningitis, pneumonia, and pyelonephritis. Salmonelloses may be severe and death dealing; or they may be mild and even inapparent.

With regard to their natural host, salmonellae are divided into the following categories: (1) those that primarily affect man, (2) those primarily affect the lower animals but may cause disease in man, and (3) those that affect lower animals only.

### SALMONELLA TYPHI (THE TYPHOID BACILLUS)

The organism *S. typhi* causes typhoid fever, which as the natural infection occurs only in man.

---

* In keeping with their role as intestinal pathogens, salmonellae do not ferment lactose.

**General characteristics.** A short, motile, non-encapsulated bacillus, S. *typhi* grows luxuriantly on all ordinary media. It grows best under aerobic conditions but may grow anaerobically. The temperature range for growth is from 4° to 40° C., and the optimum, 37° C. It ferments glucose with the production of acid but not gas. Typhoid bacilli can survive outside the body; they live about 1 week in sewage-contaminated water and not only live but multiply in milk. They may be viable in fecal matter for 1 or 2 months. Their pathogenic action relates to endotoxins.

**Portal of entry.** Any person who contracts typhoid fever has swallowed typhoid bacilli. If the bacilli enter the body by a route other than the alimentary tract, infection does not occur. The incubation period is from 7 to 21 days.

**Pathology.** Typhoid fever is an acute infectious disease characterized clinically by continuous fever, skin eruptions, bowel disturbances, and profound toxemia. Except in the first few days, leukopenia is always present in uncomplicated cases, probably because typhoid bacilli depress the bone marrow, where normal production of white blood cells occurs. Leukocytosis in the course of the disease strongly suggests a complication.

Typhoid bacilli first penetrate the intestinal lining to attack the lymphoid tissue in the wall, Peyer's patches in the small bowel bearing the brunt of the attack. From the intestinal wall the bacilli pass to the mesenteric lymph nodes draining the area, where they colonize. Passing on to the thoracic duct, they enter the bloodstream. Here many bacilli are lysed. Liberation of endotoxins brings about the manifestations of the disease. The bacilli that escape bacteriolysis tend to localize in the gallbladder, bone marrow, and spleen and have disappeared from the bloodstream beyond the first week of illness. The rose spots seen on the skin of the abdomen early in the illness contain many bacilli. As the disease progresses, the bacilli confine their activities to the intestinal wall.

Pathologically, typhoid fever is a granulomatous inflammation that involves the lymphoid tissue of the body. The hyperplastic lymphoid masses (including Peyer's patches) swell and plateau above the level of the intestinal mucosa. In most cases necrosis and sloughing take place, leaving an oval ulcer of varying depth. If a blood vessel undergoes necrosis, hemorrhage may occur, and if the ulcer extends deep enough, there is perforation of the intestinal wall. The mesenteric lymph nodes are swollen and may suppurate. The hyperplastic spleen is soft and enlarged to 2 or 3 times its normal size. The liver and kidneys show degenerative changes, and the gallbladder may be inflamed. Toxic degeneration of the myocardium may precipitate acute heart failure and death.

*Complications.* Fully three fourths of the deaths in typhoid fever result from some complication. *Hemorrhage* occurs most often during the third week; the passing of a tarry stool or clotted blood may be the first indication. *Perforation* of the bowel is usually at a single site, most often in the lower 18 inches of the small intestine. The mortality is very high. *Cholecystitis* may follow the disease, and typhoid bacilli may be found in the gallbladder years later.

**Portal of exit.** Typhoid bacilli leave the body via feces and urine and are found therein usually after the second week of illness.

**Spread.** The fundamental basis of every typhoid infection is the same. *Typhoid bacilli from the feces or urine of a carrier or a person ill of typhoid fever have reached the mouth of the victim.*

Typhoid carriers are of two types: fecal and urinary. In the more common fecal carriers the bacilli multiply in the gallbladder and are excreted in the feces. (Infection of the gallbladder with stagnation of bile predisposes to the formation of gallstones.) In urinary carriers the organisms multiply in the kidney and are excreted in the urine. From 40% to 45% of patients become convalescent carriers for 3 to 10 weeks. About 5% carry the bacilli for 1 year, and about 2% become permanent carriers. The average carrier is female and more than 40 years of age.

The most dangerous factor in the spread of typhoid fever is the carrier–food handler who prepares foods that are served raw. Carriers contaminate their fingers with their discharges and then contaminate food with their fingers. It is hard to prevent the carrier state, and treatment for it can be difficult. Removal of the gallbladder cures selected cases.

With improvements in sanitation widespread epidemics of typhoid fever from contamination of water supplies with sewage, once so common in large cities, are almost unknown. Strict laws regulate the cultivation of oysters and other shellfish eaten raw to eliminate contamination of these foods with sewage-laden water.

**Laboratory diagnosis.** The laboratory offers four procedures for the diagnosis of typhoid fever: (1) blood culture, (2) the Widal test, (3) stool culture, and (4) urine culture. Blood cultures are positive during the first week in 75% to 80% of patients. The percentage falls until not more than 10% of patients have positive blood cultures by the fourth week. The diagnosis of infection with S. *typhi* is made by isolation of the organism.

After 7 or 10 days of infection, agglutinins against typhoid bacilli appear in the patient's blood, increasing during the second and third weeks of disease. They may persist for weeks, months, or years after the patient recovers. Agglutinins also appear in the blood after typhoid vaccination and are usually found in the blood of carriers.

When an animal is immunized with typhoid bacilli and certain other actively motile organisms, two types of agglutinins are formed. One, acting on the flagella of the bacterium, is the *H (flagellar)* agglutinin. The other, acting on the body of the bacterium, is the *O (somatic)* agglutinin. The O agglutinins are thought to appear earlier in the disease and to indicate actual infection with typhoid bacilli or *closely related organisms*. If they are present in the serum of persons vaccinated, they are in small quantities and only for a short time. In addition to H and O antigens typhoid bacilli responsible for active disease or the carrier state contain a third antigen, the *Vi (virulence)* antigen. Vi antibodies are not thought to occur significantly after vaccination. *Salmonella* species other than *S. typhi* possess O and H antigens; some possess Vi antigens. The species may be divided into groups on the basis of their O antigens and further subdivided on the basis of their H antigens.

The Widal test is used to detect the presence of these agglutinins. It is said to be positive in 15% of typhoid patients during the first week of illness, with the incidence of positive results rising to 90% or more during the third week. However, there are considerable difficulties in interpretation of the Widal test. Many authorities are thoroughly disillusioned with it.

Stool and urine cultures are of value in the detection of carriers and indicate when a given patient ceases to be a source of infection. Typhoid bacilli may be cultivated from the stool in 50% of the cases by the third week. Positive urine cultures are obtained at some time during the course of the disease in 25% to 50% of patients. Convalescent carriers excrete the bacilli in their feces or urine during convalescence only, but permanent carriers continue to excrete them.

**Immunity.** In about 98% of the cases an attack of typhoid fever renders the patient immune for the remainder of his life. The production of an artificial immunity by the administration of typhoid vaccine has been one of the most important measures in the control of typhoid fever.

**Prevention.** The prevention of typhoid fever is twofold—community and personal. Community prevention means those steps taken by the community as a whole to block the spread of disease among its members; personal prevention means those taken to block the spread of infection from a person ill of the disease. The most important factors in the community program are (1) a supply of clean pasteurized milk, (2) a pure water supply, (3) efficient disposal of sewage, (4) proper sanitary control of food and eating places, (5) detection and isolation of carriers, especially food handlers, (6) destruction of flies, and (7) vaccination.*

Personal prevention depends on isolation of the patient. Isolation does not mean merely putting the patient in a room and shutting the doors but must close all the routes by which bacteria may be transmitted to others.

Preferably the patient is hospitalized and kept there until he is no longer infectious. Nurses attending a patient with typhoid fever should consider every secretion and excretion of the patient to be a living culture of typhoid bacilli and should use every means to protect themselves, members of the patient's family, and people in the community. They should have nothing to do with the preparation of food, and their hands should be disinfected after each contact with the patient or anything that either the patient or his secretions have touched. Feces and urine can be disinfected with chlorinated lime, 5% phenol, or 2% Amphyl (p. 171). Sputum should be received on disposable paper tissues and burned. Linen and bedclothes should be sterilized. Food remains should be burned, and dishes boiled. The patient's bath water can be sterilized with chlorinated lime. The sickroom should be screened, and flies that accidentally gain access to it should be killed. All rugs, curtains, and similar fabric materials should be removed from the room. Pets should not be allowed to enter. Disinfection should continue through convalescence, and no patient should be released as cured until repeated cultures of feces and urine have failed to show typhoid bacilli.

That the procedures just outlined, together with vaccination, have materially reduced the incidence of typhoid fever is proved by the following facts. In 1900 the death rate in the United States from typhoid fever was 35.9 per 100,000 persons; today less than 500 cases are reported annually (0.21 cases per 100,000 persons reported in 1974). That universal vaccination alone will materially reduce the incidence of typhoid fever is proved by the experience of the U. S. Navy during the years 1911 to 1913, a period in which no revolutionary developments in sanitation took place. In 1911 there were 361 cases of typhoid fever per 100,000 men. In 1912 universal vaccination of naval personnel was put into effect. In 1913 the rate had fallen to 34 per 100,000, a reduction of more than 90%.

---

*Currently the U. S. Public Health Service is *not* recommending typhoid immunization within the United States. The Advisory Committee does not indicate typhoid vaccination for persons going to summer camp or even for those surviving a flood disaster. Typhoid immunization is discussed on pp. 402, 416, and 417.

## PARATYPHOID BACILLI

The paratyphoid bacilli are so called because they have been isolated from paratyphoid fever in man, a disease resembling typhoid fever but milder in its manifestations and shorter in duration. Although associated with enteric fever, each of the three species causes other forms of salmonellosis.

The three are *Salmonella paratyphi*-A, *Salmonella schottmuelleri*, and *Salmonella hirschfeldii* and were formerly known respectively as the paratyphoid bacilli A, B, and C. Infections with *Salmonella paratyphi*-A occur almost exclusively in man; *Salmonella schottmuelleri* occasionally causes infections in lower animals. *Salmonella hirschfeldii* is rarely found in the United States; infections are frequent in eastern Europe, and mice are said to be its natural host. *Salmonella paratyphi*-A resembles *Salmonella typhi* more closely than does *Salmonella schottmuelleri*, but infections with the latter are more prominent.

The mode of infection, sources, laboratory diagnosis, nursing precautions, and prevention are the same as those in typhoid fever. The immunity produced by paratyphoid infection or vaccination is uncertain (see also p. 416).

## OTHER SALMONELLAE

Among the many salmonellae that primarily affect the lower animals but that may cause disease in man are *Salmonella typhimurium* (cause of a typhoid-like disease of mice; may cause gastroenteritis in man); *Salmonella cholerae-suis* (once thought to be the cause of hog cholera; can cause septicemia in man); and *Salmonella enteritidis,* known also as Gärtner's bacillus (found in hogs, horses, mice, rats, and fowls; causes infections in man). An organism primarily affecting lower animals is *Salmonella gallinarum* (cause

of fowl typhoid); it differs from other *Salmonella* species in that it is not motile.

Attacks of enteric infection are on occasion traced to salmonellae from unusual sources. Recently salmonellae were demonstrated in the small turtles given as pets to children who subsequently developed salmonellosis. Contaminated baby chicks have been a similar source for small children.

## Shigella species (the dysentery bacilli)

Dysentery is a painful diarrhea accompanied by the passage of blood and mucus and associated with abdominal pain and constitutional symptoms. It may be primary disease or secondary. When primary, it may be of protozoal, bacterial, or viral origin. Protozoal dysentery caused by an ameba is amebic dysentery (p. 342). Dysentery caused by members of the *Shigella* genus is known as bacillary dysentery. Bacillary dysentery may be epidemic or endemic, is usually acute but may be chronic, and is an important form of summer diarrhea in infants.

**General characteristics.** The *Shigella* are classified in four species, each of which is divided into several types: *Shigella dysenteriae* (7 types), isolated by Shiga in the Japanese epidemic in 1898; *Shigella flexneri* (6 types), isolated by Flexner in the Philippine Islands in 1900; *Shigella boydii* (11 types); and *Shigella sonnei* (6 types). *Shigella flexneri* and *Shigella sonnei* are worldwide in distribution. In recent years infection with *Shigella dysenteriae* has been limited to the Orient.

Dysentery caused by the Shiga bacillus (*Shigella dysenteriae*) is much more severe than that caused by the other organisms, since this bacillus produces a powerful exotoxin-like substance in addition to an endotoxin. There is no evidence, however, that this substance is actively excreted by the bacterial cell.

**Table 20-3**
Biochemical reactions of *Shigella* species

| ORGANISM | PRODUCTION OF HYDROGEN SULFIDE | LIQUEFACTION OF GELATIN | REDUCTION OF NITRATES | PRODUCTION OF INDOLE | FERMENTATION OF CARBOHYDRATES | | | | |
|---|---|---|---|---|---|---|---|---|---|
| | | | | | GLUCOSE | LACTOSE | SUCROSE | MANNITOL | DULCITOL |
| *Shigella dysenteriae* | − | − | + | − | Acid | − | − | − | − |
| *Shigella flexneri* | − | − | + | + | Acid | − | − | Acid | − |
| *Shigella boydii* | − | − | + | Variable | Acid | − | − | Acid | Variable |
| *Shigella sonnei* | − | − | + | − | Acid | − | Acid | Acid | − |

Rather, it seems to be liberated by the disintegration of the cell, and as a neurotoxin, the exotoxin-like substance acts on the nervous system, causing paralysis in the host. The endotoxin irritates the intestinal canal.

The dysentery bacilli are gram-negative, nonsporebearing rods that grow on all ordinary media at temperatures from 10° to 42° C. but best at 37° C. They are aerobic and facultatively anaerobic. Unlike most other members of the enteric group, they are nonmotile. Table 20-3 gives biochemical reactions for *Shigella* species.

**Pathogenicity.** Dysentery is a human disease, and natural infections of the lower animals do not occur. The incubation period is 1 to 7 days. Epidemic dysentery is primarily an intestinal infection. Unlike typhoid bacilli, the organisms do not invade the bloodstream and are seldom if ever found in the internal organs or excreted in the urine. They are excreted in the feces.

**Pathology.** Pathologically, bacillary dysentery is recognized as diffuse inflammation with ulceration of the large intestine and sometimes the lower portion of the small intestine. Early in the disease shallow ulcers or extensive raw surfaces that may be covered by a pseudomembrane form in the mucous membrane. In mild cases healing is complete, but in severe cases there is extensive scarring of the intestine.

**Mode of infection.** The mode of infection is practically the same as for typhoid fever; the bacilli enter the body of the victim by way of the mouth, having been transferred there from the feces of carriers or patients. Contaminated food, water, fingers, or other objects are the vehicles of spread. Contact with persons who have symptomless infections is especially important in the spread of bacillary dysentery. Flies are a factor.

**Laboratory diagnosis.** The only practical method of laboratory diagnosis is the cultivation of the organisms from the stool. Unfortunately this can be done only during the first 4 to 5 days of the disease.

**Immunity.** An attack of dysentery probably confers some degree of immunity, but the same person has been known to have two episodes in a single season.

**Prevention.** Bacillary dysentery may be checked by the sanitary measures that control typhoid fever, but it remains ready to rise in epidemic form when people are crowded together in unsanitary conditions. The feces and everything contaminated by the patient should be handled exactly as for a case of typhoid fever. Food or milk should not be carried from the premises, and persons attending the patient should not handle food for others. The patient should not be dismissed as cured until repeated feces cultures have failed to show the causative organism. After the patient has recovered, the sickroom should be thoroughly cleaned.

Preventive vaccination is not yet available. An oral attenuated vaccine against *Shigella flexneri* is being tested. One such is a "mutant hybrid," produced by "mating" *Escherichia coli* with a nonvirulent strain of *Shigella flexneri*. There is no serum therapy.

## Escherichia coli and related organisms (the coliform bacilli)

**General characteristics.** Besides *Escherichia coli*, coliform bacteria comprise members of the genera in

**Table 20-4**
Biochemical reactions of the coliforms and proteus bacilli

| ORGANISM | PRODUCTION OF INDOLE | METHYL RED TEST | VOGES-PROSKAUER REACTION | PRODUCTION OF HYDROGEN SULFIDE | LIQUEFACTION OF GELATIN (22° C.) |
|---|---|---|---|---|---|
| Coliforms: | | | | | |
| *Escherichia coli* | + | + | − | − | − |
| *Klebsiella* species | − | − | + | − | − |
| *Enterobacter* species | − | Variable | Variable | − | Variable |
| *Serratia marcescens* | − | − | + | − | + |
| *Arizona* species | − | + | − | + | Slow |
| *Edwardsiella tarda* | + | + | − | + | − |
| *Citrobacter* species | − | + | − | + | − |
| *Providencia* species | + | + | − | − | − |
| Proteus bacilli: | | | | | |
| *Proteus vulgaris* | + | + | − | + | + |
| *Proteus morganii* | + | + | − | + | − |

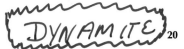 

the following groups: (1) *Klebsiella-Enterobacter-Serratia;* (2) *Arizona-Edwardsiella-Citrobacter;* and (3) the "Providence" group.

As normal inhabitants of the intestinal tract* these microbes share certain traits. They are gram-negative, short rods that do not form spores. They grow at temperatures from 20° to 40° C. but best at 37° C. A few species are surrounded by capsules. Most are motile. They are not so susceptible to the bacteriostatic action of dyes as are many other bacteria. Therefore media for the isolation of coliform bacilli can contain inhibitory dyes. Table 20-4 presents bacteriologic features of coliforms.

In a sanitary water analysis the presence of coliform bacilli indicates fecal pollution of the water supply being tested.

**Pathogenicity.** Coliform bacilli usually do not penetrate the intestinal wall to produce disease unless (1) the intestinal wall becomes diseased, (2) the resistance of the host is lowered, or (3) the virulence of the organisms is greatly increased. Under one of these conditions coliforms may pass to the abdominal cavity or enter the bloodstream. Once outside the intestinal canal and in the tissues of the body, their virulence is remarkably enhanced (Fig. 20-1).

Among the diseases that they cause are pyelonephritis, cystitis, cholecystitis, abscesses, peritonitis, and meningitis, They play a part in the formation of gallstones; they are found in the cores of such stones. In the peritonitis complicating intestinal perforation

_____
*In the adult, 30% of the dry weight of the feces is made up of bacteria.

the coliform group is joined by other organisms such as streptococci and staphylococci. From any focus of inflammation coliform organisms may enter the bloodstream to produce a septicemia.

## ESCHERICHIA COLI

An important member of the coliform group and long known as the colon bacillus (of man and other vertebrates) because of its natural habitat in the large bowel, *Escherichia coli (E. coli)* is unabashed as an opportunist when out of its natural setting. It is the commonest cause of pyelonephritis and urinary tract infections and is an important cause of epidemic diarrhea in nurseries for newborn infants. The immunologic pattern for *Escherichia* is as complex as that for *Salmonella.* Immunologic subdivision of *E. coli* is made on the basis of O (somatic) antigens, K (capsular) antigens, and H (flagellar) antigens. More than 150 serologic types are known, of which 11 have been correlated with infantile diarrhea.

**Infantile diarrhea.** Infectious diarrhea is an extremely important cause of infant death. In underdeveloped areas of the world over 5 million infants succumb to it each year. Infantile diarrhea including summer diarrhea is especially prevalent during the hot weather among bottle-fed babies who are reared in unhygienic surroundings, but it is also a problem in modern hospital nurseries. In institutional outbreaks (hospitals and orphanages) half the cases are caused by *Shigella* (especially *Shigella sonnei*), *Salmonella,* and enteropathogenic *E. coli.* Strains of enteropathogenic *E. coli* have recently been shown to release an exotoxin that acts on the wall of the small intestine to

| USE OF SIMMONS CITRATE | SPLITTING OF UREA | FERMENTATION OF CARBOHYDRATES | | | | |
|---|---|---|---|---|---|---|
| | | GLUCOSE WITH GAS | LACTOSE | SUCROSE | MANNITOL | DULCITOL |
| − | − | + | + | + | + | Variable |
| + | + | + | + | + | + | − |
| + | − | + | Variable | + | + | − |
| | (Variable) | | | (Variable) | | |
| + | Variable | + | Very slow | + | + | − |
| + | − | + | Slow | − | + | − |
| − | − | + | − | − | − | − |
| + | Variable | + | + | Variable | + | + |
| + | − | Variable | − | Variable | Variable | − |
| Variable | + | + | − | + | − | − |
| − | + | + | − | − | − | − |

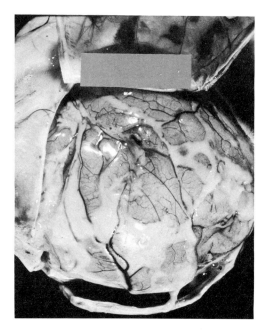

**Fig. 20-1.** *Escherichia coli* as cause of meningitis in 24-day-old premature infant. Note immature brain with coating of pus over outer surface and prominent vascular markings. Skull flaps are laid back; brain is seen in cranial cavity.

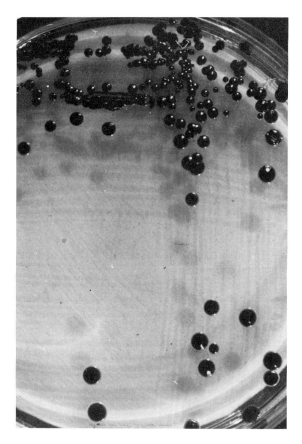

**Fig. 20-2.** *Serratia marcescens.* Colonies of pigmented strain on nutrient agar plate. Characteristic red suggested by dark appearance.

cause movement of fluid and electrolytes across the mucous membrane into the lumen. The presence of an "enterotoxin" correlates with severe watery diarrhea. Other causative agents include *Proteus, Pseudomonas, Staphylococcus,* cholera-like vibrios, and enteroviruses. A significant number of cases are related to the enteroviruses.

In the hospital nursery, care in the preparation of infant formulas and the sterilization of bottles and nipples are essential to prevent this disorder, which is uncommon in the breast-fed baby. Fluorescent antibody technics detect the serotypes of *E. coli* in stools or rectal swabs from the babies and help to trace carriers among the personnel of the nursery.

### KLEBSIELLA-ENTEROBACTER-SERRATIA

The biologic qualities of *Klebsiella* indicate a relationship to the coliforms; the disease-producing capacities, a kinship to respiratory tract pathogens. *Klebsiella* are nonmotile, gram-negative, aerobic organisms surrounded by a broad, well-developed polysaccharide capsule. They are differentiated from *E. coli* biochemically (Table 20-4). The type organism is *Klebsiella pneumoniae* (Friedländer's bacillus). A hazard to the chronic alcoholic, pneumonia caused by Friedländer's bacillus may be either lobar or lobular,

is very severe, and is frequently fatal. Middle ear infections and meningitis may complicate it. Friedländer's bacillus is also responsible for septicemia.

The genus *Enterobacter* includes the organisms formerly known as *Aerobacter aerogenes.* These bacilli are found in the soil, water, dairy products, and the intestines of animals, including man. As opportunists, they play a part in urinary tract infection and rarely cause more serious conditions—endocarditis, suppurative arthritis, and osteomyelitis. The type species is *Enterobacter cloacae.*

*Serratia marcescens* is a small, free-loving, ubiquitous rod celebrated for the red pigment (prodigiosin) produced in cultures (Fig. 20-2). Since it has emerged as a sometime formidable pathogen, investigators have found that only a small number of the organisms are chromogenic. The pigment-producing strains do so at room temperature, seldom at incubator temperatures. As is true for other coliforms, infections with this organism (serratiosis) complicate surgical procedures and antibiotic therapy, especially in elderly, debilitated patients in the hospital. The results may be urinary tract infections, pneumonia, empyema, meningitis, or wound infections, to mention but a few.

Bacteriologically the organisms in the genera *Klebsiella, Enterobacter,* and *Serratia* are similar. However, when they are grown on a modified deoxyribonuclease (DNase) agar containing toluidine blue as indicator, colonies of *Serratia* may be distinguished from those of the other organisms. A bright pink zone around *Serratia* indicates that this organism elaborates deoxyribonuclease. The clear blue color of the other colonies indicates that these organisms do not.

### ARIZONA-EDWARDSIELLA-CITROBACTER

Formerly known as paracolon bacilli, these organisms ferment lactose very slowly, if at all.

Arizonae are short rods similar to the salmonellae and in the eighth edition of *Bergey's Manual* are classified in genus *Salmonella,* subgenus III. From 7 to 10 days may be required for them to ferment lactose. The type species is *Arizona hinshawii* (or Bergey's *Salmonella arizonae*). They are found in human infections and cause disease in dogs, cats, and chickens.

Because of their pattern of biochemical reactivity, certain motile rods were separated into the genus *Edwardsiella.* The type species *Edwardsiella tarda* was given a name implying a kind of biochemical *in*activity. *Edwardsiella tarda* has been isolated from man and animals, especially snakes. In fact, snake meat is postulated to be a source of infection. In man the infections are similar to the salmonelloses: (1) bacteremia with coexisting localization away from the gastrointestinal tract, (2) gastroenteritis, (3) typhoid-like disease, (4) wound infections, and (5) the establishment of a carrier state.

*Citrobacter* are motile rods fermenting lactose. The type species is *Citrobacter freundii.* They may be confused with *Salmonella* and *Arizona* organisms. Certain strains possess the Vi antigen found in S. *typhi. Citrobacter* is differentiated from *Arizona* and *Salmonella* by its ability to grow in the presence of potassium cyanide (positive KCN test).

### "PROVIDENCE" ORGANISMS

Also known as paracolons, these organisms are free-living, lactose-negative, and biochemically related to *Proteus.* The type species is *Providencia alcalifaciens.* (In the eighth edition of *Bergey's Manual of Determinative Bacteriology,* they are classified within the genus *Proteus.*) Ordinarily nonpathogenic, they have been recovered from cases of human diarrhea and urinary tract infections.

## Proteus species (the proteus bacilli)

The proteus bacilli comprise a genus of motile organisms that resemble, and yet differ from, the other enteric bacilli in many ways (Table 20-4). They are gram-negative, do not form spores, and are normal inhabitants of feces, water, soil, and sewage. They grow rapidly on ordinary media and, being very actively motile (Fig. 20-3), tend to "swarm" over the surface of cultures on solid media. As a consequence, colonies do not remain discrete. Growth from the colony edge in time extends over all available surface area as a thin, translucent, bluish film. The bacilli can be seen microscopically to break away, migrating over the agar surface. This property poses problems to the isolation of *Proteus* from mixed cultures, although generally with care it can be done.

*Proteus* is pathogenic for rabbits and guinea pigs. The primary pathogenicity of these organisms is slight, but as secondary invaders they are vigorous. The type species is *Proteus vulgaris,* which is remarkably resistant to antimicrobial drugs. Proteus bacilli in the stool often increase in number after diarrhea caused by other organisms, especially when antibiotics have been given for the diarrhea.

*Proteus* species rank next to *E. coli* in importance as a cause of urinary tract infections and pyelonephritis. They are important in wound infections and are a rare cause of peritonitis. *Proteus morganii* is thought to cause infectious (summer) diarrhea in infants.

It is a peculiar fact that although proteus bacilli do not cause typhus fever or act as secondary invaders, the serum of a patient with typhus fever agglutinates certain strains of proteus bacilli. This is the basis of the Weil-Felix reaction for typhus fever.

## Endotoxin shock (septic shock)

Endotoxin shock (bacteremic shock, gram-negative shock, gram-negative sepsis) is a very serious complication of bacteremia with gram-negative enteric bacilli, notably *Pseudomonas aeruginosa** (85% mortality), *Proteus,* and coliforms of the genera *Klebsiella, Enterobacter,* and *Serratia.* The mortality is over 50%. The dramatic clinical picture is drawn by the precipitous development of chills, fever, nausea, vomiting, diarrhea, and prostration. There is a sharp drop in blood pressure, and the state of shock is profound.

The combination of events appears to result directly from the action of the lipopolysaccharide endotoxin released into the circulation and there activated by certain components of the plasma including complement. Endotoxin effects constriction of small blood vessels and in so doing sets off a series of events lead-

---

*See p. 258.

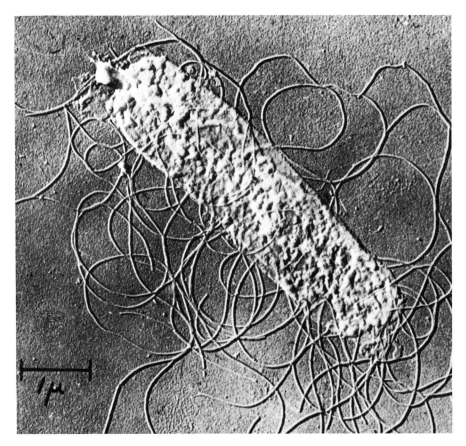

**Fig. 20-3.** *Proteus vulgaris.* Electron micrograph of the actively motile bacterium. Note flagella all over bacterial cell. (Courtesy J. B. Roerig Division, Pfizer Inc., New York.)

ing to the shock state—increased peripheral vascular resistance, pooling of blood in the capillary circulation, hypotension, and shutdown of kidney function. The presence of the inciting gram-negative bacteria in the bloodstream also plays a part in pathogenesis.

This kind of bacteremia is especially prone to complicate infections where enteric bacilli are already entrenched, such as those of the genitourinary tract, lungs, intestinal tract, and biliary tract. Instrumentation or an operative procedure on the infected area favors the release of organisms into the bloodstream. In diseases such as leukemia where host resistance is low, the organisms flood the bloodstream from no apparent focus.

### Enteric bacilli in nosocomial (hospital-associated) infections

In a study it was estimated that about 6% of all patients admitted to the hospital of today would acquire an infection there. Since around 30 million persons are admitted to hospitals annually, this means that more than a million and a half hospital patients develop an infection they did not themselves bring there. The predominating organism in hospital-associated (-acquired) infections has been *Staphylococcus aureus.* (It is still important, accounting for about one fifth.) Today most observers unanimously agree that the prime offender is the gram-negative enteric bacilli as a group (*E. coli,* other coliforms, *Proteus, Pseudomonas*). Such enteric bacilli easily account for two thirds of nosocomial infections. Other important agents are enterococci, pneumococci, and other streptococci.

Most hospital-associated (-acquired) infections with enteric bacilli seem to occur in the very young or the very old patient. They tend to complicate chronic debilitating diseases, diseases that alter the patient's resistance to infection, and diseases treated with antibiotics to which the gram-negative bacilli have or easily acquire resistance. Most infections are endogenous; that is, they are caused by organisms available from a plentiful supply within the gastrointesti-

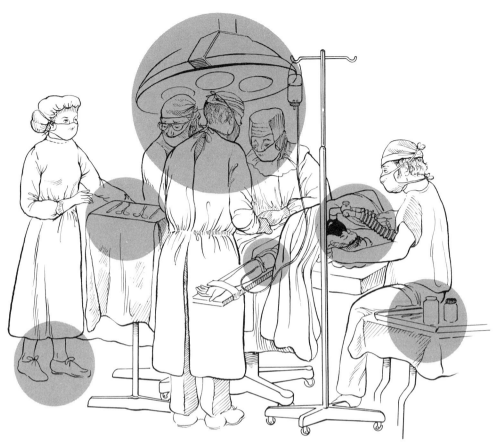

**Fig. 20-4.** Sources of infection in hospital setting. Note hazards in operating room. How many areas in this picture can you identify as potential foci of infection? What precautions would you advise?

nal, respiratory, or urinary tract of a given patient.

Around 90% of the time there is a surgical wound infection (especially where the operation was done on the alimentary tract), a urinary tract infection, or respiratory tract infection such as bronchopneumonia.

It is to be reemphasized that varied pathogens exist everywhere in the hospital environment (Fig. 20-4), in foci one would least suspect—faucets, flower vases, soaps, and lotions, for examples. The role of the more sophisticated items indigenous to a hospital is often overlooked—urethral catheters, intravenous catheters, respirators, reservoir nebulizers, and so on. Much current thought is going to measures designed to reduce the hazards.

## Questions for review

1 Classify the enteric bacilli.
2 Comment on the various ways to identify enteric bacilli.
3 Briefly characterize organisms of the genus *Salmonella*.
4 Name the three major types of salmonellosis.
5 Name and describe the organism causing typhoid fever.
6 Draw a diagram tracing the spread of typhoid infection from person to person.
7 Discuss the nursing precautions in typhoid fever and other infections of the alimentary tract.
8 What is the laboratory diagnosis of typhoid fever?
9 Name and describe the organisms causing bacillary dysentery.
10 Which of the *Shigella* causes the most severe disease and why?
11 Briefly comment on the pathogenicity of *Shigella* species.
12 Name the members of the coliform group of microorganisms.
13 Under what conditions can coliform bacilli invade the tissues of the body?
14 Discuss infantile diarrhea. Give causes.
15 What is the basis of the Weil-Felix reaction for typhus fever?
16 Compare proteus bacilli with coliforms.
17 How does enteropathogenic *E. coli* produce disease?
18 Briefly discuss nosocomial infections.
19 What is meant by gram-negative sepsis?
20 Make a list of opportunist pathogens you have studied.

**References on pp. 276 to 280.**

# CHAPTER 21

# Small gram-negative rods

The microbes of this chapter are tiny gram-negative bacilli or coccobacilli, which considered together hardly measure 1 $\mu$m. in greatest dimension. Three of the seven genera discussed are strict aerobes; the rest are facultative anaerobes. With one exception, the genera presented are those of uncertain affiliation in Part 7 Gram-Negative Aerobic Rods and Cocci and Part 8 Gram-Negative Facultatively Anaerobic Rods of the eighth edition of *Bergey's Manual*. The exception from Part 8 is *Yersinia*, Genus XI of Family I Enterobacteriaceae.

## Brucella species (the agents of brucellosis)

The genus *Brucella* includes three intracellular parasites that attack lower animals primarily, from which they are transmitted to man to cause *brucellosis*. One, known as *Brucella melitensis*, produces Malta fever in goats and sheep, with prolonged fever, arthritis, and a tendency to abort. Another, known as *Brucella abortus*, causes contagious abortion, or Bang's disease, in cattle. Contagious abortion of cattle is characterized by a tendency to abort, retention of placentas, sterility, and death of newborn offspring. The third, known as *Brucella suis*, causes contagious abortion in hogs. Male hogs are affected by brucellosis even more often than female hogs, and in the females the tendency to abort is less than in cows. Brucellosis sometimes attacks animals other than the ones just mentioned. The disease known as poll evil in horses is caused by brucellae. A newly recognized strain, *Brucella canis*, infects dogs.

*Brucella melitensis* was discovered in Malta in 1887 by Sir David Bruce (1855-1931), a surgeon in the British army, and *Brucella abortus* was discovered in Denmark by Bernhard L. F. Bang (1848-1932), in 1897. In 1918 and 1925, Alice C. Evans proved that these organisms are closely related. *Brucella suis*, discovered in infected hogs in the United States, was found to be closely related to the other two, and all three were placed in the genus *Brucella*, honoring Bruce, the discoverer of *Brucella melitensis*. *Brucella*

*melitensis* and *Brucella suis* probably represent variations of *Brucella abortus*, the result of its adaptation to the goat and hog, respectively.

**General characteristics.** Brucellae are small, nonmotile, ovoid, gram-negative, nonsporeforming coccobacilli. Some form capsules. Brucellae elaborate an endotoxin. As is true of other gram-negative organisms, their cell wall is made up of a lipoprotein-carbohydrate complex. Being so closely related to each other, they cannot be differentiated by ordinary cultural methods. Special methods using to advantage the action of dyes such as basic fuchsin and thionine on the different species of *Brucella* effect separation. The production of hydrogen sulfide is another differential point. Brucellae grow best on enriched media, but growth is slow. *Brucella melitensis* and *Brucella suis* grow in atmospheric oxygen. For the primary isolation of strains of *Brucella abortus* the presence of 5% to 10% carbon dioxide in the atmosphere is necessary. The agglutination test separates *Brucella melitensis* from *Brucella abortus* and *Brucella suis* but not *Brucella abortus* from *Brucella suis*. Table 21-1 summarizes important differential features in the genus *Brucella*.

Brucellae are destroyed within 10 minutes by a temperature of 60° C. Fortunately they are quickly destroyed by pasteurization. They can remain alive and virulent for as long as 4 months in dark, damp surroundings.

**Pathogenicity.** *Brucella melitensis* is more pathogenic for man than *Brucella suis*, and the latter is more pathogenic than *Brucella abortus*. Animals may be infected with any one of the three. Domestic animals that are pregnant are more likely to be infected than are young animals or nonpregnant adults, and abortion is probable when the infection is acquired during the pregnancy.

Brucellae can attack every organ and tissue of the human body. For this reason a person with brucellosis may seek as his initial consultant almost any medical specialist—an internist, a surgeon, or other.

Infections in man follow five patterns. The com-

**Table 21-1**

Differential patterns of *Brucella* species

| CHARACTERISTICS | ORGANISM | | |
| --- | --- | --- | --- |
| | **BRUCELLA ABORTUS** | **BRUCELLA MELITENSIS** | **BRUCELLA SUIS** |
| Culture in medium containing dyes | | | |
| 1. Thionine | Growth inhibited | No effect | No effect |
| 2. Basic fuchsin | No effect | No effect | Growth inhibited |
| Exposure to atmosphere of 10% carbon dioxide | Required for best growth | Not required | Not required |
| Production of hydrogen sulfide | For 2 to 4 days | None | For 6 to 10 days |
| Hydrolysis of urea (urease test) | None (or very slowly) | None (or very slowly) | Rapid |
| Lysis by phage | Yes | None | None at routine test dilution (RTD) Yes at 10,000 × RTD |
| Agglutination reaction | Differentiates this organism from Brucella melitensis but not from Brucella suis | Differentiates this one from other two | Differentiates this one from *Brucella melitensis* but not from *Brucella abortus* |
| Biotypes | Nine | Three | Four |
| Most common host reservoir | Cattle | Goats (also sheep) | Pigs (also hares, reindeer) |

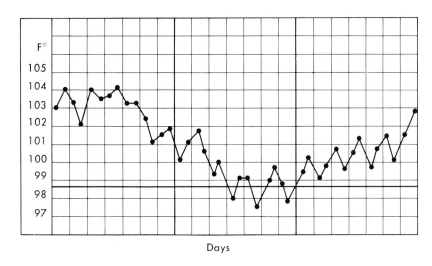

**Fig. 21-1.** Undulant fever curve.

monest form of brucellosis is a long-continued fever or cycles of fever alternating with afebrile periods (Fig. 21-1), pronounced weakness, and profuse sweating. The other four are variants. The incubation period varies from 5 to 30 days (sometimes longer). *Melitensis* infections are common in the Mediterranean basin. Imported goats brought the infection from this area to the southwestern United States. *Brucella abortus* and *Brucella suis* infections are widespread in the United States.

Various names are applied to the disease in man— Malta fever (because of its prevalence on the island of Malta), undulant fever (because of the clinical fever curve, Fig. 21-1), and brucellosis. In southwest Texas it is goat fever and Rio Grande fever.

**Sources and modes of infection.** Infection is widespread among goats, cattle, and hogs. In cattle, brucellosis ranks with tuberculosis as a source of economic loss. Infection is transmitted from animal to animal by food contaminated with the urine, feces, or lochiae of infected animals and by contact with infected placentas or fetuses. Suckling animals may become infected by the milk of infected mothers. Cows become carriers and excrete the organisms in their milk for as long as 7 years.

Human infections are common but often overlooked. In man, as in animals, infection enters via the gastrointestinal tract or through the skin. Most of the time, the infectious material is derived from the excreta of living animals or the blood or tissues of dead animals, and the organism penetrates cuts or abrasions of the skin. It is thought that these virulent pathogens can pass the unbroken skin or mucous membrane. Packinghouse workers, butchers, farmers, stockmen, and veterinarians can get the infection by handling infected cows or hogs and the meat of these animals. Man can become infected by eating dairy products from infected cows. Infection with *Brucella melitensis* is contracted by the consumption of unpasteurized milk from infected goats. Dust containing the organisms may be infectious. Transfer of the infection directly from person to person is very rare.

**Laboratory diagnosis.** Laboratory aids in the diagnosis of undulant fever are an agglutination test, blood cultures (about one-third positive), animal inoculation, feces cultures, urine cultures, cultures of bone marrow (taken by sternal puncture), and cultures of material aspirated from lymph nodes. The last two are important because, after the bacilli have spread through the body, they localize in the bone marrow, liver, spleen, and lymph nodes. Positive cultures confirm the diagnosis, but *Brucella* often cannot be cultured, even with definite disease. Therefore one must usually rely on the agglutination test, done with a carefully standardized antigen. (It also may be negative, even with definite disease.) Persons who have received cholera vaccine may develop agglutinins against *Brucella,* a point to be remembered in the investigation of suspected cases of undulant fever.

Patients recovering from one attack of brucellosis may continue to show agglutinins for months or years. If symptoms reappear and the disease seems to be coming back, the determination of the nature of that person's immunoglobulins is significant. If immunoglobulins are 7S, even in low titers, active disease is a good bet. If they are 19S in type, it is not. Also used in the laboratory diagnosis of brucellosis are a modified Coombs' test (helpful in chronic cases), a complement fixation test, and fluorescent antibody technics. Veterinarians use the milk ring test, an agglutination test using the whole milk instead of serum as the source of antibodies.

Guinea pigs may be inoculated with blood or cream from a suspect cow. The skin test to detect hypersensitivity to *Brucella* is performed by injecting bru-

cellergen, a crystalline polypeptide extract of the killed organisms, between the layers of the skin. If positive, the skin test indicates infection at some time past or present. A negative skin test eliminates that possibility. The skin test is comparable to the tuberculin skin test and as informative. However the antigen for intradermal testing is no longer commercially available.

**Immunity.** Children under 10 years of age seldom contact brucellosis. Men are more often attacked than are women (4:1), probably because of greater exposure. One attack may confer permanent immunity, although the disease is not self-limited. After an acute attack, a person may be well, but there is reason to think that the organisms remain alive but quiescent in lymph nodes and spleen.

**Prevention.** Vaccines may provide temporary protection for humans but are still experimental. An avirulent live strain of *Brucella* can be used to vaccinate cattle.

All milk (including goat's milk) and milk products should be pasteurized. All dairy cattle should be tested for brucellosis, and infected animals removed from the herd. Those who work with animals must know how the disease is spread and what precautions to take to avoid contact with the flesh or excreta of infected animals. The strict application of sanitary and hygienic measures helps to minimize the occupational hazards.

The excreta of a patient with undulant fever should be disposed of as though from a patient with typhoid fever.

## Hemophilic bacteria

The hemophilic (blood-loving) bacteria include diverse organisms sharing the following characteristics: (1) their growth depends on, or is aided by, hemoglobin, serum, ascitic fluid or certain growth-accessory substances; (2) they are small; (3) they are gram-negative and nonmotile; and (4) they are strict parasites. Two factors in blood aiding their growth are X and V. Factor X (hemin) withstands the temperature of the autoclave, but since factor V (coenzyme 1) is heat labile, it must be supplied by potatoes or yeasts in culture media. Some hemophiles depend on both factors for continued multiplication; others rely on only one; and still others require neither. One genus name for some of these organisms is *Bordetella*. Another genus in this category, *Haemophilus,* indicates by the name its members to be well known as "blood-loving" bacteria. (See Table 21-2 for comparisons.)

### BORDETELLA SPECIES (THE AGENTS OF PERTUSSIS)

**The disease.** *Whooping cough (pertussis)* is a communicable disease of 1 or 2 months' duration that chiefly affects children. It is a catarrhal inflammation of the respiratory tract with a paroxysmal cough that ends in a whoop. (The whoop may be absent in adults and very young children.) The incubation period is 5 to 21 days. A widespread and dangerous disease, it is one of the major causes of death in young children, and 90% of the deaths occur in children under 5 years of age. The danger lies in the frequency with which bronchopneumonia, malnutrition, or such chronic diseases as tuberculosis follow in its wake. In the 25% of children who have whooping cough before they are 1 year old (in 75% of cases, the child is older), bronchopneumonia is the usual cause for the deaths that occur.

**The agents.** The causative organism was first observed in the sputum of patients with whooping cough by Jules Jean Baptiste Bordet and Octave Gengou in 1900. Often spoken of as the Bordet-Gengou bacillus, it is properly known as *Bordetella pertussis* and is the agent in most cases of the disease.

In possibly 5% of the patients a disease clinically indistinguishable from whooping cough has been related to an organism other than *Bordetella pertussis,* known as *Bordetella parapertussis. Bordetella parapertussis* is similar to *Bordetella pertussis* in its growth patterns. It can be separated biochemically and by the production of a brown pigment. It can be identified serologically.

**The Bordet-Gengou bacillus.** A small gram-negative bacillus, *Bordetella pertussis (Haemophilus pertussis)* shows polar staining, often forms capsules, is nonmotile, and does not form spores. It grows strictly in the presence of oxygen. When freshly isolated from the body, all pertussis bacilli are alike, but on cultivation they resolve into four phases. Phase I represents the freshly isolated pathogen, phase IV is the completely nonpathogenic form, and phases II and III are intermediate.

Freshly isolated from the body, *Bordetella pertussis* grows only on special media containing blood. One especially suitable is glycerin-potato-blood agar, on which it grows slowly, with 2 or 3 days for visible growth. If repeatedly cultured on media in which the amount of blood is decreased stepwise, *Bordetella pertussis* is able to grow on blood-free media. With prolonged cultivation *Bordetella pertussis* loses its dependence on both the X and V factors, and when this occurs, it loses pathogenicity.

**Pathogenicity.** In the respiratory system of man the bacilli aggregate in large masses among the cells lining the wall of the trachea and bronchi. They do not invade the bloodstream. The action of *Bordetella pertussis* is, at least in part, the effect of a toxic substance it produces. This substance appears to be both endotoxin and exotoxin. One fraction is thermolabile, destroyed by a temperature of 56° C. for 30 minutes. The other is thermostable. *Bordetella pertussis* is distinctly pathogenic for lower animals, especially rabbits and guinea pigs.

**Modes of infection.** Whooping cough is one of the most highly communicable of all diseases. It is usually transmitted by droplet infection and direct contact but may be transmitted by recently contaminated objects. The disease is communicable during any stage and often during convalescence. The child is most likely to spread the infection just before the whoop appears and for about 3 weeks thereafter. The bacilli enter the body by the mouth and nose and are thrown off in the buccal and nasal secretions and in the sticky sputum that is coughed up. With the exception of those who have been closely associated with the disease or patients convalescent from the disease, carriers do not exist. Convalescent carriers become noninfectious soon after the disease subsides.

**Laboratory diagnosis.** Two culture methods for the bacteriologic diagnosis of whooping cough are the cough plate method and the nasal swab method. In the first, an open Petri dish containing glycerin-potato-blood agar is held in front of the child's mouth during a paroxysm of coughing. The organisms are sprayed on the medium in droplets from the mouth and nose. In the second, a nasal swab is passed through the nose until it touches the posterior pharyngeal wall. After the swab is withdrawn it is passed several times through a drop of penicillin solution on the surface of a plate of Bordet-Gengou medium. The

## Table 21-2
Biologic features of some hemophilic bacteria

| ORGANISM | HEMOLYSIS | CAPSULE | PRODUCTION OF INDOLE | FACTOR REQUIRED FOR GROWTH | |
|---|---|---|---|---|---|
| | | | | X | V |
| *Bordetella pertussis* | + | + | − | − | − |
| *Haemophilus influenzae* | − | + | + or − | + | + |
| *Haemophilus ducreyi* | Slight | − | − | + | − |
| *Haemophilus aegyptius* | − | − | − | + | + |
| *Haemophilus parainfluenzae* | − | + | + or − | − | + |

penicillin solution destroys many species of contaminating bacteria. Then the material is spread over the surface of the medium with a platinum loop. The cultures made by either method are incubated for about 3 days for visible growth. Identification of the bacilli may be made also in nasopharyngeal smears stained by fluorescent antibody technics.

A peculiar white blood count is found in pertussis (leukocytes 15,000 to 30,000 per cubic millimeter, of which 80% are lymphocytes), and in many cases it suggests the correct diagnosis.

**Immunity.** Man possesses no natural immunity to whooping cough. However, an attack is usually followed by permanent immunity. Second attacks, except in the aged, are usually mild. Even though immune herself, a mother does not transmit immune bodies to her offspring. Therefore the newborn child is not protected. Some degree of immunity may be conferred on the baby if the mother is immunized during the latter months of pregnancy.

**Prevention.*** Whooping cough itself cannot be prevented completely by our present public health methods, but its death rate can be reduced to a remarkable degree. Mothers should be taught how deadly a disease whooping cough is among young children and the value of immunization. The unvaccinated child should be protected from exposure. The infected child should be isolated and remain so for several weeks after the whoop has disappeared. However, the child need not be kept in bed but may be allowed to play in the sunshine and fresh air.

## HAEMOPHILUS INFLUENZAE (THE INFLUENZA BACILLUS)

In 1892, Richard F. J. Pfeiffer (1858-1945) described a bacillus, now known as Pfeiffer's bacillus or *Haemophilus influenzae* (*H. influenzae*), which he found in the sputum of patients with influenza. Until the 1918-1919 pandemic this bacillus was regarded as the sole cause of influenza. Now we know that the cause of influenza is a virus. *H. influenzae* maintains an important position as secondary invader in influenza and many other respiratory diseases as well. It may be the primary cause of a purulent meningitis in young children and of subacute bacterial endocarditis. It may be one of the primary pathogens in mixed infections of the upper respiratory tract and bronchopneumonia.

**General characteristics.** The smallest known pathogenic bacillus, *H. influenzae* grows best in the presence of oxygen but may grow without it. Nonmotile and nonsporeforming, it does not occur outside the body and is very susceptible to destructive in-

fluences. There are two forms, the encapsulated and the nonencapsulated. The encapsulated form has been divided into types a, b, c, d, e, and f. Most infections are caused by encapsulated type b organisms.

Influenza bacilli grow only on special media such as chocolate agar or hemoglobin oleate agar. Both factors V and X are required for growth, which is often more luxuriant about an organism such as *Staphylococcus aureus*. Some staphylococci and certain other bacteria produce factor V. The vigorous growth of bacteria in proximity to colonies of another organism is the *satellite phenomenon*. *H. influenzae* forms a toxic substance, which resembles an exotoxin though not a true one, and is moderately pathogenic for the lower animals, especially the rabbit.

By immunofluorescent microscopy, the influenza bacilli may be identified in cerebrospinal fluid taken from children with meningitis. Diagnostic serologic tests available include complement fixation and agglutination.

*H. influenzae* is found in the throats of about 30% of normal persons. Adult human beings show bactericidal substances for *H. influenzae* in their blood; such substances are not found in young children. Therefore infection is much more serious in children. *H. influenzae* meningitis, the most frequent form of nonepidemic meningitis, occurs in children between 2 months and 3 years of age in 85% of the cases. Of these, 90% are caused by type b bacilli, against which an anti–*Haemophilus influenzae* serum has been made in rabbits. Modern methods of treatment have considerably reduced the death rate in influenzal meningitis which used to be uniformly fatal. *H. influenzae* is also responsible for an obstructive inflammation of the larynx, trachea, and bronchi that begins suddenly with great severity. Breathing is blocked. If the obstruction is not relieved, death may occur in 24 hours.

A vaccine to *H. influenzae* type b is being field tested. The antigen is type b capsular polysaccharide.

## HAEMOPHILUS DUCREYI (DUCREY'S BACILLUS)

*Haemophilus ducreyi*, or Ducrey's bacillus, is the cause of *chancroid*, a local, highly contagious, venereal ulcer with no relation to the chancre, the initial lesion of syphilis. It begins as a pustule that ruptures, exposing an ulcer with undermined edges and a gray base. There are usually multiple ulcers that spread rapidly. Unlike chancres, they do not have indurated edges; hence chancroids are spoken of as soft chancres. The infection spreads to the inguinal lymph nodes to form abscesses known as buboes. *Haemophilus ducreyi* may be detected in smears made di-

---

*For immunization see pp. 400, 402, 409, and 411.

rectly from the edges of the lesions or cultivated from the lesions if some of the exudate is inoculated into sterile rabbit blood. But smear and culture sometimes fail to demonstrate the organisms.

The chancroid must be differentiated from the chancre of syphilis, and the buboes from those of lymphopathia venereum. It is not uncommon for a chancroid and a syphilitic chancre to occupy the same site. The chancroid appears first and heals, after which the chancre presents, or the chancre may appear before the chancroid heals. About one half of venereal ulcers are syphilitic chancre mixed with chancroid. Chancroid is usually transmitted by sexual intercourse but may be transmitted by surgical instruments or dressings.

A skin test for the diagnosis of chancroid has been devised and used extensively in European countries. It consists of the intradermal injection of a saline suspension of *Haemophilus ducreyi*. A positive result is an area of redness and induration at the site of injection. The reaction reaches its maximal intensity at the end of 48 hours.

### HAEMOPHILUS VAGINALIS

*Haemophilus vaginalis* is a small, nonmotile, non-encapsulated, facultatively anaerobic, gram-negative rod, which although placed with other species in the genus *Haemophilus* is not comparable to them in its traits. Exacting in its growth requirements, the microbe grows slowly and forms small colonies. It is a low-grade pathogen related primarily to human vaginitis, but sometimes to cervicitis, and, in males, to mild prostatitis and nongonococcal urethritis.

The diagnosis is easily made from a gram-strained smear of the associated vaginal discharge (the leukorrhea). One notes that lactobacilli of normal vaginal flora have been replaced by the small rods and that squamous cells are covered with myriads of the tiny microorganisms (the "clue cells").

### HAEMOPHILUS AEGYPTIUS

The Koch-Weeks bacillus, as *Haemophilus aegyptius* is also known, is the cause of pinkeye, a highly contagious conjunctivitis prone to epidemics. It is well named because of the intense inflammation of the conjunctival linings, which imparts a brilliant pink color to the white of the eyes. There is intense itching, but rubbing the eyes aggravates the situation. A yellow discharge forms, dries, and crusts on the eyelids. The disease is transferred by hands, towels, handkerchiefs, and other objects that contact the face and eyes. Other names for the bacillus are *Haemophilus Koch-Weeks* and *Bacillus conjunctivitidis*. Since 1950 it has been renamed *Haemophilus aegyptius*.

### HAEMOPHILUS SUIS

*Haemophilus suis* in combination with a virus causes swine influenza (p. 306).

### HAEMOPHILUS PARAINFLUENZAE

Very similar to *H. influenzae* is *Haemophilus parainfluenzae*, which may cause subacute bacterial endocarditis, but usually it is a nonpathogenic microbe in the upper respiratory tract.

## Yersinia species

The genus *Yersinia* includes *Yersinia (Pasteurella) pestis*, the cause of plague, and two causes of yersiniosis, *Yersinia enterocolitica* and *Yersinia pseudotuberculosis*.

### YERSINIA PESTIS (THE PLAGUE BACILLUS)

Plague is an infectious disease of rodents, especially rats, and is transferred from them to man. First described in Babylon, it has been a devastating pestilence for more than 3000 years. Pandemics in the past have swept over great areas of the world, with a terrifying mortality rate (50% or more). Hundreds of years ago the Chinese related the disease to rats by using the term "rat pestilence." That this disease still exists over the world at all times must be remembered in these days of extensive travel and commerce. In our own country plague has been encountered in Texas, Louisiana, and many states in the far west. The disease is endemic (enzootic) among the wild rodents of the southwestern United States, especially ground squirrels, and this focus of infection is an ever-present and increasing threat. Among wild rodents it is known as sylvatic plague (Latin *silva*, forest).

**General characteristics.** *Yersinia (Pasteurella) pestis* (discovered in 1894) is small, aerobic or facultatively anaerobic, and gram-negative and does not form spores (Table 21-3). It grows on all ordinary media. Growth on agar containing from 3% to 5% salt is a specific feature in its identification.

Plague bacilli may live in the carcasses of dead rats, in the soil, and in sputum for some time. They retain their vitality for months in the presence of moisture and in the absence of light. Phenol, 5%, or Amphyl solution, 2%, destroys them in 20 minutes.

Plague bacilli are highly pathogenic for many animals—monkeys, rats, mice, guinea pigs, and rabbits. They owe their action to toxic substances, one of which is an endotoxin similar to other bacterial endotoxins in both structure and physiologic effects.

**Clinical types.** Plague occurs in three patterns: bubonic, septicemic, and pneumonic. The first is the most frequent. In bubonic plague the organisms enter through the skin and are carried by the lymphatics to the lymph nodes draining the site of infection, com-

**Table 21-3**

Biochemical patterns of some small gram-negative bacilli

| ORGANISM | OPTIMAL TEMPERATURE FOR GROWTH | FERMENTATION OF SUGARS | | | | PRODUCTION OF INDOLE | PRODUCTION OF HYDROGEN SULFIDE | OXIDASE REACTION |
|---|---|---|---|---|---|---|---|---|
| | | GLUCOSE | MALTOSE | SUCROSE | LACTOSE | | | |
| *Yersinia pestis* | 28° C. | Acid | Acid | – | – | – | – | – |
| *Francisella tularensis** | 37° C. | Acid | Acid | – | – | – | + | – |
| *Pasteurella multocida* | 37° C. | Acid | – | Acid | – | + | + | + |

*Note again the hazard of handling cultures of this organism. In routine identification, biochemical differentiation is not necessary.

monly in the inguinal region. Here the bacilli multiply and form abscesses of the nodes (buboes). The bubo is extremely painful; a severe cellulitis surrounds it. Secondary buboes are formed in the nodes draining the primary buboes, and the bacilli finally move into the bloodstream, causing septicemia. The hemorrhages in bubonic plague that result in black splotches in the skin gave the name "black death" to the plague during the Middle Ages. (From 1347 to 1349 A.D. the black death killed 25 to 40 million persons.)

Pneumonic plague manifests as bronchopneumonia, and the bacilli are abundant in the sputum. Only a very small percentage of cases in the average epidemic take the pneumonic form (or that of a meningitis), but epidemics strictly of pneumonic plague may occur. Septicemic plague is a highly virulent form in which the patient dies before buboes can develop.

**Modes of infection.** Although many rodent species may be infected by *Yersinia (Pasteurella) pestis,* the most important source of primary infection is the rat, and as a rule, epidemics of human plague closely follow epizootics of rat plague. Plague is transmitted from rat to rat by the bite of the rat flea. Man contracts the bubonic form of plague by the bite of a flea that has previously fed on an infected rat or, rarely, on an infected person. The reason for epidemics of human plague occurring *after* epizootics of rat plague is that an epizootic destroys the rat flea's food source of first choice—the rat. The flea must then seek his food source of second choice—man. Unless infection is mechanically transferred by blood adherent to the mouthparts, the flea spreads the infection 4 to 18 days after biting an infected animal or person. Plague bacilli are found in the intestine of the flea, where they live for a long time and multiply rapidly, and the bacilli are introduced into the human body by material regurgitated from the flea while it is biting. The flea may die of the infection or become a carrier. The incubation period in man is 2 to 6 days.

Pneumonic plague may result from involvement of lungs during the course of bubonic plague (primary pneumonic plague) or from the inhalation of particles of sputum thrown off by a person with pneumonic plague (secondary pneumonic plague). Epidemic pneumonic plague is of the secondary type.

Plague may occasionally be acquired by the handling of infected rodents. The disease is transmitted from locality to locality by infected rats. Dozens of wild and domestic rodents other than rats may contract plague naturally—ground squirrels, voles, prairie dogs, chipmunks, marmots, and guinea pigs. The black house rat is more dangerous to man than other types because this one lives in dwellings, and therefore its fleas are more likely to bite a human being. The common gray sewer rat and the Egyptian rat can be infected.* Bedbugs and the human flea may transmit plague from person to person. Recently carriers (without symptoms) have been found to harbor *Yersinia (Pasteurella) pestis* in their throats.

**Laboratory diagnosis.** The important methods of laboratory diagnosis are the agglutination test on the patient's serum and the demonstration of the bacilli in the lesions by smears, cultures, and animal inoculation. There is a fluorescent antibody test to identify the organisms in sputum.

**Immunity.** An attack of plague usually brings about a state of permanent immunity.

**Prevention.†** The prevention of plague depends on the eradication of rats and rat fleas. Patients with plague should be isolated in well-screened, vermin-free rooms. (The technic of quarantine was first used

---

*Today in Southeast Asia conditions are favorable for outbreaks of plague. A large infected rat population with the right number of rat fleas exists alongside a dense, nonimmunized human population in a humid, wet (not hot) climate. During the wet season, the monsoons cancel out the effect of insecticides and force the rats into human shelters. The natives kill the rats with sticks, and the fleas move onto their new, human hosts.

†For immunization see pp. 402, 416, and 417.

with plague.) Although seldom do patients with bubonic or septicemic plague transmit the infection to others, no chance can be taken. They should be nursed with the same precautions as are patients with typhoid fever. The sputum from patients with pneumonic plague should receive special care. The sickroom should be dusted with the insecticide DDT to eliminate the vector flea. Attendants should be protected with plague vaccine. A live, attenuated plague vaccine is being tested in monkeys.

Measures designed to block the transport of rats from infected to noninfected localities by trains, aircraft, and ships are imperative. Rat-infested ships should be fumigated with a potent rodenticide. Maritime rat-control measures are in force in most parts of the world. Relatively few rats are found on ships today. Because the rats can be trapped, fumigation is rarely necessary.

### OTHER YERSINIAE

*Yersinia pseudotuberculosis* and *Yersinia enterocolitica* cause yersiniosis in man and animals, in which fever is prominent. Acute mesenteric lymphadenitis and enteritis with chronic arthritis are manifestations of infection with these two.

## Francisella tularensis (the agent of tularemia)

*Francisella (Pasteurella) tularensis* causes tularemia (rabbit fever), an acute infectious disease of wild animals, especially rodents, transferred from animal to animal by the bite of an insect. It may be transmitted from animal to man by insect bite, but human infections usually come from contamination of the hands or conjunctivae by the tissues or body fluids of an infected animal or insect.

**General characteristics.** The organism *Francisella (Pasteurella) tularensis* derives its name from Tulare County, California, where the disease was first observed. *Francisella tularensis* is a small, gram-negative, nonsporeforming, nonmotile organism varying considerably in size. Enormous numbers fill the phagocytic cells of the body. It grows on cystine agar (not on ordinary agar) and is easily demonstrated in the lesions of the disease by animal inoculation.

**Clinical types of tularemia.** Tularemia is a febrile disease accompanied by severe constitutional manifestations, pain, and prostration. The incubation period is usually 1 to 10 days. The clinical types are (1) the ulceroglandular (there is an ulcer at the site of infection with involvement of regional lymph nodes, (2)

*[handwritten marginal note: sulfur contains. Amino acid bound in skin tough pliable Elastic]*

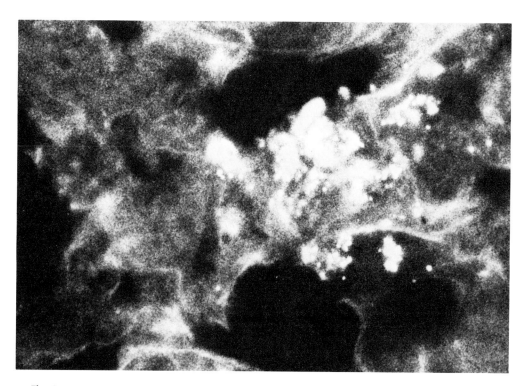

**Fig. 21-2.** *Francisella tularensis* identified by fluorescent antibody staining. Glow of bacterial immunofluorescence apparent even in black and white photomicrograph. (From White, J. D., and McGavran, M. H.: J.A.M.A. **194:**294, 1965.)

the oculoglandular (the pattern is similar to the ulceroglandular type, with the conjunctiva as primary site), (3) the glandular (the lymph nodes are involved but ulceration is absent), and (4) the typhoid (neither ulceration nor lymph node involvement is present). Death occurs in about 5% of the patients. Those who recover are incapacitated for weeks or months. (Clinically tularemia may be confused with cat-scratch disease.)

**Modes of infection.** Tularemia is most prevalent in cottontail rabbits, jack rabbits, snowshoe rabbits, and ground squirrels. Certain birds have tularemia, and the disease is not unknown in cats and sheep. The water of streams inhabited by infected animals (beavers and muskrats), once contaminated, may remain a source of infection for a long time. Epidemics caused by pollution of streams have been reported. In Russia human infections are often contracted from a species of fur-bearing water rat. More than forty-five species of wild animals are known to be infected. Tame rabbits are susceptible but ordinarily do not contract the disease, since they do not harbor the small parasites that transmit the infection among animals.

The insects that transmit tularemia in animals are wood ticks, rabbit ticks, lice, horseflies, deer flies, and squirrel fleas. Wood ticks, dog ticks, horseflies, deer flies, and squirrel fleas may sometimes transmit the infection to man. Rabbit ticks, rabbit lice, and mouse lice, important agents in transferring the disease from rodent to rodent, do not bite man.

In our country man usually contracts tularemia by handling infected rabbits, and, of these, about 70% are cottontails. Cold-storage rabbits remain infectious for 2 to 3 weeks, and if kept frozen, they may be a source of infection for 3½ years. The disease may be contracted if insufficiently cooked rabbit meat is eaten.

Inhalation of organisms can result in disease. The ocular type of tularemia usually results from a person rubbing his eye with contaminated fingers. Tularemia is not transmitted directly from man to man.

*Francisella (Pasteurella) tularensis* is the most easily communicable of all organisms, and many laboratory workers who have investigated tularemia have contracted the disease. Some have died.

**Laboratory diagnosis.** The laboratory diagnosis of tularemia depends on the agglutination test, immunofluorescence (Fig. 21-2), Foshay's antiserum test, the tularemia skin test, and the inoculation of guinea pigs or rabbits with material from the lesions. Cultures are too dangerous to be handled routinely.

**Immunity.** An attack of tularemia is followed by permanent immunity.

**Prevention.** The nature of the infection and its modes of transfer render the preventive measures obvious. Tularemia vaccine is a lyophilized, viable, attenuated strain of *Francisella tularensis*. Vaccination is indicated for those at risk.

## Pasteurella species

The genus *Pasteurella* (named for Louis Pasteur) includes a group of pasteurellae causing disease in animals but seldom attacking man.

### PASTEURELLAE OF HEMORRHAGIC SEPTICEMIA

Certain members of the genus *Pasteurella* cause hemorrhagic septicemia (pasteurellosis), a disease of cattle, horses, swine, bison, and poultry, characterized by septicemia, petechial hemorrhages of mucous membranes and internal organs, edema, and changes in the lungs. The mortality is high. The most important ones are *Pasteurella multocida* (cause of fowl cholera and shipping fever of cattle) and *Pasteurella haemolytica* (cause of pneumonia in sheep and cattle). *Pasteurella multocida* can infect man.

**Microbiology of dog and cat bites.** Over half a million persons, principally children, are bitten by animals each year in the United States. Most of the bites come from cats and dogs, with cats heading the list. Generally such wounds heal without complications,

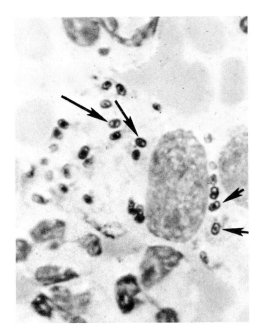

**Fig. 21-3.** Donovan bodies in cytoplasm of phagocytic cell. Note "safety pin" appearance of dark bipolar bodies. Clear surrounding areas correspond to capsules about microorganisms. (From Davis, C. M.: J.A.M.A. **211:**632, 1970.)

but they can be infected by microorganisms passed by the animal in biting.

Since it is normally found in the nose and throat of cats and dogs, *Pasteurella multocida* is an offender. Other organisms encountered, usually in mixed culture, include *Staphylococcus aureus* and alpha and beta hemolytic streptococci. The lesion produced may be a cellulitis, an abscess, or, about the extremities, a tenosynovitis. Osteomyelitis can complicate a deep-seated bite, and there is always the danger of bacteremic spread. Resolution of the tissue injury from the bite can be slow. Scarring results from the damage to tissue, and the distortion from scar about the head and neck is disfiguring.

### Calymmatobacterium granulomatis

*Calymmatobacterium granulomatis,* the only species in the genus, causes granuloma inguinale, one of the venereal diseases. This is an ulcerative infection in the skin and subcutaneous tissues of the groin and genitalia. In the lesions, encapsulated, oval, rodlike bodies with a unique "safety pin" appearance are found within the cytoplasm of large mononuclear phagocytic cells (Fig. 21-3). These are the agents also known as Donovan bodies.

The laboratory diagnosis of this disease rests on microscopic demonstration of Donovan bodies in Wright-stained smears made of material taken from the lesions.

## Questions for review

1 Name the species of *Brucella*. How are they alike and how do they differ?
2 Comment on the laboratory diagnosis of brucellosis, making mention of difficulties encountered.
3 How is whooping cough transmitted? What are the dangers of the disease?
4 Give the laboratory diagnosis of pertussis.
5 List features shared by hemophilic bacteria.
6 What is the importance of factors V and X?
7 Briefly discuss the pathogenicity of the influenza bacillus.
8 List five animals (other than man) that contract tularemia. Name five vectors associated.
9 Give clinical types of plague and tularemia.
10 What is the reservoir of plague? How is it conveyed to man?
11 What are Donovan bodies? Where found?
12 Briefly discuss microbiology of dog and cat bites.
13 Describe the condition pinkeye. What organism usually causes it?
14 What is chancroid? What causes it? How does it differ from chancre?

**References on pp. 276 to 280.**

# CHAPTER 22

# Anaerobes in disease

*free oxygen, produce spores*
*Gram + saprophytic pathogenic*

## General discussion

**Definition.** Generally speaking, anaerobes are bacteria that must have a low or zero oxygen tension for their continued growth and are sensitive to the action of oxidizing agents such as peroxide. Indeed, some are so fastidious that for their cultivation or manipulation in the laboratory, oxygen must be meticulously eliminated every step of the way. However, within such a large group of complex microorganisms one would expect varying degrees of tolerance, and this is the case.

The preceding definition suggests that anaerobes in their native habitats might in some way influence their surroundings. Studies show that most do synthesize regulatory substances like certain organic acids or particular enzymes, which act to keep the oxidation-reduction potential of the milieu at the required low level. For instance, one bacterial enzyme, superoxide dismutase, is known to neutralize the toxic by-products from various oxidative processes. It belongs to anaerobes.

The upsurge of interest in anaerobic bacteriology is another example of progress in a field following hard on the heels of advancements in technology. Now we can view anaerobes realistically, and with the greatly increased concern about them, the confusion that clouds so many of their biologic attributes is clearing.

**Pertinence.** Important to a consideration of anaerobes in disease is the knowledge of their position in health. It is amazing to realize that this poorly understood category must make a sizable contribution to man's well-being, since in great abundance they are intimately bound to him. The vast majority are indigenous to man (in space age lingo, "Life on man is—anaerobic"). They are the predominant population group of his resident microflora, and their myriads occupy his intestinal tract, oral and nasal cavities, genital tract (especially in the female), respiratory tract, and skin. In most areas anaerobes outnumber aerobes 10 to 1; in the large intestine, 1000 to 1 (*Bac-teroides* species, the anaerobe; *Escherichia coli*, the aerobe).

The more sophisticated technics of isolating, identifying, and studying anaerobes soon showed us that they had capabilities for severe disease and that under the right circumstances they expressed them. The restrained indigenous one of great potential quickly became the unleashed opportunist of inordinate vigor.

Many observers state that anaerobes cause practically any type of disease known to man, and currently, of specimens from cases of infectious disease submitted to clinical laboratories properly equipped to deal with them, anaerobes are found in 40% or more.

**Pathogenicity.** The key to the reversal of the biologic role of the normally saprophytic anaerobe is the level of tissue oxidation. As this level is crucial for normal growth, so it can, if lowered, further enhance growth. At the same time, the level of tissue oxidation is also important to the function of body defense mechanisms such as that of certain bactericidal systems. What expands microbial growth also diminishes body resistance.

The most common reason for lower tissue oxygen potential is the pathologic state of tissue anoxia regularly accompanying many pathologic processes that impair the circulation to a given area. Other factors operating are (1) the presence of dead tissue from whatever cause—trauma, injection of drugs, and others; (2) the growth of aerobic microbes; and (3) the presence of ionized calcium salts. The last-named factor favors especially infections of wounds contaminated with well-tilled topsoil (containing the anaerobes).

Most anaerobes are destructive. The type lesion can be said to be tissue necrosis. Two other features of their infection, sometimes dramatic, are the foul odor to the discharges and purulent drainages and the manifestation of gas in the soft tissues (crepitation) (Fig. 22-1).

The pattern for disease is obviously a diffuse one.

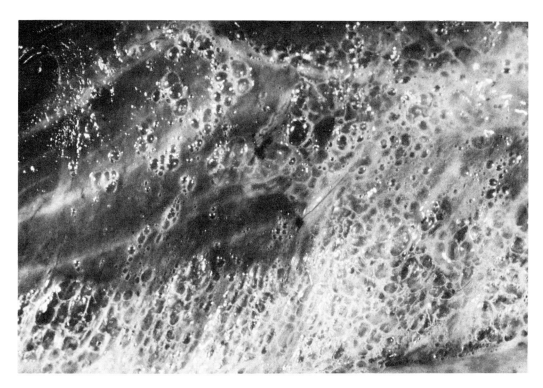

**Fig. 22-1.** Gas formation in soft tissues, as seen in certain anaerobic infections.

There is a long list of possibilities. To emphasize the more important is to list septicemia with metastatic suppuration; intra-abdominal abscesses with peritonitis; infections of female genital tract like endometritis, tubo-ovarian abscess, pelvic cellulitis, and post-surgical wound infections; pleuropulmonary disease with empyema and abscess; and skin and soft tissue infections.

**Laboratory diagnosis.** Because of the ubiquity and profusion of anaerobic species, specimens for microbiologic study are taken directly only from a site that is normally sterile. Otherwise, special collection technics are used (p. 80). Important sources for test material include wounds, abscesses, the blood, abdominal discharges, and such. Getting the test materials to the laboratory may necessitate transport in a special carbon dioxide–filled container; the specimen requires immediate attention on arrival at its destination.

For the isolation and identification of anaerobic species, three cultural methods have been standardized. (1) In the *roll-streak tube system,* PRAS (pre-reduced, *a*naerobically *s*terilized) media are prepared in anaerobic culture tubes, stored, inoculated (rolled to distribute inoculum), and manipulated under a stream of oxygen-free gas. (2) The *anaerobic glove box* or chamber houses cultures and cultural materials in an oxygen-free environment yet allows the technician access to contents of chamber through openings (ports) sealed off with gloves. (3) In the *anaerobic jar system* (Fig. 22-2), plates are kept during incubation in an atmosphere made appropriate by a specially devised elimination-replacement (of gases) scheme.

Colony growth is usually slow, several days required for visible signs. For identification of species, the organisms recovered are gram-stained for morphology and subjected to selected biochemical reactions for metabolic patterns (all under oxygen-free gas, the pH of reactions checked by pH meter). Gas-liquid chromatography may be performed to measure acid and alcoholic products. Antibiotic susceptibility testing is done by a pour plate method.

**The approach.** A broad division of the total array of anaerobic microbes into two major categories on the basis of endospore formation is a convenient approach to the discussion of particular ones. The first such category would contain the sporeformers of a single genus, *Clostridium,* a fairly homogeneous group with several unifying features, a well-known and long-studied group, and one wherein the saprophytes exist in the external environment (although some are part of the intestinal flora of man and animals). A fund of knowledge has accumulated on these,

225

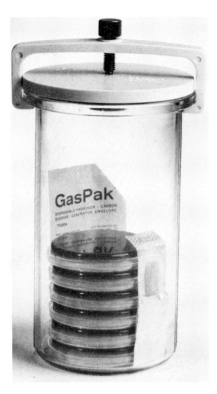

**Fig. 22-2.** GasPak 100 anaerobic jar system (self-contained, evacuation-replacement system). Anaerobic conditions are induced when water is added to GasPak envelope to form hydrogen, which reacts with atmospheric oxygen on palladium catalyst to form water. Carbon dioxide is also generated to produce growth of fastidious anaerobes. (Courtesy BioQuest, Division of Becton, Dickinson & Co., Cockeysville, Md.)

their patterns for clinical disease are classic for the most part, and in some instances a great deal has been accomplished in the related areas of preventive medicine.

The second category, nonsporulating microbes, is not a straightforward one. It gathers essentially all the rest, a more heterogeneous complex with few, if any, unifying features among the species other than their anaerobic specifications. There is no backlog of knowledge on these microorganisms; in fact, up to recent past, information has been sketchy. Today technology makes the difference. (Technology, although designed for the basic characteristic of both categories, has had a much greater impact for the nonsporeformers than the sporeformers.) These of the second category are the microorganisms from within, predominant in the internal environment of man. They operate from a more strategic position in the body than sporeformers. Their patterns for clinical

disease are diffuse and diverse, ranging from minor superficial infections to septicemic dissemination.

Infections associated with anaerobes of whatever category are generally quite serious and carry a high mortality. Some of the more important genera and species now pass muster.

## Clostridium species

Certain sporulating anaerobes of genus *Clostridium* (Family Bacillaceae), known for a long time, are the large bacilli peculiarly distorted by their heat-resistant spores and producing potent exotoxins and enzymes.

### CLOSTRIDIUM TETANI (THE BACILLUS OF TETANUS)

**The disease.** Tetanus, or lockjaw, is a disease worldwide in distribution, with manifestations in the central nervous system produced by the potent exotoxin of *Clostridium tetani (Cl. tetani)*. There are classic muscular spasms in tetanus involving the face, neck, and other parts of the body that are provoked by the slightest sort of stimulation (noise, movement, touch). These are very painful. Severe ones may compromise respiration. The name *lockjaw* comes from the muscular contractions that rigidly close or lock the jaws together. The corners of the mouth are turned up and the eyebrows peaked, so that a characteristic facial expression is produced, referred to as *risus sardonicus* (sardonic grin).*

The tetanus bacilli do not invade but remain at the site of infection, where they elaborate their powerful poison. The disease comes from infection of a wound and is not transmitted from person to person.

**General characteristics.** The tetanus bacillus is an anaerobic sporeformer. Biologically a saprophyte, it probably never infects a wound that does not contain some dead tissue. *Cl. tetani* stains with ordinary stains and is gram-positive. The vegetative forms are slightly motile; the sporulating forms are nonmotile.

---

*"They [the spasms] are characterized by a violent rigidity, usually sudden in onset but sometimes working up to a crescendo, with every single voluntary muscle in the body thrown into intense, painful tonic contraction. The eyes start, the jaw clenches, the tongue is bitten, the neck is retracted, the back arched, and opisthotonus is extreme. Often there is a muffled inspiratory cry, as the diaphragm contracts and draws air through the apposed vocal cords. Finally laryngeal spasm becomes complete, the chest fixed, and respiration ceases from muscle spasm. At the same time there is a gross outpouring of secretion, with profuse perspiration and foaming at the mouth." (From Ablett, J. J. L.: Tetanus and the anaesthetist; review of symptomatology and recent advances in treatment, Br. J. Anaesth. **28:**288, 1956.)

The spore is situated in one end, giving the bacillus an appearance of a round-headed pin or a drumstick. Growth is fairly luxuriant on all ordinary media if anaerobic conditions are maintained (Table 22-1). The optimum temperature for growth is 37° C. In both cultures and infected wounds, the presence of certain aerobic bacteria accelerates the growth of tetanus bacilli. Young cultures contain numerous vegetative bacilli. Old cultures are composed chiefly of sporulating organisms. The bacilli are seldom demonstrated in cultures from infected wounds because so few bacilli are present.

The vegetative bacilli are no more resistant to destructive influences than are other vegetative bacilli. The spores, however, are very resistant. They withstand boiling for several minutes, pass through the intestinal canal unaffected, and when protected from the sunlight, remain infective for years.

**Distribution.** Tetanus bacilli are common residents of the superficial layers of the soil. Since they are normal inhabitants of the intestine of horses, cattle, and other herbivores, they are always found where manure is freely used as fertilizer, and barnyard soils are heavily contaminated. They are found in the intestinal canal of about 25% of human beings. Tetanus spores may be spread over a wide area by flies and high winds.

**Extracellular toxin.** If it were not for their toxin, infection with tetanus bacilli would be without effect. Tetanus toxin is one of the most powerful poisons known, second only to that of botulism in potency. This explains why a comparatively few bacilli at the site of infection can induce such profound changes. The toxin of tetanus is a simple protein of a single antigenic type with a molecular weight of 67,000. It is a neurotoxin, that is, one with a specific affinity for the tissues of the central nervous system. From the site of infection the toxin travels to the central nervous system along the axis cylinders of the motor nerves, where it is specifically and avidly bound to the gray matter. Its action is central but also on the peripheral nerve endings.

Besides the important neurotoxin, the tetanus bacilli elaborate small amounts of a toxic substance that destroys red blood cells and injures the heart. Taken orally, tetanus toxin is harmless.

**Pathogenicity.** Tetanus in man is a lethal disease. Horses, cattle, sheep, and hogs may become infected.

Tetanus occurs in two clinical forms: one associated with a short incubation period (from 3 to 21 days), an abrupt onset, severe manifestations, and a high mortality; the other characterized by a longer incubation period (from 4 to 5 weeks), less severe manifestations, and a lower mortality. Rapidly fatal tetanus is more likely to follow wounds about the head and face, that is, near the brain.

**Pathology.** The action of the toxin of *Cl. tetani* is directly on the central nervous system. The characteristic muscle spasm, from which the disease got its name, and the convulsive seizures originate in the central nervous system, and the impulses are transferred to the muscles by the motor nerves.

In this kind of disease process, the pathologic changes are functional, not structural. There is no typical lesion. Even after death, no organic lesions are seen. The cerebrospinal fluid is normal.

**Sources and modes of infection.** Tetanus is practically always caused by spores introduced into a wound. Whether a given wound is complicated by tetanus depends on the type of wound, the chance of contamination with tetanus spores, the presence of dead tissue, and secondary infection. Deep puncture wounds are dangerous because they provide anaerobic conditions for the growth of the bacilli. In lacerations, gunshot wounds, compound fractures, wounds containing foreign bodies, and infected wounds, the presence of dead tissue and certain other bacteria favors the growth of tetanus bacilli. If such wounds are contaminated by soil, especially heavily manured soil, the chances of tetanus infection are greatly increased. It is not surprising that war wounds are often followed by tetanus. Rusty nail wounds may be so complicated, not because the nail is rusty but because rusty nails are usually dirty nails and tetanus spores are likely to be in the dirt.

In narcotic addicts injection-related tetanus is a public health problem. The rapidly progressive and highly fatal disease in the drug addict is another, even more terrifying expression of tetanus. It is seen in the large metropolitan centers of the United States, especially in black women. The narcotic, usually heroin, has been given by the subcutaneous route of injection. Quinine, the adulterant, favors the growth of the bacilli by promoting anaerobic conditions in the tissues, enhancing the disease.

Puerperal tetanus exists in tropical countries. Infection from bacilli inhabiting the intestinal canal may rarely follow intestinal operations. Tetanus of the newborn, *tetanus neonatorum*, is caused by infection through the navel and is still seen in the Americas in certain black and Spanish-speaking groups where neonatal medical care remains primitive. At the extremes of life the mortality rates are high. Elderly persons may be exposed to tetanus-prone injuries in their gardening activities.

Although tetanus is more likely to occur under the conditions just enumerated, it may follow trivial wounds inflicted by apparently clean objects.

## Table 22-1
Bacteriologic patterns of clostridia

| ORGANISM | GROWTH IN LITMUS MILK | GROWTH IN COOKED MEAT | GELATIN LIQUEFACTION | SYNTHESIS OF LECITHINASE |
|---|---|---|---|---|
| *Clostridium tetani* | Soft clot | Gas, slow blackening | + (Blackening) | No |
| *Clostridium perfringens* | Stormy fermentation | Gas | + (Blackening) | Yes |
| *Clostridium novyi* | Acid, no clot | Gas | + | Yes |
| *Clostridium septicum* | Slow clot, gas | Gas | + (Gas) | Yes |
| *Clostridium botulinum* | Acid | Gas, blackening, digestion | + | Yes |

**Prevention of tetanus.*** Any wound suggesting the least danger from tetanus should be treated surgically. Puncture wounds should be widely opened and thoroughly cleaned for two reasons: tetanus bacilli and other organisms are removed, and oxygen antagonistic to the growth of tetanus bacilli is allowed access. Mangled wounds should be thoroughly cleaned, and all dead tissue removed. Proper wound care cannot be overstressed, since tetanus organisms do not multiply in a surgically clean, aerobic wound with a good blood supply. Antibiotics help to control associated pyogenic infections that damage tissues. *Cl. tetani* is sensitive to penicillin, but no amount of antibiotic has any effect at all on toxin released into the body from the wound site.

Active immunization for every member of the community cannot be too strongly recommended. In special need of protection are those workers in industry or agriculture whose occupation predisposes them to wounds easily contaminated with tetanus bacilli, all allergy-prone individuals, and even all recipients of a driver's license. All athletes must be fully immunized. (Football players suffer more abrasions and minor injuries from sliding and falling on artificial turf than on sod fields, although artificial turf is a less likely source of tetanus spores.)

Active immunization is practiced on a large scale in the armed forces of both the United States and England. That this has been effective is proved by the fact that only 12 cases of tetanus appeared among 2,785,819 hospital admissions of military personnel for war wounds and other injuries during World War II. Of the 12 tetanus patients, 6 had not been adequately immunized and 2 failed to get the booster dose of toxoid at time of injury.

*See also pp. 397, 398, 402, 403, 409, and 416.

## CLOSTRIDIUM PERFRINGENS, NOVYI, AND SEPTICUM (THE CLOSTRIDIA OF GAS GANGRENE)

**The organisms.** Gas gangrene (clostridial myonecrosis) is a highly fatal disease caused by the contamination of wounds with one alone or any combination of certain anaerobic, toxin-producing, sporeforming, gram-positive bacteria (Table 22-1). (Less than half the time there is only one organism.) All exist as saprophytes in the soil and as normal inhabitants of the intestinal canal of man and animals. Infection happens when soil contaminated by feces gets into a wound. Most important are *Clostridium perfringens* (formerly *Clostridium welchii*, Welch's bacillus), *Clostridium novyi* (formerly *Clostridium oedematiens*), and *Clostridium septicum* (formerly *Vibrion septique*). *Clostridium sporogenes*, considered a nonpathogenic organism, is often present also.

The single most significant of the gas gangrene clostridia is *Clostridium perfringens* (*Cl. perfringens*), related to 75% of all cases of gas gangrene and responsible for practically all instances in civilian life. In one third of cases it is the sole pathogen.

Aerobic pus-producing microbes and certain proteolytic organisms without effect on clean wounds often produce considerable destruction of tissue in wounds infected with gas bacilli. Aerobes in the wound facilitate the germination of clostridial spores and their vegetative growth by reducing the oxidation-reduction potential. In most cases of gas gangrene two or more clostridial anaerobes are associated with one predisposing aerobe.

**The disease.** The organisms responsible for gas gangrene grow in the tissues of the wound, especially in muscle, releasing exotoxins and fermenting the muscle sugars with such vigor that the pressure of accumulated gas tears the tissues apart. The air-filled

| NITRATE REDUCTION | FERMENTATION | | | HEMOLYTIC | SPORES | MOTILITY |
|---|---|---|---|---|---|---|
| | GLUCOSE | LACTOSE | SUCROSE | | | |
| − | − | − | − | + | Round, terminal | + |
| + | + | + | + | + | Rare | − |
| − | + | − | − | + | Ovoid, eccentric | + |
| + | + | + | − | + | Ovoid, eccentric | + |
| − | + | − | − | ± | Ovoid, eccentric | + |

(emphysematous) blebs of the wound give the name *gas gangrene* (Figs. 22-3 and 22-4). The exotoxins cause swelling and death of tissues locally, breakdown of red blood cells in the bloodstream, and damage to various organs over the body. The bacteria enter the blood just before death. Clinically there is profound toxemia. (The incubation period is 1 to 5 days.)

*Cl. perfringens* elaborates several hemolysins and an extracellular proteolytic enzyme, collagenase, that facilitates the spread of gas gangrene organisms through tissue spaces, since it is active against the fibrous protein supports of the body tissues. *Clostridium perfringens, novyi,* and *septicum* elaborate lecithinase; species *histolyticum* and *sporogenes* do not. The potent lecithinase (the alpha-toxin) of *Cl. perfringens* is both hemolytic and necrotizing in its effects on tissues.

Lacerated wounds, compound fractures, wounds with extensive death of tissue, and war wounds are likely sites of gas gangrene. Injuries acquired in the vicinity of railroad tracks tend to be so complicated. Clostridial infection rarely complicates gangrenous appendicitis, strangulated hernia, and intestinal obstruction in the abdominal cavity.

Skin samples taken from the thighs, groins, and buttocks of hospitalized patients sometimes yield a heavy growth of *Cl. perfringens*. To eliminate this kind of contamination, compresses of povidone-iodine or 70% alcohol may be applied. The presence of the organisms of gas gangrene in a wound does not invariably mean gas gangrene.

**Clostridial infection and malignancy.** *Clostridium septicum* is important in wartime gangrene but rarely complicates infection in otherwise healthy civilians. If the person's defenses are weakened, the situation may be reversed. This organism is acquiring some

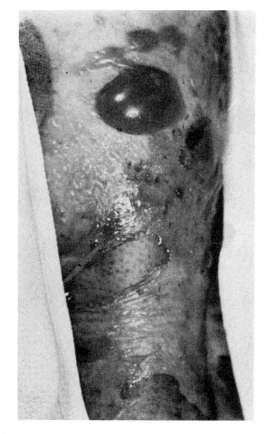

**Fig. 22-3.** Gas gangrene in 16-year-old boy, complicating compound fractures of leg sustained in motorcycle accident. Organism is *Clostridium perfringens*. Note blisters and discoloration. (From Altemeier, W. A., and Fullen, W. D.: J.A.M.A. **217:**806, 1972.)

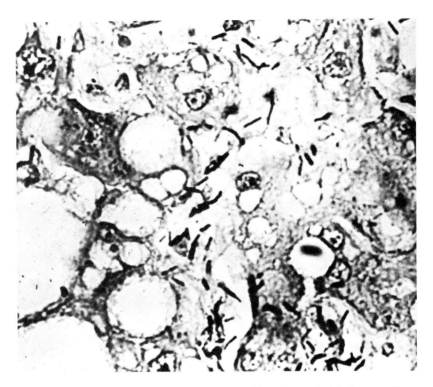

**Fig. 22-4.** Gas gangrene in Gram-stained tissue section of liver. Large air-filled spaces disrupt structure. Large gram-positive rods are present. Patient had leukemia. (Courtesy Dr. R. C. Reynolds, Dallas.)

notoriety currently by complicating cases of leukemia and intestinal cancer with clostridial septicemia.

**Prevention.*** Prevention of gas gangrene depends on the proper surgical care of wounds. With established disease there must be free incision to open the wound as widely as possible, all devitalized tissue must be excised, foreign bodies must be removed, and adequate drainage of the wound instituted.

Gas gangrene antitoxin has been prepared against the organisms important in causing gas gangrene, but its efficacy today is challenged. Toxoids for *Clostridium perfringens* and *Clostridium novyi* are experimental.

## CLOSTRIDIUM BOTULINUM (THE BACILLUS OF BOTULISM)

**Nature of botulism.** Botulism is a specific intoxication caused by the ingestion of foods in which *Clostridium botulinum* (*Cl. botulinum*) has grown and excreted its toxin. The toxin, not the bacillus, is responsible for the disease. Like tetanus, it is a poisoning instead of an infection. The foods most often linked to botulism are sausage (the disease derives

*See also p. 397.

its name from the Latin word *botulus*, sausage), pork, and canned vegetables such as beans, peas, and asparagus. Cases have been traced to ripe olives and tuna. Most of the foods incriminated have shared one feature: they were processed (improperly!) in the home by canning or pickling weeks or months before.

In the last decade there have been 78 outbreaks of botulism in the United States, plus nearly 200 individual cases. The most serious ones of our times, those in 1963, resulted from the consumption of commercially processed foods. From eating such foods as liver paste, tuna fish, salmon eggs, and smoked white-fish products, 46 persons were poisoned and 14 died of a disease ordinarily quite rare.

The disease develops as follows. Since the organism is widely distributed in nature, food is easily contaminated. If it is not canned or otherwise preserved properly, the spores are not destroyed. In the interval between preservation and use, the spores revert to the growing stage, and the bacilli multiply and excrete their toxin into the food. (Toxin remains potent in canned foods for 6 months or more.) If the contaminated food is not heated sufficiently for consumption, toxin has not been inactivated. When such food is ingested, the toxin is absorbed through the intestinal wall to exert its effects. Toxic signs usually appear within 24 to 48 hours and consist of generalized weakness, disturbance of vision (often double vision), thickness of speech, nausea and vomiting, and difficulty in swallowing. There is no fever. Death from asphyxia usually occurs between the third and seventh day. The mortality ranges from 50% to 100%.

Natural food poisoning of this type occurs among certain wild animals (if toxin is swallowed with their food). Examples are limberneck of chickens, fodder disease of horses, and duck sickness.

**The organism.** The microbe *Cl. botulinum* is also an anaerobic, gram-positive, sporeforming bacillus (Table 22-1). A common inhabitant of the soil, the usual source from which foods are contaminated, *Cl. botulinum* is primarily a saprophyte. (Infections of laboratory animals have been caused experimentally.) Generally, the organism is unable to grow inside the body of a warm-blooded animal. *Cl. botulinum* and its toxin are destroyed in 10 minutes at the temperature of boiling water, but the "hard shell" spores must be held at a temperature of 120° C. (249° F.) for 15 minutes to be killed. Spores can withstand more than 2000 times the radiation lethal to a human being.

The toxin of *Cl. botulinum* is the most deadly of poisons, the mere tasting of food having been known to cause death. One ounce could exterminate all the people in the United States, and a mere half pound of botulinal toxin could wipe out the population of the world. (Botulinal toxin has been classified as an agent for chemical warfare.) It is 10,000 to 100,000 times more potent than diphtheria toxin or animal venoms. It differs from diphtheria and tetanus toxins in that it causes disease when swallowed and is more resistant to heat. A fast-acting neurotoxin, it affects the central nervous system, paralyzing the muscles of vision, swallowing, and respiration. It dilates blood vessels, and hemorrhages occur in different parts of the body. The toxin's effect is a specific one at the neuromuscular junction. Mental faculties are not impaired, and there are no sensory disturbances.

There are six *toxigenic* types of *Cl. botulinum*: A, B, C, D, E, and F. All these toxins resist the intestinal juices, and the action of type E toxin can be increased 50 times by trypsin. In man, botulism almost always results from ingestion of toxin from types A, B, E, and F. C and D toxins cause disease in animals. Most A and B toxins are found in home-preserved vegetables and fruit (food of plant origin). Recent outbreaks of botulism have pointed to the presence of *Cl. botulinum*, type E, in water and marine wildlife. Therefore type E toxin is found in fish and marine products. Type E spores can germinate at refrigerator temperatures and form toxin. Type F toxin has been reported in home-processed venison jerky.

There is good evidence that toxigenicity of clostridial species and even the type of toxin depend on the presence of specific bacteriophages or bacterial viruses (lysogeny). For instance, if *Cl. botulinum*, type C, is "cured" of its phage, it loses its toxin. A startling fact is that experimentally the right phage can then convert it to a different clostridial species, also toxigenic, and producing that specific toxin.

**Laboratory diagnosis.** The laboratory diagnosis of botulism is made by (1) finding the toxin in the patient's serum (toxemia may persist for prolonged periods), (2) isolating the microbes, and (3) identifying the toxin in the food ingested. The mouse is a suitable test animal for inoculation. Being highly susceptible to the effects of the toxin, the mouse succumbs to even the small amounts of circulating toxin in the blood sample received from the patient. Identification of the toxin as to type in suspected foods may be made by mouse tests. For type A toxin there is also a radioimmunoassay.

**Prevention.*** Prevention of botulism depends primarily on (1) heating foods to a temperature of 120° C. for at least 15 minutes in the canning process (or steam-cooking under adequate pressure, especially for low-acid foods)† to destroy any spores present, (2) boiling canned foods for 15 minutes immediately before they are eaten, to destroy heat-labile toxins, and (3) proper refrigeration of foods after cooking. In the canning of high-acid foods such as tomatoes and fruits, botulinal spores can be killed by a temperature of 120° C. for 15 minutes. For the processing of low-acid foods (beets, beans, corn, and meats) steam pressure methods are imperative. Note the hazard for botulism at high altitudes—the boiling temperature is too low to destroy spores.

Do not so much as taste canned food until it has been fully heated. Remember: the poison is odorless and tasteless!

If fowls that have been eating discarded food develop limberneck and if the responsible food can be traced, persons known to have eaten the same food should receive botulinal antitoxin. If a case develops in a group of people who have eaten the same food, the members of the group should be given the antitoxin.

Round the clock help—available antisera, consultation, laboratory assistance to establish the diagnosis—can be obtained from the U. S. Public Health Service Center for Disease Control in Atlanta, Ga. (telephone: 404-633-3311).

---

*See p. 396 for passive immunization.
†If food were boiled, at least 3 hours would be required.

## Bacteroides species

The Family Bacteroidaceae contains the obligate anaerobes, the natural inhabitants of the natural cavities of man, animals, and insects. The serious anaerobic infections in the hospital today come from the gram-negative members of this family.

Bacteria of the genus *Bacteroides* are mostly non-motile, nonsporeforming, usually gram-negative, very pleomorphic rods. They reside in the colon, oral cavity, genital tract, and upper respiratory tract in man. *Bacteroides* species make up 95% of the bacterial content of the stool and 20% by weight.

Outside their native haunts, they are astounding pathogens, feared for the hemolytic and necrotizing lesions of bacteroidosis. The expected portal of entry is the gastrointestinal tract, the female genital tract, or areas of decubitous ulceration and of gangrene. They are found in mucosal ulcers and may form foul-smelling abscesses in the lung and other organs, often together with other microbes. They are prone to complicate abdominal surgery, alcoholic liver disease, diabetes mellitus, and malignancy.

Most human infections come from *Bacteroides fragilis*, the type species, and *Bacteroides melaninogenicus*. *Bacteroides melaninogenicus* elaborates a melanin-like pigment that makes its colonies brown or black.

## Fusobacterium species

Members of the genus *Fusobacterium* (also in Family Bacteroidaceae) are characteristically long, slender, spear-shaped bacilli with tapered ends and are sometimes incriminated in suppurative and gangrenous lesions. The species of note include *Fusobacterium nucleatum,* the type species, and *Fusobacterium necrophorum (Sphaerophorus necrophorus)* (name means "necrosis producing"). *Fusobacterium fusiforme* has been reclassified to fit into the third genus *Leptotrichia* of the Family Bacteroidaceae as *Leptotrichia buccalis.*

## Other anaerobes

The significance of a host of anaerobes is increasing in relation to disease. Mention is made of only a few being incriminated with greater regularity.

Gram-positive cocci of the genera *Peptococcus* and *Peptostreptococcus* are important in anaerobic infection of the female genitalia. Small gram-negative capnophilic cocci of the genus *Veillonella,* found ordinarily in the mouth, possess endotoxins. Species of gram-positive, nonsporeforming bacilli, notable for their output of organic acids, include *Propionibacterium acnes* and *Eubacterium limosum. Propionibacterium acnes,* based on the skin, is a troublesome contaminant of blood cultures. *Eubacterium limosum* resides in the intestinal tract and is known to synthesize vitamin $B_{12}$.

## Questions for review

1 Define anaerobes.
2 Discuss anaerobes as organisms indigenous to man.
3 How do anaerobes produce disease? Give four factors relating to their pathogenicity.
4 List diseases produced by anaerobes.
5 Outline briefly the laboratory diagnosis of anaerobic infections.
6 What has been the effect of technological developments in anaerobic microbiology?
7 Name and describe the causative agents for tetanus, gas gangrene, and botulism.
8 What is the derivation of the word botulism?
9 What is the effect of tetanus toxin? Of diphtheria toxin? Of botulinal toxin? Compare the three as to potency.
10 List types of wounds likely contaminated with *Clostridium tetani.*
11 What types of wounds are most likely infected with clostridia of gas gangrene.
12 What measures other than immunization help to prevent tetanus and gas gangrene?
13 Briefly describe the disease tetanus.
14 What are the circumstances producing botulism? What are the main preventive measures?
15 Why is botulism a risk at high altitudes?
16 Briefly characterize *Bacteroides* species. What is their importance today in hospital infections?

**References on pp. 276 to 280.**

# CHAPTER 23

# Spirochetes and spirals

Spirochetes are actively motile, flexible, spiral bacteria found in contaminated water, sewage, soil, decaying organic matter, and within the bodies of animals and man (Fig. 23-1). They may be free-living, commensal, or parasitic. Spiral microorganisms vary in length from only a few to 500 $\mu$m. and move by rapidly rotating about their long axis, by bending, or by "snaking" along a corkscrew path. They are aerobic, facultatively anaerobic, or anaerobic, with no flagella and no endospores. Many of them are best visualized by phase-contrast and dark-field microscopy.

Within Bergey's Order I, Spirochaetales, Family I, Spirochaetaceae, contains slender spiral bacteria in five genera. They include nonpathogenic spirochetes often found on the mucous membranes of the mouth, about the teeth, and on the genitals, and three significant pathogens. The pathogenic spirochetes are found in Genus III, *Treponema,* containing the organisms responsible for syphilis and yaws; Genus IV, *Borrelia,* with the organisms responsible for relapsing fever; and Genus V, *Leptospira,* with the organism responsible for infectious jaundice (Weil's disease) and other forms of leptospirosis.

Other spiral-shaped bacteria with slightly different properties fall into another division (Part 6) of Bergey's classification. In Family I, Spirillaceae, are the spirilla —spirally twisted rods. These are rigid, possess one flagellum or a tuft of flagella, and are actively motile, swimming in straight lines in corkscrew fashion. They may be saprophytes or pathogens. Genus I, *Spirillum,* contains the organisms of one form of rat-bite fever.

## Treponema pallidum (the spirochete of syphilis)

Syphilis *(lues venerea)* is an infectious disease caused by *Treponema pallidum (T. pallidum).* Clinically it may be either *acquired* or *congenital,* that is, incurred after or before birth; the former is more usual. The historic origin of syphilis is a debated question. Many observers believe that Columbus's sailors introduced it into Europe on their return from the New World. About that time the disease did spread over certain parts of Europe in virulent epidemic form.

*T. pallidum* (the pale spirochete) (Fig. 23-2) is an actively motile, slender, corkscrewlike organism that, when properly searched for, can be found in practically every syphilitic lesion. It is especially abundant in chancres and mucous patches (lesions of the skin and mucous membranes found early in the disease). It has six to fourteen spirals and rotates on its long axis. Usually rigid, it may bend on itself. In addition to its rotary motion, it has a slowly progressive motion.

*T. pallidum* is very difficult to stain with ordinarily used bacteriologic dyes and is best demonstrated by dark-field microscopy in syphilitic chancres and mucous patches. Since the organisms are examined in

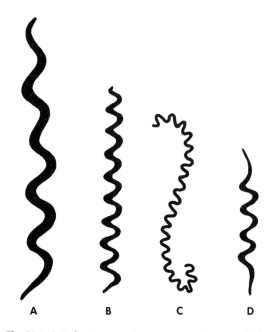

**Fig. 23-1.** Spiral microorganisms, comparative morphology. **A,** *Borrelia.* **B,** *Treponema.* **C,** *Leptospira.* **D,** *Spirillum.*

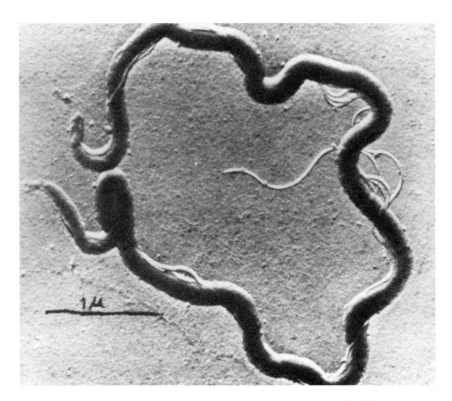

**Fig. 23-2.** *Treponema pallidum,* electron micrograph. (Courtesy Technical Information Services, State and Community Services Division, Center for Disease Control, Health Services and Mental Health Administration, Department of Health, Education, and Welfare, Atlanta.)

the living state by this method, the diagnostic features of motility and shape are seen.

*T. pallidum* can live outside the body under suitable conditions for 10 to 12 hours but is killed within 1 hour by drying. It does not occur outside the body except very briefly on objects contaminated with syphilitic secretions. In whole blood or plasma at refrigerator temperature it remains viable for 24 hours but dies within 48 hours.

Under natural conditions *T. pallidum* infects man only, but anthropoid apes, monkeys, rabbits, and guinea pigs may be infected artificially. The disease in rabbits and monkeys resembles the human disease in many but not all respects.

### ACQUIRED SYPHILIS

**Mode of infection.** Syphilis is caused by a microorganism that is not borne by food, air, water, or insect. Man is its only reservoir. To contract the disease, a human being must be in close and intimate contact with an infectious person. Acquired syphilis therefore is contracted in the great majority of instances by sexual intercourse. In a few cases it is contracted by other types of direct contact of skin or mucous membranes, such as kissing, if the patient has lesions in

his mouth. It is but rarely spread by contaminated objects such as drinking cups or towels. Physicians, dentists, and nurses may become infected in the examination of a syphilitic patient.

With modern blood banks and blood banking methods the danger of transferring syphilis by blood transfusion is minimal. Blood that comes into a modern blood bank is routinely tested by a standard serologic test for syphilis. If the result is positive, that blood is not released for transfusion.

**Evolution of a typical case.** The course of syphilis is outlined in Table 23-1.

*Incubation stage. T. pallidum* is a highly invasive organism. When introduced into the human body, it begins to multiply. Many of the treponemes migrate via the lymphatics to the regional lymph nodes. From the thoracic duct they enter the bloodstream and rather quickly spread over the entire body. Some continue to multiply at the original site. From 2 to 6 weeks later an inflammatory reaction at the site of inoculation develops, and the primary lesion, the *chancre,* forms.

*Primary stage.* The chancre is the first clinical sign of infection. It usually appears on the genitals, where in the male it is readily detected. In the female,

**Table 23-1**
Evolution of a typical case of syphilis

| STAGE | DURATION | CLINICAL DISEASE | ACTIVITY OF *TREPONEMA PALLIDUM* | DIAGNOSIS | TISSUE CHANGE |
|---|---|---|---|---|---|
| Incuba-tion | 2 to 6 weeks (most often 3 to 4 weeks) | None | Spirochetes actively pro-liferate at entry site, spread over body | Identification of *Treponema pallidum:*<br>a. Dark-field microscopy<br>b. Fluorescent antibody technic | Chancre appears at inoculation site |
| Primary | 8 to 12 weeks | 1. Chancre present at inoculation site<br>2. Regional lymph-adenopathy | Chancre teeming with them | 1. Dark-field microscopy of chancre<br>2. STS* become positive | Chancre present |
| Primary latent | 4 to 8 weeks | None | Inconspicuous | STS positive | None demonstra-ble; chancre has healed with little scarring |
| Secondary | Variable over period of 5 years (latent periods with recur-rences) | 1. Skin and mucosal lesions ("mucous patches")<br>2. Generalized lymphadenopathy | Skin and muco-sal lesions rich in spirochetes (highly in-fectious) | 1. Dark-field microscopy of lesions<br>2. STS positive | 1. Infection active:<br>a. Vascular changes<br>b. Cuffs of in-flammatory round cells about small blood vessels<br>2. Resolution spontaneous—little scarring |
| Latent | Few months to a lifetime (average 6 to 7 years) | None | Inconspicuous | STS positive (can be nega-tive) | |
| Tertiary | Variable—rest of patient's life | Related to organ system diseased and the incapacity thereof | Paucity of spiro-chetes in clas-sic lesions | 1. STS positive or negative<br>2. Special silver stains of tissue lesions may show spiro-chetes | 1. Gumma<br>2. Definite pre-dilection to heal in lesions<br>3. Scarring<br>4. Tissue dis-tortion and abnormal function |

*Serologic tests for syphilis.

the chancre, if on the cervix, is so located as to escape detection. Some 10% or more of chancres are extragenital, being found on the face, lips, tongue, tonsils, breasts, or fingers.

The *chancre* presents beneath the mucous membrane or skin as a small nodule having the feel of a shot. It breaks down, forming a shallow ulcer with indurated edges and a hard, clean base. There is little pain or discharge unless secondary infection occurs. Chancres are usually single but may be multiple. They vary in size but are seldom more than ½ inch in diameter. After a few days the lymph nodes draining the site enlarge. Pain is absent, and the nodes show no tendency to suppurate.

After the chancre has persisted for 4 to 6 weeks, it heals. For the next 4 to 8 weeks (prior to the secondary stage) the patient shows no signs of disease. This is the *primary latent period*.

*Secondary stage (stage of systemic involvement).* The manifestations of secondary syphilis may recur over a period of 5 years. They are (1) skin lesions, (2) lesions of the mucous membranes, (3) generalized rubbery lymphadenopathy, and (4) an influenza-like syndrome. The variable skin eruption is usually symmetrically arranged, macular, and copper colored and seldom itches or burns. A patchy loss of hair, even that of the eyebrows, is associated. Known as mucous patches and most often found in the mouth, the mucosal lesions are painful superficial ulcers with a white raised surface. They are swarming with treponemes.

*Latent stage.* Following the secondary stage is a period during which the patient shows no signs, the disease being recognized only by serologic tests. This stage may last a few months, but in 25% to 50% of patients it lasts a lifetime. It may at any time become active.

For some patients there is no latent period, the tertiary stage appearing right after systemic manifestations have disappeared. In those patients in whom the chancre and secondary manifestations are not present or not detected, the whole course of the disease may be of the latent type. Lesions of primary and secondary syphilis may be atypical and inconspicuous. Many patients are unaware of or ignore the signs of the disease in these stages. Latent syphilis probably represents a biologic balance between the disease-producing powers of *T. pallidum* and the defensive forces of the body.

*Tertiary stage.* The hallmark of *tertiary* syphilis is the destructive *gumma*, a firm, yellowish white central focus surrounded by fibrous tissue. The tertiary lesions involve the deeper structures and organs of the body and interfere materially with the functions of the internal organs. Syphilis seems to have a predilection for the cardiovascular system and the central nervous system, but other organ systems are vulnerable. Trepo-

nemes are sparse in tertiary lesions, and the tissue reaction is usually attributed to some form of allergic response.

Syphilis has been called the "great imitator." There is practically no organic disease whose manifestations it cannot copy, and no other disease assumes so many clinical expressions with progression.

*Cardiovascular syphilis* is tertiary stage syphilitic involvement of the heart and blood vessels. It results in inflammation of the aorta (syphilitic aortitis), aneurysmal dilatation of the thoracic aorta, and distortion of the aortic valve to produce aortic insufficiency (one form of valvular disease of the heart). Syphilis also predisposes to arteriosclerosis in the aorta.

*Neurosyphilis* is syphilitic involvement of the central nervous system. When syphilis becomes generalized during its early stages, the central nervous system seldom escapes invasion. In many patients treponemes die without causing any damage there, but in some 30% to 40% of the patients they remain alive and initiate tertiary stage lesions that come to light weeks, months, or years later. Depending on the anatomic site, neurosyphilis takes three forms: (1) syphilitic meningitis or meningovascular syphilis, (2) tabes dorsalis, or (3) general paresis. In addition, gummas occur as isolated lesions in various parts of the central nervous system.

A regular manifestation of neurosyphilis, *syphilitic meningitis,* more properly called *meningovascular syphilis,* is inflammation of the meninges of the central nervous system with or without involvement of the brain itself. The meninges are variably thickened, and typical changes occur in the walls of meningeal blood vessels. Although not all patients with syphilis develop meningovascular disease, a good percentage do. It usually develops within the first 5 to 6 years after infection but may appear as early as 2 months or as late as 40 years.

*Tabes dorsalis* or *locomotor ataxia* is a degeneration of the posterior columns of the spinal cord and the posterior nerve roots and ganglia caused by *T. pallidum*. Since the sensory pathways of the spinal cord are involved, the disease is chiefly one of muscular incoordination and sensory disturbances.

*General paresis* (general paralysis of the insane; paralytic dementia) is a diffuse meningoencephalitis characterized by progressive mental deterioration, insanity, and generalized paralysis, terminating in death. About 3% of patients with syphilis are affected. Paresis prefers the highly civilized to the primitive races, better educated to less well-educated persons, and is five times more frequent in males than in females.

Neurosyphilis may simulate almost any disease of the central nervous system, but a careful history with a correct interpretation of laboratory tests on the blood and spinal fluid usually makes the differentiation.

**Immunity.** Although antibody formation comparable to that in typhoid fever does not occur in syphilis, the victim develops some kind of resistance. A person with syphilis is not susceptible to superimposed syphilitic infection. If he is completely cured, however, susceptibility becomes as great as ever.

The serum of a patient with syphilis (cerebrospinal fluid in neurosyphilis) contains an antibody substance not found in normal blood or spinal fluid, which can combine with an antigen prepared as a lipid extract of normal tissues, for example, cardiolipin from the heart muscle of an ox. On this phenomenon are based the serologic tests for syphilis, since this kind of antigen-antibody combination can be demonstrated to destroy complement or cause visible aggregation in a colloidal suspension of antigen.

There has been much speculation about this antibody substance. Because of its uncertain nature it is called *reagin*. According to some observers a syphilitic infection causes a breakdown of the patient's tissue cells, releasing fatty substances. These combine with the protein of the treponemes to form an antigen that stimulates the formation of antibodies to both lipids and treponemes. This explains why lipid extracts of heart muscle may be used as the antigen in the different serologic tests for syphilis and why it is possible to use treponemes as the antigen in the *Treponema pallidum immobilization test* (TPI).

There is no definitive method of artificially producing an active or passive immunity against syphilis. Inadequate early treatment may be of greater harm than good because it fails to effect a cure and at the same time retards the establishment of any degree of immunity.

**Laboratory diagnosis.** The laboratory has at its disposal two important approaches to the diagnosis of syphilis: (1) the demonstration of the organisms in the lesions by dark-field microscopy or by immunofluorescence, and (2) serologic testing for syphilis (STS), notably the use of complement fixation and flocculation tests. The serologic tests include *nontreponemal* tests to demonstrate reagin (performed on serum and cerebrospinal fluid) and *treponemal* tests to detect the antigens of *T. pallidum* (performed on serum as the direct source of the specific antibodies).

The dark-field microscope to demonstrate *T. pallidum* is most practical in the investigation of suspected chancres and mucous patches. Fluorescent antibody technics can also be used on exudates therefrom.

During the first few days of a chancre the organisms are found in almost all patients. As it ages, *T. pallidum* gradually disappears. Serologic tests are seldom positive during the first few days of the chancre but usually become positive before the appearance of the secondary stage. In neurosyphilis, serologic tests on both blood and cerebrospinal fluid are positive in the great majority of patients.

The complement fixation (nontreponemal) test, regardless of the technic, is referred to as the Wassermann test because August von Wassermann (1866-1925) first applied in 1906 the principle of complement fixation to the diagnosis of syphilis. The test has been so much improved that of the original, only the principle and the name remain. Two modifications of the Wassermann test in routine use are that of Kolmer and that of Eagle.

Precipitation (or flocculation) tests are the Kline, Kahn, Eagle, Hinton, Mazzini, RPR (rapid plasma reagin), and VDRL (Venereal Disease Research Laboratory) tests. The VDRL is probably the most widely used and exclusively so for testing cerebrospinal fluid. The Kahn presumptive test and the Kline exclusion test are highly sensitive and can detect amounts of syphilitic reagin much less than the smallest amount that the so-called standard or diagnostic tests can. These sensitive tests have the disadvantage that positive results may often be obtained in perfectly healthy persons or persons who at least do not have syphilis. Therefore they are more significant when negative than when positive and are used for *screening*. A positive result is then followed by other serologic tests, and for the laboratory diagnosis of syphilis positive results are required from two or more tests less sensitive than the screening test.

Nontreponemal flocculation and complement fixation tests for syphilis may give negative results in the presence of syphilis and sometimes give positive results in its absence.* Such results are called false negative and false positive reactions. False negatives may be caused by technical errors or by undetectably small amounts of syphilitic reagin in the blood. False positives come from technical error, or they may be biologic false positives (BFP). BFP results are occasionally or uniformly found in certain diseases such as yaws, infectious mononucleosis, malaria, leprosy, and rat-bite fever, and in drug addicts. Partly to eliminate the biologic false positive, developments in serologic research have largely been concerned with the production of tests utilizing either the organisms themselves, dead or alive, or chemical extracts of the organisms as antigens.

The TPI test, a treponemal test in which *T. pallidum* itself is immobilized in the presence of guinea pig complement and serum from a person with syphi-

---

* A serologic test for syphilis cannot diagnose disease. It only gives immunologic information; none devised so far is absolutely specific.

lis, is negative with serums giving BFP reactions. Its clinical usefulness depends on this fact. As specific as, and more sensitive than, the TPI test is the FTA-ABS (fluorescent treponemal antibody absorption) test, considered to be the best of the treponemal tests today. Some authorities believe it is 99% accurate. As the name indicates, test serum is absorbed of non-specific (confusing) antibodies. It is then brought into contact with *T. pallidum* and fluorescein-tagged anti-human globulin in a special way so that the combination may be viewed microscopically. Antibodies to the spirochetes, if present, attach to the organism, the antihuman globulin in turn uniting with them. When seen through the ultraviolet microscope, the result glows beautifully.

Other treponemal tests are the *Treponema pallidum* complement fixation test and the Reiter protein complement fixation test (RPCF).

*Remember that the diagnosis of syphilis must be made only after careful evaluation of both clinical features and laboratory findings.*

**Prevention.** The patient is most likely to convey syphilis during the primary and secondary stages because chancres and mucous patches are living cultures of syphilitic organisms. Attendants of patients with these lesions should be careful not to contact the patient's secretions. Certain manual examinations must always be made with gloves because a patient may show no evidence of syphilis but at the same time be capable of transmitting the infection.

People should still be educated as to the universal prevalence of syphilis and the danger of syphilis not only to the person who has it but also to his marriage partner and his children. Today a growing public health problem, the disease is significant among young adults and especially teenagers, in whom there has been better than a 200% increase in the incidence of syphilis over the last decade.

Considerable thought today is going to the development of a syphilitic vaccine. One under investigation is the gamma-irradiated Nichols strain of *T. pallidum*, nonvirulent but antigenic.

### CONGENITAL (PRENATAL) SYPHILIS

*Congenital syphilis* refers to the disease acquired before birth. As a result of the upsurge in the incidence of venereal disease including syphilis, over 2000 babies will be born this year in the United States with congenital syphilis. For this form of syphilis to occur, the mother must be infected. The treponemes are blood-borne to the maternal side of the placenta and deposited there. Syphilitic foci develop in the placenta, and the organisms spread through to the fetal circulation. A syphilitic father can transmit the infection to his child only indirectly, that is, by infecting the mother.

The shorter the time elapsing between infection of the mother and conception, the more likely will the unborn baby be infected. If adequate treatment of the mother is instituted before the fifth month of pregnancy, the child should be born free of syphilis. The requirements by law in many states for premarital examination for syphilis and for prenatal serologic testing for syphilis have been important public health measures in the prevention of this form of the disease.

Congenital syphilis usually appears at birth or within a few weeks thereafter, but it may appear years later. The child of a syphilitic mother may be (1) born dead, (2) born alive with syphilis, (3) born apparently in good health but show evidence of syphilis several weeks or months later, or (4) entirely free of the disease.

The placenta of a syphilitic child is large for the weight of the child. In stillborn infants the lungs fill the entire thoracic cavity, are grayish white, and are incompletely developed. This condition, known as white pneumonia or *pneumonia alba*, is pathognomonic for congenital syphilis. Congenital neurosyphilis simulates the acquired form and may appear in early life or be delayed to adolescence.

Infants born with active syphilis are undersized and look strikingly like an old man. A vesicular skin eruption and persistent nasal discharge (*snuffles*) are often present. The child may have linear scars at the angles of the mouth (*syphilitic rhagades*). Among the late manifestations of congenital syphilis are poorly formed, small, peg-shaped permanent teeth. The upper central incisors are wedge shaped and show a central notch (*Hutchinson's teeth*). Other late manifestations are interstitial keratitis, anterior bowing of the tibia (saber shin), dactylitis, and neurosyphilis.

To detect congenital syphilis in a newborn baby with no outward signs, a modified FTA-ABS test is applied. Specific antihuman immunoglobulin tagged with fluorescein indicates the presence of 19S immunoglobulins (IgM antibodies). Unlike the smaller 7S immunoglobulins, which are formed by the mother, these macroglobulins cannot cross the intact placenta and must be formed by the baby. Their presence indicates the baby's reaction to *his* disease, not his mother's.

### SYPHILIS AND YAWS

Yaws or frambesia, a tropical disease closely akin to syphilis, is caused by *Treponema pertenue*, a spirochete that cannot be differentiated serologically from *T. pallidum* and that, like *T. pallidum*, is susceptible to arsenic and penicillin. Yaws may be a special form of syphilis; however, most observers believe that they are distinct.

Yaws is nonvenereal and does not occur in the congenital form. Skin and bone lesions are prominent.

When the yellowish crusts covering the large pustules are removed, the slightly bleeding surface looks exactly like a raspberry stuck on the skin, hence the name frambesia or raspberry disease.

## Borrelia species

Members of the genus *Borrelia* are helical cells with coarse, uneven coils. They are anaerobic parasites found on mucous membranes, and some cause disease in man and animals (for example, avian and bovine spirochetosis in animals).

**Disease in man.** Relapsing fever is an acute infectious disease caused by several species of spirochetes in the genus *Borrelia* (Fig. 23-1) and is characterized clinically by alternating periods of febrile illness with apparent recovery. The incubation period is 3 to 10 days. The spirochetes are found in the peripheral blood during the fever and are transferred from man to man by body lice (*Pediculus humanus* subsp. *humanus*) and from rodent to man by ticks (*Ornithodoros*). Thus there are two types of relapsing fever—that borne by the louse and that borne by the tick. The former occurs as epidemic relapsing fever in the general pattern of louse-borne diseases, and the spirochete causing it is *Borrelia recurrentis*. Tick-borne relapsing fever does not occur in epidemics. It is endemic relapsing fever caused by other species of *Borrelia*. It is the only type found in North America. Infected ticks may transmit the infection to their offspring for generation after generation. Body lice do not thus transmit it. Rodents such as the ground squirrel and prairie dog are the main reservoir of the tick-borne disease. A wide variety of animals may be infected with borreliae, including armadillos, bats, dogs, foxes, horses, rabbits, and porcupines.

**Laboratory diagnosis.** Actively motile spiral organisms, borreliae differ from *T. pallidum* in that they take the usual laboratory stains. They may be detected in the Wright-stained smears of peripheral blood or by dark-field illumination. Blood from a patient may be inoculated into a white mouse or young rat. Wright-stained films made from the tail blood 1 to 4 days later will show the organisms. *Borrelia* species can be grown in the chick embryo.

## Leptospira species

Leptospires are tightly and finely coiled spiral bacteria with one or both ends bent characteristically to form a hook. Some are free-living; others are parasitic or pathogenic in vertebrates. Only one species of the genus *Leptospira* is recognized in Bergey's recent classification (1974)—*Leptospira interrogans* (*Leptospira icterohaemorrhagiae*). There are serotypes as yet incompletely defined. Taxonomic data in this genus are incomplete at present.

**The disease.** Leptospirosis is an acute febrile disease caused by spirochetes in the genus *Leptospira*, the best known of which is *Leptospira interrogans*. There are various names for this condition, including swamp fever, swineherd's disease, infectious jaundice, spirochetal jaundice, and Weil's disease. Weil's disease represents the most severe form.

Clinically, leptospirosis is characterized by high fever, muscular pains, redness of the conjunctivae, jaundice (not invariable), and aseptic meningitis. An attack is followed by a lasting immunity. Inapparent infections also occur.

Leptospires (Fig. 23-1) are found in wild and domestic animals all over the world. Disease is mainly zoonotic; man is only accidentally infected. In animals the spirochetes localize in the kidney and are excreted profusely in the urine. They can survive if urine is discharged to neutral or slightly alkaline water, sewage, or mud. Man probably acquires the infection through the skin from soil contaminated with the urine of infected rats or through the mouth by food or water that has been contaminated in the same way. The organisms enter the animal or human body through the abraded skin and the mucous membranes of the eye, nose, and mouth. Leptospirosis is important as an occupational disease. Especially vulnerable to it are workers in rat-infested mines, rice fields, and sewage disposal plants.

**Laboratory diagnosis.** The spirochetes are found in the blood early in the disease and in the urine after the seventh day. Leptospires of typical shape and motility are best seen by dark-field examination of blood and urine. They may be recovered from blood cultures and from the peritoneal cavity of a guinea pig inoculated with blood or urine. A microagglutination test is diagnostic.

## Other spirochetes and associated organisms

*Treponema buccale* and *Treponema denticola* are nonpathogenic saprophytes found in the mouth. Their presence may cause confusion in the examination of material from the mouth suspected of containing the spirochete of syphilis. *Treponema refringens* is part of the normal flora of the male and female genitalia and may be associated with *Treponema pallidum* in various syphilitic lesions.

**Vincent's angina (fusospirochetal disease).** In Vincent's infection (fusospirochetal disease), a grayish white pseudomembrane forms in the throat or mouth, beneath which ulceration occurs. When the gums and mouth are primarily involved, the disease is known as *trench mouth*. When the throat and tonsils are ulcerated, it is called *Vincent's angina* (Fig. 23-3). The disease is more properly called acute necrotizing ulcerative gingivitis. The disease is important within itself and because the membrane may be mistaken for

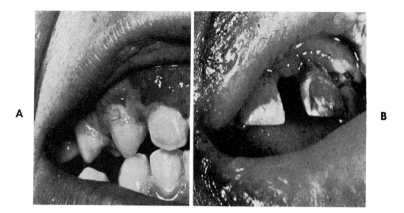

**Fig. 23-3.** Vincent's angina (necrotizing gingivitis). **A,** Early stage. **B,** Late stage with marked destruction of tissues. (From Bhaskar, S. N.: Synopsis of oral pathology, ed. 4, St. Louis, 1973, The C. V. Mosby Co.)

a diphtheritic membrane. The extensive ulceration may cause the disease to be confused with syphilis.

Associated together in the lesions are two organisms: (1) a large, gram-negative, cigar-shaped, anaerobic "fusiform" bacillus and (2) a gram-negative spirochete, *Treponema (Borrelia) vincentii*. Vincent's infection is thought by some to be caused by *Bacteroides melaninogenicus,* found in the mouth and pathogenic usually in association with other kinds of organisms. Early the cigar-shaped bacilli are more numerous, whereas later on in the disease, spirochetes are. These two do not cause this condition, and most workers believe that they are only secondary invaders. They grow symbiotically here as opportunists, being already in the mouth. Their mere presence is not enough to cause disease. This must be triggered by some unusual circumstance, such as an injury to the mouth or decreased oral resistance. Vincent's angina (fusospirochetal disease) accompanies malnutrition, debilitating states, viral infections, and poor oral hygiene.

Fusospirochetal organisms are identified directly on a crystal violet–stained smear of the membranous exudate.

## Spirillum minor

There are two clinical entities known as rat-bite fever that are conveyed by the bite of a rat or other rodent. One, known in Japan as sodoku, is caused by *Spirillum minor*. This small and rigid spiral microbe (Fig. 23-1) is found primarily in wild rats and is spread from rat to rat and from rat to man by the bite of the rat (the healthy carrier). The features of the disease are ulceration of the bite, fever, and a skin eruption. The spirilla may be seen in material from the ulcer ex-

amined in stained smears or by dark-field illumination, and a guinea pig may be inoculated with blood or tissue from lymph nodes to isolate the organisms. Rat-bite fever of this type is uncommon but is worldwide in distribution.

The other entity is streptobacillary rat-bite fever (Haverhill fever), caused by *Streptobacillus moniliformis* (formerly *Actinomyces muris ratti*), an actinomycete-like, necklace-shaped bacterium found in the mouth and nasopharynx of normal rats, among which it causes widespread epidemics. Man contracts the infection from the bite of a rat. The disease is a febrile one with manifestations similar to those of rat-bite fever caused by *Spirillum minor*. Both resemble tularemia clinically. *Streptobacillus moniliformis* is identified by fluorescent antibody technics.

## Questions for review

1 Name and describe the causative agent of syphilis.
2 Outline the evolution of a typical case of syphilis.
3 Characterize congenital syphilis. What are its hazards?
4 How is syphilis transmitted?
5 Outline the laboratory diagnosis of syphilis. Briefly discuss the serologic tests.
6 Classify spiral bacteria. Present salient features.
7 Comment on the pathogenicity of *Treponema pallidum*. Why is it called the "great imitator"? What is a gumma?
8 How does the causative agent of yaws compare with that of syphilis?
9 Name two vectors of relapsing fever and possible rodent reservoirs.
10 Characterize leptospirosis.
11 Give the names of the two microbes causing rat-bite fever.
12 How is Vincent's angina diagnosed bacteriologically?

**References pp. 276 to 280.**

# CHAPTER 24

# Actinomycetes
## including corynebacteria

## Corynebacteria

The coryneform group of bacteria takes the lead position in the discussion of microbes gathered into Part 17 of *Bergey's Manual,* eighth edition, which is entitled "Actinomycetes and related organisms." The term *coryneform* is a working concept to sidestep for the time being unresolved problems in classification. Genus I, *Corynebacterium* (club bacteria), includes one dreaded pathogen—*Corynebacterium diphtheriae,* the type species.

### CORYNEBACTERIUM DIPHTHERIAE (THE BACILLUS OF DIPHTHERIA)

Six or seven decades ago diphtheria, or membranous croup as it was called, was a major cause of death. Since the causative organism, *Corynebacterium diphtheriae (C. diphtheriae),* was first discovered by Edwin Klebs (1834-1913) in 1883, the epidemiology has become known, methods of producing a permanent immunity have been devised, and the mortality has been reduced from nearly 50% to such a level that death seldom occurs in patients who are adequately treated during the early days of the disease.* Few diseases have been so well studied and are today so well understood as diphtheria.

The causative agent belongs to the genus *Corynebacterium* of gram-positive, unevenly staining bacteria with clubbed or pointed ends. (*Coryne* signifies clubbed.) *C. diphtheriae* is often called the Klebs-Löffler bacillus because it was discovered by Klebs and first grown in 1884 in a pure culture by F. A. J. Löffler (1852-1915). The word *diphtheria* is derived from a Greek word meaning leather. The disease was so named because of the leathery consistency of the diphtheritic membrane.

**General characteristics.** *C. diphtheriae* is distinct

for its variation in size, shape, and appearance (pleomorphism). The bacteria may be straight or curved and may be swollen in the middle or clubbed at one or both ends. When division occurs, the bacteria remain attached at the point of separation in a V-shaped arrangement (snapping). Stained organisms may have a granular, solid, or barred appearance and deeply staining granules (metachromatic granules) are characteristic. Granules at the ends of the bacilli are known as *polar bodies.*

*C. diphtheriae* is a gram-positive nonmotile, strictly aerobic microbe that does not form spores. It grows best at 35° C. on almost all ordinary media, but growth is most luxuriant on Löffler's blood serum and media containing potassium tellurite. Potassium tellurite inhibits the growth of many organisms found in the throat, and colonies of diphtheria bacilli assume a typical appearance on media containing it. The morphologic features of the organisms are best preserved on Löffler's blood serum.

Based on cultural characteristics, fermentation tests, and immunologic reactions, *C. diphtheriae* has been divided into three types: *gravis* (meaning severe), *intermedius* (meaning of intermediate severity), and *mitis* (meaning mild). Epidemics are most often caused by the *gravis* type, and the manifestations are the most severe.

For man and some laboratory animals *C. diphtheriae* is highly pathogenic. In nature the disease is restricted to man. The incubation period of diphtheria is 2 to 6 days.

Diphtheria bacilli are fairly resistant to drying but are easily destroyed by heat and chemical disinfectants. Boiling destroys them in 1 minute. They may remain alive in bits of diphtheritic membrane for several weeks.

**Extracellular toxin.** Diphtheria bacilli owe their pathogenicity to their extracellular toxin. The bacilli do not invade the tissues but grow superficially in a restricted area, usually on a mucous membrane. The

---

*Within the last 3 decades an especially severe type of diphtheria has appeared in different parts of the world, one that is difficult to treat and often seen in adults.

exotoxin formed is released into the bloodstream and circulated. As a result of its primary action in blocking the cellular synthesis of protein, toxin produces cellular injury, leading to systemic disturbances, and degenerative changes in the organs of the body. It affects certain nerves, the heart muscle, the kidneys, and the cortex of the adrenal gland. The features of the disease relate directly to the exotoxin; that is, it is a toxemia and a molecular disease.

In 1951 the remarkable discovery was made that exotoxin can be elaborated only by lysogenic strains of *C. diphtheriae*, that is, strains infected with certain bacteriophages (bacterial viruses) carrying the *tox* gene. If the specific phage is lost to the bacterium, the quality of toxigenicity goes also, and conversely a nontoxigenic strain may be converted to a lysogenic and toxigenic strain if treated (infected) with the proper phage. The tox gene programs the structure of exotoxin, but biosynthesis is enacted by the bacterial cell. The amount of inorganic iron in the external and internal milieu is a critical factor regulating toxin production, which is depressed until that level of iron is critically reduced.

Soluble exotoxin released into media is concentrated to yield the diphtheria toxin of commerce. Such preparations contain 200 to 1000 MLD (p. 395) per milliliter. The toxin can be separated from the medium and purified. It deteriorates with age and is destroyed by a temperature of 60° C.

Not all diphtheria bacilli produce toxin. Toxigenic organisms cannot be distinguished from nontoxigenic ones by microscopic appearance or by cultural characteristics. Differentiation is made by animal inoculation. A small amount of a liquid culture of the bacilli is injected either beneath or between the superficial layers of the skin of two guinea pigs, *only one* of which has been protected by a dose of diphtheria antitoxin. If the bacilli are toxigenic, a zone of inflammation appears at the site of inoculation in the unprotected pig, but there is no reaction at the site in the protected pig. If the bacilli are not toxin producers, neither pig shows a reaction. This is the *guinea pig virulence test*. Virulence tests may be carried out on rabbits. The technic differs somewhat from that in guinea pigs, but the underlying principle is the same. Eight or ten tests may be carried out at one time on the same rabbit. A cultural method, the in vitro gel diffusion test, has also been devised whereby the virulence of diphtheria bacilli may be determined.

**Pathogenicity.** Diphtheria is an acute infectious disease caused by the extracellular toxin of *C. diphtheriae*. There is a characteristic inflammatory change at the site of infection, and systemic disturbances accompany it.

Pathologically, the type lesion of diphtheria is the *pseudomembrane,* a superficial lesion occurring on mucous membranes. The first stage in its formation is degeneration of the epithelial cells of the affected area. This is followed by an abundant fibrinous exudation onto the surface. As the fibrin precipitates, it entraps leukocytes, red blood cells, bacteria, and dead epithelial cells to form a thick tough membranelike structure anchored to the underlying tissues. When the pseudomembrane is pulled off, a raw bleeding surface is left, but a new pseudomembrane soon forms. In the absence of antitoxin it persists for 7 to 10 days and then disappears. It may obstruct breathing, and in some patients tracheotomy or intubation is required to prevent suffocation.

The most frequent sites for pseudomembrane formation are the tonsils, pharynx, larynx, and nasal passages. The diphtheritic membrane or pseudomembrane usually begins on one or both tonsils and spreads to the uvula and soft palate. Less often diphtheria attacks the vulva, conjunctiva, middle ear, and skin and infects wounds. Skin infections were prevalent among soldiers of World War II. Organisms other than *C. diphtheriae* may produce pseudomembranes, and in a few patients with diphtheria pseudomembranes do not form.

Diphtheria occurs in three clinical patterns: (1) *faucial,* in which the membrane forms on the tonsils and spreads to other parts of the pharynx (Fig. 24-1); (2) *laryngeal,* in which the membrane may easily cause suffocation; and (3) *nasal,* in which the membrane is often not associated with severe disease because the toxin is poorly absorbed by the lining of the nose. Bronchopneumonia is an important complication.

The really serious effects of diphtheria stem from the action of the toxin. The damage done to the heart may precipitate heart failure, even after other manifestations of the disease have subsided and sometimes in comparatively mild cases. Sudden death has been reported several weeks after apparent recovery. Degeneration of the peripheral nerves induced by the toxin leads to late paralysis, particularly of the soft palate.

**Sources and modes of infection.** The sources of infection in diphtheria are persons with typical cases, persons with mild undetected cases, and carriers. Ordinarily the bacteria enter and leave the body by the same route, the mouth and nose. They may be transferred directly from person to person by droplets expelled from the mouth and nose or indirectly by cups, toys, pencils, dishes, and eating utensils contaminated by buccal or nasal secretions. The direct method of transfer is the more important.

Nasal diphtheria is an important source of infection because it is often overlooked. Diphtheria

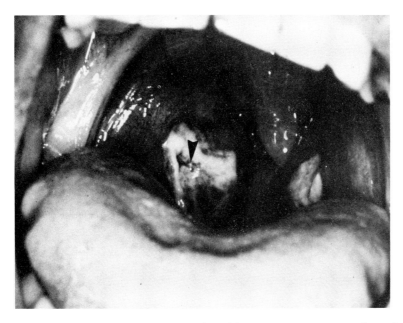

**Fig. 24-1.** Diphtheria in 43-year-old man; fourth day of disease. Arrow is over membrane in tonsillar area of throat. (From McCloskey, R. V., and others: Ann. Intern. Med. **75:**495, 1971.)

bacilli can be spread from skin infections appearing to be less serious ailments. In epidemics, such skin sources have figured significantly. Cutaneous diphtheria in indigent adults is a significant reservoir. A few milkborne epidemics have been reported. Such are usually caused by the contamination of the milk by a person working in the dairy who either is a carrier or may have a mild case of disease. He transfers his buccal or nasal discharges by his hands. The rather prevalent idea that cats convey diphtheria is not true.

Over the last decade or so in this country diphtheria has continued to occur in the economically depressed areas of the South where living conditions are crowded, medical care lacking, hygiene poor, and immunization inadequate.

*Diphtheria carriers.* In about one half of patients with diphtheria the bacilli leave the body within 3 days after the membrane disappears, and in four fifths of the patients they have disappeared within 1 week; but sometimes they persist for a longer period, and the patient becomes a carrier. Also, certain persons in contact with a diphtheria patient or a carrier become carriers themselves without contracting the disease. It has been estimated that from 0.1% to 0.5% of the population are carriers of virulent diphtheria bacilli. The percentage increases during epidemics and in crowded communities during cold weather.

Most carriers harbor the bacilli a short time only (from a few days to a few weeks), but a few harbor them permanently and remain carriers in spite of intensive treatment. Because a high percentage of organisms with the morphology and cultural characteristics of diphtheria bacilli in normal throats are nontoxigenic and are therefore not dangerous, virulence tests should always be done on diphtheria bacilli from suspected carriers. If a suitable antibiotic such as erythromycin or penicillin is given in conjunction with antitoxin during the acute stage of the disease and continued during the period of convalescence, the carrier rate is reduced.

**Bacteriologic diagnosis.** The laboratory diagnosis of diphtheria is made by culture of the organisms (Table 24-1). Some of the material from the pseudomembrane is removed with a sterile swab; a slant of Löffler's blood serum or tellurite medium is inoculated and incubated from 12 to 14 hours. Smears made from the culture are stained with Löffler's methylene blue or one of the special stains for diphtheria bacilli. A diagnosis may sometimes be made by finding the bacilli in smears made directly from the pseudomembrane, but failure to find them in no manner indicates that the patient does not have the disease. Antiseptics, gargles, or mouthwashes must not be used before cultures are taken because they may prevent the proper growth of the bacteria. Antibiotics given 5 to 7 days previously may inhibit bacterial growth on the culture medium. If possible, cultures should be taken before antibiotics are given. Care should be taken to bring the swab in contact only

**Table 24-1**
Bacteriologic diagnosis of diphtheria

| ORGANISM | MOR-PHOLOGY | GROWTH ON BLOOD TELLURITE | HYDROL-YSIS OF UREA | REDUCTION OF NITRATE | FERMENTATION OF CARBOHYDRATES | | | | TOXIGENICITY |
|---|---|---|---|---|---|---|---|---|---|
| | | | | | TREHALOSE | GLUCOSE | MALTOSE | SUCROSE | |
| *Corynebacterium diphtheriae* | Pleo-morphic | Gray to black colonies | − | + | − | + | + | − | + |
| *Corynebacterium pseudo-diphtheriticum* (example of a diphtheroid) | More uniform | Opaque grayish | + | + | − | − | − | − | − |

with the site of disease, and cultures should be made from both throat and nose.

In a patient with an ulcerative or membranous inflammation of the throat, both cultures for *C. diphtheriae* and smears for the organisms of Vincent's angina should be made. The two conditions may be easily confused. If only a culture is made, an infection with the organisms of Vincent's angina could be missed because these organisms do not grow in cultures, and diphtheria could be missed if smears alone are examined. Moreover, the two diseases can coexist.

The finding of diphtheria bacilli in the throat does not necessarily mean the patient has diphtheria; he may be a carrier. Remember that membranous infections of the throat may be caused by organisms other than *C. diphtheriae* and that nonmembranous infections with *C. diphtheriae* occasionally occur. If streptococcal infection is suspected, a blood agar plate is inoculated.

*Diphtheroid bacilli.* The diphtheroid bacilli, a heterogeneous group, bear a close microscopic resemblance to *C. diphtheriae* and are sometimes confused with it on throat smears. They are numerous and have been isolated from many different sources such as the skin, nose, throat, urethra, bladder, vagina, and prostate gland. They reside in soil and water as saprophytes, do not produce toxins, and are nonpathogenic for man except under exceptional circumstances. They have recently been reported as rare causes of wound infections, meningitis, osteomyelitis, and hepatitis.

**Immunity.** Immunity to diphtheria results from the presence of diphtheria antitoxin in the blood. Newborn babies of immune mothers receive a passive immunity because of the transfer of antitoxin from the maternal to the fetal circulation via the placenta. In breast-fed infants this immunity is augmented by antibodies in the milk of the mother. This immunity is usually lost by the end of the first year,

and from this time to the sixth year most children are susceptible. Minor infections with *C. diphtheriae* reestablish an immunity during late childhood.

About 60% of adults are immune, a figure once considerably higher. The reduction in the incidence of diphtheria, the decreased likelihood of minor infections, and the institution of vaccination during childhood (which does not give the permanent immunity that repeated minor infections do) have meant a decrease in adult immunity. The presence of from $1/500$ to $1/250$ unit of diphtheria antitoxin per milliliter of blood renders a person immune.

The *Schick test* purports to determine whether a person has sufficient diphtheria antitoxin in his blood for immunity. One-fiftieth MLD of diphtheria toxin (0.1 ml. of diluted toxin) is injected into the skin of one arm of a subject, and a control dose of toxoid into the other. The skin sites on both arms are read 4 days later. In principle, if the subject's blood contains sufficient antitoxin for protection against diphtheria, no reaction occurs (negative test). An insufficient amount of antitoxin (positive test) is indicated by the appearance within 24 to 36 hours of a firm red area, 1 to 2 cm. in diameter, persisting 4 or 5 days. In the past the Schick test has been used to detect persons lacking immunity and to determine the efficacy of active immunization once given. Since the highly purified, adult-type toxoids have become available the need for routine Schick testing is largely eliminated. Active immunization is desirable, and difficulties encountered with the Schick test are bypassed.

An attack of diphtheria is usually followed by a fair degree of immunity, which may be temporary or permanent. In a few patients immunity does not seem to develop. Most carriers of virulent diphtheria bacilli are immune to the diphtheria toxin.

**Prevention and control of diphtheria.*** All per-

---

*For immunization in diphtheria see pp. 395-397, 403, 409, 410, 411, and 416.

sons ill of diphtheria should be isolated, and neither they nor their close contacts should be released until it is proved that they harbor no virulent diphtheria bacilli in their noses and throats. The mouth secretions and all objects so contaminated should be disinfected. The eating utensils used by patients should be boiled. Nurses must be careful that they do not contaminate their hands with the mouth and nose secretions of patients so as to infect themselves. Persons known or presumed to be susceptible who contact a diphtheria patient should receive diphtheria toxoid (for active immunization) and antibiotics. If they cannot be seen daily by the physician, they may be temporarily immunized with 10,000 units of diphtheria antitoxin intramuscularly. Remember that the administration of antitoxin can set the stage for an anaphylactic reaction should another agent containing horse serum be given to that person.

The general measures that cause the greatest reduction in incidence of diphtheria are (1) the detection and treatment of carriers and (2) the production of an active immunity in all susceptibles—children under 6 years of age and all older children and adults, especially physicians and nurses, not previously immunized.

## Actinomycetes

Actinomycetes are now classified as bacteria. For a long time these microbes, because of their similarities to both the true bacteria and the true fungi, were thought of as intermediates between the two, were sometimes called "higher bacteria," but were usually included in a discussion of medical mycology.

Within Part 17 of the eighth edition of *Bergey's Manual*, Order I, Actinomycetales, contains grampositive, sometimes acid-fast, mostly aerobic bacteria forming branching filaments that in some of the families develop into a mycelium. Some members are pathogens of man, animals, and plants.

In this classification of funguslike bacteria, there are four families of note. The family Mycobacteriaceae comprises the genus *Mycobacterium* of acid-alcohol–fast microbes,* of which *Mycobacterium tuberculosis* is the type species (Chapter 25). The family Streptomycetaceae is medically very significant because the actinomycetes of genus *Streptomyces* provide us with many important pathogenic antibiotics. Two families of actinomycetes, each with an important genus, are Actinomycetaceae of nonacid-fast, diphtheroid-shaped bacteria with no mycelium, and Nocardiaceae of variably acid-fast organisms with variable mycelial development. The genera are *Actinomyces* and *Nocardia*,

---

*Mycobacteria are not referred to as actinomycetes as are members of the other three families.

respectively, and the diseases, actinomycosis and nocardiosis. Species of genus *Actinomyces* are anerobic or microaerophilic, whereas species of genus *Nocardia* are aerobic. The acid-fast species of genus *Nocardia* may be confused with *Mycobacterium tuberculosis*.

The actinomycetes (including streptomycetes) resemble the fungi in that they may have a mycelium of masses of branched filaments, but their "hyphae" are much slenderer than those of true fungi. The filaments of actinomycetes fragment into spherical or rod-shaped segments that function as spores and in turn develop into new hyphae. Spore formation comparable to that in bacteria is seen in the hyphae of the genus *Streptomyces*, wherein development of a mycelium is complete.

Actinomycetes are widely distributed in nature and play a vital part in changes in organic material of the soil. This activity is more crucial to man than any disease-producing capacity.

### ACTINOMYCOSIS

Actinomycosis is an infectious disease of lower animals (especially cattle) and man caused by several species of bacteria belonging to the genus *Actinomyces*. Of these, *Actinomyces bovis* (bovine actinomycosis) and *Actinomyces israelii* (human actinomycosis) are the most important. Actinomycosis is typified clinically by the formation of nodular swellings that soften and form abscesses, discharging a thin pus through multiple sinuses. The disease in man is in three patterns: (1) cervicofacial, (2) thoracic, and (3) abdominal. The cervicofacial type is described by

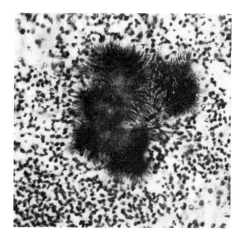

**Fig. 24-2.** *Actinomyces* sulfur granule (colony) in a microscopic field of pus. Club-shaped processes are at periphery. (From Bauer, J. D., and others: Clinical laboratory methods, ed. 8, St. Louis, 1974, The C. V. Mosby Co.)

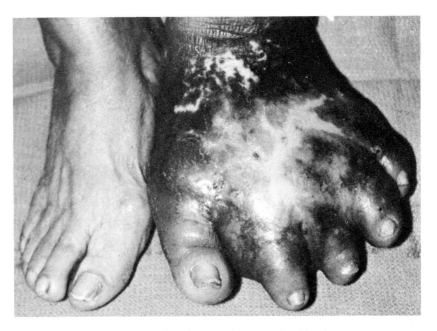

**Fig. 24-3.** Madura foot (maduromycosis of foot).

swelling and suppuration of the soft tissues of the face, jaw, and neck. It is the usual type (about half the cases) and the least dangerous. It appears to have a special association with dental defects. The thoracic type is characterized by multiple small cavities and abscesses in the lungs. The abdominal type usually begins about the appendix or cecum. In advanced thoracic and abdominal disease, sinus tracts extend to the surface. The disease in cattle is known as lumpy jaw.

The etiologic agent is found in the pus or in the walls of abscesses as small, yellow granules about the size of a pinhead, the sulfur granules. When a sulfur granule is placed on a microslide and a cover glass is pressed down on it, a distinct microscopic picture is seen—a central threadlike mass from which radiate many clublike structures (Fig. 24-2). For this reason *Actinomyces* have been called ray fungi. The clubbed appearance is not very pronounced in cultures. The laboratory diagnosis of actinomycosis is made by finding objects in the discharges that are both grossly and microscopically sulfur granules or by demonstrating the organisms in sections of tissue taken from the lesions. Cultural methods help, but serologic and skin tests contribute little.

Pathogenic actinomycetes are normal inhabitants of the mouth of cattle and man, probably existing in an attenuated state. There is no evidence that the organisms are saprophytic outside the animal body. Infection occurs in the event of injury to the mouth, tooth decay, or some other abnormal state. Such conditions favor invasion of the tissues. There is no evidence of direct transmission from animal to animal or from animal to man. People who pursue nonagricultural occupations are as likely to contract actinomycosis as are farmers and stockmen.

## NOCARDIOSIS

*Nocardia asteroides*, an aerobic actinomycete found free in nature, is responsible for a variety of infections in man, designated nocardiosis. It is one cause of *mycetoma* or "Madura foot," a localized involvement usually of the foot (Fig. 24-3). After initial injury in this condition, the organisms invade to produce in time a network of interlocking abscesses and granulomas in the soft tissues and bones of the foot. The organisms of actinomycotic mycetoma (or maduromycotic mycetoma, if certain fungi are operative) can be identified in the purulent discharge from the draining sinus tracts.

*Nocardia* may be responsible for infections of the lungs (pulmonary nocardiosis) and other internal organs. Brain abscess commonly complicates systemic infection. Nocardiosis (like cryptococcosis), with an affinity for the lungs, accompanies malignant diseases of the reticuloendothelial system—Hodgkin's disease, lymphosarcoma, and leukemia. Steroid hormones enhance infection.

## Questions for review

1 What are actinomycetes? Their importance?
2 Briefly indicate what is meant by actinomycosis, toxigenicity, sulfur granule, Madura foot, mycetoma, nocardiosis, mycelium, lumpy jaw, ray fungus, diphtheroid bacilli, tox gene.
3 What does the word diphtheria mean?
4 Name and describe the bacterium causing diphtheria.
5 What are the clinical patterns in this disease? Characterize the pseudomembrane.
6 Explain the pathogenicity of the diphtheria bacillus. What is the mechanism for exotoxin formation?
7 Briefly discuss virulence tests in diphtheria.
8 Outline the laboratory diagnosis of diphtheria.

**References on pp. 276 to 280.**

# CHAPTER 25

# Acid-fast mycobacteria

Non–acid-fast bacteria are easily stained with basic dyes, but the color is quickly removed when the microorganisms are treated with acid-alcohol. Acid-fast bacteria, on the other hand, are so resistant to the penetration of basic dyes that in order to color them, the stain has to be either gently heated or applied for a long period of time. Once stained, however, they are not easily decolorized with acid-alcohol.

The acid-fast bacteria are classified in the genus *Mycobacterium,* the members of which are straight or curved acid-fast rods that may show branching or irregular forms. Those of greatest importance and pathogenic to man are *Mycobacterium tuberculosis,* the cause of tuberculosis in man*; *Mycobacterium bovis,* the cause of tuberculosis in cattle, also in man; *Mycobacterium leprae,* the cause of leprosy; and certain species of atypical, formerly "unclassified" mycobacteria, the cause of mycobacteriosis and various other infections. In addition to these acid-fast organisms, forty or more species exist. Most of them are saprophytes and nonpathogenic, but they may gain access to milk, butter, or other dairy products and be mistaken for *Mycobacterium tuberculosis.* Some are pathogenic for lower animals; for example, one, *Mycobacterium paratuberculosis* (Johne's bacillus), causes a granulomatous enteritis in cattle, known as Johne's disease.

## Tuberculosis

**Importance.** In 1900, tuberculosis (a preventable disease) was the leading cause of death in the United States, as it was throughout the civilized world. (In the tropics it ranked second to malaria.) Since that time it has dropped from first place in this country but still remains a major cause of chronic disability and ill health produced by a communicable disease. In the

United States each year some 30,000 new cases and slightly less than 4000 deaths are reported.

Tuberculosis, a lifelong disease, is a health hazard of the lower socioeconomic groups, densely populated areas, persons over 50 and under 5 years of age, and the chronically ill. Over the world it is still a principal cause of death, ranking with malaria and malnutrition; there are at least 15 million persons with active tuberculosis, and 3 million die annually of the disease. Throughout the world (as well as in this country), it is the most frequent *infectious cause* of death. The mortality is highest in the Orient, Asia, Africa, and Latin America.

**Etiologic agents.** Three species of genus *Mycobacterium* are important causes of tuberculosis. They are *Mycobacterium tuberculosis* (the human bacillus; primary host, man), *Mycobacterium bovis* (the bovine bacillus; primary host, cattle), and *Mycobacterium avium* (the avian bacillus; primary host, birds)—the human, bovine, and avian variants. The three resemble each other rather closely but may be differentiated by animal inoculation and cultural procedures.

## MYCOBACTERIUM TUBERCULOSIS (THE HUMAN TUBERCLE BACILLUS)

*Mycobacterium tuberculosis* (*M. tuberculosis*)—the tubercle bacillus of common parlance—attacks all races of man, other primates, and some domestic animals, such as swine* and dogs. Wild animals living in their natural surroundings do not have tuberculosis but may contract it when placed in captivity.

**General characteristics.** The organism *M. tuberculosis* is a slender, rod-shaped, nonmotile, nonsporeforming bacillus, often beaded or granular in appearance on acid-fast smears. Tubercle bacilli are more resistant than are other nonsporeforming organisms to the deleterious effects of drying and germicides.

---

*Tuberculosis has claimed the lives of many great writers, painters, and musicians—Keats, Chopin, Goethe, Poe, Gauguin, Paganini, Molière, and many others. In fact, no other disease has had such a significant relation to literature and the arts.

---

*A small percentage of hogs slaughtered for food shows evidence of tuberculosis. Hogs are susceptible to the bovine, avian, and human bacilli.

They remain alive in dried sputum or dust in a dark place for weeks or months and in moist sputum for 6 weeks or more. Direct sunlight kills them in 1 or 2 hours. Sufficiently susceptible to heat, however, they are destroyed by the temperature of pasteurization. Phenol, 5%, kills them in sputum in 5 or 6 hours. Tubercle bacilli are not affected by the routinely used antibiotics but are susceptible to streptomycin, dihydrostreptomycin, para-aminosalicylic acid, rifampin, and isoniazid. *M. tuberculosis* tends to develop a resistance to these antimicrobial agents, and toxic effects are sometimes observed after their use. However, their value in treatment and in modifying the course of the disease has been considerable.

*M. tuberculosis* grows only on special media. Even then, growth is slow, and 2 to 4 weeks often elapse before any growth is visible (ordinary bacteria display colonies on routinely used media within 24 to 48 hours). Body temperature (37° C.) is best, but the tubercle bacillus may grow at a temperature as low as 29° or as high as 42° C. Although tubercle bacilli are aerobic, 5% to 10% carbon dioxide enhances growth, and the presence of glycerin in the medium accelerates it for the human bacillus. A bacteriostatic dye such as malachite green, added to the culture medium, suppresses the more rapid growth of contaminants. Note: the human tubercle bacillus is more readily cultivated than is the bovine bacillus.

**Toxic products.** Tubercle bacilli do not produce exotoxins, hemolysins, or comparable substances, but poisonous products partly responsible for the clinical features of tuberculosis are liberated when the bacilli disintegrate.

When *M. tuberculosis* is grown artificially, the culture medium contains a product known as *tuberculin*, without effect on a nontuberculous animal (no history of contact with the tubercle bacillus) but with powerful effects in the body of a tuberculous animal. These effects come from surprisingly small doses, and if the dose is large enough, the results are disastrous.

There are more than fifty methods of preparing tuberculin, and the nature of each tuberculin depends to some extent on the method. The best known and, in the past, the most extensively used tuberculin is Koch's original (or old) tuberculin, often spoken of simply as OT. It is prepared from a culture of tubercle bacilli in 5% glycerin broth that is concentrated and filtered. This bacteria-free filtrate of tuberculin contains bacterial distintegration products, substances formed by the action of the bacilli on the culture medium, and concentrated culture medium.

The tuberculin used today in the tuberculin test is known as PPD (purified protein derivative). It consists chiefly of the active principle of tuberculin without extraneous matter. It is more stable than OT and gives less variable results.

**Sources and modes of infection.** The sources of infection in tuberculosis are the sputum of patients with pulmonary disease and discharges from other tuberculous foci. The patient discharging tubercle bacilli in the sputum is by far the most important reservoir of infection. The bacilli have no natural existence outside the body and are transmitted from source to destination by some form of direct or indirect contact. Droplet infection is the commonest mode of spread. Droplets from the mouth of the tuberculous patient or dust containing the partly dried but still living bacilli are inhaled. The size of the infectious droplet in tuberculosis has been determined at 5 to 10 $\mu$m. ($\mu$); such a particle can remain suspended indefinitely. It is thought that just one bacillus can cause disease.

The next most common mode is the transfer of the bacilli to the mouth by contaminated hands, handkerchiefs, or objects. The infant crawling on the floor may contract tuberculosis by contaminating his hands with tuberculous material and then placing them in his mouth. Unless properly washed and sterilized, the eating utensils used by a tuberculous patient may be a source of infection. The milk of a tuberculous mother may rarely convey the infection to her nursing child.

The avenues of exit for tubercle bacilli depend on the part of the body infected. In pulmonary tuberculosis they are cast off in the sputum, although tubercle bacilli may sometimes be found in the feces of persons who swallow their sputum. In intestinal tuberculosis they are discharged in the feces, and in tuberculosis of the genitourinary system they appear in the urine. Tubercle bacilli may be found in discharges from abscesses and in lesions of the lymph nodes, bones, and skin.

**Pathogenicity.** Tuberculosis is the chronic granulomatous infection caused by *M. tuberculosis*. Although almost any tissue or organ of the body may be affected, the parts most often involved are the lungs, intestine, and kidneys in adults and the lungs, lymph nodes, bones, joints, and meninges in children.

**Pathology.** The reticuloendothelial system of the body provides the main line of cellular defense, and the term *tuberculosis* is derived from the small nodules of reticuloendothelial cells (tubercles), the unit lesions produced by *M. tuberculosis*.

*Primary tuberculosis (childhood type).* When tubercle bacilli first enter the body, the ensuing infection lasts several weeks, during which time the individual develops considerable immunity and a state of specific hypersensitivity to the tubercle bacillus. As a result, his tuberculin test becomes positive and remains so for his lifetime. The sequence of events in the first infection is termed the *primary complex*, and it may occur in the lungs (most commonly), in the intestinal tract, in the posterior pharynx, or in the skin (rarely). In the average person the primary complex is benign on the whole. The lesions in the lung heal or become latent without treatment. Most of these cases show residual calcification.

A feature of the primary complex is the extension of tubercle bacilli to the regional lymph nodes. With a primary complex in the lung the chest nodes are infected, as are the mesenteric nodes from the mucosal focus in the small bowel and the cervical lymph nodes from the mucosal focus in the tonsils, throat, or nasopharynx. Tuberculosis of the lymph nodes of the neck, or *scrofula*, is typically produced by the bovine tubercle bacillus as part of the primary complex it sets up in this area.

*Chronic pulmonary tuberculosis (adult type).* Chronic tuberculosis, adult type, from exogenous reinfection is considered to be quite rare. It may come from the progression of the primary infection. In a few persons, after a period of latency following the first infection, there is reactivation of dormant foci to produce the pattern of chronic disease. According to recent studies 5% of children with inactive untreated primary infection will develop the chronic pulmonary or extrapulmonary infection after the age of puberty, especially during adolescence.

Chronic tuberculosis is common in the lungs but may involve other sites in the body.

*The lesions.* The reactions obtained in a positive tuberculin test and the responses in sensitized tissues depend on the hypersensitive (allergic) state developed. As a consequence, lesions are produced that are typical of tuberculosis and not exactly duplicated in any other disease.

The reticuloendothelial system responds to the presence of tubercle bacilli by sending out macrophages to engulf them and to form restricting barriers around them. In their attack on the bacilli the macrophages form firm, round or oval, white, gray, or yellow nodules from 1 to 3 mm. in diameter, which are the *tubercles*. Microscopically a tubercle contains tubercle bacilli, epithelioid cells, and giant cells surrounded by a narrow band of lymphoid cells and encapsulated by fibrous tissue. Epithelioid cells are macrophages altered on contact with the fatty substances contained in the tubercle bacillus. The merging together of many macrophages results in a giant cell.

A tubercle may enlarge singly, or a number of small tubercles may coalesce to form a *conglomerate tubercle*. Because of the cellular reaction at the periphery of the tubercle, blood vessels are compressed, and the nutrition of the tubercle is disturbed. This

plus the lethal action of the tubercle bacilli themselves leads to a peculiar type of change in the center of the tubercle known as *caseation*, from the dry, granular, cheesy quality of the dead tissue.

Such a caseous focus may remain unchanged for a long time, or it may be altered pathologically. It may calcify. Calcification, the deposit of lime salts in dead tissue, is a reparative process. The caseous nodule may be organized, in which event the dead tissue is at least partially replaced by connective tissue. The end stage of organization is a scar. On the other hand, the caseous nodule may soften, and necrotic (dead) material may dissect through the tissues to form a so-called *cold abscess*. A caseous focus in the lung may release its contents into the lumen of a bronchus, forming a *cavity*. If a caseous area is situated near a body surface or a mucous membrane, the discharge of caseous material onto that surface leaves a *tuberculous ulcer*.

*Spread.* Tubercle bacilli may be spread in the lymph or bloodstream to different parts of the body. Infection may permeate adjacent tissues, move along natural passages (from the kidneys to the bladder via the ureters), and expand over a surface. Spread by blood and lymph is the usual way. Occasionally material heavily laden with tubercle bacilli (for example, the liquefied center of a tubercle) is discharged into a blood vessel, and infection is seeded widely over the body. Many small tubercles resembling millet seeds form in the lungs, spleen, liver, and various organs throughout the body. This is *miliary tuberculosis*. Discharge of the tuberculous material into the pulmonary artery seeds one or both lungs; extrusion into the portal vein seeds the liver. In these areas miliary tuberculosis is *localized*.

*Tuberculosis of the lungs. Pulmonary tuberculosis* (Fig. 25-1) is the usual form of the disease caused by the human bacillus. In hypersensitive adults tuberculosis involves the upper and posterior portions of the upper lobes, especially on the right side. This is *apical tuberculosis*.

Cavity formation is an important development in the course of pulmonary tuberculosis in adults. A tuberculous cavity may be only 1 or 2 cm. in diameter, or it may excavate a whole lobe of the lung. A cavity is formed when caseous material from a tuberculous focus is discharged into the lumen of a bronchus to be either coughed up or dispersed in the tracheobronchial tree. With a communication established between the excavated tuberculous focus and a bronchus, the newly formed cavity enlarges and becomes secondarily infected. Secondary infection is most often caused by streptococci or staphylococci and is frequently responsible for the hectic fever occurring in tuberculosis. Hemorrhage comes from

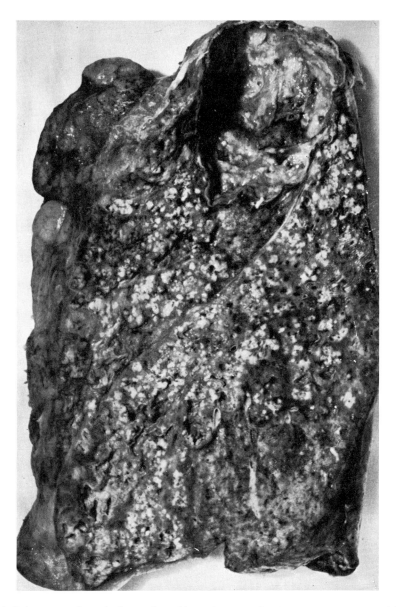

**Fig. 25-1.** Pulmonary tuberculosis, section of lung. Large cavity at apex; numerous grayish white tuberculous foci throughout rest of lung. (From Anderson, W. A. D., and Scotti, T. M.: Synopsis of pathology, ed 9, St. Louis, 1976, The C. V. Mosby Co.)

the erosion of a blood vessel in the wall of the cavity.

The body's attempts to check and heal even a progressively destructive tuberculous focus such as a cavity are reflected in a buildup of fibrous and scar tissue in the adjacent pulmonary tissues. Scar tissue replaces functioning pulmonary tissue, and contraction of the scar effects great shrinkage of the affected lung.

An acute form of pulmonary tuberculosis, *tuberculous pneumonia*, results from the sudden spilling of tuberculosis exudate into the sensitized air sacs of a large lung area. It is a manifestation of allergy.

*Tuberculous pleurisy* or *pleuritis* is secondary to tuberculosis of the lungs. Pleural effusion (collection of fluid in the pleural cavity) often accompanies it. *All unexplained pleural effusions should be considered of tuberculous origin until proved otherwise.*

*Tuberculosis of the intestine.* Tuberculosis of the intestine and regional mesenteric lymph nodes in adults is secondary to pulmonary tuberculosis. It develops because human tubercle bacilli are swallowed in the sputum raised from the tuberculous focus in the lung. (In children it is usually a primary infection caused by the ingestion of bovine bacilli in unpasteurized milk from tuberculous cows.) Intestinal tuberculosis affects the lower end of the ileum and the cecum. Tubercles and caseous foci form in the solitary lymphoid follicles and in Peyer's patches. The overlying epithelium breaks down, forming ulcers that tend to encircle the intestine. Perforation is not common, but the peritoneal surfaces of the ulcers become adherent to adjacent structures. Contraction of the scars formed in the healing of ulcers may lead to obstruction of the intestine.

*Tuberculous meningitis.* See p. 622.

**Laboratory diagnosis.** Direct microscopic examination of suspect material after it has been stained with an acid-fast stain is the first method to be used in the laboratory diagnosis of tuberculosis. *M. tuberculosis* is the only acid-fast organism regularly found in sputum. The failure to find tubercle bacilli in sputum does not rule out pulmonary disease, since the bacilli may not appear in the sputum until the disease is advanced. Moreover, they may occur plentifully in one specimen and be scanty or absent in the next. Tubercle bacilli are especially hard to find in smears of urine, cerebrospinal fluid, pleural fluid, joint fluid, and pus because of the relatively small number of organisms present, sometimes even with advanced disease. Various methods of concentration may be applied to the test material, especially sputum, if direct smears fail to reveal the bacilli.

The second step in the laboratory diagnosis of tuberculosis is the culture of suspicious material on special media devised for the growth of the tubercle bacillus, regardless of whether acid-fast organisms were demonstrated in the stained smear. The best media are the egg-containing ones, which are opaque, and those made of oleic acid agar, which are translucent. Earlier detection of colonies is possible on translucent media. Cultural methods require a number of days or weeks for the dry, crumbly, colorless colonies to form, sometimes even 10 to 12 weeks. When bacilli are not demonstrated directly in suitably prepared smears, they may frequently be found in cultures or by animal inoculation, the third step in laboratory diagnosis.

Some of the test material is injected subcutaneously into the groin of the extremely susceptible guinea pig.* If tubercle bacilli are present, the guinea pig becomes infected; the tissues about the site of inoculation thicken and may ulcerate; the inguinal

---

*Guinea pigs are very susceptible to both the human and bovine tubercle bacilli but are unaffected by the avian bacilli.

lymph nodes enlarge; a generalized tuberculosis develops; and the animal dies about 6 weeks after the inoculation. As a rule, the guinea pig is not allowed to die but is killed at a stated time and an autopsy performed when the disease is known to be far advanced.

Infection of a guinea pig with a given acid-fast bacillus may be used to indicate the virulence of that organism; this is the *guinea pig virulence test.* If it produces disease in the animal, it is, for practical purposes, the pathogenic *M. tuberculosis.* If it fails, it is a nonpathogenic acid-fast organism, with certain important exceptions (p. 256).

The bovine bacillus is more pathogenic for ordinary laboratory animals than is the human bacillus. When inoculated into a rabbit, the bovine bacillus kills the animal in 2 to 5 weeks, whereas the human bacillus kills it in about 6 months, and in some cases death does not occur at all.

There is presently a fluorescent antibody test in human tuberculosis that is applied to the serum (indirect fluorescent antibody).

**Tuberculin tests.** The tuberculin test depends on the fact that persons infected with tubercle bacilli are allergic to the tubercle bacillus and its products (tuberculin). If a scratch is made on the arm of a person at some time infected with tubercle bacilli and tuberculin is rubbed into the scratch (the *von Pirquet test*) or if some of the diluted tuberculin is injected *between the layers of the skin* (the *Mantoux test*), an area of redness and swelling appears at the site of inoculation. If the person has never been infected, no reaction occurs. In the patch test (the *Vollmer test*) a drop of ointment containing tuberculin or a small square of filter paper saturated with tuberculin is placed on the properly cleaned skin and held in place with adhesive tape for 48 hours. A positive test is indicated by redness and papule formation at the site of application.

The multiple-puncture technic (tuberculin *tine test*) applies tuberculin *transcutaneously.* Tuberculin four times the standard strength of old tuberculin is dried onto the tines of a small, specially constructed metal disk, backed by a plastic holder. It is packaged commercially as a sterile disposable unit. After the skin has been cleaned, the disk is applied briefly to the test area of skin with firm downward pressure, allowing the prongs to pierce the skin. Reactions to this technic are seen in Fig. 25-2.

The Mantoux test, performed with serial dilutions of tuberculin beginning with a high dilution (which contains less tuberculin) and descending to lower dilutions (which contain more tuberculin), is considered the most reliable of the tuberculin tests. The dose of tuberculin used in the Mantoux may be

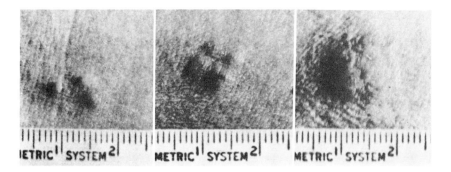

**Fig. 25-2.** Tine test—typical reactions with old tuberculin (OT). At 48 to 72 hours, readings should be made in good light with forearm slightly flexed. By inspection and gentle palpation, induration is determined, and diameter of largest single area taken in millimeters. Results: 5 mm. or more of induration—positive reaction; 2 to 4 mm.—doubtful reaction; and 2 mm. or no induration—negative. (Courtesy Lederle Laboratories, Pearl River, N.Y.)

given by jet gun. The intradermal wheal produced should be 6 to 10 mm. in diameter. In case-finding, multiple-puncture tests are practical and satisfactory for screening large groups, but a positive tine test, unless strongly reactive, should be confirmed with a Mantoux test.

The appearance of a positive tuberculin reaction indicates that tuberculous infection has occurred. Since many reach adulthood today in this country with a negative reaction, the circumstances under which there is conversion to a positive reaction may be known and the time that the infection was incurred approximated. The timing of the infection is important because it is in the early stages that tubercle bacilli proliferate very actively. Since infection *is* a recent event, a positive tuberculin reaction is a serious finding in the infant or young child. For all persons of any age with a positive tuberculin reaction, the best thinking is that a course of antituberculous therapy is advisable for at least 1 year. After a preliminary chest film, the individual is given isoniazid (see also p. 155) either singly or in combination with pyridoxine hydrochloride. In an adult where the presence of calcified lymph nodes in the chest indicates a process of long standing, such therapy is recommended because of the 5% to 10% hazard that this person will have active tuberculosis during his lifetime.

Positive reactions in the tests just described are known as *local* reactions. If tuberculin is given *beneath the skin*, two other reactions may occur, the *focal* and the *constitutional*. By focal reaction one means acute inflammation around a tuberculous focus in the body. This may have serious consequences; for instance, if the tuberculous focus is in the lung, a hemorrhage may result. By constitutional reaction one means systemic reaction with a sharp

rise in temperature and a feeling of malaise lasting for several hours.

**Immunity.** Whites possess considerable inherent resistance to tuberculosis but never complete immunity. The incidence of tuberculosis in blacks is high, averaging in proportion to population eight cases to one in whites. Not only is this true, but when the black contracts tuberculosis, the average time that he will live, if untreated, is about one-sixth that of the white who contracts tuberculosis. The American Indian and Mexican are also very susceptible to tuberculosis. The incidence of tuberculosis tends to be increased among doctors, nurses, and persons working directly with the disease.

Persons who live in isolated communities seem to be more vulnerable when exposed for the first time during adult life than are those who have been reared in closely crowded and highly infected communities.

Not so very long ago it was thought that tuberculosis was hereditary and ran in families, but tuberculosis runs in families because closely associated members of the family pass it to each other. Children of tuberculous parents may inherit certain predisposing factors, but a child born of tuberculous parents and at once removed to infection-free surroundings has a better chance of escaping tuberculosis than one born of healthy parents but reared in contact with tubercle bacilli.

The defensive factors that operate in a given infection depend on whether infection has occurred before. Most observers think that a degree of protection against subsequent infections is afforded the individual by the first infection. Whether a given infection means active disease depends on (1) the number of bacilli, (2) their virulence, (3) the state of allergy, and (4) the resistance of the subject. Conditions that lower body resistance are malnutrition, crowded housing, and predisposing diseases such as measles, whooping cough, and diabetes mellitus.

**Prevention.*** Since tuberculous sputum is the chief source of infection with human bacilli, it should be disposed of carefully. It should not be allowed to dry, for then it may be blown from place to place and the germs spread over a wide area. Sputum should be received in suitable covered containers and burned. Promiscuous spitting should be taboo. The patient must cover his mouth when he coughs. A tuberculous mother should not nurse her child. The woodwork of a room occupied by a tuberculous patient can be washed with soap and water, and a suitable disinfectant, usually one of the phenol derivatives, applied.

Eradication of tuberculous cows and the universal use of pasteurized milk control infection with the bovine bacillus.

In communities with the best type of health supervision there has been a decided decrease in the incidence of tuberculosis because of several factors, among which are better living conditions and medical prophylaxis. Mass surveys of the population by chest x-ray examination have been of great value in detecting pulmonary tuberculosis and other lung lesions as well. Radiographs of the chest at regular intervals are recommended for individuals whose work brings them into contact with active cases of tuberculosis.

## MYCOBACTERIUM BOVIS (THE BOVINE TUBERCLE BACILLUS)

*Mycobacterium bovis (M. tuberculosis* var. *bovis)* is highly virulent for man. Human infections caused by bovine bacilli were once very common in children and young people and affected the cervical lymph nodes (scrofula), intestines, mesenteric lymph nodes, and bones. Bovine bacilli cause pulmonary tuberculosis in cattle and can cause it in man. However, practically all pulmonary infections in children and adults result from the human bacillus.

The infection is acquired from the milk of tuberculous cows. In the cow, tuberculosis usually attacks the lungs, but since the cow swallows her sputum, the bacilli are excreted in the feces. The udder and flanks of the cow become contaminated, and the bacilli gain access to the milk, which, if consumed unpasteurized, is a source of infection. Sometimes the bacilli are excreted in the milk as it comes from the udder. This may occur without demonstrable tuberculous lesions in the udder.

The tuberculin reaction is of inestimable value in

---

*For BCG vaccination see pp. 399 and 414.

detecting tuberculous cows. Routine tuberculin testing of cattle by the U.S. Department of Agriculture and elimination of infected cattle from the herd, plus the pasteurization of milk, have practically eliminated bovine infection in the United States. In countries where no such safeguards exist, the bovine bacillus is responsible for 15% to 30% of the cases of tuberculosis in the young ages.

## Leprosy

Leprosy* is a chronic communicable disease caused by *Mycobacterium leprae* (Hansen's bacillus)* that involves skin, mucous membranes, and nerves. Leprosy has affected man from the beginning of history, and descriptions of it occupy a prominent place in the Old Testament and other ancient writings. It is estimated that presently there are about 15 million patients with leprosy in the world, with approximately 2000 in the United States.

## MYCOBACTERIUM LEPRAE (THE LEPROSY BACILLUS)

*Mycobacterium leprae (M. leprae)* is an acid-fast organism closely resembling *M. tuberculosis*. It occurs abundantly in the lesions of leprosy. The bacillus of leprosy has been cultivated in the ears and rear footpads of white mice and hamsters, sites chosen as the largest and coolest parts of the experimental animal. After many months mild changes detectable with the microscope occur at the sites of inoculation, but there is no gross advanced disease. The bacillus has also been grown in tissue culture.

**Mode of infection.** The imagination of man has clothed leprosy with many attributes it does not possess. One is that it is a highly communicable disease. This is not true. Man contracts leprosy only after prolonged and intimate contact, and even then he often escapes infection. The bacilli leave the body in great numbers from degenerating lesions of the skin and mucous membranes, and spread is directly from person to person. Nose and mouth discharges are especially dangerous because lesions are very common in these locations. The portals of entry are probably skin and mucous membranes. Small breaks in the skin may admit organisms discharged from a patient with the disease. Although the bacteria prefer certain cool sites, they are spread widely over the body. They may be found in feces and urine. The

---

*Discovered in Norway by Gerhard Hansen (1841-1912) in 1874, *Mycobacterium leprae* was actually the first bacterium implicated as a cause of human disease. For nearly a century it remained the only one known to infect man that could *not* be cultured in the laboratory and that did not produce progressive disease if inoculated into a test animal.

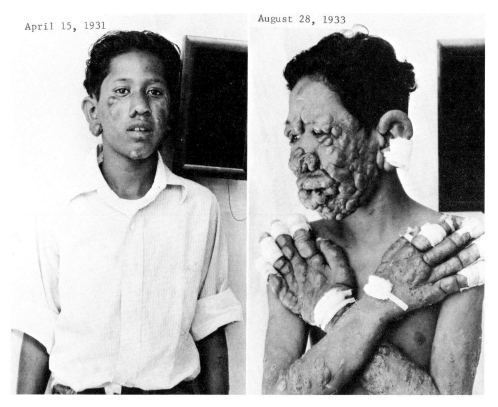

**Fig. 25-3.** Leprosy. Progression in a teen-aged Filipino. (Note dates—this occurred before sulfone drugs were available.) (Courtesy Dr. C. Binford, Washington, D.C.)

disease is not hereditary, but since children are un-usually susceptible, the percentage of infection in children associated with leprous parents is very high (30% to 40%). The highly variable incubation period is usually estimated from 5 to 15 years.

**Pathogenicity.** Leprosy (Fig. 25-3) belongs with the infectious granulomas (diseases in which a de-fensive multiplication of reticuloendothelial cells occurs at the site of infection). Although it is general-ized with a variety of changes, there are two con-spicuous patterns. One, the *lepromatous* or *nodular* form, is marked by tumorlike growths of the skin and mucous membranes. The other, *tuberculoid* or *anes-thetic* leprosy, is manifest by involvement of peripheral nerves, with localized areas of skin anesthesia. The end stages of the disease are associated with extensive deformity and the destruction of tissue (Fig. 25-3).

The earliest lesion in leprosy may be diagnostic in that it contains acid-fast bacilli. Since it may not indicate the subsequent course of the disease, it is referred to as an *indeterminate* lesion. *Dimorphous leprosy* refers to the coexistence of the two forms—lepromatous and tuberculoid.

**Laboratory diagnosis.** The organism *M. leprae*

occurs abundantly in the lesions of leprosy. A diag-nosis of leprosy is most often made with scrapings from the nasal septum or in biopsies of the skin of the ear that have been stained for acid-fast bacilli. Fluorochrome staining (Fig. 25-4) can be done on leprae bacilli. The bacilli in large numbers are found within phagocytic cells packed together like packets of cigars. Bacilli may also be demonstrated in acid-

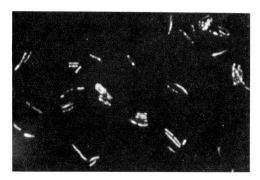

**Fig. 25-4.** *Mycobacterium leprae,* fluorescent staining. Note morphology. (×1000.) (Courtesy Dr. R. E. Mansfield, Can-ton, Ill.)

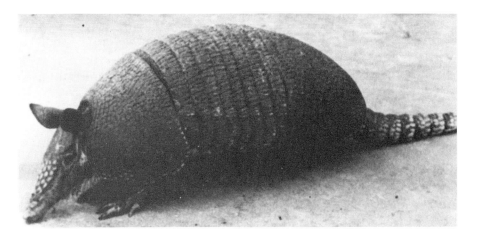

**Fig. 25-5.** Armadillo (nine-banded), *Dasypus novemcinctus* Linn. (Courtesy Dr. E. E. Storrs, New Iberia, La.)

fast stained material from lesions elsewhere in the skin and lymph nodes. Leprosy and tubercle bacilli are separated by guinea pig inoculation, since leprosy bacilli have no effect on the animal.

No animal shares a susceptibility to leprosy comparable to man except the armadillo (Fig. 25-5). The discovery has been made only recently that this creature develops leprosy some 3 years after initial infection and it plays host to an enormous profusion of organisms. The experimental animals also succumb to a more severe disease, showing involvement of the central nervous system and lungs, areas spared in human beings.

*Lepromin* is a suspension of killed leprosy bacilli used in a skin test to detect susceptibility to this disease.

**Prevention.** Leprosy is best prevented by good living conditions. Prolonged and intimate contact with patients is hazardous. Strict isolation with segregation has not proved completely successful as a method of control, but most persons in the United States discharging *M. leprae* are referred to the national leprosarium, the U.S. Public Health Service Hospital at Carville, Louisiana.

A patient who has improved and has failed to discharge the bacilli for a period of 6 months may be paroled. Paroled patients should be examined twice yearly. Back home, the patient should be semisegregated, with his own room, linens, and dishes. His discharges, cooking utensils, and linens should be carefully disinfected. No children or young people should live in the house. Children of lepers should be separated from their parents at birth because the chances of infection are much greater in infants and young children. All persons who contact a patient should be examined every 6 months.

Results of clinical trials in eastern Uganda in Africa indicate that BCG vaccine protects children against leprosy. The possibility of such a surrogate vaccine strengthens the case for a cross immunity among mycobacteria.

## Mycobacteriosis
### OTHER MYCOBACTERIA (ATYPICAL, ANONYMOUS, UNCLASSIFIED MYCOBACTERIA)*

**The organisms.** In tuberculosis hospitals over the United States unusual acid-fast bacilli are found in the sputum of patients with a typical setting for tuberculosis and cavitary disease by x-ray examination. Although they are able to cause pulmonary disease mimicking tuberculosis (*mycobacteriosis*), these acid-fast organisms differ sharply from the tubercle bacillus. They can also cause infection in lymph nodes and skin. Infections are usually chronic, variably destructive granulomas.

**Classification.** These mycobacteria are differentiated from *M. tuberculosis* by their colonial characteristics, biochemical reactions,† susceptibility to antituberculous drugs, and animal pathogenicity. Although species identification is important here, these organisms are commonly considered in four categories (Table 25-1). In group I the photochromogens produce yellow-orange colonies in the light. *Mycobacterium kansasii* ("yellow bacillus"), the representative

---

*"MOTT" bacilli (*m*ycobacteria *o*ther *t*han *t*ubercle bacilli). They have been referred to as anonymous or unclassified because most of them up until recently were not adequately identified to permit assignment to a definite species.
†In the clinical setting, production of niacin (p. 71) by an acid-fast bacillus identifies it as the human tubercle bacillus.

**Table 25-1**

Pathogenicity of anonymous mycobacteria

| GROUP AND COMMON NAME | SOME SIGNIFICANT MEMBERS | NIACIN TEST* | PATHOGENICITY FOR | | |
|---|---|---|---|---|---|
| | | | MAN | GUINEA PIG | MOUSE |
| I Photochromogens | *Mycobacterium kansasii* | Negative | + | − | + |
| | *Mycobacterium marinum (balnei)* | | | | |
| II Scotochromogens | *Mycobacterium scrofulaceum* | Negative | + | − | − |
| III Nonphotochromogens | *Mycobacterium intracellulare* | Negative | +,− | − | +,− |
| | *Mycobacterium xenopi* | | | | |
| IV Rapid growers | *Mycobacterium fortuitum* | Negative | +,− | − | +,− |
| | *Mycobacterium chelonei* | | | | |

*Niacin test positive with *Mycobacterium tuberculosis.*

of this group, is a respiratory pathogen. Group I members are most closely associated with human pulmonary disease.

The scotochromogens of group II produce a yellow to orange pigment in the dark as well as in the light. *Mycobacterium scrofulaceum* is the example. It causes cervical lymphadenitis in children.

Not affected by light, the nonphotochromogens of group III form buff-colored colonies, soft in consistency by comparison with the rough ones of the tubercle bacillus. These include the Battey bacillus (*Mycobacterium intracellulare*) and other respiratory pathogens.

The rapid growers of group IV form colonies on simple media within a short time, even at room temperature. Their nonpigmented colonies most closely resemble those of the tubercle bacillus. The pathogen of note here, among many saprophytes, is *Mycobacterium fortuitum*. Group IV mycobacteria produce subcutaneous abscesses following trauma to the skin.

*Mycobacterium smegmatis* (the smegma bacillus) is an acid-fast bacillus widespread in dust, soil, and water. It is of no importance as a disease producer, but because it is a normal resident of the prepuce and vulva, it may gain access to urine and be mistaken for *M. tuberculosis* unless the specimen is properly collected. Smegma bacilli are sometimes found in feces. They are differentiated from tubercle bacilli by their growth pattern and by the fact that they do not produce disease in guinea pigs. They are now placed in group IV.

The pathogenicity of members of groups I, III, and IV is established; that of group II less definite. All the mycobacteria except those in group II cause disease in the mouse; none is pathogenic for the guinea pig.

The tuberculin test in mycobacteriosis is negative or weakly positive. A tuberculin reaction less than 10 mm. in diameter may represent the cross reaction to "unclassified" mycobacterial sensitivity.

**Transmission.** Much remains to be learned of the mode of spread and the source of these mycobacteria. Their tolerance for adverse environments and their survival in sparse media are consistent with their wide dispersion in nature. Man's environment probably serves as the source of the organisms. A wide host range of wild and domestic animals may exist. Some of the group I mycobacteria are found in raw milk and can survive the temperature of pasteurization. The Battey bacilli may spread to man from the soil. Mycobacteriosis is not contagious.

## Questions for review

1 What are the salient features of acid-fast organisms?
2 Name and describe the acid-fast bacilli causing human tuberculosis.
3 Classify acid-fast bacteria and indicate their pathogenicity.
4 Discuss the sources of infection in tuberculosis.
5 Outline the laboratory diagnosis of tuberculosis.
6 Give the technics for and the significance of the tuberculin test.
7 How should tuberculin tine tests be evaluated?
8 Compare the tubercle bacillus with mycobacteria of mycobacteriosis.
9 Compare the tubercle bacillus with Hansen's bacillus.
10 Briefly characterize leprosy.
11 What provision does the United States Public Health Service make for the care of patients with leprosy?
12 Define: tuberculin, tubercle, scotochromogen, cavity, infectious granuloma, scrofula, miliary, "MOTT" bacilli, smegma bacilli, primary complex, Battey bacilli, "yellow bacillus," tuberculoid leprosy, lepromatous leprosy, lepromin.

**References on pp. 276 to 280.**

# CHAPTER 26

# Miscellaneous microbes

## Pseudomonas species

The family *Pseudomonadaceae* of strictly aerobic, straight or curved rods contains the genus *Pseudomonas* of soil and water bacteria, notable among which are the water-soluble, fluorescent pigments of some species. The genus *Pseudomonas* contains some pathogens for animals and man, producing a variety of diseases, and many pathogens for plants.

### PSEUDOMONAS AERUGINOSA

**The organism.** The organism of blue pus, *Pseudomonas aeruginosa*, is an actively motile, gram-negative, nonsporeforming, oxidase-positive bacillus (Fig. 26-1). When stained with simple stains, it resembles *Corynebacterium diphtheriae*. It is unique for the diffusion of a blue pigment (pyocyanin and fluorescein) through the medium on which it is grown, and the same color is seen in the purulent discharges it produces in disease. Green pigment belongs to several species of bacteria, but the blue color seems to be specific for *Pseudomonas aeruginosa*.* Aging, surface-grown cultures of *Pseudomonas aeruginosa* display a diffuse bright iridescence (metallic sheen) over the growth. Varied explanations are given for the *iridescent phenomenon*, including the one that it reflects phage action, but the mechanism is not understood. Cultures of this microbe have an odor like that of fermented grapes.

**Its potential.** *Pseudomonas aeruginosa* is widely found in water and soil and often as a normal inhabitant of the skin and intestinal tract in man and animals. Ordinarily it is but mildly pathogenic and causes primary infections only when the resistance of the host is lowered. However, it is a problem in young infants (Fig. 26-2) and the aged and, as a secondary invader, often delays the repair of wounds. Among the diseases that it may effect are otitis media, abscesses, wound infections, sinus infections, and

bronchopneumonia (Fig. 26-3). It is also an important cause of gram-negative shock (mortality, 80%), urinary tract infections, and the sepsis complicating severe burns. The way *Pseudomonas aeruginosa* brings about disease is unclear. It is known to possess an endotoxin and to produce certain extracellular substances including a collagenase, lecithinase, lipase, and hemolysin. The necrosis of tissue, a striking feature of infection with this microbe, is thought related to its necrotizing proteolytic enzymes (proteases).

This organism is more resistant to the chemical disinfectants usually employed than are other gram-negative bacilli, but it can be killed by exposure to a temperature of 55° C. for 1 hour. In the treatment of *Pseudomonas* infections polymyxin and colistin, rather toxic drugs, are often the only antibiotics to which the organisms are susceptible. Since *Pseudomonas aeruginosa* is resistant to the action of most antibiotics, it tends to become the dominant organism in a diseased area after extended antimicrobial therapy has eliminated the primary ones. Then it takes on a vigorous disease-producing quality and is responsible for significant destruction of tissue, especially with lowered host resistance. Such infections with *Pseudomonas aeruginosa* are formidable. Microscopically, there is massive overgrowth of the organisms in the areas of dead tissue.

The sources of *Pseudomonas aeruginosa* in hospital-acquired infections are many, but especially the pieces of equipment that are hard to clean and sterilize, such as face masks, certain kinds of humid rubber tubing, water containers, nebulizers, and parts of the intermittent positive-pressure breathing machines. A source easily overlooked is the hospital supply of distilled water. This is a serious hazard because of the widespread need for distilled water in preparation of various hospital solutions—detergents, disinfectants, and even parenteral medications. Pseudomonads have been demonstrated not only to survive but also to multiply rapidly in distilled water and seem to have a greater resistance to antimicrobial

---

*Pathogenic pseudomonads produce a great deal of fluorescein. With the Wood's ultraviolet light, this pigment is readily detected even under the black, silver-stained eschar of a burn wound that has been treated with silver nitrate.

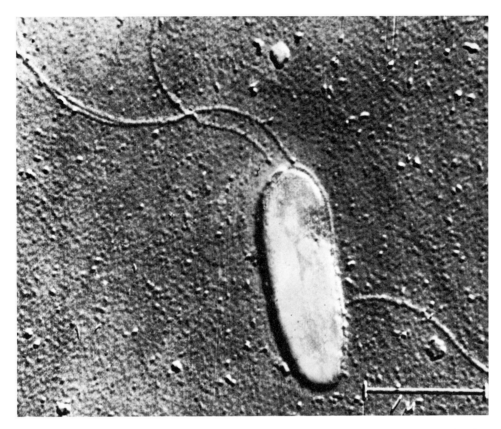

**Fig. 26-1.** *Pseudomonas aeruginosa,* electron micrograph. Note flagella. (Courtesy J. B. Roerig Division, Pfizer Inc., New York.)

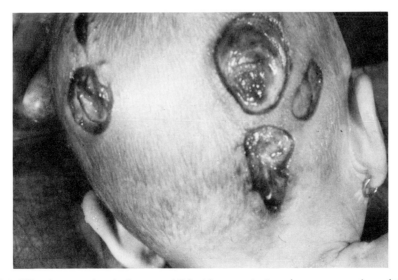

**Fig. 26-2.** Skin ulcers on head of young child with systemic *Pseudomonas aeruginosa* infection.

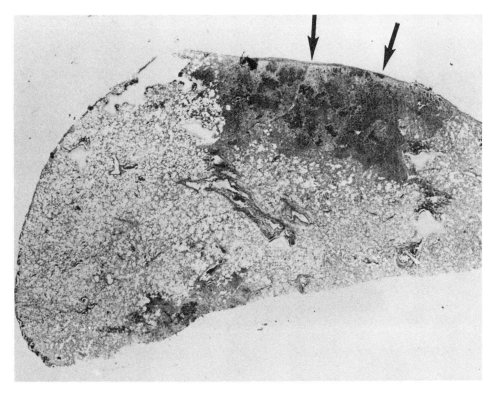

**Fig. 26-3.** Bronchopneumonia caused by *Pseudomonas aeruginosa*. A well-defined, solidified, darkened portion is sharply distinct in thin slice of air-containing lung. Focus of disease is hemorrhagic and partly necrotic.

agents than do the ones recovered from laboratory media.

Patients with 40% or more burned surface area are vulnerable to *Pseudomonas* sepsis. Administration of a septivalent *Pseudomonas* vaccine to these seriously burned persons is a great advance in the management of their injury. It dramatically reduces the mortality.

### PSEUDOMONAS PSEUDOMALLEI

The pseudomonad, *Pseudomonas pseudomallei* is a gram-negative, motile, nonpigmented bacillus that produces *melioidosis*, an uncommon tropical disease of man and animals. Its pulmonary manifestations are easily confused with those of tuberculosis. There may be a septicemia, with widespread lesions over the body. Nicknamed the "Vietnamese time bomb," the disease can be dormant for a number of years only to appear suddenly, become active, and lead to death within days or weeks. The disease is endemic in Southeast Asia, where the organism is saprophytic in surface waters, soil (notably the rice fields), and organic matter. The epidemiology and transmission of the disease are not known. The or-

ganisms are thought to enter the body by way of the mouth and nose or through open wounds in the skin.

Growth of the bacilli is characteristically crinkly in cultures. A hemagglutination test is available for diagnostic study.

### PSEUDOMONAS MALLEI

Glanders (farcy) is primarily a disease of horses, mules, and donkeys, which may be transmitted to man. Cattle are immune. It is characterized by the formation of ulcerating, tubercle-like nodules in the lungs, superficial lymph nodes, and mucous membranes. If lymph nodes are affected, the disease is known as *glanders;* if mucous membranes, it is *farcy*. With the replacement of the horse by the automobile, this once prevalent disease is now rare.

The cause, *Pseudomonas (Actinobacillus) mallei*, is a narrow, sometimes slightly curved, small bacillus, that is gram-negative, nonmotile, nonencapsulated, nonsporeforming and has little resistance to physical and chemical agents. Man is easily infected if he contacts tissues or excreta of diseased animals, since these contain virulent bacilli. The microbes enter the body by a wound, scratch, or abrasion of the skin.

**Laboratory diagnosis.** Glanders is diagnosed in man and animals by the isolation of the bacilli from the lesions or in blood cultures. There is a complement fixation test. The skin test utilizes *mallein,* a product of *Pseudomonas mallei,* injected subcutaneously in animals. Mallein tablets are placed in the conjunctival sac. If infectious material is injected intraperitoneally into a male guinea pig, the testicular swelling and generalized reaction within 3 or 4 days give the *Straus reaction.*

**Prevention.** No immunity exists to glanders. Control depends on destruction of animals with clinical or occult disease and on disinfection of stables, blankets, harnesses, and drinking troughs used by sick animals.

## Vibrio species

In the family Vibrionaceae are rigid, gram-negative, straight or curved rods, facultatively anaerobic, found in fresh water and seawater. In its member genus *Vibrio* are the agents of cholera and vibriosis.

### VIBRIO CHOLERAE (THE COMMA BACILLUS)

**The organism.** Cholera is caused by *Vibrio cholerae* (*V. cholerae*). Formerly known as *Vibrio comma,* the comma bacillus is a small, comma-shaped, motile, gram-negative rod. It multiplies rapidly in the lumen of the small bowel and produces a powerful exo-enterotoxin that acts on the lining of the bowel to induce copious loss of water and essential salts. This explains the fecal discharges being described as "rice water"—clear, not malodorous, with flecks of mucus. Organisms abound in the stools. There are three immunologic types, the Inaba, Ogawa, and Hikojima.

The cholera vibrio grows aerobically on routine laboratory media. If a few drops of sulfuric acid are added to a growth of cholera vibrios in nitrate-peptone broth, a red color develops, the *cholera red reaction.*

**The disease.** Asiatic cholera is a specific infectious disease that affects the lower portion of the intestine and is described by violent purging, vomiting, burning thirst, muscular cramps, suppression of urine, and rapid collapse. Untreated, it can be a terrifying disease with a 70% or more mortality. Only plague causes as much panic. With massive diarrhea the patient's fluid losses are enormous—10 to 20 quarts a day. With severe rapid dehydration death comes within hours. Four great pandemics spread over the world during the eighteenth century, and on two occasions in the nineteenth century the disease invaded the United States: in 1832 in New York City and in 1848 in New Orleans, whence it spread up

the Mississippi Valley. The disease is endemic in India and China. The "scourge of antiquity," it originated in India in the vicinity of Calcutta and on the delta of the Ganges River, where it was known at the time of Alexander the Great.

**Mode of infection.** The disease is contracted by the ingestion of water or food contaminated by the excreta of persons harboring the bacilli. Man is the only host. The bacilli leave the body in the feces, urine, and secretions of the mouth. As a rule, the feces become free of bacilli during the last days of the disease, but some patients become convalescent carriers. Permanent carriers do not occur.

Cholera today is rampant in the areas of the world occupied by better than half the world's population where, because of low standards of sanitation, human excrement easily contaminates the waterways and surface wells that are sources of drinking water. Vibrios may live in water for as long as 2 weeks.

As a disease cholera should be only a historical note. Modern sanitation can eliminate waste-contaminated water supplies, the primary source of infection, and modern medical treatment can effectively deal with it.

**Immunity.** The immunity occurring after an attack of cholera is short-lived. The risk of reinfection is only slightly less than that of the initial infection. Although vaccination is done against cholera, to date, a truly effective vaccine would still be an experimental

**Table 26-1**

Classic cholera vibrio compared with El Tor biotype

| | VIBRIO CHOLERAE | VIBRIO CHOLERAE BIOTYPE *ELTOR* |
|---|---|---|
| Voges-Proskauer test | − | + |
| Production of indole | + | + |
| Liquefaction of gelatin | + | + |
| Production of hydrogen sulfide | − | − |
| Cholera red reaction | + | + |
| Fermentation of glucose | + | + |
| Fermentation of lactose | Slow | Slow |
| Hemolysis of sheep (or goat) cells | − | + |
| Hemagglutination of chicken cells | − | + |
| Phage lysis | Susceptible | Resistant |

one and therefore not widely available. An experimental "toxoid" has been put to field trial.

### Vibrio cholerae biotype eltor

A biotype to *V. cholerae*, more resistant to physical and chemical agents and in itself quite virulent, is *Vibrio cholerae* biotype *eltor* (*Vibrio El Tor*). Unlike the classic cholera vibrio, the El Tor vibrio produces a hemolysin that lyses the red cells of sheep and goats. (See Table 26-1 for comparison of the two.) It causes cholera and in recent times has been more significant than the classic vibrio as the cause of pandemics in South and Southeast Asia. The current one is the seventh resulting from this biotype.

### VIBRIO PARAHAEMOLYTICUS

A vibrio like the classic one, *Vibrio parahaemolyticus* is a major cause of a gastroenteritis with manifestations similar to the classic disease (a vibriosis). In countries such as Japan it is responsible for 50% to 60% of cases of "summer diarrhea." Widely distributed as a marine microorganism, it is an important cause of "food poisoning" where seafood has been consumed, and it can infect wounds incurred along the seashore. It is a small halophilic vibrio giving a negative cholera red reaction. Present vaccines are of no effect against it.

## Bacillus anthracis (the anthrax bacillus)

Known since antiquity, anthrax (charbon) is an acute infectious disease caused by *Bacillus anthracis* (*B. anthracis*). It is primarily a disease of lower animals, especially cattle and sheep, but it is easily communicated to man. Horses and hogs may become infected. Anthrax is worldwide in distribution but, with the exception of certain restricted areas, is unusual in the United States.

In man anthrax presents in two forms: *external* (malignant pustule or carbuncle and anthrax edema) and *internal* (pulmonary anthrax or woolsorters' disease and intestinal anthrax). External anthrax is the more common. Because of the fever and enlargement of the spleen that accompany the disease, anthrax is often called splenic fever. The incubation period for external anthrax is 1 to 5 days.

In the body of an animal dead of acute disease, there is little change other than the dark blood and a swollen spleen.

**General characteristics.** The organism *B. anthracis* is quite large, in fact one of the largest bacterial pathogens. It forms spores and is gram-positive. The swollen and concave ends of the bacilli give the chains of bacilli the appearance of bamboo rods. The organism grows in the presence of oxygen and also in its absence. It is the only sporeforming aerobic pathogenic bacterium and, unlike most sporeforming aerobic bacteria, is nonmotile. Since spores are not formed in the absence of oxygen, they are not formed in the animal body. In the blood and tissues of infected animals, the anthrax bacillus is surrounded by a capsule. Growth is luxuriant on all ordinary culture media. Spores retain their vitality for years and are extremely resistant to heat and chemical disinfectants in the concentrations ordinarily used. They are fairly susceptible to sunlight.

*B. anthracis* is of historic interest because it was the first pathogenic organism to be seen under the microscope, the first one *proved* to be the cause of a specific disease, the first one to be grown in a pure culture, and the organism that Pasteur used in his classic experiments on artificial immunization.

**Modes of infection.** Animals usually become infected via the intestinal route while grazing in infected pastures. Buzzards carry the infection long distances and contaminate soil and water with organisms on their feet and beaks. Dogs discharge spores in their feces after eating the carcasses of infected animals. This disease is sometimes transmitted from animal to animal or from animal to man by greenhead flies and houseflies.

In man, anthrax is primarily an occupational disease confined to those who handle animals and animal products, such as hair and hides. Imported animal products are of special danger. The commonest route of infection is through wounds or abrasions of the skin (cutaneous route of infection). In numerous cases of anthrax, infection of the face by the bristles of cheap shaving brushes has been reported. The pulmonary form of anthrax is caused by inhalation of dust containing the spores (respiratory route of infection) and endangers those who handle dry hides, wool, or hair. The intestinal form of anthrax is acquired by ingestion of infected milk or insufficiently cooked food (intestinal route of infection). The bacilli leave the body in the exudate of the local lesion (malignant pustule) and in the sputum, feces, and urine.

**Prevention.** Patients with anthrax should be isolated. The dressings of external lesions should be burned, and the person doing the dressings should wear gloves. The feces, urine, sputum, and other excreta should be disinfected at once to prevent the formation of spores. The disinfectant should be strong and applied for a long time. Phenol, 5%, is probably the best one. The local lesions of anthrax should not be traumatized as by squeezing, since this may cause the bacilli to invade the bloodstream.

The possibility of confusing a malignant pustule with an ordinary boil is so important that a description of the former is not out of place. A malignant pustule begins as a small, hard, red area; a small vesicle soon develops in the center. The area increases in size, vesicles develop at the periphery, and the surrounding tissues become swollen. The center of the lesion softens, and a dark eschar forms. Pain is not present, and the draining lymph nodes are swollen.

Infected animals should be separated from the herd. The bodies of animals dead of anthrax should be completely burned if possible. Their blood should not be allowed to escape, and their bodies should not be opened for autopsy except by an experienced veterinarian, since the bacilli form spores when exposed to the air. If the body is buried, it should be packed with lime and buried at least 3 feet in the ground. When infection occurs in a herd, the pasture must be changed, and the herd quarantined. A sharp watch should be kept for new cases, and the quarantine should not be lifted until 3 weeks after the last case. Cattle that have been vaccinated and survive an epidemic must not be taken to slaughter for 42 days. Milk from infected herds should not be used. Hides, hair, and shaving brushes should be sterilized. If the soil becomes contaminated, it remains infectious for years. The best soil disinfectant is lye. Anthrax spores from buried animals have been brought to the surface by earthworms.

Prophylactic vaccination of animals against anthrax must be carried out with vigor. Cattle and sheep may be actively immunized with a vaccine that contains living but attenuated bacteria. Dead bacteria are without effect. A therapeutic serum has been prepared by immunizing horses against anthrax bacilli.

An anthrax vaccine prepared from a culture filtrate of an avirulent strain is available for laboratory workers at risk and for workers in occupations exposed to the disease.

## Lactobacillus species (the lactobacilli)

The lactobacilli are gram-positive, microaerophilic rods that produce lactic acid from carbohydrates and are able to live in a more highly acid environment than most other bacteria. They are widely distributed in nature and out of character as disease producers. Many are normal inhabitants of the alimentary tract. Most are nonmotile. Since they require many essential growth factors for their metabolism, they are used commercially in the bioassay of the B complex vitamins and certain amino acids. They are a more sensitive index than current chemical methods. They also are used extensively in the fermentation and dairy industries.

Some of the noteworthy members* of the genus are *Lactobacillus delbrueckii,* *Lactobacillus acidophilus,* *Lactobacillus bulgaricus,* and *Lactobacillus casei.* *Lactobacillus delbrueckii* is the type species. *Lactobacillus acidophilus,* a normal inhabitant of the intestinal tract, is increased by a diet rich in milk or carbohydrates. The *Boas-Oppler bacillus,* found in the stomach in gastric cancer, is most likely the same organism. *Lactobacillus bulgaricus* was isolated from Bulgarian fermented milk and is the organism that Metchnikoff thought would prevent intestinal putrefaction and thereby increase length of life. *Lactobacillus casei* is most often used in the bioassay of vitamins and amino acids. *Lactobacillus* species make up the normal flora of the vagina during a woman's active reproductive years, where they are referred to collectively as *Döderlein's bacilli.*

---

*\*Lactobacillus bifidus,* found in the intestine of breast-fed infants, is now classified as *Bifidobacterium bifidum,* the type species of that genus.

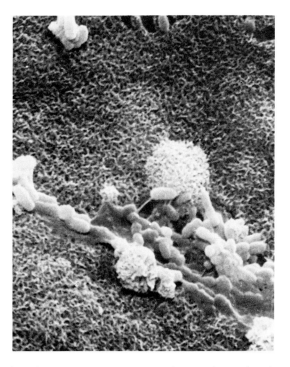

**Fig. 26-4.** *Streptococcus mutans* in experimental cariogenesis, scanning electron micrograph. Note cocci attached to toothlike surface, "mesh" of which corresponds to salivary pellicle, the thin surface film of adsorbed glycoproteins from saliva. After bacteria caught to pellicle were incubated in 1% glucose, they synthesized glucan, the extracellular glue of the micrograph. (Courtesy Dr. W. B. Clark, Boston.)

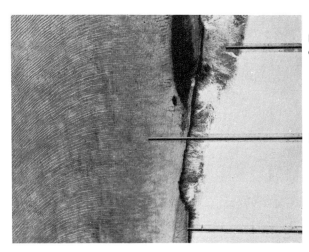

Plaque (microbial growth, debris, desquamated cells)

Dentin (ivory of tooth)

Thin layer of cementum covering dentin

**Fig. 26-5.** Early dental decay (plaque), microscopic section. Microbial growth is associated with debris, mucus, and desquamated cells. The action of acid-producing bacteria, including lactobacilli, on sugars in the food results in an accumulation of lactic acid, believed to trigger process of decay by decalcifying enamel of tooth. (From Bhaskar, S. N.: Synopsis of oral pathology, ed. 3, St. Louis, 1969, The C. V. Mosby Co.)

**Dental caries.** Dental caries (tooth decay) is one of the most widespread of disorders; it is estimated that every American has at least 3. The factors implicated in the pathogenesis of caries and determining their severity are (1) individual susceptibility, (2) presence of bacteria capable of producing organic acids, and (3) presence of carbohydrates to support the cariogenic activities of the acid-producing microorganisms. Some of the lactobacilli and certain acid-producing streptococci, notably *Streptococcus mutans,* are found in the mouth associated with tooth decay, and most observers believe that they play a role, especially *Streptococcus mutans,* whose cariogenic property is nicely shown in experimental animals (Fig. 26-4). The first attack on tooth structure is postulated to come from the acid-producing bacteria. *Streptococcus mutans* produces an enzyme, dextran-sucrase, that converts sucrose of food eaten to dextran. Dextran combines with salivary proteins to create on tooth surfaces a sticky, colorless film called a plaque (Fig. 26-5). Plaque piles up continuously on teeth, reforming after removal at any given time. The plaque provides a haven for bacteria from which they can undermine and demineralize the enamel of a tooth. Subsequently with breakdown of tooth enamel, the typical cavity appears. Fragments of debris found therein support continued bacterial growth and thus tend to perpetuate the process of decay.

## Listeria monocytogenes

*Listeria monocytogenes* is a small (less than 2 $\mu$m. [$\mu$] long), gram-positive, aerobic to microaerophilic, nonsporeforming, motile coccobacillus that affects man and a great variety of animals. The coccobacillus causes disease (listeriosis) characterized by an increase in large mononuclear leukocytes (monocytes) in the bloodstream. It produces an encephalitis or an encephalomyelitis, especially in ruminant animals. In man the most prominent manifestation is a purulent meningitis. Infection can also be widely disseminated. Listeriosis is seen as encephalitis, conjunctivitis, endocarditis, urethritis, or septicemia with multiple abscesses. Untreated, it is fatal in 90% of cases. Involving the fetus and newborn infant, *granulomatosis infantiseptica* is an intrauterine listerelial infection associated with widespread necrosis of the internal organs and hemorrhagic areas in the skin. The newborn infant usually dies within 2 or 3 days. Although human listeriosis is rare, the number of cases in man and in poultry and livestock is increasing. It is a hazard to the compromised host, especially the baby and the old person.

From specimens of blood, spinal fluid, and pus the organism can be identified by cultural methods in the laboratory. It produces beta hemolysis and is novel in that it can grow at the temperature of the refrigerator. A highly specific test for identification of the organism utilizes the rabbit; the everted eyelid of the animal is swabbed with the culture. Typically the reaction to the presence of *Listeria* is the development of purulent keratoconjunctivitis. *Listeria monocytogenes* is widely distributed in nature and can be recovered from such diverse sources as man and animal feces, ferrets, insects, sewage, silage, and decaying vegeta-

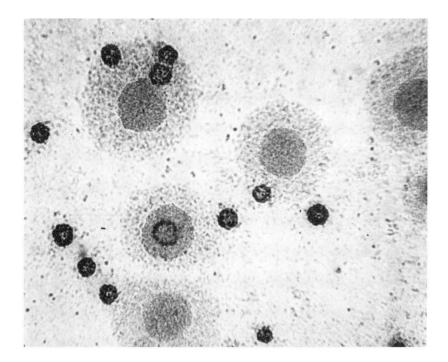

**Fig. 26-6.** Mycoplasmas. Mixture of classic *(Mycoplasma hominis)* colonies and smaller, very dark colonies of T (T-strain) mycoplasmas. Direct test for urease (that of Shepard and Howard) has been applied to this preparation. Colonies of T-strain mycoplasmas are urease-positive, showing dark bronze color of reaction product. Note fried-egg appearance of classic colonies. (×300.) (From Shepard, M. C., and Howard, D. R.: Ann. N.Y. Acad. Sci. **174:**809, 1970.)

tion. The transmission of listeriosis in man and animals is not known.

## Mycoplasma species

Mycoplasmas are out of the ordinary. They do not have a cell wall, and because they do not, they demonstrate a set of remarkable and unusual features. In the recent edition of *Bergey's Manual,* they are segregated into Part 19. The classification begins with Class Mollicutes to encompass the delicate coccoid to filamentous procaryotic microbes with a "pliable cell boundary." Gram-negative, nonmotile, tiny, some are so small as to be ultramicroscopic (about 200 nm.). Order I, Mycoplasmatales, and Family I, Mycoplasmataceae, gather the ones needing sterol for continued growth. Mycoplasmas are everywhere. They are saprophytes, parasites, and pathogens for a wide range of hosts.

**General characteristics.** Mycoplasmas (pleuropneumonia-like organisms, PPLO's) are smaller than ordinary bacteria and about the size of the larger viruses; in fact, they are the smallest microorganisms that can be cultivated on cell-free media (Fig. 26-6). They possess soft, fragile cell bodies and lack a rigid

cell wall.* Hence they are highly pleomorphic. They contain both DNA and RNA and some metabolic enzymes. Like viruses, they are filtrable and, in the animal body, intracellular parasites. Also they are sensitive to ether and insensitive to many antibiotics. Their ability to induce cytopathogenicity in tissue cultures is a nuisance. The type species is *Mycoplasma mycoides,* the cause of pleuropneumonia in cattle.

**Pathogenicity.** In addition to bovine pleuropneumonia, mycoplasmas cause contagious mastitis in sheep and goats and respiratory disease in poultry. Dogs, rats, and mice may become infected with them. In man they are linked to infections of the genitourinary tract and the upper and lower respiratory passages, and rarely to other systemic disorders.

*Primary atypical pneumonia. Mycoplasma pneumoniae* (the Eaton agent) is the smallest known pathogen that can live outside of cells. It causes primary atypical pneumonia, and acute febrile, self-limited disease of man that begins as an upper respi-

---

*Since they have no cell wall, they would have to be gram-negative.

ratory tract infection and spreads to the lungs. It was among the most common respiratory tract infections of World War II, and today the Eaton agent can still be recovered from a large number of military recruits. The manifestations of the disease including headache and malaise are fairly severe. The cough is paroxysmal, but little sputum is raised. The lungs may be extensively involved, although in most patients only one lobe is affected. The attack lasts 2 to 3 weeks. Recovery is gradual. The disease, though prevalent, does not occur in widespread epidemics. Epidemics occur among persons living in crowded conditions and have been reported among newborn infants. Milder respiratory disease or even inapparent infection ("walking pneumonia") may be associated with *Mycoplasma pneumoniae*.

Primary atypical pneumonia is not very contagious, although apparently it can be spread directly from one person to another. Very likely the disease is transmitted by oral or nasal secretions, and the portal of entry is the upper respiratory tract. *Mycoplasma pneumoniae* is easily recovered from the throats of convalescent patients. The disease is not always followed by immunity.

The classic case of primary atypical pneumonia is associated with an increased number of cold agglutinins[*] for red blood cells in the patient's serum. In recent studies over half of mycoplasmal pneumonias had demonstrable cold agglutinins. In the serums of some convalescent patients agglutinins develop to *Streptococcus* MG (from the name McGuinness of the patient from whom it was originally recovered), an alpha hemolytic streptococcus now classified as *Streptococcus anginosus*. There is also a complement fixation test.

An alum vaccine prepared from formalin-killed organisms has been tested experimentally in animals and man. A live mycoplasma vaccine is also in process.

**T mycoplasmas.** "T" strains of mycoplasmas, "tiny forms," or "T-form" PPLO colonies represent human mycoplasmas with a distinct growth pattern. T strains produce very small colonies on their agar media (only a few micrometers in diameter). Colonies of the "classic" organisms, first studied, are much larger, many micrometers in diameter, even up to 0.75 mm. (Fig. 26-6). (Both "tiny form" and "large form" colonies must be viewed with a microscope.) Moreover, T strains are unique among mycoplasmas in being sensitive to therapeutic agents not affecting the classic ones and in possessing an active urease system.

---

[*]These are agglutinins that clump human type O, Rh-negative erythrocytes at low temperatures (5° to 20° C.) but not at body temperature. They are found in several unrelated diseases.

Mycoplasmas are common parasites of the genital tract. Colonization therein is related to sexual activity. In fact, they are considered part of the normal flora of sexually active males and females. However, there is reason to think that genital mycoplasmas—both T strains and *Mycoplasma hominis*—are not always benign. Postulated to be agents of venereal infection, T strains produce nongonococcal urethritis (NGU) and prostatitis in the male, and in the female, cause cervicitis, cystitis, endometritis, and contribute to infertility and premature births. Classic mycoplasmas are also implicated in so-called reproductive failure.

**Laboratory diagnosis.** The laboratory diagnosis of the presence of mycoplasmas is made by cultural methods adapted to their size and peculiar growth requirements. Mycoplasmas tend to grow down into a solid medium and in a distinctive fashion produce a colony with a "fried egg" appearance. They proliferate also in tissue culture and in the developing chick embryo. Serologic identification is practical because mycoplasmas are vulnerable to neutralizing antibodies and induce hemagglutination and hemadsorption reactions. Since many normal persons demonstrate circulating antibodies to them, it is the *rising* titer that is of diagnostic significance.

## Questions for review

1  What is the relation of acid-producing bacteria such as lactobacilli to dental caries?
2  What is the significance of *Pseudomonas aeruginosa* in clinical medicine? Why is it so hard to deal with?
3  What is melioidosis? Name and describe the causative microbe.
4  Briefly characterize mycoplasmas. How is the laboratory diagnosis made for mycoplasmas?
5  List diseases caused by *Pseudomonas*.
6  State the practical importance of lactobacilli. List important members of the genus *Lactobacillus*.
7  Define listeriosis. What forms of human listeriosis are significant?
8  Compare mycoplasmas with viruses.
9  Give the role of T-strain mycoplasmas in human disease.
10  Outline the salient features of primary atypical pneumonia.
11  What are Döderlein bacilli?
12  Give the method of spread of glanders. How may this disease be controlled?
13  Compare the classic cholera vibrio with its biotype El Tor.
14  How is Asiatic cholera transmitted? How can it be prevented?
15  Explain the pathogenic mechanism for the diarrhea in cholera. State the serious consequences of this.
16  Describe the organism causing anthrax.
17  Discuss the proper disposal of the bodies of animals dead of anthrax.
18  Why is the anthrax bacillus of historic interest?

**References on pp. 276 to 280.**

# CHAPTER 27

# Rickettsias
## including chlamydiae*

## General discussion

Rickettsias are known for a distinct, selective type of parasitism of cells in disease and for a special relation to an arthropod, be it vector or host. Long thought of as occupying an intermediate position between bacteria and viruses, these procaryotic microbes are now recognized as bacteria.

In Bergey's Part 18, one finds Order I, Rickettsiales, with two such families. The members of Family I, Rickettsiaceae, parasitize tissue cells (excepting the red blood cells) of a vertebrate host, and within Tribe I, Rickettsieae, of microbes adapted to existence in arthropods, there are three genera of medical importance—*Rickettsia, Rochalimaea,* and *Coxiella.* The members of Family II, Bartonellaceae, affect both red blood cells and tissue cells; one genus, *Bartonella,* causes disease in man.

**Special properties.** Rickettsias of Family I are small, pleomorphic, bacillary or coccobacillary forms named in honor of Dr. Howard T. Ricketts, of Chicago, who lost his life in the scientific investigation of tabardillo. They occur singly or in pairs, chains, or irregular clusters. The electron microscope indicates that they have an internal structure much like that of bacteria and that they divide by binary fission. Most rickettsias are held back by bacteria-retaining filters. They are close to the size of some of the larger viruses, being 0.3 $\mu$m. ($\mu$) in their smallest dimension. They are nonmotile, gram-negative, and stain with difficulty. They are obligate intracellular parasites. With rare exception, they do not multiply in the absence of living cells; the pathogenic forms grow only in the cells of infected animals. Some grow only in the cytoplasm, but others grow in both the cytoplasm and the nucleus of the infected cell. The fragments of enzyme systems that rickettsias possess allow them a range of metabolic activity. Their resistance to deleterious influences such as heat, drying, and chemicals is about the same as that of most bacteria.

The rickettsial diseases are transmitted to man by insects, the natural and primary hosts of the rickettsias.

**Pathogenicity.** When rickettsias invade man, they attack the reticuloendothelial system, colonizing the endothelial lining cells of the walls of small blood vessels (small arteries, arterioles, and capillaries). Within these cells they induce a vasculitis (inflammation of the blood vessel) that is distributed all over the body as the small blood vessels are. The consequence is disease in many anatomic areas in the body. A characteristic skin rash and a whole host of pathologic changes occur. Rickettsial diseases can be quite serious and many times life-threatening in spite of the best available therapy.

An attack of rickettsial disease is usually followed by a lasting immunity.

**Laboratory diagnosis.** Rickettsias can be cultivated in the yolk sac of the chick embryo (provided the hen did not receive antibiotics) or in tissue cultures. Recovery of the microorganisms may be made when blood and suitable specimens from a patient are inoculated into laboratory animals such as guinea pigs, mice, and rabbits.

The most important rickettsial diseases are associated with a positive *Weil-Felix reaction.* This is an agglutination test similar to the Widal test for typhoid fever except that the test serum is mixed with different types of *Proteus* bacilli. The Weil-Felix is a heterophil antibody reaction, since *Proteus* bacilli *do not* cause any of the rickettsial diseases or even act as secondary invaders. Complement fixation tests are of value in differentiating the rickettsial diseases.

---

*Within Part 18, the Rickettsias, of the recent Bergey classification, there are two orders. The first classifies microbes traditionally thought of as rickettsias; the second, those better known as chlamydiae or bedsoniae.

**Table 27-1**
Rickettsial infections in man

| GROUP | AGENT | WEIL-FELIX REACTION | | | COMPLE-MENT FIXATION* | RESERVOIR IN NATURE | VECTOR | GEOGRAPHY |
|---|---|---|---|---|---|---|---|---|
| | | OX-19 | OX-2 | OX-K | | | | |
| **Typhus fevers** | | | | | | | | |
| Epidemic typhus | *Rickettsia prowazekii* | ++ | | | + (specific) | Man | Body lice | Worldwide |
| Murine typhus | *Rickettsia typhi (mooseri)* | ++ | | | + (specific) | Rats | Rat fleas | Worldwide |
| Brill-Zinsser disease | *Rickettsia prowazekii* | | | | | Man | — | Worldwide |
| **Spotted fevers** | | | | | | | | |
| Rocky Mountain spotted fever | *Rickettsia rickettsii* | + | + | — | + | Wild rodents | Ticks | Western hemisphere |
| Rickettsialpox | *Rickettsia akari* | — | — | — | + | House mice | Mites | United States, Russia, Korea |
| Fièvre boutonneuse | *Rickettsia conorii* | + | + | + | | Small wild mammals | Ticks | Mediterranean coast, Middle East |
| Scrub typhus | *Rickettsia tsutsugamushi* | — | — | ++ | ± | Wild rodents | Mites | Asia, Australia, Pacific Islands |
| Trench fever | *Rochalimaea quintana* | | | | | Man | Body lice | Europe, Mexico, Africa |
| Q fever | *Coxiella burnetii* | — | — | — | + | Ruminants, small mammals, domestic livestock | Ticks—animals —airborne animal products—man | Worldwide |

*Cross reactions between Rocky Mountain spotted fever and rickettsialpox.

**Classification.** Rickettsial diseases may be divided into the following groups:

1. Typhus fevers
2. Spotted fevers
3. Scrub typhus
4. Trench fever
5. Q fever

Table 27-1 indicates epidemiologic features of these groups. Rocky Mountain spotted fever, rickettsialpox, and Q fever are the three prevalent in North America.

## Rickettsial diseases
### TYPHUS FEVER GROUP

**General considerations.** The typhus fever group includes epidemic typhus, murine typhus, and Brill-Zinsser disease. Clinically the different types of typhus fever closely resemble each other but vary in severity. They usually begin with severe headache, chills, and fever. A rash develops about the fourth day and persists throughout the course of the disease. Mentally the patient is dull and stuporous. This feature of the disease gave origin to the name *typhus*, which is derived from the Greek word *typhos*, meaning smoke or vapor. The course of the disease varies from 3 to 5 weeks. The mortality varies from 5% to 70%.

*Epidemic (classic, European, Old World, louseborne) typhus.* Epidemic typhus is caused by *Rickettsia prowazekii** and is spread from person to person by the body louse *Pediculus humanus corporis* (Fig. 27-1). Head lice (*Pediculus humanus capitis*) can transmit the disease but seldom do so. No animal reservoir has been found. Epidemic typhus is an acute and severe disease with a high mortality rate (10% to 40%) that has been known to spread over the world

*The species name *Rickettsia prowazekii* is derived from Stanislas von Prowazek (1876-1915), an early investigator who lost his life in the study of typhus.

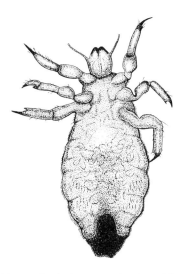

**Fig. 27-1.** Human body louse, vector in epidemic typhus fever, louse-borne relapsing fever, and trench fever. With heavy infestation, one may recover 400 to 500 lice per person.

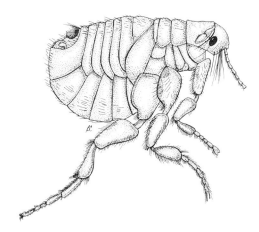

**Fig. 27-2.** Cosmopolitan rat flea (1500 species of rodent fleas). Vector in murine typhus and plague.

in devastating epidemics. It is a disease of overcrowding, famine, filth, and war. (It is also known as jail fever, war fever, and famine fever.)

When a louse bites a person with epidemic typhus, the rickettsias are taken into the stomach of the louse and invade the cells lining the intestinal tract. They multiply to such an extent that the cells become greatly swollen, burst, and liberate the rickettsias into the feces of the louse. When a louse bites a person, it defecates at the same time. The site of the bite itches, and that person introduces the infectious material into his skin by scratching. Infected lice die within 8 to 10 days after infection, from intestinal obstruction caused by parasitism of the lining cells.

*Murine (endemic, New World, flea-borne) typhus.* Murine typhus fever, caused by *Rickettsia typhi,* is relatively mild. A natural infection of rats, less often of mice, it is transmitted from rat to man by the rat flea (Fig. 27-2) and from rat to rat by the rat louse and the rat flea. The rats do not die of the disease, nor do the fleas or lice that infest them. Murine typhus may be transmitted from man to man by the body louse and become epidemic in louse-infested communities. In man the mortality is about 2%. The endemic typhus fever of Mexico is known as *tabardillo* (from the Spanish word *tabardo,* meaning a colored cloak, to designate the mantlelike spotted rash of the disease).

*Brill-Zinsser disease (recrudescent typhus).* Brill-Zinsser disease is a mild form of typhus existing along the Atlantic coast and occurring in persons who have had classic typhus fever many years before.

**Laboratory diagnosis.** The typhus fevers all are identified by a positive Weil-Felix reaction (agglutination in serum of the bacteria known as *Proteus* OX-19). Although the Weil-Felix reaction may be detected as early as the fourth day, it is strongly positive about the eighth day. The Weil-Felix reaction does not differentiate the typhus fevers from Rocky Mountain spotted fever, but it does separate them from certain other rickettsial infections. Fluorescent antibody technics can be used in the diagnosis of the typhus fevers. The epidemic and endemic forms of the disease may be distinguished and the rickettsias demonstrated if blood from a patient is inoculated into a male guinea pig.

**Immunity.** If a person recovers from either epidemic or endemic typhus, he is immune to both types, but a vaccine prepared against one type of the disease protects against only that type. Vaccines seem to be rather effective in preventing the typhus fevers, and when disease does occur in spite of vaccination, the severity is lessened and the mortality reduced.* In only a few cases is recovery from epidemic or endemic typhus not followed by permanent immunity.

**Prevention.** Prevention of epidemic typhus fever depends on (1) isolation of the patient in a vermin-free room, (2) use of insecticides on clothing and bedding, with destruction of insect eggs (nits) attached to hair, (3) quarantine of all susceptible persons if many lice are in the vicinity of the patient, (4) systematic delousing and vaccination of susceptible persons, and (5) general improvement of living and sanitary conditions. The control of the endemic form depends on ratproofing buildings and destroying rodents with their louse and flea populations.

---

*For immunization see p. 407.

## SPOTTED FEVER GROUP

**Rocky Mountain spotted fever.** Recognized as one of the most severe of all infectious diseases, Rocky Mountain spotted fever is like typhus fever and is caused by a similar organism, *Rickettsia rickettsii.* In areas where it is well known, it is often referred to as tick fever. (This should not cause it to be confused with relapsing fever, also known as tick fever.) It occurs in the Rocky Mountain states, many cases being found in Idaho and Montana, but is becoming increasingly prevalent on the Atlantic seaboard, chiefly east of the Appalachian Mountains. For this reason two types of the disease are designated: the western type (the original Rocky Mountain spotted fever) and the eastern type. The difference rests mainly on geographic distribution and mode of spread. The disease does show, however, great variation in severity. In Idaho the mortality varies from 3% to 10%, whereas in the Bitter Root Valley of Montana it may reach 90%. In the eastern states the disease is comparatively mild, and the mortality is about 20%.

The western variety is transmitted by the Rocky Mountain wood tick *(Dermacentor andersoni),* and the eastern variety is transmitted by the American dog tick *(Dermacentor variabilis).* In the southwestern United States the disease is transmitted by the Lone Star tick *(Amblyomma americanum).* Several species of hard-shell ticks (Ixodidae) (Fig. 27-3) are infected. The male tick can infect the female, and the female is able to transmit the infection to her offspring. With fluorescent antibody technics it can be shown that infected female ticks may pass rickettsias to all their progeny. This is an example of *transovarian* infection.

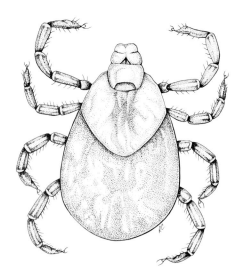

**Fig. 27-3.** Hard-shell tick, vector in Rocky Mountain spotted fever and tularemia.

The infection may be retained in the ticks through many generations. The tick is therefore able to maintain the disease in nature without either rodent or human help. A reservoir of infection appears to exist among a variety of rodents, particularly jackrabbits and cottontail rabbits. The disease is transmitted from rabbit to rabbit by the rabbit tick, a tick that does not bite man. It is also maintained in birds and in large wild and domestic animals.

The rickettsias of Rocky Mountain spotted fever differ from those of typhus fever in that they invade both the cytoplasm and nucleus of the infected cell. An attack renders a person immune for life. The serum from persons with Rocky Mountain spotted fever agglutinates *Proteus* OX-19 (positive Weil-Felix reaction), but the agglutination is not so strong as in typhus fever. *Proteus* OX-2 also may be agglutinated. A complement fixation test is highly specific. The patient's blood may be inoculated into a male guinea pig and organisms recovered from the animal.

Suspect ticks may be examined microscopically for the presence of rickettsias. A tick engorged from feeding is dissected from its shell, fixed in a suitable solution, and stained with Giemsa stain. If infectious, the tick will contain rickettsias within the nuclei of cells of the salivary glands.

Health officials advise persons going into tick-infested areas to wear protective clothing such as high boots and afterward to examine clothing and their bodies carefully for ticks. It is said that the time required for rickettsias to be transmitted from the attached tick to the human being on which it is feeding is 2 hours or more. Dogs and other pets should be inspected daily. Infective ticks are likely to be found in underbrush, tall grasses, and weeds. It is advisable to clear out such from an area where children may be playing or else to keep the children away from that area.

**Rickettsialpox.** Rickettsialpox is an acute mild febrile disease characterized by the appearance of a red papule at the site of inoculation, followed later by a skin rash. The disease is caused by *Rickettsia akari.* The house mouse is the reservoir of infection, and the bite of the house mouse mite conveys the infection from mouse to mouse and from mouse to man. The serum of those ill with or convalescing from the disease does *not* give a positive Weil-Felix reaction. Clinically, rickettsialpox may be mistaken for chickenpox. The primary lesion at the site of inoculation often resembles the vesicle resulting from a smallpox vaccination. The destruction of mice and their mites eliminates this disease. Rickettsialpox has been found among apartment dwellers of the northern United States.

**Other fevers.** Included with the spotted fevers

are tick-borne typhus fevers—fièvre boutonneuse, Queensland tick typhus, South African tick-bite fever, and tick-bite rickettsioses of India.

These illnesses are nonfatal and only moderately severe. They are caused by rickettsias related to the agent of spotted fever. Each can be traced to the bite of an ixodid tick. Fièvre boutonneuse is the most widespread and the prototype; it is caused by *Rickettsia conorii*. In this disease there is an initial lesion, the *tache noire* (an ulcer covered by a black crust is the black spot), which is followed by a generalized rash. The Weil-Felix reaction is positive but not strongly so.

## SCRUB TYPHUS

Scrub typhus, known also as tsutsugamushi (dangerous bug) disease and mite typhus, is so called because the mites that transmit the disease to man are found in scrubland, land covered by a stunted growth of vegetation. The disease attacked thousands of soldiers in the southwest Pacific area during World War II. It is an acute febrile disease with a rash, generalized lymphadenopathy, and lymphocytosis. The disease may simulate infectious mononucleosis. The mortality is from 0.5% to 60%. The disease resembles Rocky Mountain spotted fever clinically, except that in scrub typhus there is a primary sore at the site of the mite bite. The name of the causative rickettsia is *Rickettsia tsutsugamushi*.

Scrub typhus is a disease primarily of mites and wild rodents. It is transmitted from rodent to rodent and from rodent to man by mites. Two types of mites are known to transmit the disease to man. The rodents and mites that take part in the propagation of the disease probably differ in various parts of the world. The mites grow on short blades of grass and in the top layers of the soil. Persons who contact the soil are therefore likely to contract the infection. There is no evidence that the disease spreads from man to man. The serum of persons who have the disease agglutinates *Proteus* OX-K, but not OX-19. There is an indirect fluorescent antibody test, and inoculation of a mouse may be done.

Prevention depends on the destruction of the mites in the soil by insecticides and the application of insecticidal chemicals to clothing. There is as yet no effective preventive vaccine.

## TRENCH FEVER

Trench fever is a remittent or relapsing fever that affects soldiers on trench duty, but it may occur in civilian life when people live under conditions comparable to those of the trenches. It was prevalent during World War I but has since almost passed out of existence. It was infrequent during World War II. *Rochalimaea quintana* is the causative agent and is transmitted by the body louse. Unlike other rickettsias, man is its primary host, and the rickettsias of the genus *Rochalimaea* can be cultured in host cell–free media.

Although trench fever is never fatal and recovery is usually complete, it may recur, and in some cases it is followed by a state of chronic ill health with pain in the limbs, mental depression, and circulatory disorders. An attack does not confer immunity.

## Q FEVER

Q fever is a febrile disease of short duration caused by *Coxiella burnetii*. Rickettsias of the genus *Coxiella* are set apart from other rickettsias by their amazing resistance outside cells to heat, drying, and sunlight. The usually mild respiratory symptoms of the disease make it similar to primary atypical pneumonia or influenza. It differs from most of the other rickettsial diseases in that it is not transmitted to man by an insect vector, there is no rash, and the serum of an infected person does not agglutinate *Proteus* bacilli. The disease was first observed in Queensland, Australia, but the place of discovery did not give origin to the term "Q fever"—Q indicates "query."

Q fever is worldwide in distribution and is prevalent in the United States, especially in certain areas along the west coast. It is a disease of animals (a zoonosis). Man becomes infected by residence or occupation that brings him in contact with infected livestock —cattle, sheep, and goats. Most human infection is acquired by breathing contaminated air such as the dust from dairy barns and lambing sheds. Infected cattle and sheep may shed infected placentas and fluids at time of parturition. About one half of the cows harboring this rickettsia discharge it in their milk. Ingestion of the milk of infected cows or goats is a source of infection. Although the rickettsias of Q fever are fairly resistant to heat, they are effectively destroyed in milk by the high-temperature, short-time method of pasteurization. Infection is especially common among packinghouse employees and laboratory workers. In some instances mass aerial infection of large groups has occurred. Such an instance happened to more than 1600 soldiers who were returning from Italy to the United States and who apparently received their infection from winds blowing at an airport.

A capillary tube agglutination test is used to detect the presence of antibodies in serum from human beings and animals. Blood from a patient may be inoculated into a male guinea pig.

## RICKETTSIAL DISEASES IN ANIMALS

A list of rickettsial diseases in animals follows.

Heartwater disease of cattle
Rickettsiosis of cattle
Febrile disease of dogs and sheep
Salmon disease of dogs and foxes

## Bartonella bacilliformis

The intracellular parasites of the genus *Bartonella* (in Family II) are small, gram-negative, flagellated, and very pleomorphic coccobacilli. They can be cultivated on cell-free media, unlike other rickettsias. All infect red blood cells as well as endothelial cells of liver, spleen, and lymph nodes. They are transmitted by the night bite of the sandfly (*Phlebotomus*). The one species of the genus, *Bartonella bacilliformis,* is the cause of the South American disease known as Carrión's disease (Oroya fever, verruga peruana), which is characterized by an acute anemia with fever followed by a verrucous, or wartlike, skin eruption. *Salmonella* species are prone to complicate. Infection with *Bartonella* is endemoepidemic in the Andean valleys of the Peruvian sierra. This is a South American parasite.

*Bartonella bacilliformis* is easily recognized in Wright-stained films of peripheral blood and in material from skin lesions because of its unique microscopic appearance.

## Chlamydiae (bedsoniae)

In Bergey's Order II of Part 18, Chlamydiales, are placed gram-negative, intracellular pathogens of vertebrates with an intracellular pattern for reproduction peculiarly their own.

**Description.** The name *chlamydiae** (bedsoniae) is applied to a large group of microorganisms (psittacosis group) that have comparable design and make-up and cause several important diseases. Chlamydiae multiply within the cytoplasm of the cell attacked and form characteristic cytoplasmic inclusion bodies. The infectious particle is known as an elementary body, and the mature inclusion body contains a host of them. Their life cycle is a complex one.

For a long time chlamydiae were thought of as large viruses and were classified and referred to as basophilic viruses and mantle viruses. Like viruses they are obligate intracellular parasites, but there are important points of difference (see also Tables 28-1 to 28-4). Unlike viruses they possess enzymes and both DNA and RNA. They have no capsid symmetry, and they are susceptible to some of the antimicrobial drugs (very sensitive to tetracyclines). The patterns of their diseases differ in many ways from those of viruses.

---

*From the Greek, *chlamys,* "cloak." Each organism is surrounded by a dense cell wall in part of its life cycle.

Recent studies indicate that these parasites are better separated from true viruses and considered as small bacteria (Fig. 27-4). They are comparable to rickettsias but are still distinct. The name *Bedsonia* was given in honor of Sir Samuel Bedson (1886-1969), who studied them extensively. However, many microbiologists believe the genus name should be *Chlamydia,* and therefore these microbes are most often called chlamydiae. They are nonmotile, reproduce by binary fission, and have an outer cell wall chemically similar to that of gram-negative bacteria, from which they were probably derived.

**Laboratory diagnosis.** Many of the procedures used in the laboratory diagnosis of viral infection are applicable to these organisms (p. 289). They grow in the fertile hen's egg and express in tissue culture their distinct cytopathogenicity. They are easily stained with basophilic dyes (hence the term "basophilic viruses"), and because of their unique staining qualities, they can be visualized readily in suitable specimens by technics of light or fluorescent microscopy. There are diagnostic serologic tests, and the Frei test for lymphopathia venereum is a well-known skin test.

**Importance.** The genus *Chlamydia* of Family I, Chlamydiaceae, comprises only two known species, but their diseases sort out ecologically into three categories: (1) man—oculogenital and respiratory; (2) birds—respiratory and generalized; and (3) nonprimate mammals—respiratory, placental, arthritic, enteric, and so on. *Chlamydia trachomatis* is responsible for trachoma, lymphopathia venereum, inclusion conjunctivitis, urethritis, and proctitis in man. *Chlamydia psittaci* causes ornithosis and psittacosis in birds and various other diseases in animals.

The as yet undefined agent of cat-scratch fever is postulated to belong with the chlamydiae.

## Chlamydial infections
### TRACHOMA

Although rare in the United States, trachoma, one of the oldest diseases known to man, afflicts more than 500 million persons in the world. The causative organism, one of the chlamydiae, specifically attacks the lining cells of the cornea and the conjunctival membrane of the eye. Growth in these cells produces very distinctive inclusion bodies. As is often the case with viral diseases, bacterial infection is superimposed to intensify the injury already done. The inflammatory changes are pronounced, and the scar tissue formed over the cornea, ordinarily transparent, results in impaired vision. The name "trachoma" is derived from a Greek word meaning "rough" to set forth the pebblelike appearance of the infected conjunctival membrane (Fig. 27-5). This disease is the world's

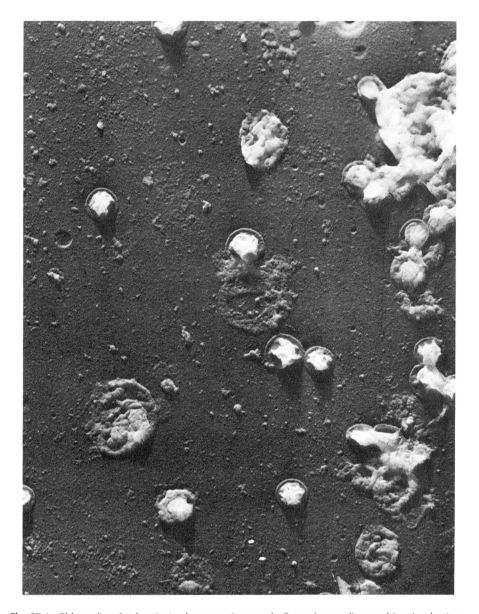

**Fig. 27-4.** Chlamydiae (bedsoniae), electron micrograph. Extensive studies on this microbe (meningopneumonitis agent) were important to the conclusions that these basophilic organisms, now termed chlamydiae, were *not* viruses. (×28,000.)

leading cause of blindness (in some 20 millions or more with the disease).

**Spread.** Trachoma is endemic in the large underprivileged areas of the tropics and subtropics; in some countries 75% of the population may suffer. Transmission requires close personal contact, and for this reason the disease is often passed from mother to child. Flies can carry the infection mechanically. Chlamydiae may be spread by contaminated fingers and articles of clothing.

**Laboratory diagnosis.** The diagnosis is made by identification of the typical inclusion bodies in scrapings made from the conjunctival membranes and by means of a complement fixation test.

**Control.** The agent has been grown in fertile eggs, and an effective vaccine prepared. The prognosis in this disease has been greatly improved with the use of antibiotics alone, and the incidence of the disease has been shown to drop simply with improvements in living conditions.

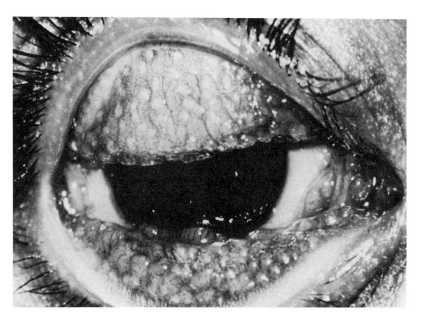

**Fig. 27-5.** Trachoma. Note inflammatory nodules spread over thickened conjunctival membrane of eye of Pima Indian (from tribe of southern Arizona and northern Mexico). Trachoma is prevalent among Indians of Southwest. (Courtesy Dr. Phillips Thygeson, Los Altos, Calif.)

## LYMPHOPATHIA VENEREUM

Lymphopathia venereum (venereal lympho-granuloma, lymphogranuloma venereum, lymphogranuloma inguinale), formerly known as climatic bubo, is a venereal disease of chlamydial etiology. It seems to be increasing in this country and all over the world.

**Pathology.** In the male it starts with a primary ulceration on the external genital organs. The infection extends to the inguinal lymph nodes, where buboes are formed. In the female, infection extends from the primary lesion to the lymph nodes within the pelvis, where the chronic inflammation set up may lead to stricture of the rectum. The disease involves mainly the lymphatics in each sex. The scar tissue associated with long-standing lymphangitis results in striking deformity of the external genitalia in both sexes.

Lymphopathia venereum should not be confused with *granuloma inguinale*, also a venereal disease but caused by a different etiologic agent (p. 223).

**Laboratory diagnosis.** Lymphopathia venereum is detected by the Frei test, which consists of the intradermal injection of material prepared by growing the agent in the yolk sac of a developing chick embryo. The development of a bright red papule at the site of inoculation constitutes a positive test. There is also a diagnostic complement fixation test. Inclusion bodies may be seen in suitably stained smears of pus from the buboes.

## PSITTACOSIS (PARROT FEVER) AND ORNITHOSIS

Psittacosis (parrot fever) is a chlamydial infection so named because it affects primarily the psittacine birds, most often parrots and parakeets. Ornithosis is the corresponding disease in domestic fowl and birds other than those of the parrot family—chickens, turkeys, pigeons, and sea birds. Psittacosis is important because of its worldwide distribution. The number of human beings attacked, however, is small.

**Transmission.** Psittacosis is widespread among the birds just named, the sources of most human infections. Man may contract the disease from birds through (1) handling of sick birds or their feathers, (2) transmission of the agent through the air, (3) contact with materials contaminated by infected birds, and (4) bites or wounds inflicted by sick birds. Sick birds show the agent in their nasal discharges and feces. Birds may become carriers. In birds the gastrointestinal tract is primarily affected. In man the infection enters by way of the respiratory tract, and infection is localized there. In a few cases the infection is transmitted directly from man to man. The onset of the disease in man may be sudden, and the mortality high. Explosive outbreaks sometimes occur in poultry-processing plants.

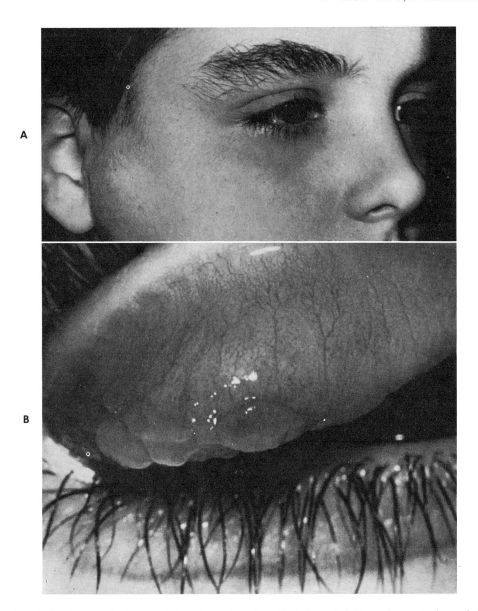

**Fig. 27-6.** Cat-scratch disease. **A,** Lymph node regional to inflamed right eye (preauricular node) is swollen and tender. **B,** Upper eyelid everted to show inflammatory swelling and congestion of blood vessels. A purulent exudate is present. Not only did this patient have a cat, but his cat-scratch antigen test was positive. (From Donaldson, D. D.: Atlas of external diseases of the eye, vol. 1, St. Louis, 1966, The C. V. Mosby Co.)

**Laboratory diagnosis.** The disease may be diagnosed by injecting some of the patient's sputum into a mouse and observing the development of the disease in the mouse. A complement fixation test is available.

**Prevention.** The sick patient should be isolated, and all discharges disinfected. A vaccine has been prepared against psittacosis, but how effective it is in the control of the disease, is undetermined.

## CAT-SCRATCH FEVER

Cat-scratch fever (benign lymphoreticulosis) is a febrile illness that may come after scratching, biting, or licking by a cat. It is characterized by a purulent lesion at the site of infection, and 2 or 3 weeks later the lymph nodes draining the area enlarge (Fig. 27-6). Incubation time from injury to illness is usually 3 to 10 days. As a rule, the disease is mild. Cats are mechanical vectors and do not show related illness.

It is possible that animals other than cats carry the infection, including birds and insects, but the monkey is the only animal artificially infected.

**Laboratory diagnosis.** Antigen for the skin test is prepared from the purulent material aspirated from the lesions. The causative chlamydial agent has not been isolated, but elementary bodies similar to those of psittacosis may be seen in stained sections of affected lymph nodes.

**Prevention.** The only preventive measure known is the avoidance of cats.

### CHLAMYDIAL INFECTIONS IN ANIMALS

The following list gives examples of chlamydial (bedsonial) diseases in animals:

Feline pneumonitis
Conjunctivitis and keratitis of sheep, cattle, goats, and chickens
Pneumonitis in mice
Stiff-lamb disease (polyarthritis)—one form
Sporadic bovine encephalomyelitis

## Questions for review

1 What are rickettsias? How did they get their name? Give their characteristics.
2 What is the Weil-Felix reaction? Its importance?
3 Into what five groups may rickettsial diseases be classified?
4 Give the laboratory diagnosis of rickettsial infections.
5 Briefly discuss Q fever.
6 Explain the pathological changes in rickettsial diseases.
7 State special properties of chlamydiae. Compare them with other microbes.
8 Give examples of chlamydial diseases with diagnostic inclusion bodies in parasitized cells.
9 What disease is responsible for most of the world's blindness? Give its salient features.
10 What is the cause of Carrión's disease?

**REFERENCES** (Chapters 18 to 27)

Adams, M. M. E.: Cholera: new aids in treatment and prevention, Science **179:**552, 1973.
Allison, F., Jr., and Sanders, C. V.: The extragenital manifestations of gonococcal infection, South. Med. Bull. **59:**38, April, 1971.
Altemeier, W. A.: The significance of infection in trauma, AORN J. **15:**92, March, 1972.
Altemeier, W. A., and Fullen, W. D.: Prevention and treatment of gas gangrene, J.A.M.A. **217:**806, 1971.
Anderson, D. R.: The organisms called *Mycoplasma,* Bull. Pathol. **9:**2, 1968.
Anthony, B. F., and others: Nursery outbreak of staphylococcal scalded skin syndrome, Am. J. Dis. Child. **124:**41, July, 1972.
Armstrong, D., and Kaplan, M. H.: Sepsis: a pictorial guide to some important clinical signs and initial laboratory studies, Hosp. Med. **8:**22, July, 1972.

Astor, G.: Plague, American-style, Today's Health **50:**54, Aug., 1972.
Bailey, W. R., and Scott, E. G.: Diagnostic microbiology, ed. 4, St. Louis, 1974, The C. V. Mosby Co.
Balows, A., and others, editors: Anaerobic bacteria: role in disease, Springfield, Ill., 1974, Charles C Thomas, Publisher.
Barrett-Connor, E.: Gonorrhea and the pediatrician, Am. J. Dis. Child. **125:**233, 1973.
Barton, F. W.: Venereal disease (editorial), J.A.M.A. **216:**1472, 1971.
Barua, D., and Burrows, W., editors: Cholera, Philadelphia, 1974, W. B. Saunders Co.
Beam, W. E., and others: An evaluation of the FTA-ABS test for syphilis, Am. J. Clin. Pathol. **47:**404, 1967.
Benenson, A. S.: Cholera today (editorial), Arch. Environ. Health **18:**305, 1969.
Benenson, A. S., editor: Control of communicable diseases in man, ed. 11, Washington, D.C., 1970, American Public Health Association, Inc.
Berger, S. A., and others: Bacteremia after the use of an oral irrigation device, a controlled study in subjects with normal-appearing gingiva: comparison with use of toothbrush, Ann. Intern. Med. **80:**510, 1974.
Bisno, A. L., and Ofek, I.: Serologic diagnosis of streptococcal infection, Am. J. Dis. Child. **127:**676, 1974.
Bloch, M.: The royal touch: sacred monarchy and scrofula in England and France, London, 1973, McGill-Queens University Press.
Blount, J. H.: A new approach for gonorrhea epidemiology, Am. J. Public Health **62:**710, 1972.
Bowen, W. H.: Dental caries, Arch. Dis. Child. **47:**849, 1972.
Bowen, W. H.: Prospects for the prevention of dental caries, Hosp. Pract. **9:**163, May, 1974.
Bowmer, E. J.: Salmonellae: ubiquitous pathogens of animals and man (editorial), Can. J. Public Health **59:**408, Oct., 1968.
Branson, D.: Timely topics in microbiology: enterics, Am. J. Med. Technol. **34:**120, 1968.
Branson, D.: Timely topics in microbiology, mycobacteria, 1968-1971, Am. J. Med. Technol. **38:**13, 1972.
Brown, W. J.: Acquired syphilis, drugs and blood tests, Am. J. Nurs. **71:**713, 1971.
Brown, W. J., and Kraus, S. J.: Gonococcal colony types, J.A.M.A. **228:**862, 1974.
Burgoon, C. F., Jr.: Acne, Mod. Med. **40:**57, April 17, 1972.
Busch, L. A.: Human listeriosis in the United States, 1967-1969, J. Infect. Dis. **123:**328, 1971.
Butler, T., and others: Bubonic plague: detection of endotoxemia with the limulus test, Ann. Intern. Med. **79:**642, 1973.
Caldwell, J. G.: Congenital syphilis: a nonvenereal disease, Am. J. Nurs. **71:**1768, 1971.
Chapman, J. S.: Atypical mycobacterial infections, Med. Clin. North Am. **51:**503, 1967.
Chapman, J. S.: The atypical mycobacteria, their significance in human disease, Am. J. Nurs. **67:**1031, 1967.
Chapman, J. S.: Ecology of atypical mycobacteria, Arch. Environ. Health **22:**41, 1971.
Charles, A. G., and others: Asymptomatic gonorrhea in pre-

natal patients, Am. J. Obstet. Gynecol. **108:**595, 1970.

Cherington, M.: Botulism, Arch. Neurol. **30:**432, 1974.

Cherubin, C. E., and others: Investigations in tetanus in narcotic addicts in New York City, Am. J. Epidemiol. **88:**215, 1968.

Chow, A. W., and Guze, L. B.: Bacteroidaceae bacteremia; clinical experience with 112 patients, Medicine **53:**93, 1974.

Christy, J. H.: Pathophysiology of gram-negative shock, Am. Heart J. **81:**694, 1971.

Cohen, J. O., editor: The staphylococci, New York, 1972, John Wiley & Sons, Inc.

Convit, J., and Pinardi, M. E.: Leprosy: confirmation in the armadillo, Science **184:**1191, 1974.

Cooke, E. M.: Escherichia coli and man, New York, 1974, Longman, Inc.

Copps, S. C., and others: A community outbreak of *Mycoplasma* pneumonia, J.A.M.A. **204:**123, 1968.

Corman, L. C., and others: The high frequency of pharyngeal gonococcal infection in a prenatal clinic population, J.A.M.A. **230:**568, 1974.

Costerton, J. W., and others: Structure and function of the cell envelope of gram-negative bacteria, Bacteriol. Rev. **38:**87, March, 1974.

Crowder, J. G., and White, A.: Teichoic acid antibodies in staphylococcal and nonstaphylococcal endocarditis, Ann. Intern. Med. **77:**87, 1972.

Davis, B. D., and others: Microbiology including immunology and molecular genetics, New York, 1973, Harper & Row, Publishers.

deLouvois, J., and others: Frequency of *Mycoplasma* in fertile and infertile couples, Lancet **1:**1073, 1974.

Diagnostic standards and classification of tuberculosis, New York, 1969, National Tuberculosis and Respiratory Disease Association.

Dillon, H. C.: Impetigo contagiosa: suppurative and nonsuppurative complications, Am. J. Dis. Child. **115:**530, 1968.

Dillon, H. C., Jr., and Derrick, C. W.: Streptococcal complications: the outlook for prevention, Hosp. Pract. **7:**93, Sept., 1972.

Dryden, G. E.: Sources of infection in the surgical patient, AORN J. **13:**64, May, 1971.

Dull, H. B., and others: Jet injector tuberculin skin testing: a comparative evaluation, Am. Rev. Resp. Dis. **97:**38, 1968.

Duma, R. J.: Management of hospital infections, GP **39:**106, Jan., 1969.

Duncan, W. C., and others: The FTA-ABS test in dark-field-positive primary syphilis, J.A.M.A. **228:**859, 1974.

Dunton, E. A., and Raymond, O. C.: The ramifications of salmonellosis, Can. J. Public Health **59:**246, 1968.

Edwards, P. R., and Ewing, W. H.: Identification of Enterobacteriaceae, rev. ed. 3, Minneapolis, 1972, Burgess Publishing Co.

Epidemic plague (editorial), J.A.M.A. **205:**871, 1968.

Erdtmann, F. J., and others: Skin testing for tuberculosis, **228:**479, 1974.

Fasal, P., and others: Leprosy prophylaxis, J.A.M.A. **199:**905, 1967.

Favero, M. S., and others: *Pseudomonas aeruginosa:* growth in distilled water from hospitals, Science **173:**836, 1971.

Feeney, R.: Preventing rheumatic fever in school children: Am. J. Nurs. **73:**265, 1973.

Feinstein, A. R.: A new look at rheumatic fever, Hosp. Pract. **3:**71, March, 1968.

Fekety, F. R., Jr., and others: Bacteria, viruses and mycoplasmas in acute pneumonia in adults, Am. Rev. Resp. Dis. **104:**499. 1971.

Feldman, H. A.: Some recollections of the meningococcal diseases, J.A.M.A. **220:**1107, 1972.

Feldman, S., and Pearson, T. A.: *Limulus* test and gram-negative bacillary sepsis, Am. J. Dis. Child. **128:**172, 1974.

Finegold, S. M., and others: Scope monograph on anaerobic infections, Kalamazoo, Mich., 1974, The Upjohn Co.

Fisher, M. W.: Development of immunotherapy for infections due to *Pseudomonas aeruginosa,* J. Infect. Dis. **130:**s149, 1974.

Fleming, W. L., and others: Clinical gonorrhea in the female: laboratory findings, South. Med. J. **65:**890, 1972.

Freedman. S. O.: Tuberculin testing and screening: a critical evaluation, Hosp. Pract. **7:**63, May, 1972.

Gangarosa, E. J., amd Faich, G. A.: Cholera: the risk to American travelers, Ann. Intern. Med. **74:**412, 1971.

Gilardi, G. L.: Practical schema for the identification of non-fermentative gram-negative bacteria encountered in medical bacteriology, Am. J. Med. Technol. **38:**65, March, 1972.

Goldmann, D. A., and others: Guidelines for infection control in intravenous therapy, Ann. Intern. Med. **79:**848, 1973.

Goldsmid, J. M., and Mahomed, K.: The use of the microhematocrit technic for the recovery of *Borrelia duttonii* from the blood, Am. J. Clin. Pathol. **58:**165, 1972.

Goodgame, R. W., and Greenough, W. B., III: Cholera in Africa: a message for the West, Ann. Intern. Med. **82:**101, 1975.

Gorbach, S. L.: The toxigenic diarrheas, Hosp. Pract. **8:**103, May, 1973.

Gorbach, S. L., and Bartlett, J. G.: Anaerobic infections, N. Engl. J. Med. **290:**1177, 1974.

Gorbach, S. L., and Bartlett, J. G.: Anaerobic infections: old myths and new realities (editorial), J. Infect. Dis. **130:**307, 1974.

Greenberg, J. H., and Madorsky, D. D.: Young physicians' knowledge of venereal disease (editorial), J.A.M.A. **220:**1736, 1972.

Greenfield, S., and Feldman, H. A.: Familial carriers and meningococcal meningitis, N. Engl. J. Med. **277:**497, 1967.

Greenwood, B. M., and others: Countercurrent immunoelectrophoresis in the diagnosis of meningococcal infections, Lancet **2:**519, 1971.

Hand, W. L., and Sanford, J. P.: *Mycobacterium fortuitum*—a human pathogen, Ann. Intern. Med. **73:**971, 1970.

Handsfield, H. H., and others: Neonatal gonococcal infection. I. Orogastric contamination with *Neisseria gonorrhoeae,* J.A.M.A. **225:**697, 1973.

Harner, R. E., and others: The FTA-ABS test in late syphilis, J.A.M.A. **203:**545, 1968.

Hassell, T. A., and Stuart, K. L.: Rheumatic fever prophylaxis: three-year study, Br. Med. J. 2:39, 1974.

Hattwick, M. A., and others: Surveillance of Rocky Mountain spotted fever, J.A.M.A. 225:1338, 1973.

Hofer, J. W., and Davis, J.: Survival and dormancy of Clostridia spores, Tex. Med. 68:80, Feb., 1972.

Holdeman, L. V., and Moore, W. E. C., editors: Anaerobe laboratory manual, Blacksburg, Va., 1972, Virginia Polytechnic Institute Education Foundation–Anaerobe Laboratory Fund.

Holmes, O. W.: The contagiousness of puerperal fever, N. Engl. Quart. J. Med. Surg. 1:503, 1843.

Hughes, A. E., and others: Nurses at Carville, Am. J. Nurs. 68:2564, 1968.

Hull, F. E.: Tuberculin tine test, J.A.M.A. 203:562, 1968.

Hussey, H. H.: Mycoplasmas in arthritis and urethritis (editorial), J.A.M.A. 227:194, 1974.

Iannini, P. B., and others: Bacteremic Pseudomonas pneumonia, J.A.M.A. 230:558, 1972.

Isenberg, H. D.: The ecology of nosocomial disease, ASM News 38:375, 1972.

Janeff, J., and others: A screening test for streptococcal antibodies, Lab. Med. 2:38, July, 1971.

Jawetz, E., and others: Review of medical microbiology, Los Altos, Calif., 1974, Lange Medical Publications.

Jelinek, G.: Gonorrhoeae, Nurs. Mirror 137:30, July 20, 1973.

Johanson, W. G., Jr., and others: Nosocomial respiratory infections with gram-negative bacilli, the significance of colonization of the respiratory tract, Ann. Intern. Med. 77:701, 1972.

Joint FAO/WHO Expert Committee on Brucellosis: Fifth report, WHO Techn. Rep. Ser. No. 464, Geneva, 1971, World Health Organization.

Jordan, G. W.: Bacteriologic and clinical features of Edwardsiella tarda, Bull. Pathol. 10:249, 1969.

Kahn, S. P., and others: Clostridia hepatic abscess: unusual manifestation of metastatic colon carcinoma, Arch. Surg. 104:209, 1972.

Kaiser, A. B., and Schaffner, W.: Prospectus: the prevention of bacteremic pneumococcal pneumonia, a conservative appraisal of vaccine intervention, J.A.M.A. 230:404, 1974.

Kampmeier, R. H.: The matter of venereal disease in 1971 (editorial), Ann. Intern. Med. 75:793, 1971.

Kampmeier, R. H.: Final report on the "Tuskegee syphilis study," South. Med. J. 67:1349, 1974.

Kaplan, K., and Weinstein, L.: Diphtheroid infections of man, Ann. Intern. Med. 70:919, 1969.

Kauffmann, F.: Serological diagnosis of Salmonella species, Kauffmann-White schema, Baltimore, 1972, The Williams & Wilkins Co.

Kinnear-Brown, J. A., and others: BCG vaccination of children against leprosy in Uganda: results at end of second follow-up, Br. Med. J. 1:24, 1968.

Klein, J. O.: Mycoplasmas, GU tract infections and reproductive failure, Hosp. Pract. 6:127, Jan., 1971.

Krolls, S. O., and others: Oral manifestations of syphilis, Hosp. Med. 8:14, July, 1972.

Krugman, S., and Ward, R.: Infectious diseases of children and adults, ed. 5, St. Louis, 1973, The C. V. Mosby Co.

Kubica, G. P., and Dye, W.: Laboratory methods for clinical and public health mycobacteriology, Washington, D.C., 1967, U.S. Government Printing Office.

La Force, F. M., and others: Tetanus in the United States (1965-1966): epidemiologic and clinical features, N. Engl. J. Med. 280:569, 1969.

Lancefield, R. C.: Current problems in studies of streptococci, J. Gen. Microbiol. 55:161, 1969.

Leino, R., and Kalliomaki, J. L.: Yersiniosis as an internal disease, Ann. Intern. Med. 81:458, 1974.

Lennette, E. H., and others: Manual of clinical microbiology, Washington, D.C., 1974, American Society for Microbiology.

Lenz, P. E.: Women, the unwitting carriers of gonorrhea, Am. J. Nurs. 71:716, 1971.

Levin, J., and others: Detection of endotoxin in the blood of patients with sepsis due to gram-negative bacteria, N. Engl. J. Med. 283:1313, 1970.

Luby, J. P., and others: Jet injector tuberculin skin testing: a comparative evaluation, Am. Rev. Resp. Dis. 97:46, 1968.

Mackey, D. M., and others: Specificity of the FTA-ABS test for syphilis, J.A.M.A. 207:1683, 1969.

Maki, D. G., and others: Infection control in intravenous therapy, Ann. Intern. Med. 79:867, 1973.

Maniar, A. C., and Fox, J. G.: Techniques of an "in vitro" method for determining toxigenicity of Corynebacterium diphtheriae strains, Can. J. Public Health 59:297, 1968.

Mansfield, R. E., and others: Evaluation of earlobe in leprosy, Arch. Dermatol. 100:407, 1969.

Marcuse, E. K., and Grand, M. G.: Epidemiology of diphtheria in San Antonio, Tex., 1970, J.A.M.A. 224:305, 1973.

Marlow, F. W., Jr.: Syphilis then and now, J.A.M.A. 230:1320, 1974.

Martins, R. R., and others: The production of type-specific antibody for the identification of mycobacteria, Lab. Med. 4:28, Feb., 1973.

McGowan, J. E., and others: Meningitis and bacteremia due to Haemophilus influenzae: occurrence and mortality at Boston City Hospital in twelve selected years, 1935-1972, J. Infect. Dis. 130:119, 1974.

Medical News: Rocky Mountain spotted fever case numbers rise, J.A.M.A. 230:1503, 1974.

Merson, M. H., and others: Current trends in botulism in the United States, J.A.M.A. 229:1305, 1974.

Meyers, B. R., and others: Infections caused by microorganisms of the genus Erwinia, Ann. Intern. Med. 76:9, 1972.

Meyers, W. M.: Leprosy—some immuno-pathologic considerations, Intern. Pathol. 9:57, July, 1968.

Mitchell, R. S.: Medical progress: control of tuberculosis, N. Engl. J. Med. 276:842, 1967.

Morehead, C. D., and Houck, P. W.: Epidemiology of Pseudomonas infections in pediatric intensive care unit, Am. J. Dis. Child. 124:564, 1972.

Moser, R. H.: Ruminations: holy man and his disease, J.A.M.A. 228:78, 1974.

Moulder, J. W.: Intracellular parasitism: life in an extreme environment, J. Infect. Dis. 130:300, 1974.

Mudd, S.: Resistance against *Staphylococcus aureus*, J.A.M.A. **218**:1671, 1971.

Munford, R. S., and others: Diphtheria deaths in the United States, 1959-1970, J.A.M.A. **229**:1890, 1974.

Norins, L. C.: The case for gonococcal serology (editorial), J. Infect. Dis. **130**:677, 1974.

Nosocomial bacteremias associated with intravenous fluid therapy—USA (epidemiologic notes and reports), Morbid. Mortal. Wk. Rep. **20**(9) (special supp.):1, 1971.

Owen, R. L., and Hill, J. L.: Rectal and pharyngeal gonorrhea in homosexual men, J.A.M.A. **220**:1315, 1972.

Owens, D. W.: General medical aspects of atypical mycobacteria, South. Med. J. **67**:39, 1974.

Palmer, D. L., and others: Clinical features of plague in the United States, 1969-1970 epidemic, J. Infect. Dis. **124**: 367, 1971.

Pappenheimer, A. M., Jr., and Gill, D. M.: Diphtheria, Science **182**:353, 1973.

Pariser, H., and Farmer, A. D.: Diagnosis of gonorrhea in the asymptomatic female: comparison of slide and culture technics, South. Med. J. **61**:505, 1968.

Pavlech, H. M.: Reusable laboratory glassware or disposable glassware, ASM News **40**:275, 1974.

Perkins, J. E.: Airborne infection and tuberculosis, Arch. Environ. Health **16**:738, 1968.

Peterson, J. C.: Congenital syphilis: a review of its present status and significance in pediatrics, South. Med. J. **66**: 257, 1973.

Piggott, J. A., and Hochholzer, L.: Human melioidosis, Arch. Pathol. **90**:101, 1970.

Powell, S., and McDougall, A. C.: Clinical recognition of leprosy: some factors leading to delays in diagnosis, Br. Med. J. **1**:612, 1974.

Quinn, R. W.: Epidemiology of gonorrhea, South. Med. Bull. **59**:7, April, 1971.

Rammelkamp, C. H., Jr.: Rheumatic fever: advances and problems (editorial), Hosp. Pract. **3**:9, March, 1968.

Rapkin, R. H., and Bautista, G.: *Haemophilus influenzae* cellulitis, Am. J. Dis. Child. **124**:540, 1972.

Reichman, L. B.: Tuberculosis care: when and where? Ann. Intern. Med. **80**:402, 1974.

Reif, J. S., and Marshak, R. R.: Leptospirosis: a contemporary zoonosis (editorial), Ann. Intern. Med. **79**:893, 1973.

Rensberger, B., and Roueché, B.: When Americans are a swallow away from death, Today's Health **49**:40, Sept., 1971.

Reyes del Pozo, E.: Bartonellosis or Peruvian verruca, J. Am. Med. Wom. Assoc. **24**:422, 1969.

Rhamy, R. K.: Gonococcal complications in genitourinary system of the male, South. Med. Bull. **52**:29, April, 1971.

Rhodes, L. M.: Why cholera is the disease nations try to hide, Today's Health **49**:51, June, 1971.

Riley, H. D., Jr.: Meningococcal disease and its control, South. Med. J. **66**:107, 1973.

Rocky Mountain spotted fever (editorial), J.A.M.A. **225**: 1372, 1973.

Rodman, M. J.: Drugs for treating tetanus, RN **34**:43, Dec., 1971.

Rosebury, T.: Microbes and morals: the strange story of venereal disease, New York, 1971, The Viking Press, Inc.

Rosenthal, S. R., and others: Tuberculin tine test in infection and disease, South. Med. J. **60**:1336, 1967.

Ross, S., and others: Staphylococcal susceptibility to penicillin G, the changing pattern among community strains, J.A.M.A. **229**:1075, 1974.

Rowley, D.: Endotoxins and bacterial virulence, J. Infect. Dis. **123**:317, 1971.

Rubio, T., and Riley, H. D., Jr.: Serious systemic infection associated with the use of indwelling intravenous catheters, South. Med. J. **66**:633, 1973.

Runyon, E. H.: Identification of mycobacterial pathogens utilizing colony characteristics, Am. J. Clin. Pathol. **54**:578, 1970.

Runyon, E. H.: Whence mycobacteria and mycobacterioses? (editorial), Ann. Intern. Med. **75**:467, 1971.

Russell, P., and Altschuler, G.: Placental abnormalities of congenital syphilis, Am. J. Dis. Child. **128**:160, 1974.

Sanders, D. Y.: Complications of ear piercing, Wom. Physician **26**:459, 1971.

Sanders, W. E.: Diphtheria: "From miasmas to molecules" revisited (editorial), Ann. Intern. Med. **75**:639, 1971.

Schroeder, S. A.: Interpretation of serologic tests for typhoid fever, J.A.M.A. **206**:839, 1968.

Schroeter, A. L., and Pazin, G. J.: Gonorrhea, Ann. Intern. Med. **72**:553, 1970.

Schultz, R. C., and McMaster, W. C.: The treatment of dog-bite injuries, especially those of the face, Plast. Reconstr. Surg. **49**:494, 1972.

Shepherd, M. C.: Nongonococcal urethritis associated with human strains of "T" mycoplasmas, J.A.M.A. **211**:1335, 1970.

Small, N. N.: Evaluation of PathoTec™ strips in diagnostic bacteriology, Am. J. Med. Technol. **34**:65, Feb., 1968.

Smilack, J. D.: Group Y meningococcal disease, Ann. Intern. Med. **81**:740, 1974.

Smith, B. B.: After the nail it's too late, Today's Health **48**: 30, Aug., 1970.

Smith, D. T.: Isoniazid prophylaxis and BCG vaccination in the control of tuberculosis, Arch. Environ. Health **23**: 235, 1971.

Smith, J. W.: Tetanus, Tex. Med. **66**:52, Sept., 1970.

Smith, J. W.: Leprosy, Tex. Med. **67**:58, July, 1971.

Smith, L.: The pathogenic anaerobic bacteria, Springfield, Ill., 1974, Charles C Thomas, Publisher.

Snape, P. S.: Rocky Mountain spotted fever in southeastern United States: a review of eighteen cases from Greenville, South Carolina, South. Med. J. **66**:765, 1973.

Sommers, H. M.: Are we recognizing most cases of clinical botulism? Lab. Med. **1**:41, Aug., 1970.

South, M. A.: Enteropathogenic *Escherichia coli* disease: new developments and perspectives, J. Pediatr. **79**:1, 1971.

Spaeth, R.: Tetanus and how to fight it, RN **28**:63, July, 1965.

Spitz, B.: In the hospital a bug is no joke, Hosp. Top. **50**:42, Jan., 1972.

Status of immunization in tuberculosis in 1971: report of a conference on progress to date, future trends and research needs, by the John E. Fogarty International Center for Advanced Study in the Health Sciences, (Bethesda, Oct., 1971), Washington, D.C., 1972, U.S. Government Printing Office.

Storrs, E. E., and others: Leprosy in the armadillo: new model for biomedical research, Science **183**:851, 1974.

Sullivan, R. J., Jr., and others: Adult pneumonia in general hospital, Arch. Intern. Med. **129**:935, 1972.

Sulzer, C. R., and Jones, W. L.: Evaluation of hemagglutination test for human leptospirosis, Appl. Microbiol. **26**:655, 1973.

Sutter, V. L., and others: Anaerobic bacteriology manual, Los Angeles, 1972, UCLA Extension Division.

Syphilis: the same old disease (editorial), South. Med. J. **65**:250, 1972.

Taylor, A.: Botulism and its control, Am. J. Nurs. **73**:1380, 1973.

Tempel, C. W.: Tuberculosis prevention; the child-centered program, GP **37**:99, May, 1968.

The two faces of pathogenic *Escherichia coli* (editorial), J.A.M.A. **180**:248, 1971.

Thomas, B. J.: Leprosy, an ancient scourge—a continuing problem, RN **38**:47, March, 1975.

Thompson, T. R., and others: Gonococcal ophthalmia neonatorum, J.A.M.A. **228**:186, 1974.

Tillotson, J. R., and Lerner, A. M.: *Bacteriodes* pneumonias: characteristics of cases with empyema, Ann. Intern. Med. **68**:308, 1968.

Tong, M. J.: Septic complications of war wounds, J.A.M.A. **219**:1044, 1972.

Top, F. H., Sr., and Wehrle, P. F., editors: Communicable and infectious diseases, ed. 7, St. Louis, 1972, The C. V. Mosby Co.

Top, F. H., editor: Control of infectious diseases in hospitals, New York, 1967, American Public Health Association, Inc.

Torphy, D. E.: Bacteriology of dog and cat bites, Bull. Pathol. **10**:276, 1969.

Tyeryar, F. J., and others: DNA base composition of rickettsiae, Science **180**:415, 1973.

Vandermeer, D. C.: Meet the VD epidemiologist, Am. J. Nurs. **71**:722, 1971.

Van Ness, G. B.: Ecology of anthrax, Science **172**:1303, 1971.

Von der Muehll, E., and others: A new test for pathogenicity of staphylococci, Lab. Med. **3**:26, Jan., 1972.

Walsh, H., and Dowd, B.: Tonsillectomy and rheumatic fever, Med. J. Aust. **2**:1121, 1967.

Wannamaker, L. W., and Matsen, J. M., editors: Streptococci and streptococcal diseases; recognition, understanding, and management, New York, 1973, Academic Press, Inc.

Wapen, B. D.: Wound botulism, a case report, J.A.M.A. **227**:1416, 1974.

Washington, J. A., II: Useful laboratory procedures: gram-negative bacilli other than Enterobacteriaceae, Bull. Pathol. **10**:316, 1969.

Weed, L. A.: Useful laboratory procedures: brucellosis, Bull. Pathol. **10**:120, 1969.

Weg, J. G.: Tuberculosis and the generation gap, Am. J. Nurs. **71**:495, 1971.

White, P. C., Jr., and others: Brucellosis in Virginia meat-packing plant, Arch. Environ. Health **28**:263. 1974.

Williams, C. P. S., and Oliver, T. K., Jr.: Nursery routines and staphylococcal colonization of newborn, Pediatrics **44**:640, 1969.

Willis, A. T.: Anaerobic bacteriology in clinical medicine, Washington, D.C., 1964, Butterworth, Inc.

Woodward, T. E.: A historical account of the rickettsial diseases with a discussion of unsolved problems, J. Infect. Dis. **127**:583, 1973.

Yow, M.: Group B streptococci: a serious threat to the neonate (editorial), J.A.M.A. **230**:1177, 1974.

# CHAPTER 28

# Viruses

## General considerations

**Definition.** Viruses are agents that cause infectious disease and that can only be propagated in the presence of living tissues (that is, they are obligatory intracellular parasites). If we say that the least requirement for life is the ability of a living organism to duplicate or reproduce itself, viruses are the smallest known living bodies. Most of them are so small that they cannot be seen with an ordinary light microscope, and some are so small that they approximate the size of the large protein molecules. Viruses seem to lie in a partially explored twilight zone between the cells that the biologist studies, on the one hand, and the molecules with which the chemist deals, on the other, being smaller than the smallest known bacterial cells and just larger than the largest macromolecules.* (It would take 2500 poliovirus particles to span the point of a pin.) Viruses can pass through filters that retain all ordinary bacteria and for many years were called filtrable viruses.

Our knowledge of the nature and structure of viruses and their disease-producing potential has increased greatly in the last several decades, especially since the invention of the electron microscope, the introduction of the ultracentrifuge, the development of modern cell (tissue) culture technics, and the applications of immunofluorescence and cytochemistry. As a result many viruses previously unknown have been isolated and identified—in the last 15-20 years over a hundred. Also, more has been learned about the natural history or *life cycle* of a virus.

**Structure.** Viruses are particulate and vary considerably in size (Table 28-1) and shape. (See Fig. 28-1.) Generally the viruses of man and animals are spherical, those of plants are rod-shaped or many-sided, and those of bacteria (bacterial viruses or *bacteriophages*)

are tadpole-shaped. Once thought to be fairly simple, today viruses are known to be highly complex structures in which viral components are fitted together into rigid geometric patterns with mathematical precision. In fact, a highly purified preparation of virus is referred to as a virus crystal (Fig. 28-2). There are three basic forms in viral structure—the icosahedral, the helical, and the complex-enveloped. The *icosahedron*, a crystal, is a solid, many-sided geometric form with 20 triangular faces and 12 apexes. The *helical* form indicates a spiral tubular structure bound up to make a compact long rod. The *complex-enveloped* form is enclosed by a loose covering envelope, and because the envelope is nonrigid, the virus is highly variable in size and shape.

**Table 28-1**

Relative sizes of viruses

| BIOLOGIC UNIT | APPROXIMATE DIAMETER (OR DIAMETER × LENGTH) IN nm. (mμ)* |
|---|---|
| RED BLOOD CELL | 7500 |
| CHLAMYDIAE† | 300-800 |
| Poxvirus | 230×300 |
| Rhabdovirus | 60×225 |
| Coronavirus | 80-160 |
| Paramyxovirus | 100-300 |
| Myxovirus | 80-120 |
| Herpesvirus | 110-200 |
| Bacterial viruses | 25-100 |
| Adenovirus | 70-80 |
| Leukovirus | 100 |
| Reovirus | 70-75 |
| Rubella virus | 50-60 |
| Papovavirus | 40-55 |
| Arbovirus (togavirus) | 40 |
| Picornavirus | 18-30 |
| Parvovirus (picodnavirus) | 18-24 |
| Certain plant viruses | 17-30 |
| SERUM ALBUMIN MOLECULE | 5 |

*1 nm. (mμ) = 1/1000 μm. (μ) = 1/1,000,000 mm.
†See p. 272.

---

* Dr. Wendell Meredith Stanley (1904-1971), biochemist and virologist, defined viruses as follows: "The virus is one of the great riddles of biology. We do not know whether it is alive or dead, because it seems to occupy a place midway between the inert chemical molecule and the living organism." (From Alvarez, W.: Mod. Med. **35:**78, Jan. 30, 1967.)

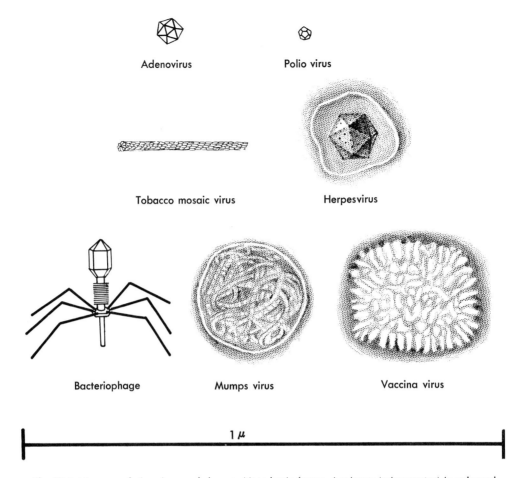

Adenovirus

Polio virus

Tobacco mosaic virus

Herpesvirus

Bacteriophage

Mumps virus

Vaccina virus

1 μ

**Fig. 28-1.** Viruses, relative sizes and shapes. Note basic forms. A micron (micrometer) is enlarged 175,000 times.

In the simplest viruses there is a long coil of nucleic acid sufficient for several hundred genes, the *chromosome* of the virus, tightly folded and packed within a protein coat called the *capsid*. The capsid is made up of subunits or *capsomeres* (aggregates of oligopeptides) arranged in precise fashion around the nucleic acid core. In the larger viruses, the more complicated chemical envelope is seen, wherein fatty substances and complex sugars (but no enzymes) are linked to the protein coat. The viral particle as a unit is a *virion*.*

---

*A *viroid* is a new kind of agent recently described. Said to be like a virus, it is a self-replicating, infectious entity 1/80 the size of the smallest known virus and is thought to be single-stranded, free RNA of low molecular weight. It may be the responsible agent in some forms of cancer, but presently its importance is as cause for certain plant diseases (examples: potato spindle tuber disease and citrus exocortis disease).

Cells of bacteria, plants, and animals contain both deoxyribonucleic acid (DNA) and ribonucleic acid (RNA). True viruses, however, contain only one. DNA serves as the genetic material in complex viruses such as vaccinia and bacteriophages, as it does for all other living things. RNA is the genetic material not only in complex viruses such as the influenza viruses but also in some of the simplest and smallest such as the polioviruses. The DNA or RNA may be either single-stranded or double-stranded.

Table 28-2 highlights some of the differences between viruses and other microbes.

**Life cycle.** The life cycle of a virus may be briefly sketched as follows. A virus contacts and parasitizes a susceptible cell in a given host. In some way the protein coat of the virion seems to be able to find just the right cell. Besides protecting the viral particle during its extracellular existence, the protein coat can attach to the cell under attack. Next the protein coat

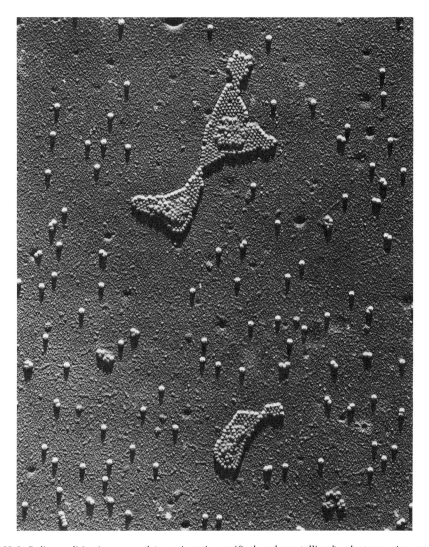

**Fig. 28-2.** Poliomyelitis virus crystal (type I strain purified and crystallized), electron micrograph. Individual viral particles are 28 nm. in diameter. In absence of any immunity one crystal of poliovirus contains enough particles to infect population of world. (×64,000.) (Courtesy Parke, Davis & Co., Detroit, Mich.)

is stripped off, and viral nucleic acid only (the chromosome of the virus) penetrates the parasitized cell, probably aided by enzymes from that cell. This kind of phagocytosis is called *viropexis*. The dissembled virus appears to vanish into the cytoplasmic maze of the cell.

Invasion of the cell by the virus is an act of piracy. Because a virus contains such a small number of proteins, it cannot do much, if any, metabolic work. It is not capable of independent reproductive activity. It must seek out an environment in which chemical building blocks and energy for work are provided, conditions existing only inside a cell. A virus must take nourishment from the parasitized cell, and it can multiply only within the confines of that cell. Since its genetic material is carried into the cell, the information needed to make new viruses inside that cell is available.* In fact, viral RNA can initiate the life cycle of the virus from which it was isolated even when chemically separated from the protein coat. The entry of viral nucleic acid into the host cell results in an infected cell that is then immune; it cannot be reinfected by the same or related viruses.

A variable period of time (the eclipse) elapses after

---

*Viruses act as independently existing genes.

**Table 28-2**
Comparison of viruses with other infectious microbes*

| AGENT | PRESENCE OF NUCLEIC ACIDS | REPRODUCTION | POSSESSION OF METABOLIC ENZYMES | OBLIGATE INTRACELLULAR PARASITE | RIGID CELL WALL | ANTIBIOTIC SUSCEPTIBILITY |
|---|---|---|---|---|---|---|
| Viruses | Either DNA or RNA (not both) | Replication (synthesis, then assembly of subunits) | None | Yes | None | None |
| Chlamydiae (bedsoniae) | DNA and RNA | Binary fission | Yes (parts of enzyme systems present) | Yes | May be present | Yes |
| Rickettsias | DNA and RNA | Binary fission | Yes | Yes | Yes | Yes |
| Mycoplasmas | DNA and RNA | Binary fission | Yes | No | None | Yes |
| Bacteria | Dna and RNA | Binary fission | Yes | No | Yes | Yes |

*Modified from Moulder, J. W.: The life and death of the psittacosis virus, Hosp. Pract. **3:**35, June, 1968.

**Table 28-3**
Inclusion bodies in infections with intracellular parasites

| DISEASE | ETIOLOGIC AGENT | LOCATION OF INCLUSION* | NAME OF INCLUSION BODY OR COMMENT |
|---|---|---|---|
| Rabies | Virus | Cytoplasm | Negri bodies |
| Yellow fever | Virus | Cytoplasm | Councilman bodies; areas of necrosis in cell |
| Cytomegalic inclusion disease | Virus | Nucleus, also cytoplasm | Cytomegalic inclusions; prominent in enlarged cells |
| Molluscum contagiosum | Virus | Cytoplasm | Molluscum bodies; elementary bodies are Lipschütz bodies |
| Varicella-zoster | Virus | Nucleus | Prominent inclusions |
| Herpes simplex | Virus | Nucleus | Prominent inclusions |
| Vaccinia-variola | Virus | Cytoplasm | Guarnieri bodies; elementary bodies are Paschen bodies |
| Adenovirus pneumonia | Virus | Nucleus | Inclusions of rosette type |
| Measles giant cell pneumonia | Virus | Nucleus, also cytoplasm | Prominent within syncytial giant cells |
| Trachoma | Chlamydia | Cytoplasm | Prominent |
| Psittacosis | Chlamydia | Cytoplasm | Psittacosis bodies |
| Lymphopathia venereum | Chlamydia | Cytoplasm | Gamna-Favre bodies |
| Granuloma inguinale | Bacterium | Cytoplasm | Donovan bodies |

*Note that what is called an inclusion body is a body visible with the *compound light microscope.* The electron microscope visualizes viral particles throughout the cell even in instances where there is a characteristic inclusion body in only one area.

the resources of the cell have been commandeered before new viral particles are released. At the end of this phase, swarms of full-grown viruses appear and escape from the cell. (In the case of poliovirus [Fig. 28-2] in only a few hours a single parasitized cell has produced 100,000 poliovirus particles.) When released, the new generation of viruses is able to survive outside the cell until it can reach the susceptible cells of another host, but it must find new living quarters.

**Pathogenicity.** In many instances little or no harm is occasioned to the host in the life cycle of a virus, and many viral infections are silent, inapparent ones. For example, unrecognized infection with polioviruses is hundreds of times more common than the clinical disease. Some infections are latent ones, undetectable until activated by the proper stimulus; for example, infections with herpes simplex. However, if the cells are damaged by the viral attack, disease exists, and the signs of viral infection naturally reflect the anatomic location of the cells.

The pathology of viral diseases relates primarily to the visible effects of intracellular parasitism. When cells that have been specifically attacked by a virus show changes that directly reflect cell injury, the sum total of these is designated the *cytopathogenic* or *cytopathic effect* (CPE), an especially useful concept in cell (tissue) cultures.

In some cells small, round or oval bodies known as *inclusion bodies* will be formed as a manifestation of the cytopathic effect. Inclusion bodies are typical in size, shape, and intracellular position for a given virus. They are emphasized by the pathologist, since they are usually easily visualized in the compound light microscope. In stained preparations inclusion bodies are commonly about the size of a red blood cell and rounded. Some viruses produce inclusion bodies in the cytoplasm of the parasitized cell, and some in the nucleus; others produce them in both cytoplasm and nucleus. At times, within the inclusion bodies still smaller units known as *elementary bodies* are seen. The elementary bodies are the virus particles, and an inclusion body with its elementary bodies may be likened to a colony of bacteria. Table 28-3 lists some infections where an intracellular parasite is related to an inclusion body.

Another reflection of cytopathogenic effect of virus is the formation of a giant cell or syncytium. This is prominent in measles and cytomegalic inclusion disease (Fig. 28-3).

Mechanisms of viral injury to the infected cell are not well understood. There are several possibilities. Viral particles may interfere with cell function by altering protein synthesis, or they may cause chromosomal changes, even to incorporating viral nucleic acid into the host cell genome. The presence of virus

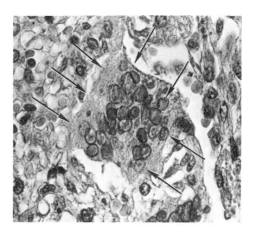

**Fig. 28-3.** Inclusion bodies of measles virus within nucleus of multinucleated giant cell (arrows), as seen in cell cultures and lymphoid tissues of patients with measles. (Microscopic section of lung from patient with rare measles giant cell pneumonia.) Note many nuclei piled upon one another in murky cytoplasm. In each, chromatin is displaced to nuclear membrane by inclusion body. Viral particles in cytoplasm are not shown in routine hematoxylin-eosin stain. (×800.)

may mean a direct injurious effect. Certain viruses such as poliovirus can activate and release enzymes contained in the lysosomes of the cell. In whatever way sustained, progressive injury to a parasitized cell may mean that the cell is either partly or completely destroyed.

There is an opposite effect that viruses at times produce on parasitized cells, an effect not seen in relation to any other known living agent. Viruses can stimulate the parasitized cells to increase their numbers in a way that the cells would not do if they did not contain virus. Such an increase in the number of cells is referred to as *hyperplasia* (virus-induced). It is this tissue response of cells parasitized by certain viruses that implicates viruses as a possible cause of cancer in human beings. Viruses may not only destroy cells or stimulate them to proliferate but may also induce a reaction in parasitized tissue cells that combines features of both destruction and hyperplasia.

Two factors influencing the response of cells to viral injury are (1) the rapidity with which a virus produces its effects—the more rapid its action, the more likely are cells to be damaged severely—and (2) the power of the cells injured to multiply. Nerve cells regulating sensory and motor function in the body cannot duplicate themselves (*regenerate*); if parasitized, they tend to be killed in the process. Cells lining the skin possess great powers of regeneration; therefore viral lesions in the lining cells of the skin may result in a piling up of increased numbers of epithelial cells at the site of injury. If not followed by any kind of cellular deterioration, viral-induced hyperplasia is not accompanied by any detectable inflammation.

There is often little in the way of measurable inflammatory response in viral infection. Where there is cell destruction, the tissues may show a minimal to moderate infiltration of inflammatory cells (lymphocytes and mononuclear cells, a few neutrophils) and vascular changes (edema and hyperemia) of limited extent.

Viruses are responsible for more than eighty diseases of plants and many diseases of lower animals. Practically all plants of commercial importance are attacked by them.* Viruses also attack insects. Of some 550 viruses known, more than 200 produce better than fifty viral diseases in man, some of which are the most highly communicable and dangerous diseases known. Today the prevalent infections in man are viral.

**Classification.** At present, most virologists seem to favor a classification system based on major biologic properties such as nucleic acid present, size, structure (geometric pattern of capsid and number of capsomeres), sensitivity to physical and chemical agents (ether and chloroform), immunologic aspects, epidemiologic features, and pathologic changes. Consistent with this, most animal viruses fall into 13 groups, 8 with a DNA core (deoxyriboviruses) and 5 with an RNA one (riboviruses). The important groups (corresponding to genera) are outlined as follows:

1. Poxviruses
2. Herpesviruses
3. Adenoviruses
4. Papovaviruses
5. Parvoviruses (picodnaviruses)
6. Myxoviruses
7. Paramyxoviruses
8. Rhabdoviruses
9. Arboviruses (togaviruses)
10. Reoviruses
11. Picornaviruses
12. Leukoviruses
13. Coronaviruses
14. Unclassified viruses

*Poxviruses.* The largest and most complex of the animal viruses, these brick-shaped, enveloped, double-stranded DNA viruses form characteristic inclusions in the cytoplasm of parasitized cells. Poxviruses may be categorized into three groups: (1) poxviruses of mammals, (2) poxviruses of birds, and (3) oncogenic

poxviruses (myxoma and fibroma). There are 22 members whose action may either destroy cells or stimulate them to proliferate. The skin is a prime target, and viruses included are those of smallpox (variola), vaccinia, molluscum contagiosum, and cowpox.

*Herpesviruses.* These medium-sized, ether-sensitive, enveloped, double-stranded DNA viruses, like poxviruses, often parasitize lining cells of skin and can pass from cell to cell without killing. The characteristic viral inclusions are found in the nucleus. The protein shells of herpesviruses show cubic symmetry, with 162 capsomeres. Latent infections with these agents may endure a lifetime. There are 20 members including varicella-zoster virus, herpes simplex virus types I and II, Epstein-Barr (EB) virus, and cytomegaloviruses (some oncogens are found here).

*Adenoviruses.* These medium-sized, ether-resistant, double-stranded DNA viruses may persist for years (latent) in human lymphoid tissue. Adenoviruses have cubic symmetry, with 252 capsomeres. There are 31 human, 12 simian, and 2 bovine types. Adenoviruses produce characteristic cytopathogenic changes in tissue culture, and their inclusion bodies are within the nucleus. These agents produce a range of diseases; some cause tumors in animals.

*Papovaviruses.* These small, ether-resistant, nonenveloped, double-stranded DNA (circular) viruses are notable for producing neoplasms in animals (oncogenic). Their growth cycles are relatively slow, and they replicate in the nucleus of the parasitized cell. Capsid symmetry is cubic. Papovaviruses include the *pa*pilloma viruses of man, the rabbit, cow, and dog; the *po*lyoma virus of mice, and the *va*cuolating virus of monkeys (SV/40), all known oncogenic (tumor-producing) agents. There are at least 11 of them.

*Parvoviruses (picodnaviruses).* These are small, ether-resistant DNA viruses. Capsid symmetry is cubic. Certain adeno-associated or adenosatellite viruses (defective viruses not able to replicate without adenovirus) and certain viruses of hamsters, rats, and mice are found here. They can produce latent infections in animals.

*Myxoviruses.* These medium-sized, spherical, ether-sensitive, enveloped, single-stranded RNA viruses have helical symmetry and replicate in the nucleus of the parasitized cell. Viral particles are pleomorphic, sometimes filamentous. Members of the myxovirus group agglutinate red blood cells of many mammals and birds. This hemagglutination is associated with the viral particle itself and inhibited by antibody acting against it. Some contain an enzyme, neuraminidase, capable of splitting neuraminic acid from mucoproteins. Myxoviruses (or orthomyxoviruses) include the influenza viruses A, B, and C, the virus of swine influenza, and that of fowl plague.

---

*Viruses have been known to attack the fungus from which penicillin is derived, thereby interfering with its manufacture. Fungal viruses are common among the fungi.

*Paramyxoviruses.* These medium-sized, ether-sensitive, enveloped, single-stranded RNA viruses have helical symmetry. They are similar in appearance to but somewhat larger than myxoviruses. Paramyxoviruses appear to be antigenically stable, and certain ones hemagglutinate red blood cells, as do myxoviruses, with or without hemolysis. Replication in cell cultures occurs within cytoplasm. Some cause multinucleated giant cells to form in tissue cultures and sometimes in human tissues (example: measles virus). Distinctive inclusion bodies are seen with certain ones. Within this category are the parainfluenza viruses (4 types), respiratory syncytial viruses, and the viruses of measles and mumps in man and of Newcastle disease and distemper in animals.

*Rhabdoviruses.* These ether-sensitive, single-stranded RNA viruses have helical symmetry. Members of this group have an unusual appearance. Mature virions are shaped like bells or bullets. Intracytoplasmic inclusions, the Negri bodies, are seen with the rabies virus. The rhabdoviruses include the viruses of rabies and vesicular stomatitis of cattle, some insect viruses, and 3 important plant viruses.

*Arboviruses (togaviruses\*).* These small, ether-sensitive, enveloped, RNA viruses (*arthropod-borne*) have a complex life cycle involving biting (hemophagous) insects, especially mosquitoes and ticks. Arboviruses (togaviruses) can multiply in many species—man, horses, birds, bats, snakes, and insects. With the exception of dengue fever and urban yellow fever, man is only an accidental host. They are most prevalent in the tropics, notably in the rain forests. Three disease patterns are prominent; one is fairly mild, the other two are severe and often fatal. They include (1) fever (denguelike), with or without skin rash, (2) encephalitis, and (3) hemorrhagic fever, as its name suggests, with skin hemorrhages and visceral bleeding.

Presently, on the basis of antigenicity, arboviruses, now togaviruses, are laid out in groups A and B. Other arthropod-borne viruses resembling togaviruses such such as the Bunyamwera supergroup and the arenaviruses are tentatively aligned with them. Groups A and B togaviruses are best known. Included in group A are the viruses of western equine encephalitis, eastern equine encephalitis, and Venezuelan equine encephalitis, and in group B are Japanese B encephalitis, St. Louis encephalitis, Murray Valley encephalitis, West Nile fever, dengue fever, and yellow fever. Bunyamwera supergroup comprises 100 viruses or more, including that of California encephalitis. Arenaviruses (enveloped, single-stranded RNA viruses) were so designated because of their unique electron

---

\* Note the new taxonomic designation for arboviruses.

microscope appearance. They include the Tacaribe viruses of South American hemorrhagic fevers, and the viruses of Lassa fever and lymphocytic choriomeningitis.

The ecologic hodgepodge of this total group with over 220 members is reflected by the names of many exotic diseases described, such as Bwamba fever, Singapore splenic fever, Kyasanur Forest disease of India, and O'nyong-nyong infection in Uganda.

*Reoviruses.* These are medium-sized, ether-resistant RNA (uniquely double-stranded as a group) viruses. Capsid symmetry is cubic, with 92 capsomeres. Reoviruses replicate within the cytoplasm. The three members in this group were originally so named because of their presence in the respiratory tract and the enteric canal and because of their orphan status (*r*espiratory *e*nteric *o*rphans). (Orphans are not known to produce disease.) The term *diplornavirus* is suggested to take in the reoviruses of mammals, wound tumor virus of plants, Colorado tick fever virus, and certain arboviruses with double-stranded RNA. A number of reovirus strains have been recovered from patients in Africa with Burkitt's lymphoma. They are excellent inducers of interferon.

*Picornaviruses.* These include the smallest known, simplest, and most readily crystallizable RNA viruses. The term *picorna* was coined to designate enteric and related viruses. *Pico* is for very small viruses, and *rna* indicates their nucleic acid. In addition, *p* is for polioviruses, the first known members of the group; *i* is for insensitivity to ether, a distinguishing feature of the group; *c* is for coxsackieviruses; *o* is for orphan or echoviruses; and *r* is for rhinoviruses, further indicating the membership of the group. Capsid symmetry is cubic, with 32 capsomeres.

The nearly 200 members are subdivided into (1) enteroviruses, including polioviruses (3 types), coxsackieviruses (30 types), and echoviruses (31 types); and (2) rhinoviruses (100 or more types), the major causes of the common cold. A rhinovirus in cattle causes foot-and-mouth disease. Picornaviruses produce a wide range of diseases in many areas of the human body, the best known of which is poliomyelitis.

*Leukoviruses.* Also called C-type particles, these small, ether-sensitive, enveloped RNA viruses of known structure are the member viruses of the avian leukosis complex and the viruses of murine and feline leukemias. No such viruses have yet been identified in man.

*Coronaviruses.* Ether-sensitive RNA viruses, the members of this group are similar to myxoviruses. Symmetry is helical, and the surface projections are petal-shaped. Replication is cytoplasmic. In this group are included the viral agents of avian infectious bronchitis, mouse hepatitis, and certain human respiratory viruses.

*Unclassified viruses.* These include viruses on which pertinent information is lacking. This category includes the agents of well-known diseases such as rubella and viral hepatitis, types A and B. Rubella virus, a small, ether-sensitive, enveloped RNA virus, does not seem to fit readily into existing schemes; only one antigenic type has been detected.

**Categories as to source.** When viruses are emphasized as to their source, the following three categories are named: (1) enteroviruses, or those isolated from the alimentary tract, (2) respiratory viruses, or those isolated from the respiratory tract, and (3) arboviruses (arthropod-borne), or those isolated from insects. (The term arbovirus emphasizes a biologic feature, that of insect transmission.)

Sometimes in the classification of viruses, emphasis is given to the anatomic area in the body where the virus produces its dramatic effects. Viruses so distinguished include (1) those whose typical lesions appear on the skin and mucous membranes—*dermotropic viruses* of smallpox, measles, chickenpox, and herpes simplex; (2) those related to acute infection of the respiratory tract—*pneumotropic viruses* of the common cold, influenza, and viral pneumonia; (3) those that primarily affect the central nervous system —*neurotropic viruses* of rabies, poliomyelitis, and encephalitis; and (4) those in a miscellaneous group with no common organ system (each virus having its own special affinity for a given organ)—*viscerotropic viruses* of viral hepatitis (liver), mumps (salivary glands), and other diseases. This restricted scheme of classification, although of some interest to the pathologist, is far from rigid, since certain viruses or groups of viruses induce various disease processes. In some instances a virus may invade the body without necessarily attacking the part that it ordinarily does. Further knowledge of viruses is revealing the fact that certain viruses thought limited in their preference for certain cells can infect a number of different cells in man and animals. The viruses of poliomyelitis, thought to be highly neurotropic for many years, are now known to be more flexible, with all three types growing well in tissue cultures of many different cells.

Viral diseases may be either generalized or localized. In *generalized* infection the virus is disseminated by the bloodstream over the body but without significant localization, even though a skin rash may be present. Examples of generalized infections include smallpox, vaccinia, chickenpox, measles, yellow fever, rubella, dengue fever, and Colorado tick fever. In some viral diseases there is restriction of viral effect to a particular organ, to which the virus travels by the bloodstream, peripheral nerves, or other body route.

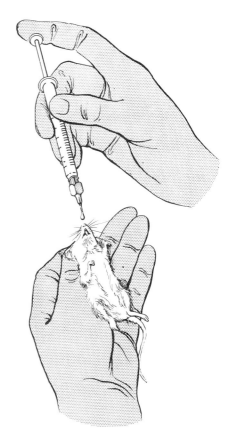

**Fig. 28-4.** Mouse inoculation with virus-containing material, intranasal route.

Examples of *localized* virus infections include poliomyelitis, the encephalitides, rabies, herpes simplex, warts, influenza, common cold, mumps, and hepatitis.

**Cultivation.** To repeat, viruses multiply only inside living cells. Viruses in virus-containing material may be artificially brought into contact with living cells by (1) inoculation of a susceptible animal such as a suckling mouse (Fig. 28-4), (2) inoculation of cell (tissue) culture systems, and (3) inoculation of the membranes or cavities of the developing chick embryo.

The chick embryo method (Fig. 28-5) is carried out in the following manner. A fertile egg is incubated for 7 to 15 days. With a syringe and needle the virus-containing material is injected into the membranes of the embryo or into one of the cavities connected with its development (yolk sac, amniotic cavity, or allantoic sac). This may be done through a window made in the shell of the egg over the chick embryo or through a hole drilled in the shell. Of course, *aseptic technic is mandatory.* After inoculation the egg is incubated for 48 to 72 hours, the time for the virus to multiply. The material in which the virus has multiplied is then re-

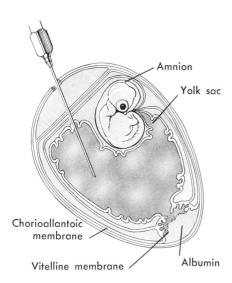

**Fig. 28-5.** Injection of yolk sac in hen's egg containing embryo, schematic drawing.

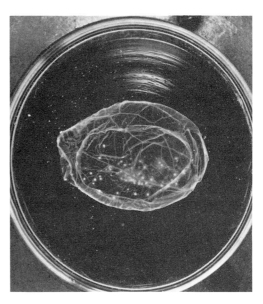

**Fig. 28-6.** Chorioallantoic membrane, showing whitish plaques (pocks) produced by smallpox virus. (From Hahon, N., and Ratner, M.: J. Bacteriol. **74:**696, 1957.)

moved; it is used for the study of the virus or sometimes purified, processed, and employed as a vaccine.

One of the most widely used laboratory methods of growing viruses today is the cell (tissue) culture method, which has come into its own within the last four decades. It has been made possible because of discoveries in basic technics, such as the preparation of improved culture media for living cells. The use of antibiotics has eliminated bacterial contamination, and the recognition of cytopathogenic effect has furnished a measure of viral injury in growing cells, where cytopathic changes indicate that virus is living and growing.

Formation of plaques in the cell culture under a layer of agar may also reflect viral growth, as does the phenomenon of hemadsorption. In certain instances, either guinea pig or chicken erythrocytes incubated in the given culture system will adhere in clumps to the infected host cells. There are three standard cell culture systems, using (1) human fibroblasts from the embryo lung, (2) a neoplastic line of cells, or (3) primary monkey kidney.

Both the chick embryo and cell culture enable the laboratory worker to obtain large quantities of virus for study and for vaccine production.

**Laboratory diagnosis of viral infections.** Many procedures are available for the laboratory diagnosis of viral infections, although some are most efficiently carried out in specially equipped laboratories. These include (1) technics for isolation and identification of

the virus, (2) serologic tests done serially during the course of infection, (3) fluorescent antibody technics to detect viral antigen directly in lesions, (4) microscopic examination of the lesions by smears, imprints, scrapings, or diseased tissues, and (5) skin tests.

Test material may be inoculated into the embryonated hen's egg, cell culture, or a susceptible laboratory animal (mouse, guinea pig, cotton rat, rabbit, monkey), from which the virus is recovered and identified. The appearance of typical lesions or inclusion bodies may be diagnostic. (See Fig. 28-6.)

Important in the identification of virus are several serologic procedures, of which the virus neutralization, hemagglutination-inhibition, complement fixation, and precipitin reaction tests are especially valuable. For the serologic evaluation of a patient's serum it is important that *paired samples* of blood be taken. The first is collected as early as possible in the acute stages of disease, and the second is drawn 2 to 4 weeks later during convalescence. The significant finding is at least a fourfold increase in the content of antibodies between the specimens.

Viruses contain good antigens in their makeup (that is, in the capsid) and, as a result, stimulate antibody formation. One of the most important antibodies formed in man and animals with viral infection is the virus-neutralizing antibody, which neutralizes or obliterates the infective and destructive capacity of the virus. This humoral antibody is an important constituent of immune serum given for viral infection. To

## Table 28-4
Skin testing in viral and chlamydial diseases—demonstration of allergy to agent

| DISEASE | TEST MATERIAL | INTERVAL BETWEEN INJECTION AND EVALUATION | INTERPRETATION |
|---|---|---|---|
| Mumps | Infected allantoic fluid | 24 and 48 hours | Past or present infection |
| Herpes simplex | Infected amniotic fluid | 48 hours | Past or present infection |
| Smallpox | Vaccinia virus vaccine | 48 hours | Immunity |
| Cat-scratch disease* | Lymph node extract | 48 hours | Past or present infection |
| Lymphopathia venereum* | Lymph node extract or chick embryo vaccine | 48 hours | Past or present infection |

*Chlamydial disease.

measure its activity, suitable mixtures of serum and virus preparation are inoculated into white mice susceptible to the pathogenic effect of the virus, and the protective quality of the test serum is titrated. To gauge the protective effects of the combination, either cell cultures or chick embryos may also be used. This is the virus neutralization test.

*Hemagglutination testing,* important in the identification of a given virus, is valid because most of the disease-producing viruses exert a direct or indirect action on red blood cells of man and other animals to clump them. Viral hemagglutination may be blocked by the action of specific antibodies found in immune or convalescent serum. This is the basis of the hemagglutination-inhibition (HI) test.

Many viruses induce the formation of complement-fixing antibodies. Precipitin reactions are associated with several viruses and are analogous to those observed with soluble products and toxins of bacteria.

The fluorescent antibody technic can be used to demonstrate viral antigens in specimens from patients or diseased animals. A diagnosis may sometimes be made within a few hours. In rabies, for example, the fluorescent antibody is applied to thin sections or smears of brain or salivary gland, and fluorescence is observed within a few hours if viral antigen is present.

Direct microscopic examination may be made of suitable preparations such as smears, imprints, scrapings, or tissue sections. In certain viral diseases inclusion bodies (viral aggregates) and cellular reactions are easily recognized in thin sections of diseased tissue with the compound light microscope (Table 28-3). The electron microscope is being used for an increasing number of viral diseases to show viral particles both in body fluids and secretions and in the *ultra*thin sections of tissue. Negative staining with an electron-dense material such as phosphotungstic acid is a technic used in the preparation of electron micrographs of viruses (Fig. 6-8).

A skin test is available to aid in the diagnosis of some viral diseases, as indicated in Table 28-4.

Table 28-5 shows how the laboratory is used in the diagnosis of viral disease.

**Spread.** The most important of the viral diseases are caused by organisms that have as their natural host man himself. Spread from man to man is either by direct or indirect contact, especially by means of nose and throat secretions, fecal material, and articles so contaminated. Droplet infection is very common. Some viral diseases are spread to man by insect vectors (flies, cockroaches, mosquitoes, or ticks) from a reservoir of infection in either a lower animal or in the insect. One viral disease (rabies) is transmitted directly by the bite of the affected animal; another (cat-scratch disease) is transmitted by the bite or scratch of an infected cat. Viral diseases are transmitted by water (hepatitis, enterovirus infections), and instances of milk- or food-borne epidemics are occasional (hepatitis, poliomyelitis, enterovirus infections). Human carriers, except in enteric infections, are not important in the spread of viral diseases.

**Immunity.** In many viral diseases (mumps, smallpox, measles) one attack confers lifelong immunity. In others (common cold, influenza) no immunity of any appreciable duration is produced. Where immunity is short-lived, the incubation period has been short, viruses have not circulated in the bloodstream, and the antibody-forming tissues have failed to receive adequate stimulation. In most persons in whom immunity lasts, antibodies in the serum of that person may be demonstrated for many years, and it has been postulated that virus, inactivated and non–disease-producing, has remained within his body.

The mechanisms of natural resistance are poorly understood. Newborn mice are extremely susceptible to coxsackievirus and easily infected, whereas adult mice are quite resistant under ordinary conditions. The virus of chickenpox is pathogenic only for man; other animals are completely resistant.

An *interference phenomenon* unlike immunologic mechanisms for other microbes is observed with viruses. A plant or animal cell exposed to a given virus

**Table 28-5**
Laboratory diagnosis of selected viral diseases in man

| AGENT | TEST SPECIMEN | ANIMAL INOCULATION | CHICK EMBRYO CULTURE | CELL CULTURE—CYTOPATHIC EFFECT | COMPLEMENT FIXATION | HEMAGGLUTINATION-INHIBITION | VIRUS NEUTRALIZATION | FLUORESCENT ANTIBODY | INCLUSION BODIES |
|---|---|---|---|---|---|---|---|---|---|
| **Viruses in respiratory disease** | | | | | | | | | |
| Influenza viruses | Nose and throat secretions | | × | | × | × | | × | |
| Adenoviruses | Throat secretions, fecal material, eye fluid, cerebrospinal fluid | | | × | × | × | × | | |
| **Viruses in central nervous system disease** | | | | | | | | | |
| Polioviruses | Throat secretions, rectal swabs, blood, urine, cerebrospinal fluid | × | | × | × | | × | × | |
| Encephalitis viruses | Blood, throat swabs, cerebrospinal fluid, urine, brain; other tissues if illness fatal | × | | × | × | × | × | | |
| Rabies virus | Saliva, throat swabs, eye fluid, cerebrospinal fluid | × | | | × | | × | × | × |
| **Viruses in skin disease** | | | | | | | | | |
| Variola virus | Material from vesicle, pustule, or scab | | × | × | × | × | × | × | × |
| Rubeola virus | Blood, urine, throat swabs, eye fluid | | | × | × | × | × | | |
| Rubella virus | Blood, urine, throat swabs | × | × | | × | | × | × | |
| **Other** | | | | | | | | | |
| Colorado tick fever virus | Blood, throat swabs, fecal material | × | × | × | × | × | × | | |

subsequently develops a resistance to infection by a closely related strain of the same or another closely related virus. There is this kind of interference between the viruses of yellow fever and dengue fever in the body of their insect vector, the mosquito *Aedes aegypti*. Such a mosquito cannot spread more than one of these diseases at the same time.

*Interferon* or the interferon system is thought of as a broad-spectrum antiviral agent, a soluble, nontoxic, nonantigenic protein (or family of proteins), smaller in size than antibodies. It is elaborated in small amounts by a normal body cell under attack from an invading virus. Interferon is cell-specific (including species specificity), *not* virus-specific. Present within the specific cell, it is able to block the effect of the virus by stopping the synthesis of nucleic acid for the virus and thereby breaking into its life cycle. The action of interferon is a manifestation of viral interference and is a most important part of the body's defense against viral infection—part of nature's first line of defense. A patient with agammaglobulinemia who is plagued with repeated infections caused by bacteria seems to recover uneventfully from those caused by viruses, perhaps because of interferon. Practically every class of animal virus has been associated with its formation. Only a few viruses are resistant to it.

There is a great deal of interest in interferon inducers, substances stimulating the endogenous production of interferon and thereby active against viral infection. A well-known one in the investigational field is polyinosinic:polycytidylic acid (poly I:C), a synthetic, double-stranded RNA.

**Prevention of viral diseases.** Immunization procedures prevent viral diseases (Chapters 36 and 37), as do proper technics of sterilization (p. 164). Effective disinfectants to inactivate or destroy viruses are formalin, dilute hydrochloric acid, organic iodine, and 1% phenol. Roentgen rays and ultraviolet light destroy viruses, but the effective dose varies with different viruses. Most viruses, except those of hepatitis, are destroyed in pasteurized milk. Influenza viruses are readily destroyed by soap and water.

Except to treat bacterial complications that are prone to follow viral diseases, the antimicrobial drugs are generally of no value in the management of diseases caused by true viruses.

## Bacteriophages (bacterial viruses)

**General characteristics.** In 1917, d'Herelle discovered that a bacteria-free filtrate obtained from the stool of patients with bacillary dysentery contained an agent that when added to a liquid culture of dysentery bacilli, caused the bacteria to dissolve. If but a minute portion of the dissolved culture were added to another culture of dysentery bacilli, the bacteria in the second culture were likewise dissolved. This transfer from culture to culture could be kept up until the bacteria in hundreds of cultures were dissolved, which proved that the agent was not consumed in the process but apparently increased in amount. This agent d'Herelle called *bacteriophage,* meaning bacteria eater. We know bacteriophages today as viruses that attack bacteria—*bacterial viruses.*

In recent years viruses infecting many strains of bacteria have been isolated, and it has been demonstrated that a given phage acts only on its own particular species or group of species of bacteria. In fact, their highly specific nature has made them useful to the epidemiologist in typing or classifying bacteria; for example, the phage typing of pathogenic staphylococci is important in the epidemiologic study of hospital-acquired staphylococcal infections.

Tending to occur in nature with their specific hosts, bacteriophages are found most plentifully in the intestinal discharges of man and the higher animals or in water and other materials contaminated with these discharges. They also are found in pus and even in the soil. When phages are named, reference is made to the specific hosts, as with coliphages, staphylophages, cholera phages, and typhoid phages. A very few bacteria such as the pneumococci apparently do not possess phages. Of all the viruses known, bacterial viruses are the most easily studied in the research laboratory, and the ones most thoroughly investigated have been those related to the enteric group of microorganisms. As obligate intracellular parasites they resemble closely other viruses in their biologic properties.

**Life cycle.** With the aid of the electron microscope, phages are seen to be tiny tadpole units possessing a head, which is either rounded or many-sided, and a tail, which is a specialized structure for attachment. Like other viruses, a phage particle is composed of nu-clear material (DNA) encased in a protein coat (Fig. 28-7).

Although appearing to be harmless, a bacteriophage in its virulent form can literally blow its bacterium to bits in a matter of minutes. The attack on the specific bacterium occurs in a fantastic series of steps. Seeking out the susceptible bacterial cell, the virus fixes itself tail first to the cell (Fig. 28-8). By chemical action it drills out a tiny hole in the cell wall, the tail penetrating the plasma membrane to the interior of the cell. The head changes shape, and soon the DNA of the virus flows through the tail into the cell. The bacteriophage seems to work like the world's smallest syringe and needle when it injects its nuclear DNA into the bacterial cell. Once the fatal injection is made, drastic changes occur. The DNA takes command of the vital forces of the microbe and in a matter of minutes imposes the synthesis of hundreds of bacterial viruses exactly like the one originally invading the injured bacterial cell. The deranged cell swells and shatters, setting free a multitude of new viruses able to seek out a new host and repeat the cycle. This rapid destruction of a bacterium is *lysis.*

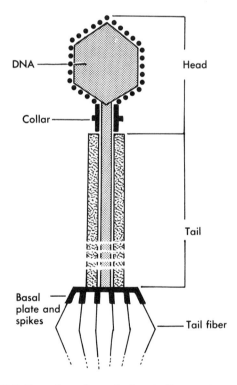

**Fig. 28-7.** Phage (mycobacteriophage), diagram. Large dots about head are protein coat. Measurements of this phage: head about 950 Å, tail about 3000 Å, and tail fibers 1500 Å. (From Arnett, R. H., Jr., and Braungart, D. C.: An introduction to plant biology, ed. 3, St. Louis, 1970, The C. V. Mosby Co.)

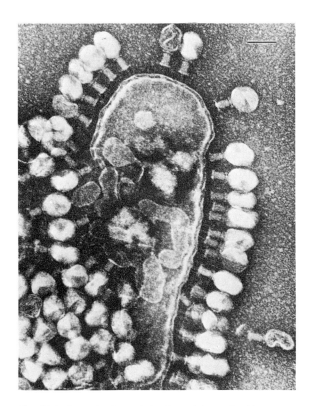

**Fig. 28-8.** Bacteriophage infection of bacteria. Numerous specific phages are adsorbed on *Escherichia coli*. Distance between baseplates of phage particles and cell wall is 300 to 400 Å. (Negative staining.) (From Simon, L. D., and Anderson, T. F.: Virology **32**:279, 1967.)

Lysis is not the invariable result of bacteriophage action. When certain phages infect, they do not destroy but seem to be able to establish a relatively stable symbiotic relation with the host that they have parasitized. The host bacterium continues to grow and multiply, carrying the virus in its interior in a noninfective condition more or less indefinitely, and the virus meantime multiplies at the same rate. This kind of phage is referred to as a *prophage,* and this condition of mutual tolerance is termed *lysogeny* or *lysogenesis.* Lysogeny is widespread in nature. That the process is not without effect is seen in changes in physiologic characteristics in the infected bacteria. Phages may even be responsible for the conversion of an avirulent strain to a virulent one.

**Laboratory diagnosis.** Bacteriophages may be isolated and studied in the laboratory. If they are taken from a source in nature, they must be separated from bacteria by filtration. When they are added to a growing culture of specific bacteria, their action to block bacterial growth may be nicely shown. In a liquid culture medium, clearing indicates bacterial lysis. On a solid culture medium, lysis by virulent phages is seen in zones, usually circular, where bacterial growth has disappeared (clearing of bacterial growth). These zones are called *plaques* (Fig. 28-9). Each plaque contains many particles that, in turn, can form plaques. Pure preparations of phage may be obtained by picking material from well-isolated plaques.

**Importance.** Bacteriophages may be of practical importance. In certain of the fermentation industries

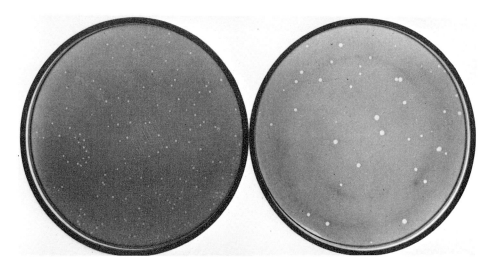

**Fig. 28-9.** Phage plaques. Small plaques (zones of clearing) in assay plate on left are *Staphylococcus aureus* phages; those on right are *Staphylococcus epidermidis* phages. In preparation of an assay plate, a mixture of test phages and microorganisms is poured over nutrient base. After plate has been incubated, plaques are evaluated and counted. (Courtesy Drs. E. D. Rosenblum and B. Minshew, Dallas.)

**Table 28-6**
Patterns of tumor viruses

| CATEGORY | NUCLEIC ACID | APPROXIMATE SIZE IN nm. | MEMBER VIRUSES | NATURAL HOST | TUMORS PRODUCED | EXPERIMENTAL HOSTS |
|---|---|---|---|---|---|---|
| Papovaviruses | DNA | 45 | Polyoma | Mouse | Solid tumors in many sites of animal body | Mouse, hamster, guinea pig, rat, rabbit, ferret |
| | | | SV/40 | Rhesus monkey | Sarcomas | Hamster |
| | | | Papilloma Human | Man | Common warts (papillomas) | Man |
| | | | Rabbit | Rabbit | Papillomas | Rabbit |
| | | | Bovine | Cow | Papillomas | Cow, hamster, mouse |
| | | | Dog | Dog | Papillomas | Dog |
| Poxviruses | DNA | 250 × 200 | Yaba | Monkey | Benign histiocytomas | Monkey |
| | | | Fibroma | Rabbit, squirrel, deer | Fibromas, myxomas | Rabbit, squirrel, deer |
| | | | Molluscum | Man | Molluscum contagiosum | Man |
| Adenoviruses | DNA | 80 | Types 3, 7, 12, 18, 31 | Man | Sarcomas, malignant lymphomas | Hamster, mouse, rat |
| Herpesviruses | DNA | 100 | Lucké | Leopard frog | Renal adenocarcinoma | Leopard frog |
| | | | Marek's disease | Chicken | Neurolymphoma (Marek's disease) | Chicken |
| | | | *Herpesvirus saimiri* | Squirrel monkey | Melendez' lymphoma of owl monkey | Owl monkey, marmoset |
| | | | Herpesvirus of rabbit | Rabbit | Hinze's lymphoma | Cottontail rabbit |
| | | | EB (Epstein-Barr) | Man | Burkitt's lymphoma (?), nasopharyngeal carcinoma (?) | |
| | | | *Herpesvirus hominis,* type II | Man | Carcinoma of cervix of uterus (?) | |
| Myxovirus-(like) particles | RNA | 70-110 | Rous sarcoma | Chicken | Sarcomas, leukemias, adenocarcinoma of kidney | Chicken, turkey rat, monkey, hamster, guinea pig |
| | | | Avian leukosis complex* | Chicken | Leukemias, sarcomas | Chicken |
| | | | Murine leukemia complex*; 14 strains, including Gross, Friend, Graffi, Rauscher, Moloney | Mouse | Leukemias, malignant lymphoma | Mouse, rat, hamster |
| | | | Milk factor or Bittner virus (mouse mammary tumor) | Mouse | Mammary carcinoma | Mouse |

*Leukoviruses.

in which the commercial product is dependent on bacterial action (examples: streptomycin, acetone, and butyl alcohol), an "epidemic" of viral infection in the large vats used to grow the microorganisms can be of grave economic concern.

## Viruses and teratogenesis

See p. 439.

## Viruses and cancer*

Experimental evidence indicates that filtrable viruses do cause several kinds of cancerous growth in lower animals—in rabbits (Fig. 46-4), mice, chickens, hamsters, rats, dogs, frogs, monkeys, horses, squirrels, and deer. Cancer is induced in all major groups of animals (including subhuman primates). Table 28-6 emphasizes certain features of viruses known to cause tumors.

*See also p. 509.

## Questions for review

1 State briefly the salient features of viruses. Compare them with other microbes.

2 Sketch the life cycle of viruses (including bacterial viruses).

3 What are inclusion bodies? Their importance? Their specificity?

4 What is meant by the cytopathic effect of viruses? How is this used in virology?

5 Give the two major pathologic effects viruses produce on cells they parasitize.

6 How may viruses be cultivated in the laboratory?

7 Discuss briefly the spread of diseases caused by viruses.

8 Outline the laboratory diagnosis of viral infections.

9 Comment on the nature and importance of interferon and viral interference.

10 Classify broadly the viruses. Indicate the most widely used system.

11 Discuss the role of viruses in teratogenesis (see p. 439).

12 What is the importance of the nucleic acids in viruses?

13 State the case for viral oncogenesis.

14 Define or briefly explain: bacteriophage, arbovirus, enterovirus, virion, viropexis, capsid, picorna, virology, lysogeny, papovaviruses, viral hemagglutination, plaque, icosahedron, hyperplasia, dermatropic, prophage, capsomere, life cycle, helix, regeneration, virus neutralization.

**References on pp. 322 and 323.**

# CHAPTER 29
# Viral diseases

## Skin diseases
### MEASLES (RUBEOLA)*

Measles is an acute communicable disease associated with a catarrhal inflammation of the respiratory passages, fever, constitutional symptoms, a skin rash, and a distinct predilection for grave complications. Among these are streptococcal or pneumococcal bronchopneumonia, encephalitis, otitis media, and mastoiditis. The incubation period is 10 to 12 days. One of the most common diseases, measles is said to be responsible for about 1% of deaths occurring in the temperate zones.

Only 1 immunologic type of measles virus (a paramyxovirus) is known. The virus of measles is thrown off from the body in the lacrimal, nasal, and buccal secretions and enters by the mouth and nose. It is found in the blood, urine, secretions of the eyes, and discharges of the respiratory tract. The infection is usually transmitted directly from person to person. Healthy carriers are unknown. The time that an object contaminated by the secretions of a patient with measles remains infectious is short. Measles is not transferred by the scales from the skin. Measles virus may be spread a considerable distance through the air. Measles is most highly communicable during the 3 to 4 days preceding the skin eruption. It is not transmitted after the fever has subsided. Epidemics tend to recur every 2 or 3 years and are likely to break out when young adults from rural communities come together in large groups, such as when armies are mobilized. The disease is especially virulent in populations native to the tropics or in primitive races anywhere with no ethnic history of previous exposure. Children of mothers who have had measles are immune to the disease until they are about 6 months old. An attack of measles almost invariably produces a permanent immunity.

Measles depresses allergic conditions and immune processes. It renders the tuberculin and agglutination tests less positive or even negative. The Dick and Schick tests may become more strongly positive, and eczema and asthma often disappear during or after the attack.

The measles patient should be isolated and protected against streptococcal infections, staphylococcal infections, and common colds. Discharges from the nose, mouth, and eyes should be disinfected. When measles appears in army camps, daily inspections of personnel should be made, and persons having conjunctivitis, colds, or fever should be isolated. Bear in mind that patients with measles are vulnerable to pneumonia and other serious complications.

### RUBELLA (GERMAN MEASLES)*

German measles (3-day measles) is a mild but highly prevalent disease described by fever, enlargement of lymph nodes, mild catarrhal inflammation of the respiratory tract, and a skin rash similar to that of measles (rubeola) or scarlet fever (Fig. 29-1). The incubation period is 14 to 21 days. Transmission is airborne from person to person. A common source is someone with an inapparent infection. The cause is a medium-sized, spherical unit, an extremely pleomorphic virus that, isolated from throat washings and the blood of patients, has been grown in cell cultures. This peculiar virus, as yet unclassified, with an RNA core is about the size of a myxovirus but it behaves somewhat like a togavirus. There is no insect vector. Only 1 antigenic type is known.

Rubella is important because approximately one out of four children born to mothers contracting German measles during the first 4 months of pregnancy has congenital defects or is malformed. If rubella is contracted during the first 4 weeks of pregnancy, approximately half the children born will be deformed.

From the mother's blood the rubella virus crosses the placenta into the developing tissues of the new individual, where it can persist throughout gestation

---

*For a discussion of measles vaccines and immunization procedures see pp. 400, 404, and 415.

*For immunization see pp. 400, 406, and 412.

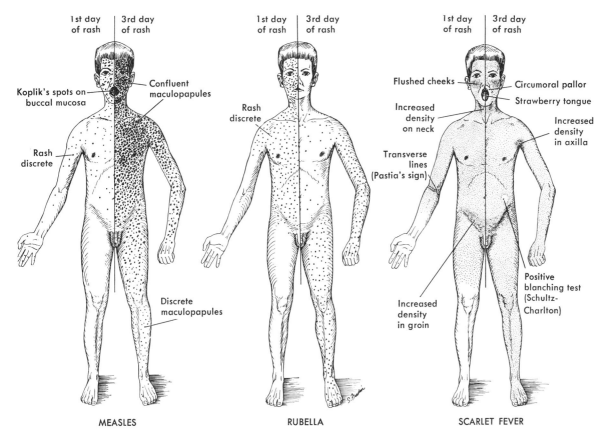

**Fig. 29-1.** Skin rashes in measles, rubella, and scarlet fever, sketch. (From Krugman, S., and Ward, R.: Infectious diseases of children, ed. 5, St. Louis, 1973, The C. V. Mosby Co.)

and into the neonatal period. The unborn child is infected at the same time as his mother, and since the viral injury leads to irregularities in the development of one or more organs, malformations result. The defects are common in the eyes, ears, heart, and brain. Examples are microcephaly (extremely small head), deaf-mutism, cardiac defects, and cataracts.*

Viral injury in rubella is unique. In keeping with the mild nature of the infection, the virus neither destroys nor invigorates. It merely slows things down. The cells it parasitizes continue to grow and multiply but at a decreased rate. The embryo and fetus of the first 3 to 4 months of pregnancy are in a period of development during which the anatomic units define their shapes, take their places, and lay out their interconnections. Timing here is as critical as it is with a trapeze artist.

_____

*As a result of the epidemic of 1964 in the United States, there were 20,000 stillbirths and 30,000 babies born with congenital anomalies to mothers whose pregnancies were complicated early by rubella.

When infection with this virus persists after birth, the baby is born with *congenital rubella*, the manifestations of which may be mild or severe. There may be a single serious defect or multiple ones in a small undersized baby. The *rubella syndrome* indicates active infection in the newborn, which is easily demonstrated by recovery of the rubella virus from nasopharyngeal washings, conjunctivae, urine, and spinal fluid.

**Laboratory diagnosis.** As a routine, virus isolation is impractical. The following serologic procedures are available for the laboratory diagnosis of rubella infection: virus neutralization, complement fixation, hemagglutination inhibition (HI), and immunofluorescence.

The hemagglutination-inhibition test is the most sensitive and most widely done. With a single specimen of serum this test indicates immunity in the presence of HI antibody. With paired serums spaced 1 or 2 weeks apart and a fourfold increase in the HI titer, it can make the diagnosis. If a woman is exposed to a possible case of rubella during her pregnancy, the

HI test may be used to determine both in the pregnant woman and in the contact whether the exposure is to rubella and what the woman's immune status is to rubella. For the diagnosis of congenital rubella there is the determination of rubella-specific immunoglobulin M in the baby. (This is an antibody that does not cross the placenta and that therefore could not be derived from the baby's mother.)

**Immunity.** An attack of German measles is followed by permanent immunity. Girls should have German measles if possible before the childbearing years, and a pregnant mother should avoid exposure to the disease. This is true even in women supposed to have had an attack, because an erroneous diagnosis is often made. Although the newborn baby possesses virus-neutralizing antibodies in high titer, he may continue to harbor virus and to shed it, even for several years, thus constituting an important reservoir and source of infection to susceptible individuals in his environment.

## SMALLPOX (VARIOLA)*

Smallpox, one of the most highly communicable diseases, is characterized by severe constitutional symptoms and a rash (Figs. 29-2 and 29-3) that goes through a typical evolution to become hemorrhagic in the severest cases. The incubation period is 12 days. Before the days of vaccination, smallpox spread over the world in devastating epidemics. It has been estimated that in some of these, 95% of the population was attacked and 25% died.

Smallpox is the most infectious of diseases, and the death rate in unprotected individuals is high. Although today in the United States death from smallpox is almost unheard of, thousands of persons succumb each year to the disease in countries such as India and Pakistan. In the 1960s, an unsuspected case in a Pakistani girl initiated an epidemic of smallpox in Great Britain, with at least thirteen deaths resulting. With the modern jet plane an area in which smallpox is prevalent is less than a day away from this country.

There are 2 types of smallpox virus (a poxvirus). One causes the severe form, *variola major*. *Variola minor*, or *alastrim*, the other type, is mild.

**Transmission.** Smallpox is transmitted directly from person to person by droplet infection. Man alone carries the infection. It may sometimes be conveyed by objects such as handkerchiefs and pencils that have been contaminated with the nasal and buccal secretions of a person ill of the disease. It may also be transmitted from pustules by the hands. Persons immune by virtue of vaccination or an attack of the disease may become contact carriers and disseminate

virus for a short period. The infectious agent is generally thought to enter the body by the respiratory tract and leave by the buccal and nasal secretions. The virus may be found in the blood, skin lesions, and secretions of the mouth and nose. It may remain active for a long time in the dried crusts of skin lesions. Even the dead body may be a source of infection.* A mother with smallpox may infect her child in utero, and the child may be born with a typical smallpox eruption.

An attack of smallpox usually renders the patient immune for the remainder of his life.

**Laboratory diagnosis.** The elementary bodies of the smallpox virus may be seen microscopically within cells of a stained preparation of scrapings taken from a lesion. In material suitably prepared, the virus may also be identified in an electron micrograph, usually within a few hours. A smallpox gel precipitin test has been developed.

**Prevention.** Patients with smallpox should be isolated. The nurse should be isolated and, of course, vaccinated or revaccinated at once. All objects in contact with the patient should be sterilized, preferably by heat (burning, high-pressure steam, boiling). If this cannot be done, they should be soaked in a 2.5% saponated cresol solution. The feces and urine should be disinfected with chloride of lime. Sputum and discharges from the mouth and nose should be received on tissues and burned. The patient should not be released until desquamation is complete.

### Vaccinia

Smallpox and vaccinia or cowpox are caused by poxviruses with similar biologic properties. Both can be grown on the chorioallantoic membrane of the chick embryo. The virus of vaccinia produces a mild disease either in man or in cattle (its natural host), and its importance is that it can be used to produce immunity against the more severe disease, smallpox.

## MOLLUSCUM CONTAGIOSUM

Molluscum contagiosum is a skin disease characterized by the presence of small, pink, wartlike lesions on the face, extremities, and buttocks. It is spread from person to person by direct and indirect contacts. The cause is a large poxvirus that produces very dramatic intracytoplasmic inclusions in the squamous cells lining the affected skin site.

---

*For immunization see pp. 402, 406, 411, and 416.

*In the smallpox epidemic in the United Kingdom the body of a victim was thoroughly sprayed with 5% Lysol, placed in a plastic bag, wrapped in a rubber sheet, placed on a Lysol-soaked bed of sawdust, and sealed in an airtight, watertight casket. Cremation was urged. The health officers caring for the body wore full protective clothing.

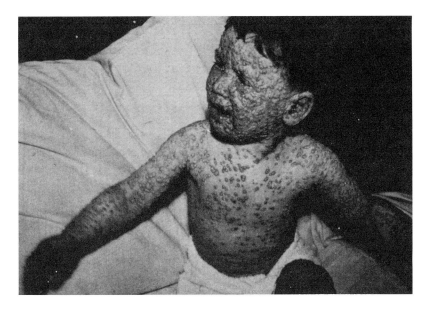

**Fig. 29-2.** Smallpox in unvaccinated 2½-year-old boy on eighth day of illness. Attack was severe, but boy recovered. (Courtesy Dr. Derrick Baxby, University of Liverpool, England.)

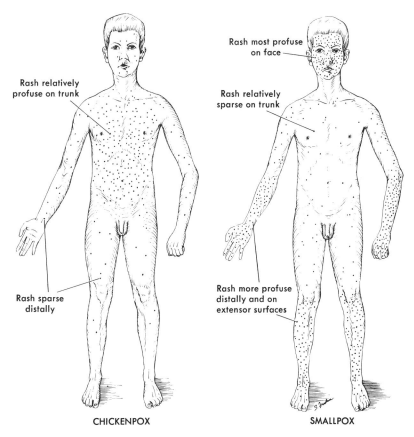

**Fig. 29-3.** Skin rashes in chickenpox and smallpox, sketch. (From Krugman, S., and Ward, R.: Infectious diseases of children and adults, ed. 5, St. Louis, 1973, The C. V. Mosby Co.)

## CHICKENPOX AND SHINGLES
## (VARICELLA–HERPES ZOSTER)

The two diseases, chickenpox (varicella) and shingles (herpes zoster), represent two phases of activity of a single virus (a herpesvirus), referred to as the varicella-zoster or VZ virus. The first invasion of the body by the virus produces chickenpox, the generalized infection. Shingles, a localized infection, represents the reinvasion of an immune or partially immune host.

Varicella, usually a mild disease of childhood, presents a typical (teardrop) vesicular rash that although generalized in the skin and mucous membranes, is concentrated on the trunk (Fig. 29-3). The incubation period of chickenpox is 14 to 16 days. Herpes zoster, on the other hand, is a disease of adults. It is characterized by the appearance of a vesicular eruption, the individual blisterlike lesions of which are similar to those of varicella but whose distribution is quite different. In shingles, vesicles occur on one side of the chest, following the course of the peripheral nerves supplying that part of the chest. They may occur in other parts of the body, but since the primary involvement is in the ganglion of the posterior nerve root, they always follow the course of the nerve or nerves supplying the affected part. Shingles may cause prolonged suffering because the skin eruption is associated with intense burning pain.

In the blisterlike lesions of the skin in either disease there are typical reddish inclusion bodies in the nuclei of injured epithelial cells. The virus is present in the fluid of the vesicles in either disease (Fig. 29-4). The moist crusts of chickenpox are infectious, whereas the dry ones are not. Chickenpox is transmitted by direct contact with a patient. Frequently it has been observed that herpes zoster in adults has served as a source of varicella in children.

No immunity to chickenpox is conferred by the mother on her newborn infant, and convalescent serum is of little value in preventing or modifying the

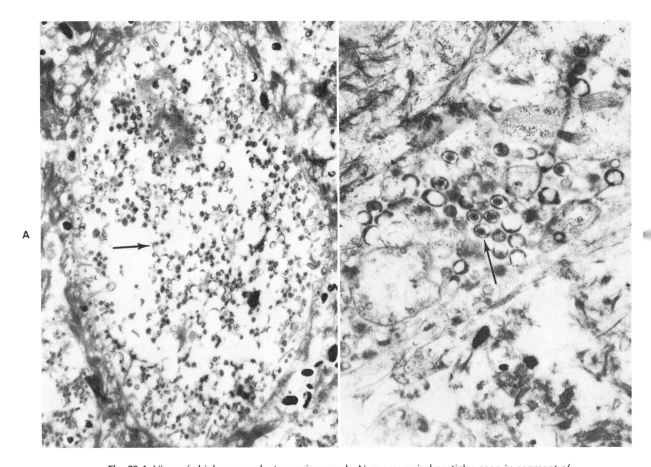

**Fig. 29-4.** Virus of chickenpox, electron micrograph. Numerous viral particles seen in segment of squamous cell from skin. (**A,** ×15,000; **B,** ×30,000.)

disease. A vaccine for chickenpox is in the experimental stage, but any licensed vaccine goes well into the future.

## HERPES SIMPLEX

Infection with herpes simplex virus (HSV; *Herpesvirus hominis*) is related to either of 2 recognized serotypes, each with unique biologic features. The more common HSV type I is responsible for the familiar fever blisters (herpes simplex) and cold sores found about the mouth and lips (herpes labialis). Type I lesions include recurrent labialis, gingivostomatitis, corneal lesions in the eye, and eczema herpeticum. This type is probably spread via the respiratory route and occurs in older children and adults.

Type II is found about the genital organs. Spread as a venereal disease through sexual contact, it produces skin and mucosal lesions below the waist (herpes progenitalis). (Type I tends to produce lesions above it.) Because patients with cancer of the mouth of the womb (cervix uteri) show statistically significant evidence for having had type II infection previously, this herpesvirus has recently been implicated in the causation of this form of cancer.

In most instances the first infection with herpesvirus is an inapparent one; clinical signs of disease occur in only about 10% to 15% of persons infected. Saliva and genital secretions are probable sources of infection. The incubation period is 2 to 12 days. It is believed that thereafter the virus exists in the body as a latent infection and that when the body resistance is weakened from any cause, the virus is reactivated. Recurrent herpes simplex often accompanies febrile illness, exposure to cold or sunlight, fatigue, mental strain, or menstruation. (See Schema 6.) Unlike other viral infections, the host's humoral antibodies apparently give no protection against subsequent lesions.

One very serious complication of herpes progenitalis is infection of the newborn. By contacting a herpetic lesion in his mother's birth canal, the baby acquires the infection. In 1 to 3 weeks he becomes gravely ill with generalized herpesvirus infection and usually succumbs. Herpetic lesions can be found in all organs including the brain.

The virus can be cultivated in cell cultures and recovered from newborn mice. It forms characteristic intranuclear inclusion bodies in multinuclear giant cells, which may be identified by the light or the electron microscope in suitable preparations of the fluid from the superficial vesicles (Figs. 29-5 and 29-6). Fluorescent antibody technics are used in the diagnosis of this infection, and there are neutralization and complement fixation tests.

## CYTOMEGALIC INCLUSION DISEASE

Cytomegalic inclusion disease (salivary gland disease) is infection caused by the ubiquitous cytomegaloviruses (salivary gland viruses). The pathologic lesions are striking in nature. Large, well-defined viral inclusions are seen in the nucleus, and smaller ones are found in the cytoplasm of the injured cells, which are enlarged (*cytomegaly* means cell enlargement) (Fig. 29-7). In fatal cases the cell changes are seen in the gastrointestinal tract, lung, liver, spleen, and other organs. In nonfatal cases, inclusions may be found in epithelial cells from the kidney shed into the urinary sediment.

In its overt form, cytomegalic inclusion disease is seen in the newborn as a congenital infection acquired from a mother who was probably asymptomatic (latent infection) and in an older individual as a complication of a preexisting disease state. In the infected newborn, cytomegalovirus is the cause of birth defects, especially in the central nervous system (examples: microcephaly, hydrocephaly, blindness). Mal-

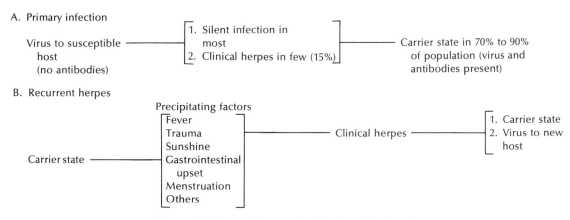

**Schema 6.** Schema of herpes simplex virus infection in man.

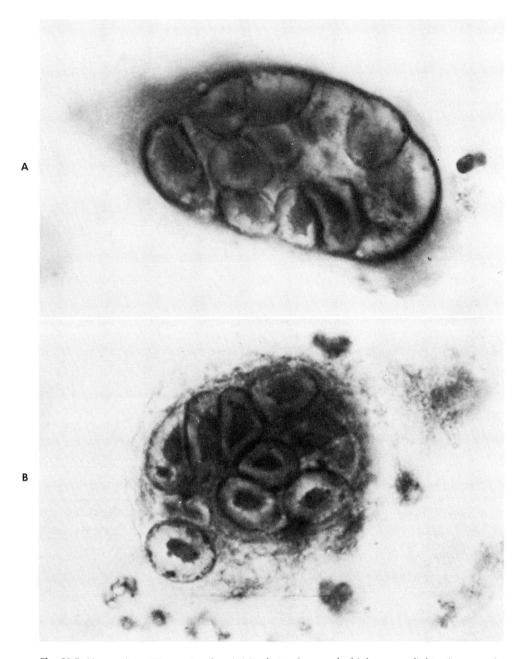

**Fig. 29-5.** Herpesvirus *(Herpesvirus hominis),* photomicrograph (high-power, light microscope). Inclusion bodies within nuclei of multinucleated squamous cell from skin. **A,** Early stage in formation of inclusion bodies. **B,** Inclusion bodies well defined.

formed babies exhibit the viral inclusions. In modern clinical medicine the patient on immunosuppressive therapy after organ transplant and the leukemic patient receiving cancer chemotherapy are vulnerable for cytomegalovirus pneumonia. Cytomegalic inclusion disease is associated with the postperfusion syndrome. This is an infectious mononucleosis–like syndrome following perfusion of fresh blood in patients undergoing open heart surgery with cardiopulmonary bypass.

The viral inclusions are readily visualized and diagnostic. Serologic technics used are those of neu-

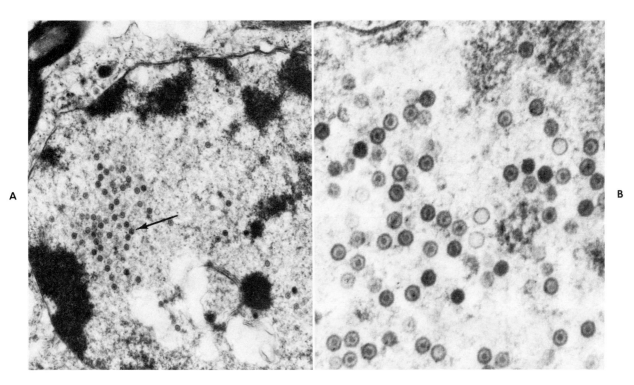

**Fig. 29-6.** Herpesvirus *(Herpesvirus hominis),* electron micrograph. Numerous viral particles in one nucleus of squamous cell from skin. (**A,** ×20,000; **B,** ×56,000.)

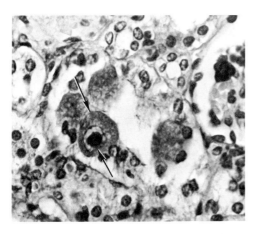

**Fig. 29-7.** Cytomegalic inclusion disease of kidney, microscopic section. Arrows spot enlarged renal tubular cell. Note large intranuclear inclusion body of cytomegalovirus. (×800.)

tralization, complement fixation, and immunofluorescence. There are 2 distinct antigenic types of cytomegalovirus (a herpesvirus) from man. Virus has been propagated in cell culture. There is an experimental vaccine.

## Respiratory diseases
### INFLUENZA

Influenza* is a highly communicable disease occurring in epidemics that are characterized by explosive onset, rapid spread, involvement of a high percentage of the population, and frequency of serious secondary bronchopneumonia. An influenza pandemic occurs every 10 to 14 years. The name *influenza* comes from Italian astrologers of long ago who believed that the periodic appearance of the disease was in some way related to the *influence* of the heavenly bodies.

One of the world's greatest catastrophes occurred in the pandemic of 1918-1919. Although other epidemics have had higher death rates, on the basis of total number of deaths this was the worst pestilence that civilization had ever experienced. It is estimated that there were 200 million cases with 20 million

*For immunization see pp. 404, 415, and 416.

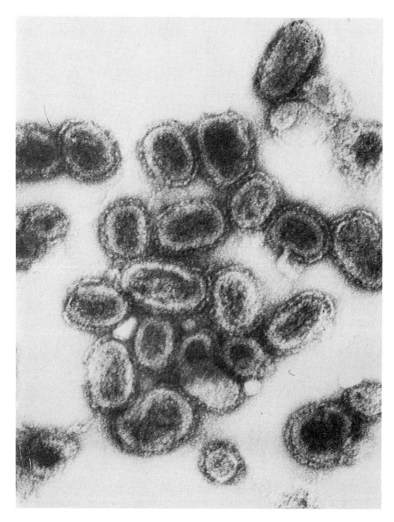

**Fig. 29-8.** Influenza virus negatively stained ($A_2$/Aichi/68 or "Hong Kong" virus), electron micrograph. (×303,100.) (Courtesy Dr. C. A. Baechler, Parke, Davis & Co., Detroit, Mich.)

deaths over the world. In the United States alone there were 850,000 deaths, a figure greater than that for the combined battlefield losses of World Wars I and II and the Korean War. And this occurred within the twentieth century.*

Influenza is caused by a myxovirus† (so tiny that 29 to 30 million of them could rest on the head of a pin), and like many viral diseases, it seems to potentiate serious bacterial infection, mostly broncho-

pneumonia. The mortality of the 1918 pandemic was largely the result of the severe, complicating bronchopneumonia produced by virulent streptococci.

**The agent.** Three types of influenza virus are known today: A, B, and C. Of these A and B have been best studied. They are alike in many ways but differ serologically. Each includes numerous distinct strains. Influenza A strains (Figs. 29-8 and 29-9) have figured much more frequently in epidemics than those of type B, the strains of which are considered to be less virulent than those of type A. The pandemic of 1918-1919 is thought to have been caused by type A. The epidemic of 1947 was caused by a strain of virus A designated as A′; Asian strains of virus A were responsible for the pandemic of 1957, and a variant also in the A group—$A_2$ Hong Kong/68—caused the Hong

---

*Only two places in the world allegedly escaped the pandemic—St. Helena, an island in the South Atlantic, and Mauritius, one in the Indian Ocean.

†It was originally thought that *Haemophilus influenzae* was the cause of influenza. This organism is an important *secondary* invader in this and other respiratory diseases.

**304**

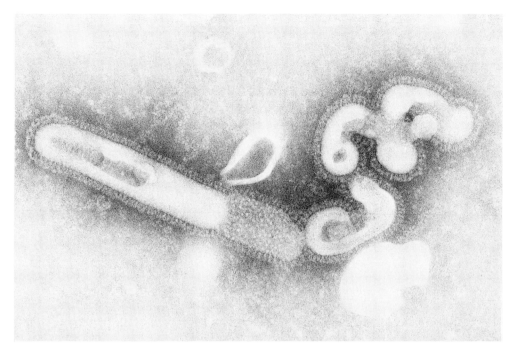

**Fig. 29-9.** Influenza virus, negatively stained (A/Hong Kong/1/68), electron micrograph. Note filamentous and pleomorphic particles. Virus isolated from throat of newborn baby. (×200,000.) (From Bauer, C. R., and others: J.A.M.A. **223**:1233, 1973.)

Kong pandemic of 1968. An unexpected event was the emergence of another $A_2$ virus—the $A_2$/England/42/72 strain as the predominant one and the cause of "London flu" in 1972-1973. At this date it has been superseded by the Port Chalmers (A/Port Chalmers/1/73) strain, called after the town in New Zealand from where it has spread slowly since it was first isolated in 1973. There have also been scattered outbreaks of influenza B in the last several years.

**Epidemiology.** The clinical manifestations of influenza remain fairly constant throughout the years although caused by an agent capable of remarkable changes. It has been said that it is an "unvarying disease caused by a varying virus." The infectious agent of influenza enters the body by the mouth and nose and leaves by the same route. Recently influenza virus has been recovered from anal swabbings. Influenza has been produced artificially in chimpanzees, ferrets, and mice by injection of filtrates of nose and throat washings from known human cases.

The disease is spread by direct and indirect contact, including droplet infection. An epidemic is usually of short duration and quickly subsides, to be followed after several weeks by a secondary wave, a free period, and a tertiary wave. Never does the infection spread faster than people travel. What happens to

the virus between epidemics remains still a mystery, although the relationships of influenza viruses to animals are becoming more apparent. There is good reason to think that in the interval the virus resides in animals, multiplies, and changes genetically, possibly by genetic recombination of human strains with those from the lower animals, thus becoming infective for man again. An epidemic seems to depend on the emergence of the new strain; since this organism possesses a continuing and dramatic tendency to change its chemical and genetic nature, that is, to mutate, new variants of the virus types arise constantly from the major antigenic shifts. Flu virus mutates to a magnitude not found for any other infectious agent. If the majority of persons do not possess the immune mechanisms to meet the new variation, then far-reaching epidemics and pandemics threaten. (See Fig. 29-10.)

The explosive outbreak may be explained by the high communicability of the disease, the great number of susceptibles, and the fact that during the early days of the attack the patient is not confined to bed but mingles freely with other people. The average duration of an epidemic in a community is from 6 to 8 weeks. In secondary and tertiary outbreaks the number of people attacked is less than in a primary outbreak, but the disease tends to be severe, complica-

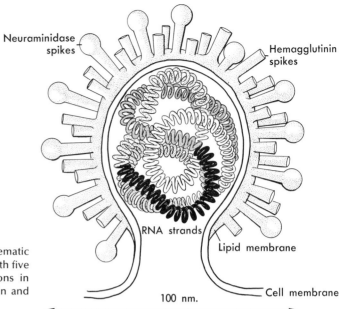

**Fig. 29-10.** Influenza virus emerging from cell, schematic drawing. Note unusual nature of viral nucleic acid with five discrete segments. Mutations result from alterations in biologically active surface proteins of hemagglutinin and neuraminidase spikes.

tions are more common, and the mortality is higher. Interepidemic cases are usually mild.

**Recent epidemics.** In early 1957 influenza appeared out of north China and within the next several months spread all over the world. There were millions of cases over a wide area of the Far East. Referred to as Asian flu, it quickly spanned the extent of the United States.

The virus was found to comprise new strains of influenza virus type A, designated the Asian strains, and cultures were established in embryonated eggs. On the whole, the mortality rate of this pandemic was low; in areas where notable, it was associated with severe staphylococcal pneumonia.

In the summer of 1968 another pandemic of influenza came out of the Orient, starting in Hong Kong with close to half a million cases. Hong Kong influenza was caused by a virus not completely different from the Asian flu virus of 1957, and the clinical disease was similar to that of the prior decade. During the last 3 months of 1968 it was estimated that 30 million persons were stricken. There were more deaths with Hong Kong influenza than with Asian influenza, especially among chronic invalids. *Staphylococcus aureus* and *Pseudomonas aeruginosa* were the complicating bacterial infections.

Since the 1968 pandemic, epidemics have tended to occur annually. Asian strains could dominate the influenza picture for a period of time, until the level of immunity in the general population has risen significantly.

**Immunity.** Part of the population apparently possesses natural immunity to influenza, because during an epidemic some persons do escape infection. There is reason to think that natural immunity acquired from an attack of the disease protects against a repeat attack by the same or very closely related strain. However, there is no protection against the new strains that are appearing. Little success has been obtained in producing passive immunity by means of convalescent or immune serum.

**Laboratory diagnosis.** The diagnosis of influenza can be confirmed only by isolation of the virus or serologic studies. The virus can be grown in cell cultures or in the embryonated egg. The serologic tests include hemagglutination-inhibition, hemadsorption-inhibition, neutralization, and complement fixation.

**Prevention.** When an epidemic of influenza strikes, all the methods known to preventive medicine fail to check it. Wholesale isolation seems to be of little value and is almost impossible to achieve. Nurses attending patients with influenza should disinfect the mouth and nasal secretions of the patient and should avoid exposing themselves to droplet infection.

### SWINE INFLUENZA

Swine influenza is a severe respiratory infection of hogs caused by the combined action of a myxovirus and a bacterium, *Haemophilus suis*. The bacterium is closely related to *Haemophilus influenzae*, and the virus is closely related to that of human influenza. The diseases differ in that the human virus can pro-

**Table 29-1**
Respiratory illnesses related to known respiratory viruses

| ILLNESS | VIRUS |
|---|---|
| Influenza | Influenza viruses A, B, C |
| Common cold of adults | Rhinovirus (Salisbury)—100 or more types |
| | Coronavirus—3 types |
| Acute respiratory syndromes* | Influenza viruses A, B, C |
|   Common cold syndrome in children, some adults | Parainfluenza viruses 1, 2, 3, 4 |
|   Rhinitis | Respiratory syncytial virus |
|   Pharyngitis and nasopharyngitis | Adenoviruses—10 types |
|   Tonsillitis | Echovirus—6 types |
|   Laryngitis | Coxsackievirus A—23 types |
|   Tracheitis | Coxsackievirus B—6 types |
|   Bronchitis | Poliovirus—types 1, 2, 3 |
|   Bronchiolitis | Reovirus—types 1, 2, 3 |
|   Bronchopneumonia | |
|   Pneumonitis | |
|   Croup (acute laryngotracheobronchitis) | |
| Viral pneumonia (primary atypical pneumonia) | Influenza viruses A, B, C |
| | Parainfluenza viruses 1, 2, 3, 4 |
| | Adenoviruses—2 types |
| | Respiratory syncytial virus (in children) |
| | Measles virus |
| | Varicella virus |
| | Vaccinia virus |
| | Rubella virus |
| Pharyngitis (part of poliomyelitis) | Poliovirus—types 1, 2, 3 |
| Pharyngitis (part of infectious mononucleosis) | Epstein-Barr virus |

*No specific constant relation between given disorder and viral agent. See text.

duce the complete disease whereas the virus of swine influenza alone produces only a mild form. Swine may become infected with the strains of type A virus that happen to be prevalent in the human population at a given time. The Asian strains of the 1957 epidemic were recovered from hogs in Japan.

## ACUTE RESPIRATORY SYNDROMES

A recent national health survey reflected that acute viral infection of the respiratory tract is one of the most common causes of illness in man. It is responsible for approximately one third of all days lost from work and two thirds of days missed from school. Acute respiratory infection of the viral type is not a single disease but a spectrum of such entities as rhinitis, pharyngitis, tonsillitis, laryngitis, and bronchitis (Table 29-1). These inflammatory processes can occur singly, but combinations are frequent.

**Clinical features.** Viral infection of the lining of the nose results in a reddened mucous membrane and a hypersecretion of mucus—hence the well-known runny nose. A sensation of stuffiness comes from

nasal congestion and blockage. When the throat is involved, it is reddened, tonsils and other lymphoid masses are enlarged, and there is soreness. Hoarseness may result from inflammatory swelling of the larynx. Other clinical features associated in whole or in part with acute respiratory disease include low-grade fever, cough, pain and discomfort in the chest, headache, sensations of chilliness, and sometimes enlargement of cervical lymph nodes. Droplet infection accounts for spread; respiratory diseases are prevalent in cool months; and the epidemic pattern is a familiar one.

The disease influenza was originally considered to be part of the general complex of respiratory disorders. With a typical pattern for recurrent epidemics, influenza could be easily separated when the causative virus was discovered. Primary atypical pneumonia emerged in part from the respiratory assortment in World War II because of the characteristic findings in the lungs of soldiers. A mycoplasma (pleuropneumonia-like organism), *Mycoplasma pneumoniae*, not a virus, is responsible for a significant number of these cases (p. 265). In Great Britain certain viruses have been recovered from adults with the common cold (acute coryza), and the infection transferred to a chimpanzee, the only animal susceptible to the particular agents. The experimental studies suggest that the common cold may well have unique features.

**Relation of viruses.** By the early 1950s, tissue (cell) culture technology was developed to a high degree of efficiency. Viruses were recognized and recovered in such rapid succession as to incur a kind of viral explosion. So many were identified that proper assimilation and definition of medical importance have not yet been made. Regarding respiratory infections, it soon became clear that an array of viral agents were associated with a variety of clinical infections, with no fixed or specific relationship between the ailment and the virus. Viruses were recovered singly or together from the respiratory tract, both in health and in disease. Many observers prefer the term *syndrome*, the sum total of the clinical features of an illness, to emphasize the lack of a specific correlation between any precise agent and the clinical manifestations. In the light of present knowledge of viruses associated with respiratory disease the best we can do is to present certain viruses as being found in respiratory secretions and tissues and to point out the variety of associated syndromes. Table 29-1 lists the viral agents recovered from acute respiratory syndromes.

**Respiratory viruses.** From the known acute respiratory infections, viral agents have been recovered in a majority of instances. Viruses that cause respiratory disease are spoken of collectively as *respiratory viruses,* and as an entity they encompass several major groups of viruses, including the myxoviruses (influenza viruses), the paramyxoviruses (parainfluenza viruses and the respiratory syncytial virus), the picornaviruses (enteroviruses and rhinoviruses), the adenoviruses, and the reoviruses.

*Parainfluenza viruses,* classified as paramyxoviruses, were first recognized in 1957. The 4 antigenic types are more stable than the influenza viruses; they do not mutate so often. Parainfluenza viruses are present in the community most of the year. The typically mild, first-contact infection usually comes early in life. These viruses enter by way of the respiratory tract, and except in infants and young children, inflammation is usually confined to the upper part. They cause a number of illnesses, primarily in infants and young children, ranging in severity from mild upper respiratory infection to croup and pneumonia. The clinical features of their infections are not distinct; the majority are clinically inapparent.

*Respiratory syncytial (RS) virus,* also a paramyxovirus, infects a child before the age of 4 years. It is probably the most important cause of acute respiratory

disease in infants and young children. A formalin-killed vaccine containing the respiratory syncytial and types 1, 2, and 3 parainfluenza viruses from kidney cell cultures is being field-tested.

Among the *picornaviruses,* certain of the *enteroviruses* are respiratory pathogens. All the coxsackieviruses and some of the echoviruses (p. 315) are believed to cause respiratory disease. Coxsackieviruses have been isolated from nasal and pharyngeal secretions, and coxsackievirus A, type 20, has been studied in its relation to an acute upper respiratory coldlike illness. The respiratory agents among the echoviruses probably infect through the respiratory tract. They are known to multiply in the pharynx, producing a pharyngitis, and most likely are transmitted in respiratory secretions. Upper tract infections of echovirus are generally mild; the syndrome is many times that of the common cold. Echovirus types 11 and 20 have been specifically observed in such infections.

*Adenoviruses,** also known as adenoidal-pharyngeal-conjunctival (APC) viruses, were first discovered in adenoids removed surgically from persons without any detectable clinical disease. To date, 31 types have been isolated from human beings. Although these viruses may be recovered from persons without disease, some do cause acute infection of the respiratory mucous membranes and the conjunctival membranes. Adenoviruses are related to a striking variety of clinical conditions, such as acute respiratory disease, febrile pharyngitis or pharyngoconjunctival fever (especially in children), acute follicular conjunctivitis, epidemic keratoconjunctivitis (shipyard eye), tracheobronchitis, bronchiolitis, and pneumonitis. Types 3, 4, and 7 are related to epidemics of respiratory disease. Type 8 virus is the major cause of epidemic keratoconjunctivitis. Type 3, sometimes found in swimming pools, is the cause of pharyngoconjunctival fever.

In civilian groups, only a small percentage of acute viral respiratory diseases are caused by adenoviruses, but this group, particularly types 3, 4, 7, 14, and 21, is of special importance to the Armed Forces. It incapacitates many of the recruits inducted in the fall and winter about 8 weeks later. Immunization of military inductees therefore is highly desirable.

Man is the only known reservoir of adenoviruses, and the virus is transmitted in respiratory and ocular secretions. The fact that the conjunctival inflammation often precedes the respiratory infection indicates the eye to be a significant portal of entry. Epidemics of pharyngoconjunctival fever and conjunctivitis have been traced to dissemination of the virus in swimming pools.

---

*For immunization see p. 404.

**Table 29-2**

Comparison of viral infection of the respiratory tract in children and adults

|  | CHILDREN | ADULTS |
| --- | --- | --- |
| Type of infection | Primary contact often | Inactivation of latent virus often; rarely, primary contact |
| Degree of involvement | Severe; infection may be fatal; mild cases also seen | Mild (except in elderly and debilitated) |
| Clinical picture | Spectrum of respiratory disease | Common cold and related syndromes prominent |
| Causative viruses | Parainfluenza viruses, adenoviruses, and respiratory syncytial virus (viruses of childhood) | Cold viruses (coronaviruses and rhinoviruses) important; parainfluenza viruses, adenoviruses, and enteroviruses implicated |

The respiratory and ocular involvement, often combined in adenovirus infection, is associated with enlargement of the lymphoid tissue in the respiratory passages and of the lymph nodes in the neck.

Adenoviruses cannot be studied by their effects in animals, since they do not produce disease in the routinely used laboratory animals, nor do they grow on the membranes of the fertile egg. However, they can be demonstrated nicely in cell cultures in which certain human and monkey cells are used (Fig. 34-2). In virus-infected cells examined with the electron microscope, viral particles can be seen. This group shares a common antigen demonstrable in the serum of an infected person by means of a complement fixation test. The breakdown of the group into the different types is done by means of the virus neutralization test.

*Reoviruses,* viruses of undetermined pathogenicity and ubiquitous in nature, have been recovered from the respiratory and alimentary tract in man, in health and disease. Respiratory disease from all 3 types is usually low grade.

In the early stages of certain viral diseases—for example, poliomyelitis and infectious mononucleosis—involvement of the upper respiratory tract figures prominently.

**Influence of age.** The patterns of respiratory disease in adults and children are basically similar in many respects. Influenza, for example, is much the same at any age. Yet there are points of contrast. These are presented in Table 29-2.

## COMMON COLD (ACUTE CORYZA)

The common cold is said to be the most commonly occurring ailment of mankind and to disable temporarily more people than any other infectious disease. The characteristic nasal discharge of only a few days' duration is spread by direct contact, and a cold is most communicable in the early stages. The incubation period is 2 to 3 days. The agent enters the body by way of the upper respiratory tract. In sneezing and coughing, the affected person spreads not only his disease but also the bacteria he may be carrying in his throat. As with other viral diseases, the cold is often complicated by more serious bacterial infections such as pneumonia.

Some persons appear comparatively resistant to colds, whereas others are relatively susceptible. Factors said to predispose to colds are exposure to chilling and dampness, sudden changes in temperature, dusty atmospheres, drafts, loss of sleep, overwork, and lowered bodily resistance. Most colds occur between October and May, and preschool children have the greatest number. Immunity after an attack is brief. An individual may average two to four colds a year. The development of a vaccine is still experimental.

**Cold viruses.** In patients with the syndrome of the common cold, adenoviruses, certain enteroviruses, respiratory syncytial virus, influenza viruses, and parainfluenza viruses have at times been incriminated specifically. A true cold may be caused by one or more than one virus. The designation "cold viruses," however, usually applies to rhinoviruses and coronaviruses.

Echovirus 28, reclassified as rhinovirus type 1 (p. 308), was the first to be implicated as a "cold virus." Later pathogenic strains referred to as *rhinoviruses* or *Salisbury viruses* (100 or more rhinoviruses recognized, 75 characterized) were found in persons with colds, and were grown in cell cultures containing cells from lungs of human embryos. Rhinoviruses are responsible for more colds than is any other known agent. Another group of cold viruses, the *coronaviruses,* is made up of at least 10 serotypes. It is so named because of a segmented ring about the virion.

The cold caused by coronaviruses has a longer incubation period and a shorter sequence of illness than is seen with rhinoviruses.

### VIRAL PNEUMONIA*

Viral pneumonia is a clinical syndrome—*not* a single specific disease—acute, infectious, and self-limited. It is similar in its manifestations to primary atypical pneumonia, also a syndrome. Viruses implicated include the influenza viruses, the parainfluenza viruses, the adenoviruses, and in infants the respiratory syncytial virus.

## Diseases of central nervous system
### RABIES (HYDROPHOBIA)†

**The disease.** Rabies is an acute, paralytic, ordinarily fatal, infectious disease of warm-blooded animals, including man. Rabies has been recognized for 2000 years and has changed little in that period of time. It is primarily a disease of the lower animals, and dogs are chiefly responsible for its propagation in civilized communities. Other domestic animals that contract rabies are cats, horses, cows, sheep, goats, and hogs. When the disease occurs in wildlife, it is referred to as sylvatic rabies or wildlife rabies. Wild animals that often contract it are wolves, foxes, skunks, coyotes, raccoons, and hyenas. The rabid skunk is most dangerous to man or other animals, since the saliva of the skunk carries 100 to 1000 times the amount of virus carried by the dog. Skunks are more susceptible than are dogs and spread the disease among themselves. The skunk is said to be the commonest rabies carrier in the United States today. In certain parts of the world (South America, West Indies, Central America, and Mexico) the vampire bat transmits the disease to horses and other livestock. This is a serious veterinary problem because the vampire bat differs from other animals in that it does not succumb to the disease but becomes a symptomless carrier, remaining infective a long time. Bats are dangerous carriers of rabies because of their habits and close contact with man's dwellings. They are more likely to be found in barns and in deteriorating houses than out in the wilds. They migrate constantly and thus evade man. The disease has been recognized in certain insect-eating bats in parts of the United States (Florida, Texas, Pennsylvania, California, Montana), in the Caribbean area, and in Europe. No instance of the transmission of the disease from man to man has been recorded. Rabies in dogs is declining in incidence, but the disease in wild animals is definitely on the increase. It is rare in rodents (rats, mice, squirrels) and almost unheard of in laboratory animals (hamsters, gerbils, guinea pigs).

Rabies in animals occurs in two forms, the *furious* and the *dumb.* In the former a stage of increasing excitability is followed by a stage of paralysis ending in death. The animal fearlessly* attacks anything that it encounters; it drools saliva because its throat is paralyzed. In the dumb rabies, paralysis and death supervene without a preceding stage of excitement. The animal neither bites nor attacks. Except that its lower jaw drops down, it may show little sign of illness. It often hides and may be found dead. In either form of rabies there is no fear of water, and the animals do attempt to drink. The human patient, however, avoids fluids because of painful spasms in the throat muscles induced with the act of swallowing. This explains the name *hydrophobia* for the disease. It has been said that the agony of the spasms of the victim of rabies possibly exceeds all other forms of human suffering.

**The virus.** The bullet-shaped rabies virus (rhabdovirus) (Fig. 29-11) is found in the nervous system and saliva of infected animals. It is transmitted in the saliva introduced into the body through a wound, which is usually the bite of a rabid animal. If a wound such as a cut or abrasion becomes accidentally contaminated with the saliva of a rabid animal, infection is as likely to occur as if the animal had inflicted the wound. Rabid animals can transmit infection to others for several days before they show signs of the disease. When a person or animal becomes infected, the infectious agent passes from the site of inoculation along the nerve trunks to the central nervous system. When the virus reaches the brain, the manifestations of rabies appear. About 30% to 40% of the people and 50% of the dogs bitten by rabid animals develop rabies. *Once the disease develops, it is almost invariably fatal.*†

Rabies virus in the brains of animals naturally infected is known as street virus. If some of the emulsified brain containing street virus is inoculated into the brain of a rabbit, that rabbit will develop rabies within 15 to 30 days. If some of the emulsified brain of this rabbit is injected into a second rabbit, the second rabbit will contract rabies in a slightly shorter time. When the virus has been passed through a series of some ninety rabbits, it becomes highly virulent for the rabbit, producing rabies in 6 days. At the same time it has, to some extent, lost its virulence for all other species of animals. It is now *fixed* virus

---

*See the discussion on primary atypical pneumonia, p. 265.
†For immunization see pp. 398, 405, and 412.

*Absence of fear in a wild animal is abnormal.
†The first time anyone has survived the disease has been in a recent case in the United States given extensive coverage by the news media.

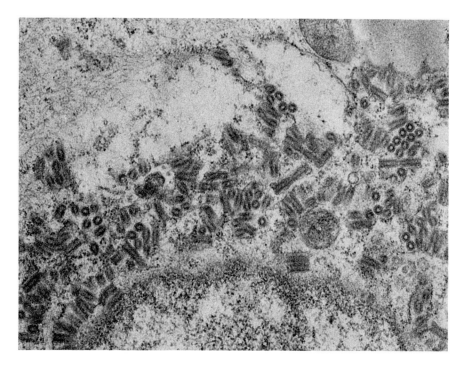

**Fig. 29-11.** Bullet-shaped rabies virus particles from hamster kidney cells shown in clusters, electron micrograph. (Courtesy Dr. K. Hummeler, Philadelphia.)

because of this loss of virulence. Further passage through rabbits does not reduce the time required for rabies to occur. This virus, treated with phenol, is the Semple vaccine used in the Semple method of antirabies vaccination. This vaccine has been replaced by improved preparations.

**Incubation period.** The period of incubation of rabies is remarkable for its length. In man it can vary from 10 days to 1 year, with an average of 2 to 6 weeks. In dogs it varies from 8 days to 1 year, with an average of from 2 to 8 weeks. The nearer the site of inoculation to the brain, the shorter is the period of incubation. It is also shorter in children than adults.

**Laboratory diagnosis.** Adelchi Negri (1876-1912) discovered certain inclusions in the brain cells of animals with rabies. These *Negri bodies* store ribonucleoprotein and virus antigen and are found in almost 100% of patients when disease is fully developed. By finding them, the laboratory diagnosis of rabies is most quickly made. The fluorescent antibody examination of brain tissue is the preferred diagnostic method.

Infant mice are susceptible to rabies virus and may be infected by intracerebral inoculation of suspect material; the virus is then identified by immunologic methods or by demonstration of Negri bodies in brain tissue.

**Prevention.** *If a person is bitten by an animal sus-pected of having rabies, the animal should not be killed but should be placed in the hands of a competent veterinarian for observation.* If the animal has rabies, the disease will be sufficiently developed within a few days for a definite diagnosis to be made. If the dog is well 10 days after biting a person, the person is in no danger from the bite. If, on the other hand, the animal is destroyed at the time of the bite, examination of the brain may fail to show Negri bodies because they are often absent in the early stages of the disease.

If examination of the brain of the animal fails to show Negri bodies, six or eight mice should be inoculated intracerebrally with an emulsion of the brain. If the animal had rabies, the mice may show Negri bodies in their brain tissue as early as 6 days and will exhibit signs of the disease on the seventh or eighth day. If the mice survive the twenty-first day, the animal may be considered not to have had rabies.

Local treatment of wounds inflicted by rabid animals is very important in the prevention of the disease. Adequate first aid treatment is crucial. Immediate and thorough cleansing of superficial wounds with tincture of green soap or benzalkonium chloride solution may inactivate the virus. (Even tap water has merit.) An antiseptic may be applied and the wound dressed. If a wound is deeply placed and washing by soap and water is not feasible, it is then considered advisable to cauterize the wound with fuming (concentrated) nitric acid. Antiserum may be injected into the base of the wound. Dogs, cats, and other pets bitten by rabid animals should be destroyed at once or, otherwise, vaccinated and kept in strict isolation for 6 months.

Persons who work with the disease are often confronted with the question of what course to take when a person drinks the milk or eats the flesh of a rabid animal. Eating or handling infected flesh or drinking contaminated milk can produce rabies if there is an open lesion on the skin or in the alimentary tract.

The nursing precautions in rabies are rather simple. All that is necessary is to sterilize the secretions from the mouth and nose of the patient and articles so contaminated. Rabies can be eradicated from civilized communities by measures designed for intensive control of stray dogs, immunization of resident dogs, and elimination of any reservoir of infection in wild animals of the area.

## VIRAL ENCEPHALITIS AND ENCEPHALOMYELITIS

The term *encephalitis* (pl., *encephalitides*) means inflammation of the brain, but by common usage it is applied to inflammatory conditions of the brain accompanied by degenerative changes instead of suppuration (pus formation). When the brain is involved, the spinal cord usually is also—hence the term *encephalomyelitis*. Encephalitis and encephalomyelitis indicate disease primarily of the central nervous system.

Animal viruses carried in the body of an insect vector are *arboviruses,* a simplification of "*a*rthropod-*bo*rne viruses." Arboviruses, or togaviruses, are the most numerous of the viruses infecting man. Important forms of encephalitis are caused by neurotropic arboviruses, the *arboviral (togaviral) encephalitides.* Two other noteworthy forms of encephalitis are *epidemic encephalitis,* or *encephalitis lethargica,* and *postinfection encephalomyelitis.* Neither is produced by a neurotropic virus or transmitted by an insect.

### Arboviral (togaviral) encephalitides

Arboviral infections occur principally in mammals or birds, and for most, man is only an accidental host. Arboviral infections are the largest group of zoonoses. The mosquito is an important insect vector, although arbovirus (togavirus) is found in ticks and mites. Although the arboviral encephalitides are similar in many respects, the causative agents are immunologically distinct, and the geographic distribution of disease is clear-cut.

*Equine encephalomyelitis,* a disease of horses and mules, secondarily of man, occurs in three types, each with its own virus: the eastern type (EEE) in the southern and eastern United States, the western type (WEE) in the western United States and Canada, and the Venezuelan type (VEE) in South America and Panama. *St. Louis encephalitis* (SLE), so named because it was first recognized in an epidemic in the vicinity of St. Louis in 1933, is a disease widespread in the United States. It occurs only in man. *Japanese B encephalitis* is found in the Far East, and *Murray Valley encephalitis* is found in Australia.

The eastern type of equine encephalitis is a severe form of disease with a mortality rate up to 70%. The death rate is much lower in the western form and St. Louis encephalitis. Young persons, particularly infants, have an increased susceptibility to western equine encephalomyelitis, and St. Louis encephalitis has its greatest incidence in persons of middle age or older. The incubation period for the different encephalitides ranges from 5 to 15 days.

The epidemiologic pattern for the different forms of arboviral encephalitis is reasonably consistent, with but slight variations. Arbovirus resides and multiplies in wild birds, its natural and primary hosts, and occasionally in domestic fowl. Venezuelan equine encephalomyelitis multiplies best in a reservoir of mammals; the eastern equine encephalomyelitis virus multiplies in both mammals and birds. From its natural reservoir arbovirus is transmitted from fowl to fowl (or mammal to mammal) and from bird to horses and man (terminal hosts) mainly by the mosquitoes of the genus *Culex.* There is no known instance of direct person-to-person transmission of encephalitis.

Encephalitis is a disease of warm weather and the summertime. In nontropical areas snakes and other cold-blooded animals harbor the virus for the cold months of the year. When snakes come out of hibernation, they seek out areas that also shelter large numbers of wild birds. Virus circulates in the bloodstream of snakes, as it does in birds, so that in the early spring mosquitoes can pick up the virus from such an overwintering host and carry it straight to the wild bird reservoir. Once infected, a mosquito remains so for life.

For mosquito-borne encephalitis to reach epidemic proportions a combination of factors is required, including a large wild bird population, favorable breeding sites for mosquitoes in stagnant pools and puddles, a high temperature, and susceptible terminal hosts.

The laboratory diagnosis of encephalitis is made on recovery of the virus from suitable specimens and its proper identification. Clotted whole blood or serum, throat washings, cerebrospinal fluid, urine, and in fatal cases brain tissue are specimens for virus isolation. Young or newborn mice are inoculated and observed. Serologic tests for identification of virus or its presence are the neutralization test, the complement fixation test, and a hemagglutination-inhibition test.

Effective vaccines made by growing the equine viruses in a chick embryo confer immunity in horses lasting from 6 months to 1 year or longer. A vaccine prepared against eastern equine encephalitis is suitable for use in human beings, but the vaccine for the western form of the disease is given only in special circumstances to individuals at high risk because of contact with the exotic and virulent form of the disease. The practical approach to the control of the disease is eradication of the mosquito vector.

### Epidemic encephalitis (von Economo's disease)

Epidemic encephalitis is probably an old disease, but it did not become prominent in medicine until a great outbreak followed the influenza pandemic of 1918-1919. Sometimes called sleeping sickness, it is described by lethargy and drowsiness that gradually pass into coma. The varied nervous system manifestations are severe. Although the early epidemics seemed to follow in the wake of influenza, the relation of the two diseases is not known. It is assumed that the disease is caused by a virus, but one has never been identified. It is believed that epidemic encephalitis is spread by droplets of buccal and nasal secretions and that the virus gains access to the central nervous system via the nasopharynx. The disease may be epidemic or sporadic, and institutional outbreaks occur. Peculiarly, the patient's family is not especially vulnerable, although the incidence among doctors and nurses is rather high. There is no known treatment for established disease and no known method of preventing or controlling an outbreak. Fortunately no epidemics have occurred since 1926.

### Postinfection (demyelinating) encephalomyelitis

Postinfection encephalomyelitis (allergic encephalomyelitis) is an acute disease of the central nervous system that occasionally arises during convalescence from infectious diseases or follows vaccination against such. The diseases are most often viral diseases, important among which are measles, German measles, smallpox, and influenza. Vaccination for smallpox and rabies is complicated by this type of encephalomyelitis. Postinfection encephalomyelitides resemble the viral encephalitides, not from the pathologic but from the clinical standpoint.

Most encephalomyelitides following smallpox vaccination (postvaccinal encephalomyelitis) occur in children and young adults who have never been vaccinated. Infants seem to be resistant. The incidence of postvaccinal encephalomyelitis is less than 1 in 33,000 vaccinations.

The following theories are offered to explain postinfection encephalomyelitis: (1) it is caused by the virus that produced the primary disease; (2) vaccina-

tion activates some latent virus in the body; and (3) the disease reflects an allergic reaction to the virus causing the preceding infection or to the patient's own nervous tissue now altered by a virus. Currently this last, the autoimmune, approach is favored.

### Slow virus infections

In some chronic diseases of animals and man, there is experimental evidence that the end-stage changes in the tissues, particularly in the central nervous system, are the result of a slowly progressive and damaging proliferation of a virus. In such diseases there is a long incubation period (years), a slow start, a protracted course, fatal outcome, no demonstrable formation of antibodies, no fever, and no inflammatory changes. *Scrapie*, a slowly developing, fatal neurologic disease of sheep, is an example of a "slow virus" infection. An example in man is *kuru*, a neurologic disease found in certain cannibals in New Guinea, transmitted by the ingestion of undercooked brain tissue containing the agent. In the chronic disorder in man, subacute sclerosing panencephalitis, an agent resembling measles virus has recently been cultured from affected brain tissue. Slow viruses may also be implicated in arthritic and rheumatic diseases and in the autoimmune diseases. Slow viruses are so designated because of their very long developmental cycles during which they are masked or inapparent. There is a definite possibility that some so designated may not be viruses at all. To date they have not been isolated. The current interest in slow virus infections stems from the suggestions they give as to the cause of many poorly understood central nervous system diseases in man.

### POLIOMYELITIS (INFANTILE PARALYSIS)*

**Poliovirus infection.** Poliomyelitis is an acute infectious disease that in its severest form affects the brain, the spinal cord, and certain nerves (Fig. 29-12). Poliomyelitis occurs in four forms:

1. Silent or asymptomatic infection. Any symptoms present are so mild as to be overlooked by the infected person. Such a person is a healthy carrier. Infection of the human alimentary tract by the poliovirus is exceedingly common all over the world. From the alimentary tract the virus at times enters the blood or the lymph stream. Silent infection exists among the members of a family with a clinical case of poliomyelitis.

2. Abortive infection. Findings referable to the nervous system are absent, although the affected person has a brief febrile illness, such as

---

*For immunization see pp. 400, 405, 414, and 416.

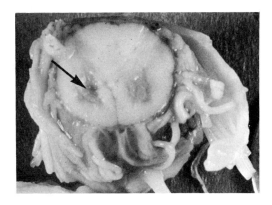

**Fig. 29-12.** Poliomyelitis, cross section of spinal cord from patient with paralytic poliomyelitis. (Paralysis results when motor neurons of anterior horns of spinal cord are destroyed by poliovirus.) Arrow points to anterior horn on left, a softened, depressed area of dead tissue, focally hemorrhagic. Anterior horn on right is similarly involved. (Courtesy Dr. B. D. Fallis, Dallas.)

a mild respiratory infection or a simple gastrointestinal upset. Most cases are abortive.

3. Nonparalytic infection. Findings point to the nervous system, but no residual paralysis develops.
4. Paralytic infection. Paralysis persists.

**Polioviruses.** There are 3 serologic types of poliomyelitis virus designated type I (Brunhilde), type II (Lansing), and type III (Leon). These viruses, among the smallest in size, may be grown in monkeys and chimpanzees.

Cell cultures of monkey kidney sustain a generous growth, as do certain human cell cultures. Polioviruses are pathogenic for man, monkeys, chimpanzees, and apes. As far as we know, man is the only animal subject to the disease; no reservoir of infection has been demonstrated in animals.

Polioviruses can be inactivated by ultraviolet irradiation, by drying, and if in a *watery* suspension, by a temperature of 50° to 55° C. for 30 minutes. Inactivation is slow with disinfectant alcohol and unsatisfactory with many bacterial germicides in wide use.

**Transmission.** The incubation period ranges from 3 to 35 days. The infected person is most likely to pass the virus to a noninfected person during the latter part of the incubation period and the first week of the clinical illness, the time at which the virus is present in his throat. Before the onset of symptoms in infected persons poliovirus is found in the secretions from the mouth and throat and in the feces. Today the poliovirus is believed to enter the body at the upper end of the alimentary tract and to leave through either the upper or the lower end.

Poliovirus has been recovered in large amounts from sewage, and milk-borne epidemics have been recorded. But the epidemiologic pattern for poliomyelitis is not that for the enteric infections. The most important mode of spread seems to be the direct one from person to person. It has been said that poliomyelitis "travels with a crowd." Houseflies, filth flies, and cockroaches can be contaminated with virus, especially during an epidemic, but the role of these agents in transmission is undefined.

**Epidemiology.** Poliomyelitis occurs sporadically but tends to be epidemic. Infantile paralysis is not a good name for the disease, since it occurs in adults and paralysis may be absent. In the early epidemics the disease chiefly attacked children less than 5 years of age, but then, in time, the children affected were older, and the number of adult cases increased.

The disease is thought to be increasing in severity and is worldwide. All races and classes of people can be affected. In temperate climates poliomyelitis appears in early summer. The number of patients and the severity of disease increase, a peak is reached in late summer and early fall, and the disease subsides after the first frost. Occurrence in more than one member of a family is frequent. There is an increased incidence in pregnant women because they are more susceptible to the disease, and there have been cases of congenital poliomyelitis reported in which the mother had had the disease late in pregnancy.

Radical changes have occurred in the epidemiology of poliomyelitis with the use of the polio vaccines. In 1957, for the first time, all the states and territories of the United States were free of epidemics. For the year 1957 less than 6000 cases of poliomyelitis were reported to the U. S. Public Health Service, of which about 2500 were paralytic. A decade later, in 1967, there were 44 cases (29 paralytic), mostly in nonimmunized or inadequately immunized children. Compare these figures with over 57,000 cases (21,000 paralytic) reported for the prevaccine year of 1952.

**Immunity.** Infection with one type of virus does not confer immunity for the other types. Poliomyelitis confers lasting immunity only for the viral type responsible. A high percentage of adults have virus-neutralizing substances in their blood. Infants can inherit an immunity from their mothers by placental transfer.

**Prevention.** Preferably the patient with poliomyelitis is isolated, although with widespread distribution of the virus, real insulation from contacts is impossible. Cross infections between patients probably are inconsequential in hospitals where no attempt to isolate is made. However, the disease is apparently sometimes spread from patient to attendant, nurse, or physician. On the whole, contacts, especially between children, should be minimized during epidemics, and in an epidemic such public health measures as the closing of public swimming pools are not inadvisable. Tonsillectomies should not be done during epidemics or in the season of the year when the incidence of the disease is highest. There is a greater risk for the severe form of the disease in persons who have recently had their tonsils removed. Healthy children may carry the virus in their throats, and it has been demonstrated in surgically excised tonsils.

## Other enterovirus diseases
### INFECTIONS WITH COXSACKIEVIRUSES

The coxsackieviruses are worldwide in distribution and have been frequently associated with epidemics of poliomyelitis. They were named after the town in New York where the first such virus was identified as research work was being done on poliomyelitis. They resemble the viruses of poliomyelitis in many respects, including their epidemiology. They are found in the nasopharynx and feces and at times in other parts of the body. They have never been found in the cerebrospinal fluid.

They are divided into groups A and B. Within each group are a number of types, of which at least 30 are known. These viruses possess an unusual pathogenicity for infant mice and hamsters but none for the adult animals. Group B is the more important in man. Coxsackieviruses produce such conditions as aseptic meningitis, epidemic pleurodynia (group B), herpan-gina (group A), vesicular pharyngitis, encephalitis, hepatitis, orchitis, an influenza-like fever, 3-day fever, pericarditis, and a severe form of myocarditis in infants. Group A viruses are usually associated with infections of the mouth. Most illnesses produced by coxsackieviruses present in children. Neutralizing antibodies to the viruses are found in the convalescent serum of patients recovering from diseases listed.

Modern classification of viruses assigns the coxsackieviruses to the category of picornaviruses, along with the polioviruses and the echoviruses. Most strains of coxsackieviruses and echoviruses can cause a disease closely resembling either nonparalytic or paralytic poliomyelitis.

### INFECTIONS WITH ECHOVIRUSES

Echoviruses were found by accident during epidemiologic studies of poliomyelitis. They were recovered from human fecal material in cell cultures. Their destructive effect on tissue culture cells and the fact that any disease to which they were related was unknown at first led to the designation of *echo*—*e*nteric, *c*ytopathogenic, *h*uman *o*rphan viruses. Some 31 members of this group have been so far classified. Many of these viruses may be harmless parasites, but some cause epidemics of aseptic meningitis, summer diarrhea in infants and young children, and febrile illness, with or without a rash. To date, the echoviruses have been found to be etiologic agents only in clinical syndromes (not specific diseases) that may be

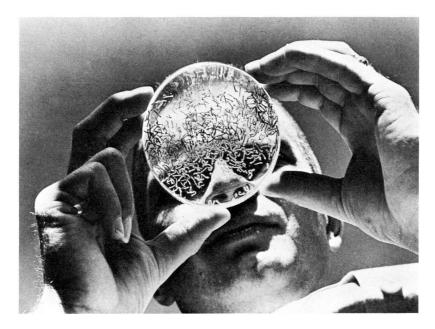

**Fig. 29-13.** *Aedes aegypti* mosquito, larval forms in Petri dish. (From Med. World News **6:**168 [Nov. 12], 1965; courtesy Eli Lilly & Co., Indianapolis, Ind.)

produced also by a number of other viruses (and bacteria as well). For example, aseptic meningitis, their chief central nervous system manifestation, is a syndrome, not a distinct disease.

## Other arthropod-borne viral diseases
### YELLOW FEVER*

Yellow fever, a mosquito-borne hemorrhagic fever once known as yellow jack, is an acute infectious disease defined by an abrupt onset, a rapid course, and a high mortality. The most characteristic feature is the rapid and extensive destruction of the liver. Prominent features are jaundice (yellow color to the skin and mucous membranes), albumin in the urine, hemorrhage, and vomiting.

The virus of yellow fever is transmitted by the mosquito *Aedes aegypti* (Fig. 29-13), which also transmits dengue fever. The mosquito bites a person during the first few days of illness and becomes infected. The virus multiplies in the body of the mosquito and reaches the salivary glands at the end of about 12 days; the mosquito remains infective the remainder of *her* life. (Only the female transmits the disease.) When a nonimmune person is bitten by an infected mosquito, manifestations of yellow fever develop in 3 to 5 days. The virus is found in the bloodstream during the first 3 days of the disease.

Yellow fever still remains endemic in many parts of the world. We must always guard against it because an epidemic requires but three things: a person ill of the disease, mosquitoes to be infected, and susceptible recipients. The transport of infected mosquitoes by airplanes and ships must be prevented.

A source of yellow fever in tropical Africa and Latin America is jungle yellow fever, found in monkeys. It is transmitted from animal to animal and from animal to man by forest mosquitoes (genus *Haemagogus*) living high in treetops. Epidemics appear in monkeys. The causative virus seems to differ in no respect from that producing ordinary yellow fever. If man becomes infected, the infection is transmitted from him by *Aedes aegypti*.

An active immunity to yellow fever can be established. The value of convalescent serum is undetermined.

### DENGUE FEVER

Dengue or breakbone fever is an acute disease lasting about 10 days and depicted by sudden onset of paroxysmal fever, intense joint pain, skin rash, and mental depression. It is caused by a virus that is found in the bloodstream during the early days of the attack and transmitted by the *Aedes aegypti* mosquito,

which, once infected, remains so for the rest of her life. When dengue fever is introduced into a community, a high percentage of the population contract the disease. An attack is followed by immunity that may persist for 1 or 2 years or for the remainder of the patient's life.

There are 4 distinct immunologic types of the virus, of which types 1 and 2 are most often responsible for the disease in the western hemisphere. The dengue viruses can be grown in cell cultures. Type 1, live virus, weakened by repeated passages through mouse brain is an effective vaccine in the clinical trials to date. Neutralizing and complement fixing antibodies may be demonstrated in the serum of a patient following infection.

### COLORADO TICK FEVER

An arboviral infection carried by an insect vector other than the mosquito is Colorado tick fever, caused by a single, small virus transmitted by the wood tick, *Dermacentor andersoni*. A mild febrile, diphasic illness, it is found largely in the western states, the natural habitat of the tick vector. Patients usually have been in a tick-infested area 4 to 6 days before becoming ill, and ticks are even found still attached to their bodies. The onset of disease is sudden, with chills, fever, and bodily aches that continue for 2 days or so. Then follows a period wherein the patient is essentially free of clinical manifestations. The fever returns to last for several days more before the disease has run its course. There are no complications. The disease has not been fatal, and the pathology is not known.

**Laboratory diagnosis.** Colorado tick fever virus may be recovered from the patient in specimens of blood, throat washings, and stool. It grows in tissue culture and in the fertile hen's egg. When inoculated into young mice, it produces paralysis. There are complement fixation, virus neutralization, and hemagglutination-inhibition tests for serologic diagnosis.

**Immunity and prevention.** Infection is thought to produce lasting immunity. Prevention depends on the avoidance of tick-infested areas or the wearing of adequate protective clothing. The body should be regularly inspected for ticks, and any present should be detached. Effective vaccines have been prepared by growing the virus in chick embryos.

## Diseases of liver (viral hepatitis)*

There are two viral diseases of the liver of special interest. They closely resemble each other in their clinical manifestations, yet because of certain sup-

---

*For immunization see pp. 406, 416, and 417.

*Viruses that may cause hepatitis include arbovirus, myxovirus, adenovirus, herpesvirus, coxsackievirus, reovirus, cytomegalovirus, and the Epstein-Barr virus.

posed differences in their epidemiology and mode of onset, they have been defined as distinct clinical entities. One, viral hepatitis type A, has been known as infectious hepatitis, catarrhal jaundice, epidemic jaundice, and short-incubation hepatitis; the other, viral hepatitis type B, as serum hepatitis, homologous serum jaundice, transfusion jaundice, posttransfusion jaundice, and long-incubation hepatitis. The virus postulated to cause the first has been referred to as virus A, and the agent for the second as virus B.

As a frame of reference a traditional consideration of these two is presented herein (Table 29-3). With the impact of new discoveries related to viral hepatitis and its causation, our concepts are drastically changing. Conventionally both are acute or subacute infections of the liver found only in man.* Note that the pathologic changes in the injured liver

_____

*Recently it has been reported that hepatitis B has been transmitted to nonhuman primates.

**Table 29-3**
Comparison of the traditional two types of viral hepatitis

|  | VIRAL HEPATITIS TYPE A (INFECTIOUS HEPATITIS, CATARRHAL JAUNDICE, EPIDEMIC JAUNDICE) | VIRAL HEPATITIS TYPE B (SERUM HEPATITIS, HOMOLOGOUS SERUM JAUNDICE, POSTTRANS-FUSION HEPATITIS) |
|---|---|---|
| Agent | | |
|   Virus | A (?) | B (Au + Dane particle?—see discussion) |
| Epidemiology | | |
|   Transmission | Fecal-oral route; also parenteral | From blood and blood products—parenteral; also oral, contact; insect? |
|   Experimental inoculation | Oral, parenteral | Parenteral |
|   Incubation period | Around 25-30 days (15-50 days) | 30 to 180 days |
|   Age preference | Young adults, 15-24 yr.; also children | 15-24 yr. (but all ages) |
|   Duration of infectivity | Virus in feces and blood 1 to 2 weeks before disease; remains 3 to 4 weeks longer | Virus in blood 3 months before disease; asymptomatic carrier for as long as 5 years |
|   Virus present | Feces, blood | Blood (thought to be in feces) |
| Clinical features* | | |
|   Onset | Acute | Slow, usually insidious |
|   Fever | Common before jaundice | Less common |
|   Jaundice | Rare in children, commoner in adults | Rare in children, commoner in adults |
|   Severity of disease | Less severe | More severe |
|   Prognosis | Good | Less favorable |
| Pathologic changes in liver | Same for both forms | |
| Laboratory evaluation | | |
|   Thymol turbidity† | Increased | Normal |
|   Abnormal SGOT‡ | Transient; 1 to 3 weeks | Prolonged; 1 to 8 or more months |
|   IgM levels | Increased | Normal |
| Prevention and control | | |
|   Prophylactic effect of gamma globulin | Good | Present but poor (questionable) |
|   Nursing precautions and control | 1. Isolation of patient<br>2. Sterilization of contaminated items | 1. No isolation of patient needed<br>2. Sterilization of permanent medical apparatus in contact with blood<br>3. Use of disposables (needles, syringes, tubing) for all patients |

*Many clinical features are the same.
†Test of liver function.
‡The enzyme serum glutamic oxaloacetic transaminase, which is elevated with liver disease.

are the same. The true overall incidence of viral hepatitis is unknown, since subclinical infection occurs without jaundice. It has been estimated that 80% to 90% of the cases go unrecognized. Immunity from an attack of one form of disease has been thought to result in immunity to that form only.

There is now good reason for believing that the agents, presumably viruses, causing both type A and type B hepatitis have at last been identified and that clear-cut serologic differentiation between the two has been made.

**Australia antigen.** As a population geneticist was working with the blood of an Australian aborigine in 1964, he found a new antigen, which he called the *Australia antigen (Au)*. As it turned out, his was a most significant discovery.*

Australia antigen is tightly linked to acute and chronic hepatitis (although it is also found in diseases such as Down's syndrome and leukemia, wherein immune mechanisms have gone awry). Its role in hepatitis rests on observations such as the following. More than half the patients with hepatitis B have the antigen in their blood. It can be recovered from liver cell nuclei, urine, and feces. If it is given experimentally to a group of human beings, the majority will come down with viral hepatitis type B. Antibodies develop in some persons who remain asymptomatic. Clearly not all viral hepatitis is associated with this antigen. All agree that there is an Au-positive and an Au-negative hepatitis.

The immediate application of this is in the blood bank to screen blood donors. The incidence of viral hepatitis among patients receiving blood containing Australia antigen is five times greater than it is among those patients given Au-negative blood. Already a number of tests have been designed to detect the Australia antigen in blood for transfusion. In rapid succession many are still coming onto center stage. Technics include those of complement fixation, immunoelectrophoresis, hemagglutination inhibition, reversed passive hemagglutination, and the widely acclaimed radioimmunoassay. Something is being done to minimize a very serious risk.

**The Dane particle.** Shortly after its discovery, Australia antigen was visualized with the electron microscope as a very small, spherical, viruslike particle about 200 Å in diameter, with knoblike units on its surface. Its identity as a virus was challenged, in part because of its rather simple outlines. In 1970 the

Dane particle was discovered, a structurally more complex particle with a 70 Å outer coat and a 420 Å internal core. It could be shown to synthesize DNA and to be clearly associated with Au. Au is recognized as the surface antigen of the virus of hepatitis B and designated HB$_s$Ag. The evidence is accumulating that the Dane particle plus HB$_s$Ag represents the complete virus.

## VIRAL HEPATITIS TYPE A

Viral hepatitis type A is usually spread directly from person to person. The principal pathway is the fecal-oral route. Poor sanitation favors its spread. Water, milk, and food can be sources of infection. Recent outbreaks have occurred in persons who have eaten raw shellfish contaminated by sewage. The cockroach and fly may be vectors. The virus is present in the feces and blood of infected persons. With technics of immune electron microscopy, a serologically distinct, exceedingly small, picornavirus-like agent, one millionth of an inch in diameter, has been recovered from a case of hepatitis A and postulated to be the etiologic agent, virus A.

The mortality of type A hepatitis is not high. Widespread immunity does exist, probably gained from inapparent childhood infection. Gamma globulin given as late as 6 days before the onset of the disease may protect a person for as long as 6 to 8 weeks.

The patient with recognized disease should be isolated. Diligent handwashing, wearing of protective gowns, and autoclaving of articles contaminated by the patient are necessary.

## VIRAL HEPATITIS TYPE B

Viral hepatitis type B is carried by human serum (or plasma) and may complicate blood transfusion or the administration of convalescent serum, vaccines, and other biologic products containing human serum. Needles, syringes, and tubing sets for transfusions and stylets for finger puncture are important conveyors of the infection when soiled by blood or blood products.* *As little as 0.000025 ml. of blood contaminated with B virus (0.01 ml. with A virus) has been shown to cause disease.* For this reason the disposable needles, disposable stylets for finger puncture, and disposable syringes, all now commercially available, are strongly recommended. Disposable units of plastic tubing suitable for blood transfusion are now in wide use.

Hepatitis B represents an occupational hazard among medical personnel working with blood or serum, including laboratory technologists, blood bank

---

*The research from which this discovery "fell out" was a basic type, not goal-oriented at all. The importance of the finding and the way in which it was made reemphasize the continuing need for the "basic" approach to scientific matters.

---

*For sterilization technics to prevent the spread of the hepatitis viruses see p. 168.

workers, physicians, nurses, and dentists. Surgeons are at high risk because of the possibility of accidental self-inoculation. Persons so exposed should observe rigid asepsis. The attack rate is high in the renal dialysis unit, and, paradoxically, the hepatitis is much more severe among the nurses and other personnel than it is in the patients. The disease is also prevalent among drug addicts who share their unsterilized and contaminated hypodermic needles. Heroin addicts are especially notorious for "passing the needle." Epidemiologic changes in viral hepatitis within the last five years reflect the increase of illicit drug use and its patterns. There have been shifts in seasonal and age incidences, a trend from rural to urban cases, and more of hepatitis B than of hepatitis A.

## Miscellaneous viral infections
### MUMPS (EPIDEMIC PAROTITIS)*

Mumps, or epidemic parotitis, is an acute contagious disease prevalent in winter and early spring and accompanied by a painful, inflammatory swelling of one or both parotid glands (Fig. 29-14). It is easily recognized because of the typical appearance of the patient. (A child may look like a chipmunk with nuts in his cheeks.) Caused by a paramyxovirus, it occurs most often between the fifth and fifteenth years.

*For immunization see pp. 400, 405, and 412.

Adult epidemics may occur in military organizations and are extremely difficult to control.

The period of contagion begins before the glandular swelling and persists until it subsides. The incubation period is usually 14 to 21 days. Mumps is mostly transferred directly from person to person by droplets of saliva, but indirect transfer by contaminated hands or inanimate objects may occur. An estimated 30% to 40% of persons infected with the mumps virus have a silent infection followed by permanent immunity. During the course of the inapparent infection these individuals may pass the virus to others.

The virus is thought to enter the body by way of the mouth and throat and probably reaches the salivary glands via the bloodstream. Viremia is responsible for such complications as orchitis, oophoritis, encephalitis, and pancreatitis. Inflammation of the testicle (orchitis), usually one sided, occurs in 20% of adult males with this disease. If, as is rarely the case, both testicles are involved, sterility may result. The mumps virus is an important cause of the aseptic meningitis syndrome. Inflammation in the central nervous system can be present with or without parotitis.

**Laboratory diagnosis.** Mumps virus may be recovered from the urine, saliva, or blood; in cases of central nervous system disease it is found in the cerebrospinal fluid. The chick embryo and cell cultures

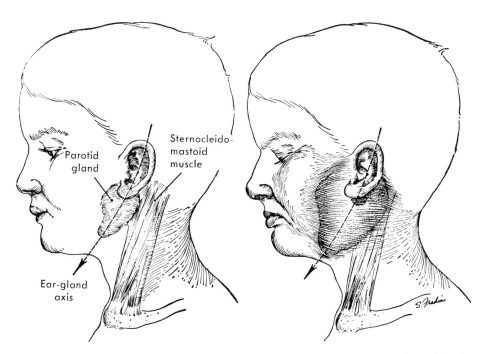

**Fig. 29-14.** Mumps, changes in the parotid gland, sketch. (From Krugman, S., and Ward, R.: Infectious diseases of children and adults, ed. 5, St. Louis, 1973, The C. V. Mosby Co.)

are used for its identification. The virus agglutinates red blood cells of the chicken and of the human blood group O. A skin test, not widely used, is available. The antigen for the test is killed virus from fertile eggs. Inflammation at the site of injection 18 to 36 hours later indicates the presence of immunity in the absence to sensitivity to egg protein.

**Immunity.** A passive immunity is given by an immune mother to her baby and persists for about 6 months. Convalescent serum given from 7 to 10 days after exposure protects a high proportion of children from infection. An attack of mumps is followed by permanent immunity, and contrary to lay belief, the same immunity follows either unilateral or bilateral involvement.

## INFECTIOUS MONONUCLEOSIS

Infectious mononucleosis or glandular fever is an acute infectious disease characterized by enlargement of the lymph nodes and spleen, sore throat, and mild fever. It is transmitted as an airborne infection. The total number of leukocytes is increased, and distinctive white blood cells (lymphocytes of unusual or atypical appearance) appear in the peripheral circulation. Rarely fatal, it may occur in epidemic form or sporadically. It usually attacks children and young adults (to 30 years of age). The incubation period is unknown but is thought to be 4 to 14 days or longer; some say 5 weeks. The disease may last 1 to 6 weeks, sometimes longer.

Infectious mononucleosis is important because it may be mistaken for diphtheria (sore throat) and such a serious disease as lymphatic leukemia. Nonsyphilitic patients may give positive serologic tests for syphilis during the disease and for several weeks after recovery. The heterophil antibody or Paul-Bunnell test is important in the diagnosis.

**Epstein-Barr virus (EB virus).** Infectious mononucleosis has long been considered a viral disease, the course of the disease suggesting that it should be. But a specific virus was not pinpointed for a long time.

In the mid-1960s a brand new member of the herpesvirus group was found under circumstances linking it first to Burkitt's lymphoma (p. 511) and then even more significantly to infectious mononucleosis. The virus was named Epstein-Barr virus after the tissue culture cell line from which it was first isolated. (It is freely called the EB virus.)

There are good reasons for thinking that the EB virus causes infectious mononucleosis, with only a few reservations. For one thing, serologic studies comparing antibodies to EB virus with the diagnostic heterophil antibodies in the course of the disease correlate well. One can demonstrate that antibodies to EB virus and heterophil antibodies come in and

peak at about the same time in a given case. Three months later heterophil antibodies drop out; EB virus antibodies remain. One important reservation is that Koch's postulates have not been satisfied. Infectious mononucleosis has not as yet been transmitted to healthy human volunteers.

Infection with EB virus must be widespread. The virus is everywhere and very common. Most infections are postulated to occur early in life, presenting themselves as either silent inapparent ones or at most as mild upper respiratory tract ailments. There are immunofluorescent and complement fixation tests for EB virus, but these are not offered in routine clinical laboratories.

## CONDYLOMA ACUMINATUM

Condyloma acuminatum is a cauliflower-like mass of coalescent warty excrescences formed on the external genitalia and about the anal region in either sex (Fig. 29-15). The growths are often multiple and vary much in size. The lesion is called a venereal wart and is transmitted as a venereal disease. The incubation period is 1 to 6 months. Large and bulky warts cause considerable discomfort and are associated with a disagreeable odor. The cause of this condition is a virus, either the same or an allied strain of the one causing the human wart so familiar in its extragenital setting. Encouraging results in treatment are reported with the use of autogenous vaccines.

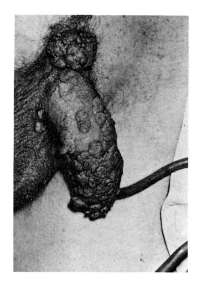

**Fig. 29-15.** Condylomata acuminata of skin of penis. Note confluence of wartlike growths. A giant condyloma acuminatum is present at penile-abdominal junction. (From Winter, C. C.: Practical urology, St. Louis, 1969, The C. V. Mosby Co.)

## FOOT-AND-MOUTH DISEASE (RHINOVIRUS OF CATTLE)

Foot-and-mouth disease, worldwide in distribution, is an acute infectious process in animals characterized by the formation of vesicles in the mouth, on the udder, and on the skin about the hoofs. One of the most contagious of all diseases, it primarily affects cloven-footed animals (cattle, sheep, swine, and goats). Horses are immune, and man seldom contracts the disease. Within the last few years it has been present in Mexico.

The disease is readily transmitted by direct contact or indirectly by contamination of fodder with infectious discharges. The disease has been transferred to man by contact with infected animals, by the milk of infected animals, and by contaminated material.

Control of the disease depends on the slaughter of all exposed animals, with burial or cremation of their bodies, disinfection of pens, and proper quarantine. There is no specific treatment. A diagnosis may be established by injecting suspicious material into the footpads of a guinea pig. Typical lesions will be produced if rhinovirus is present.

## DISTEMPER OF DOGS AND CATS

Canine distemper and feline enteritis (cat distemper) are important diseases of young dogs and cats. They are caused by two entirely different viruses. The distemper of dogs affects primarily the respiratory and nervous systems. In cat distemper the intestinal tract is primarily involved. Canine distemper is spread by food and water contaminated with the virus and to a lesser degree via the respiratory tract. Feline distemper is spread by direct contact and probably by fleas. Canine distemper affects dogs and related species. Feline distemper affects cats and raccoons. Neither affects man. Highly successful vaccines have been prepared against both diseases.

## ADDITIONAL DISEASES CAUSED BY VIRUSES

In the following lists are viral diseases that affect man, animals, plants, and insects, respectively.

### Man

| | |
|---|---|
| Hemorrhagic fevers (Omsk, Crimean, Bolivian, Indian, and Korean types; hemorrhagic nephrosonephritis; Kyasanur Forest disease) | Bwamba fever |
| | Lassa fever |
| | Rift Valley fever |
| | West Nile fever |
| Warts (verrucae) | Semliki Forest disease |
| Lymphocytic chorio- | Louping ill |
| meningitis | Russian spring-summer |
| Phlebotomus (sandfly) fever | encephalitis |

### Animals

| | |
|---|---|
| Pox of horses, sheep, goats, swine, buffalo, and camels | Infectious pancreatic necrosis of trout and Atlantic salmon |
| Rinderpest | Louping ill of sheep |
| Ectromelia | Fowl plague |
| Vesicular stomatitis | Fowl pox |
| Orf | Newcastle disease of chickens |
| Infectious canine hepatitis | Mengo fever |
| Aleutian disease of mink | Visna in sheep |
| Hog cholera | Duck virus enteritis |
| Rift Valley fever of sheep | |

### Plants

| | |
|---|---|
| Tobacco mosaic | Barley stripe mosaic |
| Tomato bushy stunt | Turnip yellow mosaic |
| Tobacco necrosis | Tomato spotted wilt |
| Peach yellows | Lettuce necrotic yellows |
| Curly top of sugar beet | Potato X |
| Swollen shoot | Striate mosaic of wheat |
| Wound tumor | Alfalfa mosaic |
| Tobacco rattle | |

### Insects (mostly larval stage actively diseased)

| | |
|---|---|
| Chronic bee paralysis | Polyhedrosis of spruce sawfly |
| Silkworm jaundice | Other polyhedroses |
| *Tipula* iridescence | |
| Granuloses | |

# Questions for review

1 Make a chart showing the causative agent, clinical features, laboratory diagnosis, transmission, and prevention of smallpox, measles, German measles, mumps, influenza, poliomyelitis, rabies, yellow fever, dengue fever, Colorado tick fever, infectious mononucleosis.

2 Discuss briefly the relation of chickenpox to shingles.

3 Outline the logical procedure to follow when a person is bitten by an animal suspected of having rabies.

4 Briefly compare hepatitis A with hepatitis B.

5 Explain the occurrence of fever blisters.

6 Briefly characterize adenoviruses, coxsackieviruses, echoviruses, arboviruses, rhinoviruses, reoviruses, enteroviruses, coronaviruses, cytomegaloviruses, herpesviruses, cold viruses.

7 Give the significance of the Australia antigen and the Dane particle.

8 What is meant by a syndrome? Briefly discuss acute respiratory syndromes.

9 Define or briefly explain: alastrim, variola major, variola minor, microcephaly, pustule, coryza, rhinitis, encephalomyelitis, yellow jack, silent infection, SGOT.

10 What is the current importance of the Epstein-Barr virus?

11 What serious effect may rubella have in a pregnant woman? Explain congenital rubella.

12 It is superstition among laymen that if the eruption of shingles encircles the body, death occurs. Explain why the eruption does not do this.

13 Discuss sylvatic or wildlife rabies and its implications for the spread of disease.

14 What is meant by slow virus infection? What is the implication?

## REFERENCES (Chapters 28 and 29)

Adams, J. M.: Persistence of measles virus and demyelinating disease, Hosp. Pract. **5:**87, May, 1970.

Alter, H. J., and others: Viral hepatitis, light at the end of the tunnel, J.A.M.A. **229:**293, 1974.

Andrewes, Sir C., and Pereira, H. G.: Viruses of vertebrates, ed. 3, Baltimore, 1972, The Williams & Wilkins Co.

Bedson, S., and others: Virus and rickettsial diseases of man, ed. 4, Baltimore, 1967, The Williams & Wilkins Co.

Behbehani, A. M.: Human viral, bedsonial and rickettsial diseases, a diagnostic handbook for physicians, Springfield, Ill., 1972, Charles C Thomas, Publisher.

Behbehani, A. M., and Marymont, J. H., Jr.: The role of the hospital laboratory in the diagnosis of viral diseases. I. Basic concepts, Am. J. Clin. Pathol. **53:**43, 1970.

Belsky, J. L., and others: Persistence of hepatitis-associated antigen within fixed population, Arch. Environ. Health **25:**420, 1972.

Benbassat, J., and others: Hepatitis in selective IgA deficiency, Br. Med. J. **4:**762, 1973.

Bishop, R. F., and others: Virus particles in epithelial cells of duodenal mucosa from children with acute nonbacterial gastroenteritis, Lancet **2:**1281, 1973.

Blumberg, B. S., and others: Australia antigen and hepatitis, Cleveland, 1972, CRC Press.

Bolivian hemorrhagic fever (editorial), J.A.M.A. **200:**716, 1967.

Bugg, R.: On the way: vaccines to snuff out sniffles, Today's Health **47:**36, Dec., 1969.

Bugg, R.: The flu that few will forget, Today's Health **47:**24, April, 1969.

Burkitt, D. P., and Wright, D. H.: Burkitt's lymphoma, Baltimore, 1970, The Williams & Wilkins Co.

Carter, W. A., and De Clercq, E.: Viral infection and host defense, Science **186:**1172, 1974.

Chang, T. W., and others: Genital herpes, some clinical laboratory observations, J.A.M.A. **229:**544, 1974.

Cohen, E. P.: What you should do when the flu bug bites, Today's Health **53:**16, Feb., 1975.

Cooper, L. Z.: German measles, Sci. Am. **215:**30, July, 1966.

Culliton, B. J.: Cancer virus theories: focus of research debate, Science **177:**44, 1972.

Docherty, J. J., and Chopan, M.: The latent herpes simplex virus, Bacteriol. Rev. **38:**337, 1974.

Dueñas, A., and others: Herpesvirus type 2 in a prostitute population, Am. J. Epidemiol. **95:**483, 1972.

Feinstone, S. M., and others: Hepatitis A: detection by immune electron microscopy of a viruslike antigen associated with acute illness, Science **182:**1026, 1973.

Fenner, F., and others: The biology of animal viruses, ed. 2, New York, 1973, Academic Press, Inc.

Finter, N. B., editor: Interferons and interferon inducers, New York, 1973, American Elsevier Publishing Co.

Fisher, M. M., and Steiner, J. W., editors: Proceedings of the Canadian Hepatic Foundation 1971 International Symposium on Viral Hepatitis, Can. Med. Assoc. J. **106:**417, 1972.

Gavrilă, I., and others: Hepatitis-associated antigen and specific antibodies in sera of convalescents and patients with viral hepatitis, J. Infect. Dis. **126:**200, 1972.

Gillette, R.: VEE vaccine: fortuitous spin-off from BW research, Science **173:**405, 1971.

Gregg, M. B.: The current status of influenza in the United States (editorial), South. Med. J. **66:**1085, 1973.

Gross, L.: Oncogenic viruses, New York, 1970, Pergamon Press.

Grossman, R. A.: Influenza, Milit. Med. **134:**8, Jan., 1969.

Hakosalo, J., and Saxen, L.: Influenza epidemic and congenital defects, Lancet **2:**1346, 1971.

Halberstam, M.: The "kissing disease" that isn't so romantic, Today's Health **52:**44, Dec., 1974.

Henle, G., and Henle, W.: EB virus in the etiology of infectious mononucleosis, Hosp. Pract. **5:**33, July, 1970.

Henry, J. B., and Widmann, F. K.: The Australia antigen: where do we stand? Part I, Postgrad. Med. **5:**167, Dec., 1971; Part 2, **51:**257, Jan., 1972.

Horne, R. W.: Virus structure, New York, 1974, Academic Press, Inc.

Horstmann, D. M.: Rubella: the challenge of its control, J. Infect. Dis. **123:**640, 1971.

Horta-Barbosa, L., and others: Chronic viral infections of the central nervous system, J.A.M.A. **218:**1185, 1971.

Hummeler, K., and Koprowski, H.: Investigating the rabies virus, Nature **221:**418, 1969.

Hunter, J., and others: Australia (hepatitis-associated) antigen among heroin addicts attending London addiction clinic, J. Hyg. (Camb.) **69:**565, 1971.

Inclusion bodies in measles encephalitis (editorial), J.A.M.A. **195:**307, 1966.

Interferon (editorial), J.A.M.A. **213:**118, 1970. .

Interferon: 1973 (editorial), South. Med. J. **67:**1, 1974.

Is monkey pox a reservoir of smallpox? (editorial), J.A.M.A. **222:**1645, 1972.

Jacobs, J. W., and others: Respiratory syncytial and other viruses associated with respiratory disease in infants, Lancet **1:**871, 1971.

Kaplan, A. S., editor: The herpesviruses, New York, 1973, Academic Press, Inc.

Kaplan, M. M.: Epidemiology of rabies, Nature **221:**421, 1969.

Katz, S. L., and Griffith, J. F.: Slow virus infections, Hosp. Pract. **6:**64, March, 1971.

Kilbourne, E. D.: The molecular epidemiology of influenza, J. Infect. Dis. **127:**478, 1973.

Kohn, A., and Klingberg, M. A., editors: Immunity in viral and rickettsial diseases, New York, 1972, Plenum Publishing Corp.

Kok-Doorschodt, H. J. Van K., and others: Determination and distribution of two types of hepatitis-associated antigens, J. Infect. Dis. **126:**117, 1972.

Koplan, J. P., and Hicks, J. W.: Smallpox and vaccinia in the United States—1972, J. Infect. Dis. **129:**224, 1974.

Krech, U., and others: Cytomegalovirus infections of man, White Plains, N.Y., 1971, Albert J. Phiebig.

Krugman, S.: Viral hepatitis and Australia antigen, J. Pediatr. **78:**887, 1971.

Langmuir, A. D.: Influenza: its epidemiology, Hosp. Pract. **6:**103, Sept., 1971.

Lennette, E. H., and Schmidt, N. J.: Diagnostic procedures for viral and rickettsial infections, Washington, D.C., 1969, American Public Health Association, Inc.

Lewis, J. H., and others: Hepatitis B: study of 200 cases positive for hepatitis B antigen, Am. J. Dig. Dis. **18:**921, 1973.

Lewis, T. H., and Brannon, W. L.: Poliomyelitis in an isolated Amerindian population, J.A.M.A. **230:**1295, 1974.

Lindsay, M. I., Jr., and Morrow, G. W., Jr.: Primary influenzal pneumonia, Postgrad. Med. **49:**173, May, 1971.

Lucas, C. J., and others: Measles antibodies in sera from patients with autoimmune diseases, Lancet **1:**115, 1972.

Luria, S. E., and Darnell, J. E., Jr.: General virology, New York, 1967, John Wiley & Sons, Inc.

Macintyre, E. H.: Oncogenic viruses and human neoplasia, J. Am. Med. Wom. Assoc. **23:**520, 1968.

Maramorosch, K., and Kurstak, E., editors: Comparative virology, New York, 1971, Academic Press, Inc.

Marymont, J. H., Jr., and Behbehani, A. M.: The role of the hospital laboratory in the diagnosis of viral diseases. II. Technics, Am. Clin. Pathol. **53:**51, 1970.

Marx, J. L.: "Viroids": a new kind of pathogen, Science **178:**734, 1972.

Marx, J. L.: Slow viruses: role in persistent disease, Science **180:**1351, 1973.

Marx, J. L.: Slow viruses (II): the unconventional agents, Science **181:**44, 1973.

Masland, R. L.: Tracking down the causes of birth defects, Today's Health **44:**60, Aug., 1966.

Maugh, T. H.,II: Hepatitis: a new understanding emerges, Science **176:**1225, 1972.

Maugh, T. H., II: Influenza. II. A persistent disease may yield to new vaccines, Science **180:**1159, 1973.

Melnick, J. L., editor: Progress in medical virology, vol. 17, White Plains, N.Y., 1974, Albert J. Phiebig.

Merigan, T. C., Jr.: Interferon and interferon inducers: the clinical outlook, Hosp. Pract. **4:**42, March, 1969.

Miller, G.: The oncogenicity of Epstein-Barr virus, J. Infect. Dis. **130:**187, 1974.

Miller, L. W., and others: Poliomyelitis in a high-risk population, Pediatrics **49:**532, 1972.

Moloney, J. B.: What is a virus? Hosp. Pract. **1:**36, Nov., 1966.

Monif, G. R. G., and others: The correlation of maternal cytomegalovirus infection during varying stages in gestation with neonatal involvement, J. Pediatr. **80:**17, 1972.

Morley, D.: Severe measles in the tropics, I, Br. Med. J. **1:**297, 1969; II, **1:**363, 1969.

Myocarditis, endocarditis, and viral infection (editorial), J.A.M.A. **202:**139, 1967.

Nahmias, A. J., and Roizman, B.: Infection with herpessimplex virus 1 and 2, N. Engl. J. Med. **289:**667, 719, 781, 1973.

Palmer, E. L., and others: Increased antibody to herpes simplex virus in patients with cancer, J. Infect. Dis. **126:**186, 1972.

Paul, J. R.: A history of poliomyelitis, New Haven, Conn., 1971, Yale University Press.

Phillips, D. F.: Hepatitis. 2. The scientific advances, Hospitals **45:**48, 1971.

Reed, W. D., and others: Exposure and immunity to hepatitis B virus in liver unit, Lancet **1:**581, 1974.

Rhodes, A. J., and van Rooyen, C. E.: Textbook of virology, ed. 5, Baltimore, 1968, The Williams & Wilkins Co.

Rhodes, L. M.: Killer on the rampage: the great flu epidemic, Today's Health **45:**24, Oct., 1967.

Rogers, R. S., III, and Tindall, J. P.: Herpes zoster in the elderly, Postgrad. Med. **50:**153, Dec., 1971.

Rose, H. M.: Influenza; the agent, Hosp. Pract. **6:**49, Aug., 1971.

Rosen, P., and Hajdu, S.: Cytomegalovirus inclusion disease at autopsy of patients with cancer, Am. J. Clin. Pathol. **55:**749, 1971.

Rosenburg, J. L., and others: Viral hepatitis: an occupational hazard to surgeons, J.A.M.A. **223:**395, 1973.

Sauer, G. C.: Skin diseases due to viruses, Hosp. Med. **7:**82, Aug., 1971.

Singer, D. B., and others: Pathology of congenital rubella syndrome, J. Pediatr. **71:**665, 1967.

Steele, J. H.: Canine and wildlife rabies in the United States, Bull. Pathol. **8:**264, 1967.

Subak-Sharpe, G.: The venereal disease of the new morality, Today's Health **53:**42, March, 1975.

Sulkin, S. E., and Allen, R.: Virus infections in bats, White Plains, N.Y., 1974, Albert J. Phiebig.

Theiler, M., and Downs, W. G.: The arthropod-borne viruses of vertebrates: an account of the Rockefeller Foundation virus program 1951-1970, New Haven, Conn., 1973, Yale University Press.

Timbury, M. C.: Notes on medical virology, ed. 5, New York, 1974, Longman, Inc.

Vaisrub, S.: Expect the unexpected in hepatitis (editorial), J.A.M.A. **230:**1020, 1974.

Vianna, N. J., and Hinman, A. R.: Rocky Mountain spotted fever on Long Island: epidemiologic and clinical aspects, Am. J. Med. **51:**725, 1971.

Ward, C., and Ward, A. M.: Acquired valvular heart disease in patients who keep pet birds, Lancet **2:**734, 1974.

Weller, T. H.: Cytomegaloviruses: the difficult years, J. Infect. Dis. **122:**532, 1970.

Wenzel, R. P., and others: Clinical application of Australia/hepatitis-associated antigen, South. Med. J. **66:**186, 1973.

Zeman, W., and Lennette, E. H.: Slow virus diseases, vol. 3, Baltimore, 1974, The Williams & Wilkins Co.

Zollar, L. M., and others: Microbiologic studies on young infants with lower respiratory tract disease, Am. J. Dis. Child. **126:**56, 1973.

# CHAPTER 30

# Fungi
## medical mycology

### Fungi in profile

Molds, yeasts, and certain related forms constitute the organisms in the plant kingdom known as *fungi*. From this group come those whose presence is a common sight on stale bread, rotten fruit, or damp leather. Be it fuzzy or sooty, green, black, or white, the growth on moldy food and clothing is familiar to everyone. Fungi (100,000 species or more*) are among the most plentiful forms of life—they powder the earth and dust the atmosphere. Their science is *mycology*.

Fungi do not contain chlorophyl and are probably degenerate descendants of chlorophyl-bearing ancestors, most likely the algae. Being unable to make their own food by photosynthesis as the higher plants do, they must either exist on other living organisms as parasites or avail themselves of the dead remains as saprophytes. Within the protoplasm of saprophytic fungi are elaborated chemical substances and enzymes that diffuse into the environment, changing what complex substances are there (wood, leather, clothing, bread, and dead organic plant or animal matter) to simpler substances that can be used for their food. The chemical processes of digestion are completed outside the organism, and the end products are then absorbed by the fungus.

**Structure.** Fungi vary in size. Some, the mushrooms and toadstools, are large and easily visible to the naked eye, but most of the ones of medical importance are microscopic or at least so small that the microscope is necessary for their complete investigation. A given fungus may be a single cell, or it may be composed of many cells laid out in a definite pattern. This distinction is not always a sharp one, for the two forms may represent different phases of fungous growth; for example, certain important pathogenic

---

*Less than a hundred can invade man or animals, and less than a dozen can infect and kill.

fungi produce disease in the body tissues as single cells but, when cultured in the laboratory, present a complex multicellular arrangement. In this chapter, however, to describe fungi, we shall separate them loosely on this basis, designating the unicellular forms as *yeasts* and *yeastlike* organisms and the multicellular ones as *molds* and *moldlike* forms.

The unicellular fungi or yeasts are nonmotile round or oval organisms, most of which reproduce by a characteristic process of budding. They vary considerably in size, depending on age and species, but all are microscopic. Nuclei may be demonstrated by a suitable stain.

The multicellular fungi, the molds and related forms, present typical structures associated with nutrition and reproduction. Most molds are made up of a *mycelium*, a network or matlike growth of branched threads bearing fruiting bodies. A rudimentary plant known as a *thallus* (see also p. 4) (no root, stem, or leaf) is formed. The individual threads of the mycelium are known as *hyphae*. In some fungi, nonseptate hyphae consist of single threads containing many nuclei spaced along the thread. In most, septate hyphae are divided by cross walls, or *septae,* into distinct cells, each containing a nucleus. The hyphae have thin walls to allow for ready absorption of food and water. This fact helps to account for the rapid growth of fungi. The portion of the mycelium concerned with nutrition is referred to as the *vegetative* mycelium. The part that usually projects into the air is the *aerial* or *reproductive* mycelium.

**Reproduction.** Multicellular fungi reproduce by the conversion of a spore into a vegetative fungus. Spores are formed in a great variety of ways from the reproductive mycelium, depending on the species. In some molds the spores are simply attached to the hyphae; in some the hyphae bear little pods or sacs in which the spores rest (Fig. 30-1, *A*); in others the

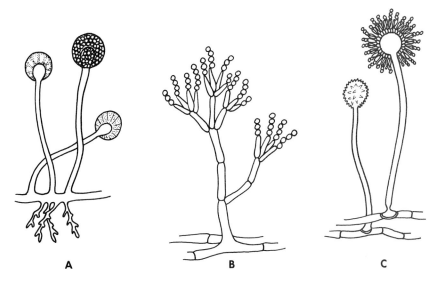

**Fig. 30-1.** Well-known saprophytic fungi. Note fruiting bodies in which asexual reproductive spores form. **A,** Genus *Rhizopus*, black mold. **B,** Genus *Penicillium*, green mold. **C,** Genus *Aspergillus*, gray-green mold.

hyphae are branched to form brushlike processes, each of which bears a spore (Fig. 30-1, *B*); and in still others the hyphae produce heads from which radiate fine chains of spores (Fig. 30-1, *C*). In most cases the spores separate from the hyphae before reproduction.

If a spore is formed after the nuclei of two hyphae have contacted and fused or after an association of a specialized structure on the mycelium with the nucleus of another specialized structure developed close by, that spore is designated a *sexual* spore. When there is no fusion of nuclei and the spore is simply formed as a swollen body at the end of the hypha, it is called an *asexual* spore. Asexual spores are formed in great numbers, sexual spores only occasionally. The fungi that produce only asexual spores are referred to as *Fungi Imperfecti* or imperfect fungi. (Fungi producing sexual spores are perfect fungi.) The Fungi Imperfecti are important because the pathogenic fungi are concentrated in this division.

Spores* are resistant to drying, cold, and moderate heat and may maintain their vitality for a long time. They are constantly present in the air. When they contact food or other material supplying the necessary elements for growth, they develop into new fungi.

___
*The spores of fungi should not be confused with bacterial spores, the resistant bodies formed by bacteria for survival, not for reproduction. Only one spore forms from one bacterial cell.

Unicellular fungi, thought of as yeasts, may reproduce by spore formation. The cell enlarges slightly, and the nucleus becomes converted into a definite number of spores. However, *budding,* considered by some as a simple type of spore formation, is more common. In the process of budding, the nucleus moves toward the edge of the cell and divides into two daughter nuclei. A knoblike protrusion of the cytoplasm forms at this point, and one of the nuclei passes into it. The protrusion increases in size and becomes constricted at its base until there is only a narrow connection between the protrusion and the parent cell. Finally the two separate, and the protrusion or bud, now a small yeast cell, continues to grow until it reaches full size; then the process is repeated.

Multiplication by simple fission, characteristic of some yeasts, resembles the process in bacteria. The yeast develops to its full size, and a membrane forms across the middle of the cell. A dividing wall forms, and the two parts separate.

**Conditions affecting growth.** Fungi grow best under much the same conditions as do bacteria, that is, in warm, moist surroundings. They can grow in the presence of much acid and large amounts of sugar, which bacteria cannot do. Most do not grow in the absence of free oxygen, and large amounts of carbon dioxide are harmful to them. (Only a few are anaerobic.) Many grow best at temperatures somewhat lower than body temperature. At low temperatures metabolic activities may be slowed, but the organisms do not die. In fact, they are rather resistant to cold; many of the commonly encountered ones survive freezing temperatures for long periods of time (months or years). Some can even grow at temperatures below freezing. To prevent the growth of mold, meats and certain food products must be refrigerated at temperatures less than 20° F. (−6.67° C.). On the other hand, fungi are quite susceptible to heat, being easily killed at high temperatures. Most species are little affected by light, being able to grow either in the light or in the dark.

**Classification.** The Eumycetes are the true fungi, the organisms without chlorophyl ordinarily thought of as yeasts, molds, and related forms. On the basis of morphology—the appearance of the colony, spores, and mycelium—the true fungi are placed in three classes and one form-class (the imperfect fungi) as follows:

1. Phycomycetes, or water molds. These grow on water plants and fish. Included are the ubiquitous bread molds of genera *Rhizopus* and *Mucor* and other widespread contaminants. (The hyphae of the water molds are nonseptate; in the other three classes the hyphae of the mycelium, where present, are septate.)
2. Ascomycetes, or sac fungi. These constitute the largest order. Sexual spores are formed within a specially developed sac or *ascus*. Included here are single-celled yeasts of the genus *Saccharomyces*, crucial to the brewing, baking, and wine industries, as well as the multicellular molds *Aspergillus* and *Penicillium* (Fig. 30-2). The common contaminant

*Aspergillus* is a sometime pathogen, and *Penicillium* species are the source of the antibiotic penicillin. Certain pathogenic Ascomycetes can cause maduromycosis. (See p. 247.)

3. Basidiomycetes, or club fungi. These fungi encompass the large fleshy toadstools, puffballs, and mushrooms as well as the small plant smuts and rusts. Certain members produce poisons toxic to man. None is infectious.
4. Fungi Imperfecti, or Deuteromycetes. These lack sexual spores. Asexual spores are formed on or from filaments in a special way. The important pathogens of this class will be discussed in their role as disease producers.

**Laboratory study.** Fungi may be studied and identified in a number of ways.

*Direct visualization.* Stained or unstained material may be observed directly with the microscope. Usually a wet mount is prepared. The specimen—a bit of fungous growth, sputum, pus, skin scrapings, or infected hairs—is placed in a drop of mounting fluid on a glass slide, covered with a cover glass, and examined under the microscope. It is important that the illumination of the specimen be reduced by lowering the intensity of light from the source.

Yeasts may simply be suspended in water. Material containing molds is placed in a 10% to 20% solution of potassium hydroxide. The specimen is cleared when left in contact with the alkali for 10 to 15 minutes or longer; that is, it becomes more transparent and is more easily defined microscopically.

Microscopic identification of a given fungus rests on the study of its structure, especially the kind of spores and their relation to the hyphae.

The phenomenon of fluorescence is important in the study of superficial fungous infections. For example, infected hairs often fluoresce under a filtered source of ultraviolet light.

*Culture.* Both pathogenic and saprophytic fungi are highly resistant to acid environments, and both prefer large amounts of sugar in their food supply. Consistent with these requirements, the French mycologist Sabouraud, around the turn of the century, devised a culture medium of maltose, peptone, and agar still in widespread use today. A fungous culture on Sabouraud's agar is incubated at room temperature (20° C.). Blood agar may also be inoculated but is incubated at body or incubator temperature (37° C.). Littman's oxgall agar is frequently used. Fungi do particularly well when portions of raw or cooked vegetables are added to nutrient media. Potato and carrot combinations and cornmeal agar are valuable. Antibiotics added to fungous culture media suppress bacterial growth. Fungi grow slowly, and cultures must be kept 1 or 2 weeks. If set up as a slide culture,

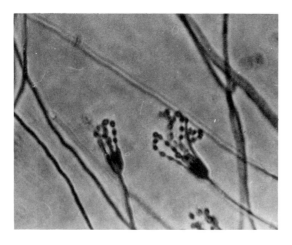

**Fig. 30-2.** Blue-green mold *Penicillium* (wet mount). Note conidia (specialized hyphae) and conidiospores (asexual spores). (From Noland, G. B., and Beaver, W. C.: General biology, ed. 9, St. Louis, 1975, The C. V. Mosby Co.)

fungous growth may be observed daily under the microscope.

In a liquid culture medium bacterial growth is dispersed; few bacteria form the characteristic sheet or pellicle on the surface of the liquid that is seen with the growth of fungi. If the very center of the agar medium in a Petri dish is inoculated, a giant colony grows out to the edge, covering the surface of the dish. The gross appearance of the colony is usually typical for a specific organism.

As with bacteria, fermentation reactions are important in identification of fungi, and animal inoculations are performed.

*Immunologic reactions.* Serologic studies in the laboratory evaluation of fungous diseases include agglutination, precipitation, and complement fixation tests and immunofluorescent and immunoelectrophoretic technics. These are generally positive with active disease. Skin testing is of great value.

**Pathology of fungous disease.** Fungi are important causes of disease in man and animals and one of the chief causes in plants. In man, *mycoses* (fungous infections) are of two types: superficial and systemic. Superficial fungi (in the skin, hair, and nails) causing the *dermatomycoses* spread from animal to man or man to man, even cause epidemics, but do not invade. Systemic fungi contact man from his environment—from the soil, vegetation, bird droppings, and so on. Ordinarily they are very insidious in their approach. They gain a foothold in the body but progress rather leisurely. (Regression seems slow also in mycoses.)

The body's response to the intrusion is granulomatous inflammation, that is, a reaction in which the macrophages of the reticuloendothelial system are seen microscopically to be numerous and conspicuous in characteristic arrangements and appear to be the main participating cells. Tissue damage comes after the state of allergy has been set up in the host to the proteins of the fungus. In many respects the pathology of the mycoses is similar to that of tuberculosis. Usually the etiologic agent can be demonstrated in sections of infected tissues or in fluids therefrom; *its presence makes the diagnosis.*

Systemic mycoses fall into three categories: (1) *primary* infections, usually with a geographic pattern; (2) *secondary* infections or "superinfections," and (3) *complicating* infections.

Most of the fungous diseases discussed in this chapter are systemic, including the important primary mycoses. The four major ones are blastomycosis, coccidioidomycosis, cryptococcosis, and histoplasmosis.

Secondary mycoses develop during the course of a bacterial or viral disease for which antibiotics are being given. (Bacteria help to control fungi in nature.) The single most important example is candidiasis. Superinfection of this kind, often hospital-acquired, is produced by both fungi and a number of bacteria—many gram-negative bacilli, including the enterics, and staphylococci.

Complicating infections appear after special therapeutic procedures such as peritoneal dialysis or the prolonged use of a catheter indwelling a blood vessel. They are a distinct hazard in the management of the "compromised host," that patient with severe, chronic, debilitating disease for which antibiotics, steroid hormones, or immunosuppressive agents are required. They also follow close on disturbances of the immune mechanisms such as are seen in cancer of the lymphoid system and bone marrow failure.

Certain fungi (example: *Cryptococcus*) are readily pathogenic either as primary or secondary invaders. Others (examples: *Candida, Aspergillus* [Fig. 30-3], *Mucor,* and *Rhizopus*), benign in nature, seize on the "opportunity" with an inordinate vigor.

**Importance.** Fungi are important in the processes of nature, agriculture, manufacturing, and medicine. Commonly encountered molds can injure woodwork and fabrics and spoil food. They destroy food during its growth, in the process of manufacture, and after it has reached the consumer. Foods most vulnerable are bread, vegetables, fruits, and preserves. Molds are an important factor in the decay of dead animal and vegetable matter; complex organic compounds, broken down into simple ones, are returned to the soil to be used as food by the green plants. Some fungi (example: certain mushrooms) are sources of food for man. Molds are used commercially in the manufacture of beverages and to give flavor to certain kinds of cheese (Roquefort, Camembert). Penicillin, an effective antibacterial substance, is derived from a common mold, *Penicillium notatum.*

Yeasts are economically important because they ferment sugars. The fact that they convert sugars by enzymatic action into alcohol and carbon dioxide is practically applied in the manufacture of alcoholic beverages and in baking. In the manufacture of alcoholic beverages, carbon dioxide is a by-product, whereas in baking it is the essential factor (p. 374). In the preparation of commercial yeast the cells are grown in a suitable liquid medium, separated from the liquid by centrifugation, mixed with starch or vegetable oil, and then molded and cut into cakes. Yeast is a source of vitamin B and of ergosterol, from which vitamin D is obtained.

## Diseases caused by fungi

*Medical mycology* treats of the fungi that bring about disease.

## SUPERFICIAL MYCOSIS
### Dermatomycoses

Superficial fungous infections of the skin, hair, and nails, generally called *ringworm* or *tinea,* are known as dermatomycoses or dermatophytoses. Fungi causing dermatomycoses and showing no tendency to invade the deeper structures of the body are called *dermatophytes.* There are three important genera: (1) *Microsporum,* (2) *Trichophyton,* and (3) *Epidermophyton.* The dermatophytes are closely related botanically.

The genus *Microsporum* is the most frequent cause of ringworm of the scalp and may give rise to ringworm in other parts of the body. Hairs removed from the affected regions are surrounded by a coat of spores, and scales of skin show many branched mycelial threads. *Trichophyton* causes ringworm of the scalp, beard, skin, or nails. The organisms are found as chains of spores, inside or on the surface of affected hairs, or as hyphae and characteristic spores in skin scrapings. *Trichophyton schoenleini* is the cause of almost all cases of favus. The spores and mycelial threads are found in the favus crusts. Hairs in the affected areas are filled with vesicles and channels from which the mycelia have disappeared. *Epidermophyton* is largely responsible for ringworm of the body, hands and feet. Epidermophyta appear as interlacing threads in the skin. They do not invade hairs.

Ringworm of the scalp *(tinea capitis),* seen most often in children, is a common and highly communicable disease. It may be spread directly from person to person or by articles of wearing apparel. It occurs in domestic animals, from which it may be transmitted to man. Ten to thirty percent of ringworm infections occurring in cities and 80% of those in rural areas are so transmitted, either by direct or indirect contact with the animal. Pets (dogs and cats) readily pass the ringworm fungi onto their human masters.

Favus usually affects the scalp, with the formation of yellowish, cup-shaped crusts, or *scutula,* about the mouths of the hair follicles. These crusts consist of masses of spores and mycelial threads mixed with leukocytes and epithelial cells. Favus may be transmitted directly or indirectly from person to person and tends to run in families.

Ringworm of the beard *(tinea barbae)* is known as *barber's itch.* Ringworm of the groin is known as *tinea cruris* or *dhobie itch.* Ringworm of the feet is known as *tinea pedis* or *athlete's foot.* It has been thought for years that athlete's foot is contracted from footwear, lockers, and floors, but experiments indicate that exposure to the pathogenic dermatophytes in public swimming pools or shower stalls plays a minor role. These fungi are everywhere, even on the feet of noninfected individuals. The lesions of athlete's foot most probably appear because of a factor of decreased resistance in the skin to contact with the disease-producing fungi.

Laboratory diagnosis of the dermatomycoses depends on demonstration of fungi in the hair and skin scrapings by direct microscopic examination or by cultural methods.

Control of the dermatomycoses is very difficult. It consists of the proper sterilization of clothing, bathing suits, and objects subject to frequent handling. Hygiene of the feet is extremely important.

## SYSTEMIC MYCOSIS
### Aspergillosis

Aspergillosis is an infection most often produced by *Aspergillus fumigatus,* a gray-green mold growing in the soil. This fungus may cause various types of infection in chickens, ducks, pigeons, cattle, sheep, and horses. Animals usually contract the disease from moldy feed.

In man the disease generally occurs as an infection of the external ear (otomycosis). The infection may be superficial and mild, or it may cause ulceration of the membrane lining of the ear and perforate into the middle ear. Infection most likely comes from fungi living saprophytically on the earwax. Other types of infection in man are pulmonary infections, sinus infections, and infections of the subcutaneous tissues. Aspergillosis as a superinfection complicating antibiotic therapy affects the lungs (Fig. 30-3). Aspergilli can no longer be passed off simply as "weeds" in the laboratory, likely to contaminate any culture.

Aspergillosis may be caused by aspergilli other than *Aspergillus fumigatus.* Among these are *Aspergillus nidulans, Aspergillus niger,* and *Aspergillus flavus.* Certain strains of *Aspergillus flavus* (and also *Penicillium puberulum*) elaborate *aflatoxins,* toxic substances that can cause cancer in the liver of animals ingesting them. Animals contact these mycotoxins (fungous toxins) in the mold produced by *Aspergillus* on peanuts and other animal foods. Aflatoxins are exceedingly potent in this respect, cancer formation requiring an amount no more than 0.05 p.p.m. (They are also natural mutagens.)

Serologic aids to the diagnosis of aspergillosis include a complement fixation test, a double-diffusion in agar gel technic, and the indirect fluorescent antibody determination.

### Blastomycosis

There are two types of blastomycosis—the North American and the South American. *North American blastomycosis,* known as *Gilchrist's disease* after its discoverer, is a granulomatous and suppurative in-

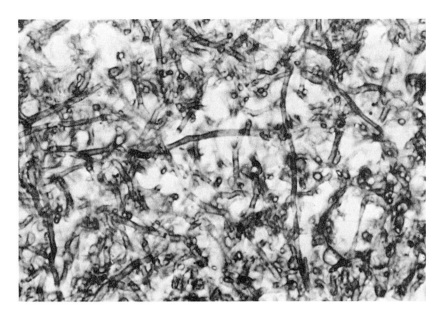

**Fig. 30-3.** *Aspergillus,* demonstrated in microsection of lung with special stain. Abundant growth of this opportunist occurred in diabetic patient. Note typical branching of hyphae. (From Zugibe, F. T.: Diagnostic histochemistry, St. Louis, 1970, The C. V. Mosby Co.)

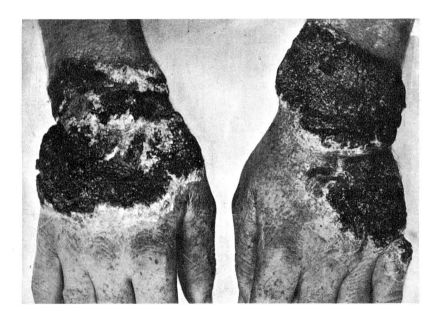

**Fig. 30-4.** Blastomycosis in farmer from Minnesota. Note verrucous or warty nature and sharp margins.

flammation. Multiple abscesses form in the skin and subcutaneous tissues (blastomycetic dermatitis) or in the internal organs of the body (systemic blastomycosis). The cutaneous form of blastomycosis is more often seen than the systemic form (Fig. 30-4). The lesions of blastomycetic dermatitis may be mis-

taken for cancer or tuberculosis. With systemic disease pulmonary blastomycosis is most likely, closely resembling pulmonary tuberculosis.

North American blastomycosis, confined almost exclusively to the United States and Canada, is caused by *Blastomyces dermatitidis.* The organisms are dem-

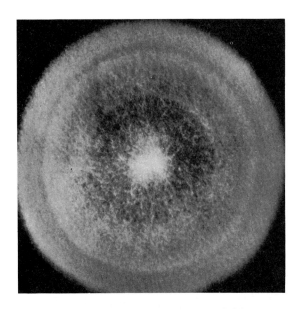

**Fig. 30-5.** *Blastomyces dermatitidis,* giant colony, showing abundant fluffy mycelial growth. (Photograph by Dr. R. H. Musgnug, Haddonfield, N.J.; from Musgnug, R. H.: Med. Tribune **3:**16, May 28, 1962.)

onstrated by direct microscopic examination of pus from the lesions or by cultural methods (Fig. 30-5). In pus they are round or oval granular yeast forms, varying from 8 to 15 $\mu$m. ($\mu$) in diameter. They are surrounded by a thick refractile wall, which makes them doubly contoured, and single budding forms are present (Fig. 30-6). The organisms grow characteristically in the mycelial phase on all media, but isolation is often complicated by the overgrowth of bacterial contaminants from the lesion.

Transmission of human infection is unsolved. Accumulated evidence indicates that cutaneous blastomycosis results from infection through wounds (Fig. 30-4). The finding of a primary focus in the lungs in systemic blastomycosis indicates that systemic infections are probably acquired via the respiratory tract. In some cases of systemic blastomycosis, infection may come from the skin.

Although fungi are weak antigens, infections with these organisms are nevertheless associated with a degree of allergy useful in the laboratory diagnosis. For North American blastomycosis there is both a complement fixation test and a skin test (the blastomycin test). The first test is specific. Cross reactions may occur with the skin test for blastomycosis and that for histoplasmosis. (An individual with histoplas-

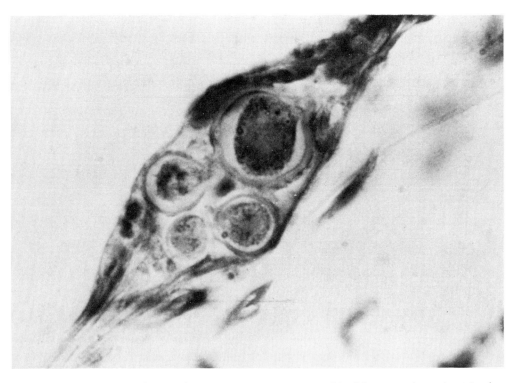

**Fig. 30-6.** *Blastomyces dermatitidis,* microscopic appearance of budding yeast forms in stained smear of sputum.

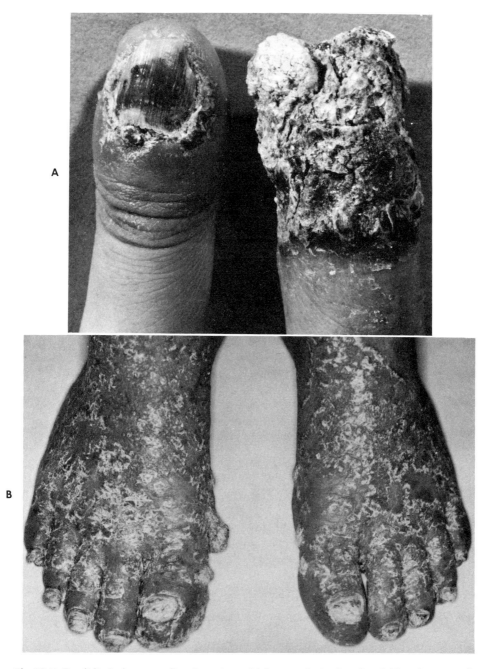

**Fig. 30-7.** Candidiasis, long-standing, in patient with immunologic disorder. **A,** Thumbs—note destruction of nails with accumulation of horny material. **B,** Feet—note changes in skin and nails. (From Kirkpatrick, C. H., and others: Ann. Intern. Med. **74:**955, 1971.)

mosis may appear to give a positive test for blastomycosis.) Skin testing may be done with *Blastomyces dermatitidis* vaccine, considered a more effective antigen than blastomycin.

*South American blastomycosis* is similar to the North American type. Caused by *Blastomyces (Paracoccidioides) brasiliensis*, it is known also as *paracoccidioidal granuloma*. The fungus enters the body by way of the mouth, where it localizes and causes ulcers and granulomas. From these lesions the fungi spread to the lungs and other parts of the body. The disease may terminate fatally. Most cases have been reported in Brazil.

### Candidiasis (moniliasis)

*Candida (Monilia) albicans* is a budding yeastlike organism, worldwide in distribution. Its relationship to disease is often hard to determine. It is found on the mucous membranes of the mouth, the intestinal tract, and the vagina and on the skin of normal persons with no disease.* It is also found in association with known pathogens in persons with known illness but in whom there is no reason to suspect its pathogenicity. In making the diagnosis of candidiasis, *Candida albicans,* the chief pathogen of the genus, must be repeatedly isolated from the lesions to the exclusion of better defined agents.

Two infections of *Candida albicans* have been with us for a long time. One, on the mucous membranes of the mouth, is known as *thrush.* The other, involving the mucous membranes of the female genitalia, is *vulvovaginitis* or *vaginal thrush.*

Thrush is characterized by many small, milk-like flecks that may coalesce and cover the entire lining of the mouth. Beneath these patches on the inside of the lips, on the hard palate, and on the tips and edges of the tongue are areas of catarrhal inflammation. Thrush is an especially troublesome infection in newborn infants in hospital nurseries. It is thought that the baby acquires the organism from the vagina of the mother during the birth process, and it is believed that the organisms can be spread from person to person by contaminated fingers, utensils, and nipples. Thrush tends to be rare after the newborn period in healthy subjects of any age but is comparatively common in poorly nourished children and in chronically ill and aged adults.

Vulvovaginitis is a thrushlike infection associated with a typical vaginal discharge. The sugar content of the urine in pregnancy and uncontrolled diabetes may be a contributing factor. Vulvovaginitis is associated with oral contraceptives. Today vaginal thrush has taken on the proportions of venereal disease.

Candidal infections are found in those individuals, such as fruit canners, who by occupation must keep their hands constantly soaked in water. *Candida albicans* is an important cause of chest disease. The manifestations of bronchopulmonary or pulmonary candidiasis vary from a mild inflammation to a severe infection like tuberculosis.

Systemic candidiasis is encountered increasingly today. It is prone to follow persistent skin or mucosal lesions in a person with lowered resistance or altered immunologic mechanisms (Fig. 30-7). *Candida* easily gains the ascendancy when dosage with a broad-spectrum antibiotic is prolonged, since the normal bacterial flora is thereby depressed. Overgrowth of *Candida* for any reason is an ominous event. If the organisms circulate in the bloodstream (a fungemia), they set up a serious toxic reaction and are widely disseminated in the body (Fig. 30-8). The patient at greatest risk is the one with leukemia, some kind of bone marrow failure, or an organ transplant. Other pathologic conditions over which the threat of candidiasis hangs are diabetes, chronic alcoholism, endocrine disorders, malnutrition, and certain kinds of cancers. Under the right circumstances *Candida* can strike as a formidable pathogen.

The laboratory demonstration of *Candida (Monilia) albicans* is easily made either by direct microscopic examination of unstained or stained material or by culture. In the exudate from a lesion or in sputum the organisms appear as oval, budding yeasts with scattered hyphal segments. Serologically there are the hemagglutination test, the precipitin reaction, an indirect immunofluorescent technic, and counter-electrophoresis. Inoculation of the chorioallantoic membrane of the chick embryo, with visible lesions appearing 72 to 96 hours later, is a good test for the pathogenicity of *Candida.* With oidiomycin, an extract of the organism, a skin test may be done to indicate past or present infection.

### Coccidioidomycosis (coccidioidal granuloma)

Coccidioidomycosis, one of the most infectious of the fungous diseases, exists in two forms—the primary (usually self-limited) and the progressive. In the primary form the lesions are confined to the lungs, giving pulmonary symptoms of varying severity. Sometimes there is cavitation in the lungs. As a rule, the infection ends in recovery, but in a small percentage of cases the process spreads from the lungs to produce the progressive form. This happens more in blacks and the darker-pigmented races than in whites.

In the progressive form, the disease spreads to

---

*Only a few fungi such as *Candida albicans* are normal inhabitants of the human body; most belong to the environment.

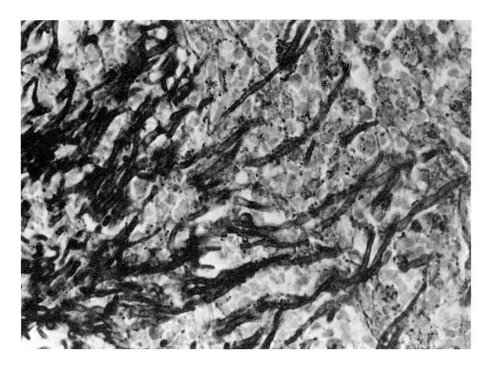

**Fig. 30-8.** Candidiasis of spleen in disseminated disease. Note abundant mycelial filaments of *Candida albicans.* (×800.)

the skin, subcutaneous tissues, bones, meninges, and internal organs. The lesions in the skin resemble those of blastomycosis. In other parts of the body they resemble the lesions of tuberculosis. The mortality is high. This is the form of the disease designated *coccidioidal granuloma.*

Coccidioidomycosis is endemic in the desert valleys of California and the dry, dusty areas of southwestern United States, especially in Arizona, New Mexico, Texas, and part of Mexico. It is most likely that man and animals are infected by the inhalation of spore-bearing dust. The infection is found in cattle, sheep, dogs, and certain wild rodents. There may be a reservoir of infection in small wild rodents, and these animals could pass the spores in their feces to contaminate the soil, after which the spores would be spread by the wind. The rather frequent dust storms of the Southwest might carry these organisms long distances.

The cause is *Coccidioides immitis.* Diagnosis is made by finding it in the disease. The appearance of the fungus in the lesions differs from its appearance on culture media. In the body tissues and exudates one sees yeastlike forms—large, thick-walled, nonbudding spherules 20 to 60 $\mu$m. in diameter and filled with endospores 2 to 5 $\mu$m. in diameter (reproduction by endosporulation) (Fig. 30-9). As many as 1000 endospores may be released from a single spherule.

In laboratory cultures growth is that of a mold, and one sees a fluffy, cottony white colony.

The *coccidioidin test,* a test of sensitivity to an extract of the organism, is of value. (Cross reactions may occur with the skin tests for histoplasmosis and blastomycosis, however.) Immunofluorescence can be used to identify the infection, as can precipitation, latex agglutination, and complement fixation tests and quantitative immunodiffusion. These serologic tests are used to follow the course of the infection in a given patient. Currently a coccidioidal vaccine made from formalin-inactivated spherules has been successful in trial runs on human beings.

**Cryptococcosis (torulosis)**

*Cryptococcus neoformans (Torula histolytica)* is a yeastlike organism that usually infects the lungs and central nervous system but may attack other parts of the body (Fig. 30-10). *Cryptococcus* is the only encapsulated yeast to invade the central nervous system. In the disease multiple small nodules form, with the gross and microscopic appearance of tubercles. In infection of the central nervous system the meninges are thickened and matted together, and the brain is invaded. In the patient with preexisting malignancy of the reticuloendothelial system this agent is an important opportunist.

Man becomes infected through the skin, mouth,

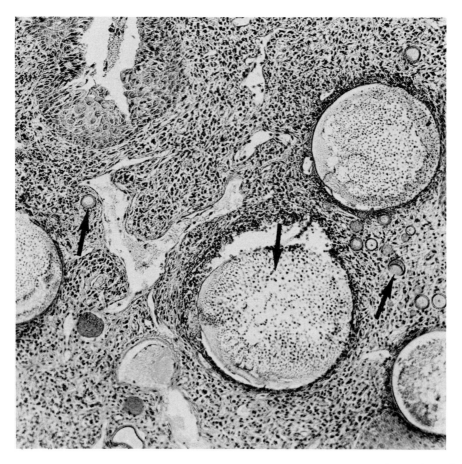

**Fig. 30-9.** *Coccidioides immitis* spherules (arrows) in tissue microsection; reproduction by endosporulation. Large balloonlike structures (note central arrow) contain myriad endospores that they release into tissues spaces. Doubly refractile capsule seen about varying-sized spherules.

nose, and throat. Transmission from man to man or from animal to man has not been recorded. This fungus, saprophytic in nature, has been found in cattle, horses, dogs, and cats. Birds are not its hosts, but the organism is a saprophyte in pigeon droppings, and cases of cryptococcal meningitis have been traced to the vast pigeon populations found in many large cities. Pigeons are mechanical vectors; they carry the organisms on their feet and beaks. Pigeons are not affected, probably because of their high body temperature. *Cryptococcus neoformans* has a definite predilection for pigeon droppings, which are rich in creatinine. Creatinine is assimilated by this organism only and not by other species of cryptococci or other fungi.

Since *Cryptococcus neoformans* is known also as *Torula histolytica,* infections with it may be referred to as either *cryptococcosis* or *torulosis.* Torulosis, or cryptococcosis, can be diagnosed with certainty only

by finding the budding organisms in the affected tissues, pus, sputum, or cerebrospinal fluid. In wet mounts (prepared with nigrosin) the cryptococci are ovoid to spherical budding yeast forms, 5 to 15 $\mu$m. in diameter. With fluorescent antibody technics, the diagnosis may be made within hours. Agglutination tests are sensitive and specific.

**Histoplasmosis**

Histoplasmosis, sometimes called *Darling's disease,* is an infection caused by *Histoplasma capsulatum,* a diphasic organism—a single, budding yeast at body temperature and a mold at room temperature and in nature. The fungus attacks primarily the reticuloendothelial system, where it parasitizes the component cells. Like coccidioidomycosis, the disease exists in the primary and the progressive forms. The primary form involves the lungs but usually heals, leaving many small calcified areas in the

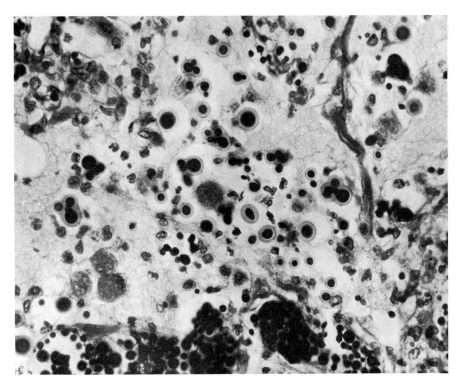

**Fig. 30-10.** *Cryptococcus neoformans (Torula histolytica)* among partially hemolyzed red cells in air sacs of lung. Wide gray capsules encompass budding yeast forms in this specially stained microsection. (From Kent, T. H., and Layton, J. M.: Am. J. Clin. Pathol. **38:**596, 1962.)

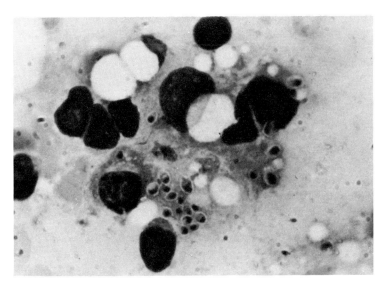

**Fig. 30-11.** Histoplasmosis of bone marrow, Wright-stained smear examined microscopically. (×950.) (From Anderson, W. A. D., editor: Pathology, ed. 6, St. Louis, 1971, The C. V. Mosby Co.)

lungs and lymph nodes of the chest. In the progressive disseminated form, ulcerating lesions are found in the nose and mouth, and there is enlargement of the spleen, liver, and lymph nodes (Fig. 30-11). The progressive form is generally fatal.

Man probably contracts the disease by inhalation of spores of organisms growing in the soil. Infection of the soil comes from the excreta of a variety of birds and bats in which the organisms have been found. No intermediate host is identified. Spores may be carried by prevailing winds and even by tornadoes. Outbreaks of the disease have been traced to the inhalation of dust from caves. Histoplasmosis is referred to as cave sickness, or *speleonosis*. Victims of histoplasmosis, and blastomycosis as well, tend to be outdoor types—construction workers, farmers, spelunkers, and so on. The disease is encountered in the central Mississippi Valley and the Ohio Valley and in widespread areas of the world.

To identify the organisms, stained smears and imprints (as well as cultures) are made of peripheral blood, bone marrow, aspirated material from lymph nodes, and sputum. To aid in the diagnosis and follow-up of histoplasmosis, the laboratory offers a skin test (the histoplasmin test or the histoplasmin tine test) and 5 serologic tests—precipitation, agglutination, complement fixation, fluorescent antibody detection, and immunodiffusion.

### Phycomycosis

Phycomycosis or mucormycosis can be an overwhelmingly acute and fatal infection. It is caused by species of *Mucor* and *Rhizopus* and other normally harmless phycomycetes of the soil and decaying organic matter.

Diabetes, untreated and out of control, is the most important forerunner; the ketoacidosis rather than the hyperglycemia is thought to trigger the process. Along with disease in the lungs and central nervous system, an intraorbital cellulitis is a prominent feature. In the tissues the hyphae abound, very broad and branching, especially within walls and lumens of blood vessels. No spores are seen, and there is little if any inflammation. In tissue section, hyphae are easily identified as belonging to the Phycomycetes because they are nonseptate and coenocytic, that is, contain many nuclei within a continuous mass of cytoplasm. The term mucormycosis is often used simply to indicate infections in which such hyphae are seen.

### Sporotrichosis

Sporotrichosis is a fungous disease caused by *Sporotrichum schenckii*. It may affect man, lower animals, or plants. *Sporotrichum* is widely distributed in nature as a saprophyte on vegetation. Man usually acquires the infection from plants, especially barberry shrubs and certain mosses, which seem to harbor the fungi. The fungi are introduced into wounds (inoculation infection) by infected plants or vegetable matter. The agent is thought to be a normal inhabitant of the alimentary and respiratory tracts in man, and in a few instances the disease has been transferred from man to man. Transmission of the infection from lower animals to man by bites or indirect routes has been noted. Recently sporotrichosis was reported as a complication of catfish stings. Animals most often affected are horses, mules, dogs, rats, and mice. The majority of cases occur in the United States, especially in the Missouri and Mississippi valleys.

The disease occurs as a chronic infection usually limited to the skin and underlying tissues and is accompanied by the formation of nodular masses that slowly undergo softening and ulceration. In typical cases the first evidence of the disease is seen at the site of some trivial injury, usually on the fingers. The wound does not heal, and an ulcer appears, to be followed by nodular corklike swellings in chain formation up the forearm. The disease seldom extends farther than to the regional lymph nodes, but secondary foci may sometimes crop up in other parts of the body such as the lungs, spleen, liver, and other organs.

The oval or cigar-shaped fungus of sporotrichosis, resident with mononuclear cells, is very rarely found in smears from the pus of a skin lesion or in sections of tissue taken from the lesions. As a rule, it is demonstrated only in cultures (Fig. 30-12). Fluorescent antibody technics detect the microorganisms in exudates from the lesions.

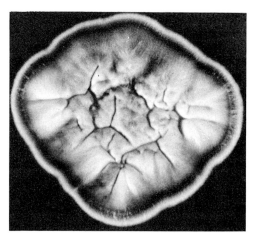

**Fig. 30-12.** *Sporotrichum schenckii*—giant colony. (Courtesy Dr. R. H. Musgnug, Haddonfield, N.J.)

## OTHER FUNGOUS DISEASES OF MAN

The following are other fungous infections, infrequent in man:

1. Rhinosporidiosis (caused by *Rhinosporidium seeberi*)
2. Geotrichosis (caused by one or more species of *Geotrichum*)
3. Chromoblastomycosis (caused by three different fungi)
4. Penicilliosis (caused by certain species of *Penicillium*)
5. Piedra (caused by two different species of fungi)
6. Otomycosis (caused by species of *Penicillium* and other fungi)

## FUNGOUS DISEASES OF LOWER ANIMALS

Fungous infections are very important to the veterinary microbiologist, such as the following:

1. Ringworm of the horse (caused by *Trichophyton equinum*); may occur in man
2. Ringworm of horses, cattle, dogs, and possibly sheep and hogs (caused by *Trichophyton mentagrophytes*); infection possible in man
3. Ringworm of cats and dogs (caused by *Microsporum canis*)
4. Epizootic lymphangitis of horses (caused by *Blastomyces farciminosus*)
5. Favus of chickens (caused by *Trichophyton gallinae*)
6. Coccidioidomycosis of cattle, dogs, horses, and sheep (caused by *Coccidioides immitis*); same organism causes the disease in man
7. Aspergillosis of wild and domestic fowl (caused by *Aspergillus fumigatus*)
8. Candidiasis of poultry (caused by *Candida albicans*)
9. Histoplasmosis of dogs, cats, cattle, sheep, swine, poultry, and horses (caused by *Histoplasma capsulatum*)
10. Cryptococcosis (mastitis) of cattle (caused by *Cryptococcus neoformans*)

## FUNGOUS DISEASES OF PLANTS

Molds and yeasts are economically important for they cause so many diseases of plants. Plants and vegetables imported from other countries are rigidly inspected upon arrival in our seaports and points of entry. If a fungous infection is found, the plant or plant product is not allowed entry. Among important plant diseases caused by molds are:

1. Brown rot of peaches and plums
2. Chestnut blight
3. Mildew of grapes
4. White pine blister rust
5. Rust of oats, wheat, and barley
6. Smuts of various grains
7. Potato rot
8. Corn leaf blight

**Ergotism.** Ergot, a drug whose derivatives are widely used to check hemorrhage after childbirth, is composed of several alkaloidal poisons (mycotoxins) produced by the growth of a mold *Claviceps purpurea* in the grains of rye, wheat, and barley. The fungus (also referred to as ergot) grows as a purple-black, slightly curved mass that replaces the infected grain and converts it to a black sclerotium, from which the drug is extracted. An enzyme secreted by the hyphae is contained in a thick honeydew that attracts insects and helps to spread the fungus. When bread made from infected grain is eaten, the condition known as *ergotism* develops. Ergotism is characterized by gangrene of the extremities, abortion, and convulsions. It was at one time most prevalent in central Europe.

A specific component of the pharmacologically potent alkaloids produced by the fungus ergot is lysergic acid. A well-known derivative is the hallucinogen lysergic acid diethylamide, or LSD.

## Questions for review

1. Give the general characteristics of fungi.
2. Name the science that treats of fungi.
3. What is a fungous infection called?
4. Make the distinction between molds and yeasts. Is it a clear one?
5. How do fungi perpetuate themselves?
6. What are the dermatomycoses? Name three major dermatophytes.
7. Outline the laboratory diagnosis of fungous disease.
8. Name and briefly describe the chief diseases caused by fungi.
9. What is ergotism? What is the pharmacologic nature of LSD?
10. Classify fungi.
11. Make pertinent comments regarding the pathology of fungous disease.
12. What threat does fungous infection pose to the "compromised host"? Cite the common offenders.
13. Briefly define: speleonosis, torulosis, mycotoxin, Madura foot, tinea, superinfection, complicating infection (in fungous disease), mycelium, aflatoxins, favus, otomycosis, thallus, cave sickness.

**REFERENCES** (Chapter 30)

Artman, S. J.: Permanent slides from fungus preps, Lab. Med. **3:**36, Sept., 1972.

Baker, R. D., editor: Human infection with fungi, actinomycetes, and algae, New York, 1971, Springer-Verlag New York, Inc.

Ballou, C. E., and Raschke, W. C.: Polymorphism of the somatic antigen of yeast, Science **184:**127, 1974.

Basler, R. S. W., and Friedman, J. L.: Mucocutaneous histoplasmosis, J.A.M.A. **230:**1434, 1974.

Beneke, E. S.: Scope monograph on human mycoses, Kalamazoo, Mich., 1968, The Upjohn Co.

Beware the Sporothrix (editorial), J.A.M.A. **215:**1976, 1971.

Buechner, H. A., and others: The current status of serologic, immunologic and skin tests in the diagnosis of pulmonary mycoses, Chest **63:**259, 1973.

Candidiasis: colonization vs. infection (editorial), J.A.M.A. **215:**285, 1971.

Caplan, R. M.: Medical uses of the Wood's lamp, J.A.M.A. **202:**1035, 1967.

Conant, N. F., and others: Manual of clinical mycology, ed. 3, Philadelphia, 1971, W. B. Saunders Co.

Deppisch, L. M., and Donowho, E. M.: Pulmonary coccidioidomycosis, Am. J. Clin. Pathol. **58:**489, 1972.

Dolan, C. T.: Evaluation of various media for growth of selected pathogenic fungi and *Nocardia asteroides,* Am. J. Clin. Pathol. **58:**339, 1972.

Dolan, C. T., and Stried, R. P.: Serologic diagnosis of yeast infections, Am. J. Clin. Pathol. **59:**49, 1973.

Edds, G. T.: Acute aflatoxicosis: review, J. Am. Vet. Med. Assoc. **162:**304, 1973.

Emmons, C. W., and others: Medical mycology, ed. 2, Philadelphia, 1970, Lea & Febiger.

Field, M. H.: Opportunistic fungal infections, J. Am. Med. Wom. Assoc. **23:**529, 1968.

Goldblatt, L. A.: Aflatoxin, scientific background, control, and implications, New York, 1969, Academic Press, Inc.

Goodwin, R. A., Jr., and Des Prez, R. M.: Pathogenesis and clinical spectrum of histoplasmosis, South. Med. J. **66:**13, 1973.

Hatcher, C. R., Jr., and others: Primary pulmonary cryptococcosis, J. Thorac. Cardiovasc. Surg. **61:**39, 1971.

Hoffman, H.-P., and Avers, C. J.: Mitochondrion of yeast: ultrastructural evidence for one giant, branched organelle per cell, Science **181:**749, 1973.

Jones, H. E., and others: Apparent cross-reactivity of airborne molds and dermatophytic fungi, J. Allergy Clin. Immunol. **52:**346, 1973.

Koneman, E. W., and Fann, S. E.: Practical laboratory mycology, New York, 1971, Medcom Books, Inc.

Lenoir, E., and Carson, P.: A rapid screening test for the identification of *Candida albicans,* Lab. Med. **4:**28, Dec., 1973.

Maddy, K. T.: Epidemiology and ecology of deep mycoses of man and animals, Arch. Dermatol. **96:**409, 1967.

Miller, D. L., and others: Preparation of permanent microslides of fungi for reference and teaching, Am. J. Clin. Pathol. **59:**601, 1973.

Moore-Landecker, E.: Fundamentals of the fungi, Englewood Cliffs, N. J., 1972, Prentice-Hall, Inc.

Moss, E. S., and McQuown, A. L.: Atlas of medical mycology, ed. 3, Baltimore, 1969, The Williams & Wilkins Co.

Myrvik, Q. N., and others: Fundamentals of medical bacteriology and mycology for students of medicine and related sciences, Philadelphia, 1974, Lea & Febiger.

Nime, F. A., and Hutchins, G. M.: Oxalosis caused by *Aspergillus* infection, Johns Hopkins Med. J. **133:**183, 1973.

Orr, E. R., and Riley, H. D., Jr.: Sporotrichosis in childhood: report of 10 cases, J. Pediatr. **78:**951, 1971.

Parkhurst, G. F., and Vlahides, G. D.: Fatal opportunistic fungus disease, J.A.M.A. **202:**279, 1967.

Reynolds, R. C., and others: Plastic tissue-culture dishes in diagnostic mycology, Am. J. Clin. Pathol. **41:**385, 1964.

Richards, R. N., and Talpash, O. S.: Sporotrichosis, Can. Med. Assoc. J. **106:**1097, 1972.

Richter, H. S.: Coccidioidomycosis, a report of 300 new cases, GP **39:**89, Feb., 1969.

Richter, M. W., and Amsterdam, D.: Plate-slide for the culture and morphological observation of fungi, Appl. Microbiol. **24:**667, 1972.

Robinson, H. M., Jr., editor: The diagnosis and treatment of fungal infections, Springfield, Ill., 1974, Charles C Thomas, Publisher.

Smith, J. W.: Coccidioidomycosis, a review, Tex. Med. **67:**117, Nov., 1971.

Smith, J. W., and Utz, J. P.: Progressive disseminated histoplasmosis, Ann. Intern. Med. **76:**557, 1972.

Snell, W. H., and Dick, E. A.: Glossary of mycology, ed. 2, Cambridge, Mass., 1971, Harvard University Press.

Spickard, A.: Diagnosis and treatment of cryptococcal disease, South. Med. J. **66:**26, 1973.

Sutaria, M. K., and others: Focalized pulmonary histoplasmosis (coin lesion), Chest **61:**361, 1972.

Swartz, J. H., and Medrek, T. F.: Rapid contrast stain as diagnostic aid for fungus infections, Arch. Dermatol. **99:**494, 1969.

Taschdjian, C. L., and others: Serodiagnosis of candidal infections, Am. J. Clin. Pathol. **57:**195, 1972.

Werner, S. B., and others: Epidemic of coccidioidomycosis among archeology students in northern California, N. Engl. J. Med. **286:**507, 1972.

Wiegand, S.: Ink blue agar for recognition of dermatophytes, Bull. Pathol. **10:**68, 1968.

Young, R. C., and others: Species identification of invasive aspergillosis in man, Am. J. Clin. Pathol. **58:**554, 1972.

# CHAPTER 31

# Protozoa
## medical parasitology

Parasites are generally defined as organisms that require living matter for their nourishment; that is, they must live within or on the bodies of other living organisms. According to this definition a parasite may be a bacterium, a virus, a rickettsia, a protozoon, a plant (example: mistletoe), or an animal. However, by common usage *medical parasitology* refers to animal parasites of medical interest and their diseases.

The animal within or on which a parasite lives is the *host*. All stages of the parasite's development may take place in the same animal host. On the other hand, a parasite may have one or more hosts. It undergoes its larval stage in the *intermediate* host and its adult stage in the *definitive* host. A parasite that lives within the body of the host is known as an *endoparasite;* one that lives on the outside of the body is an *ectoparasite*. A tapeworm is an example of an endoparasite; a louse is an ectoparasite.

## General characteristics

The animal kingdom is divided into two great divisions: the Protozoa, unicellular organisms and the lowest form of animal life, and the Metazoa, multicellular organisms (Chapter 32). Protozoa are more complex in their functional activities than are bacteria or the average cell of a multicellular organism. Each is a complete, self-contained unit, with special structures known as *organelles* to carry out such functions as nutrition, locomotion, respiration, excretion, and attachment to objects. The vast majority are of microscopic size. As a rule, the pathogenic ones are smaller than the nonpathogenic ones. They may be spherical, spindle, spiral, or cup shaped. In medical parasitology, identification of a given animal parasite is of paramount importance. Practically, this is done by the recognition of specific structural (morphologic) details in the makeup of the given parasite. There are many species, but only about thirty affect man.

**Structure.** Protozoa are units of protoplasm differentiated into cytoplasm bounded by the cell or plasma membrane and a nucleus encased by the nuclear membrane. Some have more than one nucleus. The cytoplasm is separated into a homogeneous ectoplasm and a granular endoplasm. The *ectoplasm* helps form the various organs of locomotion, contraction, and prehension, such as pseudopods, flagella, cilia, and suctorial tubes. In certain species of protozoa the ectoplasm contains a definite opening or portal for intake of food. The *endoplasm* digests food materials and surrounds the nucleus.

Many protozoa, especially the pathogenic ones, absorb fluid directly through the plasma membrane. The majority take in solid particles and digest them enzymatically. Because their food consists chiefly of bacteria, protozoa may be important in limiting the bacterial population of the universe. Waste material is excreted through the cell membrane or, in some cases, through an ejection pore.

**Locomotion.** All protozoa possess some type of motility. It may be by pseudopod formation or by the action of flagella or cilia. (See Fig. 31-1.) For locomotion by *pseudopod* (false foot) formation a sharp or blunt ectoplasmic process flows forward, pulling the rest of the organism after it. *Flagella* are whip-like prolongations of the protoplasm that propel the organism with their lashing motions. Some protozoa have only one flagellum; others have several. Some of the flagellate protozoa also have an *undulating membrane* to help in locomotion. This is a fluted membranous process attached to one side of the organism. *Cilia* are similar to flagella except that they are shorter, more delicate, more plentiful, and attached to the entire outer surface of the organism. Individually they are less powerful than flagella, but the synchronous action of the many cilia present accomplishes the most rapid motion of which unicellular organisms are capable.

**Cyst formation.** When protozoa are subjected to adverse conditions, they become inactive, assume a more or less rounded form, and surround them-

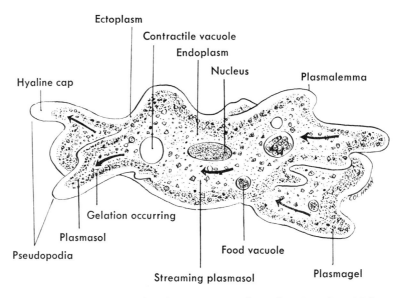

**Fig. 31-1.** Active locomotion in an ameba, sketch. Arrows indicate direction. (From Hickman, C. P.: Integrated principles of zoology, ed. 4, St. Louis, 1970, The C. V. Mosby Co.)

selves with a resistant membrane (cell wall), within which they may live for a long time and resist various destructive forces in their environment. This is *cyst* formation. When conditions suitable for growth are reestablished, the cyst imbibes water, and the protozoon returns to the vegetative state. Sometimes cyst formation precedes reproduction. Since vegetative protozoa are very susceptible to deleterious influences and cysts are very resistant, it is the cysts that are usually responsible for the spread of protozoan infections.

**Reproduction.** In protozoa, reproduction may be either sexual or asexual. In some (example: *Plasmodium* of malaria) the sexual cycle occurs in one species of animal and the asexual in another. The sexual cycle occurs in the *definitive* host, and the asexual in the *intermediate* host. Protozoan cells capable of sexual reproduction are known as *gametes*. The cell formed by the union of two gametes is a *zygote*. Asexual reproduction occurs in amebas and flagellates. Lengthwise or crosswise division of the protozoon yields two new members of the species.

**Classification.*** In the phylum Protozoa there are six classes of organisms of medical interest in man. The method of locomotion varies in each.

*Rhizopodea.* Locomotion is characterized by pseudopod formation, and the cytoplasm is divided into

---

*Classification taken from Faust, E. C., and others: Craig and Faust's clinical parasitology, ed. 8, Philadelphia, 1970, Lea & Febiger.

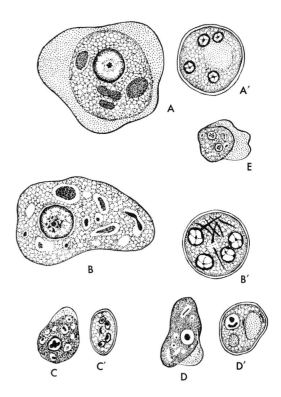

**Fig. 31-2.** Protozoa—pathogenic and nonpathogenic amebas, sketch. Note rounded cyst to right of trophozoite in **A′, B′, C′,** and **D′. A-A′,** *Entamoeba histolytica* (the pathogen). **B-B′,** *Entamoeba coli.* **C-C′,** *Endolimax nana.* **D-D′,** *Iodamoeba bütschlii (williamsi).* **E,** *Dientamoeba fragilis.*

ectoplasm and endoplasm. This includes the pathogenic and nonpathogenic amebas (Fig. 31-2).

*Zoomastigophorea* (commonly called flagellates). Movement is by means of flagella and an undulating membrane. Flagellates have two nuclei, and the cytoplasm is not differentiated into endoplasm and ectoplasm. Cell bodies are often pear-shaped and fixed in outline. The most important flagellates medically are in the genera *Trypanosoma*, *Leishmania*, *Trichomonas*, *Giardia*, and *Chilomastix* (Fig. 31-3, *A* to *C*).

*Telosporea.* There are no external organs of locomotion. These organisms live within the cells, tissues, cavities, and fluids of the body and are represented by the *Plasmodium* of malaria.

*Ciliatea.* Cilia are present for locomotion. The only pathogenic member of this group is *Balantidium coli* (Fig. 31-3, *D*).

*Toxoplasmea.* There are no external organs of locomotion. The protozoa move by bending and gliding movements of their bodies. The representative pathogen here is *Toxoplasma gondii.*

*Haplosporea.* There are no flagella, but pseudopodia may form. The parasite here is *Pneumocystis carinii.*

**Laboratory diagnosis.** The structure of many protozoan parasites makes it easy for them to be identified microscopically in suitably prepared clinical specimens such as blood or stool. At times, however, a morphologic diagnosis is not possible in parasitic infections.

Fortunately parasites possess a variety of antigens within their makeup and therefore lend themselves nicely to serologic testing. The immunodiagnostic tests that have been standardized for the identification of the protozoa of this chapter and the metazoa of the next include complement fixation, indirect hemagglutination, latex agglutination, indirect fluorescent anti-

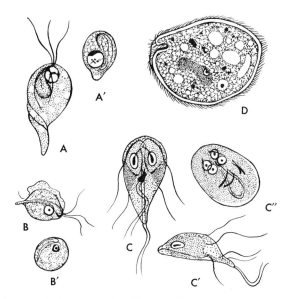

**Fig. 31-3.** Protozoa—flagellates and ciliate, sketch. Note rounded or ovoid cyst with trophozoite in **A′**, **B′**, and **C″**. **A-A′**, *Chilomastix mesnili.* **B-B′**, *Trichomonas hominis intestinalis*). **C** to **C″**, *Giardia lamblia.* **D**, *Balantidium coli.*

body, countercurrent electrophoresis, bentonite flocculation, double diffusion, and intradermal ones. For most situations there is not necessarily one best test; it may be that two or more may have to be used for clinical evaluation. Tables 31-1 and 32-2 show the applications of the various ones to diseases for which they are useful. Within the last few years a number of reagents and tests have been packaged commercially; there are kits and reagents for the protozoan diseases, amebiasis and toxoplasmosis, and for the metazoan diseases, echinococcosis and trichinosis.

**Table 31-1**

Serologic tests of value in protozoan diseases*

| IMMUNODIAGNOSTIC TEST | AMEBIASIS | CHAGAS' DISEASE | AFRICAN TRYPANO- SOMIASIS | LEISHMANIASIS | MALARIA | TOXOPLAS- MOSIS | PNEUMO- CYSTOSIS |
|---|---|---|---|---|---|---|---|
| Intradermal | | | | × | | × | |
| Complement fixation | × | × | | × | | × | × |
| Indirect hemagglutination | × | × | | × | × | × | |
| Indirect fluorescent antibody | × | × | × | | × | × | × |
| Precipitin | | | × | | | | |
| Immunoelectrophoresis | × | | | | | | |
| Double diffusion | × | | × | | × | | |

*Modified from Kagan, I. G.: Current status of serologic testing for parasitic diseases, Hosp. Pract. **9:**157, Sept., 1974.

× indicates an accepted test for routine use.

# Diseases caused by protozoa
## AMEBIASIS

The term *amebiasis* indicates an infection with *Entamoeba histolytica*. The disease occurs in two forms: acute amebiasis (amebic dysentery), characterized by an intense dysentery with bloody, mucus-filled stools, and chronic or latent amebiasis, described by vague intestinal disturbances, muscular aching, loss of weight, even constipation. In some cases of chronic amebiasis, manifestations are absent. The chronic form of amebiasis is more common than the acute. An estimated 5% to 10% of persons in the United States are affected.

**The organism.** The organism *Entamoeba histolytica* exists as a vegetative ameba or *trophozoite* and as a cyst. Vegetative trophozoites possess an active type of ameboid motion on a warm microscopic stage. Microscopically one sees the pseudopods, a characteristic nucleus, and red blood cells within the cytoplasm of the trophozoite. Vegetative amebas are very susceptible to injurious agents. In an unfavorable environment they quickly succumb; therefore they do little to transmit the disease. The cysts are smaller than vegetative amebas, nonmotile, and surrounded by a resistant wall.

**Life history.** The life cycle of *Entamoeba histolytica* begins with the cysts, by which the disease is spread from person to person. After the cysts are passed in the feces, they remain infectious for several days if not destroyed by heat and drying. When the cysts are swallowed by a new host, they pass through the stomach unchanged. The shells are dissolved by juices of the small intestine, and the vegetative forms are liberated. The trophozoites pass to the large intestine to attack the mucous membrane and produce ulceration. The vegetative amebas multiply in the ulcers; some escape into the lumen of the intestine. If diarrhea is present, they are swept out of the intestinal tract. If diarrhea is not present, they multiply one or more times and then encyst. Encystment does not occur outside the body. Cysts are excreted in the feces.

**Sources and modes of infection.** The life cycle of *Entamoeba histolytica* reveals three facts: (1) infection can be acquired only by swallowing cysts, (2) infection comes from the feces of a person excreting cysts, and (3) acute cases are of little danger. The feces of patients with acute amebiasis contain largely vegetative parasites that die quickly; they could not survive the acid gastric juice should they accidentally be ingested. Infection is usually acquired by the eating of uncooked food contaminated with feces containing cysts. The most important single source of infection is the food handler with chronic amebiasis, especially the one preparing uncooked foods. Other sources of infection are vegetables fertilized with human excreta and drinking water contaminated with sewage. Apparently the latter was the cause of the Chicago epidemic of 1933, in which there were 1409 cases with 98 deaths. The water in two hotels had been contaminated by sewage. Flies and other insects may spread the cysts mechanically.

**Lesions.** In the majority of cases there seems to be a state of balance between the amebas and the host. The patient experiences mild disturbances or none at all and is able to repair the ulcers almost as fast as they are formed. This is chronic or latent amebiasis.

If the resistance of the host is lowered or massive infection occurs, the host is unable to repair the ulcers as fast as they are formed, and the increasing ulceration causes a violent dysentery in which the stools consist entirely of blood and mucus. This is acute amebiasis or amebic dysentery. Occasionally, intestinal perforation occurs.

Sometimes amebas penetrate deeper into the intestinal wall and enter tributaries of the portal vein to be carried to the liver, where they produce amebic hepatitis or liver abscess (Fig. 31-4). Amebic abscesses can occur in the lungs or brain.

**Laboratory diagnosis.** The laboratory diagnosis of amebiasis necessitates the examination of *fresh warm* stools for vegetative amebas and the examination of ordinary specimens for cysts. The examination of iron hematoxylin–stained smears of specimens is helpful. Although morphologic recognition of *Entamoeba histolytica* under the microscope is the prime concern of the laboratory, serologic tests are used to advantage to identify this parasite. These include a complement fixation test, hemagglutination tests, an indirect fluorescent antibody test, and an agar gel double-diffusion technic.

**Prevention.** The prevention of amebiasis depends on the proper control of carriers, proper sanitary supervision of foods, and general cleanliness.

In addition to *Entamoeba histolytica,* several other amebas may be found in the intestinal canal, but *Entamoeba histolytica* is the only one that causes disease. *Entamoeba coli* is notable because it must be distinguished from *Entamoeba histolytica.*

## TRYPANOSOMIASIS

Trypanosomes (hemoflagellates) (Fig. 31-5), of which there are many species, are spindle-shaped protozoa that enter the bloodstream of many different species of animals. They are found in the plasma, not within the blood cells. Infection with trypanosomes is known as *trypanosomiasis*. The types important to man are African trypanosomiasis or African

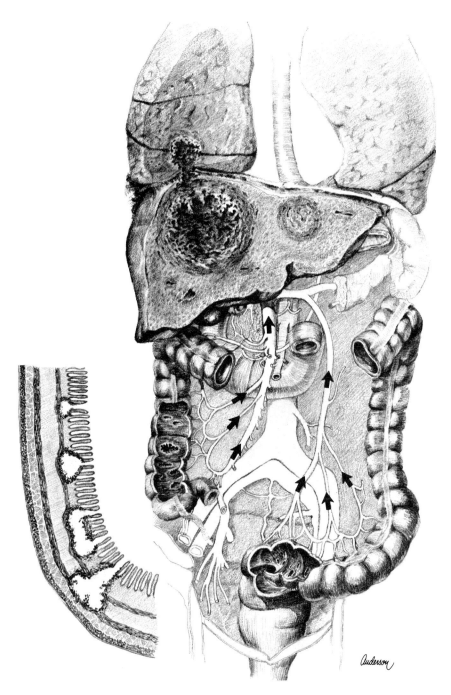

**Fig. 31-4.** Major pathology of amebiasis. Invasion of intestinal mucosa occurs most commonly in the cecum and next most commonly in rectosigmoid area. Passage of trophozoites via portal circulation may result in liver abscess formation. Metastasis through diaphragm may result in secondary abscess formation in lungs. Trophozoites carried in bloodstream may cause foci of infection anywhere in body. (From Beck, J. W., and Barrett-Connor, E.: Medical parasitology, St. Louis, 1971, The C. V. Mosby Co.)

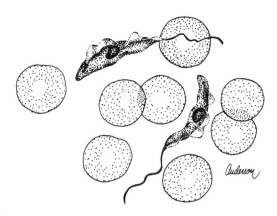

**Fig. 31-5.** *Trypanosoma gambiense* in blood smear, sketch. (From Beck, J. W., and Barrett-Connor, E.: Medical parasitology, St. Louis, 1971, The C. V. Mosby Co.)

sleeping sickness, and South American trypanosomiasis or Chagas' disease.

Abastrin, a substance elaborated by *Trypanosoma*, has some antimicrobial activity.

**African trypanosomiasis.** African trypanosomiasis occurs in two forms: Gambian trypanosomiasis (agent, *Trypanosoma gambiense*) and Rhodesian trypanosomiasis (agent, *Trypanosoma rhodesiense*). Each is transmitted by a species of the tsetse fly. The fly becomes infected by ingesting the blood of a person with the disease, and the parasite undergoes a cycle of development in its body. When the parasites develop to a certain point, they invade the salivary glands of the fly, from which they are transferred to persons bitten. Cattle, swine, and wild game animals, especially antelope, may harbor the parasites and be a source of human infection. Rhodesian trypanosomiasis is more virulent than the Gambian form. Early in the course of either form of trypanosomiasis there are acute episodes of fever and inflammation of lymph nodes as the trypanosomes multiply in the bloodstream. The Rhodesian form is usually fatal within a matter of months and rarely progresses to the chronic stages of the Gambian form. In the end stages of the disease invasion of the brain and its coverings produces the celebrated and uncontrollable sleepiness.

**South American trypanosomiasis.** South American trypanosomiasis, caused by *Trypanosoma cruzi*, is transferred to man by small, bloodsucking, cricket-like insects from a reservoir in man and domestic and wild animals such as dogs, cats, rats, armadillos, and opossums. Infection results from contamination of the skin with insect feces and is not transferred by the actual insect bite. South American trypanosomiasis differs from African trypanosomiasis in that the parasites multiply in the tissues rather than in

the blood. They reappear in the blood to be picked up by the vector. If the patient survives the acute stage, the disease becomes chronic, with the trypanosomes localized in various organs.

An experimental vaccine has been prepared by killing the microorganisms of a culture by physical means—subjecting the trypanosomes to high-frequency sound waves, to pressure, or to the mechanical forces evoked when the culture is shaken with glass beads. It has been used only in mice.

**Laboratory diagnosis.** During the fever, trypanosomes of the African disease may be demonstrated in Giemsa-stained films of peripheral blood. Concentration technics for peripheral blood facilitate the search for parasites. Smears and imprints of lymph nodes may contain them. *Trypanosoma cruzi* is identified in material aspirated from spleen, liver, lymph nodes, and bone marrow.

## LEISHMANIASIS

Leishmaniasis is a protozoan disease caused by what is probably man's most ancient parasite. It occurs in two forms: the visceral and the cutaneous.

**Visceral leishmaniasis (kala-azar, dumdum fever).** The visceral form of leishmaniasis is characterized by fever, enlargement of the spleen and liver, progressive emaciation, weakness, and, in untreated patients, death. The agent, *Leishmania donovani*, is transmitted from man to man by the bite of sandflies of the genus *Phlebotomus*. The disease is endemic among dogs, which may be a source of infection. It occurs in countries bordering the Mediterranean Sea, in India, in the Middle East, in China, and in parts of Africa.

**Cutaneous leishmaniasis.** Cutaneous leishmaniasis is described by the presence of nodular and ulcerating lesions in the skin. There are two types: one, known as Oriental sore, Aleppo button, or Delhi boil, is caused by *Leishmania tropica;* the other, known as American leishmaniasis or espundia, is caused by *Leishmania braziliensis.* Cutaneous leishmaniasis is transmitted, as is the visceral disease, by sandflies. The individual lesions on the skin represent the bites of insects or the mechanical transfer of infection by scratching or some form of abrasion. This disease is seen in the same parts of the world as visceral leishmaniasis, but the two forms of leishmaniasis are said not to occur in exactly the same localities. Cutaneous leishmaniasis is occasionally seen in the United States in persons coming from endemic areas.

**Laboratory diagnosis.** In all forms of leishmaniasis the diagnosis is made by demonstrating the organisms in smears from lesions or in biopsies of involved tissues.

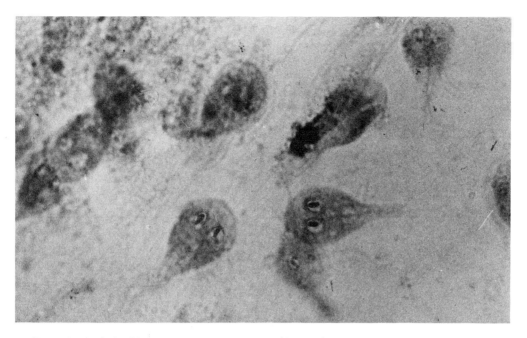

**Fig. 31-6.** *Giardia lamblia* in gastric aspirate processed for cytologic examination, photomicrograph.

## TRICHOMONIASIS

Trichomoniasis occurs as a widespread infection of the genitourinary tract caused by *Trichomonas vaginalis.* In women it is an intractable vaginitis with a profuse, cream-colored, foul-smelling discharge in which the trichomonads abound. In men they are found in the prepuce and prostatic urethra, but symptoms seldom occur. The infection is transmitted by sexual intercourse and is a venereal disease of generally unrecognized significance. The trichomonads are readily identified in vaginal discharges from the female and in urine or prostatic discharges from the male.

## INFECTIONS WITH INTESTINAL FLAGELLATES

The most important intestinal flagellates found as cysts and trophozoites in stool specimens are *Giardia lamblia, Trichomonas hominis,* and *Chilomastix mesnili.* The latter two are not considered as pathogenic agents by most protozoologists. The presence of *Giardia lamblia* in the upper part of the small intestine in man is usually associated with mild disturbances of the bowel. Giardiasis, infection with the organism, is related to persisting diarrhea, malabsorption, and inflammatory changes in the lining of the small intestine (Fig. 31-6).

## MALARIA

Malaria is an acute febrile disease caused by the malarial parasite, a protozoon belonging to class Telo-sporea and genus *Plasmodium.* The word *malaria* is derived from the Italian for "bad air," and the disease got its name in the eighteenth century because of its association with the ill-smelling vapors from the marshes around Rome.

Malaria, one of the most widely prevalent diseases in the world, remains the number one public health problem globally. More people have malaria than any other disease. It is a constant threat to more than 1 billion human beings. Prior to America's civil and military involvement in Southeast Asia, malaria was infrequently seen in the United States (60 cases reported in 1961). In 1970 there were over 3500 cases, mostly in individuals returning from Southeast Asia. Malaria has been a scourge of war and of mankind throughout the ages. The Army Medical Corps states that this disease can put more men out of action than battle casualties. In World War II there were over 490,000 cases of malaria with 8 million man-days lost.

**Types.** Malaria occurs as three distinct types (each caused by its own species of *Plasmodium*) characterized as follows*:

1. *Tertian*—by a paroxysm of chill and fever every 48 hours; cause, *Plasmodium vivax;* the most common type

---

*A fourth parasite is *Plasmodium ovale,* whose appearance and life cycle are very much like those of *Plasmodium vivax.* Infection with this parasite, tertian malaria, is usually mild. It is not widely distributed over the world.

2. *Quartan*—a paroxysm of chill and fever every 72 hours; cause, *Plasmodium malariae;* the least common type
3. *Estivoautumnal* or *malignant*—irregular paroxysms; cause, *Plasmodium falciparum*\*

The first two types are known as *regular intermittent* types. After the paroxysm of chill and fever, temperature returns to normal, and the patient is fairly comfortable until the next paroxysm. In the third or *remittent* type the fever varies in intensity, but the patient does not become completely afebrile.

---

\*Ninety percent of malaria in Southeast Asia is caused by *Plasmodium falciparum*. Although this is true, 85% of malaria in returnees is caused by *Plasmodium vivax*. In the Korean conflict malaria was almost entirely vivax. This is less severe clinically but is more likely to lie dormant only to recur many months after the initial episodes. There is little tendency for relapses with falciparum malaria.

Estivoautumnal (also called pernicious) malaria is the most severe in its consequences and is the treacherous form. Its clinical picture is diverse, sometimes obscure, oftentimes dramatic, and it can be rapidly fatal. Death, it is said, may come within a matter of hours. If there is mixed infection, falciparum is the dominant form.

**Modes of infection.** The different species of malarial parasites are closely related and are transmitted in the same way—by the bite of a female mosquito of the genus *Anopheles*. Of this genus, nearly a hundred species may transmit the infection naturally. Man is the main reservoir of infection. In malaria-infected countries many of the inhabitants become asymptomatic carriers (they harbor the parasites in their blood [parasitemia] and tissues without manifesting the disease). Repeated attacks seem to give the patient some immunity. Unrecognized infections

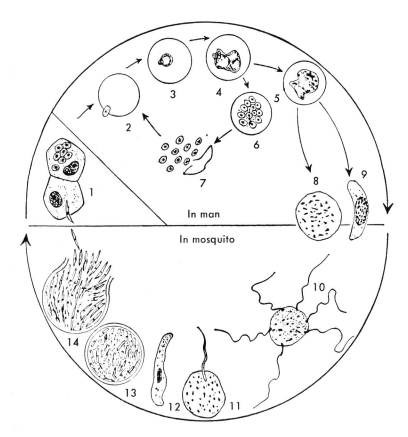

**Fig. 31-7.** Malarial merry-go-round—life cycle of malarial parasite. *Preerythrocytic phase: 1,* Sporozoite entering liver cell. *Erythrocytic phase: 2,* Merozoite entering red blood cell; *3,* trophozoite or ring form; *4,* growing trophozoite; *5,* preschizont; *6,* schizont (segmentation stage); *7,* liberated merozoites; *8,* microgametocyte (male sexual parasite); *9,* macrogametocyte (female sexual parasite); *10,* exflagellation of microgametocyte, with microgametes attached; *11,* fertilization of macrogamete by microgamete; *12,* ookinete; *13,* immature oocyst; *14,* mature oocyst discharging sporozoites.

and insufficient treatment lead to the carrier state, so important in the spread of malaria.

The disease is occasionally transferred by the use of contaminated hypodermic syringes, as is common among heroin addicts, or by blood transfusion. There is an increased awareness of this hazard in blood banking, partly because of the likelihood of the source of infection being a blood donor who is a drug addict.

A reservoir of malaria exists in monkeys, from which the infection is transmitted to man and other primates by certain forest species of *Anopheles*.

**Life story of parasite.** There are two major events in the complicated life story of the malarial parasite.

*Asexual development in man.* When young malarial parasites (*sporozoites*) are introduced into the bloodstream by the mosquito bite, they localize in the cells of the liver, where they multiply. This is the *preerythrocytic* phase. (See Fig. 31-7.) (Some 500,000 parasites must be injected by the mosquito for a human being to be infected.) After 6 to 9 days young parasites (*merozoites*) are released into the bloodstream. The *erythrocytic phase* begins when each one bores into a red blood cell on which it feeds and where it continues to develop. The parasite does not fully utilize the hemoglobin of the red cell. Because of this, granules of pigment (an iron porphyrin hematin) accumulate within the red cell cytoplasm. This residual product is the malarial pigment; it is not a normal breakdown product of hemoglobin. When the parasite reaches maturity, it is known as a *schizont*. Within the red cell the mature schizont arranges

itself into a number of segments. Suddenly the segments separate, releasing another generation of merozoites and destroying the red cell. This process is *segmentation*. Some of the merozoites are destroyed by white blood cells, but the majority bore into red blood cells to repeat the process of asexual growth and segmentation. In estivoautumnal malaria two or even three or four parasites invade a single red cell.

About 2 weeks (sometimes longer) after the infecting mosquito bite, enough parasites are present for the red blood cell destruction to cause trouble. The *incubation period* covers the initial preerythrocytic phase and the first 2 weeks or so of the erythrocytic phase. The time elapsing between the entrance of a parasite into a red blood cell and its segmentation is the periodicity of the parasite. For *Plasmodium vivax* it is 48 hours; for *Plasmodium malariae*, 72 hours. For *Plasmodium falciparum* it is usually 48 hours, but not regularly so. (See Figs. 31-8 to 31-10.)

The paroxysms of chills and fever in malaria stem from the liberation of metabolic by-products from the parasite and toxic breakdown products from the disrupted blood cell. Sharp paroxysms occur in tertian and quartan malaria because all the parasitized cells rupture at about the same time. In estivoautumnal infections some of the parasitized cells rupture ahead of time, and some rupture behind time, so that several hours are required for the whole brood of parasites to be released. This explains why chills are usually absent and the fever may be continuous.

Some of the parasites do not repeat the asexual

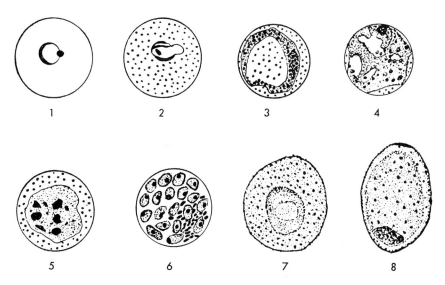

**Fig. 31-8.** *Plasmodium vivax* (parasite of tertian malaria), development in red blood cell. *1*, Young ring form (trophozoite); *2* to *5*, successive stages; *6*, mature schizont (made up of many segments or merozoites); *7*, microgametocyte (male sexual parasite); *8*, macrogametocyte (female sexual parasite).

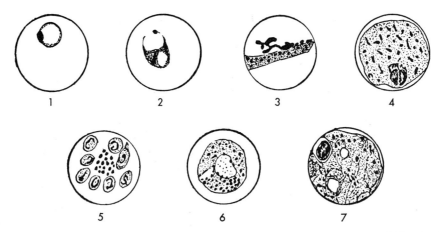

**Fig. 31-9.** *Plasmodium malariae* (parasite of quartan malaria), development in red blood cell. *1,* Young ring form (trophozoite); *2* to *4,* successive stages; *5,* mature schizont (made up of merozoites); *6,* microgametocyte; *7,* macrogametocyte.

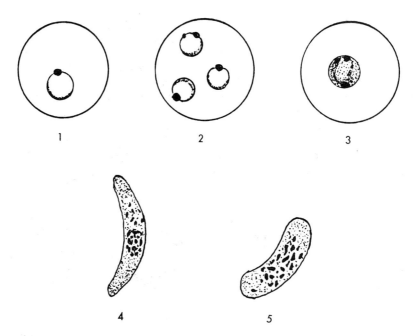

**Fig. 31-10.** *Plasmodium falciparum* (parasite of estivoautumnal malaria), development in red blood cell. *1,* Trophozoite; *2,* three trophozoites (multiple infection characteristic of *Plasmodium falciparum*) in red blood cell; *3,* schizont, early formation and production of pigment (seldom found in peripheral blood); *4,* macrogametocyte; *5,* microgametocyte.

cycle of development but produce male and female sexual forms or *gametocytes,* the sexual development of which is completed within the stomach of an *Anopheles* mosquito. Sexual forms do not appear in the blood until the infection is of 2 or 3 weeks' duration.

*Sexual development in the mosquito.* When a fe-

male *Anopheles* mosquito ingests male and female sexual parasites from the blood of an infected person, a rather complicated sexual cycle begins in its stomach. First, the female parasite or *macrogamete* is fertilized by flagellar structures, *microgametes,* that break away from the male parasite or *microgametocyte* by a process of exflagellation. These structures correspond to spermatozoa in the higher forms of life. The fertilized parasite or *ookinete* bores into the stomach wall, becomes encysted (the *oocyst*), and divides into many small, spindle-shaped parasites or *sporozoites*. The cyst ruptures, and the sporozoites are carried by the lymphatic system to the salivary gland of the mosquito, which is so constructed that the parasites are ejected in the saliva when the mosquito bites.

**Pathology.** The chief pathologic changes in malaria relate to destruction of red blood cells (hemolysis). Hemolysis leads to different degrees of anemia and jaundice. The parasitic infection seems to make the blood more viscous, and the sticky parasitized cells plug and obstruct small blood vessels. This is prone to occur with falciparum malaria and accounts for its worst complication, cerebral malaria. The liver and spleen enlarge (hepatosplenomegaly), partly because the presence of the malarial pigment stimulates the reticuloendothelial system to activity. Reticuloendothelial cells ingest the pigment and deposit it in liver, spleen, and bone marrow. In acute malaria the spleen is moderately enlarged, soft, and friable. In chronic malaria it is enlarged and markedly fibrotic. Such a spleen easily ruptures as the result of a blow or fall, or even spontaneously.

A dreaded complication is blackwater fever, which develops in certain cases with acute and massive hemolysis. Large amounts of hemoglobin are released into the plasma (hemoglobinemia), spilling over into the urine (hemoglobinuria). There is a severe kind of acute renal failure associated with the passage of reddish black urine.

On a worldwide basis malaria results in a greater morbidity and mortality than any other infectious disease.

**Laboratory diagnosis.** Malarial parasites may be easily seen in the red cells of properly prepared (and stained) thin smears of peripheral blood taken just before or at the peak of the paroxysm. Wright's and Giemsa's stains are most often used. The young parasites, seen as blue rings with a red chromatin dot attached, have a signet ring appearance. The quartan ring is thicker than the tertian, and the estivoautumnal ring is thin and hairlike. The latter often has two chromatin dots. Full-grown malarial parasites almost completely fill the red cell and contain numerous red granules. Just before the red cell is ruptured, the parasites assume a segmented or rosette pattern. Socalled malarial crescents are sausage-shaped gametocytes with a chromatin mass near their center and are the sexual parasites of estivoautumnal malaria. They are frequently seen in the blood, whereas the fully developed parasite or schizont is seldom seen in this form of malaria.

At times, when organisms are too few to be seen in thin smear, a sample of blood may be smeared thickly on a glass slide. This thick smear is treated to remove hemoglobin from the erythrocytes and then stained. The disadvantage of the thick smear is that the shape and appearance of the parasites are altered in preparation. Its advantage is that a much greater volume of blood may be examined within a given length of time.*

Fluorescent antibody technics are also used to stain the malarial parasite specifically. A soluble antigen fluorescent antibody (SAFA) diagnostic test fills a need in the blood bank in the screening of donors.

A small dose of quinine or other antimalarial drug will drive the parasites out of the peripheral blood; therefore, it is practically useless to examine the blood for malaria right after these drugs are given.

The laboratory diagnosis of malaria *does not consist only in finding the parasites but includes the determination of the species.*

**Mosquitoes transmitting malaria.** Malaria is transmitted by various species of *Anopheles* mosquitoes. It is transmitted only by the female because the male lives on fruits and vegetables (instead of blood). Since the common house mosquito (*Culex*) does not convey malaria, it is important to differentiate it from *Anopheles*. The *Culex* mosquito bites during the daytime, the *Anopheles* at night or about dusk. The wings of *Anopheles* are spotted, whereas those of *Culex* are not. When *Culex* is resting on a wall, its body is almost parallel to the wall; the body of *Anopheles* stands at an acute angle.

**Prevention.** Prevention of malaria depends on blocking the transfer of infection from person to person by mosquitoes. Recommended for this purpose are (1) screening of houses, (2) draining and oiling of ponds of water to prevent mosquito breeding and using minnows to destroy the larvae, (3) proper treatment of patients with antimalarial drugs, and (4) detection and cure of carriers.

The presence of an animal reservoir greatly complicates the problem of malarial control in those countries where the jungles swarm with monkeys and other primates.

Development of a vaccine for malaria is still experimental. Partially purified material from the malarial plasmodium is used.

## BALANTIDIASIS

*Balantidium coli* is the most important intestinal ciliate and the largest protozoon to invade man. It is seen in two life stages: the cyst and the motile

---

*In falciparum malaria thick smears may not show parasites for several days after the onset.

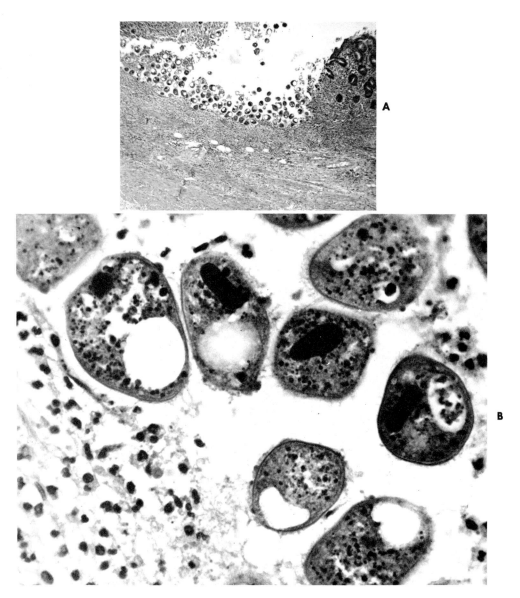

**Fig. 31-11.** *Balantidium coli,* stained tissue section (hematoxylin and eosin [H & E]). **A,** Balantidiasis of the appendix. In crater of ulcerated area of appendiceal wall are numerous organisms cut in cross section. (×35.) **B,** Cross-sectional areas of *Balantidium coli* as seen with higher microscopic magnification. (×430.) (From Anderson, W. A. D., editor: Pathology, ed. 6, St. Louis, 1971, The C. V. Mosby Co.)

trophozoite. (See Fig. 31-11.) In some cases it seems to be a harmless inhabitant of the large intestine, but usually its presence is associated with diarrhea. It may invade the intestinal wall and produce ulceration or abscesses, with intense dysentery that may even cause death.

*Balantidium coli* is a normal inhabitant of the large intestine of the domestic hog. Man is probably infected by ingesting cysts passed by the hog. The laboratory identification of cysts and trophozoites in the stool or in the exudate from intestinal ulcers makes the diagnosis.

## TOXOPLASMOSIS

*Toxoplasma gondii,* the cause of toxoplasmosis, is a delicate, boat-shaped, obligate intracellular para-

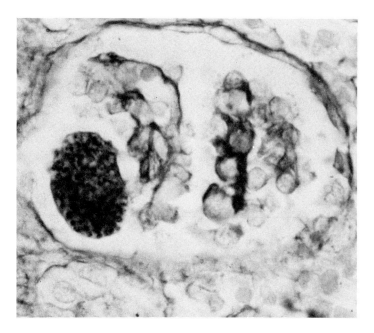

**Fig. 31-12.** *Toxoplasma* cyst (left) seen in microsection of kidney from infant dead of disease. (Courtesy Dr. J. S. Remington, Palo Alto, Calif.; from Feldman, H. A.: Hosp. Pract. **4:**64, March, 1969.)

site, somewhat similar to *Leishmania*. It is easily killed by physical agents. It is a cosmopolitan sporozoan, being found in animals and birds all over the world.

**The disease.** The organism can invade practically any tissue cell and is especially prone to affect the cells of the reticuloendothelial system, including the lining cells of the blood vessels. Within a cell the organisms rapidly proliferate in a typical fashion, forming a rosette that may become a cyst containing some 3000 parasites (Fig. 31-12). Inflammation may be present in the lungs, lymph nodes, eyes, and brain. Characteristic are the focal deposits of calcium in nervous tissue (especially in the fetus). In man the disease occurs in two forms: acquired and congenital. The acquired or adult form often passes unnoticed. One third of adults in the United States have been infected at some time. The congenital form is acquired in utero from a mother most probably with no history of previous infection. The newborn baby becomes very ill, develops a skin rash, turns yellow, and may convulse. If the baby survives, the damage done in the brain (associated with the calcium deposits), may cause him to be born with microcephaly, hydrocephalus, and mental retardation. *Toxoplasma gondii* produces changes in the eye that are designated as chorioretinitis, and the lesion is responsible for blindness in infants. (No effective form of treatment is known for the disease.)

Toxoplasmosis is associated with the formation of tumors in birds; in man it is seen with neoplasms of the central nervous system.

**Sources and mode of infection.** Recent evidence indicates that this sporozoan has a life cycle in cats similar to that of the malarial parasite in mosquitoes. Cats pick up the parasites when they consume the intermediate hosts—infected birds and mice. In the intestine of the cat, which provides a peculiarly suitable habitat for the parasite, the organisms go through asexual and sexual stages of development, and the oocysts are passed in the feces. After being passed into soil, sand, or litterbox, oocysts become infectious after 3 to 4 days in warm, moist surroundings. They can be recovered after many months from water or wet soil and are generally resistant to many chemical agents including ordinary disinfectants. However, drying and heat kill them. The common house cat is implicated as the primary host and a reservoir for man.

The parasite is universal. Many animals harbor it, and it may persist in the raw flesh of the slaughtered animal until killed by heat, drying, or freezing. Eating raw or undercooked meat is a principal source of human infection. The National Livestock and Meat Board recommends that all meat be heated to at least 140° F. throughout to kill the toxoplasmas. (This is the "rare" reading on meat thermometers designed for home use.) Pregnant women should be very careful in handling cats, cat feces, or articles contaminated with cat feces and should avoid altogether any contact with a strange cat or one newly brought into the household.

The organisms are taken into the human body by way of the mouth either because the individual has been in contact with an infected cat or because he has consumed infected meat. The toxoplasmas are released from the oocysts and migrate into body tissues and fluids.

For the congenital form to develop, the organisms must get into the bloodstream of the mother sometime after the first trimester of pregnancy. They establish a focus of infection in the placenta that enables them to penetrate the fetal circulation and so infect the fetus.

**Laboratory diagnosis.** These microorganisms, possessing a delicate, crescent-shaped body with tapered ends, are easily stained and identified in smears made from body fluids, exudates, and even diseased tissues. Toxoplasmas can be cultured in cell culture or in a fertile hen's egg. Serologic examinations include an indirect hemagglutination test, a complement fixation test, a neutralization test, and an immunofluorescence test. The antibodies detected by the Sabin-Feldman dye test are those preventing parasites of a laboratory culture from taking up methylene blue dye. A toxoplasmin skin test is available. A mouse can be inoculated with suspected material, and the organisms can be recovered and identified from that animal.

Toxoplasmas may be detected in the feces of a cat. Direct smears are not adequate; the fecal flotation method must be used.

## PNEUMOCYSTOSIS

*Pneumocystis carinii* causes pneumocystosis (diffuse interstitial pneumonitis, interstitial plasma cell pneumonia), an inflammatory process unique in the lungs. Little is known about the organism, and nothing is known as to the mode of infection. The organisms (Fig. 31-13) are studied in smears of material aspirated from the diseased lungs and stained by the Papanicolaou technic or in tissue sections of lung (from autopsy) stained with a special silver stain. In this disease the air sacs of the lungs are filled with a foamy, semiliquid, lightly staining material representing clustered masses of oval, minute organisms about

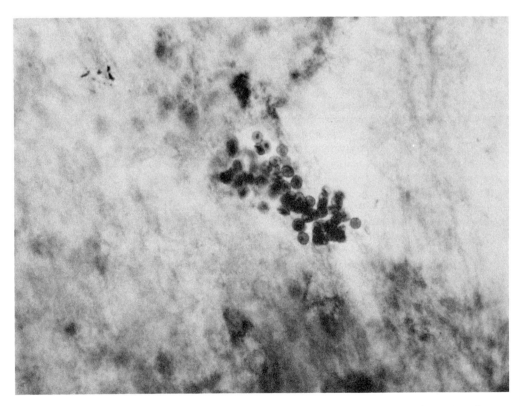

**Fig. 31-13.** *Pneumocystis carinii* in direct smear of pulmonary lavage sediment (methenamine silver stain). (×500.) (From Drew, W. L., and others: J.A.M.A. **230:**713, 1974.)

1 $\mu$m. ($\mu$) in diameter, surrounded by a thin homogeneous capsule. The walls of the air sacs are permeated by inflammatory cells.

Pneumocystosis is another, not too rare, disorder of the "compromised" host, particularly the immunosuppressed one. It was first encountered in debilitated infants. The vulnerability of much older patients stems from prolonged steroid hormone therapy, extended immunosuppresion, or the presence of leukemia or other cancer of the lymphoid system. Cortisone (a steroid hormone) is thought to enhance the growth of these organisms.

## Questions for review

1 Describe protozoa. What are their salient features?
2 Give the six classes of protozoa of medical interest. Characterize each.
3 Define: intermediate host, definitive host, organelle, pseudopod, cyst, flagella, cilia, trophozoite, parasite, endoparasite, ectoparasite.
4 How is amebiasis spread? How may it be prevented?
5 Outline the development of the malarial parasite in (a) man and (b) the mosquito.
6 Discuss the prevention of malaria.
7 Compare *Anopheles* mosquito with *Culex*.
8 Give the laboratory diagnosis for:
   a. Malaria
   b. Amebiasis
   c. Trypanosomiasis
   d. Leishmaniasis
   e. Toxoplasmosis
   f. Pneumocystosis
9 Characterize briefly: Chagas' disease, African trypanosomiasis, trichomoniasis, giardiasis, balantidiasis, toxoplasmosis, and pneumocytosis.
10 Compare the life cycle of *Plasmodium* with that of *Toxoplasma*.

**References on pp. 368 to 370.**

# CHAPTER 32

# Metazoa
## medical helminthology

## Perspectives

Among multicellular animal parasites, or Metazoa, three phyla are medically noteworthy in man: (1) *Platyhelminthes* or flatworms, which include the *Trematoda* (flukes) and *Cestoidea* (tapeworms), (2) *Nematoda* (roundworms), and (3) *Arthropoda*. Included in the Arthropoda are mites, spiders, ticks, flies, lice, and fleas. As vectors, these are medically important in the transmission of disease* (Table 32-1).

Worms are elongated, invertebrate animals without appendages or bilateral symmetry. The laboratory

---

* If the parasite is carried unchanged, the vector is a *mechanical* one. The parasite undergoes a series of developmental changes in the body of the *biologic* vector.

**Table 32-1**
Overview of Arthropoda in spread of disease

| GENUS NAMES OF VECTORS | COMMON NAMES OF VECTORS | AGENTS TRANSMITTED | EXAMPLES OF DISEASES SPREAD |
|---|---|---|---|
| *Anopheles* *Aedes* *Culex* *Mansonia* | Mosquito | Metazoa, protozoa, viruses | Malaria, yellow fever, encephalitides, filariasis |
| *Dermacentor* *Rhipicephalus* *Amblyomma* *Ornithodorus* | Tick | Bacteria, rickettsias | Spotted fevers, tularemia, Q fever, relapsing fever |
| *Trombicula* *Allodermanyssus* | Mite | Rickettsias | Scrub typhus, rickettsialpox |
| *Pediculus* | Louse | Bacteria, rickettsias | Typhus fever, relapsing fever |
| *Xenopsylla* *Pulex* | Flea | Bacteria, rickettsias | Plague, murine typhus |
| | Biting fly: | | |
| *Glossina* | Tsetse fly | Protozoa | Sleeping sickness |
| *Simulium* | Black fly | Metazoa | River blindness |
| *Phlebotomus* | Sandfly | Protozoa, bacteria | Leishmaniasis, bartonellosis |
| *Musca* | Housefly | Metazoa, protozoa, bacteria, chlamydiae, viruses | Salmonellosis, bacillary dysentery, cholera, amebiasis, poliomyelitis, trachoma, trypanosomiasis, ascariasis |
| *Triatoma* *Rhodnius* | Triatomid bug | Protozoa | Chagas' disease |

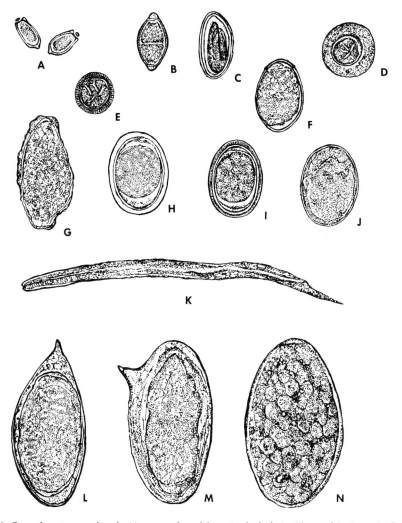

**Fig. 32-1.** Ova of metazoa, sketch. Note one larval form included. **A,** *Clonorchis sinensis.* **B,** *Trichuris trichiura.* **C,** *Enterobius vermicularis.* **D,** *Hymenolepis nana.* **E,** *Taenia solium.* **F,** *Diphyllobothrium latum.* **G,** *Ascaris lumbricoides,* unfertilized ovum. **H** and **I,** *Ascaris lumbricoides,* fertilized ova. **J,** *Schistosoma japonicum.* **K,** *Strongyloides stercoralis* larva. **L,** *Schistosoma haematobium.* **M,** *Schistosoma mansoni.* **N,** *Fasciolopsis buski.*

## Table 32-2
Serologic tests of value in metazoan diseases*

| IMMUNODIAGNOSTIC TEST | SCHISTO-SOMIASIS | CYSTICERCOSIS | ECHINO-COCCOSIS | ANCYLOSTO-MIASIS | ASCARIASIS | TRICHINOSIS | FILARIASIS |
|---|---|---|---|---|---|---|---|
| Intradermal | × | | × | | | × | |
| Complement fixation | × | × | × | | | × | × |
| Bentonite flocculation | | | × | | × | × | × |
| Indirect hemagglutination | × | × | × | × | × | × | × |
| Latex agglutination | | | × | | | × | |
| Indirect fluorescent antibody | × | | × | | | × | |
| Precipitin | | | × | | | × | |

*Modified from Kagan, I. G.: Current status of serologic testing for parasitic diseases, Hosp. Pract. **9:**157, Sept., 1974.

× indicates an accepted test for routine use.

diagnosis of metazoan, as with protozoan, infections depends most of the time on the morphologic identification of the parasite or its ova (Fig. 32-1). Table 32-2 presents serologic tests in relation to the diseases for which they are applicable. (See also p. 341.)

## Registry of pathogens
### TREMATODES (FLUKES)

The trematodes are flat, leaflike, nonsegmented parasites provided with suckers for attachment to the host. All species, except those that inhabit the bloodstream, are hermaphrodites and have operculate eggs (Fig. 32-1, *A, J, L-N*). Some have the most complicated life histories in the animal kingdom.

**Life history.** The cycle of development of flukes is briefly as follows. The egg is passed from the body of the host, and the contained embryo develops into a ciliated organism, the *miracidium* (pl., *miracidia*). If water is present, the miracidium escapes from the egg and swims (about 5 or 6 hours) until it reaches an intermediate host (certain species of water snails, Fig. 32-2). Hatching miracidia are phototrophic; that is, they swim toward light. (This phenomenon can some-

times be demonstrated in fecal or urinary specimens.) The miracidium penetrates the host snail and forms a cyst in its lungs, in which many organisms develop. These wander to other parts of the snail and develop into minute worms called *cercariae* (Fig. 32-3).

One infested snail alone can release 169 million cercariae in 1 month's time. Being phototrophic, the cercariae emerge during the hours of sunlight, and the greatest number (hence the best chance of getting the disease) is at high noon. (They seldom live more than 1 day.) They swim around until they attach themselves to blades of grass, where they encyst. Sometimes they enter other aquatic animals such as certain fishes and crabs, to encyst. When the encysted organisms are swallowed by man, the definitive host, they develop into adult flukes in his tissues. Note that the cercariae of the blood flukes gain access to the body of man through the skin. They make their way via the bloodstream to the portal venous system, where they mature to adult organisms.

**Classification.** Flukes are classified according to the area of the body in which their development into adult flukes is completed and their eggs deposited.

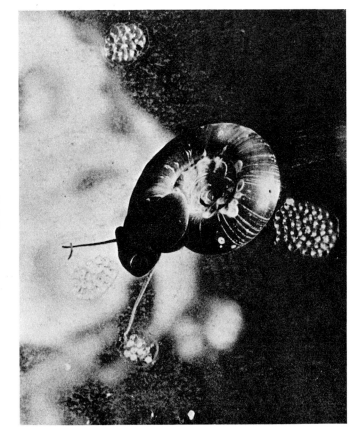

**Fig. 32-2.** *Australorbis glabratus,* snail vector for schistosomiasis in Western Hemisphere. (From Med. World News **6**:35, Dec. 3, 1965; photograph by Pete Peters.)

From the standpoint of habitat there are flukes that live in the intestine, the liver, the lungs, and the portal venous system with its tributaries. The last are called blood flukes; of special note are three: *Schistosoma japonicum, Schistosoma mansoni,* and *Schistosoma haematobium.* The large intestinal fluke is *Fasciolopsis buski; Clonorchis sinensis* and *Fasciola hepatica* are liver flukes, and *Paragonimus westermani* is the lung fluke.

**Pathogenicity.** The pathologic changes in the human body center about the eggs trapped in the tissues. Female blood flukes may migrate to the terminal vessels of the bladder and rectum to lay their eggs. (A single worm can deposit eggs in a given area for up to 20 years.) There eggs set up an inflammatory reaction in the mucous membrane. This results in papillomatous thickenings. The eggs may escape into the lumen of the bladder or rectal canal to be passed in the urine or feces. The ova of flukes that migrate to the lungs may be found either in sputum or with swallowed sputum in feces. Because of the anatomic relation of the liver to the intestine, we would expect to find the ova of flukes of this organ in the feces. It is important to look for ova in stool specimens, since practically all types may be found there, regardless of the habitat of a given fluke.

Trematode infections are prevalent in the Orient and in the tropics, where contamination of fresh water by human feces is widespread. It is estimated that blood flukes or schistosomes infest 200 million persons. Infection with blood flukes is *schistosomiasis* or *bilharziasis.* It is one of man's oldest diseases; calcified ova have been found in Egyptian mummies. Also called snail fever, schistosomiasis is one of the world's most important medical problems. As a global disease, it is second only to malaria in the geographic extent of the incapacity and morbidity produced.

As an aside, schistosomes recovered from human beings have been found to be parasitized, in turn, by salmonellae, an instance of bacterial parasitism of a parasite in man. The association and interaction may explain why chronic salmonellosis often accompanies schistosomiasis.

**Prevention.** Measures of control have been largely directed toward elimination of the intermediate host, the snail.

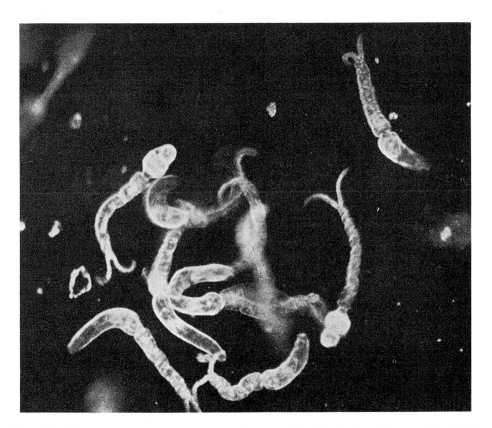

**Fig. 32-3.** Schistosome cercariae photographed by dark-field illumination. (Photograph by D. M. Blair, Salisbury, Southern Rhodesia; published by permission of F. Goodliffe, Southern Rhodesian Public Relations Department, Salisbury.)

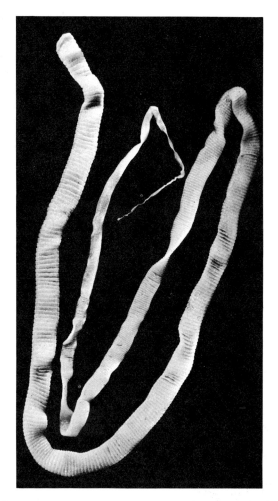

**Fig. 32-4.** Tapeworm. Note very small head and successively larger segments. Young proglottids are budded from scolex and neck (center); oldest gravid proglottids shown at upper left. (From Hickman, C. P., and others: Integrated principles of zoology, ed. 5, St. Louis, 1974, The C. V. Mosby Co.)

Experimentally it has been found that if a small, innocuous dose of *Klebsiella pneumoniae* is given to an animal infected with *Schistosoma mansoni,* the flukes die out and the host gets well. This, if feasible on a practical basis, would open a new era of *biologic* control of parasites.

## CESTODES (TAPEWORMS)

Tapeworms *(Taenia)* are typically intestinal parasites and produce digestive disturbances of variable degree.

**Anatomy.** Adult worms have a small head, which buries itself in the intestinal mucosa and anchors the worm, and a nonsegmented neck (head and neck,

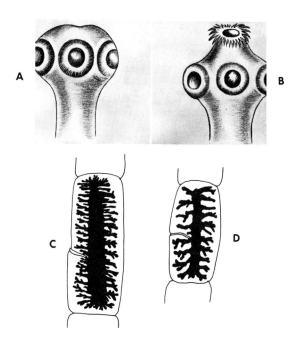

**Fig. 32-5.** *Taenia saginata* (beef tapeworm) compared with *Taenia solium* (pork tapeworm). **A,** Scolex of *Taenia saginata* with suckers only. **B,** Scolex of *Taenia solium* with apical hooks and suckers. **C,** Uterus of *Taenia saginata* with more than 14 primary lateral branches. **D,** Uterus of *Taenia solium* with less than 12.

collectively spoken of as the *scolex*), to which are attached in a line a variable number of segments *(proglottids)*. New segments are formed by a process of segmentation from the scolex: the youngest segment is the one joining the scolex, and the last segment is the oldest. Up to a certain point, the farther the segment from the scolex, the larger it is. There is no alimentary canal. Each segment obtains its nourishment from the host's intestinal juices by osmosis.

The head is extremely small by comparison with the remainder of the body, often the size of a pinhead (Fig. 32-4). It is provided with hooklets or suckers or both for attachment to the intestinal wall. (See Fig. 32-5.) The hooklets are arranged in one or more rows around a small prominence *(rostellum)* situated on the head. In at least one species, attachment is accomplished by suctorial grooves on the sides of the head. Treatment that fails to recover the head, regardless of the number of segments removed, is of no value because the head will immediately replace the lost segments. The peculiar shape, arrangement, and deeply embedded position of the hooklets often make removal of the head from the intestine difficult.

Each fully developed segment is a sexually complete hermaphrodite. From the scolex to the other end of the worm there are the following:

1. Undeveloped segments: *immature proglottids*
2. Segments with both male and female elements: well-developed *mature proglottids*
3. Segments filled by the egg-laden uterus: *gravid proglottids*
4. Degenerating gravid proglottids

In a few species the ova are extruded from the segment through a birth pore. In most species, however, no birth pore is present, and the ova escape from the proglottid through a longitudinal slit. The gravid proglottids toward the end of the tapeworm separate and may be passed in the feces. A person can harbor a tapeworm without ova appearing in the stool, since the segments may be expelled before the ova are liberated.

**Life cycle.** Tapeworms have a larval and an adult cycle of existence. (See Figs. 32-6 and 32-7.) As a rule, the cycles take place in different species of animals. The adult cycle occurs within the intestinal canal, the larval cycle within the tissues of the host.

The egg develops into an adult tapeworm as follows. Through a series of changes, an embryo is formed within the egg. After the eggs are swallowed by a susceptible intermediate host, the larvae are set

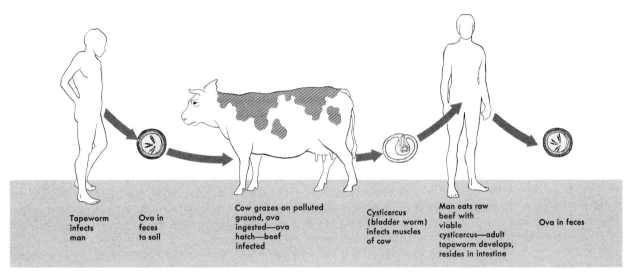

Tapeworm infects man | Ova in feces to soil | Cow grazes on polluted ground, ova ingested—ova hatch—beef infected | Cysticercus (bladder worm) infects muscles of cow | Man eats raw beef with viable cysticercus—adult tapeworm develops, resides in intestine | Ova in feces

**Fig. 32-6.** *Taenia saginata,* life cycle.

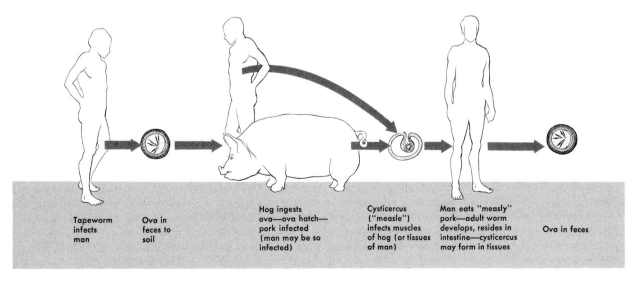

Tapeworm infects man | Ova in feces to soil | Hog ingests ova—ova hatch—pork infected (man may be so infected) | Cysticercus ("measle") infects muscles of hog (or tissues of man) | Man eats "measly" pork—adult worm develops, resides in intestine—cysticercus may form in tissues | Ova in feces

**Fig. 32-7.** *Taenia solium,* life cycle.

free. By means of their hooklets the larvae penetrate the intestinal wall and pass into the tissues, where the hooklets are lost. They then reach the bloodstream to be carried to different parts of the body to lodge and each to develop into a scolex. The irritation caused by formation of the scolex sets up a tissue reaction, and a cyst wall is formed around it. The scolex encased in the cyst is termed a *cysticercus*. When the raw or insufficiently cooked flesh of the animal containing the cyst is eaten by a susceptible host, the cyst wall is digested, the scolex attaches itself to the intestinal wall of the new host, and an adult tapeworm develops.

In worms whose eggs (Fig. 32-1, *F*) escape through a birth pore (example: *Diphyllobothrium*), the embryos become ciliated. Escaping from the egg after it is passed, they take up an aquatic existence and swim until they gain access to certain species of freshwater fish. They parasitize the fish with the help of certain species of *Cyclops* or water fleas, which act as transferring hosts. Consumption of the raw or poorly cooked fish transfers the parasite to man.

### Taenia saginata
### (beef tapeworm, unarmed tapeworm)

Infection by *Taenia saginata* is quite common. The cow and giraffe are intermediate hosts. Typically only one worm is present in man. The segments have independent motility and may escape through the anal canal.

**Anatomy.** The organism *Taenia saginata* (Fig. 32-5) ranges in length from 4 to 10 meters. The head is small (1.5 mm. in diameter), pear-shaped, and somewhat quadrangular. It has 4 suckers but no hooklets. The absence of hooklets gives it the name *unarmed tapeworm*. The neck is rather long and slender. The mature segments measure 5 to 7 mm. by 18 to 20 mm. The uterus extends along the midline and gives off twenty to thirty delicate branches on each side. The eggs are spherical or ovoid in shape and yellow or brown in color. They measure from 20 to 30 $\mu$m. ($\mu$) by 30 to 40 $\mu$m.

### Taenia solium (pork tapeworm)

Infection with *Taenia solium* is rare in America and is acquired by eating measly pork. As a rule only one worm is present, but occasionally two or more are found.

**Biologic features.** Of the two worms, *Taenia solium* (Fig. 32-5) is shorter than *Taenia saginata*, measuring 2 to 8 meters in length. The head is very dark in color and globular or quadrangular in shape. It is provided with 4 suckers and two rows of hooklets projecting from a rostellum. The neck is threadlike. The mature segments measure 5 to 6 mm. by 10 to 12 mm.

The ova (Fig. 32-1, *E*) resemble those of *Taenia saginata*. Practically, it is impossible to differentiate the two. The differentiation of the worms therefore depends on the characteristics of the uterus in the terminal proglottids. There are more branches coming from the sides of the uterus in the beef tapeworm than in the pork tapeworm. Man may also become infected by swallowing the eggs of *Taenia solium*, since it is possible for both cycles of development to occur in the human being.

### Hymenolepis nana (dwarf tapeworm)

The smallest and the one most frequently found in man, the dwarf tapeworm *Hymenolepis nana*, measures from 1 to 4 cm. in length. The head is round and provided with 4 suckers and a single row of 24 to 30 hooklets. The ova are distinctive (Fig. 32-1, *D*). As a rule, many worms and ova are present, but the worms are so degenerated as to be unrecognizable.

Infection is spread directly from one person to another; there is no intermediate host. Eggs containing a fully developed embryo are released from a disintegrating end segment and passed in the feces. The eggs hatch in the stomach or small intestine of the new host, and the larval forms released pass into the lumen to attach to the intestinal wall at a lower site, where they develop in the mucous membrane. In about 2 weeks adult worms appear.

### Dipylidium caninum (dog tapeworm)

*Dipylidium caninum* is common in cats and dogs. It is 15 to 30 cm. in length, with a small head displaying 4 suckers and about 60 hooklets arranged in four rows. The ova occur in groups and are usually passed within the segments.

### Diphyllobothrium latum
### (fish tapeworm, broad Russian tapeworm)

*Diphyllobothrium latum* usually measures 3 to 6 meters in length, but occasionally a length of 12 meters is reached. The head, flattened and almond-shaped, is provided with two lateral grooves for attachment to the intestinal mucosa of the host. The segments show a characteristic brown or black rosette formation (uterus filled with ova).

The presence of this worm gives rise to irregular fever, digestive disturbances, and a blood picture identical to that of pernicious anemia. Manifestations promptly subside after its removal.

### Echinococcus granulosus

*Echinococcus granulosus* is a tiny worm 3 to 6 mm. long with a pear-shaped head. It has 4 suckers, 30 to 36 hooklets, but only one each of immature, mature, and gravid proglottids. The adult host is the dog and

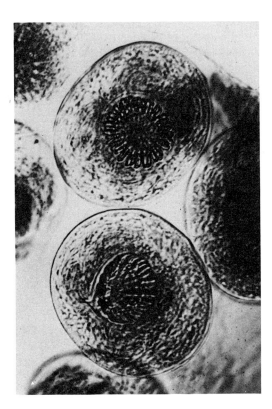

**Fig. 32-8.** Hydatid sand *(Echinococcus granulosus)*. (From Frankel, S., and others, editors: Gradwohl's clinical laboratory methods and diagnosis, ed. 7, St. Louis, 1970, The C. V. Mosby Co.)

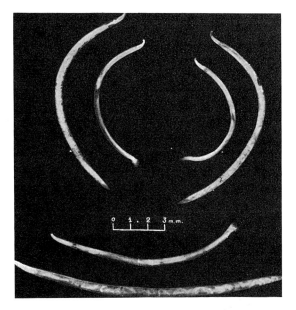

**Fig. 32-9.** Hookworms. Above, *Necator americanus* (male and female), two pairs; below, *Ancylostoma duodenale* (male and female), one pair. Note millimeter scale. (Original figure of P. Kouri.) (From Frankel, S., and others, editors: Gradwohl's clinical laboratory methods and diagnosis, ed. 7, St. Louis, 1970, The C. V. Mosby Co.)

other canines. By ingesting the eggs, man can become the larval or intermediate host, and the unique development of the scolex within the cystic cavity can occur in his organs. The cystic cavity for this parasite is termed the *hydatid cyst,* and free-floating scolices and brood capsules, structures within which scolices are formed, in cyst fluid are known as *hydatid sand* (Fig. 32-8). The liver is a favored site. The gravity of the infection in man is determined by the location and the progression of the cyst with time.

## NEMATODES (ROUNDWORMS)

Nematodes are nonsegmented worms with a flattened cylindrical body tapering toward both ends. The mouth is frequently surrounded by thick lips or papillae, and there is a complete digestive tract. The sexes are distinct. The male is shorter and more slender than the female. The adults inhabit the intestinal tract of man, and as a rule, there is no intermediate host. The nematode life cycle passes through a series of stages from the larval forms to the adult worm.

The severity of the digestive disorders related to nematode infection depends on the load of worms carried.

### Ancylostoma duodenale and Necator americanus

*Ancylostoma duodenale* and *Necator americanus* are, respectively, the Old World and New World hookworms. They resemble each other closely but differ in several important details (Fig. 32-9).

**Anatomy.** Both species are pale red and pointed at both ends. As a rule, the adult *Ancylostoma duodenale* is larger than *Necator americanus.* Its mouth has a pair of ventral hooks on each side of the midline and a pair of dorsal hooks. The mouth of *Necator americanus* is provided with plates instead of ventral hooks and has a distinct dorsal, conical toothlike structure.

The ova of the two species are practically identical, except that those of *Necator americanus* are larger. They are oval or oblong in shape but in certain positions appear spherical. They have three distinct parts—the shell, the yolk, and a clear space between the yolk and shell. (See Fig. 32-10.) The thin, smooth shell appears as a distinct line. Eggs that have been passed for 24 hours or more show well-developed embryos. The ova tend to stick to glass or other surfaces.

**361**

Advantage is taken of this trait in certain diagnostic procedures, but it makes the thorough washing of laboratory glassware imperative.

**Habitat.** The adult worms live in the small intestine, attached to the mucous membrane where their presence produces a characteristic train of events. Great numbers are usually present. They tear the tissues to get to the small blood vessels, from which blood is pumped into their intestines. However, they extravasate wastefully much of the blood into the lumen of the intestinal tract. A profound anemia is secondary to their bloodsucking activities.

**Life history.** The life history of the hookworm is as follows. After the ova are passed, development

begins with the proper temperature and moisture. The larvae hatch and undergo certain developmental changes whereby they can infect a new host. The first-stage larvae emerging are the free-living ones of distinct shape, the so-called *rhabditoid* larvae. Rhabditoid larvae can metamorphose into long, delicate, threadlike forms, the *filariform* larvae of the infective stage. When the filariform larvae contact the skin of man, they penetrate it, producing a dermatitis (ground itch). They travel by the lymph and bloodstream to the lungs. Here they gain access to the bronchi and are carried by the bronchial secretions to the pharynx, where they are swallowed. After they reach the small intestine, they develop into adult worms (Fig. 32-11). The adult worm is seldom found in the feces unless there is antihelminthic treatment. Hookworms parasitize an estimated 456 million persons.

### Strongyloides stercoralis

The adult *Strongyloides stercoralis* is only about 2 mm. long. It has a four-lipped mouth and an esophagus that extends through the anterior one fourth of the body. Male worms have not been found in man. The adult females live deep in the intestinal mucosa, where the ova are deposited. The larvae (Fig. 32-1, *K*) hatch in the intestine and are passed in the stool. (See Fig. 32-12.) Neither adult worms nor ova appear in the feces unless active purgation is present. The larvae are 250 to 500 $\mu$m. in length. They are actively motile and, when fresh, are constantly wiggling and bending but have little progressive motion. The disturbance produced in a laboratory preparation is often noticed under the microscope before the larvae are

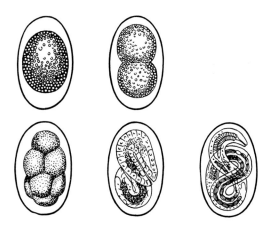

**Fig. 32-10.** Hookworm eggs, sketch. Development from earliest stage to embryo.

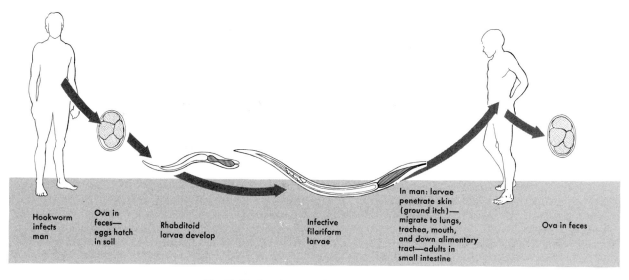

Hookworm infects man — Ova in feces—eggs hatch in soil — Rhabditoid larvae develop — Infective filariform larvae — In man: larvae penetrate skin (ground itch)—migrate to lungs, trachea, mouth, and down alimentary tract—adults in small intestine — Ova in feces

**Fig. 32-11.** *Ancylostoma duodenale,* life cycle.

located. Infection is acquired when the larvae penetrate the skin or are accidentally swallowed.

### Ascaris lumbricoides (eelworm, roundworm)

*Ascaris lumbricoides* is the largest intestinal nematode and is harbored by approximately 644 million persons. It is fusiform in shape and yellow or reddish in color. The male measures 15 to 20 cm. in length, the female 20 to 40 cm. The head is relatively small, and the oral cavity has three serrated lips. This worm looks like the ordinary earthworm but is not so red (Fig. 32-13).

The habitat of *Ascaris lumbricoides* is in the upper end of the small intestine, but it may be found in any part of the intestinal tract, free in the peritoneal cavity, or in the trachea and bronchi. Several are usually present (as many as 100 can be), clinging together to form palpable masses or even cause intestinal obstruction. Infection is most frequently seen in children under 10 years of age.

The fertilized eggs (Fig. 32-1, *H* and *I*) are oval in shape and average 48 μm. in diameter and 62 μm. in length. If only female worms are present, unfertilized eggs (Fig. 32-1, *G*) will be found. They are elongated, irregular in shape, and bear little resemblance to the fertilized egg. They frequently escape detection.

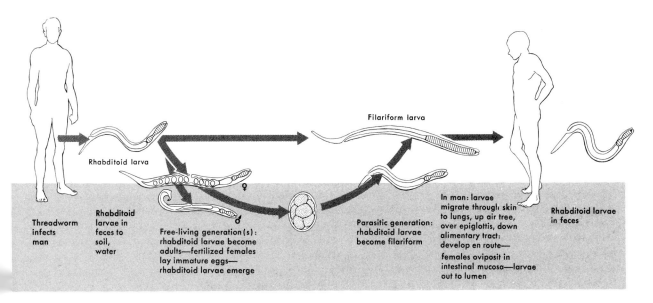

**Fig. 32-12.** *Strongyloides stercoralis,* life cycle.

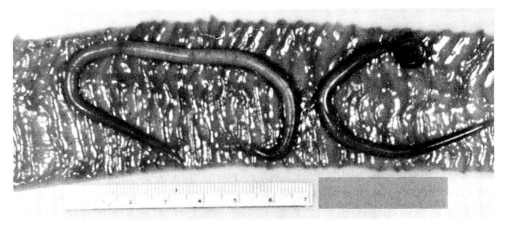

**Fig. 32-13.** *Ascaris lumbricoides* in lumen of intestine.

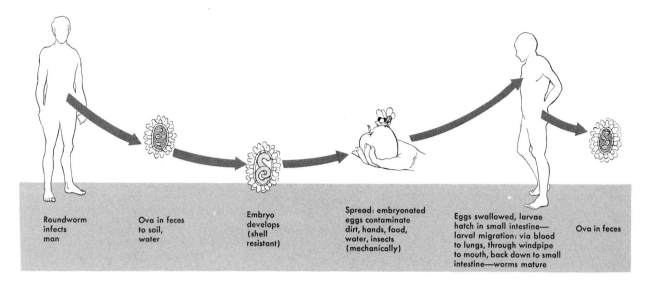

**Fig. 32-14.** *Ascaris lumbricoides,* life cycle.

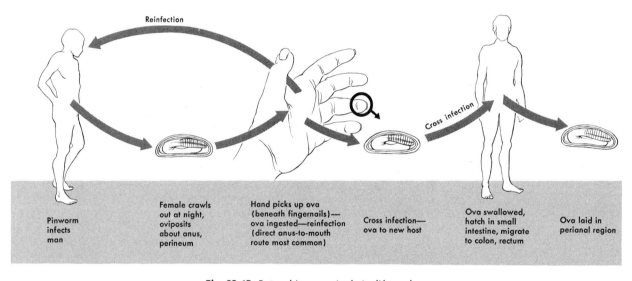

**Fig. 32-15.** *Enterobius vermicularis,* life cycle.

Adult worms appear in the feces only with active purgation. After the eggs are passed, segmentation takes place, and an embryo develops. If the mature eggs are swallowed, the embryos escape from the eggs and travel to the lungs by the bloodstream. They reach the intestines in the same manner as do hookworm larvae. (See Fig. 32-14.)

### Enterobius vermicularis (Oxyuris vermicularis, threadworm, pinworm, seatworm)

Infection with *Enterobius vermicularis* (enterobiasis) is the most prevalent worm infection of chil-

dren and adults in the United States. Over the world some 200 million persons are affected. The males of this species measure 3 to 5 mm. in length, the females about 10 mm. The adult female worms migrate through the anus and deposit their eggs on the perianal region, most frequently at night. Because of the peculiar laying habits of the female, the eggs (Fig. 32-1, C) seldom occur in the feces but are present around the anal region. They are best found by scraping this region and examining the scrapings. Eggs may be picked up from the perianal skin by means of swabs made of cellulose adhesive tape, the sticky side applied to the skin. The eggs are removed from the tape by toluene and identified under the microscope. An enema may be given, and the adult worms identified in the stool that is passed.

Deposition of eggs on the perianal skin results in intense itching. In children, pinworms should be suspected from this finding alone. The small child may maintain the infection from ova collected under his fingernails when he scratches himself (Fig. 32-15).

Infection comes from swallowing the eggs, after which male and female parasites hatch out at the lower end of the small intestine. After fertilizing the females, the males die, and the females migrate to the colon and rectum. The patient may continually reinfect himself, and parents may acquire the infection from their children. Eggs may be widely disseminated in a household or institution—in the dust, clothing, and bedding, and on furniture, doorknobs, and so on. To eliminate them is an exasperating and almost hopeless task.

The United States Public Health Service recommends that families with pinworms pay careful attention not only to general household cleanliness but also to personal hygiene among the members. It stresses the following health measures in the control of the parasites: (1) regular daily morning showers, (2) frequent handwashing, especially before food is eaten or prepared, (3) keeping of fingernails short and clean, (4) vacuuming of household surfaces and floors thoroughly and often, and (5) washing of bed linens two or three times a week in a machine in which temperature exposure is at least 150° F. for several minutes or more.

### Trichocephalus trichiurus (Trichuris trichiura, Trichocephalus dispar, whipworm)

*Trichocephalus trichiurus* is characterized by a long, threadlike neck that makes up about one half of the length of the body. The male is 30 to 45 mm. in length; the female is somewhat longer, 45 to 50 mm. The worms live in the cecum and large intestine, with the slender end of the worm embedded in the mucosa. The worms themselves are rare in the feces, and the eggs (Fig. 32-1, *B*) are not abundant. Generally symptoms are related to the number of worms in the bowel.

### Trichinella spiralis

*Trichinella spiralis* is the cause of trichinosis. It is the smallest worm, with the exception of *Strongyloides stercoralis,* found in the intestinal canal. It is barely visible with the unaided eye. The males are about 1.5 mm. in length, the females 3 to 4 mm. The posterior end of the male is bifid and has two tongue-like appendages.

The infection is primarily one of rats, propagated because rats eat their dead. Hogs acquire the infection from rats, and man becomes infected by eating insufficiently cooked pork. Pork is not the only source. Man has acquired the infection from eating bear meat. Polar bears are said to be heavily infected. The fact that it is found in the arctic region indicates that the parasite possesses a unique tolerance for cold.

**Life history.** The cycle of development of *Trichinella spiralis* is practically the same in man as in other animals. Pork containing the encysted larvae is eaten and the cyst capsule digested away. The larvae pass to the small intestine, where they mature. After copulation the males die, and the females embed in the mucous membrane, where they give birth to as many as 1000 to 1500 larvae. These larvae migrate by the lymph and bloodstream to the skeletal muscles, where they encyst, become encapsulated, and subsequently calcify. (See Fig. 32-16.)

The free larvae measure from 90 to 100 $\mu$m. in length and 6 $\mu$m. in diameter. They may be found in the blood and spinal fluid during the period of migration (6 to 22 days after infection).

After encystment the coiled embryos may be found with the low power of the microscope in a teased portion of muscle, and the diagnosis made. The cysts are most frequently found at the tendinous insertions of the muscle, and muscles most frequently infected are the pectoralis major, the outer head of the gastrocnemius, the deltoid, and the lower portion of the biceps. The cysts appear as white specks measuring 250 by 400 $\mu$m. The long axis of the cyst extends in the same general direction as the fibers of the muscle. Muscle biopsy is the surest method in diagnosis.

**Trichinosis.** When the parasites are developing in the intestines, gastrointestinal disturbances are prominent. These appear 2 to 3 days after ingestion of the contaminated pork. During this time the adult worms may be found in the feces. When the larvae migrate, fever, delirium, rheumatic pains, and labored respiration are present. This period begins at the end of 1 week after infection and lasts 1 or 2 weeks. When encystment begins, edema and skin eruptions appear. This period lasts about 1 week. After the disease becomes chronic, muscular pains of a rheumatic character may be present for months.

**Laboratory diagnosis.** Intense eosinophilia, commonly over 500 eosinophilic leukocytes per cubic millimeter of blood, is a feature of all stages of the disease. A skin test is available. A flocculation test, the Sussenguth-Kline test, becomes positive 2 to 3 weeks after infection and remains so for 10 months or longer. There are other serologic tests including complement fixation, latex agglutination, hemagglutination, and fluorescent antibody technics.

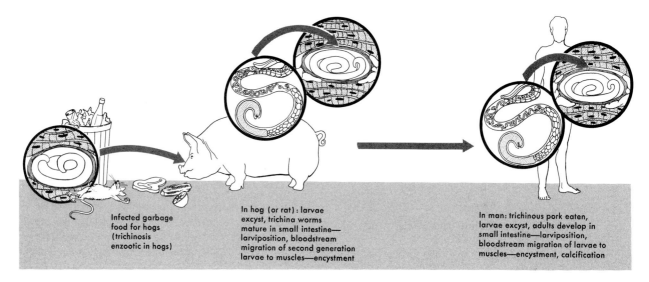

Infected garbage
food for hogs
(trichinosis
enzootic in hogs)

In hog (or rat): larvae
excyst, trichina worms
mature in small intestine—
larviposition, bloodstream
migration of second generation
larvae to muscles—encystment

In man: trichinous pork eaten,
larvae excyst, adults develop in
small intestine—larviposition,
bloodstream migration of larvae to
muscles—encystment, calcification

**Fig. 32-16.** *Trichinella spiralis,* life cycle.

Identification of the worms in feces or the larvae in other clinical specimens is usually impractical because of the course of the disease, and biopsy of a tender muscle poses difficulties. Generally the serologic tests are helpful, since they indicate recent or current infection. The skin test is consistent with more remote infection.

**Prevention.** There is no simple inspection method at a slaughterhouse for the detection of trichinas in a carcass of meat. The elimination of the disease rests practically with *adequate cooking of pork.* For example, one should cook a pork roast at an oven temperature of at least 350° F., allowing 35 to 50 minutes per pound. Smoking, pickling, heavy seasoning, or spicing does not make uncooked pork products safe. Freezing meat at −15° C. for 30 days or at −28.9° C. for 6 to 12 days eliminates the larvae.

### Wuchereria bancrofti (Bancroft's filaria worm)

*Filariasis* is infection with the filarial worms, which incorporate peculiar features in their life cycle. The best known is *Wuchereria bancrofti.* Man is its reservoir of infection, and the mosquito its vector. Of historical note is the fact that the first demonstration of the mosquito as a vector of disease was in connection with Bancroft's filaria worm, and the work suggested to Sir Ronald Ross the possibility that malaria might be similarly transmitted.

**Life cycle.** The life cycle of *Wuchereria bancrofti* (Fig. 32-17) is sketched as follows. When man, the definitive host, is infected, slender, white adult male and female worms reside in the lymphatic system. The females are 80 to 100 mm. in length and 0.24 to

0.3 mm. in diameter; the males are 40 mm. long and 0.1 mm. in diameter. Within the uterus of the adult female, embryos develop as tightly coiled threads within eggshells. About the time that an egg is laid, the embryo uncoils into a tiny, delicate, eel-like form. The eggshell remains applied about the elongated embryo, which is said to be *sheathed.* In some species of filarial worms, a naked or *unsheathed* embryo is discharged. The embryos in the lymph and bloodstream become *microfilariae* (Fig. 32-18) with remarkable habits. One is their migration into the peripheral blood at night at a time that coincides with the feeding time of the vector mosquito. During the day they are hidden away in an undetermined site.

Taken into the body of the mosquito, the microfilariae lose their sheath and further develop in a larval series. In time, infective larvae escape from the mosquito as it takes a blood meal, returning to the definitive host in whose lymphatic channels they continue their growth. Adolescent worms gather within sinuses of lymph nodes of the groin and pelvis, where they mature and mate to repeat the cycle.

**The disease.** In localizing within the human lymphatic system, the adult worms start an inflammatory process that progresses from acute to chronic stages. It is associated with tissue changes causing obstruction of lymphatic vessels, stagnation of lymph flow, and proliferation of connective tissue. The skin of the lower extremities and external genitalia becomes thickened, coarse, and redundant. The tremendous enlargement of the affected part becomes a great burden to the victim. The result of long years of infection, the end-stage lesion, is referred to as *elephan-*

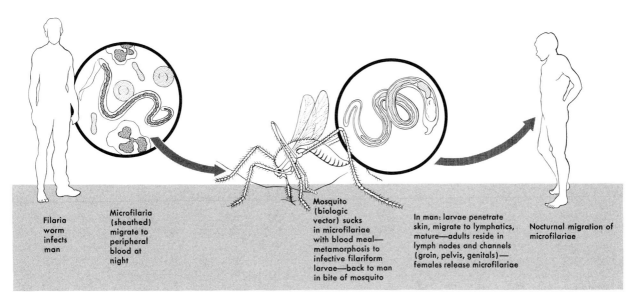

Filaria worm infects man

Microfilaria (sheathed) migrate to peripheral blood at night

Mosquito (biologic vector) sucks in microfilariae with blood meal—metamorphosis to infective filariform larvae—back to man in bite of mosquito

In man: larvae penetrate skin, migrate to lymphatics, mature—adults reside in lymph nodes and channels (groin, pelvis, genitals)—females release microfilariae

Nocturnal migration of microfilariae

**Fig. 32-17.** *Wuchereria bancrofti,* life cycle.

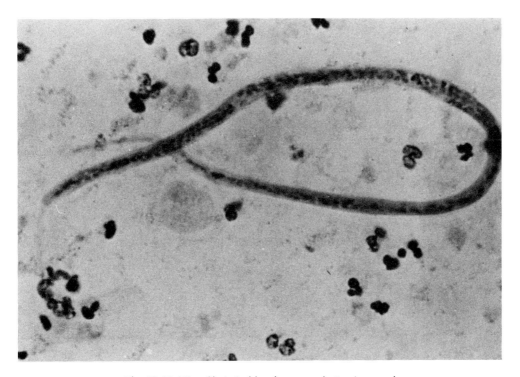

**Fig. 32-18.** Microfilaria in blood smear, photomicrograph.

*tiasis.* This disorder was well known to the ancient Hindu physicians around 600 B.C.

Filariasis is a widely distributed disease in tropical areas of the world and extends into some of the subtropical areas. Man is the only known definitive host. The appropriate mosquitoes breeding close by the dwelling places of human beings with microfilariae circulating in their bloodstream are two factors that favor the continuous spread of this disease. Therefore methods of prevention and control must be designed for treatment of the human carrier and elimination of the insect vector.

**Laboratory diagnosis.** The diagnosis of filariasis lies in the identification of microfilariae found in blood films. In a wet mount of blood they are seen to move gracefully, pushing the red blood cells gently aside. They may be seen also in a dried, fixed blood smear stained with Wright's stain. For best results with *Wuchereria bancrofti,* peripheral blood films are made between the hours of 10 P.M. and 2 A.M.

### Onchocerca volvulus

Onchocerciasis or river blindness is a disease afflicting an estimated 300 million persons in Africa and Latin America. It is produced by the filarial worm, *Onchocerca volvulus.* A hardy black fly of the genus *Simulium,* which breeds in fast-flowing, aerated mountain streams, transmits the infection as intermediate host. In the bite of the fly, larvae of the threadlike worm are deposited beneath the skin, the site of residence of the adult worms. The female worm gives birth to unsheathed microfilariae that pass into the lymphatic system. They are rarely found in peripheral blood. The microfilariae migrate throughout the body via the lymphatics. They die after reaching the eyes, but not until they have induced serious changes in the tissues of the eye that can in time lead to complete blindness. They can also produce subcutaneous nodules on the head or trunk, wherein a group of adult worms is walled off by fibrous connective tissue.

## Macroscopic examination of feces for parasites

Sometimes the nurse or medical attendant must examine feces macroscopically for parasites. In such a case the procedure is as follows.

If need be, improvise a sieve by removing both ends of a can and tying one or two layers of gauze over one opening. Allow water to run slowly over the feces and break up the masses with a glass rod or wooden applicator. Note the presence of worms. If necessary, remove worms and examine with a hand lens or the eyepiece of the microscope. Small worms may be mounted in a drop of water for macroscopic examination. If a tapeworm is present, be sure to search carefully for the head. After tapeworm treatment the entire quantity of feces passed should be saved so that the search for the head may be thorough. If it is suspected that the patient is suffering from typhoid fever or any other condition in which pathogenic bacteria appear in the feces, the washings should be received in a vessel containing a disinfectant. Needless to state, the sieve, glassware, and utensils used should be properly sterilized or carefully discarded.

**Objects likely to be mistaken for intestinal worms.** Segmented strands of mucus may be mistaken for tapeworms. The same is true of banana fibers because of their segmented structure and oval cells. Fibers of celery and green vegetables may be mistaken for roundworms, and orange fibers for pinworms.

## Questions for review

1 Define: microfilariae, hydatid sand, mechanical vector, biologic vector, ova, scolex, proglottid, ground itch, definitive host, cysticercus, hermaphrodite, operculate, phototrophic.
2 List five arthropod vectors in disease transmission. Give the diseases spread by them.
3 Briefly describe the three phyla of metazoa concerned in disease production in man.
4 Outline the life cycle of the following:
   a. Blood flukes
   b. Beef tapeworm
   c. Pork tapeworm
   d. Fish tapeworm
   e. Hookworm
   f. Pinworm
   g. Roundworm
   h. Filarial worms
5 Discuss the pathogenicity of flukes.
6 What is elephantiasis? River blindness?
7 Give the laboratory diagnosis for
   a. Schistosomiasis
   b. Trichinosis
   c. Filariasis
   d. Onchocerciasis
   e. Enterobiasis
8 List objects mistaken for worms in a *macro*scopic stool examination.
9 Comment on the control and prevention of metazoan diseases.

**REFERENCES** (Chapters 31 and 32)

Aziz, E. M.: *Strongyloides stercoralis* infestation, South. Med. J. **62:**806, 1969.

Babb, R. R., and others: Giardiasis, J.A.M.A. **217:**1359, 1971.

Barrett-Connor, E.: Amebiasis, today in the United States, Calif. Med. **114:**1, March, 1971.

Barrett-Connor, E.: Human fluke infections, South. Med. J. **65:**86, 1972.

Beck, J. W., and Barrett-Connor, E.: Medical parasitology, St. Louis, 1971, The C. V. Mosby Co.

Belding, D. L.: Textbook of parasitology, New York, 1968, Appleton-Century-Crofts.

Brown, A. W.: The attraction of mosquitoes to hosts, J.A.M.A. 196:249, 1966.

Brown, H. W.: Basic clinical parasitology, ed. 3, Englewood Cliffs, N.J., 1969, Prentice-Hall, Inc.

Cahill, K. M.: Tropical diseases in a tropical climate, Hosp. Pract. 3:56, April, 1968.

Canning, E. V., and Wright, C. A., editors: Behavioral aspects of parasite transmission, New York, 1972, Academic Press, Inc.

Carter, J. P.: Nutrition and parasitism, South. Med. Bull. 59: 31, Oct., 1971.

Crane, R. W.: Diseases we catch from animals, Today's Health 45:56, March, 1967.

Cutting, R. T.: The army malaria program—prelude to triumph, South. Med. Bull. 57:29, June, 1969.

Dangers of eating bear meat (editorial), J.A.M.A. 220:274, 1972.

DeFord, J. W.: Amebiasis: newer methods of diagnosis and treatment, South. Med. J. 66:1149, 1973.

Deller, J. J., Jr., and others: Malaria hepatitis, Milit. Med. 132:614, 1967.

Expert Committee on Malaria, Fourteenth report, WHO Techn. Rep. Ser. no. 382, 1968.

The facts about toxoplasmosis: Today's Health 50:64, July, 1972.

Fajardo, L. F., and Tallent, C.: Malarial parasites within human platelets, J.A.M.A. 229:1205, 1974.

Faust, E. C., and others: Animal agents and vectors of human diseases, ed. 4, Philadelphia, 1975, Lea & Febiger.

Faust, E. C., and others: Craig and Faust's clinical parasitology, Philadelphia, 1970, Lea & Febiger.

Febles, F., Jr.: Schistosomiasis: a world health problem, Am. J. Nurs. 64:118, Feb., 1964.

Federman, S.: Underwater weapon in war on mosquitoes, Today's Health 46:14, June, 1968.

Feldman, H. A.: Toxoplasma and toxoplasmosis, Hosp. Pract. 4:64, March, 1969.

Felsenfeld, O.: Synopsis of clinical tropical medicine—pathogenesis, clinical picture, diagnosis, prognosis, and therapy, St. Louis, 1965, The C. V. Mosby Co.

Fletcher, J. R., and others: Acute Plasmodium falciparum malaria, Arch. Intern. Med. 129:617, 1972.

Glor, B. A. K.: Falciparum malaria in Vietnam: clinical manifestations and nursing care requirements, Milit. Med. 134:181, 1969.

Gould, S. E.: Trichinosis in man and animals, Springfield, Ill., 1970, Charles C Thomas, Publisher.

Gould, S. E.: The story of trichinosis, Am. J. Clin. Pathol. 55:2, 1971.

Greenberg, J. H.: Public health problems relating to the Vietnam returnee, J.A.M.A. 207:697, 1969.

Grell, K. G.: Protozoology, New York, 1973, Springer-Verlag New York, Inc.

Hagan, A. D.: Malaria in Vietnam—1969, South. Med. Bull. 58:19, April, 1970.

Hammond, D. M., and Long, P. L., editors: The Coccidia.

Eimeria, Isospora, Toxoplasma, and related genera, Baltimore, 1973, University Park Press.

Healy, G. R.: Laboratory diagnosis of amebiasis, Bull. N.Y. Acad. Med. 47:478, 1971.

Hoare, C. A.: The trypanosomes of mammals, Philadelphia, 1972, F. A. Davis Co.

The immunology of malaria, Can. Med. Assoc. J. 106:852, 1972.

Jones, J. C.: The sexual life of a mosquito, Sci. Am. 218:108, April, 1968.

Juniper, K., Jr., and others: Serologic diagnosis of amebiasis, Am. J. Trop. Med. 21:157, 1972.

Kagan, I. G.: Current status of serologic testing for parasitic diseases, Hosp. Pract. 9:157, Sept., 1974.

Kagen, L. J., and others: Serologic evidence of toxoplasmosis among patients with polymyositis, Am. J. Med. 56:186, 1974.

Kibukamusoke, J. W.: Nephrotic syndrome of quartan malaria, Baltimore, 1973, The Williams & Wilkins Co.

Krogstad, D. J., and others: Toxoplasmosis with comments on risk of infection from cats, Ann. Intern. Med. 77:773, 1972.

Maibach, H. I., and others: Factors that attract and repel mosquitoes in human skin, J.A.M.A. 196:263, 1966.

March, C. H., and Fisher, A. A.: Man versus arthropods, GP 36:115, Oct., 1967.

Marcial-Rojas, R. A.: Pathology of protozoal and helminthic diseases, Baltimore, 1971, The Williams & Wilkins Co.

Miller, J. H., and Abadie, S. H.: Common intestinal parasites of the United States, South. Med. Bull. 59:11, Oct., 1971.

Moser, R. H.: Trichinosis: from Bismarck to polar bears (editorial), J.A.M.A. 228:735, 1974.

Peterson, D. R., and others: Human toxoplasmosis prevalence and exposure to cats, Am. J. Epidemiol. 96:215, 1972.

Quinn, R. W.: The epidemiology of intestinal parasites of importance in the United States, South. Med. Bull. 59:20, Oct., 1971.

Ramos-Morales, F., and others: Manson's schistosomiasis in Puerto Rico, Bull. N.Y. Acad. Med. 44:317, 1968.

Robson, V. L.: Malaria alert, J. Am. Med. Wom. Assoc. 22: 321, May, 1967.

Rodgerson, E. B.: The diagnosis of Trichomonas vaginalis, Woman Physician 25:576, 1970.

Seah, S. K. K., and Flegel, K. M.: African trypanosomiasis in Canada, Can. Med. Assoc. J. 106:902, 1972.

Shimada, K., and O'Connor, G. R.: Immune adherence hemagglutination test for toxoplasmosis, Arch. Ophthalmol. 90:372, 1973.

Smith, H. A., and others: Veterinary pathology, Philadelphia, 1972, Lea & Febiger.

Spencer, H., and others: Tropical pathology, New York, 1973, Springer-Verlag New York, Inc.

Teschan, P. E., editor: Panel on malaria, Ann. Intern. Med. 70:127, Jan., 1969.

Thompson, J. H., Jr.: Useful laboratory procedures. Examination of blood smears for malarial and other organisms, III, Bull. Pathol. 10:61, 1969.

Thompson, J. H., Jr.: How to detect intestinal parasites, Lab. Med. 1:31, April, 1970.

Thompson, J. H., Jr.: How to detect blood and tissue parasites, Lab. Med. **2:**42, April, 1971.

Trager, W.: Some aspects of intracellular parasitism, Science **183:**269, 1974.

Walzer, P. D., and others: *Pneumocystis carinii* pneumonia in United States, Ann. Intern. Med. **80:**83, 1974.

Wand, M., and Lyman, D.: Trichinosis from bear meat, J.A.M.A. **220:**245, 1972.

Warren, K. S.: Regulation of the prevalence and intensity of schistosomiasis in man: immunology or ecology? J. Infect. Dis. **127:**595, 1973.

Wilcocks, C., and Manson-Bahr, P. E. C., editors: Manson's tropical diseases, Baltimore, 1972, The Williams & Wilkins Co.

The worm's turn (editorial), J.A.M.A. **199:**270, 1967.

CHAPTER 33

# Microbes ubiquitous

Persons in daily contact with diseases caused by microbes are likely to look on microbes as agents of harm only, but such is not the case. *The majority of bacteria and other microbes are helpful to man, animals, and plants, all of which depend on bacteria for their very existence.* In a broad sense, microorganisms producing disease form but a small and inconspicuous group. Nothing gives us a better idea of the broad scope of microbial activity than does a consideration of how microbes affect our daily lives.

## Microbes in the processes of nature

The *microbiology of nature* defines the role that bacteria and other microbes play in the various processes of nature. Bacteria and other microbes have been said to be nature's garbage disposal system and fertilizer factory, for they are the active agents in the decomposition of dead organic matter of animal origin, releasing the elements needed for the growth of plants and returning them to the soil. Bacteria purify sewage by living on the impurities in it and converting these to inoffensive substances that serve as food material for plants. As water trickles through the soil, bacteria help to filter it. Though contaminated when it enters the earth, water may trickle out pure and clean. In short, microbes represent a major natural resource.

**Participation in the cycle of an element.** The chief elements entering the bodies of animals and plants are nitrogen, carbon, hydrogen, and oxygen, which are combined with other less common ones to form complex proteins. Animals depend on plants for these elements. Plants receive their hydrogen and oxygen from water and must obtain their carbon and nitrogen from an inorganic compound containing them. The assimilation of an element from inorganic compounds, its conversion into organic compounds to form the bodies of plants and animals, and its subsequent reappearance in the inorganic state to be used again, constitute the *cycle* of the element.

*Carbon cycle.* Plants can assimilate carbon only from carbon dioxide. Carbon dioxide is present in the air in small quantities, but the supply must be constantly renewed. This comes about as carbon dioxide, a waste product of metabolism, is constantly eliminated in the breath of all animals. (See Fig. 33-1.)

If animals were sufficiently numerous to eat all plants, converting them into carbon dioxide and excreting the gas, the supply of plant food for animals and of carbon dioxide for plants would be perfectly balanced. However, tissues of certain plants, such as wood and cellulose that contain much carbon, when eaten by animals, pass through the intestinal canal unchanged. Therefore the carbon in them is not converted into carbon dioxide and released. Other plants die with much carbon bound in their bodies. Carbon is also present in the body tissues of all animals when they die. If there were not some method of recovering this carbon in a form available for plant growth ($CO_2$), plant life would soon cease, and animal life would end shortly thereafter. To recover the carbon, fungi and bacteria attack animal excreta, dead plants, and animal bodies, and the process of decay and decomposition begins. The complex carbon compounds are broken down by microbes into carbon dioxide, which floats away in the air to become plant food.

*Nitrogen cycle.* Nitrogen is one of the most important elements in the composition of the plant body. It is abundant in the air but not in a form suitable for plant use. To be so suitable, it must be in the form of nitrates. Nitrates present in the soil in very small amounts must constantly be renewed. Microbes participate by (1) decomposing organic matter and (2) converting the nitrogen of the air into nitrates. (See Fig. 33-2.) Organic matter is broken down by different microorganisms with various actions to form simpler compounds, among which is ammonia. Ammonia is attacked by *nitrifying* bacteria (genus *Nitrosomonas*), which convert it into nitrites. Other nitrifying bacteria (genus *Nitrobacter*) then convert the nitrites into nitrates, which are absorbed by the plant roots and built into complex nitrogen compounds like those of the original organic matter.

The term *nitrogen fixation* applies to the recovery

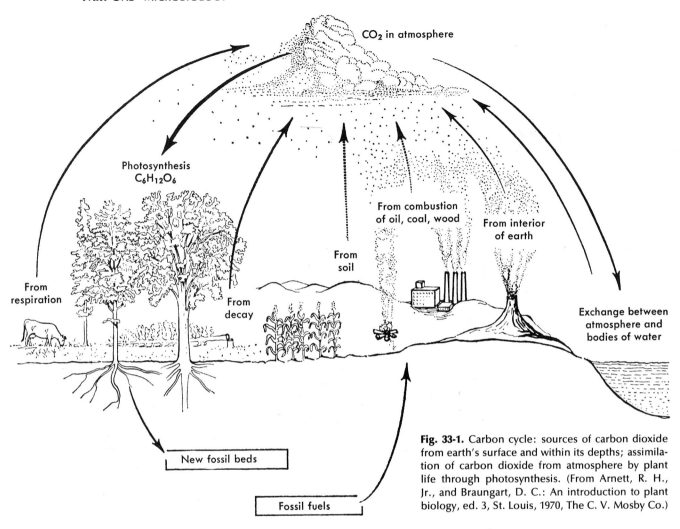

CO₂ in atmosphere

Photosynthesis
C₆H₁₂O₆

From combustion
of oil, coal, wood

From interior
of earth

From
soil

From
respiration

From
decay

Exchange between
atmosphere and
bodies of water

New fossil beds

Fossil fuels

**Fig. 33-1.** Carbon cycle: sources of carbon dioxide from earth's surface and within its depths; assimilation of carbon dioxide from atmosphere by plant life through photosynthesis. (From Arnett, R. H., Jr., and Braungart, D. C.: An introduction to plant biology, ed. 3, St. Louis, 1970, The C. V. Mosby Co.)

of free nitrogen from the air and its synthesis into nitrates for use by plants. The first step in nitrogen fixation is the formation of ammonia. This is accomplished by two groups of microorganisms. One (genus *Azotobacter*) lives in the soil. Another group (genus *Rhizobium*), penetrating the root hairs, develops symbiotically in the cells of certain legumes such as clover. It receives its nourishment from the plant and forms nodules filled with rapidly multiplying bacteria. They bind the nitrogen of the air into a compound incorporated into the bacterial body, which is removed and used by the plant. Animals eat the plants. When the plant dies and decays, the nitrogenous compounds are set free in the soil. Soils in which such products of decay are present are fertile.

Within the upper several centimeters of well tilled soil there are 300 to 3000 kg. of living microorganisms per hectare. An acre of alfalfa well nodulated by nitrogen-fixing rhizobia has the capacity to fix in the

ground 200 kg. of nitrogen from the air. The microbes in the earth's crust fix annually 10⁸ metric tons of nitrogen from the air, six times more than can be accomplished artificially in industry. *Microbiology of the soil* deals with the many aspects of the population of microorganisms, on which fertility depends.

*Other cycles.* Other elemental cycles in which microbes participate are those of phosphorus and sulfur.

## Microbes in animal nutrition

Many years ago Pasteur expressed the idea that animal life would not be possible were it not for the microbial inhabitants of the intestinal tract. "If microscopic beings were to disappear from our globe, the surface of the earth would be encumbered with dead organic matter and corpses of all kinds, animal and vegetable. . . . Without them, life would become impossible because death would be incomplete." (Louis

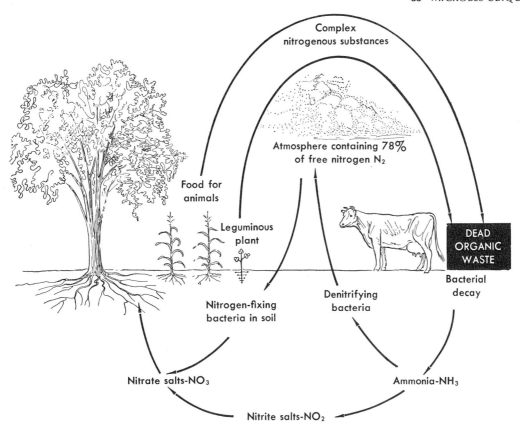

**Fig. 33-2.** Nitrogen cycle. Various sources indicated for nitrogen needed by plants and animals for protein synthesis. Note that microbes of soil convert a part of nitrogen stepwise into ammonia, nitrite, and nitrate. Nitrate is also derived from nitrogen of air by bacterial action and through oxidizing action of lightning. Nitrate from these sources is taken up by roots of plants. (From Arnett, R. H., Jr., and Braungart, D. C.: An introduction to plant biology, ed. 3, St. Louis, 1970, The C. V. Mosby Co.)

Pasteur, 1861.) Bacteria take an active part in the digestive processes of both lower animals and man. Many of the vitamins essential to animal and human nutrition are formed in the large bowel by the microbial inhabitants. Large amounts of vitamins in the B complex group are so produced. The elaboration of a certain vitamin by bacteria may constitute a major source of it, such as the production of vitamin K. Vitamin K is important in the prevention of hemorrhage in the body and is primarily supplied to the body from the lumen of the intestine, where it is manufactured by bacteria, especially *Escherichia coli*. This organism produces about 1000 units of vitamin K per gram weight of dry bacteria.

Administration of the modern broad-spectrum antibiotics (example: the tetracyclines) may so sharply reduce the microbial population of the intestinal tract as to cause a marked reduction in the production of vitamin substances there. Depletion of vitamin K is especially serious prior to surgery, and the vitamin may have to be administered to the patient as a drug to prevent hemorrhage. Microbes may have even greater importance in the physical well-being of lower animals and man than is apparent with our present state of knowledge.

## Microbes in industry

*Microbiology of industry* involves the roles that microbes play in processes of commerce and industry, such as the following.

**Manufacture of dairy products.** One of the aspects of *dairy microbiology* is the manufacture and processing of certain milk products. Broadly speaking, this subject may be included with *microbiology of agriculture*, which encompasses the relation of microbes to domestic animals and to the soil.

When it is allowed to stand, milk sours and curdles because of the conversion of lactose (milk sugar) into

373

lactic acid by bacterial action. This is known as *ripen-ing*. When milk is churned, the fat globules coalesce and take up a small amount of milk solids and water to form butter. The residue is *buttermilk*. The bacteria that play the key role in ripening are the ordinary lactic acid bacteria,* normal inhabitants of milk. Ripening is often hastened by adding cultures of these lactic acid–producers known as "starters." Originally the purpose of ripening was to preserve the milk until enough to churn had accumulated. The acidity of sour milk inhibits growth of other microbes. Now ripening is done to give flavor to the butter. Butter is usually prepared from cream instead of whole milk. Cultured buttermilk is prepared by adding ordinary butter starters to fresh sweet milk.

Cheese consists of the curd of milk separated from the liquid portion, either by the bacterial fermentation of the lactose in milk to form lactic acid or by the action of the milk-curdling enzyme, *rennin* (from the stomach of a calf). Cheese prepared by the action of lactic acid is known as cottage cheese. When rennin is the curdling agent, the water is drained away, and the curd is pressed into a block and partly dried. This is green cheese. When green cheese is set aside for a time, it undergoes changes (ripens) that give it color, flavor, and odor. Ripening is induced by the enzymes in the curd, as well as by molds, yeasts, and bacteria. The kind of cheese manufactured depends, to a great extent, on the kind of organisms that cause it to ripen. For instance, Swiss cheese is ripened by *Streptococcus thermophilus* and *Lactobacillus bulgaricus,* as starters, after which a gas-producing colony of *Propionibacterium freudenreichii* subsp. *shermanii* literally blows out the characteristic holes. In the preparation of blue cheese (example: Roquefort), the curd is sprinkled with spores of *Penicillium roqueforti* or similar mold to produce the blue green mottling. The creamy consistency of Camembert is largely due to the growth of *Penicillium camemberti,* and the strong smell of limburger cheese can be traced to the growth of yeasts and bacteria. Cheese is usually named after the locality in which it is produced, and a certain type of cheese may have several different names, depending on where it is manufactured. For instance, Cheddar (after Cheddar, England), Wisconsin, American, and brick cheeses are basically the same.

**Manufacture of alcohol and alcoholic beverages.** Alcoholic beverages are of two classes: those that are manufactured by fermentation alone and those in which the alcohol is distilled off the fermented mixture. The distillate has a higher alcoholic content than

the beverage manufactured by fermentation alone. Among the beverages manufactured by fermentation alone are wine and beer. Among those that are manufactured by distillation are commercial alcohol, whiskey, rum, and brandy. The manufacture of both fermented and distilled beverages depends primarily on the conversion of sugar into alcohol by yeasts. Commercial fermentations rely mainly on the enzymes of yeasts of *Saccharomyces* species.

Wines are made by allowing grape juice to ferment. Beer is made from grains, most often barley. Grains do not contain sugar at first, but when the grain is soaked in water, the seeds germinate and the starch-splitting enzyme known as *diastase* (amylase) is produced. It converts the starch of the grain into the sugars maltose and glucose. Grain starch that has been converted into sugar is known as *malt*. The maltose and glucose in the malt is converted into alcohol by yeasts. If the foreign organisms grow in beer, they give it an undesirable taste. This is "disease" of beer.

Purification of alcoholic beverages by distillation depends on the fact that alcohol has a much lower boiling point than water. When a fermented mixture is heated to a temperature considerably below the boiling point of water, the alcohol distills over, leaving the water behind. Commercial alcohol and whiskey are usually made by distilling fermented grains. Brandy is made by distilling fermented fruits. Rum is made by distilling fermented cane juice. The mixture of fermenting grains used in the manufacture of alcohol and alcoholic beverages is the *mash*. The mash from which rye whiskey is made contains 51% or more rye, whereas that used for the manufacture of bourbon contains 51% or more corn. The mash used in the production of alcohol is usually a mixture of corn (88.5%), barley (9.75%), and rye (1.75%), known as *spirit mash*.

Industrial alcohol (ethyl) has been for years manufactured from molasses. Alcohol may be produced by the action of bacteria on the cellulose of plants. In this method by-products of the lumber industry, such as sawdust, trimmings, and remains of trees, are used. A large amount of alcohol is obtained as a by-product when petroleum is cracked to form gasoline.

**Baking.** An essential step in baking is the same as that for the manufacture of alcoholic beverages—the conversion of sugar into alcohol and carbon dioxide by yeast. It is the carbon dioxide, not the alcohol, that plays the important role in baking. When yeasts are mixed with dough, their enzymes, notably zymase, ferment the sugar present; the carbon dioxide thus produced riddles the dough with small holes, causing it to rise. When the dough is baked, the heat volatilizes the alcohol and causes the carbon dioxide to expand and be driven off, leaving the bread light and

---

*Principal genera are *Streptococcus, Leuconostoc, Pediococcus,* and *Lactobacillus.*

spongy. Some sugar must be present or fermentation will not take place. The dough may contain a small amount of diastase, which converts some of the starch of the dough into sugar. If white flour is used in which the amylase has been destroyed in the refining process, sugar must be added.

**Manufacture of vinegar.** There are several methods of making vinegar. It may be made from wine or cider or from grains that have undergone alcoholic fermentation. In most methods the first step is the production of alcohol by fermentation, and the second step is the conversion of the alcohol into acetic acid. The first step differs in no manner from the production of alcohol for other purposes. When the alcoholic liquor is exposed to the air, a film known as mother of vinegar and containing acetic acid bacteria (genera *Acetobacter* and *Gluconobacter* [*Acetomonas*]) forms on the surface, and these bacteria convert the alcohol into acetic acid. If the process continues too long, the bacteria decompose the acetic acid into carbon dioxide and water, and the vinegar loses some of its strength.

**Production of sauerkraut.** Sauerkraut is finely shredded cabbage that has been allowed to ferment in brine formed by salt and cabbage juice. The finely shredded cabbage is placed in layers in a cask, and salt is sprinkled over each layer. The layers are packed closely together by a weight placed upon them. The salt extracts juice from the cabbage, and the bacteria present convert the sugar of the juice into lactic acid, which helps to give sauerkraut its peculiar flavor.

**Tanning.** The recently removed hide or skin of an animal must be preserved in some way, or its microbial population will destroy it. The leather is soaked and softened in numerous changes of cool water to remove dirt, blood, and nonspecific debris. Cool water retards bacterial growth. The excess flesh is trimmed from the hide or skin, and the hair is loosened. One method of loosening the hair is to soak the hide in a solution of lime. It has been found that old solutions, which contain many more bacteria, remove the hair more effectively than do fresher ones, which contain few. During the process the bacteria partially decompose and soften the leather.

After the loosened hair is scraped away, minerals are removed by washing or by chemical action. Before they are tanned, the hides of some animals are pickled. Pickling is carried out by treatment with sulfuric acid and salt. Tanning is accomplished by the use of vegetable tannins or chemicals such as alum.

**Curing of tobacco.** When tobacco leaves are cured, they change in texture and flavor and take on a brown color. These changes are accompanied by

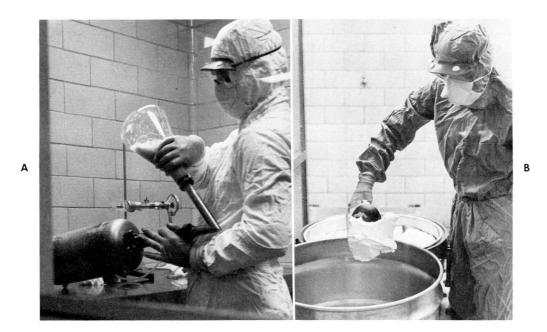

**Fig. 33-3.** Production of antibiotics. Manufacture of antibiotics is a complex process involving fermentation, filtration, extraction, and other intricate operations, many of which must be performed under sterile conditions. Antibiotic is grown in large fermentation tanks under controlled conditions, is filtered to remove impurities, and is finally recovered in crystalline form. **A,** Recharging seed tank with microbial culture in fermentation process. **B,** Handling bulk antibiotic under sterile conditions. (Courtesy Eli Lilly & Co., Indianapolis.)

a decrease in sugar, nicotine, and water. The process is apparently one of oxidation induced by fermentation.

**Retting of flax and hemp.** In flax and hemp plants the fibers are closely bound to the wood and bark of the plant by a glue-like substance. When these fibers are separated from the bark and wood, the commercial products linen and hemp are obtained. The dissolution of the pectin to effect separation is accomplished by the action of certain aerobes and the anaerobic butyric acid bacteria (organisms in genus *Clostridium*).

**Manufacture of antibiotics.** Today the manufacture of antibiotics is a major pharmaceutical activity. Over fifty are available today for plants, animals, and man. The basic materials are cultures of molds or soil bacteria. Penicillin is produced by certain molds of the genus *Penicillium,* and antibiotics such as streptomycin, and the tetracyclines are obtained from bacteria of the genus *Streptomyces.* The development of penicillin and streptomycin fermentations into industrial processes was the beginning of the field of bioengineering (Fig. 33-3). At present, antibiotic production by microbes exceeds 6 million pounds annually, and the output of penicillin alone is easily more than 1 million pounds. Within recent years the sales of internal anti-infectives in the United States have amounted to more than $500 million, and antibiotics form a large part of such sales. Prescriptions written for such pharmaceutical compounds have numbered nearly 150 million.

**Oil prospecting.** It has been found that certain types of bacteria are extremely plentiful in the soil overlying deposits of oil. This finding has been utilized to locate such deposits. The growth of bacteria is supported by gases that seep from the oil to the surface. Microbes have also been used to recover uranium compounds from low grade ores and slag of mines.

**Other industrial processes.**[*] In addition to the practical applications of microbes just given, the following may be mentioned:

1. Manufacture of acetone (fermentation of sugars—*Clostridium acetobutylicum*)
2. Manufacture of lactic acid (fermentation of molasses—lactic acid bacteria)
3. Manufacture of dextran, a plasma expander (fermentation of cane sugar—*Leuconostoc mesenteroides*)
4. Manufacture of butyl alcohol (fermentation of sugars—butyric acid bacteria)
5. Manufacture of vitamins (examples: cyanocobalamin or vitamin $B_{12}$, riboflavin or vitamin $B_2$, and vitamin C; at least 2000 pounds of vitamin $B_{12}$ made annually)
6. Microbiological assay—determination of the amount of amino acids and vitamins in tissues and body fluids (example: assay of vitamin $B_{12}$)
7. Manufacture of steroid hormones, cortisone, and hydrocortisone (action of certain molds on plant steroids)
8. Manufacture of citric acid used in lemon flavoring (oxidation of sugar—*Aspergillus niger*)
9. Manufacture of enzyme detergents (subtilisins, alkaline proteases from *Bacillus subtilis,* added to final detergent product)
10. Manufacture of insecticides (microbial insecticides or bioinsecticides—protein of *Bacillus thuringiensis* lethal to larvae [caterpillars] of serious food crop pests in order Lepidoptera)

---

[*]The theoretical study of fermentation has been constantly stimulated by the industrial values of the many end products obtained.

11. Production of food in seas and oceans (photosynthesis carried on by certain marine microbes, role similar to that of plants on land)
12. Production of ensilage for animal feed (fermentation of sugars in shredded green plants by lactic acid bacteria)
13. Manufacture of plant growth factors (example: gibberellins)
14. Manufacture of enzymes (examples: amylases, proteases, pectinases)
15. Manufacture of amino acids (examples: glutamate, lysine; 50 million pounds of glutamate and 1 million pounds of lysine produced annually in the United States, with 100,000 pounds of glutamic acid manufactured by bacterial processes for the pharmaceutical industry)
16. Manufacture of flavor nucleotides (examples: inosinate, guanylate)
17. Manufacture of polysaccharides (example: xanthan polymer)
18. Sewage disposal (see Chapter 34)

## Questions for review

1 What is meant by the cycle of an element?
2 Briefly outline the nitrogen cycle and the carbon cycle.
3 What is nitrogen fixation? Its importance?
4 What determines the fertility of the soil?
5 What causes the root nodules on clover plants? What purpose do they serve?
6 What organism is important in the synthesis of vitamin K in the intestine?
7 List 10 practical applications made of microorganisms.
8 Explain how cheese is made. What is dairy microbiology?
9 What is diastase? What is its role in fermentation?
10 Give specific examples of microbes (by name) used in industry.

**References on pp. 393 and 394.**

# CHAPTER 34

# Microbiology of water

Practically all waters under natural conditions contain microbes, including protozoa, bacteria, fungi, and viruses. Some contain many microbes; others contain few. The number and kind of microbes present depend on the source of water, the addition of excreta from man and animals, and the addition of other contaminated material.

Since sewage contains the pooled excreta from both the sick and the well, it necessarily contains pathogenic organisms, especially those that leave the body by the feces or urine. Sewage must be properly disposed of to avoid contamination of water supplies and the spread of disease by flies or other agents.

*Sanitary microbiology* (the microbiology of sanitation) pertains to drinking water supplies and sewage disposal.

**Sanitary classification.** From a sanitary standpoint waters may be classified as potable, contaminated, and polluted. *Potable* water is free of injurious agents and pleasant to the taste. In other words, it is a satisfactory drinking water. *Contaminated* water contains dangerous microbial or chemical agents. A contaminated water may be of pleasing taste, odor, and appearance. *Polluted* water has an unpleasant appearance, taste, or odor. Because of its content, it is unclear and unfit for use. It may or may not be contaminated with disease-producing agents.

The pollution of water supplies is a major health problem today. Not only sanitary sewage but also complex wastes from industry and agriculture may be discharged into water. In increasing volume such substances as plastics, detergents, insecticides, oils, animal and vegetable matter, chemical fertilizers, and even radioactive materials are released from factories, canneries, poultry-processing plants, oil fields, and farms. The persistence of synthetic detergents in wastewater and sewage reflects a failure of microbial action. Bacteria do not possess the enzymes to degrade them chemically.

Fish reflect a measure of the purity of a water supply, since they cannot live and thrive in the water of a river or lake that is heavily polluted.

**Sources of water.** Water is the most abundant of substances on the earth and is almost the only inorganic fluid found simultaneously in nature as gas, liquid, or solid. It is surprisingly difficult to obtain or keep as a pure substance. It is contaminated easily (or recontaminated after purification).

A water supply may come from (1) rain or snow, (2) surface water (shallow wells, rivers, ponds, lakes, and wastewater), and (3) groundwater (deep wells and springs) (Fig. 34-1). Generally, surface water contains more microbes than does either groundwater or rainwater. Surface water contains many harmless microbes from the soil, and in the vicinity of cities it is often contaminated with sewage bacteria (the majority of soil microorganisms are found in the upper 6 inches of the earth's crust). Surface water in sparsely settled localities may be comparatively safe, but the only safe rule is *not to use surface water without purification.*

Unless they are properly constructed, shallow wells may become contaminated with the drainage from outhouses, stables, and other outbuildings. Improperly constructed shallow wells have been responsible for many outbreaks of typhoid fever and dysentery in rural communities. For a shallow well to be safe, its upper portion must be lined with an impervious material so that water from the surface will not seep into it, and it should be located so that outhouses drain away from it. Of course it must be kept tightly closed. Shallow springs may be just as dangerous as shallow wells.

Deep-well water and deep-spring water usually contain few microorganisms because these are filtered out as the water trickles through the layers of the earth, but like shallow wells, deep wells must be protected against pollution with surface water. Microbial contamination may occur when a well is situated within 200 feet of the source of contamination, and chemical contamination may occur for a distance of 400 feet. Contamination is more likely to occur during wet weather.

**Waterborne diseases.** The sources for bacteria

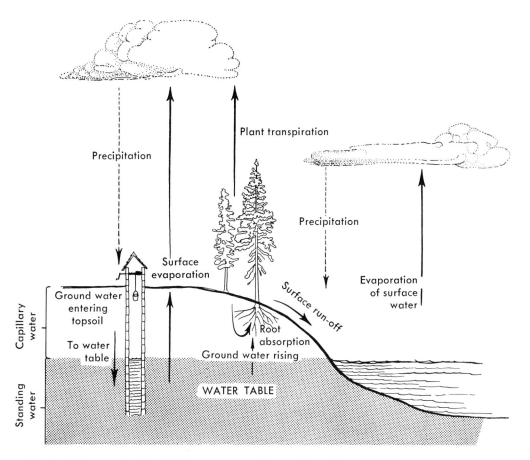

**Fig. 34-1.** Water cycle. Physical phenomena are almost independent of life, but water is necessary for metabolism in all organisms. (From Arnett, R. H., Jr., and Braungart, D. C.: An introduction to plant biology, ed. 3, St. Louis, 1970, The C. V. Mosby Co.)

in water are many—soil, air, the water itself, and the decaying bodies and excreta of man and animals. As a result, many different kinds may be found there, including well-known pathogens as well as the harmless water bacteria. There is increased concern in this country as to the presence of viruses in water, since most human ones multiply in the alimentary canal. Human enteric viruses have been recovered from a third of surface water samples examined. Groundwaters may also transmit virus.

The diseases spread by water are usually those whose causative agents leave the body by way of the alimentary or urinary tracts, and waterborne infections are mostly contracted by drinking contaminated water. They may be caused by a variety of microorganisms. When a waterborne epidemic occurs, most cases appear within a few days, indicating that all were infected at about the same time. Most important of the waterborne diseases are typhoid fever, bacillary dysentery, amebic dysentery, salmonellosis, viral

hepatitis, and cholera. Epidemics of acute diarrhea often follow heavy contamination of water with sewage. Diseases that, on occasion, are transmitted by water are tularemia, anthrax, leptospirosis, schistosomiasis, ascariasis, poliomyelitis, and other enterovirus (coxsackievirus and echovirus) infections. Pathogenic bacteria do not live long in water, and they do not multiply there; but they may persist for a time in water that is cool and contains considerable organic matter.

Certain opportunist pathogens, including many species of *Pseudomonas*, are referred to as water organisms (water bugs) since they can survive and propagate in a wet, stagnant environment. They can grow in sterile water on traces of phosphorus and sulfur and are generally resistant to antibiotics and disinfectants. In hospitals they lurk as an unsuspected source of infection in sinks, drains, faucets, and the oxygen therapy apparatus. They can gain a foothold in the air ducts, mist generators, and humidifying pans in incubators of newborn and premature nurseries. Most susceptible to these water organisms are newborn infants, patients with surgical wounds, and individuals with chronic illness. Control of this source of infection lies in heat sterilization, absolute cleanliness, and removal of the moist, stagnant areas.

Paris and numerous European cities have dual water supplies, that is, water supplies in which drinking and household water is carried in one set of mains and water for industrial purposes and fire fighting is carried in another set. This is a very dangerous arrangement because accidental cross-connections may occur between the two.

**Bacteriologic examination of water.** We know from experience that it is almost impossible to isolate from water the organisms that are responsible for the most important waterborne diseases, since few are present to begin with and they do not multiply in water. Sanitarians and public health workers therefore have concluded that the only safe method to prevent waterborne disease is to condemn any fecally polluted water as being unfit for human use. It *might* contain harmful organisms, since these practically always gain access to water in the feces or urine of man. Whether fecal pollution exists would be determined by examining the water for colon bacilli (*Es-*

*cherichia coli*), which are abundant in feces and *not* found outside the intestinal tract in nature. Certain other bacteria that resemble colon bacilli may or may not be of fecal origin. Also found in water, these bacteria ferment lactose with the formation of gas. In practical water analysis, therefore, testing includes the group spoken of as the *coliform* bacteria. (The presence of coliforms increases the likelihood of viruses being present. Note that viruses have been identified in sewage as indicated in Fig. 34-2.) The method of procedure recommended by the American Public Health Association and the American Water Works Association consists of three tests: presumptive, confirmed, and completed. The following are the tests as outlined in *Standard Methods for the Examination of Water and Wastewater.*

*Presumptive test.* The presumptive test is based on the fact that coliform bacteria ferment lactose with the production of gas. Lactose broth fermentation tubes are inoculated with 0.1, 1, and 10 ml. portions of the test water and incubated for 24 ± 2 hours at 35° ± 0.5° C. If no gas has formed, the tubes are incubated for another 24 ± 3 hours. The presence of gas is *presumptive* evidence that members of the coliform group of bacteria are present and suggests fecal contamination. The smallest amount in which the fer-

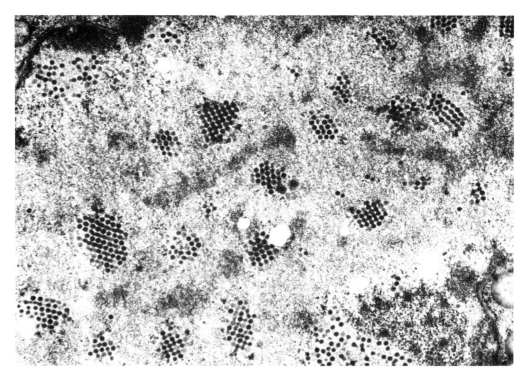

**Fig. 34-2.** Adenovirus crystals identified in sewage. (Courtesy Division of Microbiology and Infectious Diseases, Southwest Foundation for Research and Education, San Antonio, Texas.)

mentation of lactose occurs is an index of the number of organisms present.

*Confirmed test.* In the confirmed test, fermentation tubes of brilliant green lactose bile broth or solid differential media such as Endo's medium or eosin–methylene blue agar are inoculated with material from the tubes showing gas. If, when incubated at 35° ± 0.5° C., the brilliant green lactose bile broth shows gas at the end of 48 ± 3 hours or if colonies with the characteristic appearance of members of the coliform group appear on the solid medium within 24 ± 2 hours, the *confirmed* test is positive.

*Completed test.* If brilliant green lactose bile broth was used in the confirmed test, the completed test is done by streaking Endo's medium or eosin–methylene blue agar plates from the tubes showing gas and incubating them at 35° ± 0.5° C. for 24 ± 2 hours. From these plates (or the original plates if Endo's medium or eosin–methylene blue agar was used in the confirmed test) colonies typical for or similar to those of the coliform bacteria are transferred to lactose broth fermentation tubes and agar slants. These are incubated at 35° ± 0.5° C. and inspected at the end of 24 ± 2 hours and 48 ± 3 hours. After incubation, if microscopic examination of the growth on the agar slants reveals small gram-negative organisms and if the lactose fermentation is positive, the identification of coliform bacteria is said to be *completed.* At one time it was thought that when a positive test was obtained, a determination of the fecal or nonfecal origin of the bacteria should be made, but most sanitarians in the United States believe that to be satisfactory for drinking, water should be free of both fecal and nonfecal organisms.

Included in *Standard Methods for the Examination of Water and Wastewater* is the membrane filter procedure of detecting coliform bacteria. In this method, developed in Germany during World War II, the water is filtered through a thin disk of bacteria-retaining material. After filtration the disk is inverted over an absorbent pad saturated with modified Endo's culture medium and incubated for 20 ± 2 hours at 35° ± 0.5° C. All organisms that produce a dark purplish green colony with a metallic sheen are considered to be coliforms. Colonies of coliforms are counted, and an estimation of the number per 100 ml. of water sample is made.

European bacteriologists have devised systems whereby the water is also examined for *Streptococcus faecalis* and *Clostridium perfringens,* both of which are just as constantly present in the feces as the coliform organisms, but not so plentiful. Some American workers believe that fecal streptococci are more practical and reliable indicators of fecal contamination of water than are coliforms. Streptococci in the vi-

ridans group are suggested because, unlike the fecal streptococci, they strictly parasitize the alimentary tract of man and are not found in other animals or on plants. It has been suggested also that phages could be used as accurate indicators of fecal pollution of water.

**Drinking water standards.** The U.S. Public Health Service adopted certain standards for drinking water used in interstate commerce. Originally designed to protect the traveling public, these, to a great extent, have served as standards throughout the country. Included are specifications relating to (1) source and protection of the water, (2) physical and chemical properties, (3) bacteriologic content, and (4) limits on concentrations of radioactivity. Currently the Environmental Protection Agency is charged with formulation of a set of standards for safe drinking water.

Drinking water must contain no impurity that would offend sight, taste, or smell, and substances that might have deleterious physiologic effects must not be introduced.

Investigation of the problem of viruses in water is just beginning. Since minimal amounts of virus can produce infection, total removal of viruses from a water supply designed for human consumption would be indicated.

**Water purification.** Water may be purified by natural means. However natural methods are usually slow and uncertain. As water trickles through the earth, microbes are filtered out. Water standing in lakes and ponds undergoes some degree of purification because of the combined action of sunlight, sedimentation, dilution of impurities, and destruction of bacteria by protozoa. Streams may be purified as they flow along, but the possibility of contaminated material entering the stream along its course is so great that one cannot depend on self-purification of the water. In fact, all the foregoing methods of natural purification are slow and uncertain in their action. *Therefore all surface waters must be regarded as potentially dangerous unless subjected to artificial purification.**

Generally, artificial water purification (Fig. 34-3) is carried out by a combination of physical and chemical methods—sedimentation and filtration combined with the action of chemicals to soften and clarify the water, and chlorination (p. 152). *Sedimentation* is the process whereby solids in the water, such as mud and organic matter, are removed. Water is held in settling

---

*In unusual circumstances small quantities of water can be made relatively safe for drinking by the addition of 2 drops of chlorine bleach or 2 drops of tincture of iodine or Halazone, a commercial tablet, to one pint of water, provided that the mixture is allowed to stand for 30 minutes.

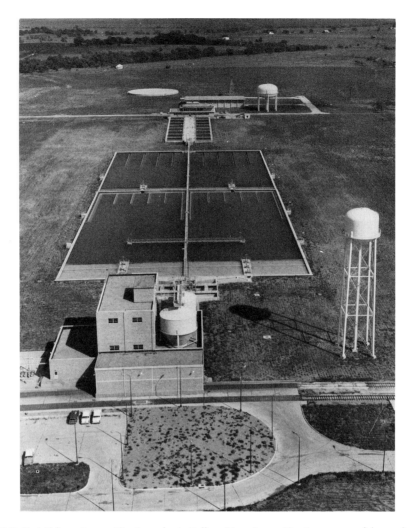

**Fig. 34-3.** East Side water purification plant, Dallas. Steps in purification proceed from chemical plant in foreground, where ferrous sulfate and lime are added to water, to pump house in background, from where water is pumped to reservoir. Between these points are rapid mixers, flocculators, settling basins, and sand filters. Water is chlorinated several times at points along way. (Courtesy Dallas Water Utilities.)

basins for a number of hours to allow the large particles to settle out. A chemical such as alum or ferric sulfate is added to coagulate the suspended organic matter and microbes present, and the precipitated coagulum is removed mechanically. Some clarification of water occurs with sedimentation. *Filtration* is the process that puts the final sparkle in the water.

The average rapid filter that is in use has the following units from the floor to the surface: (1) watertight floor with grooves and tile for draining the filtered water away, (2) layer of gravel from 12 to 18 inches thick, and (3) layer of sand. The gravel at the bottom is of such a size as to be able to pass through

a 2-inch mesh screen. The size of the gravel gradually decreases until the surface of the layer where the gravel will pass through a 1/16-inch mesh screen is approached. The sand layer is about 2.5 feet thick. Rapid sand filters can filter over 200 million gallons per day per acre of filter area. By rapid filtration 90% to 95% of all bacteria are removed more or less mechanically by the layer of sand at the top of the filter. Efficient filtration removes all pathogenic and most saprophytic organisms. Filters must be cleaned often. This is done by reversing the flow of water and agitating the upper layer of sand. In some cases air is forced through the filter from the bottom to the top. A rapid

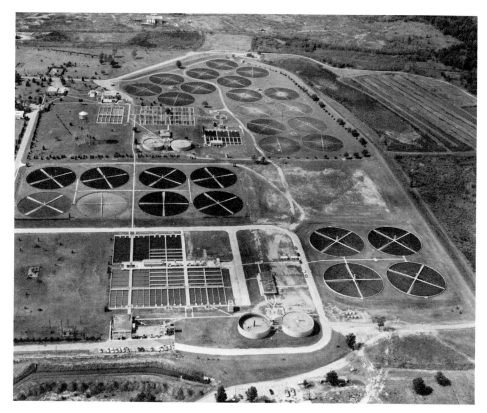

**Fig. 34-4.** Wastewater treatment plant, Dallas, aerial survey. Note layout of settling basins, microbial digestors, and trickling filters. In primary settling basins, organic wastes are oxidized by bacteria and algae growing on rocks. Sludge from primary settling basins goes to a separate group of heated tanks called digestors, where by a process of anaerobic decomposition solids are broken down by microbes. Effluent from primary settling basins goes to 29 circular trickling filters, each with a half-acre rock bed. (Courtesy Dallas Water Utilities.)

filter is made in units, so that just a part of the filter is closed for cleaning at any one time.

After filtration, water is universally chlorinated. There are three methods in common use:

1. *Simple chlorination.* This method is the addition of a standard effective amount of chlorine gas to the water. Chlorine is usually added from cylinders connected with regulating equipment to control the exact amount.

2. *Ammonia-chlorine treatment.* This treatment results in compounds called chloramines, formed when chlorine is added to water containing ammonia. Chloramines are less active as germicidal agents but are more stable than free chlorine.

3. *Superchlorination.* This process involves the addition of a much larger dose of chlorine than with simple chlorination and the removal subsequently of the excess.

Certain chemicals in hard water soften the water by removing dissolved limestone. When mixed with raw, untreated water, activated carbon absorbs odors and tastes resulting from the decaying vegetation and organic matter present.

**Fluoride content of water and tooth decay.** It is well known that the fluoride content of the drinking water of infants and children profoundly influences the development of their teeth. If too much fluoride is present (4 to 5 p.p.m. water), the condition known as fluorosis or mottled enamel develops; if too little, the incidence of dental caries is greatly increased. Adult teeth do not seem to be affected. The optimum ratio of fluoride to water for drinking by infants and young children is 1 p.p.m. When this is present, there is sufficient fluoride to retard tooth decay significantly but not enough to stain or mottle the teeth, that is, to cause fluorosis. Reduction of the incidence of tooth decay is on the order of 60% to 70%. In nature the fluoride content of water varies from much less to much more than 1 p.p.m. water, but the proper level may be maintained by adding fluoride to water whose content is low or by chemically removing fluoride from water whose content is too high.

**Ice.** When pathogenic bacteria gain access to ice, the great majority die, but a few survive. It is estimated that about 10% survive for more than a few hours. Ice that has been stored for 6 months is practically bacteria free. Few instances of the transmission of disease in ice are known. The use of water of high sanitary quality in the manufacture of ice has lessened the possibility that ice itself will act as a conveyer of disease. However, the handling of ice in the home, eating places, and cold drink stands may be a source of infection.

**Purification of sewage.** Sewage must be processed in treatment plants to render it harmless before it is discharged into a body of water such as a river or a lake (Fig. 34-4). Many methods of sewage purification are in use. The procedures involved are screening and sedimentation to remove the larger particles, chemical treatment to remove small particles, micro-

bial action to digest organic matter, aeration to induce oxidation, filtration through sand, and chlorination. There is no known way to remove all viruses from sewage (Fig. 34-2); they are not regularly inactivated by the primary and secondary treatment and easily pass into the effluent. Enteroviruses, reoviruses, and adenoviruses have been demonstrated to come through standard treatment. Parasites readily disseminated in sewage include *Entamoeba histolytica*, *Giardia lamblia*, *Ascaris*, hookworms, and tapeworms.

The breakdown of human waste in sewage by microbes is essentially the same as decay of organic material in other situations. The sanitary engineer is much concerned with this fact. He designs the sewage disposal plant to facilitate and speed up microbial activity and to ensure its completion (Fig. 34-5).

**Swimming pool sanitation.** Swimming pools may convey conjunctivitis, ear infections, skin diseases, and intestinal infections unless kept in a sanitary condition. The source of infection is a person using the pool. Swimming pool water should be kept in the same state of purity as drinking water. This is done

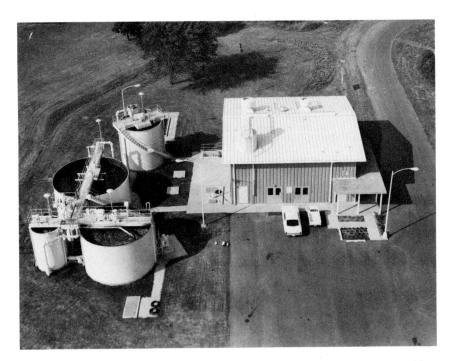

**Fig. 34-5.** Water reclamation. An "activated sludge" pilot plant in Dallas, of a type used by many cities over nation. This facility processes 1 million gallons a day. In activated sludge process, microbes are mixed with sewage to consume its organic products. Here is one large tank maintained in an aerobic state to facilitate growth of sewage microbes. It is seeded by sludge (primarily microorganisms) settled from a second large tank, the secondary clarifying tank. The input of raw sewage or sewage already settled into aeration tank provides substrate for microbial action. (Courtesy Dallas Water Utilities.)

with frequent changes of water and the use of disinfectants. Chlorine is the most widely used one. The highest practical concentration of chlorine to water should be maintained, about 1 p.p.m. (see also p. 152). A higher concentration is irritating to the eyes. Before entering the pool, each bather should take a shower bath, using soap. Persons who have infections of any kind should not be allowed to use the pool.

Some authorities prefer iodine to chlorine as a disinfectant for swimming pools. Its disinfectant action is less hindered by the presence of organic matter, and there is less eye and skin irritation than with chlorine. Bromine has also been used as a swimming pool disinfectant.

## Questions for review

1 Name the diseases that may be spread by water. Give the causal agent.
2 Discuss bacteriologic examination of water.
3 Describe the purification of water by (a) natural means, (b) artificial means.
4 List the sources of water. From a public health standpoint, how do waters from these sources differ? State the sources of the microbes in water.
5 Why is sewage of such great sanitary significance?
6 What specifications are made for drinking water standards?
7 What is the relation of the fluoride content of water to tooth decay?
8 Discuss water pollution today as a public health problem. (Consult references.)
9 Give the sanitary classification of water.

**References on pp. 393 and 394.**

# CHAPTER 35

# Microbiology of food

## Milk

If obtained in a pure state and kept pure, milk is our best single food. If improperly handled, our most dangerous one. Milk is such an important conveyer of infection because it is an excellent culture medium and is consumed uncooked. *Microbiology of dairy products* deals with (1) the microbes that make milk and milk products unfit for human consumption, (2) prevention of disease in cattle, and (3) manufacture of milk products.

**Bacteria in milk.** Bacteria gain access to milk by many different routes. Milk as secreted by the mammary glands of perfectly healthy cows is usually sterile, but as the cow is milked, bacteria from the teats and milk ducts get in. Thus by the time the milk enters the pail, contamination has taken place. Bacteria may be present within the udders of diseased cows. Unclean and unsanitary milking utensils, pasteurizing tanks, and milk containers as well as dust and manure are important sources of contamination.

Under the very best conditions the bacterial content of milk is relatively high. Some bacteria, even though they come from external sources, are so commonly present as to be regarded as normal milk bacteria; pathogenic bacteria may also be present. Normal milk bacteria help to sour milk; they also may destroy its value as a food; pathogens cause disease.

The two main sources of pathogenic bacteria found in milk are the people who handle it and infected cows. The organisms most often found in milk are staphylococci, streptococci, lactic acid bacteria, and enteric organisms.

Although it is not the only criterion, the number of bacteria in milk is the best index of its sanitary quality. The number present depends on the number originally introduced into the milk and the temperature at which the milk is kept. Many species of bacteria begin to multiply as soon as they gain access to milk. This can be largely prevented if the milk is rapidly chilled to 10° C. (50° F.) as soon as it is obtained, and kept cold. If milk is kept at that temperature, no great increase in the number of bacteria will occur, but if the

milk is allowed to warm up, there is a rapid rise in numbers.

Milk of high quality may contain only a few hundred bacteria per milliliter. Bad milk may contain millions of bacteria per milliliter. All authorities agree that a single high bacterial count does not necessarily mean that the milk is of poor quality and that, to be significant, a high bacterial count must occur day after day. The presence of coliform bacteria points to fecal contamination.

**Milk-borne diseases.*** The diseases spread by milk may be classified as (1) diseases of human origin and (2) diseases of milk-producing animals transmitted to man in their milk. Most notable of the diseases that primarily affect man and may be transmitted by milk are typhoid fever, salmonelloses, bacillary and amebic dysentery, scarlet fever, infantile diarrhea, diphtheria, poliomyelitis, infectious hepatitis, and septic sore throat. The diseases that primarily affect milk-producing animals and may be transmitted to man by the milk of the infected animal are undulant fever, Q fever, and bovine tuberculosis. Undulant fever may be contracted from the milk of infected cows or goats.

The spread of human diseases by milk usually results from contamination of the milk by the discharges of a handler who is ill of the disease or is a carrier. Milk-borne epidemics characteristically appear among the patrons of a given dairy, and the source of infection usually is traced to a food handler in that dairy.

Bovine tuberculosis, especially in children under 5 years of age, is usually caused by the ingestion of the

---

*A disease not of bacterial origin but of historic interest is *milk sickness* (called milksick by the pioneers). This disease cost the life of many midwestern pioneers including the mother of Abraham Lincoln. Milk sickness is caused by the ingestion of milk from cows that have been poisoned by eating certain species of goldenrod and the white snakeroot. The poisonous principles in these plants are excreted in the milk of the affected cow.

milk of tuberculous cows. In cattle, tuberculosis most often affects the lungs, but the sputum is swallowed and excreted in the feces. As a rule, the bacilli get into the milk by fecal contamination, but in some cases the udder becomes infected, and the bacilli are excreted directly into the milk. The milk of a single cow excreting *Mycobacterium tuberculosis* in her milk may render the mixed milk of the whole herd infectious. The danger of contracting tuberculosis through milk is completely eliminated by pasteurization of milk and the tuberculin testing of cows.

**Pasteurized milk.** *Pasteurization* is the process of heating milk to a temperature high enough to kill all *nonsporebearing pathogenic* bacteria but not high enough to affect the chemical composition of the milk. There are two methods of pasteurization. One is known as the holding method; the other as the continuous-flow, high-temperature, short-time or flash method. In the former the milk is held in tanks or vats where it is subjected to a comparatively low temperature for a comparatively long period of time while being constantly agitated. In the latter the milk is subjected to a higher temperature for a short period of time as it flows through the pasteurizing equipment.

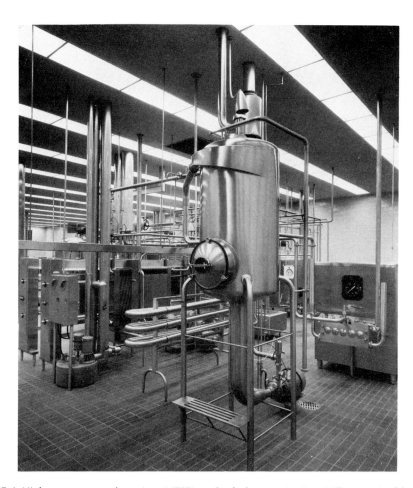

**Fig. 35-1.** High-temperature short-time (HTST) method of pasteurization. Milk is received from the dairy farm in tank trucks and placed in holding tanks. Milk is pasteurized at 175° F. for 16 seconds through a plate heat-exchanger with holding tube and timing pump. It is also clarified, standardized, homogenized, and steam heated to 190°-194° for 30 seconds, vacuum-cooled back to 175°, and cooled at 33° through a plate heat-exchanger containing cooling medium. All is done automatically from a central control panel, utilizing sanitary air-operated valves for routing the milk. Cleaning and sanitizing is also done by automatic circulation of cleaning and sanitizing compounds. Note the Vac-Heat unit in the foreground. This unit ensures the same milk flavor year-round by removing various volatile feed-off flavors, which vary during the year's four seasons. (Courtesy CP Division, St. Regis, Dallas.)

(See Fig. 35-1.) After both methods the milk should be transferred through pipes, where it is chilled, to the bottling (packaging) machines. All milk should be received into clean sanitary containers (glass, cardboard, plastic).

The *Grade "A" Pasteurized Milk Ordinance—1965 Recommendations of the Public Health Service* are that (1) in the holding method, the milk must be subjected to a temperature of *at least* 145° F. (63° C.) for *at least* 30 minutes and (2) in the continuous-flow method, the milk must be subjected to a temperature of *at least* 161° F. (72° C.) for *at least* 15 seconds. Note carefully that pasteurization does *not* completely sterilize milk and that pasteurization should never be used to cover gross negligence in sanitation and the sanitary handling of milk.

**Pasteurized versus raw milk.** Pasteurization is the single most crucial item in the maintenance of a safe milk supply. Objections to pasteurization might be that (1) it destroys vitamins, (2) dairymen may not be so careful when they know that the milk is to be pasteurized, and (3) pasteurization may be carelessly and ineffectively done. The latter two objections can be eliminated by thorough inspection systems. Vitamin C, which is destroyed, can easily be replaced in the diet or given as ascorbic acid.

The temperature of pasteurization is not high enough to affect milk and is carefully controlled during the process. Heating milk to high temperatures can drastically change it. Boiling milk causes decomposition of its proteins, changes in its phosphorus content, precipitation of calcium and magnesium, expulsion of carbon dioxide, combustion of sugar, and destruction of enzymes.

**Requirements for a safe milk supply.** To ensure a safe milk supply, the following requirements must be met:

1. The cows must be healthy, well fed, and free of diseases such as tuberculosis, brucellosis, and mastitis.
2. All individuals handling milk must be free of infectious organisms, and their hands and person must be clean.
3. The premises must be kept clean.
4. The udders and flanks of the cows must be washed before milking.
5. The milking utensils and machinery that contact the milk must be kept sterile and should be so constructed as to keep out dust and flies. (Practically all milking today in commercial dairies is done mechanically.)
6. The milk must be chilled immediately to 10° C. (50° F.) and kept cold.
7. It must be pasteurized under carefully controlled conditions and again chilled.
8. Directly after pasteurization, it must be placed into the container reaching the customer.
9. It must be delivered cold (10° C.) in refrigerated trucks and immediately refrigerated at its destination.
10. A uniform statewide sanitary milk code must provide for proper inspection of dairies and pasteurization plants.
11. Local laboratory services must check on the purity, cleanliness, and safety of the milk.

**Milk grading.** Different states have different systems of grading their milk supply, but all are based generally on the sanitation of the dairy, health of the cows, methods of handling the milk, and bacterial content. In addition to the bacterial count* of milk, testing for coliforms is done to detect contamination after pasteurization. Milk is also checked for possible adulteration.

The phosphatase test is used in grading to determine whether the milk has been adequately pasteurized. The enzyme phosphatase is mostly destroyed at the temperature of pasteurization. A significant amount detectable in milk indicates incomplete pasteurization or the presence of raw milk mixed in with a sample of pasteurized milk.

Several grades of milk are recognized by the *Milk Ordinance and Code—1953 Recommendations of the Public Health Service,* but only one, Grade A pasteurized milk, is allowed in interstate commerce for retail sale. This is milk that has been pasteurized, cooled, and packaged in accord with precise U.S.P.H.S specifications. Its bacterial content has been reduced by pasteurization from no more than 300,000 per milliliter (300,000/ml.) to no more than 20,000/ml., with coliforms no more than 10/ml.

The general improvement in milk sanitation has been such that most authorities believe there is no longer any practical necessity for special grades of milk. Therefore the present tendency is to stress the production of one standard, high-quality, safe, pure milk readily available to people in all walks of life at a reasonable cost.

**Milk formulas for hospital nurseries.** The preparation of infant milk formulas in hospitals should be

---

*Bacterial count is obtained by either the *plate count* (p. 64) or the *direct microscopic clump count.* In the direct microscopic clump count, an accurately measured amount of milk (0.01 ml.) is placed on a slide and spread into a thin smear of uniform thickness. The dried smear is stained. With a microscope calibrated so that the area of the field is known, the bacteria in a number of representative fields are counted and the number of bacteria in the whole specimen calculated. In this clump count, both individual bacteria and unseparated groups of bacteria are counted as units.

in accord with standards set by the hospital medical staff or appropriate health agency. For proper microbiologic control, the American Academy of Pediatrics in its Standards and Recommendations for the Hospital Care of Newborn Infants recommends that technics of formula preparation be checked at least once a week. As part of their surveillance plan, random samples of the ready-to-use formula are sent to the laboratory to be cultured. The limit for the bacterial plate count of a formula sample is 25 organisms per milliliter. In the identification of organisms present there should be none other than sporeformers. Otherwise a break in technic is indicated, and responsible authorities should be notified at once.

**Bacterial action on milk.** Milk may be decomposed by the action of bacteria on its carbohydrates or proteins. The former is spoken of as fermentation of milk, the latter as putrefaction of milk. Souring results from fermentation and is referred to as normal milk decomposition.

The souring of milk (lactic acid fermentation) is the result of the formation of insoluble casein by the action of lactic acid on caseinogen. Lactic acid is formed by the action of bacteria on lactose (milk sugar). *Streptococcus lactis, Lactobacillus acidophilus, Bifidobacterium bifidum (Lactobacillus bifidus), Lactobacillus casei, Lactobacillus bulgaricus, Escherichia coli,* and others are organisms responsible.

Putrefaction of milk seldom occurs, but when it does, it is a dangerous event. Putrefactive changes are caused by the action of sporebearing and anaerobic bacilli on the proteins of the milk. The milk is finally converted into a bitter liquid having little resemblance to fresh milk.

Slimy or ropy milk usually results from the action of *Alcaligenes viscolactis* or similar organisms, but it may be from other organisms such as streptococci and the lactic acid bacteria. In Norway, ropy milk is considered a delicacy. Americans consider it unfit for use.

Spontaneous alcoholic fermentation may rarely occur, but it is a feature of manufacturing processes in which sugar and yeasts or bacteria are added to milk. Among the products are kumyss or koumiss, kefir, leben, and yoghurt or matzoon. Yoghurt is the milk to which Metchnikoff referred in his book on the prolonged life of the Bulgarian tribes. Yoghurt is the forerunner of the present-day Bulgarian buttermilk.

The chief characteristic of yoghurt is its high acidity, produced by the growth of *Lactobacillus bulgaricus.* Because of this, it is considered to be one of the safest of all foods. Archaeologists working in underdeveloped areas feel that natural yoghurt, a major food item in the diet of many peoples, is always nutritious and safe to eat. Yoghurt and buttermilk are at times used in the nursing care of patients with ad-vanced cancerous growths, secondarily infected and malodorous. The alkaline medium of the cancer allows bacterial growth and fermentation activities to flourish. The application of yoghurt or buttermilk changes the tissue environment of the cancerous area to an acid one, thus inhibiting the growth of the odor-forming microbes.

Bacterial growth may color milk red, yellow, or blue.

**Ice cream.** Although ice cream is frozen, not all bacteria are destroyed. In fact, some pathogenic bacteria live longer in ice cream than in milk. Typhoid bacilli have been known to live as long as 2 years in ice cream. Outbreaks of typhoid fever, septic sore throat, diphtheria, food poisoning, and scarlet fever have been traced to ice cream. To prevent it from spreading disease, it must be made with pasteurized milk and handled properly thereafter. Proper handling means cleanliness of utensils and factory and proper health supervision of employees.

**Butter.** Although derived from milk, butter only poorly supports microbial growth because it is made up chiefly of fat and water and is deficient in protein and sugar. However, certain bacteria do grow in it and render it rancid. The ordinary saprophytic organisms found in butter are the various types of lactic acid bacteria, especially streptococci. Improperly prepared butter may contain *Escherichia coli* and various yeasts and molds. The presence of an excessive quantity of yeasts in butter indicates that proper sanitary precautions were not exercised in preparation. *Mycobacterium tuberculosis* and the atypical mycobacteria have been found in butter. Typhoid bacilli have been found, but they tend to die therein. Contamination of butter with pathogenic organisms may be eliminated by pasteurization of the cream used in making the butter, proper sterilization of utensils, and strict supervision of personnel.

## Food

The *microbiology of food* is studied from many standpoints. The soil and agricultural microbiologist thinks of the microbes (free-living and symbiotic) in the soil. These are utilized by food plants in growth and development. Microbes aid in the return of waste products of food utilization to the soil, where the waste products are used again by microbes and food plants. The food microbiologist studies the part that microbes play in (1) the manufacture of bread, butter, cheese, and many other foods and (2) the spoilage of foods, and how this may be prevented. Public health microbiologists primarily interested in the health of the community study food as to what diseases it may convey, the harmful products of its spoilage, and how both food-borne disease and food spoilage may be prevented. The diseases that food conveys are discussed here.

## FOOD POISONING

When foods are related to disease, they are considered first as carriers of infection, as given on p. 88 (examples: poliomyelitis, hepatitis).

Next comes a group of illnesses spoken of as food poisoning. By definition, food poisoning is an acute illness resulting from the ingestion of some injurious agent in food. It is classified as

1. Nonmicrobial type
   a. Individual idiosyncrasy
   b. Chemical factor from:
      (1) Foods naturally poisonous (toadstools and the like)
      (2) Poisons accidentally or intentionally added (plant sprays and the like)
2. Microbial type
   a. Food intoxications—effect of ingested toxin (example: botulism)
   b. Food infections—multiplication of ingested microorganisms
      (1) Bacterial (example: salmonellosis)
      (2) Parasitic (example: trichinosis)

A characteristic of food infections and intoxications is that many persons eat the offending food and most develop the disease. In food infection the diagnosis is made if the offending organism is cultured from the feces of the patient and from the food eaten. In food intoxication diagnostic efforts are directed toward finding the offending toxin in the food eaten. Examination of the feces of the patient is of little value.

Table 35-1 lists bacterial types of food poisoning and the prominent features of each.

Staphylococci,* *Clostridium botulinum,* and less often certain other organisms produce food intoxication. *Salmonella* species and rarely *Streptococcus faecalis* (enterococcus) cause food infection.

*Food intoxication.* Botulism is a very serious type of true food intoxication produced by the ingestion of food containing the potent exotoxin of *Clostridium botulinum* (p. 230). The major source of botulism is

---

*Food poisoning, especially infection and intoxication caused by staphylococci, was formerly known as "ptomaine" poisoning. This is incorrect because ptomaines play no part in food poisoning.

## Table 35-1

Types of bacterial food poisoning

| ORGANISM | FOODS | ONSET (AFTER FOOD EATEN) | CLINICAL FEATURES | TOXIN | OUTCOME |
|---|---|---|---|---|---|
| **Food intoxication** | | | | | |
| *Clostridium botulinum* | Canned string beans, corn, beets, ripe olives | 2 hours to 8 days | Vomiting Diarrhea Double vision Difficulty in swallowing, speaking Respiratory paralysis | Neurotoxin | Mortality high |
| *Staphylococcus* | Potato salad Chicken salad Cream fillings Milk Meats Cheese | 1 to 6 hours | Vomiting Diarrhea Abdominal cramps Prostration | Enterotoxin | Severe symptoms of short duration (death rare) |
| **Food infection** | | | | | |
| *Salmonella* | Eggs Poultry Meats | 7 to 72 hours | Diarrhea Severe abdominal pain Fever Prostration | None | Recovery—few days (death rare) |
| *Streptococcus* | Sausage Poultry dressing Custard | 2 to 18 hours | Nausea Pain Diarrhea | None | Recovery 1 to 2 days |

improperly processed home-canned vegetables of low acid content. *Before they are eaten,* such foods should always be cooked *at the temperature of boiling water for at least 15 minutes* and thoroughly stirred and mixed. Contaminated foods may have unpleasant odors somewhat characteristic for a given food, but these off-odors are not easily recognized and do not suggest spoiled food. The cans or containers holding the food do not necessarily bulge, a conventional sign of food spoilage.

Staphylococcal food intoxication is caused by the action of an enterotoxin liberated by some strains of staphylococci. The staphylococci multiply in the offending food before it is eaten and elaborate their toxin there. (They do not multiply in the intestinal tract.) Manifestations come from the ingested toxin. Staphylococci require a period of not less than 8 hours to elaborate enough toxin in food to cause symptoms. After the food is eaten, the disorder appears within 6 hours. Recovery occurs in from 24 to 48 hours. Staphylococcal food intoxication usually follows the ingestion of starchy foods, especially potato salad, custards, and pies. When the offending food is meat, it is usually ham. Many outbreaks have been traced to chicken salad. This is probably the most common type of food intoxication.

**Bacterial food infection.** Food infection is caused by the multiplication of bacteria that have been taken into the intestinal canal. The responsible bacteria are most often salmonellae. Of special concern in food infection are *Salmonella enteritidis* (Gärtner's bacillus), *Salmonella typhimurium,* and *Salmonella cholerae-suis.* Once inside the intestine, they multiply rapidly and induce widespread inflammation with severe manifestations—nausea, vomiting, diarrhea, and fever.

The disease usually occurs as an explosive outbreak following a meal attended by a large number of persons. Food cooked in large quantities is more often the source of infection than is food cooked in small quantities, since heat is not so likely to penetrate and destroy the organisms in a large quantity of food. Most outbreaks occur during the warm months. The incubation period for *Salmonella* food infection is 7 to 72 hours, and recovery occurs usually within 3 or 4 days; but in severe infections death may occur within 24 hours.

The insufficiently cooked meat of infected animals may convey the disease to man, but usually salmonellae reach the food (often, but not necessarily, meat) from outside sources. Such sources are the intestinal contents of the slaughtered animals, the intestinal contents of animals (especially rats and mice) that have contacted the food incriminated, and (probably most important) human carriers of the bacteria. *Sal-monella* infections are common in rats, and these animals often become carriers. Cockroaches have been shown to convey *Salmonella* food poisoning. Salmonellae are abundant in the intestinal tract of poultry, a very important source, and may be present on the shell of an egg. Contaminated eggs broken commercially may be a source of organisms in egg products. Food such as the meringue on pies contaminated with *Salmonella* may have no abnormal odor or taste.

Prevention of *Salmonella* food poisoning depends on cleanliness in handling food, proper cooking of food, proper refrigeration of food that has been cooked, and detection of carriers. Frequent and careful handwashing by food handlers is very important. Food that remains on their skin for a period of time provides nourishment for microbial contaminants, some foodborne, and thus contributes to their survival in the environment.

Under the provisions of the Egg Products Inspection Act of 1970, all commercial eggs broken out of the shell for manufacturing use must be pasteurized. The egg or egg product is heated to 60° to 61° C. (140° to 143° F.) and held there for 3½ to 4 minutes. The final product must be free of *Salmonella.*

Rarely streptococci may cause food poisoning of the infection type. At times the addition of large numbers of organisms to the already resident enterococci in the bowel may trigger gastroenteritis. The food usually responsible contains meat that has stood at warm temperatures for several hours, and the organism usually recovered from the feces is *Streptococcus faecalis.* The incubation period is 2 to 18 hours, and the illness lasts a very short time.

Other organisms sometimes infecting food are *Clostridium perfringens, Bacillus cereus, Proteus* species, and *Escherichia coli.* In outbreaks traced to these, it has been thought that the microbes were able to multiply in food, especially meat, that had stood at room temperature overnight or longer.

**Parasitic food infection.** For a discussion of trichinosis, see p. 365.

## MEASURES TO SAFEGUARD FOOD

To safeguard a food supply, remember that:
1. Appearance, taste, and smell are not always reliable indicators that a food is safe for consumption.
2. Any unusual change in color, consistency, or odor or the production of gas in food means that the food should be discarded *without being eaten. Note:* If *suspect* food has been tasted or eaten, it should not be discarded. It should be kept for 48 hours in the event that it might have

to be examined for the presence of *Clostridium botulinum* exotoxin.

3. Dishes, cutlery, can openers, utensils, and equipment of all kinds used to prepare, serve, and store food should be clean and sanitary.
4. Hands that prepare, serve, and store food should be clean. Preferably food is handled as little as possible.
5. Foods served raw should be washed carefully and thoroughly.
6. Bacteria grow fastest in the temperature range 40° to 140° F. Therefore:
   a. Hot food should be kept hot (above 140° F.).
   b. Cold food should be kept cold (below 40° F.). All dairy foods should be refrigerated.
   c. Cooked food that is to be refrigerated should be cooled quickly and refrigerated promptly. If cooked food is to be kept longer than a few days, it should be frozen.
   d. Perishable foods should be kept chilled if taken on a trip or picnic. Foods may spoil easily if exposed to a warmer temperature for no longer than a half hour before they are eaten.
   e. Extra care should be taken with foods easily contaminated by microbial growth—meats, poultry, stuffing, gravy, salads, eggs, custards, and cream pies.

## FOOD PRESERVATION

There are numerous methods of preserving food. The following are a few.

**Refrigerating.** Refrigeration is one of the best and most universally used methods of food preservation. It has several distinct advantages: (1) there is little change in the composition of the food, and therefore taste, odor, and appearance are preserved; (2) the nutritive value of the food is not reduced; (3) there is no decrease in digestibility; and (4) there is little effect on vitamin content. During refrigeration pathogenic bacteria are checked and many destroyed. When refrigeration is discontinued, those that remain viable begin to multiply. Some saprophytic organisms are able to multiply at refrigeration temperatures.

**Freezing.** Freezing as a way of preserving food is in widespread use today because of its application in the preparation of "convenience" food items. Quick freezing is carried out at very low temperatures ($-35°$ F. with a holding temperature of $-10°$ F.). A preliminary step to freezing is blanching. The food is heated quickly to inactivate enzymes that would break down proteins and change the texture, flavor, and appearance of the food. Blanching is followed by instant cooling in ice water. Food that is frozen retains its nutrients and is palatable. Freezing of meat kills en-

cysted larvae therein. Since cold-storage foods decompose rapidly when thawed or warmed to room temperature, they should be consumed right away.

**Drying.** Microbes are unable to multiply for lack of water.

**Smoking.** The food is dried, and preservatives from the smoke added to it.

**Pickling.** The high acid content of the medium prevents microbial multiplication.

**Salting and preserving in brine.** The osmotic pressure of the medium is so changed that microbes will not multiply. Sometimes water is extracted from the microbial cell.

**Canning.** Microorganisms are destroyed by heat. The container with its content of food is hermetically sealed to keep out contaminants. The sealing also excludes free oxygen, which would aid the growth of molds, yeasts, and most species of pathogenic bacteria.

Commercial canning is a very safe method of food preservation. It is done scientifically and under supervision by the indicated health agency. Home canning on the other hand may be done under rough and ready conditions by unskilled hands. Since there is always a possibility for food contamination, home-canned foods, especially meats and vegetables, should always be heated prior to consumption.

**Preserving.** The food is heated and sugar added. A large amount of sugar retards bacterial multiplication in the same manner as does salt. However, it does not retard the multiplication of fungi. Heating and sealing have the same effect as in canning.

**Cooking.** Microbes are killed by heat; the composition of the food is changed, and water may be removed.

**Chemicals.** The addition of chemicals such as benzoic acid in the form of the sodium salt, sodium and calcium propionates, sodium and potassium nitrites, and esters of para-hydroxybenzoic acid (parabens) to foods as preservatives is regulated by the Food and Drug Administration and by the U.S. Department of Agriculture.

**Ionizing radiation.** Ultraviolet irradiation has already been used successfully by food industries to treat the air in storage and processing rooms, to prevent the growth of fungi on shelves and walls of preparation rooms, and to destroy parasites in meat.

Cold sterilization of foods by means of ionizing radiation is under investigation by the U.S. Armed Forces and the Atomic Energy Commission, and one of the major obstacles encountered has been the terrific resistance of the spores of *Clostridium botulinum* to the effects of radiation.

**Food in vending machines.** Vending machines dispense today many foods that support the rapid growth of infectious or toxigenic microbes. The food to be safe for consumption must be prepared under sanitary conditions and be transported in properly refrigerated vehicles. In the vending machine they must be maintained at proper temperatures and replaced often.

## Questions for review

1 Name diseases spread by contaminated milk and food.
2 Give differential characteristics of milk-borne and water-borne epidemics.
3 What is meant by Grade A pasteurized milk?
4 What is flash pasteurization?
5 Give the requirements for a safe milk supply.
6 Make an outline showing the different kinds of food poisoning. Name causal agents.
7 Differentiate food intoxication from food infection. Give examples.
8 List the different methods of food preservation.
9 List practical measures to safeguard food.
10 Explain briefly: lactic acid bacteria, normal milk bacteria, yoghurt, buttermilk, holding method of pasteurization, milk sickness, phosphatase test, souring of milk, food idiosyncrasy, low-acid foods, high-acid foods, blanching of foods.
11 Indicate how a bacterial count of a milk sample is done.

**REFERENCES** (Chapters 33 to 35)

Abst, D. B., and others: Time and cost factors to provide regular, periodic dental care for children in a fluoridated and nonfluoridated area: final report, J. Am. Dent. Assoc. **80:**770, 1970.

Bauman, H. E.: Food microbiology, ASM News **38:**312, 1972.

Bell, J. A.: Viruses and water quality (editorial), J.A.M.A. **219:**1628, 1972.

Berg, G., editor: Transmission of viruses by the water route, New York, 1967, Interscience Publishers, Inc.

Brock, T. D., and Brock, K. M.: Basic microbiology; with applications, Englewood Cliffs, N.J., Prentice-Hall, Inc.

Brooks, S. M.: Ptomaine: the story of food poisoning, Cranbury, N.J., 1974, A. S. Barnes & Co., Inc.

Bulla, L. A., Jr.: Microbial control of insects: a synopsis, ASM News **39:**97, 1973.

Burt, B. A.: Fluoride—the case for hardening teeth, Nursing Times **70:**374, March, 1974.

Cairns, J., Jr., and Dickson, K. L., editors: Biological methods for the assessment of water quality, Philadelphia, 1973, American Society for Testing and Materials.

Colwell, R. R., and Morita, R. Y., editors: Effect of the ocean environment on microbial activities, Baltimore, 1974, University Park Press.

Demain, A. L.: Application of the microbe to the benefit of mankind: challenges and opportunities, ASM News **38:** 237, 1972.

Diehl, J. F.: Irradiated food, Science **108:**214, 1973.

Di Palma, J. R.: The problem of food additives, RN **33:**53, June, 1970.

Doetsch, R. N., and Cook, T. M.: Introduction to bacteria and their ecobiology, Baltimore, 1973, University Park Press.

Dugan, P. R.: Biochemical ecology of water pollution, New York, 1972, Plenum Publishing Corp.

Egeberg, R. O.: Fluoridation for all: a national priority, Today's Health **48:**30, June, 1970.

Frazier, W. C.: Food microbiology, ed. 2, 1967, McGraw-Hill Book Co.

Freese, A. S.: Salmonella: food poison plus, Today's Health **47:**34, April, 1969.

Grade "A" Pasteurized Milk Ordinance—1965 Recommendations of the United States Public Health Service, U.S.P.H.S. Bull. no. 229 (revision), Washington, D.C., 1967, U.S. Government Printing Office.

Gregory, P. H.: The microbiology of the atmosphere, ed. 2, New York, 1973, John Wiley & Sons, Inc.

Hungate, R. E.: Status of microbiological research in relation to waste disposal, ASM News **38:**364, 1972.

Kermode, G. O.: Food additives, Sci. Am. **226:**15, March, 1972.

Kilbourne, E. D., and Smillie, W. G., editors: Public health and human ecology, ed. 4, New York, 1969, The Macmillan Co.

Knutson, J. W.: Water fluoridation after 25 years, J. Am. Dent. Assoc. **80:**765, 1970.

Kretzer, M. P., and Engley, F. B., Jr.: Preventing food poisoning, RN **33:**50, June, 1970.

Marx, J. L.: Insect control. II. Hormones and viruses, Science **181:**833, 1973.

Marx, J. L.: Nitrogen fixation: research efforts intensify, Science **185:**132, 1974.

McLean, D. M.: Sewage irrigation: health benefit or hazard? Ann. Intern. Med. **82:**112, 1975.

Milk Ordinance and Code—1953 Recommendations of the Public Health Service, U.S.P.H.S. Bull. no. 229, Washington, D.C., 1953, U.S. Government Printing Office.

Mitchell, R., editor: Water pollution microbiology, New York, 1972, John Wiley & Sons, Inc.

Nickerson, W. J.: Microbial degradation and transformation of wastes, ASM News **38:**367, 1972.

Oser, B. L.: How safe are the chemicals in our food? Today's Health **44:**61, March, 1966.

Pace, W. E.: Microbiological aspects of food irradiation, Milit. Med. **134:**215, 1969.

Porter, J. R.: Microbiology and the disposal of solid wastes, ASM News **40:**826, 1974.

Porter, J. R.: Microbiology and the food and energy crisis, ASM News **40:**813, 1974.

Price, J. F., and Schweigert, B. S., editors: The science of meat and meat products, ed. 2, San Francisco, 1971, W. H. Freeman & Co.

Reimann, H., editor: Food-borne infections and intoxications, New York, 1969, Academic Press, Inc.

Rhodes, A., and Fletcher, D. L.: Principles of industrial microbiology, Elmsford, N. Y., 1967, Pergamon Press, Inc.

Rodina, A. G.: Methods in aquatic microbiology (edited, translated, and revised by Colwell, R. R., and Zambruski, M. S.), Baltimore, 1972, University Park Press.

Rose, A. H.: Industrial microbiology, Washington, D.C., 1961, Butterworth, Inc.

Schwartz, W. F.: Communities strike back, Am. J. Nurs. **71:**724, 1971.

Shea, K. P.: Infectious cure, Environment **13:**43, (Jan.-Feb.), 1971.

Sieburth, J. M.: Microbial seascapes, Baltimore, 1975, University Park Press.

Smith, E. H.: Fluoridation of water supply, J.A.M.A. **230:** 1569, 1974.

Snyder, J.: About the meat you are buying, Today's Health **49:**38, Dec., 1971.

Standard methods for the examination of dairy products, ed. 13, Washington, D.C., 1967, American Public Health Association, Inc.

Standard methods for the examination of water and wastewater, ed. 13, Washington, D.C., 1971, American Public Health Association, Inc.

Thomas, W. C., Jr., and others: Iodine disinfection of water, Arch. Environ. Health **19:**124, 1969.

Udall, S. L., and Stansbury, J.: Sewage: our most neglected resource (editorial), Ann. Intern. Med. **81:**849, 1974.

Wade, N.: Insect viruses: a new class of pesticides, Science **181:**925, 1973.

Zeikus, J. G., and Ward, J. C.: Methane formation in living trees: a microbial origin, Science **184:**1181, 1974.

# CHAPTER 36

# Biologic products for immunization*

The two terms *vaccine* and *immune serum* are often confused, any product of this nature being spoken of as a "serum." Vaccines and immune serums differ in fundamental properties, method of production, and resultant type of immunity.

A *vaccine* is the causative agent of a disease (bacterium, toxin, rickettsia, virus, or other microbe) so modified as to be incapable of producing the disease yet at the same time so little changed that it is able, when introduced into the body, to elicit the production of specific antibodies against the disease. Vaccines are always antigens; therefore they always produce active immunity. They find their greatest usefulness in the *prevention* of disease. Important vaccines are those for the prevention of typhoid fever, smallpox, poliomyelitis, diphtheria, tetanus, and rabies.

An *immune serum* is the serum of an animal (or man) that has been immunized against a given infectious disease. Its salient feature pertains to the antibodies it contains. Immune serums confer passive immunity; this immunity results from their antibodies, which do *not* stimulate further antibody production. Both vaccines and immune serums are specific in their action; that is, they induce immunity to no disease except the one for which they are prepared. Immune serums are of two types: antitoxic and antimicrobial.

## Immune serums (passive immunization)

**Antitoxins.** Antitoxins are immune serums that neutralize toxins. They may be prepared artificially, and they also develop in the body as the result of repeated slight infections. This is why some adults are immune to diphtheria. Antitoxins have no action

on the bacteria that produce the toxins. For example, diphtheria antitoxin neutralizes diphtheria toxin in the tissues and body fluids but has no effect on the diphtheria bacilli growing in the throat and producing the toxin. Neutralization of the circulating toxin in the body does favor the defense mechanisms operating to eliminate the membrane formed in the throat, however.

*Preparation.* Antitoxins can be successfully prepared only against exotoxins. The antitoxins that have been used longest and have saved most lives are those against diphtheria and tetanus toxins. Both are prepared in the same general way. The bacteria are grown in a liquid culture until the medium contains a large amount of exotoxin. The bacilli are then separated from the medium and its toxin content. It is necessary to determine the strength of each lot of toxin or antitoxin because two lots prepared exactly alike seldom have the same strength.

The unit of toxin is the *minimum lethal dose* (*MLD*). It is the amount of toxin that when injected into a test animal, will kill it within a prescribed time. For diphtheria toxin it is the amount that will kill a guinea pig weighing 250 gm. in 4 days, and for tetanus toxin it is the amount that will kill a 350 gm. guinea pig in the same length of time.* To determine the MLD, one begins with a very small dose and gives increasing amounts of toxin to a series of guinea pigs. The animals receiving small doses may not be affected or else become but slightly ill and recover; those receiving larger doses become ill, and some may die, but it is more than 4 days before death occurs. Finally, an animal receiving a still larger dose dies on the fourth day. The amount of toxin given this animal contains 1 MLD.

When the toxin is found to be of suitable strength,

---

*In this chapter are presented the biologic products that have been standardized and are available. The administration of certain of these for the production of a passive immunity is given. In the next chapter are recommended schedules for the production of active immunity.

---

*Tetanus toxin is so potent a poison that 1 ml. of a broth culture of tetanus bacilli may contain enough toxin to kill 75,000 guinea pigs.

horses* are immunized with it. First, a small dose is used; it is increased at each of several successive injections. The first dose may be preceded by an injection of antitoxin. At the time that experience has shown antitoxin production to be at its height, the horse is bled, and the antitoxin strength of its serum is tested. If the serum is found to contain sufficient antitoxin, it is further refined and purified for use. Refining serves to (1) concentrate the antitoxin and (2) eliminate horse serum protein. Horse proteins can sensitize the recipient of the antitoxin. If an immune serum is given the second time to a sensitized person, anaphylactic shock may result. It is *not* the antibodies in antitoxins and other immune serums that lead to allergic manifestations but the *serum protein* of the animal used in preparing the immune serum.

*Standardization.* There are three methods of standardizing antitoxins: (1) animal protection tests, (2) skin reactions, and (3) flocculation tests. We shall briefly describe how diphtheria antitoxin is standardized by determining its protective action against diphtheria toxin in a susceptible animal. First, there are certain definitions to be understood.

1. *Standard antitoxin*—an antitoxin of known strength prepared, stored, and distributed according to precise specifications
2. *Unit of antitoxin*—an amount of antitoxin equivalent to 1 unit of standard antitoxin†
3. *L+ dose* of diphtheria toxin—an amount of toxin that when combined with 1 unit of antitoxin, causes the death of a 250 gm. guinea pig on the fourth day

Different amounts of diphtheria toxin are mixed with 1 unit of standard diphtheria antitoxin, and the mixtures are injected into 250 gm. guinea pigs. The L+ dose of toxin as thus determined is mixed with different amounts of the antitoxin being tested. These are injected into 250 gm. guinea pigs, and the mixture that causes the death of a guinea pig on the fourth day obviously contains 1 unit of antitoxin. Tetanus antitoxin is standardized in much the same manner as diphtheria antitoxin, but different amounts of antitoxin and toxin are used. Botulism and gas gangrene antitoxins are standardized in a similar manner, but the mouse is the test animal.

Standardization of antitoxins by skin reactions is based on the same underlying principles as standardization by animal protection tests. The toxin and antitoxin are injected into the skin of rabbits or guinea pigs. The production of a skin reaction by this method has the same significance as the death of a guinea pig in the guinea pig antitoxin-toxin injection method.

The flocculation method depends on perceptible flocculation in a test tube when antitoxin and toxin are brought together in certain proportions.

Since antitoxin can be successfully prepared only against the few organisms producing extracellular toxins, the number of antitoxins is limited. Generally speaking, all antitoxins should be given *early* in the disease and in *sufficient amount* because they cannot repair injury already done.

*Listing of antitoxins.* Botulinum Antitoxin, Trivalent (Equine), types A, B, and E, is a refined and concentrated preparation distributed and stored by the Center for Disease Control in Atlanta, Georgia.* It is given to prevent damage from toxin not already taken up by the central nervous system. Therefore it is of value when given before manifestations have appeared but of little effect after that time. Antitoxin against one type of *Clostridium botulinum* is ineffective against the toxin of the other types. Therefore, to be therapeutically expedient, antitoxin must be available against toxins of the A, B, and E types of bacilli, the ones that cause disease in man.

Before he receives antitoxin, the individual must be *skin tested*—about 15% of persons receiving the antitoxin show allergic reactions. For the treatment of botulism it is best to give large doses early, with the first one given intravenously and an additional dose intramuscularly. More antitoxin is given in 2 to 4 hours if indicated. For prophylaxis in an individual who has consumed suspect food, antitoxin is given intramuscularly, and the individual watched for signs of botulism.

*Diphtheria antitoxin* (Purified, Concentrated Globulin, Equine) is a therapeutic agent that has given possibly more brilliant results than any other. By its use, much suffering has been prevented and many lives saved. In the production of diphtheria antitoxin in horses, toxoid has replaced diphtheria toxin as the immunizing agent. Refinements in manufacture give a diphtheria antitoxin that contains more than 5000 units per milliliter and is less likely to trigger serum reactions than antitoxins previously manufactured, since in production a very high proportion of the horse serum protein is removed.

---

*In a few instances cattle are used instead of horses.

†This definition is used instead of the original definition of Ehrlich—the amount of antitoxin required to neutralize 100 MLD of toxin—since toxin also contains variable quantities of toxoid. Although toxoid has no disease-producing capacity, it can combine with antitoxin. Different lots of antitoxin tested against different lots of toxin therefore have different strengths. The standard antitoxin unit used in the United States contains sufficient antitoxin to neutralize 100 MLD of the particular toxin that Ehrlich used originally in establishing his unit of antitoxin.

---

See also p. 231.

Diphtheria antitoxin is *not* effective against toxin that has combined with the body cells, and no amount of antitoxin given late in the disease can repair injury already done. For best results, the disease must be recognized early, and sufficient antitoxin must be given at once. After subcutaneous administration the antitoxin content of the blood does not reach its maximum for 72 hours. Injections must therefore be made *intravenously* (or intramuscularly).

The Committee on Infectious Diseases of the American Academy of Pediatrics *insists* that antitoxin be given as soon as the clinical diagnosis of diphtheria is made, with *no delay* even in waiting for bacteriologic results. The site of the membrane, the degree of toxicity, and the length of illness are much more reliable guidelines for determining the dose of diphtheria antitoxin than the weight and age of the patient. (Children and adults receive the same doses.) The Committee's schedule for the administration of diphtheria antitoxin is given in Table 36-1.

*Note:* When diphtheria antitoxin is given, the possibility of a *serum reaction* must always be kept in mind. This is especially true when antitoxin is given *intravenously*. Preliminary testing for serum hypersensitivity is mandatory.

Although penicillin G and erythromycin have no effect on the toxin of *Corynebacterium diphtheriae,* they attack the organism itself. The administration of these antibiotics is a valuable adjunct to serum therapy, never a substitute. It reduces the number of secondary invaders, decreases the severity and length of the illness, and helps to eliminate carriers.

*Tetanus antitoxin* (TAT) or *antitetanic serum* (ATS) is a product usually obtained from horses, but it may also be produced in cattle. Although patients have undoubtedly benefited by the use of tetanus antitoxin, in the person allergic to horse serum there is a real hazard in its use. *Tetanus immune globulin*

*(human)* (TIG) or *antitetanus globulin* (ATG) is prepared from the blood of persons actively immunized with tetanus toxoid. As a gamma globulin fraction of a hyperimmunized human being, it contains antitoxin without any foreign protein. Table 36-2 compares the human antitoxin with that of animal origin.

If the tetanus-susceptible wound is seen immediately after injury and if it can be adequately cared for by standard surgical technics and antibiotics, most authorities believe that the risk involved in giving equine or bovine tetanus antitoxin is not justified regardless of the immune status of the patient. On the other hand, if the patient delays seeking medical attention for a day or more or if the wound is one in which adequate surgical care is impossible because of its extent and nature, protection must be given to nonimmunized persons and to those patients who have failed to take their tetanus booster in the preceding 5 years.

*Gas gangrene antitoxin* is prepared against the organisms important in causing gas gangrene. Its value is questioned. Many surgeons do not give it.

**Antivenins.** Antivenins have been prepared against the venoms of snakes and the black widow spider. They are prepared in the same general way as antitoxins, that is, by immunization of a horse with serial doses of the venom of a snake or the spider. Antivenins may be prepared against a single species of snake or against a group of closely related species. Whether snake antivenin is prepared against a species or a group of species depends on the geographic location in which it is to be used. North America antisnakebite serum (also known as Antivenin [Crotalidae] and *Crotalus* antitoxin) is effective against rattlesnakes, copperheads, and cottonmouth moccasins, the most common poisonous snakes of North America. It is not effective against the venom of the coral snake. To combat the potent poison of the North American coral

## Table 36-1
Administration of antitoxin in diphtheria*

| DURATION OF ILLNESS† | 48 HOURS | | OVER 48 HOURS | |
|---|---|---|---|---|
| Lesions | Throat and larynx | Membrane in nasopharynx | Brawny swelling of neck | Extensive disease (3+ days) |
| Dose of antitoxin (units) | 20,000 to 40,000 | 40,000 to 60,000 | 80,000 to 120,000 | 80,000 to 120,000 |
| Route of administration ‡ | 1. Intravenously or 2. Intravenously up to one half; rest intramuscularly | Intravenously | Intravenously | Intravenously |

*Recommendations (1974) of the Committee on Infectious Diseases of the American Academy of Pediatrics.

†For prophylaxis, 1000 to 5000 units of antitoxin are given to the Schick-positive individual exposed.

‡Preferred route is intravenous (after eye and skin tests for hypersensitivity) to neutralize toxin rapidly. If patient reacts to antitoxin, desensitization is indicated.

**Table 36-2**
Evaluation of biologic products for passive immunization in tetanus

| POINT OF COMPARISON | TETANUS ANTITOXIN (TAT) | |
| --- | --- | --- |
| | EQUINE OR BOVINE* | HUMAN (TETANUS IMMUNE GLOBULIN—TIG) |
| Comparative effectiveness | Less effective | More effective, 10:1 |
| Dosage | Usual—3000 to 6000 units† | Usual adult dose—250 to 500 units |
| Duration of protective levels of antitoxin in recipient | 5 days | Up to 30 days (detectable levels reported to 14 weeks) |
| Danger of allergic reaction | Present; estimated 6% to 7% or more | Remote |
| Cost | Less expensive | More expensive |
| Evaluation | Not advocated if human product available | Recommended in allergic persons and generally |

*The majority of persons sensitive to horse serum are also sensitive to bovine serum.
†Recommendations vary as to administration of tetanus antitoxin.

snake, licensed antivenin (North American coral snake [*Micrurus fulvius*] Antivenin [Equine origin]) is distributed to state and local health departments through the Center for Disease Control, Atlanta.

The use of antivenin in snakebite or black widow bite should in no way replace first aid and supportive measures.

**Antibacterial serums.** Before the discovery of the antimicrobial compounds, antibacterial serums played an important part in the treatment of various infections. Among such were those against meningococci (antimeningococcal serum) and pneumococci (antipneumococcal serum). Most of these were prepared by injecting horses with the given bacteria. Rabbits were employed in the manufacture of antipneumococcal serum, and a specific serum for each known type of pneumococcus was prepared. A serum against *Haemophilus influenzae*, type b, has been prepared by injecting rabbits with the bacilli and was formerly used in the treatment of meningitis caused by *Haemophilus influenzae*, type b. Antipertussis serum has been prepared by injecting rabbits with *Bordetella pertussis* and its products. This serum has been used with success in very young children to prevent the disease in those exposed (when given early enough) and to decrease the severity of the established disease.

Antibacterial serums act to destroy bacteria. It is thought that they combine with a surface antigen, thereby rendering the bacteria more susceptible to leukocytes.

A serum that acts on several strains of bacteria is *polyvalent*, one that acts on only one strain, *univalent*. Today the treatment of disease processes with antibacterial serums has almost completely been supplanted by sulfonamide and antibiotic therapy.

**Antiviral serums.** The best known antiviral serum is *antirabies hyperimmune serum*. It is prepared by injecting horses with rabies virus. (In any serum of equine origin there is always the danger of an anaphylactic reaction or severe serum sickness.) Its purpose is to establish an immunity directly after exposure and to provide a passive immunity until an active one can be established by vaccination. See Table 37-2 (p. 413) for the recommendations of the World Health Organization.

For passive immunization in rabies, an effective human antiserum, rabies immune globulin of human origin (RIGH) has been developed, but as yet its availability is limited.

**Convalescent serum.** Convalescent serum therapy consists of the injection of the whole blood or serum of a person *recently* recovered from a disease into one ill of the disease (as a therapeutic measure) or into one exposed to the disease (as a preventive measure). By this method the blood of the convalescent patient containing antibodies confers a passive immunity on the recipient. This type of therapy has been used with good results in measles, whooping cough, and scarlet fever.

*Adult immune serum* is the serum from a person who had the disease (example: measles) many years previously. The serum of an adult recently vaccinated against the disease helps to prevent infection in those exposed and to reduce the severity of disease in those already ill. *Hyperimmune human antipertussis serum* (prepared by giving pertussis vaccine to a person who has recovered from the disease) has been used successfully in the treatment of whooping cough.

*Caution should be observed in giving convalescent serum or any human serum because it may transmit viral hepatitis.*

**Gamma globulin.** Gamma globulin is the one of several fractions of the globulin of blood plasma with which antibodies are associated. It is prepared com-

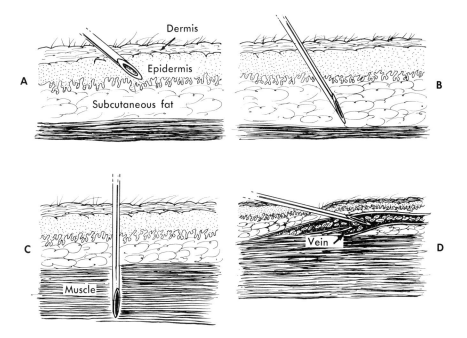

**Fig. 36-1.** Routes of injection, diagrammatic sketches. Note position and depth of needle. **A,** Intradermal. **B,** Subcutaneous. **C,** Intramuscular. **D,** Intravenous.

mercially by a series of precipitations in pooled normal adult plasma, in venous blood, or in pooled extracts of human placentas, with varying concentrations of alcohol at a low temperature. The gamma globulin fraction removed is more than forty times as rich in antibodies as the original plasma from which it is taken. Five hundred milliliters of blood yields an average dose.

Gamma globulin, usually dispensed as *immune serum globulin (human) (ISG),* is emphasized as indicated in Table 36-3. Gamma globulin is always given *intramuscularly—never intravenously.** (See Fig. 36-1.) As ordinarily given, gamma globulin is one of the benign injectables, being associated with few side reactions.

## Vaccines (active immunization)

**Bacterial vaccines.** Bacterial vaccines are suspensions of killed bacteria in isotonic sodium chloride solution. After culture for 24 to 48 hours, the bacterial growth is emulsified in sterile saline solution, and the number of bacteria in each milliliter of the washings is determined. Isotonic sodium chloride solution is added until the desired number per milliliter is obtained. The bacteria are then killed at the lowest possible lethal temperature in the shortest possible time. Without heat, they may be killed by formalin, cresol,

or Merthiolate. In some vaccines the bacteria are killed by ultraviolet light. Cultures are made from the finished product to ensure its sterility. Vaccines are usually prepared so that the number of dead microbes given at a single injection ranges from 100 million to 1 billion.

Bacterial vaccines are of two types: *stock,* made from stock cultures maintained in the laboratory, and *autogenous,* made from organisms of a specific lesion in the patient for whom the vaccine is made. A *mixed* vaccine is one containing bacteria belonging to two or more species. A *polyvalent vaccine* contains several strains of organisms belonging to the same species, for instance, one containing several strains of *Pseudomonas aeruginosa.* Bacterial vaccines show their best results in the prevention of typhoid fever, whooping cough, and plague.

Prompted by the growing resistance of bacteria to standard antibiotics, researchers are presently concentrating on the development of bacterial vaccines. As improvements in laboratory technology have come and as more is learned of the mechanisms of host immunity and how bacteria cause disease, they are accomplishing more. Major bacterial antigens, both polysaccharide and protein, have been isolated, purified, and studied, and of special interest in vaccine production, certain avirulent bacterial hybrids have been formulated.

*Listing of bacterial vaccines. BCG vaccine (bacille*

---

*The consequence can be a severe shock–like state.

**Table 36-3**

Clinical value of immune serum globulin (gamma globulin) (ISG)*

| DISEASE | INDICATIONS | PREPARATION |
|---|---|---|
| Measles† | Modification of symptoms after vaccination; use only with Edmonston live virus vaccine | Immune serum globulin (human) |
| | Prevention: | |
| | 1. Children with normal immune mechanisms | Immune serum globulin (human) |
| | 2. Children with immune system disorder | Immune serum globulin (human) |
| | Modification | Immune serum globulin (human) |
| Rubella‡ | Prevention only in female in first trimester of pregnancy | Immune serum globulin (human) |
| Varicella (chickenpox) | Modification | Immune serum globulin (human) |
| Immunologic deficiency syndromes (agammaglobulinemia, hypogammaglobulinemia, dysgammaglobulinemia)§ | Replacement therapy | Immune serum globulin |
| Rh hemolytic disease | Prevention | $Rh_0$ (D) immune globulin (human)‖ (Ortho) |
| Mumps | Prevention | Mumps immune globulin (human) (Cutter) |
| Poliomyelitis‡ | Prevention | Immune serum globulin (human) |
| Viral hepatitis type B (serum) | Prevention (value undetermined) | Immune serum globulin (human) |
| Viral hepatitis type A (infectious) | Prevention or modification in children or adults | |
| | 1. Short-term, moderate risk | Immune serum globulin (human) |
| | 2. Long-term, intense exposure | |
| | Prophylaxis (in institutions) | |
| Pertussis‡ | Prevention in infants under 2 years | Pertussis immune serum globulin (human) (Cutter) |
| | Treatment | |

*Compiled from the 1975 Physicians' Desk Reference, Oradell, N.J., 1974, Medical Economics, Inc., and the 1974 Red Book of the American Acade▪ been prepared.
†See also p. 415 for schedule of measles vaccination.
‡See also Chapter 37.
§See also p. 109 for discussion.
‖Rh immune globulin (RhoGAM) is discussed on p. 113.

| DOSE | SCHEDULE | ROUTE | COMMENTS |
|---|---|---|---|
| 0.04 ml./kg. body weight | One dose | Intramuscular | Inject measles vaccine in one arm, this in other |
| 0.25 ml./kg. body weight | | | Inject within 6 days of exposure; give live virus vaccine in 8 or more weeks |
| 20 to 30 ml. | | | |
| 0.05 ml./kg. body weight | | | Give within 6 days, if possible (rarely indicated) |
| 0.25 to 0.44 ml./kg. body weight (20 ml. total advised by some) | One dose | Intramuscular | Subject controversial |
| 0.6 to 1.2 ml./kg. body weight (20 to 30 ml. total sometimes advised) | | Intramuscular | Give within 3 days of exposure; may decrease severity of illness |
| 0.66 ml./kg. every 3 to 4 weeks Double dose at onset of therapy | One dose a month | Intramuscular | Maximum dose 20 to 30 ml. at any one time; gamma globulin deficiency here; adequate levels must be supplied to protect against infections |
| One vial | | Intramuscular | Give to nonsensitized Rh-negative mothers after delivery of Rh-positive infant or after abortion |
| 2.5 to 7.5 ml. | One dose | Intramuscular | Efficiency not known |
| 0.3 ml./kg. body weight | One dose (second dose can be given 5 weeks after first) | Intramuscular | Possible protection for 2 to 6 weeks if given before exposure or development of symptoms |
| 10 ml. | One dose within 1 week after transfusion; one dose (10 ml.) 1 month later | Intramuscular | For adults—not recommended for children; recommended for high-risk adults only; give right after transfusion |
| 0.02 to 0.04 ml./kg. body weight | One (repeat in 3 to 5 months if necessary) | Intramuscular | Give within 1 week of exposure |
| 0.06 ml./kg. body weight | One (repeat in 5 to 6 months if necessary) | | |
| 0.06 to 0.10 ml./kg. body weight | One (repeat in 5 months) | | Protection for 1 year |
| 1.5 ml. | One dose (repeat in 5 to 7 days) | Intramuscular | Product from donors hyperimmunized with pertussis vaccine; protection not reliable |
| 1.25 ml. | One dose every day for three to five doses; or 3 to 6.75 ml. at once | | Use larger doses with severe disease |

of Pediatrics. Diphtheria immune (human) globulin, zoster immune globulin (ZIG), and rabies immune globulin of human origin (HRIG) have also

*Continued.*

**Table 36-3**
Clinical value of immune serum globulin (gamma globulin) (ISG)—cont'd

| DISEASE | INDICATIONS | PREPARATION |
|---------|-------------|-------------|
| Tetanus‡ | Prevention—children and adults | Tetanus immune globulin (human) (Parke-Davis) |
| | Treatment | |
| Vaccinia-smallpox‡ | Prevention | Vaccinia immune globulin (human) (VIG) (Center for Disease Control) |
| | Protection of children | |
| | Treatment | |

*Calmette-Guérin* is made from a strain of bovine tubercle bacilli cultivated on artificial media (containing bile) for so long that they have completely lost their virulence for man. In the United States freeze-dried BCG vaccine is available in two concentrations, the higher for use in the multiple puncture technic, and the lower for intradermal inoculation. Administered orally or intradermally, BCG vaccine is given *only to persons with a negative tuberculin test.* The immunity induced lasts over a considerable number of years.

Being tested experimentally is a BCG vaccine aerosol. Persons to be vaccinated breathe in vaccine droplets suspended in a manmade mist for some 45 minutes or so.

BCG vaccine has been used extensively in European countries to immunize children. The World Health Organization in recent years has vaccinated over 250 million persons with BCG. This has been an especially worthwhile program in parts of the world where the incidence of tuberculosis is high. In the United States where the prevalence rate of tuberculosis is low, BCG vaccination, a controversial issue for nearly 50 years, has not been used widely. The U.S. Public Health Service recommends it only for those tuberculin-negative individuals in close contact with known, untreated cases of tuberculosis.

*Cholera vaccine* given to the military personnel of the U.S. Armed Forces sent to duty in cholera-endemic areas contains 8 billion killed vibrios per milliliter. Cholera vaccine is toxic and must be injected at frequent intervals to maintain immunity. A new oral vaccine that contains killed vibrios in water is being tested. It can be given daily and induces antibody formation in the intestinal tract, the actual site of involvement in the disease. Another new vaccine, a cholera toxoid (inactivated cholera toxin), will soon be available.

*Pertussis vaccine* is a saline suspension of the killed organisms. Pertussis vaccine is commonly prepared and used in the alum-precipitated and the aluminum hydroxide– and aluminum phosphate–adsorbed forms in combination with diphtheria and tetanus toxoids. Severe neurologic reactions rarely complicate administration of pertussis vaccine.

*Plague vaccine* of the U.S. Armed Forces contains 2 billion killed plague bacilli per milliliter.

*Tularemia vaccine, live, attenuated* is a lyophilized, viable, weakened variant of *Francisella tularensis.* Tularemia vaccine has also been prepared by the U.S. Army as an inhalant-type vaccine. Large numbers of persons can be vaccinated against this disease simply by marching through a room containing vaccine droplets in the atmosphere. The interest of the military in this disease stems from its possibilities in bacteriologic warfare. Airborne immunization is being evaluated experimentally in other diseases transmitted by droplet infection. *Foshay's tularemia vaccine* is made of killed organisms and produces an immunity that lasts about 1 year.

*Typhoid vaccine* for the U.S. Armed Forces is an acetone-inactivated dried strain of *Salmonella typhi* (the AKD vaccine). An oral vaccine containing live attenuated typhoid bacilli is being tested. The U.S. Public Health Service discredits paratyphoid A and B vaccines as immunizing agents and has implicated them in reactions following administration of mixed vaccines.

**Toxin-antitoxin.** A mixture of diphtheria toxin and antitoxin with a small excess of the former, *diphtheria toxin-antitoxin* has been used to produce permanent active (not passive) immunity to diphtheria. Toxin-antitoxin is unstable and may be toxic. Manufacturers have discontinued it.

**Toxoids.** *Botulinum toxoid,* an effective pentavalent preparation available for active immunization

| DOSE | SCHEDULE | ROUTE | COMMENTS |
|---|---|---|---|
| 250 to 1,500 units | One dose | Intramuscular | Product from person hyperimmunized with tetanus toxoid |
| 5,000 to 20,000 units | May be repeated 1 month later | | Active immunization should be started with tetanus toxoid |
| 0.3 ml./kg. body weight | One dose | Intramuscular | Product from blood collected from military recruits 3 to 4 weeks after reaction to smallpox vaccination |
| 0.6 ml./kg. body weight | | | |

against botulism, incorporates aluminum phosphate–adsorbed toxoids (see below) for the antitoxins of *Clostridium botulinum,* types A, B, C, D, and E. It is given in three spaced injections followed by a booster to laboratory workers at risk.

*Diphtheria toxoid* is diphtheria toxin detoxified so that it cannot cause diphtheria but can induce the formation of specific antitoxin. Formalin, 0.2% to 0.4%, is added to diphtheria toxin, and the mixture incubated at 37° C. until detoxication is complete (several weeks). This treatment, used with other bacterial toxins as well, reduces toxicity but preserves the antigenic properties of toxin. After purification to remove inert protein, the preparation is available as *plain* or *fluid toxoid.* (Fluid toxoids are used in the United Kingdom and Canada.)

Alum added to diphtheria toxoid precipitates the antigenic portion. The precipitate, after being washed and suspended in sterile physiologic saline solution, is *diphtheria toxoid, alum precipitated.* Its advantage is that the alum is not absorbed but remains at the site of injection. The toxoid slowly separates from it to give a prolonged antigenic stimulation. If aluminum hydroxide or aluminum phosphate is added to the liquid toxoid, the antigenic portion adheres to the particles of the aluminum compound. This process is known as *adsorption,* and diphtheria toxoid so treated is known as *aluminum hydroxide–* or *aluminum phosphate-adsorbed diphtheria toxoid* (depot toxoid or antigen). Its properties are similar to those of the alum-precipitated toxoid. Diphtheria toxoid should not be given to a person more than 10 to 12 years of age without preliminary sensitivity tests.

*Tetanus toxoid* establishes permanent immunity to tetanus. It is manufactured in the liquid (or fluid), alum-precipitated, aluminum hydroxide–adsorbed, and aluminum phosphate–adsorbed forms.

Most manufacturers market mixtures of diphtheria and tetanus toxoids (DT), or mixtures of diphtheria and tetanus toxoids and pertussis vaccine (DTP). Combinations are available in the unconcentrated, alum-precipitated, aluminum hydroxide–adsorbed, and aluminum phosphate–adsorbed forms. They have proved to be very satisfactory.

**Viral vaccines.** With the exception of the antibiotics, nothing has done more to protect us against infection than has the unborn chick. Viral vaccines have been possible largely because of the development of modern technics for cultivating viruses in embryonated hen's eggs and also in cell cultures, thus furnishing the large supply of virus essential to the production of vaccines. In chick embryos or in cell cultures, cultivation of a virus involving multiple transfers from one medium to another (serial passage) can alter the organism's capacity to produce disease. A normally virulent virus can thus be *attenuated* (weakened) or domesticated. Fortunately with loss of virulence there is *no* loss of antigenicity. This makes possible the production of very effective vaccines.

In a killed or *inactivated* virus vaccine the infectivity of the virus and its ability to reproduce have been destroyed by physical or chemical means, but its capacity to induce antibody formation has been preserved. Formalin is a standard inactivating agent. Killed virus vaccines must be injected in several doses, but live virus vaccines can be taken orally or inhaled (as an aerosol).

Virologists have long preferred living agents to killed or inactivated viruses for vaccines. A living agent continues to multiply in the body of the animal or man to which it is given and thus exerts a prolonged and increasingly strong stimulation to the host to make antibodies. The immunity so produced is stronger and longer lasting because the presence of the live virus simulates actual infection. The possi-

**403**

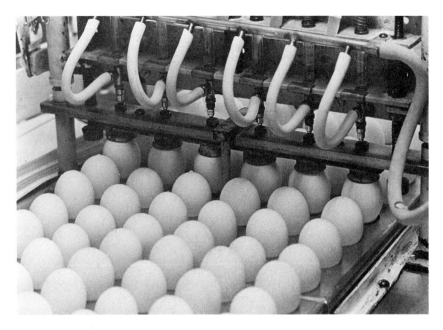

**Fig. 36-2.** Influenza vaccine, commercial production. Virus is being injected into fertile hen eggs along assembly line. (Courtesy Eli Lilly & Co., Indianapolis.)

bility that the virus will revert to its original level of pathogenicity in the vaccinated person is an obvious disadvantage to the use of the living agent. Live viral vaccines are well known in veterinary medicine. The two best known in human medicine are the measles vaccine and the live poliovirus vaccine, Sabin-type strains.

*Listing of viral vaccines. Adenovirus vaccine* has been prepared by the formalin and ultraviolet inactivation of viral types grown on monkey kidney cells. Because of the discovery that some of the *inactivated* adenovirus serotypes produced tumors in experimental animals, active immunization with these agents is suspended. Trials with *live* adenovirus types 4 and 7 vaccine given orally in an enteric-coated tablet are in operation, since live adenoviruses presumably have no capacity to cause cancers.

*Influenza vaccine* is prepared from virus grown in the fertile hen's egg, inactivated with formalin, and concentrated (Fig. 36-2).

The Bureau of Biologics, Food and Drug Administration, regularly reviews the formulation of influenza vaccines, suggesting changes as needed to take in the strains expected to cause trouble during the next flu season. Usually the strains of recent epidemics are known, and the most practical arrangement from year to year seems to be one wherein two strains recently implicated are placed in a bivalent vaccine. It is thought that a bivalent vaccine with greater

amounts of antigen is preferable to a polyvalent one containing smaller amounts of four or five strains. In the event that a large-scale epidemic is anticipated, a monovalent vaccine might be indicated.

The peculiar ability of influenza viruses to change their antigenic structure from time to time poses a problem to the manufacturer of flu vaccines. A strain against which there is no protection in an existing polyvalent vaccine can easily emerge. Great care must be taken that strains containing a wide pattern of antigenic substances are selected for vaccine production.

The production of active immunity by influenza virus vaccine has met with considerable success. However, the immunity is short-lived, the vaccine sometimes gives fairly severe reactions, and the subject can become sensitized to egg protein, as well as react to a previously existing sensitivity. Highly purified vaccines with most of the egg protein eliminated are being made available.

A viral hybrid influenza vaccine is ready for field trials; its effect is to inhibit the surface antigen, neuraminidase, thus limiting but not preventing viral replication. It is an aerosol vaccine.

*Measles vaccines* recommended for use are either (1) the *attenuated live virus vaccine* (Edmonston B vaccine) prepared from chick embryo or canine renal cell cultures of the Edmonston B strain of the measles virus (developed by John F. Enders and associates) or (2) the *live virus vaccines* (Edmonston strains) which have been further attenuated by additional chick embryo passages (the *further attenuated vaccines* of Schwarz and Moraten). Live virus vaccines give permanent protection. Inactivated virus vaccines are in disrepute. *Note:* Measles vaccines must be carefully refrigerated.

*Mumps vaccine* is an attenuated live virus vaccine adapted to the chick embryo and given in a single injection. The vaccine contains egg proteins and a small quantity of neomycin. Routine administration of mumps vaccine is contraindicated before puberty. At the present time, it is believed best to let the younger child develop his own immunity. The duration of protection afforded by the mumps vaccine is at least 4 years.

*Salk poliomyelitis vaccine* is prepared by growing all three types of poliomyelitis virus separately in tissue cultures on the kidney cells of rhesus monkeys. The viral suspensions are filtered to remove cells and other particles. Formaldehyde is added or ultraviolet irradiation used to inactivate the virus. In the last step of production the three suspensions are mixed. Salk vaccine is a highly effective vaccine judged to be 90% preventive.

*Sabin poliomyelitis vaccine* is prepared with the three types of attenuated live poliovirus grown in human (not monkey) cell culture. After the vaccine has been fed to an individual, the virus of the vaccine multiplies in the lining and in the lymphoid tissue of the alimentary tract. A satisfactory immune response from the vaccinated person occurs usually within 7 to 10 days. The implantation of the virus in the bowel blocks further infection by the same type of a wild poliovirus. This materially cuts down on the number of carriers. The fear that competition from other enteroviruses might check growth of the poliovirus in the intestinal tract has been largely obliterated by studies of children in the tropics. Their alimentary tracts swarm with viruses, and yet they show antibody responses indicating growth of poliovirus. To minimize possible interference from other enteric viruses, it is recommended that the oral vaccine be given during the spring and winter months in temperate climates.

The chief disadvantage of the Sabin vaccine is that it is difficult to preserve. It can be kept frozen for years but *only for 7 days in an ordinary refrigerator* and *3 days at room temperature!* Tap water cannot be used to dilute the vaccine since *the contained chlorine destroys the poliovirus.* Like other vaccines manufactured on monkey kidney cells, the final preparation contains traces of penicillin and streptomycin from the cell culture medium. The overall effectiveness of the Sabin vaccine is 94% to 100%.

*Rabies vaccines* are of two kinds, one made from

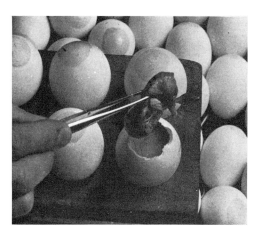

**Fig. 36-3.** Virus-laden duck embryo used for rabies vaccine. Frozen, finely ground embryonic tissue is inactivated, filtered, and dried under sterile conditions. (Courtesy Lilly Research Laboratories, Eli Lilly & Co., Indianapolis.)

nervous tissue and the other from nonnervous tissues. The first is prepared from the brain and spinal cord of rabbits suffering with rabies induced by the inoculation of fixed virus (p. 310). Just before death the brain and cord are removed under strict aseptic precautions, and the virus is inactivated. The phenol-inactivated vaccine is known as *Semple vaccine.* An emulsion is prepared by grinding the virus-containing material in water or isotonic saline solution, either during the process of inactivation or after it is complete. The fact that this vaccine contains brain and spinal cord tissue is thought to be responsible for the severe complication of encephalomyelitis that sometimes follows its administration. Probably existing on an allergic basis, complication may lead to paralysis and even death.

The other kind of rabies vaccine is free of nervous tissue. It is prepared by growing the fixed rabies virus in tissues of the embryonated duck egg (Fig. 36-3). To the suspension of embryonic duck tissue a viricidal agent, beta propiolactone, is added to inactivate the virus. The duck embryo vaccine (DEV) is dried and administered after dilution with distilled water. Because of the absence of central nervous system tissue, this vaccine is less hazardous than the one prepared from the nervous tissues of the rabbit. However, it is not quite as immunogenic. Because of the rarity of serious complications, preexposure prophylaxis with duck embryo vaccine is practical in veterinarians, animal handlers, and research workers at risk. In the United States today, 96% of rabies vaccine given is of this type.

For dogs a vaccine is grown on a series of chick embryos to reduce its virulence. Such a live virus vaccine, given in a single dose, will produce immunity of over 3 years' duration in the dog. In areas where the vampire and other bats exist it may be necessary to immunize livestock.

Currently a potent, experimental, killed-virus rabies vaccine has been grown in nonneural tissue culture. There is also work being done to minimize the amount of fat where nervous tissue is used to grow the virus.

*Rubella vaccine*, live, attenuated, exists as several preparations, three licensed and one still under investigation. One vaccine is a live virus strain originally attenuated by seventy-seven passages in green monkey kidney and then prepared in duck embryo culture. A second is the same strain prepared in dog kidney culture. The third vaccine, the Cendehill strain, was isolated in green monkey kidney and then passed fifty-one times in rabbit kidney culture. These three vaccines are effective ones. A fourth vaccine (unlicensed) has been developed in human fibroblast tissue culture.

Episodes of arthritic joint pain, found especially in the older age groups, occur with the use of the licensed vaccines, especially the dog kidney one. Although arthritis was a disturbing event when first recognized as a complication to vaccination, it has usually turned out to be mild and self-limited, without sequelae. Hypersensitivity reactions to egg protein and neomycin may occur.

*Smallpox vaccine* is prepared with cowpox (vaccinia) virus inoculated into calves or grown in the chick embryo. Female calves 6 months to 1 year old are used. After the skin of the abdomen is shaved and disinfected, it is scarified in many places, the scratches being just deep enough to bring a little blood, and cowpox virus is rubbed into these scratches. At the end of 6 days the skin of the abdomen is thickly broken out with vesicles (blisters) that contain the modified virus used for vaccination. With the most careful aseptic technic the tops of the vesicles are opened, and the sticky exudate removed. The exudate is mixed with four times its weight of glycerin and water (equal parts) containing 1% phenol for preservation. The vaccine is purified and, if found to be of sufficient potency and sterile, is ready for use. Some manufacturers add brilliant green to the vaccine to inhibit bacterial growth. They also paint the vaccinated area on the calf with this dye. This vaccine, made from the dermal lymph of the calf, is the one most widely accepted at present.

A smallpox vaccine as effective as the calf vaccine is produced by growing the vaccinia virus in bacteria-free tissues of the chick embryo. Vaccine may also be prepared by growing the virus in cell cultures.

*If smallpox vaccine is not shipped and stored at freezing temperatures, it rapidly loses its potency.* There is a lyophilized (freeze-dried) preparation that can be stored at temperatures ranging from 35° to 50° F. without losing its potency for a period of 18 months. Once this vaccine is reconstituted, it must be refrigerated.

Smallpox vaccination (see also p. 411) means infecting a person with a strain of vaccinia or cowpox virus. The viruses of cowpox and smallpox are quite similar in makeup and serologic properties. Some authorities believe that cowpox originated by the transfer of smallpox from man to the cow, with an adaptation of the virus to this animal to produce a milder disease.

*Yellow fever vaccine* is prepared by growing a strain of the virus in chick embryos. It was developed at a time when little thought was given to the avian leukosis viruses. A new strain of the virus is being tested with technics that filter out any such contaminants. It will ultimately replace the old one. For purposes of international travel, yellow fever

**Table 36-4**
Current status of common vaccines*

1. Vaccines satisfactory in:
   Diphtheria
   Measles
   Mumps
   Poliomyelitis
   Rocky Mountain spotted fever
   Rubella
   Tetanus
2. Vaccines being improved for:
   Cholera
   Influenza
   Smallpox
   Tuberculosis
   Yellow fever
3. Vaccines being developed for:
   Meningococcal meningitis
   Mycoplasma pneumonia
   Pneumococcal pneumonia
   Rabies
   Respiratory syncytial virus disease
   Shigellosis
   Streptococcal infections (group A)
4. Vaccines with improved product desired (no work in progress) for:
   Pertussis
5. Vaccines needed for:
   Varicella
   Cytomegalic inclusion disease
   Gonorrhea
   Hepatitis

*Modified from Medical World News **12:**31, Feb. 5, 1971.

vaccine must be approved by the World Health Organization and be administered at a designated Yellow Fever Vaccination Center.

**Rickettsial vaccines.** Rickettsias for vaccine production have been grown in lice, rodent lung, and cell cultures. The vaccines in use at the present time are prepared by growing the rickettsias in the yolk sac of the developing chick embryo. A vaccine so prepared is referred to as a *Cox vaccine*. Cox vaccines containing the respective rickettsias have been prepared against epidemic typhus fever, murine typhus fever, Rocky Mountain spotted fever, and Q fever. In addition, a Rocky Mountain spotted fever vaccine found to be effective has been made by grinding up the bodies of infected ticks.

Vaccination against the rickettsial diseases is advised for persons likely to contact the infectious agent because of living conditions or occupation. Protection against epidemic typhus is strongly urged for those who have been in contact with a patient. Although typhus immunization is not required by any country in the world as a condition of entry, it is nevertheless recommended to travelers when travel plans include a geographic area that is not only infected but one in which living conditions are generally poor.

**Summary.** Table 36-4 summarizes material just presented and indicates prospects for the future.

# Precautions for administration of biologic products

To ensure the development of the desired immunity and to prevent insofar as possible certain untoward side effects or complications, the following precautions in the administration of vaccines and serums are strongly advised:

1. *Read carefully the label on the package and the accompanying leaflet when any biologic product is to be given!*
2. Disinfect properly the skin at the site of injection. (Note also proper disinfection of the surface of the vial of medication.)
3. Use a sterile syringe and needle for each injection, preferably a sterile *disposable* unit. (Using several needles with the same syringe can be a way to spread viral hepatitis.)
4. When the needle is placed into the subcutaneous or intramuscular area, pull the plunger of the syringe outward to check that the needle has not inadvertently entered a vein. If it has, blood wells up in the syringe.
5. Immunize only well children. Delay any such procedure for sick children until their recovery.
6. *Anaphylactic and allergic accidents in biotherapy are unpredictable—the next one may be yours!* Carefully question the recipient of the injection as to reactions to previous doses of the same or comparable biologic products. Inquire carefully as to previous injection of horse serum, any known allergy to horse serum protein, and any history of allergic conditions such as asthma. Did the child have reactions to a previous dose, such as fever or sleeplessness? Was there an area of redness and tenderness about the injection site? If the child had only a mild reaction, the injections may be continued. In some instances the amount of the material must be reduced, and the overall number of injections increased. If the child had a severe reaction, *do not repeat* the injection. Consult the physician.
7. Ascertain the presence of allergy to egg or chicken dander if certain viral vaccines prepared in chick embryos (influenza, yellow fever, measles) are to be given. Practically speaking, if the recipient can eat eggs without event, it is safe to give the vaccine. Some of the newer vaccines may contain neomycin to which an allergic state may also exist.
8. Note these special situations:
   a. Do *not* immunize persons with altered or deficient immunologic mechanisms.
   b. Do *not* immunize persons receiving steroid hormones.
   c. Do *not* vaccinate children for smallpox who have a generalized dermatitis such as eczema, because of the danger of a generalized vaccinia. Children with skin diseases should be segregated from children being vaccinated against smallpox.
   d. Unless there is an emergency, do *not* immunize during a poliomyelitis outbreak.

**Tests for hypersensitivity.** Preliminary testing to detect hypersensitivity by all means is mandatory.

The following tests must be used discreetly, and a syringe containing 1 ml. of epinephrine 1:1000 should be handy. (See also p. 131.)

1. In the *scratch* test, a 1:10 dilution in isotonic saline solution of the biologic product (tetanus antitoxin, for example) is applied to the abraded skin.
2. In the *eye* test, one drop of a 1:10 dilution is placed in the conjunctival sac. If this is negative, the eye test may be repeated with undiluted material.
3. The *intradermal* skin test is usually carried out with 0.02 to 0.03 ml. of a 1:10 dilution. (*An intradermal test with 0.1 ml. of undiluted TAT may prove fatal.*) If indicated, skin tests may be carried out serially with 0.02 to 0.03 ml. of 1:10,000, 1:1000, 1:100, and 1:10

dilutions. The positive reaction is a hivelike wheal with redness.

4. In the *intravenous* test, the patient's blood pressure is recorded before the 5 minutes taken to inject 0.1 ml. of biologic product in 10 ml. of isotonic saline solution and every 5 minutes afterward for 30 minutes. If the blood pressure falls 20 points or more, a hypersensitive state is indicated.

**Injection site for biologic products.** The *optimal site for injection* is the outer lateral aspect of the thigh. By directing the needle downward as it enters the tissues at the junction of the upper third with the lower two-thirds, one can deliver the serum or other biologic product into the middle third of the thigh. This area is preferred because (1) in the event of an impending serum reaction a tourniquet can be placed on the thigh above the injection site and the absorption of the biologic product greatly delayed; and (2) here there are no important anatomic structures to be injured by the pressure of injected material. If speed of absorption is desired, the fascia lata, a tense band stretched across this area, facilitates it.

## Standards for biologic products

**Manufacture.** It is so important that serums, vaccines, and other biologic products, including human blood and its derivatives, meet acceptable standards of safety, purity, and potency that when offered for sale, import, or export in interstate commerce, they must be manufactured under the license and regulations of the federal government. Authority for this is delegated to the Food and Drug Administration of the United States Department of Health, Education, and Welfare.

**Label.** Each package must be properly labeled. The name, address, and license number of the manufacturer, the lot number, and expiration date must be shown.

**Date of expiration.** On the *date of issue*, the product is placed on the market. This must be within a certain time after manufacture, depending on the kind of product and the temperature of storage. The *expiration date* means the date beyond which the product cannot be expected to exert its full potency. For instance, if a package of diphtheria antitoxin has a stated potency of 10,000 units and an expiration date of Sept. 1, 1978, it means that, properly stored, the package will contain 10,000 units of diphtheria antitoxin on Sept. 1, 1978. An excess of antitoxin in the package allows for this. The expiration date of most biologic products is 1 year after manufacture or issue.

## Questions for review

1 Define vaccine, immune serum, antitoxin, antivenin, antibacterial serum, MLD, date of issue (of vaccine), expiration date (of vaccine), autogenous vaccine, lyophilized vaccine, immune serum globulin, gamma globulin.
2 Cite at least four differences between vaccines and immune serums.
3 What is the term used to designate the strength of tetanus and diphtheria antitoxins?
4 Briefly discuss the three methods of standardizing diphtheria antitoxin.
5 Name three antitoxins of importance, indicating the manufacture of one.
6 List seven diseases for which immune serum globulin may be of benefit. Indicate how gamma globulin is used to modify or prevent disease.
7 How is toxoid prepared? Name three important ones.
8 What is BCG? Comment on its usefulness.
9 Compare live virus vaccines with inactivated virus vaccines.
10 List and briefly describe the measles vaccines.
11 Name the immunizing agents used in combination.
12 How are rabies vaccines prepared?
13 List the rubella virus vaccines.
14 Give the optimal site for injection of biologic products.
15 List the tests for hypersensitivity.
16 Give precautions in the administration of biologic products.

**References on pp. 418 to 420.**

# CHAPTER 37

# Recommended immunizations

In this chapter methods of immunization for the prevention of the more important infectious diseases are given. Since opinions from public health physicians and authorizing agencies concerning the most efficacious methods of immunization are not uniform, the student will note variations in procedures endorsed in standard references.

## Recommendations of Committee on Infectious Diseases of American Academy of Pediatrics*

The Red Book of the American Academy of Pediatrics is widely accepted as a source of the best immunization procedures in both children and adults. Table 37-1 schedules the protection recommended by the Committee on Infectious Diseases for normal infants and children from 2 months of age through the sixteenth year of life (after which the immunizing procedures are those for adults).

**Combined active immunization.** In the schedule of Table 37-1, combined diphtheria and tetanus alum (depot) toxoids and *Bordetella pertussis* vaccine are preferred as primary immunizing agents over the nonadsorbed (fluid or plain) mixtures. A dose† is injected deep into the deltoid or midlateral muscles of the thigh or given by intradermal jet injection (Fig. 37-1).

The standard preparations of *combined diphtheria-tetanus toxoids (DT)* used in infants and young children contain 7 to 25 Lf. (flocculating units) diphtheria toxoid per dose. The *adult type* of *combined tetanus-diphtheria toxoids (Td)* with adjuvant used in teenagers and adults contains not more than 2 Lf. diphtheria toxoid per dose. Td contains less diphtheria antigen than DT, since fairly severe reactions in older children and adults may be associated with the increase of diphtheria antigen. Adult type toxoids are specially purified preparations.

Live oral poliovirus vaccine is recommended over the killed vaccine because it is more effective as an immunizing agent, the antibodies induced persist longer, and it is easier to give. TOPV (trivalent oral poliovirus vaccine) is the one preferred. (If monovalent virus-type feeding is carried out, the order is type 1 followed by type 3 and then type 2.)

The immunity for each disease produced by the combined method of immunization is as great as would be obtained by separate immunization against the given disease.

**Tetanus.** For individuals to whom the combined primary immunizations of early childhood do not apply, the Red Book recommends administration of alum tetanus toxoid. The total recommended dose of the manufacturer may be given in fractional doses of 0.05 or 0.1 ml. A booster (recall) injection of alum tetanus toxoid should be given 1 year later. When the child or older person sustains an injury and the wound remains clean, the Committee on Infectious Diseases believes that in a fully immunized child no booster dose is needed unless more than 10 years have elapsed since the last dose. When the child or older person incurs a contaminated wound likely to be complicated by tetanus, such as a deep puncture wound, dog bite, certain crusted or suppurating lesions, and wounds containing soil or manure, T (tetanus toxoid with adjuvant) or Td should be given regardless of the immunization status of the patient *unless* the patient is known to have received Td or T within the past 5 years. If he has, the inoculation at this time need

---

*A copy of the Red Book is obtained from the American Academy of Pediatrics, Inc., Evanston, Ill. The Academy has developed a personal immunization card, billfold size and plastic, to provide a permanent record.

†The concentration of antigens varies in various products. The package insert supplied with the vaccine should be carefully studied as to volume of dose.

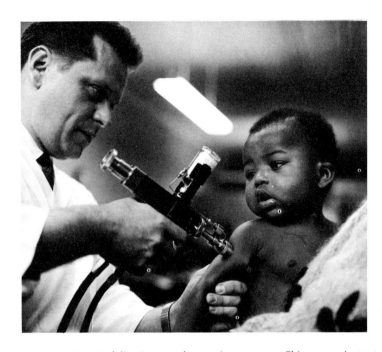

**Fig. 37-1.** Jet injector (air gun) delivering measles vaccine to young Chicagoan—instant, pain-free. This method is also used for other vaccines mentioned in text. (From Medical News, J.A.M.A. **196:** 29, May 23, 1966; courtesy American Medical Association.)

**Table 37-1**

Schedule for active immunization and tuberculin testing in normal infants and children*

| AGE | | ADMINISTRATION OF IMMUNIZING AGENTS† | | TUBERCULIN TESTING‡ |
|---|---|---|---|---|
| **MONTHS** | **YEARS** | **COMBINED VACCINES** | **OTHERS** | |
| 2 | | DTP (diphtheria and tetanus toxoids, adsorbed, and pertussis vaccine) | TOPV (trivalent oral poliovirus vaccine) | |
| 4 | | DTP | TOPV | |
| 6 | | DTP | TOPV | |
| 12 | | Measles-rubella or measles-mumps-rubella§ | Live measles vaccine (2 to 3 days after tuberculin test) | × |
| 18 | | DTP | TOPV | |
| | 4 to 6 | DTP | TOPV | |
| | 14 to 16 | Td (adult type combined tetanus-diphtheria toxoids) | | |
| | Thereafter | Td every 10 years | | |

*See also text.
†Routine smallpox vaccine no longer recommended.
‡Risk of exposure indicates frequency of tuberculin testing.
§Combined viral vaccines (single injection) can be given from ages 1 to 12.

not be given.* It has been found that the immunity conferred by tetanus toxoid is extremely long-lasting† and that frequent recall doses seem to provoke reactions.

**Pertussis.** Combined immunization as indicated in Table 36-1 is preferable, utilizing the antigens combined with adjuvant, especially when immunization is begun under the age of 6 months. Pertussis vaccine is not given beyond the age of 6 years.

When the young child has been intimately exposed to whooping cough or there is an epidemic and protective immunity must be developed as soon as possible, pertussis vaccine adsorbed should be given intramuscularly in three doses of 4 protective units each, 8 weeks apart. Routine recall injections are given 12 months later and at school age with adsorbed vaccine. Exposure recall injections indicated for children up to the age of 6 years are given with adsorbed vaccine.

**Diphtheria.** In infants and young children diphtheria toxoid is given alone *only* when there is definite reason for not using the combined immunization schedule, such as the occurrence in the child of a severe reaction following the injection of the multiple vaccines or the exposure of the child to a possible or known case of diphtheria. The toxoid with adjuvant is given in three fractional (0.05 to 0.1 ml.) doses.

*Toxoid sensitivity test (Zoeller, Moloney).* Since even small doses of diphtheria toxoid can cause a

---

*Nonimmunized individuals also require passive immunization. See pp. 397 and 402.
†The U.S. Public Health Service recommends that tetanus boosters of adsorbed toxoid be given at 10-year intervals.

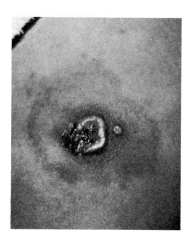

**Fig. 37-2.** Smallpox vaccination. Primary vaccinia on arm of year-old child. A red areola surrounds umbilicated, partly encrusted pustule with small satellite.

reaction in a highly sensitive person, when the adult type toxoids are not available, a toxoid sensitivity test should be done beforehand. One-tenth milliliter of *fluid* diphtheria toxoid diluted 1:50 or 1:100 in saline is injected intracutaneously. The test site is read after 18 to 24 hours. A positive reaction, indicating hypersensitivity, is a red indurated area. In that person the positive toxoid sensitivity test is presumptive evidence of immunity from natural exposure, and further toxoid should *not* under any circumstances be given. Persons with no reaction, a negative test, should receive diphtheria toxoid adsorbed as a single antigen, or diphtheria and tetanus toxoids, childhood type (DT).

**Smallpox.** The preferred method of smallpox vaccination is either the multiple pressure method or intradermal jet injection with calf lymph virus.* In the preparation of the arm acetone or ether is suitable; alcohol, especially if medicated, should *not* be used because it destroys the virus. However, no preparation at all is better than vigorous cleaning that might abrade the skin. The vaccination site† should be kept dry, preferably uncovered, until the scab falls off. The site of a primary vaccination should be inspected between the sixth and the eighth days, the revaccination site between the fourth and the seventh days.

After vaccination *primary vaccinia* (Fig. 37-2) occurs in persons with no immunity. On the fourth day a small, circumscribed, solid elevation of the skin (*papule*) appears; on the eighth day the lesion con-

---

*There are three methods for smallpox vaccination:
1. In the *multiple pressure* technic, a sterile sharp needle is held tangentially to the skin. Pressure is applied to an area about one-eighth inch in diameter. For primary vaccination in a smallpox-free area, 6 to 10 pressures within 5 or 6 seconds suffice. For revaccination 20 to 30 pressures within 30 seconds are given. A trace of blood welling up within half a minute indicates the right amount of force exerted against the drop of vaccine on the skin.
2. In the *multiple puncture* method, a forked needle dipped in vaccine is touched to the surface of the skin. The needle is held perpendicular to the skin, and (if the geographic area is free of smallpox) 2 to 3 punctures are made in an up-and-down manner within a small area about one-eighth inch in diameter.
3. The *jet injection* method requires a specially constructed injector that delivers about 0.1 ml. of a specially purified vaccine into the skin (Fig. 37-1).
†"Primary vaccination and revaccination are best performed on the outer aspects of the upper arm, over the insertion of the deltoid muscle or behind the midline. Reactions are less likely to be severe on the upper arm than on the lower extremity or other parts of the body. With proper technique, resultant scars are small and unobtrusive." (Kempe, C. H., and Benenson, A. S.: Smallpox immunization in the United States, J.A.M.A. **194:**161, 1965.)

tains fluid (*vesicle*) and has a pink areola around it that averages several centimeters in diameter. On the ninth day it is filled with pus (*pustule*) and has begun to dry up by the end of 14 days. The formation of a scar at the site is evidence of a successful vaccination.

After revaccination, the following may be seen:

1. *Major reaction**—a vesicular or pustular lesion, an area of hardening, or a reddened zone about a central crust or ulcer—indicates virus has multiplied at the site.
2. *Equivocal reaction*—any other reaction—indicates vaccination did not "take." Equivocal reactions may come as a consequence of immunity adequate to suppress the virus or may represent only an allergic reaction to an inactive vaccine.

No reaction means inactive vaccine or faulty technic. In such a case vaccination should be repeated. Vaccine virus is very susceptible to even moderate warmth and should be kept in the freezing compartment of the refrigerator. *The vaccine virus must be kept frozen.*

*Indications.* The U.S. Public Health Service currently recommends that primary smallpox vaccination be discontinued on a routine basis in the United States. The risk from the disease is small, and on occasions severe reactions present to the vaccine. Accordingly, the American Academy of Pediatrics no longer advocates this immunization routinely. It stresses vaccination in the event of exposure and in preparation for foreign travel. The U.S. Public Health Service advises personnel in medical and allied health fields to be vaccinated every 3 years because there is a potential hazard to these persons from unsuspected cases accidentally imported into the country.

All persons, including those who have had smallpox, should be vaccinated if exposed to the disease. Those who live and work under conditions of constant exposure to smallpox should be vaccinated every year. This includes laboratory workers and residents in areas of the world where smallpox is endemic and occasionally epidemic.

*Contraindications.* Children with eczema and skin lesions such as poison ivy or impetigo, extensive wounds, or burns should not be vaccinated against smallpox because generalized vaccinia, a condition resembling smallpox, may develop; nor should they be allowed to contact a person who has an active vaccination lesion. It would be dangerous to vaccinate a patient with depressed immunologic responses, either because of a disease such as dysgammaglobu-

linemia, lymphoma, leukemia, or blood dyscrasia or because of therapy being given with steroids, antimetabolites, alkylating agents, or ionizing radiation. Pregnant women must *not* be vaccinated.

**Mumps.** Live attenuated mumps vaccine given in a single 0.5 ml. subcutaneous injection or in combination with measles and rubella vaccines (Table 37-1) protects for 6 years. Febrile reactions have not been noted. The vaccine is advocated for susceptible children approaching puberty, adolescents, and adults, particularly males with no history of the disease. In special circumstances vaccination may be considered for younger children in closed populations such as special schools, camps, institutions, and so on. It should not be given to pregnant women or to children less than 12 months of age.

**Rubella.** Rubella immunization is carried out with a single subcutaneous injection of the vaccine (or given in a combined vaccine as indicated in Table 37-1). It is advocated for boys and girls between the ages of 1 year and puberty and especially for those of kindergarten age. Vaccinees will shed virus from their throats for 2 or more weeks afterward, but they are not thought to be infectious. It is felt that vaccination gives long-range protection.

Immunization is contraindicated for infants less than 1 year of age, for pregnant women, and for individuals with altered immune states (leukemia, lymphoid malignancies, recipients of immunosuppressive therapy). It should not be given routinely to adolescent girls (after the twelfth birthday) or adult women because of the danger that it might complicate a pregnancy. It is not given in severe febrile illness.

More than 32 million children have received rubella vaccine in the all-out effort to block the circulation of rubella virus in population groups and thus avoid the exposure of pregnant women to the virus.

**Rabies.** With rabies we have an exception to the rule that there is not enough time between exposure and onset of disease to establish an *active* immunity to protect the person exposed. Since the incubation period of rabies may be much longer than that of most diseases, an active immunity can usually be established before the disease begins.* The onset of the disease *must* be prevented because there is no treatment; *the disease must be considered to be 100% fatal.*

---

*The World Health Organization's Expert Committee on Smallpox defines only two responses to smallpox vaccination—"major" and "equivocal."

---

*Smallpox and rabies are the only diseases in which the exposed person can be protected against development of the disease by the production of an active immunity. In smallpox an active immunity develops very quickly. In rabies the period of incubation is so long that an active immunity can be produced before the disease takes effect.

**Table 37-2**
Recommendations for the prevention of rabies*

| EXPOSURE | CONDITION OF VACCINATED OR UNVACCINATED ANIMAL INFLICTING INJURY | | RECOMMENDED TREATMENT† |
| | AT EXPOSURE | DURING 10 DAYS' OBSERVATION | |
| --- | --- | --- | --- |
| 1. Indirect contact | Healthy or rabid | Healthy or rabid | None |
| 2. Licks | | | |
|   a. Intact skin | Rabid | | None |
|   b. Skin lesions, scratches; mucous membrane intact or abraded | 1. Healthy | Clinical signs of rabies or laboratory diagnosis of rabies made | Serum now; start vaccine at first signs of rabies in the animal |
| | 2. Signs veterinarian judges to suggest rabies | Healthy | Serum now; start vaccine; stop at 5 days if animal is normal |
| | 3. Rabid, escaped, killed, or unknown | Rabid | Serum now; start vaccine |
| 3. Bites | | | |
|   a. Mild exposure | 1. Healthy | Clinical signs of rabies or laboratory diagnosis made | Serum immediately; start vaccine at first sign of rabies in animal |
| | 2. Signs veterinarian judges to suggest rabies | Healthy | Serum and vaccine at once; stop at 5 days if animal is normal |
| | 3. Rabid, escaped, killed, or unknown | Rabid | Serum and vaccine at once |
| | 4. Wild wolf, fox, bat, skunk, other | — | Serum and vaccine at once |
|   b. Severe exposure such as multiple wounds or face, finger, and neck wounds | 1. Healthy | Clinical signs of rabies or laboratory diagnosis made | Serum at once; start vaccine at first sign of rabies in animal |
| | 2. Signs veterinarian judges to suggest rabies | Healthy | Serum and vaccine at once; stop at 5 days if animal is normal |
| | 3. Rabid, escaped, killed, or unknown | Rabid | Serum and vaccine at once |
| | 4. Wild wolf, fox, bat, skunk, others | — | Serum and vaccine at once |

*Modified from Technical Report Series No. 321 (1966), WHO Expert Committee on Rabies, Fifth Report, Geneva, 1966, World Health Organization.
†See text for the dosage and administration of vaccine and serum.

Table 37-2 outlines the recommendations of the WHO Expert Committee on Rabies for rabies prevention. Active immunization, as indicated in this table, is carried out in a series of 14 to 21 daily doses of rabies vaccine (duck embryo or brain tissue types). A booster dose is given 10 days and 20 days after the last dose.

The best prophylaxis against rabies following exposure is the use of hyperimmune serum in combination with vaccine. The hyperimmune serum (horse serum)* is given as soon as possible. Within

24 hours after the bite, 1000 units of antirabies serum per 55 pounds of body weight is given intramuscularly. If more than 24 (up to 72) hours has elapsed, two to three times this amount of serum is given. Part of the dose of rabies serum may be injected around the wound inflicted by the animal for local antiviral effect. If reexposure of an ordinary nature occurs, one booster dose of duck embryo vaccine is given. If reexposure is severe, 5 daily doses of vaccine are given followed by a booster 20 days later.

Prophylactic vaccination is now advised for laboratory workers, veterinarians, spelunkers, and others likely to contract the disease. Two subcutaneous inoculations of 1.0 ml. of duck embryo rabies vaccine

*Rabies immune globulin human (RIGH) has been developed.

413

each into the deltoid area, 1 month apart, are followed by a booster dose 6 months later. Boosters are recommended every 1 to 3 years.

The amount of protection needed from hyperimmune serum and the vaccine depends on many factors (Table 37-2) such as the type of animal, the location of the bite, the extent of injury, the protection afforded by clothing, whether rabies is present in the community, and whether observation of the animal is possible. *It is very important that the animal inflicting the bite be apprehended and kept for a 10-day period of observation.* (Rats and mice do not transmit rabies.)

Although the method of preparing antirabies vaccine differs greatly from the original method of Pasteur, the administration of antirabies vaccine is still referred to as the *Pasteur treatment*. It is fitting that his name be thus remembered.

**Tuberculosis.** BCG vaccination against tuberculosis is done as superficially as possible into the skin of the upper arm over the deltoid or triceps muscle. To the newborn infant 0.05 ml. is given; to the older tuberculin-negative individual, 0.1 ml. Tuberculin testing must be done before vaccination except in infants less than 2 months of age. A preliminary radiograph of the chest may be indicated. Two to

## Table 37-3
Administration of poliovirus vaccines

| GROUP | DOSES | POLIOVIRUS TYPE(S) | TIME INTERVAL | COMMENTS |
|---|---|---|---|---|
| *I. Administration of trivalent oral poliovirus vaccine (TOPV)* | | | | |
| Infants | First | TOPV (I, II, III) | | Primary immunization begun at 6 to 12 weeks of age; may be given with DPT |
| | Second | TOPV | 8 weeks after first dose (no less than 6 weeks) | |
| | Third | TOPV | 8 to 12 months after second dose | |
| | Booster | TOPV | | Given at time that child enters school; boosters with TOPV otherwise not indicated |
| Children and adolescents | First | TOPV | | |
| | Second | TOPV | 6 to 8 weeks after first dose | |
| | Third | TOPV | 8 to 12 months after second dose | Third dose given as early as 6 weeks after second dose in unusual circumstances |
| Adults* | First | TOPV | | Recommended for adults at high risk; pregnancy not indication or contraindication for immunization |
| | Second | TOPV | 6 to 8 weeks after first dose | |
| | Third | TOPV | 8 to 12 months after second dose | |
| *II. Administration of monovalent oral poliovirus vaccine (MOPV)* | | | | |
| All ages | First | MOPV (I) | | |
| | Second | MOPV (III) | 6 to 8 weeks after first dose | |
| | Third | MOPV (II) | 6 to 8 weeks after second dose | |
| | Fourth | TOPV (I, II, III) | 8 to 12 months after third dose of monovalent vaccine | |
| *III. Administration of inactivated poliovirus vaccine (IPV)* | | | | |
| All ages | First | IPV | | Parenteral administration; immunization series: 4 doses; for infant 6 to 12 weeks of age, IPV may be given with DPT |
| | Second | IPV | 4 weeks after first dose | |
| | Third | IPV | 4 weeks after second dose | |
| | Fourth | IPV | 6 weeks to 2 months after third dose | |
| | Booster | IPV | 2- to 3-year interval | |

*Routine immunization is not indicated for most adults residing in continental United States.

three months after vaccination, tuberculin testing is repeated, and if the test is negative, vaccination is repeated.

BCG vaccination is advised for children living or traveling in areas of the world where tuberculosis is a major health problem and for those likely to be exposed to adults with the disease. It should be carried out 2 months before exposure.

## Recommendations of U.S. Public Health Service

**Influenza.** The U.S. Public Health Service recommends annual influenza vaccination for persons over 65 years of age and for those in whom the onset of flu would represent an added health risk, such as individuals of all ages with chronic debilitating diseases (diabetes, cardiovascular ailments, pulmonary disease, and others). There is some indication for immunization of persons responsible for furnishing essential public services, such as law enforcement officers, firemen, and many others.

The primary series has traditionally been 2 doses given subcutaneously (beneath the skin) 6 to 8 weeks apart. A single dose is now considered reasonable for either the primary or annual booster vaccination. The second dose provides little extra benefit. (In the package insert supplied with the vaccine, the manufacturer gives the recommended dose for adults and children and the directions for administration.) Vaccination should be done by the middle of November.

The status of influenza immunization (both vaccine and schedule) can change rapidly. For this reason, the recommendations of its Committee on Immunization Practices are regularly published by the U.S. Public Health Service and should be consulted before any procedure is carried out.

**Poliomyelitis.** The U.S. Public Health Service is urging regular immunization against poliomyelitis for all children from early infancy. Routine immunization of infants should begin at 6 to 12 weeks of age and be completed against all three types of the virus. The schedule for oral vaccination is given in Table 37-3. Oral poliovirus vaccine (OPV) is more widely used in the United States than the inactivated poliovirus vaccine (IPV), and the TOPV has largely replaced the monovalent form in immunization programs.

Vaccination is contraindicated in patients with severe underlying diseases such as leukemia or generalized malignancy or those with lowered resistance because of therapy.

**Measles.** The U.S. Public Health Service urges immunization for all susceptible children (those not having had vaccine or natural measles). The prime target groups are children at least 1 year of age and susceptible children entering nursery school, kindergarten, or elementary school (Fig. 37-1). Protection against measles is especially needed for children in the high-risk groups, that is, children in institutions and those with chronic heart or pulmonary disease and cystic fibrosis. Vaccination of adults is not stressed because most individuals are serologically immune by the age of 15 years.

**Table 37-4**
Schedules for measles immunization

| SCHEDULE | TYPE OF VACCINE* | AGE | DOSE (SUBCUTANEOUS)† | REMARKS |
|---|---|---|---|---|
| 1. | Live, attenuated (Edmonston B strain) measles virus vaccine | 12 months and older | One | Although live attenuated viral vaccine may be given safely, many physicians may wish to add immune serum globulin (human) because of fewer clinical reactions |
| 2. | Live, attenuated (Edmonston B strain) plus immune serum globulin (human) | 12 months and older | One plus 0.01 ml. per pound of immune serum globulin (human) at different site with different syringe | |
| 3. | Live, further attenuated (Schwarz and Moraten strains) | 12 months and older | One | Clinical reactions those of schedule 2; immune serum globulin (human) *not* indicated |

*Only live, attenuated virus vaccines should be used! As soon as possible children who may have received inactivated vaccine should be revaccinated with live virus vaccine. It has been found that children having received inactivated vaccine develop a sinister illness when they are exposed to natural measles several years later.
†No booster needed.

Table 37-4 gives the currently acceptable schedules for measles immunization.

Live, attenuated vaccine should not be given to pregnant women or to patients being treated with steroids, irradiation, antimetabolites, or those agents that depress an individual's immunologic capacities. Leukemia, lymphoma, and other generalized malignancies are also contraindications, as is untreated tuberculosis.

**Typhoid and paratyphoid fevers.** The U.S. Public Health Service no longer recommends routine typhoid immunization in the United States, even for individuals in flood disaster areas. Circumstances where vaccination would be indicated include an intimate exposure to a known carrier, an outbreak of the disease in a community, or the event of travel to an endemic area. The Public Health Service does

*not* advise paratyphoid immunization because there is good evidence that paratyphoid A and B vaccines are worthless. (Schedules for typhoid immunization may be found in the Red Book of the American Academy of Pediatrics.)

## Requirements for U.S. Armed Forces

Immunization procedures for the U.S. Armed Forces are regularly evaluated and updated. So that the requirements may be precisely related to the geographic area of military duty, the world is divided into the following areas:

*Area I* (routine)—United States (includes the 50 states, District of Columbia, Virgin Islands, Puerto Rico, Wake Island, Midway Island), Canada, Greenland, Iceland, Marshall Islands, Guam, Pacific islands east of the 180th me-

**Table 37-5**
Immunizations required for U.S. Armed Forces

| IMMUNIZING AGENT | BASIC SERIES* | REQUIRED AREA I (EXCLUDING ALERT FORCES) | REQUIRED AREA II | REIMMUNIZATION AREA I | REIMMUNIZATION AREA II |
|---|---|---|---|---|---|
| Smallpox vaccine, USP (freeze-dried) | Vaccination to be read after 6 to 8 days; successful reaction required | ✔ | ✔ | 3 years | 3 years |
| Typhoid vaccine (acetone-killed, dried) | Single 0.5 ml. injection—Area I Two 0.5 ml. injections 4 weeks apart—alert forces | ✔ | ✔ | None | 0.5 ml.—3 years |
| Tetanus and diphtheria toxoids, absorbed, USP (for adult use) | Two 0.5 ml. injections 1 to 2 months apart, with third dose of 0.1 ml. 12 months later | ✔ | ✔ | 0.1 ml.—6 years; 0.5 ml. after injury or burn | 0.1 ml.—6 years; 0.5 ml. after injury or burn |
| Poliovirus vaccine, live oral, trivalent USP, types I, II, and III | Two oral doses 6 to 8 weeks apart; third dose 8 to 12 months later | ✔ | ✔ | None | None |
| Yellow fever vaccine, USP† | One 0.5 ml. injection of concentrated vaccine diluted 1:10 | | ✔ (Areas IIY, IIYC) | | 0.5 ml. of 1:10 dilution—10 years |
| Influenza virus vaccine, USP | One 0.5 ml. injection | ✔ | ✔ | 0.5 ml.—1 year | 0.5 ml.—1 year |
| Cholera vaccine, USP | 0.5 ml. injection followed by 1.0 ml. in 1+ weeks | | ✔ (Areas IIC, IIYC, IICP) | | 0.5 ml.—6 months |
| Plague vaccine, USP | Two *intramuscular* injections—1.0 ml. followed in 3 months by 0.2 ml. | | ✔ (Area IICP) | | 0.2 ml. (intramuscular)—6 months (while in area) |

*Smallpox vaccination is given either by multiple puncture technic or by intradermal jet. Plague vaccine must be given intramuscularly. Other injections are subcutaneous or intramuscular. (See Fig. 36-1)
†The vaccine listed in the United States Pharmacopeia.

ridian, North Pole, South Pole, Bermuda, Bahama Islands, Baja California, and a strip of Mexico 50 miles south of the United States border

*Area II*—All areas outside Area I

*Area IIC* (cholera)—Arabian peninsula, Afghanistan, Burma, Ceylon, Republic of China, Hong Kong, India, Indonesia, Korea, Peoples Republic of China, Macao, Malaysia, Pakistan, Philippines, Thailand, Iran, Iraq, Syria, Turkey, Lebanon, Israel, Jordan, Kuwait, African continent north of the Sahara, and Madagascar

*Area IICP* (cholera and plague)—Laos, Cambodia, and Vietnam

*Area IIY* (yellow fever)—Central America

southeast of the Isthmus of Tehuantepec, Panama, and South America

*Area IIYC* (yellow fever and cholera)—Africa south of the Sahara

Table 37-5 summarizes the immunization requirements for United States military personnel. Military dependents and civilians in the employ of the Armed Forces, or organizations serving the Armed Forces, are not required to take immunizations while within the United States or Canada. Outside the United States and Canada they are required to take essentially the same ones as members of the Armed Forces.

## International travel

**Immunizations.** The Red Book of the American Academy of Pediatrics also contains immunization

### Table 37-6

Special immunization requirements by age for international travel*

| DISEASE | TRAVEL DESTINATION | AGE | DOSES OF VACCINE | ROUTE OF INOCULATION | INTERVALS | RECALL NEEDED |
|---|---|---|---|---|---|---|
| Cholera | Asian countries Middle East | 6 months to 5 years | (1) 0.1 ml. (2) 0.3 ml. Booster: 0.1 ml. | Subcutaneously | 1 month between 1 and 2; 6+ months between 2 and 3 | 6 months |
| | | 5 to 10 years | (1) 0.3 ml. (2) 0.5 ml. Booster: 0.3 ml. | | | |
| | | 10 years and older (adults also) | (1) 0.5 ml. (2) 1.0 ml. Booster: 0.5 ml. | | | |
| Yellow fever† | Central and South America, Africa | All ages | 0.5 ml. of 1:10 dilution | Subcutaneously | | 10 years |
| Plague | High-risk area | Less than 1 year | (1) 0.1 ml. (2) 0.1 ml. (3) 0.04 ml. | Intramuscularly | 30 days between 1 and 2; 4 to 12 weeks between 2 and 3 | 6 to 12 months |
| | | 1 to 4 years | (1) 0.2 ml. (2) 0.2 ml. (3) 0.08 ml. | | | |
| | | 5 to 10 years | (1) 0.3 ml. (2) 0.3 ml. (3) 0.12 ml. | | | |
| | | 10 years and older (adults) | (1) 0.5 ml. (2) 0.5 ml. (3) 0.2 ml. | | | |
| Typhoid fever | Developing countries and those with low standards of sanitation | 6 months to 10 years | (1) 0.25 ml. (2) 0.25 ml. | Subcutaneously | 4+ weeks | 1 to 3 years if exposed (0.1 ml. intradermally or 0.25 to 0.5 ml. subcutaneously) |
| | | 10 years and older (adults also) | (1) 0.5 ml. (2) 0.5 ml. | | | |

*Based on data from the Red Book of the American Academy of Pediatrics, 1974.
†Note that yellow fever vaccination for international travel must be given at a designated Yellow Fever Vaccination Center, registered by the World Health Organization. Centers are located in 46 states, the District of Columbia, Puerto Rico, Canal Zone, and American Samoa. Yellow fever vaccination certificate is not valid until 10 days after primary immunization.

information and recommendations for international travel.* In Table 37-6, which presents vaccination schedules recommended by this organization, there is a breakdown of special travel requirements by age groups.

**Where to find a doctor.** The International Association for Medical Assistance to Travelers, Inc., 745 Fifth Avenue, New York, N. Y. 10022 (also note Intermedic, 777 Third Avenue, New York, N. Y. 10017, and World Medical Association, 10 Columbus Circle, New York, N. Y. 10019) supplies without charge a directory of English-speaking physicians available 24 hours a day in the different cities of the world. A long way from home one may also obtain medical aid from the United States embassies and consulates, the Red Cross, travel agencies, the police, medical associations, hospitals, clinics, and the U.S. Armed Forces bases and installations.

**Traveler's diarrhea.** Traveler's diarrhea is known by the many colorful synonyms—Aztec two-step, Montezuma's revenge, Cromwell's curse, Delhi belly—that mark out a widespread geographic distribution, and preventive immunization does not exist for this unpleasant complication of the initial phase of the tourists' trip abroad (or out of the country). Traveler's diarrhea is described consistently by nausea and vomiting, abdominal cramps, chills, low-grade fever, and a diarrhea productive of loose and watery, foul-smelling stools. Manifestations, though distressing and temporarily incapacitating, disappear within a few days. Relapses or sequelae are rare. Microbes found in the stools and thereby implicated include *Shigella* species, *Salmonella* species, enteropathogenic *Escherichia coli*, and *Giardia lamblia*. However, the cause is uncertain and a cure-all, nonexistent.

To minimize the hazard, especially where sanitary practices are substandard, certain precautions are stressed. The tourist can safely eat only foods thoroughly cooked or recently peeled. He can drink with impunity only boiled water, carbonated mineral water, or beverages boiled or carbonated in cans. Very hot water out of the tap is not likely to transmit viable enteric bacteria. After it has cooled, it can be used for oral hygiene and various other purposes.

**Center for Disease Control.** The responsibility for assisting the states in controlling communicable and vector-borne diseases and for participation in international programs of disease eradication rests with an agency of the U.S. Public Health Service— the Center for Disease Control (CDC). Its headquarters at Atlanta

is a vast complex of specialty laboratories and other disease control facilities, and there are field stations across the United States and Puerto Rico. Valuable advice for the traveler is given in its booklet *Health Information for International Travel.**

**World Health Organization.** The World Health Organization, or WHO as it is usually called, is an agency of the United Nations set up to provide for the highest level of health for all peoples of the world. It is composed of 135 member states and 2 associate members. It works with the United Nations, governments, and special health groups to devise standards, train personnel, carry on research, and improve public health in every way at the international level. To protect the sightseer of the jet age, WHO is concerned for uniform standards of hygiene in aviation. Guidelines are detailed for aspects of sanitation applied to aircraft and international airports, the design to provide every safety factor for the traveler in rapid transit over the globe.

For the traveler, the World Health Organization (Geneva, Switzerland) publishes the bilingual (English and French) *Vaccination Certificate Requirements for International Travelers, Situation as on 1 January, 1975.*

---

* Health information for international travel, Morbid. Mortal. Weekly Rep. **23**(supp.): Sept., 1974, Department of Health, Education and Welfare pub. no. (CDC) 75-8280.

## REFERENCES (Chapters 36 and 37)

Arteinstein, M. S.: The current status of bacterial vaccines, Hosp. Pract. **8**:49, June, 1973.

Balagtas, R. C., and others: Treatment of pertussis with pertussis immune globulin, J. Pediatr. **79**:203, 1971.

Barkin, R. M.: Measles: regaining control (editorial), J.A.M.A. **231**:737, 1975.

Barrett-Connor, E.: Chemoprophylaxis of malaria for travelers, Ann. Intern. Med. **81**:219, 1974.

Beardmore, W. B.: A new form of smallpox vaccine, J. Infect. Dis. **127**:718, 1973.

Benenson, A. S., editor: Control of communicable diseases in man, ed. 11, New York, 1970, American Public Health Association.

Brooks, G. F., and others: Tetanus toxoid immunization of adults: a continuing need, Ann. Intern. Med. **73**:603, 1970.

Brown, H.: Tetanus, J.A.M.A. **204**:614, 1968.

Byrne, E. B.: Prevention of viral hepatitis in hospital physicians, Res. Phys. **15**:62, June, 1969.

Collected recommendations of Public Health Service Advisory Committee on Immunization Practices, Morbid. Mortal. Weekly Rep. **25**(25, supp.):1, 1972.

Cooper, L. Z., and Schweitzer, M. D.: Hospital personnel: the immunization gap, Hosp. Pract. **9**:11, March, 1974.

Coriell, L. L.: Recommendations and schedules for immunization, Arch. Environ. Health **15**:521, 1967.

---

*This booklet advises suppressive medication for malaria (a major worldwide problem) prior to entry into an infected area, during sojourn there, and even for a number of weeks thereafter.

Dowling, H. F.: Diphtheria as a model, J.A.M.A. **226:**550, 1973.

Dukelow, D. A.: The AMA's continuing interest in immunization, Arch. Environ. Health **15:**515, 1967.

Edsall, G.: Diphtheria, tetanus, and pertussis immunization, Arch. Environ. Health **15:**473, 1967.

Edsall, G.: The current status of tetanus immunization, Hosp. Pract. **6:**57, July, 1971.

Eickhoff, T. C.: Committee on Immunization (Infectious Disease Society of America): Immunization against influenza: rationale and recommendations, J. Infect. Dis. **123:**446, 1971.

Eickhoff, T. C.: The current status of influenza vaccines, J.A.M.A. **230:**1046, 1974.

Fireman, P., and others: Effect of measles vaccine on immunologic responses, Pediatrics **43:**264, 1969.

Francis, B. J.: Current concepts in immunization, Am. J. Nurs. **73:**646, 1973.

Ganguly, R., and others: Rubella virus immunization of preschool children via respiratory tract, Am. J. Dis. Child. **128:**821, 1974.

Gordon-Smith, C. E.: Prospects for the control of infectious disease, Proc. R. Soc. Med. **63:**1181, 1970.

Grand, M. G., and others: Clinical reactions following rubella vaccination, J.A.M.A. **220:**1569, 1972.

Hatwick, M. A., and others: Postexposure rabies prophylaxis with human rabies immune globulin, J.A.M.A. **227:**407, 1974.

Hayflick, L.: Human virus vaccines: why monkey cells? Science **176:**813, 1972.

Hill, S. A.: Prophylaxis against tetanus in the wounded (editorial), South. Med. J. **67:**759, 1974.

Holder, A. R.: Compulsory immunization statutes, J.A.M.A. **228:**1059, 1974.

Johnson, R. H., and Ellis, R. J.: Immunobiologic agents and drugs available from the Center for Disease Control, Ann. Intern. Med. **81:**61, 1974.

Karchmer, A. W., and others: Simultaneous administration of live virus vaccines, Am. J. Dis. Child. **121:**382, 1971.

Kilbourne, E. D.: Influenza: the vaccines, Hosp. Pract. **6:**103, Oct., 1971.

Koenig, M. G.: Trivalent botulinus antitoxin, Ann. Intern. Med. **70:**643, 1969.

Kolata, G. B.: Phage in live virus vaccines: are they harmful to people? Science **187:**522, 1975.

Lane, J. M., and others: Complications of smallpox vaccination, 1968: results of 10 statewide surveys, J. Infect. Dis. **122:**303, 1970.

Lane, J. M., and others: Deaths attributable to smallpox vaccination, 1959 to 1966, and 1968, J.A.M.A. **212:**441, 1970.

Lerman, S. J., and Gold, E.: Measles in children previously vaccinated against measles, J.A.M.A. **216:**1311, 1971.

Lerner, A. M.: Committee on Immunization (Infectious Disease Society of America): Guide to immunization against mumps, J. Infect. Dis. **122:**116, 1970.

Linnemann, C. C., Jr., and others: Measles antibody in previously immunized children, Am. J. Dis. Child. **124:**53, July, 1972.

Loofbourow, J. C., and others: Rabies immune globulin (human). Clinical trials and dose determination, J.A.M.A. **217:**1825, 1971.

McCloskey, R. V., and Smilack, J.: Diphtheria antitoxin content of human immune serum globulins, Ann. Intern. Med. **77:**757, 1972.

Medical News: Immunization vs complacency: are we ready for the challenge? J.A.M.A. **229:**1557, 1974.

Medical Services, Immunization requirements and procedures; Army Regulation no. 40-562; BUMED Instruction no. 6230 1G; Air Force Regulation no. 161-13; CG COMDTINST 6230 4B, Department of the Army, The Navy, The Air Force, and Transportation, Washington, D. C., 22 March 1974.

Miller, L. W., and others: Diphtheria immunization, Am. J. Dis. Child. **123:**197, 1972.

Mumps vaccine, Ann. Intern. Med. **68:**632, 1968.

Neumann, H. H.: Foreign travel immunization manual, Springfield, Ill., 1971, Charles C Thomas, Publisher.

Ogra, P. L., and Herd, J. K.: Arthritis associated with induced rubella infection, J. Immunol. **107:**810, 1971.

Okada, N.: The eradication of infectious diseases (editorial), J. Infect. Dis. **127:**474, 1973.

Paton, B. C.: Bites—human, dog, spider and snake, Surg. Clin. North Am. **43:**537, 1963.

Physician desk reference to pharmaceutical specialties and biologicals, Oradell, N.J., 1975, Medical Economics, Inc.

Pitel, M.: The subcutaneous injection, Am. J. Nurs. **71:**76, 1971.

Plorde, J. J.: Advice to foreign travelers, Postgrad. Med. **51:** 179, 1972.

Plotkin, S. A.: Rubella vaccination (editorial), J.A.M.A. **215:** 1492, 1971.

Plotkin, S. A., and Clark, H. F.: Committee on Immunization (Infectious Disease Society of America): Prevention of rabies in man, J. Infect. Dis. **123:**227, 1971.

Rauch, P.: Avoiding injuries from injections, Nursing '72 **2:**12, May, 1972.

Recommendation of the Public Health Service Advisory Committee on Immunization Practices: Combination live virus vaccines, measles and rubella, and measles, mumps, and rubella, Morbid. Mortal. Weekly Rep. **20:** (16):145, 1971.

Recommendation of the Public Health Service Advisory Committee on Immunization Practices: Diphtheria and tetanus toxoids and pertussis vaccine, Morbid. Mortal. Weekly Rep. **20**(43):396, 1971.

Recommendation of the Public Health Service Advisory Committee on Immunization Practices: Measles vaccines, Morbid. Mortal. Weekly Rep. **20**(42):386, 1971.

Recommendation of the Public Health Service Advisory Committee on Immunization Practices: Rubella virus vaccine, Morbid. Mortal. Weekly Rep. **20**(34):304, 1971.

Recommendation of the Public Health Service Advisory Committee on Immunization Practices: Immune serum globulin for protection against viral hepatitis, Ann. Intern. Med. **77:**427, 1972.

Recommendation of the Public Health Service Advisory Committee on Immunization Practices: Influenza vaccine, Morbid. Mortal. Weekly Rep. **24**(23):197, 1975.

Recommendations of the Public Health Service Advisory

Committee on Immunization Practices: BCG vaccines, Morbid. Mortal. Weekly Rep. **24**(8):69, 1975.

Report of the Committee on Infectious Diseases, Evanston, Ill., 1974, American Academy of Pediatrics, Inc.

Rose, N. J., and others: Rabies prophylaxis, the physician's dilemma, Arch. Environ. Health **23**:57, 1971.

Rubin, R. J., and Corey, L.: Preventing rabies in humans, South. Med. J. **67**:1472, 1974.

Rubin, R. H., and others: Adverse reactions to duck embryo rabies vaccine, Ann. Intern. Med. **78**:643, 1973.

Rubin, R. H., and others: Human rabies immune globulin, J.A.M.A. **224**:871, 1973.

Sanford, J. P.: Personal communication, 1975.

Schaffner, W., and others: Polyneuropathy following rubella immunization, Am. J. Dis. Child. **127**:684, 1974.

Sever, J. L.: Present status of vaccines for rubella, Arch. Otolaryngol. **98**:265, 1973.

Sikes, R. K.: Rabies vaccines, Arch. Environ. Health **19**:862, 1969.

Stanfield, J. P., and others: Diphtheria-tetanus-pertussis immunization by intradermal jet infection, Br. Med. J. **2**:197, 1972.

Stokes, J., Jr., and others: Trivalent combined measles-mumps-rubella vaccine, J.A.M.A. **218**:57, 1971.

Suggested ordinances and regulations covering public swimming pools, Washington, D.C., 1964, American Public Health Association, Inc.

United States designated yellow fever vaccination centers, Morbid. Mortal. Weekly Rep. **20**(9, supp.):1, 1971.

Vaccination certificate requirements for international travel, Morbid. Mortal. Weekly Rep. **21**(11, supp.):1, 1972.

Vaheri, A., and others: Isolation of attenuated rubella vaccine virus from human products of conception and uterine cervix, N. Engl. J. Med. **286**:1071, 1972.

Waldman, R. H., and Coggins, W. J.: Influenza immunization: field trial on university campus, J. Infect. Dis. **126**: 242, 1972.

Wallace, R. B., and others: Joint symptoms following an area-wide rubella immunization campaign—report of a survey, Am. J. Public Health **62**:658, 1972.

Weibel, R. E., and others: Persistence of immunity following monovalent and combined live measles, mumps, and rubella virus vaccines, Pediatrics **57**:467, 1973.

Weinstein, L.: Whatever happened to the "old-time" infections, J.A.M.A. **229**:196, 1974.

White, C. S., III, and others: Repeated immunization: possible adverse effects, Ann. Intern. Med. **81**:594, 1974.

Wiktor, T. J., and others: Human cell culture rabies vaccine, J.A.M.A. **224**:1170, 1973.

Wilkins, J., and others: Live further attenuated rubeola vaccine, Am. J. Dis. Child. **123**:190, 1972.

Wilson, G. S.: The hazards of immunization, New York, 1967, Oxford University Press, Inc.

Witte, J. J.: Healthy criticism: we're not immunizing enough of our children, Today's Health **51**:4, Sept., 1973.

Woodson, R. D., and Clinton, J. J.: Hepatitis prophylaxis abroad: effectiveness of immune serum globulin in protecting Peace Corps volunteers, J.A.M.A. **209**:1053, 1969.

Wyll, S. A., and Grand, M. G.: Rubella in adolescents, J.A.M.A. **220**:1573, 1973.

Yellow fever vaccine: recommendations of the Public Health Service Advisory Committee on Immunization Practices, Ann. Intern. Med. **71**:365, 1969.

# Part two
# PATHOLOGY

**UNIT I**

General pathology: perspective

**UNIT II**

Special pathology of major
organ systems

## CHAPTER 38

# Pathology
## definition and dimension

### Definition

Pathology is the science on which the successful practice of medicine is founded. The word *pathology* is derived from two Greek words—*pathos* (meaning suffering or disease) and *logy* (meaning science). *Pathology* is therefore the science that treats of the study of disease. It considers the cause *(etiology)* of disease, the manner in which disease develops *(pathogenesis)*, and the changes and final effects brought about in the body. Its purpose is to correlate the manifestations of disease with the underlying abnormalities and physiologic disturbances. In short, pathology deals directly with all phases of disease except treatment. Although not a part of pathology, the treatment of a given disease cannot be successfully carried out without an understanding of the body changes in that disease.

### Divisions

If we define *biology* as the science that treats of the *normal* origin, structure, and functional activities of living things, *pathology* is then the science that treats of the *abnormal* origin, structure, and function of living things.

Pathology naturally falls into several subdivisions. *Gross pathology* refers to the changes in structure in the body as a result of disease that are readily seen with the unaided eye. *Microscopic pathology* (pathologic histology) deals with the changes in microscopic structure that cells, tissues, and organs undergo as a result of disease, alterations that must be viewed under the microscope. It emphasizes changes occurring in the basic unit of living things, the cell, a biologic unit too small (with a few exceptions) to be viewed except with magnification. *General pathology* surveys the field broadly, dealing with disease processes such as degenerative changes, disturbances of circulation, inflammation, tumors, and similar maladies that may affect many tissues and organs or

the body as a whole. *Special pathology* classifies the diseases of individual organs and given anatomic areas of the body. It may be subdivided more precisely with respect to a particular anatomic region. *Neuropathology* is pathology of the central nervous system; *urologic pathology* is pathology of the genitourinary system; *gynecologic and obstetric pathology* is pathology of the female reproductive system.

There are two major divisions in the science of pathology that represent and emphasize two distinct and important approaches to the study of the disease process in a given person. The first is pathologic anatomy, and the second is clinical pathology.

*Pathologic anatomy* deals practically with tissues and organs separated or removed from the living body for purposes of pathologic study. Such tissues and organs are primarily obtained in two ways: (1) as a result of a limited procedure of major or minor proportions, *surgery,* or (2) through the systematic dissection of the human body at *autopsy. Surgical pathology* is the study of tissue specimens excised surgically in a major or minor operation. *Autopsy pathology* is the study of tissue specimens from the dead individual on the autopsy table. It is quite apparent that during life direct observation of pathologic changes in the body is limited. Even surgery of the abdomen enables the operator to explore or view only the contents of the abdominal cavity; he cannot at the same time look into the chest.

Disease can be studied in the human body as it is reflected in changes in cells, tissues, and organs. It can also be studied as it induces changes in the body fluids, secretions, and excretions. A body fluid rather closely reflects the state of the organ that produces it; for example, the urine indicates disease in the kidney. This close correlation between disease processes in organs and changes produced in body fluid, secretion, or excretion is a fortunate circumstance. Such body products are easily and readily taken, often with little if any inconvenience to the person. The organized study of the composition and characteristics of body secretions, excretions, and fluids is *clinical pathology*. This branch of pathology contributes to the diagnosis of disease, the measurement of the course of disease, and the evaluation of therapy. In practice, the term *clinical pathology* refers to the various standardized procedures performed in the laboratory on body fluids, especially in the diagnosis of disease, such as urinalyses, blood examinations, and microbiologic cultures and smears of various kinds.

It is a mistake to believe that *human pathology* (pathology of the human body) is the only kind of pathology. Just as important in the scheme of things are *pathology of the lower animals* and *plant pathology*.

*Experimental pathology* is the study of disease produced in animals for the purposes of making significant correlations with the comparable disease process in the human being.

## The pathologist

A *pathologist* is a person engaged in the practice of pathology (the study of disease), and for human pathology he is a doctor of medicine with a prescribed period of special postgraduate training. The pathologist practices pathology so as to fulfill one or a combination of the three major purposes of all scientific endeavors: service, teaching, and research. That person who has emphasized the science of pathology in his postgraduate medical training may make practical application of his store of knowledge for the benefit of his medical colleagues and their patients, he may disseminate or pass on the fund of knowledge to others, or he may engage in activities that have for their primary purpose additions and contributions to the general store of knowledge of pathology. In other words, a pathologist gives service, teaches, or does research.

Because of the broad scope and fundamental importance of pathology and the fact that numerous practical applications are increasing, the pathologist may limit his activities to one of the major divisions of pathology. By the nature of pathology as a medical specialty it is usually, but not necessarily, based in an institution such as a hospital, a school of medicine or dentistry, an experimental laboratory, or a research institute.

The activities of the department of pathology in a modern hospital fall into three categories: *clinical pathology, surgical pathology,* and *autopsy pathology*. In a small hospital all three departments may be under the supervision of one pathologist. In a larger hospital each department may be under the supervision of a pathologist specially trained in the type of work done in that department. These pathologists may be aided by assistant pathologists.

Laboratory workers known as *medical technologists* are vitally related to laboratory medicine. Medical technologists are not graduates in medicine but are educated in the basic sciences of physics, chemistry, and biology and have had special training in the technics of laboratory procedure. The pathologist and his medical colleagues are dependent on their skill and experience in the actual performance of the many and variably complicated laboratory technics that are their responsibility. The medical technologist makes a major contribution not only to pathology but to all of medicine.

## CLINICAL PATHOLOGIST

The person designated a clinical pathologist is well versed in both the performance of general laboratory procedures and their interpretation. Because of the complexity and number of laboratory procedures on which modern medicine is dependent, there are subdivisions in the field of clinical pathology. In a large medical institution these are usually laid out in physically separate laboratories under the supervision of the clinical pathologist and his assistants. The departments are as follows:

1. *Hematology*. In this, laboratory blood counts are done as well as tests relating to the microscopic appearance of the blood cells, coagulation of the blood, amount of hemoglobin in the blood, and other critical factors. Hematology is an important specialty of medicine in itself, being the study of the blood in all its aspects as well as the study of the many and complex diseases of the blood and blood-forming organs.

2. *Microbiology*. In a hospital laboratory microbiologic investigation is mainly diagnostic. Suspect materials from patients are sent into this laboratory, where smears, cultures, and perhaps animal inoculations are made in an effort to isolate and identify pathogenic microorganisms. In many instances with the specific pathogen, susceptibility tests may be required to guide the physician in choosing the most effective antibiotic agent to give the patient.

3. *Clinical chemistry*. In this, laboratory chemical determinations are made of the inorganic and organic constituents of blood, urine, and other body secretions and excretions. Automation has taken over many of the technics of this laboratory.

4. *Serology and immunohematology*. Special tests are performed in this department on the serum of patients or normal persons. Generally the serum as the unknown is tested against known

antigens. The specificity of the antigen-antibody reaction makes it possible to identify an unknown antibody by this sort of testing or typing. Here are done agglutination tests to detect the presence of the causative agents of the continued fevers (or fevers of unknown origin) and complement fixation and precipitation tests to detect the presence of syphilis.

5. *Clinical microscopy.* In this, laboratory diagnostic examination is made of urine, feces, and the contents of the stomach as to composition, characteristics, presence of abnormal elements, and the possible presence of disease-producing factors.

6. *Parasitology.* This department is concerned with the demonstration, primarily in the stool, of protozoan and metazoan parasites and their ova. Sometimes the laboratory procedures to demonstrate ova or parasites are performed in the department of microbiology or in the clinical microscopy department.

Some clinical pathologists limit their practice to one special phase of clinical pathology as indicated above, for example, hematology (the study of the blood and the blood-forming organs) or serology (the diagnosis of disease by the study of reactions of the serum). The clinical pathologist is often consulted by the physician practicing in his hospital. This honor he shares with the surgical pathologist and the autopsy pathologist because it is oftentimes just as important to know the results of microbiologic cultures, the report of the urinalysis, or the chemical composition of the blood as it is to know the nature of the disease process in tissue that has been removed from the body or the cause of death as determined by the autopsy. This is as it should be, since the greater the cooperation between the physicians who have patients in the hospital and the pathologists, the better the treatment the patient receives.

## SURGICAL PATHOLOGIST

Although he may not be seen in the operating room as often as the surgeon, the surgical pathologist in modern hospitals takes part in every operation in which tissue is removed from the body, since this tissue is eventually subjected to his inspection and critical analysis. He has part of his equipment set up in the vicinity of the operating room, where he may examine portions of tissue (processed by the frozen section method) while an operation is in progress to determine how the operation should be modified or completed. For instance, the operative procedure is quite different when a tumor of the breast or another part of the body is found to be malignant from what it is when the tumor is benign.

It is interesting to note what the surgical pathologist does with tissue removed from the body. The purpose of the pathologic examination of tissue is to determine what type of disease is present—whether the tissue is inflamed, is the site of a tumor, is affected in some other manner—or, as is sometimes the case, that the tissue is entirely normal. Diagnostic examination (usually a microscopic one) is often made on a sample or a rather small portion of tissue referred to as a *biopsy*. The given area is then said to have been *biopsied*.

For proper examination tissue *must*, immediately after removal from the body, be put in a fluid that preserves the cells as nearly as possible in the natural state. This is *fixation*. One of the best fixing fluids is *formalin* (a solution of formaldehyde in water), which quickly penetrates the tissue and fixes the cells. Formalin is an inexpensive fixative and easy to prepare. One part of stock solution diluted with nine parts of water makes what is referred to as 10% formalin. (This is not exactly 10% formalin, since the stock solution is only approximately a 37% solution of the gas in water. Nevertheless, the 10% formalin solution as prepared makes an excellent fixative.) There are other standard fixatives in wide use. At times tissues are placed in isotonic saline solution right after excision; in this case *they should be promptly refrigerated.*

The first step in the routine examination of surgically excised tissues is the *gross description,* in which the pathologist describes the tissue as it is received in the laboratory, including such characteristics as size, shape, weight, color, consistency, special markings, and appearance of the outer and the cut surfaces. A deviation from normal, such as tumor formation, is precisely noted. After the macroscopic observations, the pathologist removes small blocks or slices of the tissue to be processed for microscopic study. Needless to say, the sites in tissues from which the blocks are taken are carefully selected so that all disease processes and suspicious areas are included. Surgical tissues are usually processed by one of two methods: the paraffin method or the frozen section method. The paraffin method is more often used, but the more rapid frozen section method is always used when a diagnosis on the tissue removed must be given while the operation is still in progress.

In the *paraffin method* the selected portions of tissue are fixed, dehydrated, and then embedded in paraffin (Figs. 38-1 and 38-2). After this, thin slices known as *sections* are cut from each paraffin block (Fig. 38-3). The sections must be about 8 $\mu$m. ($\mu$) or less in thickness. Obviously it would be impossible to cut such thin sections with an ordinary knife, so that the sections must be cut with a special instrument known as a *microtome*. There is a mechanism on microtomes that pushes the paraffin block forward with each stroke of the knife. By virtue of this advancing mechanism, it is possible to cut section after section of equal thinness.

In the *frozen section method* of tissue preparation the moistened, fixed or unfixed tissue is placed on the table of a freezing microtome, and carbon dioxide is allowed to enter the table through perforations on the sides. Freezing the water around the tissue attaches it to the table, and the tissue is frozen at the same time. Because of the hardness of the frozen tissue it is easily cut into thin sections. The *cryostat* is specially constructed to house a microtome that will freeze and section tissues in the cold.

After a given section has been cut, it is attached to a glass slide and stained. Staining makes the architecture of the tissue and the structure of the cells easily visible. The method used most often is the hematoxylin and eosin method, in which the tissue is first treated with the dye hematoxylin to stain the nucleus of the cells and then is treated with the dye eosin to stain the cytoplasm. The stained slide is ready for the pathologist to scrutinize under the microscope, and he can describe his findings.

The written microscopic description of a tissue is an important record. It describes the fundamental unit (the cell), its characteristics, and its architectural relations to other cells of the same kind and to cells of different origin and structure in the tissue. The microscopic description is the most important part of the pathologist's study of disease, for it is at the cellular level that disease originates. Microscopic findings may be the most crucial part of the pathologic examination, for many times disease processes are not fully manifest on gross inspection and are wholly or in part discovered only when the tissue is examined microscopically. The microscopic examination of a given tissue may be said to be the ultimate step in making the diagnosis of a given lesion. Finally, in tissue examination a pathologic report is made out, including the gross and microscopic findings and concluding with the final pathologic diagnosis.

## AUTOPSY PATHOLOGIST

Dissect in anatomy, experiment in physiology, and make necropsy in medicine; this is the three fold path without which there can be no anatomist, no pathologist, no physician.

FRANÇOIS XAVIER BICHAT

An *autopsy* is defined as the examination of the body after death. The word is derived from the Greek *autopsia* (*autos*, self, and *opsis*, sight) and in its early meaning referred to seeing with one's eyes. In modern medicine an autopsy is a scientific procedure per-

formed by a physician with special postgraduate training in the science of pathology, and it is carried out in a specified sequence (Fig. 38-4). There are two important phases—first, the gross inspection of organs and tissues at the time of dissection and second, the microscopic examination of small representative samples of tissue carefully chosen for their diagnostic value.

In order that medicine may more closely approach an exact science, it is highly desirable that the correctness of the diagnosis be proved or disproved by au-

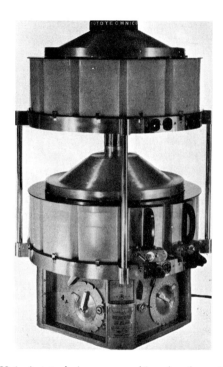

**Fig. 38-1.** Autotechnicon, a machine for the automatic fixation, dehydration, and infiltration with paraffin of specimens of tissue (paraffin method). Two decks permit simultaneous processing of two sets of specimens. Thin representative slices cut from tissue are placed in automatic processing machine, where they are changed from reagent to reagent in containers seen on each deck. After portions of tissue have been fixed, they are subjected to action of reagents such as alcohol or acetone, which remove water (dehydration). The dehydrant is then replaced by a reagent in which paraffin is soluble. For paraffin to infiltrate tissues, all reagents in which paraffin is insoluble must be removed. After having carried portions of tissue through reagents that remove the dehydrant, machine transfers them to melted paraffin, where they are kept for several hours to become thoroughly infiltrated with the paraffin. The time required for processing as described above is 12 to 14 hours. An automatic processing machine is a time-saver because specimens may be processed overnight. The Autotechnicon is also used for staining. (Courtesy Technicon Corp., Tarrytown, N. Y.)

426

topsy in every patient who dies. So important is the autopsy in medical teaching that it is requested as a matter of routine in many hospitals on all deaths regardless of whether the cause of death is obscure. Both the American Medical Association and the American College of Surgeons refuse to recognize medical institutions that fail to secure a specified percentage (20% of deaths) of autopsies.

The autopsy pathologist is responsible for doing the autopsy, for carrying out the systematic examination of tissues macroscopically and microscopically, and for summarizing his findings and diagnoses in a

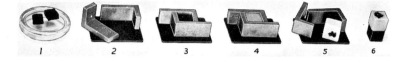

**Fig. 38-2.** Embedding. After portions of tissue have been infiltrated with melted paraffin, they are ready to be embedded. Embedding stabilizes tissue so that it can be cut into thin sections. The portions of tissue, *1*, are removed from the melted paraffin, and an embedding box, *2*, which consists of two L-shaped pieces of lead and a metal base, is assembled. *3*, Portion of tissue is placed in assembled box and covered with melted paraffin. *4*, Paraffin is allowed to cool and harden. *5*, Embedding box is then dismantled. At this point, paraffin block is shown turned on its side to give a better view of entrapped tissue. The paraffin block may be attached to a piece of wood, *6*, or a metal holder. (Infrequently tissues are embedded in celloidin.) The tissue is now ready to be cut into thin sections (Fig. 38-3).

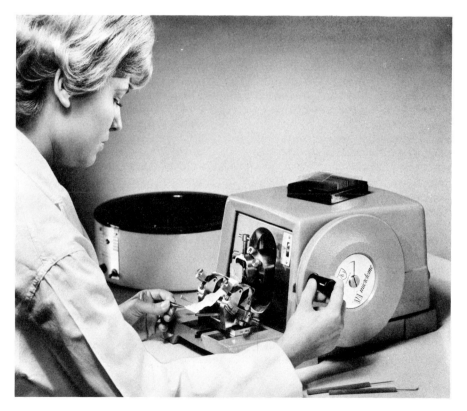

**Fig. 38-3.** Sectioning. Paraffin block containing embedded tissue is firmly secured in the microtome. The medical technologist (or histologic technician) cuts thin sections of tissue, floating them in a warm water bath to spread. From water bath (on the technologist's left) thin slices of tissue are attached to glass microslides. (Courtesy American Optical Corp., Buffalo, N. Y.)

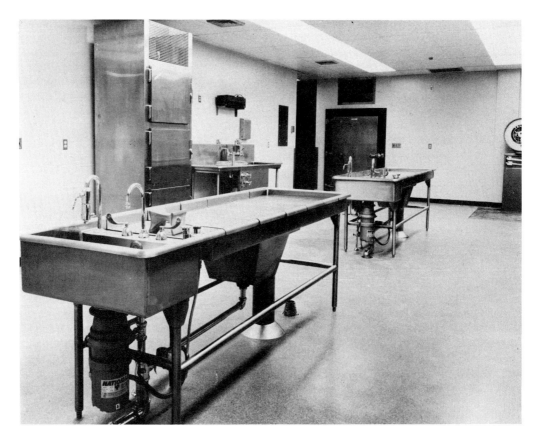

**Fig. 38-4.** Autopsy room, properly equipped and set aside in the modern hospital for this purpose. (Courtesy The Jewett Refrigerator Co., Inc., Buffalo, N. Y.)

prepared report available to the physician in attendance on the case.

Unfortunately laymen, as a rule, do not understand the importance of autopsies or how they are performed and consequently are often averse to the procedure. There are certain important arguments in favor of the autopsy. Among these are the following:

1. If the correctness or incorrectness of the diagnosis is proved in a given patient, the medical attendants are in a better position to render aid when subsequently another patient presents the same type of illness.*

2. Conditions of consequence to surviving relatives may be discovered, or, which is often as important, the surviving relatives may be comforted by finding that some disease which they thought the deceased had was not present.

3. Every person who has an autopsy done on his body makes a contribution, even in death, to the total fund of medical knowledge.

4. Rare or new diseases are often discovered by the routine performance of autopsies.

5. The autopsy yields important medical statistics.

It has been said that the general adoption of the autopsy is the mark that separates primitive from modern medicine.

Relatives of the deceased often voice certain objections, and these must be answered with assurance. The first is that an autopsy is a ghastly and mutilating procedure to which one would hesitate to subject a member of his family. Those who constantly deal with death develop a respect for the dead body that probably is not possessed by those who do not have special training, and an autopsy performed by a capable pathologist leaves no more visible mutilation than an operation on the living performed by a capable surgeon. After an autopsy has been performed, the body may be so completely restored to its original appearance that those who view the body will fail to recog-

---

*Napoleon, who suffered from cancer of the stomach, requested that an autopsy be performed on his body and that his son be given all information that might help him to escape a similar condition.

nize the fact that an autopsy has been done. A second objection is that a body on which an autopsy has been done does not embalm well. This is not true if there is cooperation between the pathologist doing the autopsy and the mortician caring for the body. Several associations of morticians are now working with medical societies to promote more autopsies.

Under present laws an autopsy cannot be performed without authorization from the next of kin of the deceased except in cases in which the detection of crime is an element.* Some states authorize an autopsy when the deceased requests it in his will. The authorization for an autopsy *must be written out* and should state whether it is to be a complete one or whether only certain parts of the body are to be examined. An unauthorized autopsy is a cause for civil action, and in some states it is a violation of the criminal code.

In many hospitals it is the duty of the autopsy pathologist to teach interns, residents, and other persons how to approach relatives of the deceased with a request for an autopsy and by whom and when the results of the autopsy should be discussed with relatives. Wherever this is done, more relatives will be tactfully approached, the results of the autopsy will be made known to them in a sympathetic and understanding manner, and the percentage of autopsies in that hospital will increase. A survey by Memorial Hospital in New York has shown that gratitude for kindly services rendered the patient, more than any other factor, led relatives to consent to the performance of an autopsy.

---

*There is no charge made for an autopsy—both the doctor and the hospital lay aside all fees for an examination that would normally cost around $500 or more.

## Pathology in patient care

Applications of the science of pathology are everywhere in the medical environment and apply directly or indirectly to all facets of the patient's welfare. There are three major aspects of patient care with which the members of the health team are concerned and to which their knowledge of pathology is applicable. First, in the *diagnosis of disease* a better understanding of basic pathology means more careful supervision of diagnostic regimens, more careful collection and processing of diagnostic specimens, and smoother relations between the clinical and diagnostic departments of the large medical institutions of today. Second, in the *treatment of disease* an appreciation of disease changes helps to explain therapeutic procedures and results and alerts the nurse or medical attendant to complications. The medical attendant who is informed of the pathology of chronic peptic ulcer is in a better position to aid in the medical or surgical management of the disease and better realizes the possibility of dangerous complications such as perforation or hemorrhage. Last, in the *supportive care* for the comfort and well-being of the patient, it is true that a better understanding of a coldly objective science can nevertheless lead to a subjective contribution of warm human sympathy, that extra measure for total patient care.

## Questions for review

1 Define pathology.
2 Discuss the divisions of pathology.
3 What are the three major purposes of all scientific endeavors?
4 What is the role of the medical technologist in the laboratory?
5 Give examples of laboratory tests performed in the following hospital departments: microbiology, hematology, clinical microscopy, and clinical chemistry.
6 Of what importance is pathology to patient care?
7 What is the value of the autopsy?

**References on pp. 434 and 435.**

# CHAPTER 39
# Nature and cause of disease

## Nature of disease

When all the cells making up a tissue or organ are functioning in a normal manner, that tissue or organ is in a state of *health*. If all or a number are impaired in function, the opposite state of *disease* exists. If changes become so extensive that the whole tissue or organ is incapable of performing its functions in a normal manner, the manifestations of disease appear.

**Cellular concept.** The biological theory that the structural unit of all plant and animal life is the cell took shape during the first half of the nineteenth century. By mid-century Rudolf Virchow (Fig. 39-1), German professor of pathology, had proposed that the cell is also the indivisible unit of disease, that all disease is brought about by changes primarily affecting the cells making up the body. This concept, with certain modifications, has withstood the test of scientific investigation, and the whole matter of disease can be summed up largely in accordance with it.

**Definition.** Disease is the abnormal performance of certain physiologic functions as a result of injury to the cells performing the functions. Arising from this abnormal performance are the outward evidences of disease. Although often studied as a static phenomenon so that it can be described objectively, disease is not stationary but is a dynamic series of changes that may end for the patient in recovery, permanent injury, or death.

According to some authorities health is defined as that condition in which there is complete harmony between the organism and its environment, both internal and external. Conversely, disease would be the opposite condition, in which the organism is out of harmony with its environment.

**Structural and functional changes.** The abnormal activity of the cells of an organ can produce both structural and functional changes. Some degree of functional change may occur without any marked change in structure, but most structural changes are associated with change in function. Sometimes functional changes first call our attention to the presence of disease, and if they are corrected soon enough, detectable changes in structure may not occur. For instance, if an obstruction to the venous outflow from an organ is discovered early and is speedily removed, the organ, although temporarily affected, may show little if any change in its structure within a short period of time. On the other hand, if such an obstruction persists, that organ shows definite related changes—an increase in connective tissue and a loss of functioning units.

**Interdependence of organs.** When an organ becomes impaired to such an extent that it is not capable of functioning normally, other organs, or even the entire body, may become involved. When the heart can no longer pump blood efficiently, changes occur in the entire body. The lungs become engorged, and the pulmonary circulation is impaired. This means decreased oxygenation of the blood in the lungs. When such a calamity occurs, many areas in the body will suffer from oxygen lack.

**Manifestations of disease.** The changes produced by disease in the tissues are known as *lesions*. The diagnostic manifestations of disease are known as *symptoms* if they are subjective, that is, experienced by the patient but not apparent to an observer (such as pain and malaise). If the manifestations are objective, that is, detected by an examiner (fever, swellings, paralysis), they are called *signs*.* A more or less sudden increase in the severity of symptoms and signs during the course of a disease is an *exacerbation*. An abatement of the severity of signs and symptoms during the course of a disease is a *remission*. Unfavorable conditions that arise during the course of a disease are *complications* (examples: hemorrhage or perforation of the intestine in typhoid fever). Remote aftereffects produced by a disease are *sequelae* (for example, chronic nephritis often follows scarlet fever).

An *acute* disease is one characterized by a swift onset and a rapid course. An acute disease that quickly proves fatal is often spoken of as a *fulminating* disease. A *chronic* disease is one of slow evolution. An

---

*The word *symptom* is commonly used to include both symptoms and signs.

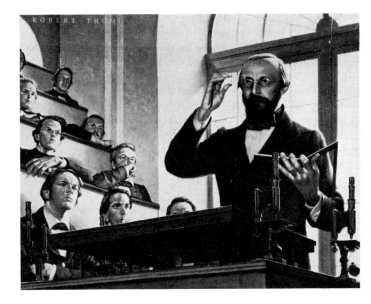

**Fig. 39-1.** Artist's concept of Rudolf Virchow (1821-1902). (Copyright 1961, Parke, Davis & Co., Detroit, Mich.)

*intercurrent* disease occurs during the course of another disease. An *idiopathic* disease is one that arises without apparent or known cause.

**Etiology and pathogenesis.** By etiology is meant the cause of disease. By pathogenesis is meant the manner of development of a disease, what causes it, what changes it produces, and how it affects the structure and the functional activities of the involved organs and the body as a whole. The prognosis and rational treatment of a disease are based on its pathogenesis.

**Predisposing factors.** Predisposing factors are those that make the body more susceptible to the development of disease, and they may significantly affect and alter the course of disease in a given person. Among the important factors are the following.

*Constitution.* By constitution is meant the sum total of those biologic characteristics that determine whether a person will find it a difficult matter to exist in his environment. Some observers consider constitution the most important factor in susceptibility and resistance to disease. How constitution plays its part we do not know. It is hereditary but can be modified greatly by environment. Persons with certain types of body build seem to be particularly susceptible to certain diseases; for instance, persons with long, thin chests seem to contract tuberculosis more readily than persons with short, broad chests. An inherited constitutional predisposition to a disease is known as a *diathesis;* a hemorrhagic diathesis means an inherited tendency for bleeding.

*Age.* There are many interesting patterns relating to age. During intrauterine life the fetus may con-

tract any of a number of diseases incident to its antenatal residence, and it is exposed to the dangers of injury and infection as it passes through the birth canal. After birth the infant may succumb to a condition that prevents the establishment of a normal extrauterine existence. Very young infants enjoy an immunity to diseases that are common in older children because of the transfer of immune bodies from the mother to the child via the placenta. These antibodies disappear from the body of the child about the time that he is 6 months old.

Tuberculosis usually begins before the end of the third decade, whereas high blood pressure, heart disease, and kidney disease usually occur after that time. Sarcomas (malignant tumors arising from connective tissue) are more common in young people, whereas carcinomas (malignant tumors arising from epithelium) are more common in older persons. Disturbances of nutrition and the manifestations of a number of diseases, especially diabetes, tuberculosis, and syphilis, differ in childhood and adulthood. In old age, atrophic changes affect the different tissues and organs of the body, and fibrotic and sclerotic changes occur in the heart and blood vessels.

*Sex.* Women and men differ anatomically, physiologically, emotionally, and constitutionally. Many diseases are less common in women than men, and the life expectancy of women is considerably greater than that of men. Excluding diseases related to the reproductive system, few major diseases are more common in women. This seems to be the result of an inherent increased susceptibility to disease on the part of males. Therefore, because of occupation and exposure, men often contract diseases that are uncommon in women.

*Race.* There is a difference in racial ability to live in different surroundings and in racial susceptibility and resistance to disease. Some races live with ease in arctic regions, others thrive equally well in torrid climates, but the majority live best in temperate zones. Blacks are very susceptible to tuberculosis but very resistant to malaria and yellow fever. They have generalized syphilis more often than whites, but their central nervous system is seldom involved. Sickle cell anemia is a disease of the blood that appears to be mostly confined to blacks, although it may be seen also in the people of countries bordering the Mediterranean Sea. The American Indian is peculiarly susceptible to tuberculosis, and the Jew, said to be resistant to tuberculosis, is especially susceptible to such metabolic diseases as diabetes.

*Nutrition.* Faulty or inadequate nutrition can lead to loss of weight and increased susceptibility to disease. Overeating leads to obesity. Fat that accumulates in the body may throw an extra burden on the circulatory system. Alterations in metabolism may lead to the development of disease, as exemplified in diabetes mellitus. The increased amount of sugar in the blood and tissues in diabetes favors the occurrence of skin infections, such as boils caused by staphylococci and other organisms that grow especially well in the presence of sugar.

*Environment.* Dark, overcrowded, damp, poorly ventilated surroundings increase the susceptibility of the inhabitants to disease. Overwork and continuous loss of sleep also decrease a person's resistance. Examples of occupational diseases are lead poisoning among workers in industries using lead compounds, silicosis among miners, and asbestosis among workers in the many industries using asbestos in the production of plastics, acoustical tiles, fire-resistant materials, and the like.

*Emotion.* Excessive emotional activity may make unusual demands on the body. "Worry is the great killer" is a saying based on a strong foundation of physiologic fact.

## Cause of disease: a classification

Although the actual cause (etiology) of some diseases is not known and that of other diseases not completely understood, it is possible, nevertheless, to outline and classify disease broadly according to the basic etiologic mechanism. We shall present this approach to disease here and shall generally follow it in our discussions in the ensuing chapters.

**Hereditary disorders and congenital anomalies.** Hereditary disorders are the disease processes that relate to the mechanisms of inheritance of character-

istics from preceding generations, and they tend to run in families. Included in this classification are those defects of development labeled congenital anomalies that result from a failure or an abnormality of development while the individual is within the uterine cavity of his mother and that are apparent shortly after birth. (See Chapter 40.)

**Circulatory disorders.** The complex arrangement of cells in the human body into an intricate physiologic system with specialization of function and division of labor among the cell groups is made possible only by communication lines between the different parts of the body. The circulatory system, a system of channels and conduits (with a central pumping station, the heart), serves not only to transport food and nutritive substances to the parts of the body and remove the waste and by-products of metabolism therefrom, but also to coordinate different parts of the body by the transportation of chemicals that relate physiologic activity in one part of the body with that in another part. If any part of the circulatory system breaks down, disease affecting wide areas of the body, even the body as a whole, results. (See Chapter 41.)

**Metabolic disorders and disturbances.** Metabolic disorders are the result of a failure, wholly or partially, in those complex enzymatic activities that occur within the cell and are concerned directly with the function of that cell. Disorders in this category produce significant diseases to which the body reacts but little. In many of these the cause and the sequence of events in between are not always well defined; yet the effects give us a well-defined pathologic change. (See Chapter 42.) There are four subdivisions in this category:

1. *Passive retrogressive or degenerative changes.* These occur as a result of certain standard conditions in the immediate environment of the cell.
2. *Deficiency states.* These result from the inadequate supply of a substance such as a vitamin or mineral that is vitally concerned in the metabolism of certain cells. There is a very obvious cause and effect here. For example, lack of a given vitamin results in a disease state; if the vitamin is supplied in adequate amounts, the disease situation is speedily cleared. (See Chapter 43.)
3. *Imbalance of hormones.* The diseases that result from an imbalance of the body hormones are included here. *Hormones* are chemical substances produced in specific glandular organs and released directly into the circulation. They generally are necessary to the physiologic well-being of cells all over the body, although they may have a target organ. There is a normal number of these that must be present in phys-

iologic amounts and proportions. With respect to hormones, diseases may be brought about in two ways—either by an excessive amount of the hormone or by an insufficient quantity. Since these substances are so necessary to well-being of cells, the state of either hypersecretion or hyposecretion means pathologic changes in cells and organs in the body. The disorders related to imbalance of hormones tie in with diseases of the glandular organs elaborating them. (See Chapter 53.)

4. *Disturbances at the molecular level.* In recent years, advances in biochemistry, genetics, and immunology have given us an insight into the relation of physical and chemical properties of molecules to the processes of life. The contribution of the biochemist has been the analysis of the protoplasm from many animal species. From this, a basic set of primary chemical building blocks for all living organisms has

emerged. The most important are the following: (a) amino acids (used to build proteins), some twenty; (b) purine and pyrimidine bases, five; (c) fatty acids, five; (d) carbohydrates, three; (e) phosphoric acid, one; (f) isoprene, one; (g) amino alcohols, three; and (h) sterol, one. These are simple, small molecules that can be built up within protoplasm into the larger, more complex *macromolecules.* In fact, in the normal state of nature many things can be done with these basic chemical units, the results of which are seen in the different biologic structures of varied functions consistent with the many kinds of biologic organisms.

*Molecular biology* is an expression used to explain life in terms of chemical molecules. *Molecular pathology,* therefore, is concerned with abnormalities of molecular structure and function and the relation to disease. By demonstrating a very complex ultrastructural organization within the cell (p. 21), the

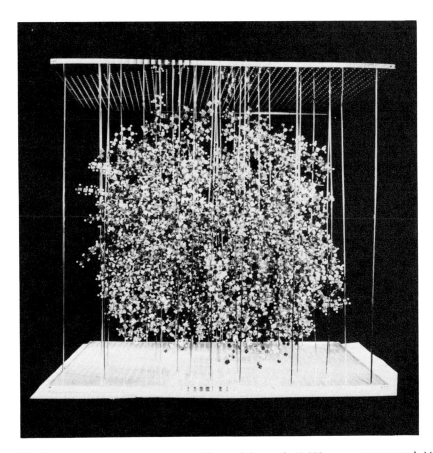

**Fig. 39-2.** Model of one molecule of normal hemoglobin with 10,000 atoms represented. Model constructed by Dr. M. Murayama, National Institutes of Health; it measures approximately 3 × 3 × 3 feet and magnifies hemoglobin molecule 127 million times. (From Lab. Med., May, 1971.)

electron microscope has helped to shape molecular pathology. As more is learned of what the ultrastructural components of the cell do, how they handle the primary chemical building blocks, how they participate in vital processes, and where macromolecules are formed, molecular pathology continues to advance as a new science and to gain in importance.

The best example of a disease caused by an abnormal chemical molecule is the hereditary blood disease of blacks, sickle cell anemia (p. 446), produced by the abnormal hemoglobin S. The departure in structure of hemoglobin S from normal hemoglobin (Fig. 39-2) is a difference of one amino acid. In this new field of molecular pathology many of the diseases have a hereditary background, but this is not invariable.

**Inflammation.** A large percentage of all diseases known to man are inflammatory. Inflammation is the sum of the body's reactions and responses to the event of injury of a part or all of the body. There is a direct sequence of events from the point of contact with the injurious agent to the resultant changes giving the full picture. A consideration of inflammation includes how the body rids itself of the injurious agent, how it resolves the effects of the total process, and how it effects healing and a return to the normal state of being. (See Chapter 44.)

**Neoplasms.** Neoplasms represent new growths of tissue within the body. It is in this category that we find cancers of the human body. Neoplasms represents a complex subject that does not lend itself easily to brief definition or description. (See Chapter 46.)

## Questions for review

1 From the standpoint of Virchow's concept of cellular pathology, explain the difference between health and disease.
2 Briefly define disease.
3 Do structural changes occur without functional changes? Do functional changes occur without perceptible structural changes?
4 Discuss the interdependence of organs.
5 What is a lesion?
6 What is the difference between signs and symptoms?
7 Briefly define acute, chronic, exacerbation, remission, sequelae.
8 What is meant by etiology of disease? By pathogenesis?
9 What factors predispose a given individual to disease?
10 What are the five major classifications of disease on an etiologic basis?
11 Briefly indicate the function of a circulation in a multicellular organism.

12 What is meant by inflammation?
13 What is meant by molecular pathology?

**REFERENCES** (Chapters 38 and 39)

Ackerman, L. V., and Rosai, J.: Surgical pathology, ed. 5, St. Louis, 1974, The C. V. Mosby Co.

Bologna, C. V.: Understanding laboratory medicine, St. Louis, 1971, The C. V. Mosby Co.

Boyd, W.: An introduction to the study of disease, ed. 6, Philadelphia, 1971, Lea & Febiger.

Bardin, J.: "Must" books for every home health library, Today's Health **50:**21, Sept., 1972.

Crowley, L. V.: A syllabus of visual aids in pathology, Chicago, 1972, Year Book Medical Publishers, Inc.

Crowley, L. V.: Introductory concepts in pathology, Chicago, 1972, Year Book Medical Publishers, Inc.

Davidsohn, I., and Henry, J. B.: Todd-Sanford clinical diagnosis by laboratory methods, ed. 15, Philadelphia, 1974, W. B. Saunders Co.

DeGraves, D., and Brondos, G. A.: A basic pathology library, Lab. Med. **4:**10, Sept., 1973.

Donnelly, A. F.: The romantic history of laboratory glassware, Lab. Med. **1:**28, March, 1970.

Environment: automated multiphasic screening, J.A.M.A. **213:**371, 1970.

Feeley, M. A.: Medical technology—a career choice, Lab. Med. **2:**19, April, 1971.

Freese, A. S.: A scientist talks about careers in science, Today's Health **47:**24, Sept., 1969.

Frumin, M. J., and Fine, E.: Post mortem or post hoc, J.A.M.A. **208:**519, 1969.

Grossman, L. W.: A primer of gross pathology, Springfield, Ill., 1972, Charles C Thomas, Publisher.

Hadley, A.: Pathology and autopsy lessons for the medical transcriber, Philadelphia, 1971, J. B. Lippincott Co.

Hathaway, B. M.: Advances in surgical pathology, J. Am. Med. Wom. Assoc. **23:**540, 1968.

Helpern, M.: Comments on the value of the autopsy, Pathologist **23:**39, Feb., 1969.

Higginson, J.: The role of the pathologist in environmental biology, Arch. Pathol. **91:**289, 1971.

Horty, J. F.: Who has the right to request an autopsy? Mod. Hosp. **110:**76, May, 1968.

King, L. S.: Signs and symptoms, J.A.M.A. **206:**1063, 1968.

King, L. S.: Organs, tissues, and cells, Lab. Med. **1:**13, Feb., 1970.

Koski, J. P.: Histochemistry in the small histopathology laboratory, Lab. Med. **2:**22, Feb., 1971.

Levinson, S. A., and MacFate, R. P.: Clinical laboratory diagnosis, ed. 7, Philadelphia, 1969, Lea & Febiger.

MacFate, R. P.: Introduction to the clinical laboratory, Chicago, 1972, Year Book Medical Publishers, Inc.

McCombs, R. P.: Fundamentals of internal medicine, ed. 4, Chicago, 1971, Year Book Medical Publishers, Inc.

Meyer, J. S., and Steinberg, L. S.: Review of laboratory medicine, ed. 2, St. Louis, 1975, The C. V. Mosby Co.

Miller, S. E., and Weller, J. M.: A textbook of clinical pathology, Baltimore, 1971, The Williams & Wilkins Co.

Moss, B. B.: Autopsy: an important medical aid, Today's Health **44:**65, May, 1966.

Neal, M. P.: The autopsy: a service and a teaching discipline, South. Med. J. **63:**47, 1970.

Reynolds, M. D.: Aim for a job in the medical laboratory, New York, 1972, Richards Rosen Press, Inc.

Peery, T. M., and Miller, F. N., Jr.: Pathology: a dynamic introduction to medicine and surgery, ed. 2, Boston, 1971, Little, Brown & Co.

Prior, J. A., and Silberstein, J. S.: Physical diagnosis—the history and examination of the patient, ed. 4, St. Louis, 1973, The C. V. Mosby Co.

Ravel, R.: Clinical laboratory medicine, ed. 2, Chicago, 1973, Year Book Medical Publishers, Inc.

Robbins, S. L.: The pathologic basis of disease, Philadelphia, 1974, W. B. Saunders Co.

Rodin, A. E.: The influence of Matthew Baillie's morbid anatomy, Springfield, Ill., 1973, Charles C Thomas, Publisher.

Sheehan, D. C., and Hrapchak, B. B.: Theory and practice of histotechnology, St. Louis, 1973, The C. V. Mosby Co.

Shivas, A. A., and Fraser, S. G.: Frozen section in surgical diagnosis, Baltimore, 1971, The Williams & Wilkins Co.

Shwachman, H.: Changing concepts of cystic fibrosis, Hosp. Pract. **9:**143, Jan., 1974.

Sisson, J. A.: The bare facts of general pathology, Philadelphia, 1971, J. B. Lippincott Co.

Sisson, J. A.: The bare facts of systemic pathology, Philadelphia, 1972, J. B. Lippincott Co.

Stenn, F.: Six hundred years of autopsies, Lab. Med. **2:**21, Jan, 1971.

Thomas, L.: The lives of a cell: notes of a biology watcher, New York, 1974, Viking Press, Inc.

Valentine, G. H.: The chromosome disorders, an introduction for clinicians, ed. 2, Philadelphia, 1971, J. B. Lippincott Co.

Wallach, J. B.: Interpretation of diagnostic tests (a handbook synopsis of laboratory medicine), Boston, 1974, Little, Brown & Co.

Ward, F. A.: A primer of pathology, New York, 1972, Appleton-Century-Crofts.

White, W. L., and others: Practical automation for the clinical laboratory, ed. 2, St. Louis, 1972, The C. V. Mosby Co.

Williams, M. R.: An introduction to the profession of medical technology, Philadelphia, 1971, Lea & Febiger.

Winsten, S., and Dalal, F. R.: Manual of clinical laboratory procedures for non-routine problems, Cleveland, 1972, CRC Press.

Woodcock, L.: Challenge and change in today's laboratory, Lab. Med. **1:**33, Feb., 1970.

Young, C. G., and Barger, J. D.: Introduction to medical science, ed. 2, St. Louis, 1973, The C. V. Mosby Co.

Zugibe, F. T.: Diagnostic histochemistry, St. Louis, 1970, The C. V. Mosby Co.

# CHAPTER 40

# Birth defects

## General considerations

A structural or functional disorder present at birth is a *birth defect.* It may be genetically determined or the result of an environmental influence during gestation.

Birth defects may be classified into three major categories: (1) *hereditary diseases* produced by disturbances in the mechanisms of inheritance; (2) *congenital disorders* related to abnormalities confined to the period of gestation (particularly the first 3 months after conception); and (3) *traumatic lesions* sustained at time of delivery. Birth trauma indicates obstetric problems such as prolonged labor and the difficulty of a large head passing through a small pelvis.

**Hereditary factors in disease.** The inherited traits of an individual are those characteristics that he has received from his ancestors and that he will transmit to his offspring. Among the many normal traits thus transmitted are body physique, color of hair and eyes, blood type, mental capabilities, and emotional makeup. Examples of abnormal traits that are inherited are color blindness, mental deficiencies, a tendency toward allergic conditions, increased susceptibility to certain drugs, and a predisposition toward metabolic diseases (diabetes or gout). Inheritable characteristics do not necessarily appear in each succeeding generation but may skip a generation before reappearing.

Inherited diseases that tend to run in families are known as *familial disorders.* Often they are seen in several members of the same family, or they may skip one or more generations. Heredity is one of the most important factors in the genesis of disease.

*Medical genetics* is the study of heredity's role in disease. It treats the disorders largely determined by changes in the normal inheritance mechanism. For many years the only source of genetic information in man was the family tree or pedigree. However, modern technics for studying the hereditary units within human cells have meant tremendous advances.

*Chromosomes.* The chromosomes carry the hereditary material, the DNA. There are two complete sets in all cells except the mature germ cells. For man, the total chromosome number is 46, with twenty-three pairs. Twenty-two pairs (44) are *autosomes,* and one pair, *sex chromosomes.*

The science studying and classifying chromosomes is *cytogenetics.* By cytogenetic technics chromosomes from rapidly growing tissues such as bone marrow can be studied in squash preparations. Fixed and stained* chromosomes are laid out so that individual ones can be paired. Paired and numbered in a standard way, the chromosomes form a pattern called a *karyotype* (Fig. 40-1). (The schematized drawing of a composite of many karyotypes is an *idiogram.*) Chromosomes are identified according to their size and shape (Table 40-1). The longest one is about 7 to 8 $\mu$m. ($\mu$) in length; the shortest, about 1 or 2 $\mu$m. Each chromosome is composed of two *chromatids* joined at the *centromere* (Fig. 40-2). According to the position of the centromere on the chromosome and the consequent length of the arms (on either side of the centromere), chromosomes are *metacentric,* arms approximately of equal length; *submetacentric,* two short and two long arms; and *acrocentric,* two very short and two very long arms.

*Sex chromosomes.* The sex chromosomes are the X and Y ones, so named because of their similarity to the letters of the alphabet. In the normal karyotype of the male the sex chromosomes are XY; in the normal female, XX. (See Fig. 40-1.)

The nuclei of cells from the female may be distinguished from those of the male by the presence of a stainable chromatin body (the Barr body) (Fig. 40-3), considered to be an X chromosome, especially well visualized in the large squamous cells lining the mouth. The chromatin body (Barr body) is referred to as *sex chromatin,* and its presence or absence helps to determine *nuclear sex.* Cells containing the sex chromatin are chromatin-positive and genetically belong to a female. Cells lacking sex chromatin are chromatin-negative and are genetically male. When the outward manifestations of sex, the secondary sex characters,

---

*A fluorescent staining technic is used effectively.

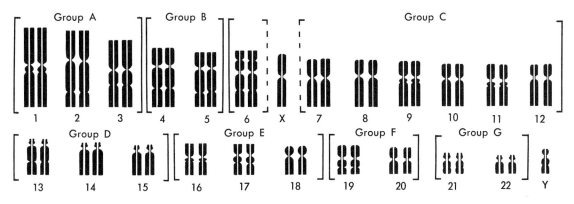

**Fig. 40-1.** Idiogram of human metaphase chromosomal pairs, showing normal male pattern (46, XY). Arbitrary divisions relate to size of chromosome and position of centromere.

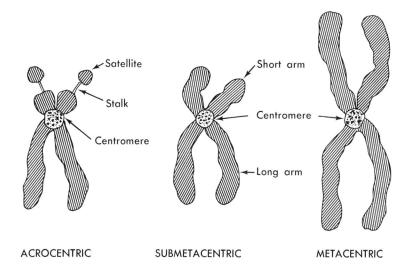

**Fig. 40-2.** Types of human metaphase chromosomes, sketch. Note different positions of centromere (primary constriction) in each of three. On left, centromere belts two chromatids together from subterminal position (just short of end of chromosome). On right, its position is median (central), and in chromosome in middle, submedian (just off-center).

## Table 40-1
Analysis of human chromosomes

| DESCRIPTION OF CHROMOSOMES | | GROUP | AUTOSOMES | SEX CHROMOSOMES | NUMBER OF CHROMOSOMES IN ALL BODY (SOMATIC) CELLS | |
|---|---|---|---|---|---|---|
| SIZE | POSITION OF CENTROMERE | | | | MALE | FEMALE |
| Large | Metacentric or submetacentric | A | 1, 2, 3 | | 6 | 6 |
| Large | Submetacentric | B | 4, 5 | | 4 | 4 |
| Medium | Metacentric and submetacentric | C | 6, 7, 8, 9, 10, 11, 12 | X | 15 | 16 |
| Medium | Acrocentric (subterminal) | D | 13, 14, 15 | | 6 | 6 |
| Small | Metacentric and submetacentric | E | 16, 17, 18 | | 6 | 6 |
| Smallest | Metacentric | F | 19, 20 | | 4 | 4 |
| Small | Acrocentric (subterminal) | G | 21, 22 | Y | 5 | 4 |
| | | | | Total | 46 | 46 |

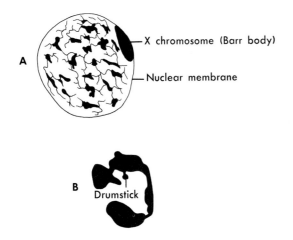

**Fig. 40-3.** Sex chromatin. **A,** X chromosome or Barr body, planoconvex body attached to nuclear membrane of body cell. **B,** Drumstick appendage from nucleus of polymorphonuclear leukocyte.

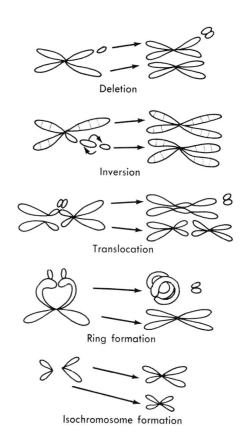

**Fig. 40-4.** Rearrangements leading to structural abnormalities in chromosomes.

are poorly developed and when the sex of an individual is reversed, nuclear testing is important. In *sex reversal* a person looks like one sex but possesses tissues of the opposite sex.

*Chromosomal abnormalities.* The science of cytogenetics effectively demonstrates many aberrations in chromosomes (Fig. 40-4). In a routine analysis, a chromosomal count is done. There may be more than the normal, fewer than normal, or a rearrangement of those normally present. Departures from the normal number and arrangement of chromosomes are usually correlated to important clinical defects.

*Genes.* Corresponding loci on the chromosomes mark the position of a pair of genes. Through their physiologic control of proteins and therefore of enzymes, genes influence the sum of the many vital activities carried out within cells to make us precisely what we are as individual human beings.

Genes are responsible directly for the traits of the individual, both the apparent ones and those less so. If genes are identical, so is their biochemical influence, and the person possessing the trait is said to be *homozygous.* If the genes of the pair are unlike, the person with those genes is *heterozygous* for the given trait. When one gene of an unlike pair is active and its influence is felt, it is said to be the *dominant* one, whereas the suppressed gene is the *recessive* one. A person may pass either the dominant or the recessive gene to his offspring.

Genetic disorders occur because of the abnormality of a single gene or of a large number of them.

**Inheritance of disease in man.** Several thousand deviations from normal in man have been investigated genetically, and for several hundred disorders a genetic basis has been established. Disease may be passed from one generation to another because of its relation to an abnormal gene that is the dominant one. Examples of dominant inheritance of disease include hereditary spherocytosis and achondroplasia. Disease may be transmitted because of its relation to recessive genes in homozygous individuals. Among the conditions transmitted by simple recessive inheritance are sickle cell anemia, phenylketonuria, galactosemia, and glycogen storage disease. Sex-linked inheritance refers to the fact that the abnormal gene is carried on the X chromosome of a female heterozygous for a sex-linked recessive disease. Examples are color blindness and hemophilia.

*Mutations.* Genetic abnormalities resulting in disease usually come about as the result of *mutations.* A mutation is an alteration of the basic hereditary material in one given gene, which is then an inheritable defect. Generally, most mutations are for the worse. Why they occur is not known. Environmental factors (temperature, atmospheric oxygen, nutrition) may be involved. Experimentally, penetrating ionizing radiation and chemicals such as formalin, mustard

**Table 40-2**
Examples of abnormalities attributed to irradiation of the human fetus

| ANATOMIC LOCATION | DEFECT |
|---|---|
| Eyes | Anophthalmia (no eyes), microphthalmia (small eyes), absence of lens or retina, open eyelids, strabismus (cross-eye), retinoblastoma (tumor), partial albinism, cataract, blindness, chorioretinitis |
| Brain | Anencephaly (no brain), microcephaly (small head), mongolism, cerebral atrophy, mental retardation, idiocy, neuroblastoma (tumor) |
| Skeleton | General stunting, skull deformities, narrow head, cleft palate, funnel chest, congenital dislocation of hips, spina bifida, overgrown and deformed feet, clubfeet, abnormal limbs |
| Other areas | Situs inversus, absence of kidney, degenerate gonad, abnormal skin pigmentation, increased probability of leukemia, congenital heart disease, deformed ear, facial deformities |

gas, and nitrogen mustard are well-known mutagens. The induction of genetic mutation is *mutagenesis*.

**Congenitally acquired disorders.** Defects resulting from a failure or an abnormality in the developmental process itself as it occurs in the embryo and that are either present at birth or shortly thereafter are spoken of as *congenital anomalies*. By definition they may but need not have a genetic basis. Examples are harelip, cleft palate, and spina bifida. More than 600 different kinds have been described, and today many new ones are defined. Congenital defects are as old as the human race. For instance, clubfoot has been recognized for centuries.

*Teratology* is the study of abnormal embryonic development resulting in these anomalies. *Teratogenesis* refers to the factors and processes involved in their production. Although little is known as to why they occur, many factors presented as causes are being carefully studied in research laboratories. Such factors include the action of drugs, the effects of radiation, and the role of viruses when viral infection complicates pregnancy.

Some malformations are related directly to genetic factors. Mongolism, for example, is a well-known disorder associated with an abnormality of chromosomes, and an extra chromosome can be demonstrated with present-day technics of cytogenetics.

There are etiologic factors for congenital anomalies that seem to relate directly to the mother of the affected infant. Congenital defects are more prevalent in older mothers. They can occur with complications of pregnancy, such as *polyhydramnios* (too much amniotic fluid). The mother's diet, her general state of nutrition, and the adequacy of her vitamin intake may have some as yet undetermined relation. Other factors implicated are the effect of toxic chemicals or drugs, the influence of hormones, and physical injury.

*Chemical teratogens.* The thalidomide tragedy taught us that some malformations are caused directly by the action of extragenetic agents (teratogens). The *thalidomide syndrome* was the conse-

quence of a teratogenic drug, which in West Germany, parts of Europe, and Canada was shown to be responsible for thousands of malformed children. Supposedly a mild and safe sedative, thalidomide was taken by pregnant women during the crucial time between the twenty-seventh and fortieth days of gestation. Of the malformations described in the infants born to these women, the most common and striking was *phocomelia*, seal limb. Previously considered an extremely rare disorder, this deformity represents failure of development of the extremities, especially the upper ones. The bones of the forearm and upper arm fail to grow so that the hands extend almost directly from the shoulders. The hands, attached directly to the body, resemble the flippers of a seal. Infants with severe involvement as a result of the thalidomide have neither arms nor legs.

In numerous studies LSD (lysergic acid diethylamide) has been shown to affect human chromosomes adversely. It is thought to do so in 75% of persons who use it. Recently, the consumption of "blighted" potatoes (potatoes bruised, discolored, or moldy) by expectant mothers has been linked to skull and spine defects in their infants.

*Physical teratogens.* Irradiation is accepted as a causal factor in congenital anomalies. Malformation rates are higher in the population of certain geographic areas where the background of natural radiation is high. Table 40-2 lists examples of radiation-induced malformations.

*Viral teratogens.* Currently, the role of viruses in teratogenesis (the production of physical defects in the offspring in utero) is being carefully studied. When the pregnant woman contracts a viral infection accompanied by viremia, the infection is often passed across the placenta to the susceptible embryo or fetus. Notable examples are measles, smallpox, vaccinia, western equine encephalitis, chickenpox, poliomyelitis, hepatitis, and coxsackievirus infection. Viral infections involving the offspring within the uterus may be more common than suspected, especially in the lower socioeconomic brackets. Although the possibilities for fetal infection are many, only three viruses have been fully qualified as teratogens. The evidence is clear cut for rubella virus, cytomegalovirus, and *Herpesvirus hominis*.

Birth defects with rubella virus (see also p. 296) have been more thoroughly examined than those with the other viruses, and most of what is known about viral teratogenesis comes from such investigations. In rubella, the teratogenic mechanism seems to stem from a direct interaction between virus and parasitized cell that continues throughout the length of gestation. That plus viral damage to blood vessels disrupts normal organ development.

The cytomegalovirus (salivary gland virus) produces a mild infection in the mother but can cause extensive and widespread damage in the neonate. (See also p. 301.) In a few instances *Herpesvirus hominis* has crossed the placenta to produce generalized infection, with documented malformations resulting in the central nervous system and in the eye. (See also p. 301.)

*Toxoplasma as teratogen.* An unborn child may acquire another infection from its mother, this time one with a protozoan parasite, *Toxoplasma gondii*. The baby shows deposits of calcium within the brain, abnormalities of brain development (microcephaly and hydrocephalus), and involvement of the eyes as a result of *congenital toxoplasmosis*.

## Catalogue of disorders
### BODY SIZE AND BUILD

**Monsters.** A monster is a grossly deformed fetus.

If a fertilized ovum starts to develop but incompletely divides into two parts, a *double monster* (instead of identical twins with complete division) is formed. Double monsters may be classified as (1) equal conjoined twins and (2) conjoined twins in which one is smaller than the other. Equal conjoined twins may be joined at the head, chest, or lower pelvic region. These combinations give various types of deformity such as (1) two well-formed bodies not extensively joined (Siamese twins), (2) one body, one set of limbs, and two heads, or (3) one head, two arms, and four legs. There are myriads of other types.

If something interferes with the development of one of the twins of a double monster, it may become attached to the larger one as a *parasitic fetus*. Fortunately, most double monsters, except the equally but not extensively joined twins, do not survive for any length of time.

The formation of double monsters represents the occurrence of identical twins gone awry. Twins are of two types, fraternal and identical. *Fraternal twins* are formed by the simultaneous fertilization of two ova.

The twins may or may not be of the same sex, and they have no more resemblance to each other than to other siblings. *Identical twins* are formed from a single ovum that in its very early stages of development becomes divided into two parts, each part developing into a child. Such twins are of the same sex and closely resemble each other in physical and mental characteristics. Triplets, quadruplets, and quintuplets may be dissimilar or identical or combinations of the two. For instance, triplets may arise from one, two, or three ova. If they arise from two ova, there will be two identical twins plus one fraternal twin.

**Achondroplasia.** Achondroplasia is a type of dwarfism recognized since ancient times by a normal sized head and trunk with very short (but functional) extremities. Such persons are healthy and intelligent and make fine acrobats and circus performers. It is thought that in this hereditary disorder the responsible gene that has undergone mutation is found in the germ cells of the father. The condition is not confined to the human race, as evidenced by the dachshund dog. (See Fig. 40-5.)

### EXTREMITIES

**Polydactylism.** By polydactylism is meant more than the normal number of fingers. The extra digit is usually a thumb or little finger. Extra fingers are often accompanied by extra toes. Webbed fingers or toes (syndactylism) are not uncommon.

**Absence of hands and feet.** Absence of hands and feet is rare. However, a family of twelve children of whom six were without hands and feet has been reported.

**Absence of arms and legs.** Rarely a person is born without arms or without legs. Sometimes both arms and legs are absent. The mermaid was probably suggested by a rare malformation in which the legs grew in a fused tapering mass, giving the body the appearance of a fish.

### HEAD AND NECK

**Shape of the face.** The most common shape of the face is such that a line drawn from the eyes to the chin is straight. A few people have a concave face (dish face). Others have a convex face. The shape of the face is greatly influenced by the chin. The protruding Hapsburg chin was characteristic of the European royal family of Hapsburg, and at least a few members of the Hohenzollern family were noted for their receding chins.

**Harelip.** In its early stages (about the second month of intrauterine life) the upper jaw of the fetus consists of three parts: a central portion bearing the incisor teeth and the two lateral portions bearing the jaw teeth. The jaw is formed when the lateral portions

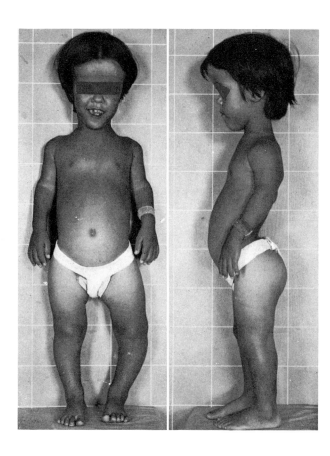

**Fig. 40-5.** Achondroplastic dwarf. At 8 years of age, her height is 37 inches (10 inches below average for her age). Typical are long torso with short extremities, "swayback," large head, saddle nose, and short thick fingers. (From Raney, R. B., and Brashear, R.: Shands' handbook of orthopaedic surgery, ed. 8, St. Louis, 1971, The C. V. Mosby Co.)

grow forward and fuse with the central portion. The roof of the mouth is made by two lateral bony portions coming together and fusing in the midline. If this fusion is imperfect, a cleft of the lip occurs. If the defect is extensive, there is also a cleft in the upper jaw and the hard palate. This is a cleft palate.

The word *harelip* is a misnomer because the cleft in the lip of a hare is in the middle, whereas with the usual harelip the cleft is on one or both sides. (See Fig. 40-6.) A harelip occurs three times more often on the left side than on the right. If the cleft is in the middle, it is caused by failure of fusion of the portions of the nose that form the upper lip. Sometimes there is a cleft palate without any change in the lip.

**Tongue-tie.** Tongue-tie is an abnormal shortness of the frenulum of the tongue. This limits the movement of the tongue, resulting in a characteristic type of speech. Tongue-tie is easily relieved by severing the frenulum.

**Fistulas and cysts in the neck.** A fistula is a tract or passageway that connects the interior of an organ with another body cavity or with the outside surface of the body. A cyst is a saccular, walled-off structure, usually round or ovoid in shape, that contains within a central cavity either fluid, a semisolid material, or a gas. With these two definitions in mind, let us consider two important sets of fistulas and cysts in the neck: the branchial fistulas and cysts and the thyroglossal duct fistulas and cysts.

During embryonic life there are structures on each side of the neck known as branchial clefts, which in mammals become obliterated and in fish persist to form gills. If one of these clefts fails to be obliterated, it persists, secreting mucus that may be discharged on the side of the neck through a *branchial fistula* or accumulated in a blind pocket to form a *branchial cyst*. Although the defect is present at birth, the accumulation of fluid is not sufficient to cause a cyst to develop until later life.

During early embryonic life there is a duct known as the thyroglossal duct, which extends from the thyroid gland to the posterior part of the tongue. It later becomes obliterated. When this duct persists in whole or in part, either a *thyroglossal duct fistula* or *cyst* is formed. Such a defect occurs in the middle of the neck. It is rarely present at birth but appears in infancy or young adulthood.

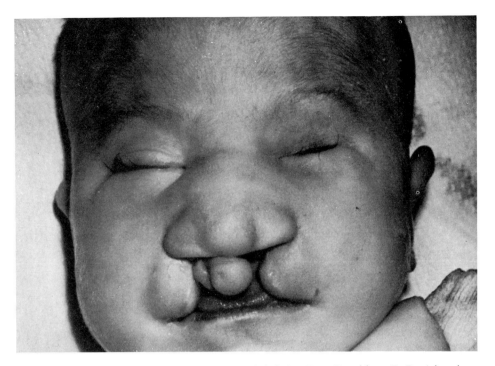

**Fig. 40-6.** Double hare-lip, cleft palate, and microophthalmia. (From Donaldson, D. D.: Atlas of external diseases of the eye, vol. 1, St. Louis, 1966, The C. V. Mosby Co.)

## SPECIAL SENSES

**Deaf-mutism.** Deaf-mutism is a congenital or acquired (in early childhood) defect of the organ of hearing that may prevent acquisition of speech. A deaf-mute is often said to be deaf and dumb. Congenital deaf-mutism may be caused by congenital syphilis or German measles. Heredity is also an important factor. Deaf-mutism is frequently associated with cretinism and goiter in certain geographic areas.

An afflicted child may learn to talk but lose his limited speech when he loses his sense of hearing. This may be prevented by cultivation of speech. The age at which deafness causes loss of speech depends upon the intelligence of the child, but on the average, unless speech is cultivated, it will be lost if deafness occurs before the seventh year.

**Color blindness.** Color blindness is a sex-linked recessive disorder in which the number of colors that may be distinguished by an individual is greatly reduced. The most common type is an inability to differentiate between reds and greens. A less common type is an inability to distinguish between blues and yellows. In the more severe and uncommon forms all objects appear to be some shade of gray. It is estimated that about 4% of males have some degree of color blindness. Total color blindness occurs one time in some 300,000 persons.

**Eyes of different color.** This rare condition may occur in each succeeding generation or may skip one or more generations.

**Cross-eye.** In cross-eye the axes of vision of the two eyes are not parallel. Either eye may look toward its fellow (convergent cross-eye) or away (divergent cross-eye). Both types may be found in the same family.

**Nearsightedness (myopia) and farsightedness (hyperopia).** The normal eyeball is practically spherical in shape. Rays of light coming from objects near the eyes are focused on the retina when the convexity of the lens becomes greater, and rays coming from faraway objects are focused on the retina when the convexity of the lens becomes less (Fig. 40-7). In a nearsighted person the eyeball is longer than normal, and since the lens is unable to flatten enough to focus the image on the retina, the image is focused in front of the retina. Biconcave glasses are used to correct this defect. In farsightedness the eyeball is so short that images of nearby objects are focused at a point behind the retina, and the lens cannot become convex enough to bring the focus sufficiently forward to make the image fall on the retina. Convex lenses help correct this defect. Both nearsightedness and farsightedness are inherited conditions.

**Cataract.** Cataract is a clouding and opacity of the

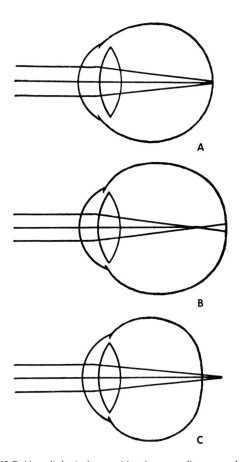

**Fig. 40-7.** How light is focused by the eye, diagrams. **A,** In the *normal* eye, light is focused on retina. **B,** In a *near-sighted* person, point of focus is in front of retina. **C,** In a *farsighted* person, point of focus is behind retina.

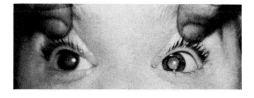

**Fig. 40-8.** Bilateral congenital cataract. (From Shirkey, H. C., editor: Pediatric therapy, ed. 4, St. Louis, 1972, The C. V. Mosby Co.)

lens (Fig. 40-8). It may be congenital or acquired. German measles during pregnancy is one cause of congenital cataract.

## SKIN AND HAIR

**Freckles.** Freckles are circumscribed areas of skin in which there is an excessive amount of skin coloring matter (melanin). They are more common in those parts of the body exposed to light (face, neck, and back of hands). Melanin (black substance) occurs in the deeper portion of the epidermis within the cytoplasm of the cells. The depth of skin pigmentation is dependent on the amount of melanin present.

**Birthmarks.** Birthmarks or *vascular nevi* (sing., *nevus*) are caused by an overgrowth and dilatation of the capillaries in the superficial layers of the skin. The color of a vascular nevus is not produced by a change in skin pigmentation but by the blood-filled vessels showing through the epidermis.

Vascular nevi occur in two types, the raised and the flat. The *raised type* usually occurs about the face. It is present at birth or appears soon thereafter. It occurs as a raised, red or bluish, spongy, circumscribed growth that is usually not more than a few centimeters in diameter. In some cases vascular nevi grow rapidly, but generally they grow slowly to a certain point and then stop. They may undergo spontaneous involution. They temporarily increase in size with crying or excitement. When occurring on the lip or ear, they may cause great deformity.

The *flat type* of vascular nevus or port-wine stain occurs chiefly on the face and back of the neck. These nevi are level with the skin and do not tend to spread as the child grows older. They are often unilateral in distribution and tend to follow the course of the sympathetic nerves. They are smooth and purplish red or violet. Their color changes with crying, coughing, or exposure to cold.

The cause of birthmarks is not known. The theory of maternal impressions is a relic of bygone days. Vascular nevi should not be confused with pigmented nevi or pigmented moles. When the word *nevus* is used without qualification, it usually refers to the latter, but it is often used as a more general term to designate any circumscribed lesion of the skin.

**Ichthyosis.** Ichthyosis ("fish scale" disease) is a congenital condition in which there is dryness of the skin associated with areas of superficial thickening. This condition is found in the fish-skinned or alligator boy of the side show.

**Increased elasticity of skin.** The skin is attached to the body by two types of fibers, elastic and nonelastic. The nonelastic fibers restrict the distance to which the skin may be pulled away from the body, whereas the elastic fibers pull the skin back to the body. If the nonelastic fibers grow to a great length, as occurs on rare occasions, the skin may be pulled a great distance from the body. This condition results in the rubber-skinned man of the sideshow.

**Congenital hypertrichosis and hypotrichosis.** Hypertrichosis is a condition in which the child is born completely or partly covered with hair. The dog-faced boy is a victim of congenital hypertrichosis.

Localized hairy growths are often seen in the lumbar or sacral regions in association with nevi. Hypotrichosis is a decrease in amount or a complete absence of hair. With complete hypotrichosis the nails are usually defective.

## BREAST (MAMMARY GLAND)

**Anomalies.** Beginning about the second month of embryonic life, the first step in the development of the breast is the formation on each side of the body of a thickened ridge of epithelium that extends from the axilla to the inguinal region. This is known as the *milk line*. The line then regresses all along its course except in the chest region in the human female, where mammary glands will later develop.

In the human female the mammary glands begin to develop at the age of puberty; in the male, they regress at puberty. One of the most common abnormalities of the mammary glands is the formation of supernumerary nipples (*polythelia*) or even complete mammary glands (*polymastia*) along the milk lines. Although the supernumerary nipples and breasts usually develop along the milk lines, they may develop in locations far removed. As a rule, supernumerary breasts are not functional, but sometimes they are. *Amastia* is congenital absence of breasts. It may be unilateral or bilateral.

## CENTRAL NERVOUS SYSTEM

**Developmental anomalies.** The central nervous system develops first by the formation of a groove, known as the *neural groove,* along the posterior surface of the embryo. As development proceeds, the neural groove deepens, and the sides fuse at the top to convert the groove into a tube within which the nervous system develops. In some cases the groove may fail to convert into a tube. In most cases, if the tube fails to close, the failure is partial and is located at the sacral or cranial end. When located at the cranial end, this condition is known as *cranioschisis* (Fig. 40-9). If this condition is extreme, there is little development of either brain or cranial bones. There is no cranial vault, and the skin passes directly from above the eyes to the occipital region, giving rise to an appearance of the head that may be described as frog-like. Fortunately these persons usually survive only a few hours or not at all.

*Microcephaly* is abnormal smallness of the head (pinhead). These unfortunate persons are usually imbeciles and, if the head is extremely small, do not live long.

In *spina bifida* the neural groove fails to close at the sacral end, and the laminae of the spinal column are absent. If there are no surface markings to indicate the defect, the condition is known as *spina bifida occulta*. In many cases there is herniation of the contents of the vertebral canal into the skin. There may be any or all of the following just beneath the skin: meninges, spinal cord, or spinal fluid.

**Pilonidal sinus\* or cyst.** Pilonidal sinus is a tract or cyst that may form in the midline of the body near the sacrococcygeal junction at the lower end of the spine. If the external opening becomes stopped up and secretions are retained, a cyst results. The tract is lined with squamous epithelium and often contains hair. The term *pilonidal* means nest of hair. A tuft of hair may project through the external opening. There are several theories explaining the formation of pilonidal sinuses and cysts. It seems likely that they are formed from remains of the neural canal, which is attached in that area.

**Hydrocephalus.** Hydrocephalus is discussed on p. 624.

**Down's syndrome.** Down's syndrome (mongolism or mongolian idiocy) is a condition in which there develops a characteristic facial appearance in a child who is an idiot. Small changes in the eyes, nose, mouth, ears, and shape of the head result in a strange facies that Europeans originally likened to that of an Asiatic, hence the term *mongolian*. Asiatics, on the other hand, consider these persons to look like Europeans. Growth is stunted, mentality is low, and susceptibility to infection is enhanced. Such a child may die early in life. The congenital defect in mongolism is a chromosomal one. There is an extra chromosome in a certain one of the autosome sets, to give a total of 47 chromosomes instead of the normal 46. The extra chromosome is postulated to come from an accident in the development of the egg, which, subsequently fertilized, formed the afflicted individual.

## INTERNAL ORGANS

**Situs inversus.** In situs inversus some or all of the organs of the body are on the side opposite that on which they normally belong. In complete situs inversus the position of the viscera is the mirror image of the normal.

**Aberrant tissues.** Tissues may be found in places other than their normal location (*ectopia* or *heterotopia*). Normal pancreatic tissues may be found in the intestinal wall or even in the stomach, with no connection to the normal organ. Most of the time such out-of-place tissue produces no symptoms and is discovered by accident, but serious disturbances are possible.

---

\*A sinus is defined as a tract that proceeds from mucous membrane, skin surface, or the interior of an organ, making no connection with any other anatomic area but ending blindly.

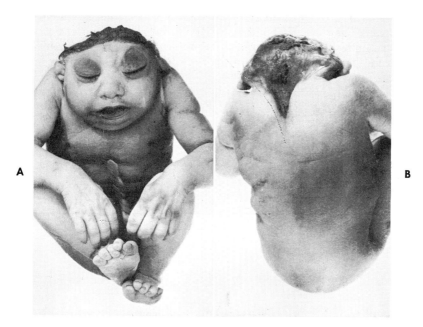

**Fig. 40-9.** Extreme cranioschisis. **A,** Anterior view. **B,** Posterior view.

**Cardiac anomalies** (see p. 528). The heart may be absent *(acardia),* may project through an anterior chest opening that has failed to close in the process of fetal development *(ectopia cordis),* or may be transposed to the opposite side of the body *(dextrocardia).* Dextrocardia usually occurs as a part of situs inversus.

**Renal anomalies.** One or both kidneys may fail to develop *(agenesis),* or they may be small and their functional capacity greatly reduced *(hypoplasia).* Bilateral agenesis or hypoplasia of any great degree is incompatible with life. Unilateral agenesis or hypoplasia is rather common and usually affects the right kidney. The opposite kidney is greatly hypertrophied.

The two kidneys may be fused at the lower poles *(horseshoe kidney)* or both kidneys may be greatly enlarged and composed of many thin-walled cysts filled with clear fluid or jellylike material *(congenital cystic kidney).* A similar condition of the liver is often associated. If extensive, the presence of multiple cysts in the organs is not compatible with life. One of the kidneys, especially the right, may be displaced downward, laterally, or forward and, because of looseness of its attachments, may exhibit considerable mobility. Kidneys showing a marked degree of mobility are known as floating kidneys.

**Exstrophy of the bladder.** A discussion of exstrophy of the bladder is given on p. 589.

**Intestinal diverticula.** Intestinal diverticula are discussed on p. 568.

**Bicornate uterus.** The vagina, uterus, and fallopian tubes are derived from the lateral fusion of two ducts known as the müllerian ducts. In animals that give birth to a single offspring, the ducts usually fuse throughout the extent of the vagina and uterus and then remain separate to form the fallopian tubes. In animals that have several offspring at a time, the tubes do not fuse except for a short distance above the vagina, and the uterus consists of two horns *(uterus bicornis).* When a similar arrangement occurs in women, a bicornate uterus results.

**Cystic fibrosis of the pancreas.** Cystic fibrosis of the pancreas (mucoviscidosis) is an inherited disorder caused by a recessive gene. The basic defect occurs in glands, especially those that secrete mucus. The pathologic effects of an abnormally thick secretion of mucus are far-reaching, especially in the pancreas and lungs. The sweat glands are also affected, and the sweat contains an excess of salt. The salt content of sweat is used as the basis of diagnostic laboratory tests. Because of the frequency of secondary infection in the lungs, chronic pulmonary disease is a problem. Digestive disturbances result from the lack of pancreatic enzymes.

## HEMATOPOIETIC SYSTEM

**Agammaglobulinemia.** Agammaglobulinemia (or, more properly, hypogammaglobulinemia) is characterized as a sex-linked recessive trait that appears only in males and is discovered early in infancy. There is a very low level of gamma globulin, a virtual ab-

**445**

sence of plasma cells (site of the formation of antibody globulin), and generalized deficiency of the lymphoid tissue. Clinically, bacterial infections are recurrent. Viral infections are usually no problem to the patient, and although antibodies cannot be demonstrated, immunity can be produced with viral vaccines.

**Hereditary spherocytosis.** Hereditary spherocytosis or congenital hemolytic anemia is a chronic familial disorder in which a defect of red blood cells is transmitted as a dominant by one parent. The normal red blood cell is a biconcave disk. The red cell of this disorder tends to be spherical, with both sides convex, and such a spherocyte is more easily trapped in the spleen and destroyed there. This congenital hemolytic anemia is usually relieved by splenectomy.

**Sickle cell anemia.** Sickle cell anemia is a prime example of molecular disease. A hereditary hemolytic anemia, it occurs almost exclusively in blacks and is caused by a gene-controlled defect in the manufacture of hemoglobin.

Hemoglobin is a conjugated protein. Heme, the nonprotein part, consists of an atom of iron in the center of the porphyrin structure. Globin, the protein part, consists of two pairs of polypeptide chains, each a spherical subunit with a specific amino acid sequence and controlled by a separate genetic mechanism. (There are four such subunits—alpha, beta, gamma, and delta.)

If a structural gene causes a substitution for an amino acid in one of the polypeptide chains of hemoglobin, an abnormal hemoglobin results (hemoglobinopathy). Sickle cell hemoglobin is an example, and its presence accounts for the manifestations of the disease. The normal amino acid sequence of peptide 4 of the beta chain of hemoglobin is as follows:

$$1 \quad 2 \quad 3 \quad 4 \quad 5$$
Valine—Histidine—Leucine—Threonine—Proline—
$$6 \quad 7 \quad 8^*$$
Glutamic acid—Glutamic acid—Lysine

The amino acid sequence for sickle cell hemoglobin is

$$1 \quad 2 \quad 3 \quad 4 \quad 5$$
Valine—Histidine—Leucine—Threonine—Proline—
$$6 \quad 7 \quad 8$$
*Valine*—Glutamic acid—Lysine

*Positions on the beta polypeptide chain of hemoglobin.

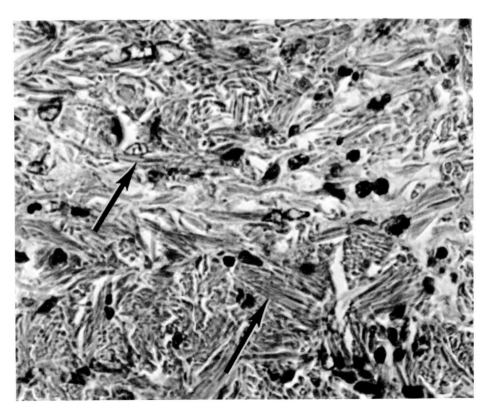

**Fig. 40-10.** Sickle cells in microsection of spleen. (×800.) Arrows point to some densely packed clumps of elongated or crescentic red cells.

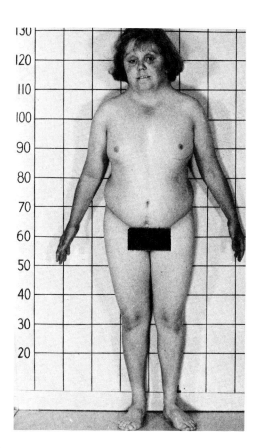

**Fig. 40-11.** Turner's syndrome (gonadal dysgenesis). Prominent features are short stature, shieldlike chest, webbing of neck, heart-shaped face, widely spaced nipples, and small breasts. Surgical scar is related to repair of coarctation of aorta. (From Goodman, R. M., and Gorlin, R. J.: The face in genetic disorders, St. Louis, 1970, The C. V. Mosby Co.)

At position 6 on the molecular chain of hemoglobin a normal gene directs the position of glutamic acid. At that same site the sickle cell gene causes the amino acid valine to be substituted. In spite of what appears to be a minor substitution of a single amino acid at one point among some 300 possibilities in the molecule, the results may be profound because the properties of hemoglobin have been significantly altered. Unoxygenated hemoglobin S (sickle cell hemoglobin) is over 100 times less soluble than is normal hemoglobin. When hemoglobin S is precipitated under unfavorable conditions, it causes the red cell containing it to assume a bizarre, crescentic shape (Fig. 40-10). Such a distorted cell is many times more vulnerable to mechanical forces within the circulation or to any factor that decreases the oxygenation of the blood. In homozygous individuals the gene produces the severe sickle cell anemia, in which more than 90% of the hemoglobin is abnormal. In an individual heterozygous for the abnormal gene the sickle cell trait is present, but appreciable amounts of normal hemoglobin also are found, and the hemolytic anemia is comparatively mild.

**Cooley's anemia.** Cooley's anemia or thalassemia is a hereditary blood disease caused by a genetic defect that by interfering with the rate of synthesis of normal hemoglobin, induces the formation of an abnormal one. Its incidence is high in Mediterranean populations, especially among southern Europeans and Arabs. The presence of the abnormal hemoglobin leads to cardiac complications, bone deformities, hepatosplenomegaly, and death, usually in the teens.

## SEXUAL ANOMALIES

**Intersex.** If the external genitals do not clearly belong to one sex or the other, the condition is referred to as intersex. In certain of these rare instances the individual is found to have an abnormal pattern of sex chromosomes different from that of the normal female

**Table 40-3**
Some patterns for sex chromosomes

| COMBINATION | SEX CHROMO-SOME FROM THE OVUM | SEX CHROMO-SOME FROM THE SPERM | MATING: SEX CHROMOSOMES OF THE ZYGOTE | RESULT |
|---|---|---|---|---|
| 1 | X | X | XX | Normal female XX |
| 2 | X | Y | XY | Normal male XY |
| 3 | XX | Y | XXY | Klinefelter's syndrome |
| 4 | X | None | XO (single X chromosome) | Turner's syndrome |
| 5 | None | Y | OY (single Y chromosome) | Lethal combination |

(XX) or the normal male (XY). Specific anomalies of the sex chromosomes cause Klinefelter's syndrome and Turner's syndrome as well as true hermaphroditism.

An individual with *Klinefelter's syndrome* possesses three sex chromosomes, XXY (total chromosome count, 47). Though appearing to be a male, he has enlarged breasts, small atrophic testes, and female nuclear chromatin in his cells. (See Fig. 40-3.)

In *Turner's syndrome,* there is only one sex chromosome. The pattern is XO, the chromosome number is 45, and sex chromatin is missing from body cells. It is found in a small woman with a webbed neck who lacks secondary sex characters. The ovaries are underdeveloped, and menstruation does not occur. (See Fig. 40-11 and Table 40-3.)

**Hermaphroditism.** A true hermaphrodite has present in the body both ovarian and testicular tissue. A pseudohermaphrodite has such imperfectly formed genitalia that they appear to belong to the opposite sex.

## INBORN ERRORS OF METABOLISM

A deficiency of a given enzyme or the absence of its action in the body can quickly halt a chain of physiologic events. If this failure is related to the action of genes, it is an inborn error of metabolism (a genetically controlled biochemical defect). Such a metabolic block can result in diverse clinical conditions of which more than 100 are known. Some examples are listed in Table 40-4.

**Albinism.** Albinism is a congenital absence of coloring matter from the skin, hair, and eyes. It may be complete (involving the whole body) or incomplete (involving only a part of the body). The *complete* albino has a white or pink skin, white hair, and pink eyes. The skin is pink because the capillaries show through the epidermis, and the lack of pigment in

**Table 40-4**
Some examples of inborn errors of metabolism

| METABOLIC DISEASE | GENETIC TRANSMISSION | PROTEIN OR ENZYME INVOLVED (DEFECT OR DEFICIENCY) | GENETICALLY PRODUCED BIOCHEMICAL STATE |
|---|---|---|---|
| Albinism | Autosomal recessive | Tyrosinase | Failure of melanin pigment production |
| Cystic fibrosis of pancreas | Autosomal recessive | Trypsin, amylase, lipase | Defect in energy release in secretory cells |
| Cystinuria | Autosomal recessive | ? | Excessive loss in urine of an essential metabolite caused by failure of tubular resorption by kidney |
| Galactosemia | Autosomal recessive | Galactose-1-phosphate uridyltransferase | Galactose of milk and milk products not metabolized to glucose |
| Gaucher's disease | Autosomal recessive and autosomal dominant | Glucocerebrosidase | Abnormal fatty substance (kerasin) deposited in reticuloendothelial system |
| Hemophilia | Sex-linked recessive | Antihemophiliac factor (globulin) | Absence of protein factor necessary for coagulation of blood |
| Hereditary spherocytosis | Autosomal dominant | Enolase | High-energy phosphate bonds of glycolysis not available |
| Infantile amaurotic idiocy (Tay-Sachs disease) | Autosomal recessive | Hexosaminidase A | Accumulation of an abnormal substance (sphingomyelin) in brain cells |
| Maple sugar urine disease | Autosomal recessive | Amino acid decarboxylase | Failure of breakdown of certain amino acids; abnormal excretion of these in urine |
| Niemann-Pick disease | Autosomal recessive | Sphingomyelinase | Lack of degradation of sphingomyelin |
| Phenylketonuria | Autosomal recessive | Phenylalanine hydroxylase | Phenylalanine not converted to tyrosine |
| Porphyria, congenital | Autosomal recessive | Porphobilinogen isomerase | Defect in metabolism of pigment related to hemoglobin |
| Von Gierke's disease (glycogen storage disease) | Autosomal recessive | Glucose-6-phosphatase | Failure of glucose formation |

the retina allows the retinal vessels to give the retina a pink color. This lack of retinal coloring matter makes the eyes very sensitive to light.

In *partial* albinism there are irregularly sized, shaped, and distributed areas of skin from which pigment is absent. This condition is known as *leukoderma,* and persons so affected are known as piebald or leopard men. The colorless areas have little tendency to enlarge. Acquired patchy loss of skin color is known as *vitiligo.*

Although albinism is more common among members of races with deeply colored skin, it is not unknown in the members of fair-skinned races. Albinism is found in practically all domestic animals and is seen in plants. Heredity is a factor in the causation of albinism, and the condition seems to run in families (Fig. 40-12).

**Phenylketonuria.** Phenylketonuria, an inborn error of metabolism, is a disorder that appears because of a specific disturbance in protein metabolism. Because of an enzyme deficiency related to a recessive gene, phenylalanine, a normal constituent of food, cannot be properly digested. As a result abnormal toxic substances accumulate in the body, which are especially toxic to the brain and nervous system. Children with this deficiency in time become mentally retarded. They may show irritability of the nervous system and may even have seizures. Growth is disturbed. Such children are striking in appearance, with blond hair and blue eyes, even children of dark-skinned races. The name of the disease comes from the presence in the urine of an abnormal product, a phenylketone (phenylpyruvic acid). It can be found in the urine of an affected infant by the age of 4 to 6 weeks.

This is an example of a biochemical disturbance for which there is treatment. Therefore, it is important that this entity be recognized as early in life as

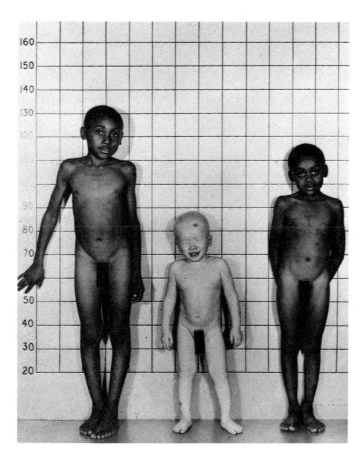

**Fig. 40-12.** Albino black boy with normally pigmented brothers. Dark spots on forehead and legs are bruises. (From Goodman, R. M., and Gorlin, R. J.: The face in genetic disorders, St. Louis, 1970, The C. V. Mosby Co.)

possible. A test for detecting the abnormal metabolite in the urine has been devised. The treatment, largely preventive, involves placing the infant on a diet that provides little or none of the offending substance that the body cannot metabolize. Results are good when the disease is treated early in life and poor if a number of years have added their toll of brain damage.

**Drugs and genes.** The term *pharmacogenetics* is used to indicate the regulatory role of genes in the metabolism of drugs in the human body. At one time in the past when large numbers of soldiers in the U.S. Army were given antimalarial medication, it was found that one drug (primaquine) produced hemolysis in a significant number of blacks. Investigation showed that the red blood cells of these persons were deficient in an enzyme, glucose-6-phosphate dehydrogenase. Because of the abnormality in the intracellular metabolism of glucose in these individuals, the enzyme defect plus the drug resulted in hemolysis (blood destruction).

The turnover of drugs by the human body involves a series of complex, enzymatically mediated reactions. It is increasingly apparent that there can be vast individual differences. Drug sensitivities and drug reactions are of major clinical importance. The individual variations, ever so subtle, in the genetic control of the clotting process might explain the slight but definitely increased frequency of clotting episodes in women taking the "pill."

## Prenatal diagnosis of genetic disorders

*Fetology* is the concept of the unborn child as a patient with a clinical condition necessitating diagnosis and management. *Amniocentesis* is the procedure whereby a needle is inserted through the abdominal wall of the baby's mother into the cavity of the gravid uterus and some of the amniotic fluid containing cells shed from the baby withdrawn. A great deal of genetic information may be obtained by chemical analysis of the fluid and cytogenetic study of the cells. The major chromosomal defects can be detected as well as certain of the genetically controlled errors of metabolism. If there is question of a sex-linked disorder, the determination of the sex of the unborn baby may be a factor to consider in genetic counseling.

## Questions for review

1 What is meant by medical genetics, cytogenetics, pharmacogenetics, fetology, teratogenesis, and mutagenesis?
2 What is the genetic code?
3 Briefly explain the karyotype and how it is prepared.
4 What is the cause of the following: leopard man, dog-faced boy, alligator boy, rubber-skinned man?
5 Outline the causes of congenital anomalies. Give examples of known teratogens.

6 Discuss the thalidomide syndrome.
7 Briefly define the following: chromosome, DNA, intersex, gene, heterozygous, homozygous, sex reversal, sex chromatin, Barr body.
8 Give the pathogenesis and importance of congenital rubella.
9 What may result if one of the branchial clefts is not obliterated? Are these clefts present during the embryonic period of growth?
10 List four abnormal traits that may be inherited.
11 List five examples of congenitally derived disorders.
12 What is an achondroplastic dwarf? What is the basic disturbance?
13 Characterize Down's syndrome.
14 Why are the eyes of an albino sensitive to light?
15 What is an inborn error of metabolism? Briefly discuss one example.
16 Define birth defects. Give the three major categories.
17 State the defect in sickle cell hemoglobinopathy.

**REFERENCES** (Chapter 40)

Aladjem, S., and Brown, A. K., editors: Clinical perinatology, St. Louis, 1974, The C. V. Mosby Co.

Apgar, V. and Beck, J.: Is my baby all right? A guide to birth defects, New York, 1973, Trident Press.

Apgar, V., and Stickle, G.: Birth defects, J.A.M.A. **204:**371, 1968.

Barrett-Connor, E.: Infections and pregnancy: a review, South. Med. J. **62:**275, 1969.

Bernsohn, J., and Grossman, H. J., editors: Lipid storage diseases: enzymatic defects and clinical implications, New York, 1971, Academic Press, Inc.

Brady, R. O.: The lipid storage diseases: new concepts and control, Ann. Intern. Med. **82:**257, 1975.

Cole, W.: The right to be well-born, Today's Health **49:**42, Jan., 1971.

Committee 17, Environmental Mutagen Society: Environmental mutagenic hazards, Science **187:**503, 1975.

Dancis, J.: The prenatal detection of hereditary defects, Hosp. Pract. **4:**37, June, 1969.

Dingle, J. T., editor: Lysosomes: a laboratory handbook, New York, 1972, American Elsevier Publishing Co.

DiPalma, J. R.: The growing new field of pharmacogenetics, RN **37:**109, Sept., 1974.

di Sant'Agnese, P. A.: Unmasking the great impersonator—cystic fibrosis, Today's Health **47:**38, Feb., 1969.

Dmowski, W. P., and Greenblatt, R. B.: Abnormal sexual differentiation, Am. Fam. Physician **3:**72, Feb., 1971.

Dumars, K. W., Jr.: Parental drug usage: effect upon chromosomes of progeny, Pediatrics **47:**1037, 1971.

Gelpi, A. P.: Migrant populations and the diffusion of the sickle-cell gene, Ann. Intern. Med. **79:**258, 1973.

German, J.: Sex chromosomal abnormalities, South. Med. J. **64** (supp. 1):73, 1971.

Goodman, R. M., editor: Genetic disorders of man, Boston, 1970, Little, Brown & Co.

Goodman, R. M., and Gorlin, R. J.: The face in genetic disorders, St. Louis, 1970, The C. V. Mosby Co.

Greenfeld, J.: Advances in genetics that can change your life, Today's Health **51:**20, Dec., 1973.

Haskins, A. L.: Early recognition of neonatal disorders, Mod. Med. **40:**103, June 12, 1972.

Hayflick, L.: Chromosomes and human disease, Hosp. Pract. **2:**54, Feb., 1967.

Hecht, F., and others: Clinical cytogenetics, Am. J. Dis. Child. **125:**319, 1973.

Hers, H. G., and Van Hoof, F., editors: Lysosomes and storage diseases, New York, 1973, Academic Press, Inc.

Hicks, C. B.: George Beadle talks about the new genetics, Today's Health **47:**44, July, 1969.

Hill, R. M.: Will this drug harm the unborn infant? The doctor's dilemma, South. Med. J. **67:**1476, 1974.

Hirschhorn, K.: LSD and chromosomal damage, Hosp. Pract. **4:**98, Feb., 1969.

Hirschhorn, K.: Human genetics, J.A.M.A. **224:**597, 1973.

Hollaender, A., editor: Chemical mutagens, principles and methods for their detection, New York, 1971, Plenum Publishing Corp.

Hsia, D. Y.: A critical evaluation of PKU screening, Hosp. Pract. **6:**101, April, 1971.

Inborn terror of metabolism (editorial), J.A.M.A. **214:**2186, 1970.

Jackson, L.: Basic chromosome abnormalities, Hosp. Top. **45:**81, Jan., 1967.

Kissane, J. M.: Pathology of infancy and childhood, ed. 2, St. Louis, 1975, The C. V. Mosby Co.

Lederberg, J.: Genetic engineering: controlling man's building blocks, Today's Health **47:**24, Nov., 1969.

Lenz, W.: How can the teratogenic action of a factor be established in man? South. Med. J. **64**(supp. 1):41, Feb., 1971.

Levine, L.: Biology of the gene, ed. 2, St. Louis, 1973, The C. V. Mosby Co.

Macintyre, M. N.: Prenatal chromosome analysis—a life saving procedure, South. Med. J. **64**(supp. 1):85, Feb., 1971.

Marx, J. L.: Drugs during pregnancy: do they affect the unborn child? Science **180:**174, 1973.

Marx, J. L.: Embryology: out of the womb—into the test tube, Science **182:**811, 1973.

Maugh, T. H., II: Marihuana. II. Does it damage the brain? Science **185:**775, 1974.

McKusick, V. A.: Human genetics, ed. 2, Englewood Cliffs, N.J., 1969, Prentice-Hall, Inc.

McKusick, V. A.: The nosology of genetic disease, Hosp. Pract. **6:**93, July, 1971.

McKusick, V. A.: Heritable disorders of connective tissue, ed. 4, St. Louis, 1972, The C. V. Mosby Co.

Milunsky, A., and Atkins, L.: Prenatal diagnosis of genetic disorders, J.A.M.A. **230:**232, 1974.

Motulsky, A. G.: Brave new world? Science **185:**653, 1974.

Nadler, H. L.: Prenatal detection of inborn errors of metabolism, South. Med. J. **64**(supp. 1):92, Feb., 1971.

Rowley, J. D.: Cytogenetics in clinical medicine, J.A.M.A. **207:**914, 1969.

Schanche, D. A.: Two facial handicaps that can be conquered, Today's Health **52:**52, Nov., 1974.

Sever, J. L.: Viral teratogens: a status report, Hosp. Pract. **5:**75, April, 1970.

Toomey, K., and Bartuska, D.: Clinical application of fluorescent staining of chromosomes, J. Am. Med. Wom. Assoc. **28:**313, 1973.

Warkany, J.: Congenital malformations: notes and comments, Chicago, 1971, Year Book Medical Publishers, Inc.

# CHAPTER 41
# Circulatory disorders

The circulatory system includes a central pumping station (heart) and a series of channels (arteries, arterioles, capillaries, small venules, and veins) through which blood is pumped all over the body, collected, and returned to the heart (Fig. 41-1). Consideration of the circulatory system includes consideration of the circulating medium, the blood. In this chapter, however, disturbances and disorders of the circulatory system are primarily those interfering with the mechanics of circulation (the coordinated functions of the separate anatomic parts). Generally disturbances of the circulation are of two kinds—those that affect restricted or localized areas of the body and those that produce generalized changes. Conditions such as hyperemia and edema may be either localized or generalized. Hemorrhage occurs locally but may have far-reaching, generalized effects.

## Hyperemia

Hyperemia or congestion means an excess of blood in a part. If caused by an increase in the amount of blood brought to the part by the arteries, it is *active* or *arterial* hyperemia; if produced by an interference with the venous return, it is *passive* or *venous* hyperemia. The excess blood is contained in capillaries, venules, or arterioles, which dilate.

**Active hyperemia.** Active hyperemia may be physiologic or pathologic. Physiologic hyperemia is established to supply increased nourishment to organs or tissues doing increased work. Active pathologic hyperemia initiates inflammation and forms one of the most important features of inflammation. The site of active hyperemia is red and warmer than normal. An example is flushing of the face provoked by emotions (blushing).

**Passive hyperemia.** Passive hyperemia is always pathologic and may occur as a localized or a generalized condition.

Localized passive hyperemia results from the obstruction of a vein by (1) a thrombus or embolus, (2) thickening of the vessel wall, or (3) pressure from an outside lesion (neoplasms, contraction of scars, or enlarged or misplaced organs). In pregnancy the enlarged uterus may press on one of the iliac veins, causing passive hyperemia of the leg on that side. For localized passive hyperemia to occur, the involved vessel must not possess a collateral circulation; otherwise, such communicating branches would shunt blood around the obstruction.

The site of passive hyperemia is bluish red, swollen, and cold. The swelling is caused by associated edema. (When blood distends the capillaries and venules, some of its constituents may leak out in the tissues.)

The cause of a generalized passive hyperemia is most often an obstruction to the passage of blood through a diseased heart. The heart may be in failure. The efficiency of the pump is impaired, and blood is dammed back into the veins draining in blood from the general circulation. Among the causes of obstruction within the heart are chronic valvular diseases such as mitral stenosis and mitral incompetency.*

In generalized venous hyperemia the effective flow of blood through the lungs is reduced; therefore, less blood in the body is oxygenated (*anoxemia*). This gives rise to shortness of breath (*dyspnea*) and results in cyanosis (a bluish discoloration of the lips, nail beds, and mucous membranes). Poorly oxygenated blood has a bluish color. Edema of the lower extremities often accompanies generalized venous hyperemia.

When heart failure develops, the heart cannot maintain an adequate circulation, and blood appears to sink or pool in the dependent areas of the body. This is *hypostatic congestion,* and the dependent parts of the lungs and the skin of the back and buttocks are chiefly affected. A frequent change of the patient's

---

*Stenosis* is a word often used in discussions of disease of the heart valves. When applied to a heart valve or certain other sites, it means a narrowing or partial closure of an opening. *Incompetency* refers to a leaky valve; synonyms for this are *insufficiency* and *regurgitation*.

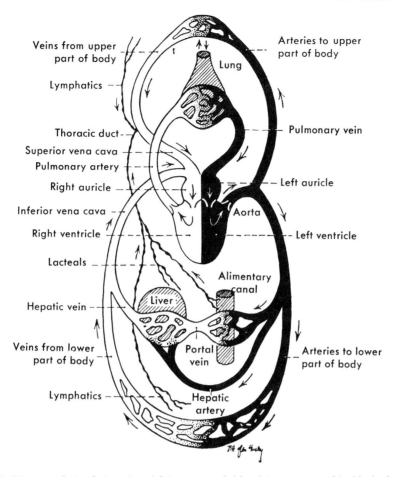

**Fig. 41-1.** Diagram of circulation. Arterial (oxygenated) blood is represented in black channels, venous blood in white. Lymphatics are outlined by thin, knotted lines.

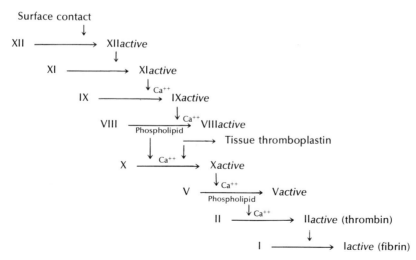

**Schema 7.** The "waterfall." (Modified from Davie, E. W., and Ratnoff, O. D.: Waterfall sequence for intrinsic blood clotting, Science **145:**1310, 1964; and Macfarlane, R. G.: An enzyme cascade in the blood clotting mechanism and its function as a biochemical amplifier, Nature **202:**498, 1964.)

position helps to prevent hypostatic congestion and its serious consequence, bronchopneumonia.

Obstruction of the portal vein leads to passive hyperemia in the portal circulation, which is associated with dilatation of esophageal, hemorrhoidal, and abdominal wall veins, ascites, and hemorrhages.

## Hemorrhage

Hemorrhage is an escape of blood from the vascular system as a result of (1) rupture of the heart or a vascular wall (hemorrhage per *rhexis*) or (2) passage of red blood cells through intact capillary walls without visible injury (hemorrhage per *diapedesis*).

**Causes.** The causes of hemorrhage are (1) mechanical injury of the heart or vessels, (2) disease or altered function of blood vessel walls, and (3) defects in factors related to the clotting of blood. Increased pressure of blood within a vessel contributes significantly to hemorrhage, particularly in the brain, where the majority of hemorrhages are caused by a combination of hardening of the arteries and high blood pressure. Conjunctival hemorrhages may follow the violent efforts of coughing, sneezing, and vomiting, if these result in a transient rise in the blood pressure within the poorly supported conjunctival vessels in the eye.

**Coagulation.** When blood comes out of a vessel, it is changed within a short period of time from a fluid to a soft, jellylike mass, a blood clot. The physiologic process whereby blood is so changed is coagulation. If the blood clot is magnified and examined, it is seen as a network of delicate fibrils in which are enmeshed the red and white blood cells. The fibrils are composed of fibrin derived from one of the plasma proteins, fibrinogen. The conversion of this protein to the solid fibrin is a complicated chemical process involving complex enzyme systems.

In recent years the enzymatic intricacies have been formalized into a "cascade" or "waterfall" scheme with at least thirteen factors involved (Schema 7). It is widely held that the different coagulation factors exist in plasma as inactive proenzymes converted to active enzymes during the clotting process. The reactants appear in a kind of sequence with the product of the first reaction operating as enzyme to catalyze the second reaction. The second reaction yields a product that is an enzyme to catalyze the third reaction, and so on. Once activated, the sequence must continue to completion.

A list of factors known to be essential parts of the complex coagulation scheme is shown in Table 41-1.

The complex process of coagulation is often greatly simplified to four stages; the first three relate to the formation of visible blood clot, the fourth to lysis of the clot. All four stages may be occurring continuously

**Table 41-1**
Coagulation factors

| FACTOR | | OTHER NAMES |
|---|---|---|
| I | Fibrinogen | |
| II | Prothrombin | Thrombogen |
| | | Serozyme |
| | | Plasmozyme |
| III | Thromboplastin | Tissue thromboplastin |
| | | Tissue factor |
| | | Thrombokinase |
| | | Cytozyme |
| IV | Calcium (ionized) | |
| V | Plasma Ac-globulin | Labile factor |
| | | Proaccelerin |
| | | Prothrombin accelerator |
| | | Thrombogen |
| VI | (Factor obsolete) | Accelerin |
| | | Serum Ac-globulin |
| VII | Proconvertin-convertin | Serum prothrombin conversion accelerator (SPCA) |
| | | Stable factor |
| | | Proconvertin |
| | | Autoprothrombin I |
| | | Serum accelerator |
| | | Cothromboplastin |
| VIII | Antihemophilic globulin (AHG) | Antihemophilic factor (AHF) |
| | | Hemophiliac factor A |
| | | Platelet cofactor I |
| | | Thromboplastinogen |
| IX | Plasma thromboplastin component (PTC) | Plasma factor X |
| | | Platelet cofactor II |
| | | Autoprothrombin II |
| | | Christmas factor |
| | | Hemophiliac factor B |
| X | Stuart-Prower factor | |
| XI | Plasma thromboplastin antecedent (PTA) | Antihemophilic factor C |
| XII | Hageman factor (HF) | Contact factor |
| XIII | Fibrin-stabilizing factor (FSF) | Fibrinase |

in minute amounts in the normal homeostasis of blood. (See Table 41-2.)

**Bleeding diseases.** Platelets (p. 547) are necessary for the coagulation of blood, since they are responsible for the production of thromboplastin. Hemorrhages that occur because of decreased numbers of platelets (*thrombocytopenia*) tend to be generalized in the skin and mucous membranes and may occur in the brain and internal organs. Sometimes

**Table 41-2**
Four stages of blood coagulation

| INTRINSIC THROMBOPLASTIN SYSTEM (THROMBOPLASTIN DERIVED FROM PLASMA) | EXTRINSIC THROMBOPLASTIN SYSTEM (THROMBOPLASTIN DERIVED FROM TISSUES) |
|---|---|
| **Stage I: Formation of thromboplastin**<br>Platelet factor (PF) released to react with AHF and PTC in presence of PTA, Hageman factor, factors V and X, and calcium ions<br>Duration: 3 to 5 minutes | Bypassed |

$$\left. \begin{array}{l} \text{AHF} \\ \text{PTC} \\ \text{PF} \\ \text{X} \\ \text{Hageman factor} \\ \text{PTA} \end{array} \right\} \quad \text{X} \xrightarrow[\text{Factor V}]{\text{Calcium}^{++}} \text{Plasma thromboplastin}$$

**Stage II: Conversion of inactive prothrombin**
Reaction requiring thromboplastin, calcium ions, and accessory factors (factors V and X for both tissue and plasma thromboplastin, factor VII with tissue thromboplastin)
*Note:* Both thromboplastin systems must function for normal coagulation
Duration: 8 to 15 seconds

$$\text{Prothrombin} \xrightarrow[\text{Calcium}^{++}, \text{V}, \text{X}]{\text{Plasma thromboplastin}} \text{Thrombin} \qquad\qquad \text{Prothrombin} \xrightarrow[\text{Calcium}^{++}, \text{V}, \text{VII}, \text{X}]{\text{Tissue thromboplastin}} \text{Thrombin}$$

**Stage III: Conversion of fibrinogen to fibrin**
As soon as any thrombin formed, soluble fibrinogen converted to insoluble fibrin
Duration: less than 1 second

$$\text{Fibrinogen} \xrightarrow{\text{Thrombin}} \text{Fibrin} \xrightarrow[\text{Calcium}^{++}]{\text{FSF}} \text{Stabilized fibrin}$$

**Stage IV: Lysis of clot**
Fibrinolysin (plasmin) acts on fibrin to dissolve it

$$\text{Fibrin} \xrightarrow[\text{Fibrinolysin (plasmin)}]{} \text{Lysis}$$

thrombocytopenia occurs without known cause (idiopathic), but it may also be associated with other blood diseases, infections, and the effects of various chemical or physical agents.

Hemorrhagic diseases may be related to a diminished level of prothrombin in the blood. Normally prothrombin is formed in the liver from vitamin K, which is absorbed from the lumen of the bowel and transported to the liver. Vitamin K is elaborated in the intestinal lumen by the action of bacteria normally inhabiting this area, and bile must be present for its absorption. Hemorrhagic diseases produced by hypoprothrombinemia may result from a failure of formation of prothrombin in the liver, a failure of absorption of vitamin K from the bowel, or a failure of the enteric bacteria to make vitamin K. In severe liver disease prothrombin is not formed. In obstructive jaundice

bile may not pass the constricting focus in the common bile duct. Lack of bile interferes with the absorption of vitamin K. Prolonged administration of excessive amounts of certain sulfonamides or antibiotics may inhibit the growth of intestinal bacteria that make vitamin K.

*Hemophilia* is a well-known bleeding disease that is inherited as a sex-linked recessive trait. The disease occurs only in males but is transmitted only by females. The clotting defect stems from a deficiency of the antihemophilic factor (AHF), a globulin normally present in blood plasma. Even minor trauma in persons affected by the disease is associated with continued oozing of blood over long periods of time. Sometimes the bleeding lasts for weeks. Hemorrhages may occur in any area of the body, but around joints they are especially severe and may be associated with

**Table 41-3**

The spectrum of hemophilia

| DESCRIPTIVE FEATURE | SEVERE DISEASE— CLASSIC HEMOPHILIA | MODERATELY SEVERE DISEASE | MILD DISEASE | SUBCLINICAL DISEASE |
|---|---|---|---|---|
| I. Laboratory testing | | | | |
|   Level of AHG | Absolute deficiency | Very low | Less than normal | Normal or slightly less |
|   Thromboplastin formation | None generated | None generated | May be normal | Normal |
|   Coagulation of whole blood | Abnormal | Normal or slightly ab-normal | Normal | Normal |
| II. Clinical feature | | | | |
|   Precipitating factor | Spontaneous— into joints, muscles, mu-cosae, internal organs | Provoked by superficial trauma | Easy bruising | Mild oozing |
|   Bleeding related to surgical procedure | Severe | Severe | Mild | Some oozing |

permanent joint deformities. Table 41-3 relates the severity of the disease to the relative deficiency of AHG.

As we learn more about the process of coagulation, we are discovering that there are a number of bleeding diseases with manifestations, on the whole, like those of classic hemophilia. Most of these, like hemophilia, are related to deficiencies of factors that enter into stage I, in which thromboplastin is generated. These bleeding diseases are sometimes designated *hemophilia-like* or *hemophilioid* diseases.

Of special importance in consideration of hemorrhagic disorders is the role of *circulating anticoagulants*. In the bloodstream these substances have a physiologic effect to prevent clotting. In certain conditions such as anaphylactoid shock and following irradiation, hemorrhage may appear because these physiologic anticoagulants are released into the bloodstream in increased amounts. One such substance is considered to be heparin-like. Anticoagulants are clinically important in the treatment of diseases characterized by an increased tendency of the blood to clot. Two anticoagulants widely used clinically to prevent abnormal clotting of blood within the lumina of blood vessels are heparin and Dicumarol.

The cause of hemorrhage is not always clear. Hemorrhage may occur even when platelets appear to be normal in number and the known necessary factors for coagulation are present in normal amounts. One explanation for such hemorrhages is given by some observers as abnormality in function of the blood vessel walls, particularly those of the capillaries. Such an alteration of function is at best ill defined.

In hemorrhage resulting from mechanical injury, clean smooth cuts are usually followed by more loss of blood than are irregular jagged ones. In the former, arterial contraction is less effective, and blood-clotting material is less abundant in the wound.

**Laboratory diagnosis.** Laboratory testing, coupled with a carefully taken history of the patient's disorder, is very important to the evaluation of bleeding diseases. Generally the laboratory tests are designed to precisely demonstrate deficiencies of factors essential to normal coagulation. A particular test reproduces a critical biochemical step in the overall clotting scheme. Known factors are checked in the patient's blood under carefully controlled conditions. Examples of tests of practical value are the thromboplastin generation test (defects in stage I of coagulation), partial thromboplastin time (PTT) (stage I), prothrombin time (stage II), platelet count (stage I), clot retraction time (platelet function), and bleeding time (integrity of blood vessels).

**Kinds.** Very small hemorrhages in the tissues are known as *petechiae* (Figs. 41-2 and 41-3), larger ones as *ecchymoses*, and tumorlike collections of blood as *hematomas*. Hemorrhages also are named according to their location. For instance, *epistaxis* is nosebleed, *hemoptysis* is blood in the sputum, *hematemesis* is vomiting of blood, and *hematuria* is the presence of red blood cells in the urine. *Apoplexy* (stroke) is commonly applied to hemorrhage and its effects within the cranial cavity. An accumulation of blood into

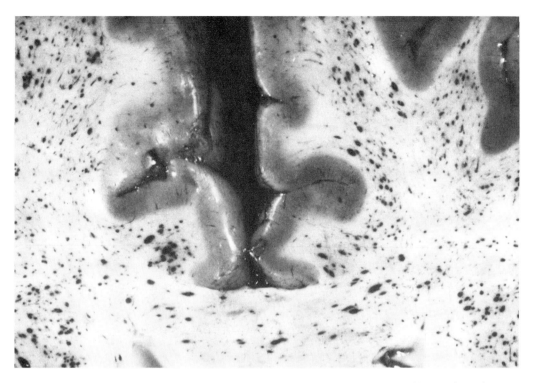

**Fig. 41-2.** Petechiae in white matter of brain, macroscopic section. Multiple small hemorrhagic foci are diffusely distributed.

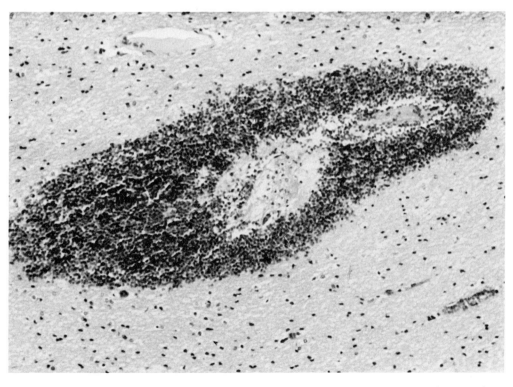

**Fig. 41-3.** Petechiae in brain, microscopic section. Note circumscribed accumulation of intact red blood cells about small blood vessel.

## Table 41-4
Aspects of blood component therapy*

| | COMPONENT | APPLICATION |
|---|---|---|
| **Cells (45% of whole blood)** | Red cells | For anemia—the reason for 30% to 50% blood transfusions given |
| | White cells | For infection—experimental only |
| | Platelets | For bleeding caused by platelet deficiency |
| **Plasma (55% of whole blood)** | Plasma | Fresh frozen—to control bleeding |
| | | Single-donor liquid plasma—to restore plasma volume |
| | Cryoprecipitate (contains antihemophilic globulin [AHG]) | For hemophiliacs (bleeders); prepared from fresh frozen plasma |
| **Plasma proteins** | Serum albumin | For treatment of shock and low blood protein |
| | Gamma globulin | For prevention of disease such as measles (p. 400) |
| | Specific immune globulins | Specially prepared gamma globulin from plasmas with specific antibodies |
| | Clotting factor concentrates Fibrinogen AHG Factor II Factor VII Factor IX Factor X | For control of bleeding caused by deficiencies of specific coagulation factors |

* From Questions and answers about blood and blood banking, Chicago, 1970, American Association of Blood Banks.

either of the pleural cavities is *hemothorax*. Blood in the pericardial cavity is *hemopericardium*. If the amount of blood in the pericardial cavity is sufficient to interfere with the action of the heart, a *cardiac tamponade* is produced. Blood in the peritoneal cavity is *hemoperitoneum*. *Menorrhagia* is excessive uterine bleeding during the menstrual period. *Metrorrhagia* is bleeding from the uterus between menstrual periods. *Purpura* is a term that refers to the presence of varying sized hemorrhages in widespread areas of the skin and mucous membranes.

**Effects.** The results of hemorrhage depend on the location, amount, and rate of blood loss. When more than one third of the total blood volume is lost rapidly, death usually occurs. Repeated small hemorrhages or continuous oozing of blood leads to anemia of varying severity.

**Blood component therapy.** Whole blood is a complex mixture of cellular and fluid constituents that may be safely and efficiently separated in the modern blood bank. Since in many instances the physiologic role of each component is known, it may be administered to a patient to fill a specific need. This is often-

times a more efficient use of a precious commodity. Not only is component therapy useful in filling a specific need, but it also allows for a concentration of the therapeutic effect not possible with whole blood transfusion. A good example of this is the treatment of the hemophiliac in a bleeding episode who needs antihemophilic globulin. The amount it takes to stop his bleeding may have to be harvested from many units of whole blood; on occasions over 100 units have been required. This much antihemophilic globulin could not be supplied to such a bleeder in whole blood units. The technic of removing plasma from a unit of blood and immediately returning the red cells to the donor is *plasmapheresis*. Table 41-4 outlines applications of blood component therapy.

### Edema

A constant amount of fluid is maintained in the tissues by the nicely balanced relation existing between the passage of fluid from the capillaries to the tissue spaces and its removal from the tissue spaces by way of the lymph channels or by its return to the capillaries. When this balance is upset, an excessive

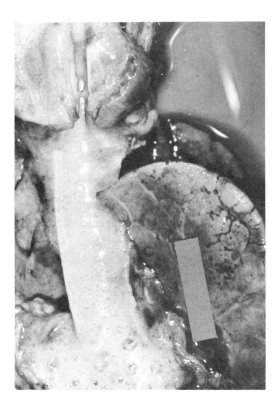

**Fig. 41-4.** Acute pulmonary edema. Frothy bubbly fluid is welling up from bronchi into trachea. Soft boggy lung is seen to sides.

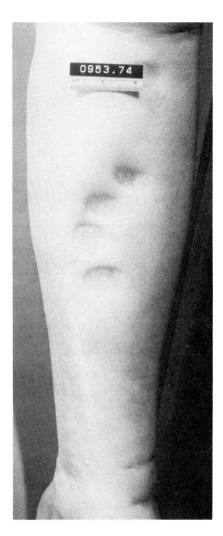

**Fig. 41-5.** Pitting edema.

amount of fluid accumulates in the tissues outside the blood vessels, giving rise to edema (Fig. 41-4). Edematous tissues are swollen, boggy, and doughy in consistency. When pressed, they retain the imprint of the finger. This is what is meant by *pitting* edema (Fig. 41-5).

*Anasarca* or *dropsy* is a generalized collection of edema fluid in body cavities. Fluid in the peritoneal cavity is *ascites;* in the pleural cavity, *hydrothorax;* and in the pericardial cavity, *hydropericardium.* Certain collections of edema fluid in the tissues or body cavities are known as *transudates.* Similar collections of an inflammatory origin are *exudates.* Transudates and exudates may be differentiated by their chemical composition.

The conditions that produce edema are weakened heart action in heart failure, venous obstruction, nephritis, nutritional factors, allergy, inflammation, and lymphatic obstruction. Edema may be localized or generalized.

Table 41-5 relates factors involved in the formation of edema to well-known types.

Although cardiac edema from a diseased heart in failure is generalized, it is best seen in the feet and ankles. Swelling subsides when the patient lies in bed, and in mild cases it may clear up entirely after a night's rest. The edema of kidney disease is notable in the eyelids. It is worse early in the morning.

## Shock

*Shock* is a general term widely used to designate the state of collapse that follows severe tissue injury. It is a disturbance of the circulation wherein there is an acute reduction in blood flow and therefore inadequate supply to body tissues. It is a dramatic event clinically for the weakness, pallor, rapid feeble pulse, and low blood pressure. *Cardiogenic* shock is directly related to cardiac malfunction. Where the pathologic processes involve the rest of the circulation, shock as

**Table 41-5**
Mechanisms in edema

| TYPE | ETIOLOGIC FACTORS | COMMENT |
|---|---|---|
| Cardiac | 1. Increased hydrostatic pressure in veins and capillaries caused by failure of pump (heart)<br>2. Oxygenation of tissues impaired—anoxia injures capillaries<br>3. Salt (sodium) retention | Generalized edema with generalized hyperemia; may involve lungs—pulmonary edema; seen best in feet and ankles |
| Inflammatory | Inflammatory injury to capillaries with loss of proteins to interstitial spaces | Localized edema at site of inflammation; swelling one of cardinal signs of inflammation |
| Renal | 1. Toxic injury to capillaries<br>2. Loss of albumin in urine (albuminuria) with lower levels of plasma proteins (hypoproteinemia)<br>3. Sodium retention<br>4. Complicating heart failure means increased hydrostatic pressure | Edema of acute or chronic kidney disease; facial edema characteristic—especially puffy eyelids; generalized anasarca—massive widespread edema with collections of fluid in body cavities characteristic |
| Allergic | Immunologic injury to capillaries | Angioneurotic edema localized; may involve lips, neck, respiratory tract |
| Lymphatic | 1. Blockage of lymphatic drainage channels<br>2. Interstitial fluid not removed | Localized edema caused by infection of lymphatics (lymphangitis) or by external pressure (tumors) |
| Nutritional | Low levels of plasma proteins | Malnutrition—inadequate food intake for proper biosynthesis |

a consequence is referred to as *peripheral circulatory collapse*. As we shall see, the conditions with which it is associated are many, varied, and quite unrelated.

Shock may be discussed as (1) primary, (2) secondary, and (3) hemorrhagic. These three categories tend to have distinct clinical and laboratory features, although the three forms can be present together.

**Primary shock.** Primary shock is comparable to syncope or fainting. It develops right after the injury, tends to be of short duration, and is usually mild. It is thought to be caused by a neurovascular reaction elicited by pain (even from such trivial injuries as the insertion of a needle into a vein), by emotion (fright), and by nerve impulses arising in injured tissues. After more severe injuries, prolonged primary shock may merge imperceptibly into secondary shock.

**Secondary shock.** Secondary shock is a state of collapse and prostration after injury, which requires an interval of time to develop. It is also referred to as surgical, wound, or traumatic shock and is more severe in its manifestations than primary shock. The patient in secondary shock is very weak but is restless and may thrash about. The pulse, if obtainable, is rapid and feeble. The body temperature is low, and the extremities are cold and clammy. The blood pressure is quite low and sometimes hard to determine. The

breathing is shallow. The face is drawn and ashen, but there is an anxious expression. The eyes appear sunken. Perspiration is profuse, and the extremities are covered with cold sweat. The patient is exceedingly thirsty. The urinary output is very small in amount (*oliguria*), or sometimes no urine at all is voided (*anuria*). If the condition is not corrected, the blood pressure drops progressively, the heart action becomes weaker, and death occurs within a relatively short time.

Secondary shock has been reported in many different clinical situations: trauma, crush injuries, burns, severe and fulminating infections (such as diphtheria, pneumonia, septicemia, gas gangrene, acute peritonitis), heatstroke, freezing injury, radiation injury, blood transfusion reactions, anaphylaxis, intestinal obstruction, bile peritonitis, myocardial infarction, anesthetic accidents, drowning, asphyxia from carbon monoxide, perforation of abdominal viscera, pancreatitis, poisonings by chemical agents, and many others.*

Secondary shock is thought to develop because of changes in the capillaries and small veins. The effect on capillaries may come directly from bacterial, chem-

---

*See also p. 211 for discussion of endotoxin shock.

ical, or other agents responsible for the background injury, or a state of anoxia produced by the original injury may increase capillary permeability. Blood is pooled in capillaries and venules and is therefore removed from the effective circulation. The fluid part of the blood leaks through altered capillaries. Soon the actual volume of blood circulating is less than the volume required to maintain an adequate flow. Less blood is returned to the heart, which pumps less effectively. A shutdown of blood flow to the kidneys means cessation of urine formation.

The pathology of secondary shock reflects changes in the capillaries. These vessels are dilated and engorged with blood. Petechial hemorrhages are seen on the serous membranes of the body, and there is edema of the soft tissues. The vital organs show degenerative changes.

**Hemorrhagic shock.** Hemorrhagic shock occurs after the sudden and rapid loss of a significant amount of blood. In its uncomplicated form it is related to loss of blood alone, but many severe traumatic injuries are associated with sizable hemorrhage so that secondary shock and this form may coexist.

## Thrombosis

Thrombosis is the formation of a solid mass, or blood clot, made up of one or more normal constituents of the blood, within the heart or blood vessels during life. The mass is known as a *thrombus.*

**Causes.** Factors operating in thrombosis are (1) injury to the lining of a blood vessel by trauma, inflammation, or degeneration, (2) slowing of the blood flow, (3) eddies in the bloodstream, and (4) diseases of the blood itself. Of these, the first is most important. Slowing of the current may be caused by enfeebled heart action or dilatation of a vessel or chamber in the heart.

Thrombi may be composed of all the constituents of the blood in about their normal proportion, or they may be composed of one or more components to the exclusion of the others; for instance, thrombi may be composed of platelets and fibrin or platelets alone. (See Fig. 41-6.) Thrombi may be attached to one spot on the wall of a vessel and protrude into the vessel for only a short distance, leaving a passageway for the blood (parietal thrombi), or they may completely occlude the vessel (obstructive thrombi).

**Sites.** The most common sites of thrombus formation are in the veins. The sudden appearance of a hemorrhoid is usually the result of the formation of a thrombus in a varicose hemorrhoidal vein. When thrombosis of an artery does occur, the cerebral arteries, aorta, or coronary arteries are most likely to be affected.

**Effects.** The local effects of arterial thrombosis are caused by the obstruction of blood flow through the

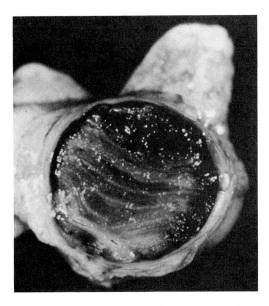

**Fig. 41-6.** Thrombus within vascular lumen seen in cross section. The white riblike markings represent layers of platelets covered with white blood cells. These are called lines of Zahn.

artery. Impairment of the circulation to a part can cause death of the tissue (p. 462). Venous thrombosis, without the establishment of a collateral circulation, can lead to passive congestion and death of the tissue. Other consequences of thrombi are (1) organization, (2) formation of sterile emboli, and (3) septic softening.

When a thrombus remains in place and is not infected, it excites an inflammatory reaction in the surrounding tissue. Proliferation of a vascular and fibrous tissue is stimulated, and the thrombus is changed into a mass of fibrous tissue. This is what is meant by *organization* of the thrombus. The capillaries taking part in the organization dilate to form new canals through which the blood can pass. This is known as *canalization.* The sequelae of the formation of sterile emboli are mainly those of sterile vascular obstruction (see the discussion of embolism that follows). When septic softening occurs, infected emboli are spread to different parts of the body, with the formation of multiple infected foci or *septic infarcts.*

Massage of a thrombosed vessel to relieve pain is dangerous because the thrombus may become detached, with most disastrous results.

## Embolism

By embolism is meant the presence of a solid (or gaseous) object floating free in the bloodstream. The object is known as an *embolus.* Emboli may consist of portions of thrombi (the most common type), clumps of fibrin from diseased heart valves, atheromatous material from a vessel wall, agglutinated bacteria, tumor cells, air, fat, animal parasites, or foreign bodies such as bullets. Emboli may be sterile or septic (contain bacteria). Embolism may follow injuries or operations, or it may be associated with certain systemic diseases.

**Effects.** In its course along a vessel an embolus may be arrested by the division of the vessel, by the narrowing of the vessel, or by projecting points. The point at which arrest occurs depends on the place of origin of the embolus. Emboli arising in the systemic veins or right heart are usually arrested in the lungs, and those arising in the left heart and aorta in the systemic circulation. The results of embolism depend on the nature of the embolus and the point of arrest. If a noninfected embolus lodges at a point supplied with a good collateral circulation, no harm results. If there is no collateral circulation, ischemia of the part occurs, and necrosis may follow. An *infarct* may form. Emboli of pathogenic bacteria set up secondary foci of infection. Emboli of tumor cells set up secondary tumor growths. Emboli in the pulmonary artery or in vessels supplying vital areas of the brain may cause

sudden death. Embolism of the arteries supplying the intestine leads to gangrene.

*Fat embolism* is caused by small droplets of fat entering the bloodstream as a result of fractures of bones or injuries to fat in any part of the body. The site of arrest is the lungs. The characteristic signs are oil droplets in the urine and sputum.

*Air embolism* follows the opening of the large veins of the neck and thorax. Negative pressure produced by the inspiratory movements of the chest sucks air into these vessels, and the air passes to the heart, where it is churned with the blood into a foamy mixture that the heart is unable to pump.

## Ischemia and infarction

The term *ischemia* refers to a crucial reduction in the arterial supply of a given part of the body. It may be produced when an artery is obstructed by (1) an embolus or thrombus, (2) external pressure, (3) a thickening of its wall, (4) nervous influences, or (5) the action of drugs or cold. For ischemia to produce its effects a collateral circulation must be lacking. An ischemic focus is reduced in size, pale and cold, and functionally less active than normal. If persisting long

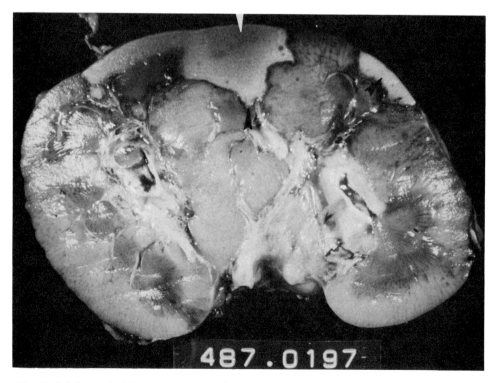

**Fig. 41-7.** Infarct of kidney. Sectioned surface shows whitish triangular areas in renal cortex, rimmed by dark hemorrhagic zone.

enough or initially severe, ischemia leads to necrosis of the involved tissue.

The term *infarction* denotes necrosis of tissue caused by an interference in blood supply. When the artery supplying an organ or part becomes occluded, as by an embolus, the area becomes necrotic (provided that there is no other source of blood supply). The necrotic tissue is called an *infarct*. As a rule, an infarct is conical in shape, corresponding to the distribution of the artery and its branches. Infarcts are best seen in organs such as the heart, spleen, kidney (Fig. 41-7), and brain, in which the arteries do not freely communicate. An infarct of the heart muscle or of certain vital areas of the brain may prove rapidly fatal.

## Gangrene

The term *gangrene* is applied when an area of ischemic necrosis (infarct) becomes the site of growth of saprophytic bacteria.

**Kinds.** Gangrene is often classified as dry and moist. *Dry* gangrene results from an interference in the arterial supply of a part without invasion by saprophytes. Strictly speaking, this condition is not true gangrene but an infarct, since bacteria play no part.

*Moist* gangrene is true gangrene because saprophytic invasion plays an important part in the process and is responsible for many of the prominent features. Dry gangrene is confined almost entirely to the extremities, whereas moist gangrene may affect either extremities or internal organs. Gangrene of the internal organs may be caused by mechanical obstruction, compression by fibrous bands, twisting of pedicles, and thrombosis or embolism of the blood vessels supplying the organs.

In dry gangrene the part becomes dry and shrinks; the skin color changes to a purplish brown or black, and complete mummification may result (Fig. 41-8). The spread of dry gangrene is slow. The irritation produced by the dead tissue causes a line of inflammation between the infarcted area and the healthy tissue. In some cases complete separation may occur along the line of demarcation. Thickened blood vessel walls and weakened circulation predispose to this type of gangrene. If bacteria invade the necrotic tissues and multiply, dry gangrene becomes moist gangrene.

In moist gangrene the part is cold, swollen, and pulseless; the skin is moist, black, and under tension; blebs form on the surface; liquefaction occurs; and a foul odor is present. The spread is rapid; there is no

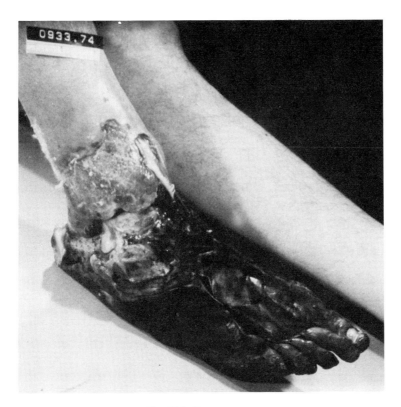

**Fig. 41-8.** Dry gangrene.

line of demarcation between the normal and diseased tissues; constitutional symptoms are severe; and death is frequent.

*Diabetic gangrene* begins as dry gangrene caused by hardening of the arteries but occurs more often in younger people than dry gangrene usually does. It extends up the lower extremity rapidly, and a line of demarcation is often absent. Because of the high sugar content of the tissues, which favors bacterial invasion, diabetic gangrene often becomes converted to the moist type.

*Gas gangrene* was discussed on p. 228.

## Fluid balance

Much attention has been given to the physiology of body fluids. It has been known for a long time that the main component of body fluids is water (about 70%) and that dissolved in it are chemical substances spoken of as *electrolytes*. With improved laboratory methods now available, disturbances in fluid and electrolyte balance are better understood in all fields of medicine.

**Fluid compartments.** For purposes of discussion the water or fluid of the body is placed into two anatomic areas: (1) *intracellular fluid* or fluid inside cells of the body, constituting about one half of the body weight, and (2) *extracellular fluid* or fluid present outside of body cells, about one fourth of the body weight. Extracellular fluid is further subdivided into *intravascular fluid,* the fluid contained within vascular channels, and *interstitial fluid,* that fluid present in the supporting connective tissues surrounding the body cells. Interstitial fluid represents the larger amount, since it is about one fifth of the body weight, whereas intravascular fluid represents only one twentieth of the body weight. For practical purposes plasma of the blood is used when intravascular fluid is studied.

The chemical composition of each fluid category is separate and distinct. However, the makeup of the intravascular fluid is so similar to that of the interstitial fluid that the two are usually designated together as extracellular fluid. Measurements easily made on the blood plasma, representing the intravascular fluid, indicate electrolyte concentrations in interstitial fluid, on which chemical analysis is made with difficulty. Extracellular and intracellular fluid, on the other hand, have quite different electrolyte patterns. However, much is still unknown as to intracellular fluid.

The electrolytes most carefully studied and of most significance clinically are sodium, potassium, bicarbonate, phosphate, and chloride. Sodium, chloride, and bicarbonate are important in the extracellular fluid; potassium and phosphate, in the intracellular

fluid. All these can be measured in the plasma of the blood by chemical analysis.

**Preservation of balance.** In the absence of disease the chemical composition and quantity of body fluid in the anatomic areas remain constant. This state of balance is maintained by certain hydrostatic and osmotic forces operating within each anatomic area. The areas are divided by biologic membranes that permit free passage of water but not of electrolytes. The cell is separated from extracellular fluid by the cell membrane. The fluid contained within vascular channels is separated from interstitial fluid by the endothelium that lines all such channels.

The most important organ in the body concerned with the regulation of the volume and chemical makeup of body fluid is the kidney. The kidney conserves or eliminates water and electrolytes in the urine. It can remove from the plasma of the blood certain chemicals that are accumulating to excess and eliminate them in the urine, or it can save for the body these or other substances for which there might be physiologic need.

**Intake of water.** In temperate climates man requires, on the average, about 1 ml. of water for each calorie contained in his food. About 50% of this is taken in as water or other liquid. About 38% is obtained from water contained in the food eaten (so-called *preformed water of food*), and 12% is made available after metabolic activity.

**Output of water.** There are several routes by which water may be lost to the body—in the urine, feces, and expired air, as sweat,* and by evaporation from the skin surface or respiratory tract. This evaporative loss is also referred to as *insensible water loss* and occurs independently of sweating. In normal persons with proper balance of intake and output of fluid, the proportions of fluid loss are as follows: 30% in the urine, 3% in the feces, 12% from the lungs as insensible loss, and 55% as sweat. These percentages, of course, are influenced by a number of factors, although there is a certain constant minimal loss of water from the body that occurs independently of the amount of water in the body. This minimum loss occurs even when there is an obvious need to conserve the fluid being lost. Some of the conditions associated with increased water loss are high fever, increase of environmental temperature, diarrhea, and vomiting.

**Disorders of fluid balance.** Disorders of fluid balance are, of course, usually the result of disease processes but may be the result of improper treatment (iatrogenic). They are most common following

---

*The average person has 17 square feet of skin and 2 or 3 million sweat glands. He perspires about 1 quart of fluid a day.

surgery and with diseases of the kidney. They are of special importance in childhood when diarrheas are frequent. They deserve special emphasis in the care of the elderly, infirm, or psychotic patient.

There are three main disturbances in fluid balance in the body: (1) changes in volume, (2) changes in osmotic concentration, and (3) changes in composition. Changes in the volume of fluids are usually expressed as deficits or excesses, depending on the decrease or increase over normal of the volume in a given area. Changes in the osmotic concentration consist of increases or decreases in the amount of a given electrolyte within the fluid. We know that sodium does not readily pass through the outer membrane of a cell. Since it does not, it exerts an effective osmotic pressure in the fluid outside the cell. Disorders of fluid balance, then, relate to variations of the sodium concentration in extracellular fluid. Changes in the composition of body fluids consist of excesses or deficits of the various chemical substances normally contained in the body fluids. Practically, these substances are measured by chemical analysis of the plasma of the blood, and therefore the disorders in this last category are usually designated as to whether the given substance is present in the blood in amounts below or above normal. Such terms as hypoglycemia and hyperglycemia, hypochloremia and hyperchloremia, hypokalemia and hyperkalemia, and hypocalcemia and hypercalcemia indicate either a decrease or an increase in glucose, chloride, potassium, and calcium, respectively.

Special instances of fluid balance disturbance follow.

*Decrease in total fluid.* A decrease in the total fluid of the body is sometimes referred to as *dehydration.* Dehydration may result not only if there is a loss of large amounts of water from the body or a failure of intake of proper amounts of water, but also if there is

a loss of considerable amounts of salt (sodium chloride). Pathologically this condition is characterized by a pronounced dryness of the skin (Fig. 41-9), mucous membranes, and surfaces of the internal organs. The serous surfaces of the internal organs no longer are glistening and moist but are opaque in appearance and sticky to the touch.

Abnormal loss of water may be the result of high fever, high environmental temperature, or diabetes insipidus, a disease that causes loss of enormous amounts of water through the kidneys. Decreased intake of water under abnormal conditions may occur in comatose patients or in persons shipwrecked or lost on a desert island. Abnormal loss of salt from the body occurs with adrenal insufficiency, as a result of metabolic disturbances, in diabetes mellitus, and in diseases associated with either severe diarrhea or vomiting.

*Increase in fluid.* The term *plethora* is used to designate an increase in the volume of blood. This may occur with an increase in both red blood cells and fluid, as is seen in polycythemia, a primary disease of the blood. When it occurs with an increase in the fluid portion alone, the increase in blood volume is referred to as *hydremic plethora.* Any condition associated with decreased excretion of water may result in this kind of plethora, particularly when no attempt is made to decrease the intake of fluid correspondingly. This is best seen in patients with nonfunctioning kidneys or renal insufficiency. Such patients may present a characteristic train of findings with headache, dizziness, vomiting, and dyspnea; and they may even develop convulsions. This clinical picture is sometimes referred to as water intoxication. Death may ensue if the derangement cannot be corrected.

Hydremic plethora sometimes results when parenteral fluids are given too rapidly by the intravenous

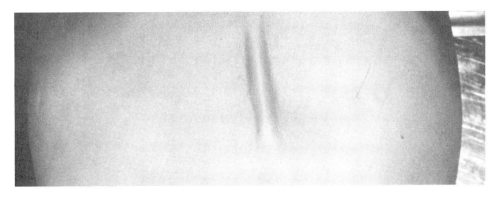

**Fig. 41-9.** Marked dehydration in 11-month-old child with gastroenteritis. Fold indicates loss of turgor in skin of upper abdomen, since normally, when pinched, skin springs back.

route. The excess of fluid tends to accumulate in the lungs, with the production of pulmonary edema. Such a sudden increase in blood volume in a person with heart disease may be fatal.

A marked increase in interstitial fluid designated as edema has already been discussed.

*Decreased osmotic concentration.* In certain occupations the laborers must work in a high environmental temperature. Consequently they sweat profusely, and the sweat as it pours from the body contains significant amounts of salt or sodium chloride. If these persons drink large quantities of water, as they tend to do, without consuming extra amounts of salt, certain changes tend to occur rather rapidly in the osmotic concentration of sodium in the extracellular fluid. The decreased osmotic concentration of sodium is associated with the development of characteristic cramps in the muscles, so-called miner's cramps or heat cramps. These muscular cramps are quickly relieved by salt.

**Diagnostic aids.** In the clinical evaluation of any fluid balance problem, it is important to have an adequate history and physical examination. In addition, the laboratory offers certain procedures that are valuable aids in diagnosis and management. These include examinations of the blood and urine. The urine specific gravity and concentration of sodium chloride may be determined. The value of sodium, potassium, chloride, and proteins in the plasma of the blood are important, as well as the carbon dioxide–combining power of the plasma of the blood and the concentration of red blood cells in the blood, or the *hematocrit*. In the management of a disorder of fluid balance it is of utmost importance to have an accurate record kept of the intake and the output of fluids by the patient, including the type and amount of oral and parenteral fluid and the type and amount of fluid lost in the urine, vomitus, and drainage from fistulous tracts. An accurate record of body weight taken daily is also valuable in cases where the patient is not too sick to be weighed.

**Acid-base balance.** Closely allied to a discussion of fluid and electrolyte balance is a consideration of the acid-base balance of the body, or the arrangement in the body whereby acid substances are counterbalanced by basic substances. This is important because normal chemical processes of metabolism result in the production of large amounts of acid substances. Some disposal of these acid substances or metabolites is made by the kidneys in the elimination of inorganic and organic acids in the urine and by the lungs in the excretion of carbon dioxide. However, before these acid substances reach either the lungs or the kidneys, there are certain chemical combinations in the body fluids, spoken of as buffers or buffer systems, that neutralize their harmful effects.

When disturbances occur in the acid-base balance of the body, they result from three situations. First, the rate of production of the acid by-products of metabolism may be speeded up as a result of disease, as in diabetes mellitus. Second, there may be impairment of the excretory process, as in advanced kidney disease with failure of renal function. Third, there may be an unchecked elimination of water and electrolytes, as in vomiting or diarrhea.

There is actually a very narrow margin compatible with life over which the ratio of acid substances to basic substances may vary in body fluids. When there is an increase in the basic components of the plasma of blood, the condition is termed *alkalosis*. If there is a decrease in these with a corresponding increase in acid metabolites, the condition is referred to as *acidosis*. Alkalosis may be associated with numbness of the fingers and face and, if severe, may lead to tetany with muscular twitchings and spasm. Acidosis is often accompanied by a type of breathing termed *Kussmaul breathing*, which is characterized by an increased depth and a slightly increased rate of respiration.

## Questions for review

1 Differentiate between active and passive hyperemia.
2 What is collateral circulation? What purpose does it serve?
3 What are the common causes of hemorrhage?
4 Define epistaxis, hemoptysis, hematemesis, hematuria, apoplexy, petechiae, ecchymosis, hematoma.
5 What is pitting edema?
6 Briefly discuss hemophilia.
7 What is the difference between a thrombus and an embolus? Compare thrombi and emboli as to composition, causes, sites of formation, and possible results.
8 What is meant by fat embolism?
9 Briefly explain acid-base balance, decreased osmotic concentration, plethora, dehydration, insensible water loss, extracellular fluid.
10 List diagnostic aids available in evaluating fluid balance problems.
11 Contrast dry gangrene with moist gangrene. Is dry gangrene a true gangrene?
12 Define anasarca, dropsy, ascites, hydrothorax, transudate, exudate.

**References on pp. 552 and 553.**

# CHAPTER 42
# Metabolic disturbances

Atrophy, degenerations, and pigmentations make up the group of passive tissue changes known as *regressive*\* tissue changes. *Necrosis* (cell death) and tissue dissolution are the final or ultimate outcomes of regressive changes that persist. Frequently, however, the process is arrested at some point short of cell destruction, and the cells and tissues are able to return to their normal state.

There are two major causes of retrogressive tissue changes: (1) reduction in the oxygen supply to the cells and (2) interference by harmful agents with cell metabolism. With progressive disease of the heart, lungs, or blood vessels the supply of oxygen so necessary for normal metabolic activity at the cellular level is decreased. Substances of a varied nature may exert a harmful influence directly on the protoplasm of living cells; these can be the by-products of bacterial metabolism, breakdown products of body tissues, and certain chemical and physical agents. (See Fig. 42-1.)

## Atrophy

Atrophy is a decrease in the size of a part or organ of the body previously of normal size; there has been a decrease in the size or number of component cells. Atrophy must not be confused with *hypoplasia,* which means that the organ or tissue has been smaller than normal from birth. When an organ undergoes atrophy, the functional tissue is primarily affected.

**Kinds.** Atrophy may be physiologic (involutional) or pathologic. Physiologic atrophy is best represented by the atrophy of the thymus gland in children, the atrophy of the mammary glands after lactation, the atrophy of the tonsils, spleen, and other lymphoid tissues after middle life, and the more or less generalized atrophy of all organs and tissues that occurs with age (senile atrophy) (Fig. 42-2).

**Causes.** The general causes of pathologic atrophy are (1) inadequate nutrition, (2) disuse, (3) pressure, (4) loss of nerve supply, and (5) lack of endocrine stimulation. When there is a serious interference

with nutrition over a considerable period of time, such as occurs in starvation and wasting diseases, the body undergoes more or less generalized atrophic change. Localized atrophy, as is sometimes seen in an extremity, may be caused by restriction of nourishment resulting from a decreased blood supply. Atrophy from disuse is most often seen in the muscles of paralyzed limbs and in muscles attached to immobilized joints. Pressure atrophy is best exemplified by the atrophy resulting from the pressure exerted by tumors and aneurysms. Bone is more susceptible to pressure atrophy than are soft tissues because it is a rigid and inelastic structure. Poliomyelitis, a disease involving the spinal cord, may cause paralysis because it causes loss of the nerve supply to the muscles of an extremity. Atrophy of the hair follicles and sebaceous glands in myxedema (caused by a deficiency in the hormone of the thyroid gland) is an example of atrophy resulting from disturbance of the endocrine glands. Atrophic organs may be irregular on the surface because of the uneven distribution of the atrophic foci within their substance.

## Degenerations

Degenerations are regressive tissue alterations characterized by swelling of the cells and chemical changes within the cell cytoplasm that lead to the appearance within the cell of substances that are normally absent, present only to a slight degree, or present and invisible. The nucleus is not so greatly affected as the cytoplasm (Fig. 42-3). The degeneration is named in accordance with the substance appearing in the cell, for example, fatty degeneration. It should be emphasized that many of the retrogressive changes are nonspecific in that they may be produced by totally unrelated agents. Degenerations have been emphasized in the pathologic literature primarily because they induce well-defined and often dramatic changes in cells, easily appreciated either microscopically or macroscopically. These changes, however, cannot be strictly correlated with functional disturbances.

---

\*Also known as retrograde or retrogressive tissue changes.

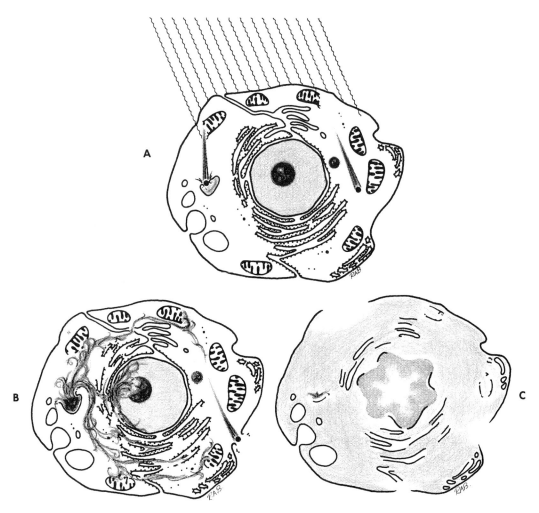

**Fig. 42-1.** Interference with cell metabolism by harmful physical agent. **A,** Radiant energy penetrates membrane of exposed cell and initiates changes in lipid metabolism. Free radicals released. **B,** Free radicals puncture lysosomes, releasing hydrolytic enzymes. Cell components and membrane disrupted. **C,** End stage—burned-out cell.

From the nature of these processes it would be expected that they would exert the maximum effects in the cytoplasm of cells said to be highly specialized, meaning that the cells possess exceedingly complex enzyme systems enabling them to carry on activities associated with the higher forms of life. Actually, these cells are more vulnerable to even minor injuries because their metabolic balance is such a delicate one. Therefore the retrogressive tissue changes are most important in the kidneys, heart, and liver, three specialized organs necessary to life and termed *vital organs.*

**Cloudy swelling.** Clouding swelling is the most common and the least damaging of the degenerations. It is a frequent accompaniment of diphtheria, typhoid fever, and pneumonia. Some degree of cloudy swelling occurs in practically all infectious diseases, follows extensive burns, and may be found with inanition. The organs most often involved are the liver and kidneys, less often the heart muscle. Basically, cloudy swelling is caused by an increased water content in the affected cells, which are enlarged; their cytoplasm is cloudy. Grossly the organs are large, pale, and plump, with the appearance of having been dipped in boiling water (parboiled). As a rule, recovery is complete, but if the causative agent is especially severe in its action or persists for a long time, cloudy swelling may change to fatty metamorphosis or even necrosis. (See Fig. 42-3.)

A condition similar to cloudy swelling is *hydropic*

*degeneration,* but in this the water content of the cell is so great that globules form which are visible microscopically in the cytoplasm.

**Fatty metamorphosis (fatty infiltration—fatty degeneration) of the liver.** The liver is an organ directly concerned with the metabolism of fats in the body, and therefore degenerative changes that result in the abnormal accumulation or distribution of visible fat in the liver cells are of special importance. Books on pathology written only a few years ago made a distinct separation between fatty infiltration and fatty degeneration of the liver. By fatty infiltration was meant the abnormal deposit within the liver cells of fat that had been brought in by the blood. Fatty degeneration was thought to be caused by the transformation of some of the cell material into fat. Actually the process is a combination of infiltration and degeneration as previously understood, with the former playing the major role. Since the two conditions often coexist, present-day treatises on pathology consider both fatty infiltration and fatty degeneration in the liver under the general term *fatty metamorphosis.* (See Fig. 42-4.) The liver cells contain deposits of fat, and the organ is enlarged, soft, and yellow. Fatty metamorphosis may follow cloudy swelling and may be present in metallic poisoning, anoxic states, chronic passive hyperemia, prolonged fevers, chronic alcoholism, malnutrition, and chronic wasting diseases. In mild cases recovery is complete. With prolonged and severe change there is cell death.

**Fatty degeneration.** Other organs, notably the heart and kidneys, may show an abnormal appearance of fat in the cell cytoplasm, or fatty degeneration, as this degeneration is termed in organs other than in the liver. This usually means a moderately severe

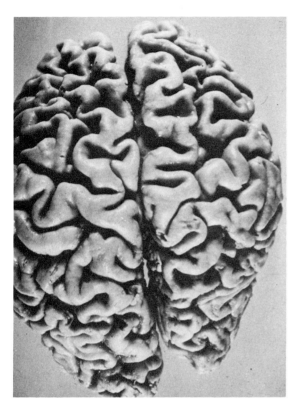

**Fig. 42-2.** Senile atrophy of brain. Convolutions narrowed, sulci widened; brain decreased in size and weight.

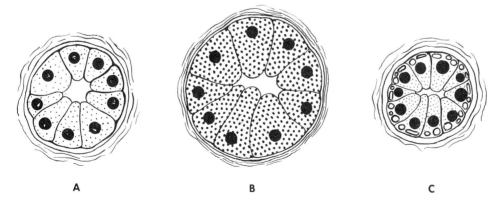

A      B      C

**Fig. 42-3.** Degenerations in cells lining kidney tubules, diagrammatic cross sections. **A,** Normal tubular epithelium. **B,** Cloudy swelling of lining cells. **C,** Fatty degeneration. Fatty droplets are seen as clear vacuolated areas beneath nucleus in cytoplasm of cells. Note how luminal area is reduced in **B** and **C.**

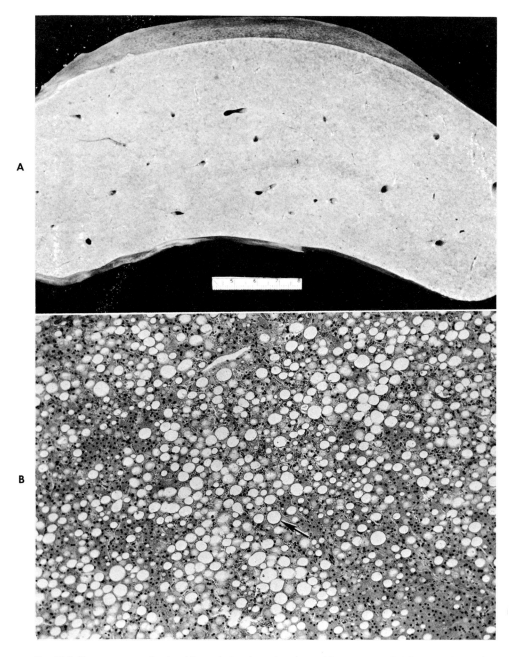

**Fig. 42-4.** Fatty metamorphosis of liver. **A,** Sectioned surface of liver (gross). **B,** Microscopic section showing vacuoles corresponding to fat dissolved out in processing. Most liver cells contain one large or several small vacuoles within cytoplasm. (×140.)

injury to the cells of these organs and may follow severe anemia, severe infections, or the ingestion of chemical poisons.

**Amyloid disease.** Amyloid disease is an unexplained accumulation of a pathologic, waxy, and starchlike protein substance, amyloid, which is formed in the body and deposited in various organs, especially the liver, spleen, kidneys, and adrenal glands. It is an accompaniment of long-continued suppurative conditions such as tuberculosis and osteomyelitis and is rare. (See Fig. 42-5.)

**Pathologic calcification.** Calcification is the deposit within the tissues of earthy salts without any consistent attempt at bone formation. It is found most

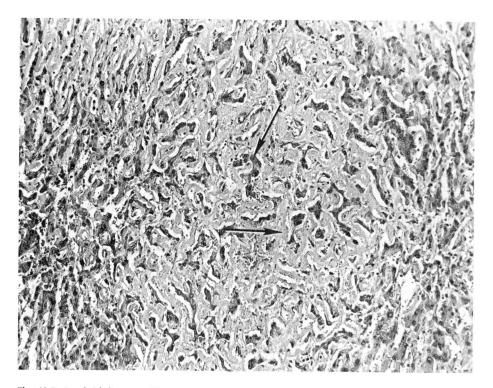

**Fig. 42-5.** Amyloid disease of liver. Note accumulation of amyloid (lower arrow) as grayish homogeneous material across middle of microscopic section, appearing to compress and push aside darker cords of liver tissue. Atrophy of liver (upper arrow) in center of section is emphasized by comparison with better preserved cells to sides. (×140.)

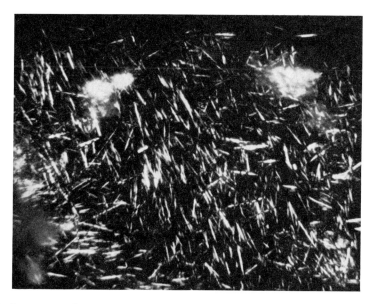

**Fig. 42-6.** Contents (sodium urate crystals) of tophus viewed under polarized light. (From Talso, P. J., and Remenchik, A. P., editors: Internal medicine—based on mechanisms of disease, St. Louis, 1968, The C. V. Mosby Co.)

often in dead or dying tissues and may be an aftermath of various types of degeneration. Among the common examples are calcification of tuberculous areas, calcification of the blood vessels in arteriosclerosis, calcification of degenerating tumors, and formation of a calcified envelope around *Trichinella spiralis* in muscle. A *lithopedion,* or stone child, is a retained fetus that has undergone calcification.

**Other degenerations.** Among the remaining degenerations are (1) *hyaline degeneration,* wherein connective tissue cells take on a glassy appearance, and (2) *mucoid degeneration,* wherein the cells of certain tumors swell and become converted into jellylike masses.

**Gout.** Gout, a metabolic disease of unknown cause, reflects an abnormality in the metabolism of uric acid (the end product of purine metabolism) in the body, with the accumulation of abnormally large amounts of uric acid and urates. Constitutional and hereditary factors seem to play a part in its development. (See Fig. 42-6.)

In this disease deposits or urates known as *tophi* (sing., *tophus*) occur in and about the joints, in the kidneys, in the cartilage of the external ear, and sometimes in the eyelid. The disease is marked by acute attacks during which there is intensely painful swelling of one or more joints, classically the metatarsophalangeal joint of the great toe. Attacks are followed by intervals of remission. Joint changes result from the deposition of sodium urate crystals in the synovial cartilages and membranes. This is accompanied by granulomatous inflammation of the foreign-body type and the accumulation of fluid within the joint cavity. In gout the amount of uric acid in the blood is invariably increased.

**Uric acid infarcts.** Because of increased uric acid excretion shortly after birth, extensive deposits of uric acid (so-called *uric acid infarcts*) may be found in the

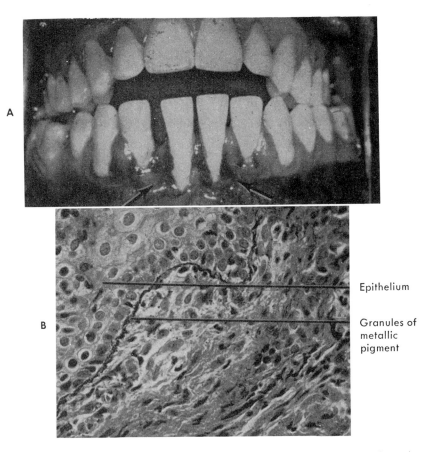

**Fig. 42-7.** Lead line. **A,** As linear dark granular areas on gums (arrows). **B,** In microscopic section as a line of pigment granules. (From Bhaskar, S. N.: Synopsis of oral pathology, ed. 4, St. Louis, 1973, The C. V. Mosby Co.)

renal tubules of the newborn infant. These have no harmful effect on the kidney and are not true infarcts.

## Pigmentations

Abnormal pigmentation may result from an increase in amount or an irregularity in distribution of the normal pigments of the body (endogenous pigments) or from the deposition within the tissues of pigments that gain access to the body from without (exogenous pigments) by way of the mouth, lungs, or skin. (See Figs. 42-7 and 42-8.)

**Endogenous pigments.** The most important endogenous pigments are melanin, hemoglobin, and the hemoglobin derivative, bilirubin. Melanin is the normal coloring matter of the skin and the choroid and iris of the eye. In the skin it is found in the cells lying in the deeper layers of the epidermis. The more melanin present, the darker is the complexion. Freckles are localized areas in which the melanin content of the skin is increased. Albinism is the congenital absence of melanin from the skin and eyes. Pigmented moles or *nevi* and the rapidly fatal tumors known as malignant melanomas are tumors made up of melanin-containing cells. *Icterus* or *jaundice* is a yellow discoloration of the skin and tissues caused by the retention within the body of bilirubin, the pigment giving color to bile (p. 578).

**Exogenous pigments.** One of the best examples of exogenous pigmentation is the yellow discoloration of the skin that may follow the consumption of large amounts of carotene-containing foods (carrots, turnips). This condition of *carotenemia* may be mistaken for jaundice. When large amounts of dust (carbon pigment or coal dust) are inhaled over long periods of time, a portion is deposited in the lungs and

in the lymph nodes receiving drainage from the lungs. This type of carbon pigmentation is known as *anthracosis*.

If medications containing silver salts are taken over a long period of time, the conjunctivae and skin may assume an ashen gray color, caused by the deposit of silver albuminate just beneath the epithelium. This condition is *argyria* and, once present, persists throughout the victim's life. Deposits of silver may occur in other parts of the body as well. The formation of a blue line (known as a lead line) along the margins of the gums is one of the diagnostic features of chronic lead poisoning *(plumbism)*. (See also p. 498.) It is much more noticeable in mouths not properly cared for and around decayed teeth. The line is produced by the combination of lead salts within the tissues and hydrogen sulfide in the decaying matter of the mouth. Similar lines are sometimes seen in chronic bismuth and mercury poisoning.

## Stones (calculi)

Concrements or calculi are solid calcific masses formed within the passages or hollow organs of the body. The important three—choleliths (gallstones), renal calculi (kidney stones), and vesical calculi (bladder stones)—are discussed on subsequent pages. Other calculi of importance are pancreatic calculi, prostatic calculi, rhinoliths, and salivary calculi. Concrements are important because they may obstruct passages and predispose to infection.

**Structure.** Most concrements have a center or nucleus made up of bacteria, necrotic body cells, inspissated mucus, or a foreign body. The remainder of the stone is composed of chemical substances, often crystalline, deposited around the nucleus in ringlike layers and derived from the lumen of the passage or from the organ in which the stone is located. Retention of secretions or excretions because of preexisting abnormality is an important predisposing cause of calculi.

**Kinds.** Concrements made up almost entirely of feces may be found in the appendix and are called *fecaliths. Prostatic calculi* are formed by the deposit of salts on corpora amylacea. *Rhinoliths* are calculi formed in the nose. *Broncholiths* are concrements formed in the bronchi. A *pneumolith* is a stone occurring in the substance of the lung. Pneumoliths and broncholiths are spoken of as lung stones.

## Necrosis

Necrosis is the death of cells, tissues, or organs while yet a part of the living body. It may be caused by (1) mechanical injury, (2) interference with nutrition, (3) extremes of heat or cold, (4) chemical or bacterial poisons, and (5) loss of nerve supply.

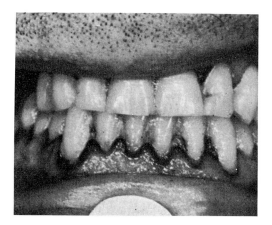

**Fig. 42-8.** Bismuth seam (chronic poisoning). Another example of metallic pigmentation. (From Thoma, K. H.: Oral surgery, ed. 5, St. Louis, 1969, The C. V. Mosby Co.)

**473**

**Kinds.** Necrotic foci may liquefy (*liquefaction* necrosis); they may be converted into a dry, firm, yellowish mass (*coagulation* necrosis); or they may be converted into a cheesy material by the admixture of fatty substances (*caseation* necrosis). An example of liquefaction necrosis is the softening of the center of an abscess with the discharge of its contents. Coagulation necrosis results from the coagulation of proteins, as is seen in infarcts. It is this type of necrosis of the mucous membrane of the stomach that occurs in carbolic acid and bichloride of mercury poisoning. Caseation necrosis is most often seen in tuberculosis. A mass of necrotic soft tissue is known as a *sphacelus;* a fragment of necrotic bone is known as a *sequestrum.*

Necrosis caused by the interruption of the blood supply to a part (*infarction*) is of special importance. When a person lies in one position for a long time, the skin and subcutaneous tissues, especially over bony protuberances, are compressed at the points of contact with the bed, and their blood supply is impaired. This leads to necrosis of the skin, with the formation of bed sores (*decubitus ulcers*) that are extremely painful. *Fat necrosis* may result from the liberation of pancreatic juice into the retroperitoneal area, with the digestion of fat therein.

## Somatic death

In the multicellular organism are three recognized forms of death—necrosis, necrobiosis, and somatic death. We have learned that *necrosis* is the death of cells, tissues, or organs while yet a part of the living body. *Necrobiosis* is death of cells, with replacement by new cells, as in the normal processes of life (example: the shedding of cells of the superficial layers of skin, with replacement by normal cells from the lower layers). By *somatic* or *total body death* is meant the cessation of all ordinarily perceived activities associated with life. Necrosis may occur without somatic death, and necrobiosis is a constant accompaniment of normal life. After somatic death a short time elapses before cellular death is complete. Cellular death following somatic death is not a progressive simultaneous affair, since the cells of some tissues die more rapidly than those of others.

**Vital organs.** Those organs that are absolutely essential to the maintenance of life are known as vital organs, and their relative importance is measured by the rapidity with which somatic death follows the complete cessation of their action. The sovereign triad of vital organ systems is the central nervous, the circulatory, and the respiratory systems. After complete obliteration of the central nervous system, death is almost instantaneous. Death usually follows within minutes after the arrest of either circulation or respiration. In both respiratory and circulatory fail-

ure the ultimate cause of death is lack of oxygen. Death follows within a period of days after the removal of both kidneys, the liver, or the pancreas. Removal of organs such as the gallbladder or spleen does not have any marked deleterious influence on health.

**Signs of death.** Usually there are changes that make the presence of death known to even the uninitiated observer, but occasionally it is difficult to differentiate apparent from true death. Apparent death is most frequently seen in partial asphyxia, catalepsy, trance, and syncope (fainting). It should be remembered that fainting is a dangerous condition that demands immediate attention.

Special signs of death occur with, or closely follow, the death struggle, and certain cadaveric changes become apparent at a later period. The special signs of death are (1) cessation of circulation, (2) cessation of respiration, (3) complete muscular relaxation, and (4) eye changes. By carefully feeling for the pulse and listening for heart sounds over a long period of time in absolutely quiet surroundings, one can determine whether there is any indication of heart action. In case of doubt, an artery may be opened. If the heart has not stopped, blood will gush out. For some time after death, blood may flow from a severed vein because of the postmortem contraction of the arteries, which drives blood into the veins and capillaries. Evidence of respiration may be sought by careful observation or by holding a mirror in front of the person's mouth and nose. If any air is expired, a fog will appear on the mirror. Peristaltic movements that sometimes continue after death should not be mistaken for respiration. Complete muscular relaxation is an essential feature of death, but in cases in which rigor mortis occurs at once, relaxation may not be detected. The eyes become glazed, noticeable especially in the corners. As a result of impaired blood flow and loss of muscular tone, the face usually but not always takes on the expression described as the *facies hippocratica*, the characteristics of which are pale ashen skin, sunken eyes, a thin prominent nose, pale thin lips, and prominent chin and cheeks.

**Cadaveric changes.** The important cadaveric changes that follow death are: (1) cooling of the body (*algor mortis*), (2) stiffening of the body (*rigor mortis*), (3) postmortem hypostasis (*livor mortis*), and (4) signs of putrefaction. In some cases there may be a postmortem rise in temperature, but in any case cooling will eventually take place. The onset and rate at which cooling takes place are influenced by so many factors that no set rules can be given. Cooling is rapid for a short time and then proceeds more slowly until about 24 hours after death, when the temperature of the surrounding air is reached. Rigor mortis is variably affected by the condition of the body just before death. As a rule, it appears at some time during the first 4 hours after death and is complete within 12 hours after onset. Rigor mortis first involves the muscles of the eyelids and jaws and then spreads from the head to the limbs. It lasts 24 to 36 hours, leaving the body in the order in which it came; when broken up by mechanical means, it never returns.

Within 1 to 6 hours after death, dark reddish blue discolorations, known as livores mortis, appear on the skin over dependent parts. These result from the pooling of blood in the capillaries, with diffusion into the tissues.

The first distinct putrefactive sign is a greenish discoloration of the abdomen caused by postmortem disintegration of blood. Some organs are much more resistant to putrefaction than are others. As a rule, the brain succumbs first.

**Time of death.** Although it is possible to arrive at an opinion as to the length of time that a body has been dead, this is sometimes a difficult matter for experts.

**Diagnosis of death in modern medicine.** It was the technical success of heart transplantation that raised the many moral, medical, and legal issues as to definition and timing of death. First of all, in the field of organ transplantation the matter is of great concern to physician and layman alike. Basic to any decision regarding transplantation from cadaver to living recipient of a viable organ (for which there is considerable demand) is the question of just when the donor became a cadaver. It is of course desirable for the transplant surgeon to have the viable organ as soon as possible. A closely related point is that in the event of a single organ transplant, especially if it be the heart or other vital organ, there will certainly be death of the donor after donation if it had not already taken place.

The time and technic of death are crucial in a second area of scientific advance. Life can now be sustained in certain instances by supportive measures long after the natural mechanisms of lungs and even the heart have failed.

Most authorities seem to feel that a cessation of activity of the brain most reliably warrants the diagnosis of death. Researchers are turning their attention to quick and sure ways of pinpointing the moment at which brain damage becomes irreversible.

## Questions for review

1 Define atrophy. How does it differ from hypoplasia?
2 Give the general causes of pathologic atrophy, with an example of each.
3 Characterize regressive tissue changes.
4 Briefly describe cloudy swelling.
5 What organs are most likely to be involved by degenerations and why?
6 What is fatty metamorphosis? What organ does it involve?
7 Distinguish between endogenous and exogenous pigmentation. Give examples of each.
8 What organs of the body may be affected by calculi?
9 Define necrosis, infarct, coagulation necrosis, caseation necrosis, liquefaction necrosis, bed sore.
10 What are the vital organs?
11 Define rigor mortis. Describe its course.
12 Name the cadaveric changes following death.

**References on p. 481.**

# CHAPTER 43

# Deficiency states

## Vitamins

**General characteristics.** That certain food principles other than proteins, carbohydrates, fats, and inorganic salts are needed for the growth, development, and continued well-being of the body was not recognized until the early part of the present century. These substances, whose mode of action is but partly understood, are known as vitamins or *food accessory factors.* With one exception they manifest themselves by a lack instead of by an excess; that is, symptoms occur only when the body is *deficient* in them. When there is a deficiency in certain vitamins, the nutrition of the body as a whole suffers, and in addition, a train of events characteristic of the deficiency of that particular vitamin occurs. Such are known as *vitamin deficiency diseases* or *avitaminoses.* A deficiency in more than one vitamin is spoken of as *polyvitaminosis.*

Most vitamins are identified by letters of the alphabet, but the letters used have no relation to the order of their discovery. We tend now to replace the alphabetical nomenclature with chemical names. The term *vitamin,* which means "life amine," is not well used because it indicates that the vitamins are amines and that they are all chemically related, neither of which is true. Chemically they may be acids, alcohols, amines, or other relatively simple molecules.

The common features are as follows: (1) all are necessary for the absorption of food and maintenance of growth and health; (2) each has its own specific action; (3) very small amounts are sufficient to meet the needs of the body*; (4) products of the vegetable kingdom, they cannot be produced by the animal body; (5) their action is similar to that of enzymes; and (6) their distribution is variable; a given vitamin may be abundantly present in one food and absent from another.

Vitamins may be defined as organic catalysts, effective in very small amounts, that are essential for the maintenance of the normal structure and function of the cells of the body. They differ from hormones in that hormones originate within the body, whereas vitamins are taken into the body from without (in some cases as precursors). A given vitamin may be required for one animal species but not for another. As a rule, vitamins taken into the body from animal sources are more potent than are those of vegetable origin. Physiologically vitamins are important components of chemical compounds (coenzymes) that activate enzymes in basic metabolic processes.

More than a dozen vitamins have been identified and studied. Of these vitamins, A, B complex, C, D, E, and K are best known. Vitamins B and C are water soluble; the others are fat soluble. Table 43-1 gives sources and deficiency states for vitamins important in human nutrition.

### Listing of vitamins

*Vitamin A.* Fat-soluble vitamin A is found in butter, codfish, egg yolk, carrots, sweet potatoes, squash, animal fats, and green leafy vegetables. In the animal body it is manufactured by the liver from the carotene of vegetable foods.

Vitamin A is necessary for the proper development of the young of the species and is concerned with the integrity of epithelial cells. When there is a deficiency in vitamin A, epithelial cells, normally moist or ciliated, revert to a flattened squamous type without protective secretion or cilia. Infection occurs more easily; hence, vitamin A has been called the anti-infective vitamin. The transformation of the epithelium of lacrimal gland ducts to a squamous type in vitamin A deficiency leads to dryness and keratinization of the conjunctiva followed by infection and corneal ulceration. This condition is known as *xerophthalmia* (dry eye). A somewhat similar condition affecting the epidermis is *phrynoderma* (toad skin). Vitamin A deficiency may also lead to keratinization of the surface epithelium and infection of the respiratory, intestinal, and genitourinary tracts. Tooth changes may occur in vitamin A deficiency. Night

*The recommended daily amounts of some thirteen vitamins necessary for health in man add up in 1 year to only 1½ ounces.

**476**

**Table 43-1**

Vitamins important in human nutrition

| VITAMIN | SOME SOURCES IN DIET | | CLASSIC DEFICIENCY STATES |
|---|---|---|---|
| | ANIMAL | PLANT | |
| A | Fish liver oils<br>Milk and milk products<br>Liver<br>Egg yolk | Yellow fruits and vegetables<br>Green, leafy vegetables | Night blindness<br>Xerophthalmia<br>Toad skin |
| B group | Liver<br>Kidney<br>Lean beef<br>Milk<br>Eggs<br>Poultry<br>Cheese | Many kinds of fresh, green<br>vegetables<br>Whole grain cereals<br>Rice polishings<br>Yeasts<br>Peanuts | Beriberi<br>Pellagra<br>Cheilosis<br>Pernicious anemia and<br>other macrocytic anemias |
| C | Lean meat | Citrus fruits<br>Berries<br>Melons<br>Green, leafy vegetables<br>Tomatoes<br>Potatoes | Scurvy |
| D | Fish liver oils<br>Liver<br>Butter<br>Egg yolk | Yeast | Rickets |
| E | | Green, leafy vegetables<br>Nuts<br>Legumes | |
| K | Liver | Cabbage<br>Spinach<br>Cauliflower | Hemorrhagic disease of<br>newborn infants<br>Certain bleeding diseases<br>associated with liver and<br>biliary tract disease |

*For this vitamin, animal sources are poor and deficiency states unrecognized.

blindness is a condition in which a person is unable to see when going from a brightly lit area into a more subdued one (as from a sunlit street into a darkened theater). It is caused by a lack of visual purple in the retina, which is related to a deficiency in vitamin A.

*Vitamin B complex.* The vitamin B group is found in wheat germ, rice polishings, and yeasts. (See also Table 43-1.) Today we have more than twenty recognized members of this group of vitamins, the important members of which are thiamine ($B_1$), niacin (nicotinic acid); riboflavin, pyridoxine ($B_6$), pantothenic acid, para-aminobenzoic acid, biotin, choline, folic acid, and vitamin $B_{12}$. At least five—thiamine, biotin, nicotinic acid, riboflavin, and pantothenic acid—are present in cell mitochondria as coenzymes, where they participate in cycles that unlock energy from sugar and fats.

Thiamine, known as the antineuritic factor and the first vitamin to be isolated, prevents *beriberi*. A deficiency of niacin leads to *pellagra* in man and blacktongue in dogs; a deficiency in riboflavin leads to *cheilosis* (sore cracked lips). Folic acid has been used effectively in the treatment of sprue (p. 572) and macrocytic anemias. Present in cereal grains, folic acid may also be found in meat and eggs. If vitamin $B_{12}$ is given in even small doses* to patients with pernicious anemia, a marked relief of symptoms occurs, and there is a pronounced hematologic response. Vitamin $B_{12}$, the antipernicious anemia principle or cyanocobalamin, is the largest, most complicated vitamin we know, and the only one containing a metal ion (cobalt). The results of deficiencies of other vitamins of the B group in man are not so striking as those given.

*Vitamin C.* Vitamin C (antiscorbutic), identified as *ascorbic acid*, is found in germinating grains and

*One microgram (one 28 millionth of an ounce) of vitamin $B_{12}$ maintains a pernicious anemia patient in good health.

the juices of citrus fruits, especially orange and lemon juices. It may be found also in lean meats, strawberries, tomatoes, and cabbage. Prolonged cooking may sharply reduce its content in food. The daily requirement of man is from 30 to 75 mg. Vitamin C assists the body's absorption of iron, plays a role in the formation of collagen, and is found in the adrenal gland in large amounts. Vitamin C deficiency classically means *scurvy*.

*Vitamin D.* Vitamin D, called the *sunray* or *antirachitic* vitamin, is a component of codfish, butter, yeast, and egg yolk and is fat soluble. Ergosterol, obtained from yeasts and other substances, develops a vitamin D potency greater than that of cod-liver oil when exposed to ultraviolet light. Such irradiated ergosterol is known as *viosterol*. Sunlight or artificial ultraviolet light increases the vitamin D content of the body by converting the ergosterol of the skin and tissues into vitamin D. Vitamin D increases the absorption of calcium from the intestine and increases phosphorus and calcium retention in the body. A deficiency leads to tooth decay and *rickets*. So far as is known, this is the only vitamin whose excess leads to bad effects. *Hypervitaminosis D* may be produced experimentally or by accidental overdosage. It results in a great increase in the calcium and phosphorus of the blood, with excessive decalcification of bone and deposit of calcium in tissues such as kidneys, arteries, and lungs, where normally no calcium is found.

*Vitamin E.* Fat-soluble vitamin E occurs principally in plant products. It is concentrated in seeds, and rich sources are wheat germ, cottonseed, and peanut and soybean oils. Experimentally, results of vitamin E deficiency in animals are many and varied, but in man little is known as to pathologic changes from a comparable lack. The vitamin is sufficiently widespread as to make unlikely any deficiency in the diet. The biochemical function of vitamin E is obscure although apparently linked to the structural integrity of muscle and to the reproductive, nervous, and vascular systems.

*Vitamin K.* Vitamin K, which is necessary for the formation of prothrombin (an essential element in blood coagulation), is ingested in the form of certain green vegetables or is formed in the intestinal canal by the action of enteric bacteria on the intestinal contents. *Hemorrhagic disease of the newborn* and the hemorrhagic tendencies in certain cases of jaundice may be explained on the basis of a deficiency of vitamin K and are easily corrected or prevented by doses of vitamin K. In the newborn infant the prothrombin received from the mother's circulation is consumed before vitamin K sufficient to furnish enough prothrombin for blood coagulation is ingested in the food

or is formed by the intestinal bacteria in the baby. In cases of jaundice of the obstructive type, vitamin K may not be absorbed from the intestinal canal because of the absence of bile, which is essential for its absorption.

## Vitamin deficiencies

**Rickets (rachitis).** Rickets is a constitutional disease of infancy that is caused, at least in part, by a diet deficient in vitamin D. It is fundamentally an overproduction of bone matrix in the skeleton that is deficient in bone salts. The growing and developing bones are incompletely and imperfectly calcified. The outstanding clinical feature of rickets is marked bony deformity, especially of the long bones and the bones of the skull.

Rickets is primarily a disease of the city. It is more common in blacks than whites because the melanin pigmentation of the black race blocks the penetration of the ultraviolet rays of the sun. Breast-fed children do not develop it as often as artificially fed babies. The disease seldom begins during the summer months, and rachitic children usually improve at this time of the year because the ultraviolet rays of sunlight produce vitamin D from the ergosterol contained in the superficial layers of the skin. Children who live in warm sunny climates are not so likely to develop rickets as are those who live in cold, dark, overcrowded surroundings. Window glass removes the ultraviolet rays from sunlight. For this reason children who stay indoors are more likely to develop rickets than are those who play outdoors.

Rickets usually begins between the sixth and eighteenth month of life and remains active for 1 or 2 years and then subsides, but the deformities produced by the disease may remain throughout life. Since the bones are deficient in lime salts, they are soft and unable to bear weight. As the disease progresses, there is even greater deformity. The ankles and wrists are greatly thickened, but the bones may be cut with a knife. Dentition is delayed, and the teeth are defective. The flat bones of the skull are thin, and the fontanels close slowly. A peculiar enlargement of the costochondral junctions between the ribs and sternum, known as the *rachitic rosary*, is a characteristic sign of rickets. Pigeon chest, bowlegs, and knock-knees are common deformities. Advanced cases show flattening of the pelvis and marked deformity of the spine. The rachitic child is often potbellied and has a large square head, and as a rule, he appears well nourished or even obese. Diffuse soreness of the body, nocturnal restlessness, slight fever, and profuse sweating of the head and neck are common findings. Complications of an infectious nature are not uncommon. In adult life the condition known as *osteomalacia* is comparable to infantile rickets.

**Pellagra.** Pellagra is a deficiency disease described by a seasonal variation, a tendency to recur, and a rather characteristic train of clinical findings consisting of a skin eruption, gastrointestinal disturbances, and nervous and mental changes. At the present time the primary factor in the production of pellagra is a diet deficient in nicotinic acid and certain other B complex vitamins, probably with some other condition a secondary factor. Depleting diseases and the prolonged and excessive use of alcohol seem to be predisposing influences.

Pellagra often begins in the spring, and recurrences are more common then. The typical manifesta-

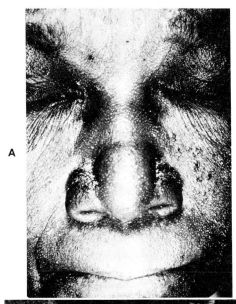

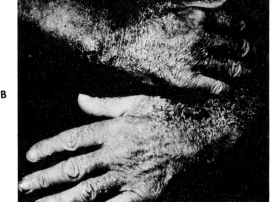

**Fig. 43-1.** Pellagra. **A,** Face. **B,** Hands. Note roughened scaly pigmented skin in both areas.

tions of the disease are frequently preceded by such prodromal signs as loss of appetite, digestive disturbances, and mental depression. A skin eruption begins on the exposed surfaces of the body and is often mistaken for sunburn, which it closely resembles at first. After a few days to several weeks the affected brown, scaly skin begins to desquamate (Fig. 43-1). The tongue and mouth are red, raw, edematous, and ulcerated. A distressing salivation may be present. The intestine is often ulcerated. Hydrochloric acid is frequently absent from the stomach, and severe diarrhea occurs in about three fourths of the patients. There is atrophy of various organs and tissues, and the patient may demonstrate a degree of emaciation seldom seen in any other disease. The central nervous system shows microscopic but no gross changes, and 40% of the patients suffer mild or severe mental disturbances. From 5% to 10% of all patients become insane. When the triad of skin eruption, gastrointestinal disturbance, and mental symptoms—that is, the three *d*'s of *d*ermatitis, *d*iarrhea, and *d*ementia—is present, the diagnosis of pellagra is easy.

**Beriberi.** Beriberi is a polyneuritis caused by a diet deficient in vitamin $B_1$ (thiamine hydrochloride). It is characterized by disturbances in sensation and motion, dropsy, and involvement of the heart. It is seen most often in countries in which the national diet consists chiefly of highly polished rice or other grains. The polishings or outer layers of the grain contain sufficient vitamin $B_1$ to prevent the disease. Beriberi occurs in two forms: *wet,* characterized by generalized edema, and *dry,* characterized by various muscular palsies. A few cases of beriberi show early and serious involvement of the heart; these may cause sudden death from acute heart failure. The clinical findings are those of neuritis or locomotor ataxia. Atrophy, degeneration of the nerves, enlargement of the right side of the heart, anasarca, and effusions in various cavities are the pathologic findings.

**Scurvy.** Scurvy is a disease caused by lack of vitamin C (ascorbic acid) brought about by the exclusion of fresh fruit or vegetables from the diet. Until modern times scurvy broke out among sailors on every long sea voyage, and in war more soldiers died from scurvy than from wounds. Since the antiscorbutic action of fresh foods, especially lemons and oranges, has become generally understood, scurvy is much less important than it was in the past. Scurvy begins with weakness, anemia, and general signs of ill health. Prominent findings are sponginess, swelling, and bleeding of the gums and capillary hemorrhages in other parts of the body, particularly the nose and kidneys. The breath becomes very foul, the teeth loosen and fall out, and the legs become swollen and so painful that the patient is incapacitated. Patients with scurvy are very susceptible to secondary infections, especially pneumonia. *Infantile scurvy (Barlow's disease)* affects children between 6 and 12 months of age. The child does not progress satisfactorily, and the appetite is poor. This is the most frequent form of scurvy.

## Other deficiencies

There are deficiency states of note other than those related to vitamins. Among them are deficiencies of protein and certain minerals, notably calcium, iodine, potassium, and iron. As with vitamin lack, the deficiency state is usually very nicely and directly relieved by administration of the specific element involved.

**Protein.** One of the consequences of starvation or subsistence on an inadequate, low-calorie diet is the development of protein deficiency. The severe state of protein-calorie malnutrition is *marasmus.* In present day Africa where protein-calorie nutrition is a serious problem, marasmus in children is correlated with the decline of breast feeding, which is a result of influences from the Western world and its "bottle feeding culture."

Pathologically, depletion of the body protein is associated with gross loss of weight and extensive loss of tissue because of atrophy, edema, and reduction of the body's lymphoid tissue. The depletion of body protein in marasmatic African children is a kind of self-cannibalism. Physiologically, depletion of body proteins adversely affects the many processes necessary for the growth, maintenance, and reproduction of the individual. Hormones, antibodies, and enzymes for the myriads of biochemical processes within cells are protein. Small wonder that without this class of chemical foodstuffs in adequate supply, the complexity of life would not exist.

Malnutrition is one of the leading health problems in the world today. (Fig. 43-2). It is said that two thirds of mankind suffers from frank hunger and starvation, protein malnutrition, or acute deficiencies of vitamins and essential elements such as iodine and iron.

*Kwashiorkor** is a special kind of protein deficiency disease seen in infants in certain tropical and semitropical areas of the world. The name tells the pathogenesis of the disorder—it is a disease of the deposed baby when the next one is born. When the baby is weaned, it is fed a maize diet of little food value. A child with kwashiorkor is very sick and edematous, with a kind of skin rash. The hair may be depigmented; in black races it assumes a reddish color. The notable pathologic finding is a fatty liver.

**Calcium.** In the human body calcium has a rather even distribution, being found in the teeth and bones, in soft tissues, and in the plasma. It is freely available in a diet containing milk, milk products, eggs, green vegetables, and nuts. The daily requirement for an average adult is 0.4 to 1 gm.; more is needed by a pregnant woman or a growing child. Physiologically calcium helps to regulate the heartbeat, enters into the formation of teeth and bones, and plays an important role in coagulation of the blood. Its metabolism is closely related to that of vitamin D and phosphorus and is regulated by the parathyroid glands (p. 600).

**Iron.** Iron is an essential component of hemoglobin. Its presence within cells is necessary to metabolic activity, since it is an important constituent of certain intracellular enzymes. The daily requirement of iron for an adult male is 10 mg.; for an adult female, 12 mg. More is required by pregnant women and growing children. Foods containing iron are red

*Kwashiorkor is a Ghana word for "deposed child disease."

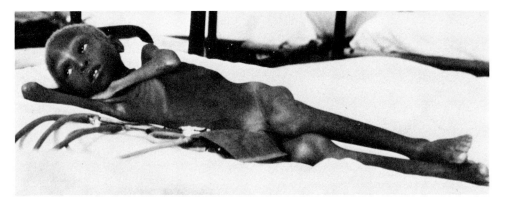

**Fig. 43-2.** Severe malnutrition in Biafran refugee child. (Courtesy Drs. Carol and Robert Master; from Silver, G. A.: Hosp. Tribune **8:**1, Oct. 14, 1974.)

meats, egg yolk, dried fruits, and green vegetables. The most dramatic consequence of iron deficiency is the development of an anemia that may be quite severe (p. 542). This may result from extensive hemorrhage or an inadequate diet. An iron-deficiency anemia is especially prone to occur in infants and very young children who persist in drinking milk to the exclusion of all other foods. (Milk is extremely poor in iron content.) Such infants appear well fed and apparently contented, but they are as pale and white as the milk that they drink. Supplying iron to the anemic individual elicits a marked response, and within a relatively short period of time the anemia is relieved.

**Potassium.** Potassium is found mostly inside cells in the body and is very necessary to vital metabolic functions. It is essential for muscular activity, including that of the heart. A deficiency of potassium is sometimes seen with the administration of steroid hormones (ACTH and the cortisone compounds), with severe states of dehydration in infants and young children, and in the clinical condition known as *familial periodic paralysis*. This is a disease characterized by recurring attacks of paralysis; potassium prevents or relieves such attacks.

**Iodine.** Iodine deficiency is closely associated with the thyroid gland (p. 598).

# Questions for review

1 Define vitamin. Give four characteristics of vitamins.
2 Briefly discuss four diseases caused by a vitamin deficiency.
3 Name four members of the vitamin B complex and tell what each prevents.
4 Briefly discuss vitamin K.
5 What is the other name for adult rickets? For infantile scurvy?
6 What deficiency disease was once associated with long sea voyages? Why?
7 Why does beriberi occur frequently in Asiatic nations?
8 Give three findings characteristic of pellagra. Of scurvy. Of rickets.
9 What is familial periodic paralysis? How is it treated?
10 Describe milk anemia in infants.
11 What is the daily requirement of calcium? Of iron?

**REFERENCES** (Chapters 42 and 43)

Altschule, M. D.: Vitamin C deficiency, Med. Sci. **16:**63, July, 1965.
Arnold, J. D., and others: Public attitudes and the diagnosis of death, J.A.M.A. **206:**1949, 1968.
Bajusz, E., and Jasmin, G., editors: Nutritional pathobiology, White Plains, N.Y., 1972, Albert J. Phiebig.
Bing, F. C.: Prevention of malnutrition, J. Am. Med. Wom. Assoc. **29:**14, 1974.

Black, M. M., and Wagner, B. M.: Dynamic pathology—structural and functional mechanisms of disease, St. Louis, 1964, The C. V. Mosby Co.
Chisolm, J. J., Jr.: The continuing hazard of lead poisoning, Hosp. Pract. **8:**127, Nov., 1973.
Chizea, D. O.: Malnutrition and infection, malaria, cholera and influenza in Africa, J. Am. Med. Wom. Assoc. **29:** 499, 1974.
Committee on Iron Deficiency: Iron deficiency in the United States, J.A.M.A. **203:**407, 1968.
Daphne, A. R.: A plague of corn: the social history of pellagra, Ithaca, N.Y., 1973, Cornell University Press.
Etheridge, E. W.: The butterfly caste—a social history of pellagra in the South, Westport, Conn., 1972, Greenwood Press, Inc.
Ford, J. A.: Asian rickets and osteomalacia, Nurs. Times **70:**49, Jan. 10, 1974.
Goldstein, S.: Biological aging, an essentially normal process, J.A.M.A. **230:**1651, 1974.
Hammar, S. L.: Obesity and the pediatrician, Am. J. Dis. Child. **125:**787, 1973.
Hankin, L., and others: Lead in pet foods and processed organ meats, J.A.M.A. **231:**484, 1975.
Kallen, D. J.: Nutrition and society, J.A.M.A. **215:**94, 1971.
Kolata, G. B.: Vitamin D.: investigations of a new steroid hormone, Science **187:**635, 1975.
Louria, D. B., and others: The human toxicity of certain trace elements, Ann. Intern. Med. **76:**307, 1972.
Martin, H.: The mad hatter visits Alice's restaurant, Today's Health, **48:**39, Oct., 1970.
Marx, J. L.: Aging research. 1. Cellular theories of senescence, Science **186:**1105, 1974.
Maugh, T. H., II: Trace elements: a growing appreciation of their effects on man, Science **181:**253, 1973.
McCarty, D. J., Jr.: Editorial: Mechanisms of the crystal deposition diseases—gout and pseudogout, Ann. Intern. Med. **78:**767, 1973.
Mennear, J. H.: Vitamins: too much of a good thing? RN **36:** 55, Oct., 1973.
Mountcastle, V. B., editor: Medical physiology, ed. 13, St. Louis, 1974, The C. V. Mosby Co.
Palmisano, P.: Vitamin D: a reawakening, J.A.M.A. **224:** 1526, 1973.
Pratt, J. M.: Inorganic chemistry of vitamin $B_{12}$, New York, 1972, Academic Press, Inc.
Sandstead, H. H.: Zinc, a metal to grow on, Nutr. Today **3:**12, March, 1968.
Schultz, D.: The verdict on vitamins, Today's Health **52:**54, Jan, 1974.
Snively, W. D., Jr.: The tiny giants, Bull. Pathol. **8:**304, 1967.
Stare, F. J., and McWilliams, M.: Living nutrition, New York, 1973, John Wiley & Sons, Inc.
Vaisrub, S.: Cellular senescence (editorial), J.A.M.A. **221:** 913, 1972.
Weinberg, E. D.: Iron and susceptibility to infectious disease, Science **184:**952, 1974.

# CHAPTER 44

# Inflammation

## General considerations

Inflammation is the sum of the reactions in the body incited by an injury. Within itself, inflammation is not a pathologic condition, but rather an exaggeration of physiologic processes set in motion by an irritant. The initial purpose of inflammation is to destroy the irritating and injurious agent and to remove it and its related by-products from the body. If this is not possible, the inflammatory process serves to limit the extension of the causative agent and its effects through the body. Finally, inflammation is the mechanism for the repair or replacement of tissues damaged or destroyed by the offending agent.

The inflammatory process consists of three parts: (1) localized vascular and cellular responses at the site of injury, (2) general body reactions (fever, leukocytosis, formation of antibodies), and (3) events designed to repair the injury done and restore the part to normal. Reparative processes are so intimately associated with inflammation that authorities consider them to be a definite part of it. Reparative processes come into play almost with the beginning of the inflammatory reaction.

**Causes.** The injury in inflammation may be produced by a great number of agents, either living or nonliving. Inflammation produced by a living agent is called *infection*. The most important living agents are bacteria. Also important, however, are viruses, rickettsias, fungi, protozoan parasites, metazoan parasites, insects, and higher plants and animals.

The nonliving inflammatory agents may be classified as (1) physical (mechanical agents of trauma such as knives, guns, blunt-edged and sharp-edged weapons; extremes of heat and cold; electricity; forms of radiant energy such as x rays, radium, ultraviolet light), (2) chemical (strong acids, alkalies, irritating gases, cauterizing chemicals), and (3) immunologic (consequent to the antigen-antibody reaction). Inflammation produced by the antigen-antibody reaction is a special category accompanying allergic and autoimmune states. Inflammation resulting from the injury to cells when the antigen-antibody reaction

occurs is responsible for the signs and symptoms of disease.

Agents causing inflammation are diverse, but basic pathogenetic mechanisms are essentially the same. The common denominator seems to be injury to body cells, with death required of a baseline number, for dying cells release at the inflammatory site certain chemical substances called *mediators*. Although the pathogenesis of inflammation is as yet incompletely understood, it can be shown experimentally that mediators do trigger key vascular and cellular components of the reaction proper. Some of the ones best studied include histamine; serotonin; the polypeptides leukotaxine, bradykinin, and kallidin; and the proteases plasmin, kallikrein, and globulin permeability factor. Mediators not only figure in local responses, but if they enter the bloodstream, they also induce certain systemic reactions.

**Local changes.** After an irritant has gained access to a tissue and injured some of the cells, the vascular response is triggered. There is a brief transient period of vasoconstriction, after which the small vessels and capillaries dilate and become filled with blood as the speed of the blood current increases. The increased velocity of blood that occurs with the dilatation of the small vessels results from a more direct transmission of arterial pressure to these vessels. The current of blood then slows because of an increased viscosity of the blood and swelling of the endothelial cells lining the small vessels. At about this time, the walls of the vessels have begun to leak the cellular and liquid constituents of the blood.

When the blood is flowing normally, the red cells and leukocytes travel along in an axial stream surrounded by a zone of plasma, but when the current slows, the leukocytes fall out peripherally into the plasma zone and adhere to the vessel wall. By their ameboid activity the polymorphonuclear neutrophilic leukocytes pass between the poorly cemented endothelial cells to initiate the cellular response. Once outside the vessel, they travel in the tissue spaces toward the injurious agent. Red blood cells, platelets, and plasma also escape from the vessels. One of the plasma proteins, fibrinogen, precipitates from the plasma to form fibrin. An *inflammatory exudate* soon surrounds the irritant agent. It is formed by the accumulation of cells and fluid from the lumen of blood vessels of the injured area, and each component plays its own specific part in the ensuing battle. The polymorphonuclear neutrophils remove bacteria, cellular debris, and solid particles by phagocytosis. The plasma (known as serum after fibrin has formed) brings antibodies to the scene, dilutes toxins that microbes produce, and floats away particles of debris. Wandering reticuloendothelial cells attracted to the site and certain leukocytes other than polymorphonuclear cells clear the ground for repair; fibrin forms a restraining wall around bacteria and acts as a framework for the repair of the destroyed tissues.

At the beginning of the inflammatory reaction the flow of lymph away from the site of inflammation is increased but is later decreased. The lymph vessels may bear microbes or other inflammatory agents to the regional lymph nodes, where they set up inflammatory reactions. The layman often refers to these swollen lymph nodes as kernels.

A *localized* inflammation is one that is restricted to a small area. A *generalized* inflammation is more widely distributed in the body.

**Timing in inflammation.** As to duration, inflammation may be classified as acute, subacute, or chronic. An *acute* inflammation lasts for only a few days to a few weeks. A *chronic* inflammation lasts for many months to many years, indicating that the causative agent is able to persist partly unchecked by the body for an indefinite period of time. A *subacute* inflammation is intermediate between the two forms, being a few weeks to a few months in duration. An acute inflammation may become chronic, or an inflammation may be chronic from the beginning.

The polymorphonuclear neutrophilic leukocyte is the characteristic cell of the exudate in acute inflammation, whereas in chronic inflammation the cells of the exudate are chiefly lymphocytes and plasma cells, with little fluid and no fibrin associated. Proliferation of the connective tissue cells in the vicinity of the inflammatory process is a prominent feature of chronic inflammation, whereas it is a negligible feature in acute inflammation. The exudate of subacute inflammations is intermediate in character between acute and chronic.

**Kinds of exudates.** The series of vascular changes is designed so that an inflammatory exudate is formed as quickly as possible. The composition of an exudate may vary. Depending on the constituent that predominates, inflammatory exudates may be classified as serous, fibrinous, purulent, catarrhal, pseudomem-

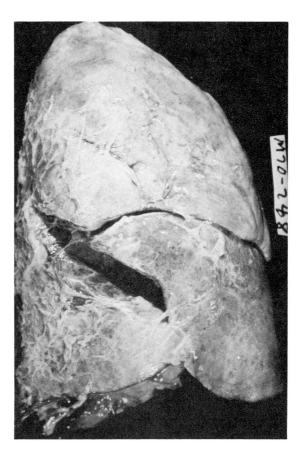

**Fig. 44-1.** Fibrinous exudate (fibrinous pleuritis) on outer pleural surface of right lung (three lobes). Note adhesions of fibrin between lobes.

branous, or hemorrhagic (sanguineous). If two components of the exudate are prominent, the inflammatory exudate is so designated (examples: serofibrinous, fibrinopurulent).

A *serous* exudate is one composed chiefly of the liquid portion (serum) of the blood, with few cells and little fibrin. *Fibrinous* exudates are characterized by the presence of a large amount of fibrin. They occur most frequently on the serous surfaces of body cavities (pleural, peritoneal, pericardial) and often lead to permanent fibrous adhesions, since fibrin once deposited in such a serous cavity is poorly reabsorbed by the body (Fig. 44-1). A *purulent* exudate is one composed chiefly of polymorphonuclear neutrophilic leukocytes (pus cells). Purulent exudates are most often caused by pyogenic organisms (streptococci, staphylococci, pneumococci, meningococci, and gonococci). A *hemorrhagic* exudate contains many red blood cells (Fig. 44-2). When there is necrosis of an epithelium, when fibrin is deposited on the epithelial

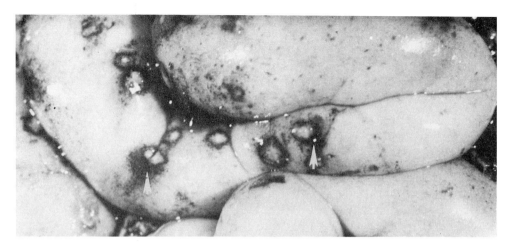

**Fig. 44-2.** Acute hemorrhagic and necrotizing inflammation from *Pseudomonas* enteritis complicating burn injury. Focal dark areas (arrows) represent hemorrhagic exudate encircling small infarcts.

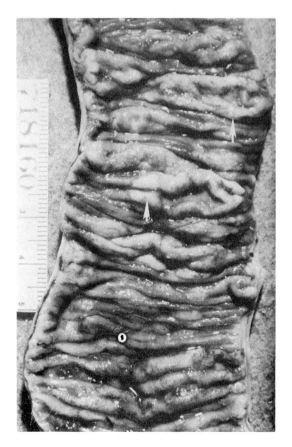

**Fig. 44-3.** Acute pseudomembranous enteritis. Mucosal folds of intestine swollen and overlain with pseudomembranous exudate (arrows).

surface, and when many leukocytes, dead epithelial cells, and bacteria are enmeshed in the fibrin threads, the exudate is described as *pseudomembranous* (Fig. 44-3). A good example of this is the pseudomembrane of diphtheria, which usually forms in the throat. Inflammations of mucous surfaces accompanied by a great outpouring of mucus, as in a cold, are spoken of as *catarrhal* inflammations. (The microbe causing an infection plays an important part in determining the nature of the exudate.)

The inflammatory exudates described as being serous, fibrinous, purulent, and hemorrhagic are associated with acute inflammations, the exudate being better defined in acute than in chronic inflammations. A chronic inflammation may be associated with pus formation, in which case it is described as a chronic *suppurative* process. The terms *productive* and *fibrous* in connection with chronic inflammations emphasize the proliferation of connective tissue cells, an unsuccessful attempt on the part of the body to resolve and heal.

**Signs.** From ancient times we have known the cardinal signs of inflammation: redness *(rubor)*, heat *(calor)*, pain *(dolor)*, swelling *(tumor)*, and *loss of function*. *Swelling* of the inflamed area is caused chiefly by the presence of the inflammatory exudate and, to a less extent, the increased amount of blood. *Heat* results from the increase in amount of blood in the part and its increased rate of flow. *Pain* is caused by pressure and the action of toxic substances on sensory nerve endings. The more solid and inelastic the tissue, the more severe will be the pain. Anyone who has had a severe toothache will readily agree with this statement. The throbbing quality that the pain may have results from the increased pressure transferred from the blood vessels with each heartbeat to the nerve endings at the site of the inflammatory exudate. *Disturbance of function* may be caused by pain, interference with nerve supply, limitation of movement because of the inflammatory exudate, and destruction of tissue.

**Outcome.** In a previous paragraph, we left an irritant surrounded by the inflammatory exudate. What happens subsequently in the inflamed tissue depends on whether the protective powers of the exudate prevail against the destructive agent. If the exudate quickly overcomes the injurious agent and too much tissue has not been destroyed, the rate of blood flow returns to normal, the caliber of the vessels is restored to normal, the fluid of the exudate is absorbed, and the fibrin, red blood cells, and dead tissue cells are removed by leukocytes entering the lymph stream. The area has returned to its natural state. This type of repair is known as *resolution.*

If the injurious agent gains the upper hand, there is death of the tissue, with or without suppuration (pus formation).* Suppuration, which means a measurable degree of tissue necrosis, contributes to the progress of the injurious agent. It may gain access to the lymphatics or bloodstream and spread to distant parts of the body. Fortunately, in the average case the defensive forces of the body eventually take over, and healing follows.

**Suppuration (pus formation).** The suppurative focus consists initially of a central mass of dead tissue cells and dead leukocytes surrounded by a zone of active leukocytes, wandering cells, and proliferating connective tissue. The surrounding leukocytes and wandering cells attempt to separate the dead cells from the living; the dead tissue cells liberate enzymes, as do leukocytes, that liquefy dead tissue cells. Because of the action of these enzymes the inflammatory focus undergoes liquefaction. The liquefied material is known as *pus,* and the chief cell of pus is the polymorphonuclear neutrophilic leukocyte. In addition to leukocytes, dead tissue cells, and red blood cells, bacteria are present in pyogenic infections. The evacuation of pus is beneficial because it releases tension and removes dead cells and inactivated liquid portions of the exudate, thus making room for new and active tissue that the vascular system is ready to supply.

When neither the injurious agent nor the bodily defenses can quite completely gain the ascendency, then what started out as an acute inflammation merges into one that is chronic. For instance, in the preceding paragraph the formation of pus in a given area and the resolution of the suppurative pro-

cess were discussed. If, however, there is no provision for release of the pus or if the agent can persist in causing pus to form, then a chronic suppurative focus has been set up. Pus formation can be progressive but still effectively limited by the body mechanisms responsible for the proliferation of a connective tissue wall and barrier about the focus. Such a lesion is simultaneously characterized by progressive destruction and by productive reactions that are attempts at healing. A peculiar kind of balance has been struck, and in the case of certain chronic inflammations this state of affairs may persist for many years.

**Inflammatory lesions.** An *abscess* is a circumscribed collection of pus surrounded by a wall of inflammatory tissue. If an abscess is located near the surface, the presence of pus is indicated by a yellow or green area on the surface near the center. As abscesses enlarge, they attempt to open onto a surface or into a cavity by extending (pointing) in the line of least resistance. In this way they may travel great distances, such as along muscle sheaths. Abscesses may reach the surface by the formation of narrow tracts known as *sinuses.* Sinuses become lined with granulation tissue but do not heal until the area which they drain has healed. A *phlegmon* (or *cellulitis*) is a diffuse, noncircumscribed, inflammatory infiltration of the tissues that spreads along fasciae and in spaces between muscles.

*Boils* or *furuncles* are abscesses located in the deeper layers of the skin and the subcutaneous tissue. The condition of generalized boils is known as *furunculosis.* Boils and furuncles often occur in poorly nourished persons, and they frequently complicate diabetes. A *carbuncle* consists of several communicating boils draining through separate openings and is often located deep in the subcutaneous tissues of the neck.

An *ulcer* is a circumscribed area of necrosis of the epithelium of the skin or mucous membrane that is often, but not always, caused by infection. A tuberculous ulcer has thin undermined edges; a syphilitic ulcer has a punched-out appearance. A serpiginous ulcer is one that heals in one portion and spreads in another. An indolent ulcer has a dry appearance and exhibits little tendency to heal.

A *granulomatous* inflammation is characterized by the formation of *granulomas.* These are tiny nodules formed by an ovoid arrangement of mononuclear macrophages, derivative cells of the reticuloendothelial system. Granulomas are usually associated with a proliferation of fibrous connective tissue cells that wall off the focus from the surrounding tissues. Granulomatous inflammation is chronic. The most characteristic granulomas are found in tuberculosis, but granulomas also are associated with other diseases such as syphilis, leprosy, and certain fungous

---

*In times before antiseptic surgery, pus formation ("laudable pus") was considered a normal part of wound healing.

diseases. The granuloma of tuberculosis is the *tubercle;* of syphilis, the *gumma;* of leprosy, the *leproma.*

**Repair.** When the injurious agent has been overcome and dead tissue cells, dead leukocytes, and other casualties are being removed from the scene, reparative processes, though active before, assume the place of greatest prominence. If the walls of the injured area are not too far apart, the gap is filled in with elements of the exudate, chiefly plasma and interlacing strands of fibrin. Small capillaries grow into the fibrin, become filled with blood, and form a network between the walls. The connective tissue of the walls proliferates and forms young cells known as fibroblasts that grow into and completely replace the framework of fibrin, which is absorbed. Because of the reddish granular appearance, this youthful tissue, composed of capillaries and fibroblasts, is known as *granulation tissue.** This method of repair is known as *primary union.*

If the wound is so large that the gap cannot be filled with exudate, the capillaries grow into the exudate formed on the sides and bottom of the wound. Failing to find anchorage beyond the surface of the exudate, the capillaries form branches that join similar branches from other capillaries to form arc-like structures extending from capillary to capillary. The arcs are filled with blood. Fibroblasts lay down fibrous tissue as usual, and the exudate is converted into granulation tissue. The layers of granulation grow inward and upward until they fuse. This is known as *secondary union* and is most common in wounds complicated by bacterial infection. When a certain point is reached in the healing of surface wounds by either primary or secondary union, the epithelium at the edges of the wound proliferates and covers over the gap. If a scab forms in the early part of the healing process, it should not be removed, since it protects the underlying epithelium.

Regardless of location or type of healing, there is a time when the fibroblasts contract, the capillaries are absorbed, and a white, bloodless glistening scar (cicatrix) remains. Scars do not contain hair follicles, sweat glands, sebaceous glands, or sensory nerve endings.

**Complications of healing.** There are two unfavorable conditions complicating the healing process: (1) the formation of permanent fibrous adhesions and

---

*Granulation tissue is a very delicate tissue, and it may be destroyed or its purpose defeated by vigorous cleaning, strong antiseptics, or frequent dressings. Overtreatment, infection, or any unhealthy condition of the tissue may stimulate the granulation tissue to such activity that it overfills the wound and protrudes beyond the surface as exuberant granulations or proud flesh.

(2) the contraction of scars. Adhesions occur where two surfaces are in contact, and as a result of the healing process the fibrinous deposits connecting them become replaced by the more dense fibrous tissue. This occurs most often in the pleural cavity when the visceral and parietal pleura become adherent (pleurisy with adhesions), in the pericardial cavity when the epicardium and pericardium become adherent (pericardial adhesions), and in the abdominal cavity when the omentum and coverings of the viscera adhere in many different ways. Abdominal adhesions may lead to vague or distinct symptoms of discomfort, or in extreme cases they may cause intestinal obstruction.

Contraction of a scar may limit the functions of an organ, cause stricture, and produce marked disfigurement. In some cases when a scar is kept tense, it stretches. This is one of the causes of postoperative hernia.

**Regeneration.** The complete restoration of destroyed tissue to normal depends on a number of factors, the most important of which is the ability of the tissue to regenerate, that is, to reproduce tissue of its exact kind. The regeneration of cells destroyed by the natural wear and tear of life is known as *physiologic regeneration;* the regeneration of tissues destroyed by disease or injury is *pathologic regeneration* (Fig. 44-4). When tissues that have little or no regenerative capacity are destroyed, the defect is repaired by proliferation of nature's omnipresent repair material—connective tissue. The same kind of repair usually takes place when there is *extensive* destruction of tissue having well-developed regenerative capacity. Naturally, in a large wound several different kinds of tissues having different powers of regeneration are involved.

The powers of regeneration, as a rule, are more highly developed in the lower forms of life—for example, if an earthworm is severed, the result is two earthworms; when a newt loses a leg, another leg grows in its place.

In man connective tissue and capillary endothelium, which are the body's repair tissues, regenerate with extreme ease. Next to these, surface epithelium possesses the greatest regenerative capacity. This applies not only to the epithelium covering the surface of the body but also to that covering mucous membranes such as the lining of the gastrointestinal, respiratory, urinary, and genital tracts. Accessory skin structures (hair follicles, sweat glands, sebaceous glands) do not regenerate when completely destroyed. This is why scars are dry and hairless. If remnants of these structures remain, regeneration will take place. Periosteum and bone regenerate well, else healing of fractures would be impossible.

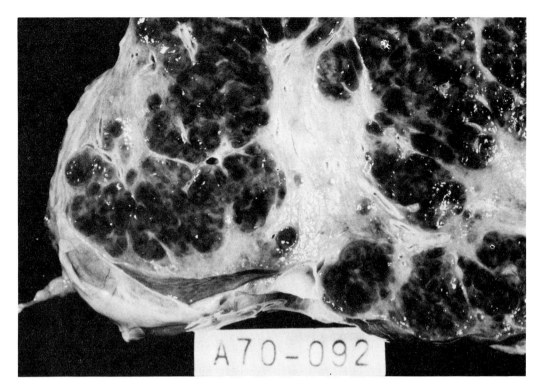

**Fig. 44-4.** Regeneration of liver after injury (postnecrotic cirrhosis, p. 577). Note many varying-sized nodules (darker) of liver tissue, with broad bands of whitish, fibrous scar tissue interspersed on sectioned surface. Well-defined liver cells are seen in nodules microscopically but without normal anatomic connections to blood vessels and collecting ducts.

Muscle regenerates poorly, and wounds of muscle are usually repaired by the formation of scar tissue. Nerve cells never regenerate when destroyed, but their processes may regenerate, provided that the cell body has not been injured. Regeneration is more active in childhood than in old age.

**Terminology of inflammation.** The following listings give the name of the inflammatory process in a given anatomic area. Usually the suffix *itis* is added to the anatomic name.

**Nervous system**

Encephalitis (brain)
Encephalomyelitis
Myelitis (spinal cord)
Meningitis

Meningoencephalitis
Poliomyelitis
Neuritis

**Respiratory system**

Rhinitis (nose)
Nasopharyngitis
Pharyngitis
Sinusitis
Tonsillitis
Laryngitis

Adenoiditis
Tracheitis
Tracheobronchitis
Bronchitis
Bronchiolitis
Pneumonitis

Pneumonia
Pleuritis

Mediastinitis

**Digestive system**

Stomatitis (mouth)
Glossitis (tongue)
Cheilitis (lips)
Gingivitis (gums)
Periodontitis (tissues
   about tooth)
Sialitis (salivary gland
   or duct)
Sialadenitis
   (salivary gland)
Sialodochitis
   (salivary ducts)
Sialoductilitis
Esophagitis
Gastritis

Duodenitis
Jejunitis
Enteritis
Colitis
Enterocolitis
Proctitis (rectum)
Peritonitis
Pancreatitis
Hepatitis
Cholecystitis
Choledochitis
   (common duct)
Appendicitis
Diverticulitis
   (diverticulum)

**Skin and skeletomuscular system**

Dermatitis (skin)
Folliculitis
Hidradenitis (sweat gland)

Panniculitis (subcutaneous
   tissue)
Fasciitis (fascia)

### Skin and skeletomuscular system—cont'd

Myositis
Dermatomyositis
Osteitis (bone)
Osteomyelitis (bone and
    bone marrow)
Periostitis (periosteum)
Arthritis

Synovitis (joint lining)
Tenosynovitis
    (tendon sheath)
Chondritis (cartilage)
Spondylitis (vertebrae)
Bursitis

### Genitourinary system

Nephritis (kidney)
Pyelitis (kidney pelvis)
Pyelonephritis
Glomerulonephritis
Ureteritis
Papillitis (papillae
    of kidney)
Cystitis (urinary bladder)
Urethritis
Orchitis (testis)
Epididymitis
Balanitis (glans penis)
Seminal vesiculitis
Prostatitis

Oophoritis
Salpingitis (fallopian tube)
Endometritis
    (lining of uterus)
Perimetritis
Myometritis
    (uterine muscle)
Endocervicitis
Cervicitis
Vaginitis
Mastitis
Amnionitis
Perioophoritis

### Endocrine system

Thyroiditis

### Vascular (blood and lymphatic) system

Carditis (heart)
Pericarditis
Epicarditis
Myocarditis
Endocarditis (valves
    of heart)
Arteritis
Aortitis
Phlebitis (veins)

Thrombophlebitis
Angiitis
Lymphangitis
Endarteritis
Polyarteritis
Lymphadenitis
    (lymph node)
Splenitis
Periarteritis

### Special sense organs

Otitis (ear)
Mastoiditis
Conjunctivitis
Retinitis (retina)
Iridocyclitis (iris and
    ciliary body of eye)
Iritis
Ophthalmitis (eye)

Panophthalmitis
Endophthalmitis
Scleritis
Episcleritis
Choroiditis (choroid)
Chorioretinitis
Uveitis (uveal tract of eye)

## Infection

An infectious disease represents a combat between two living forces—the organism *invading* and
the organism *invaded*. Fig. 44-5 summarizes the sequence of inflammatory events in an infection. Since
variability is a characteristic of living organisms, the

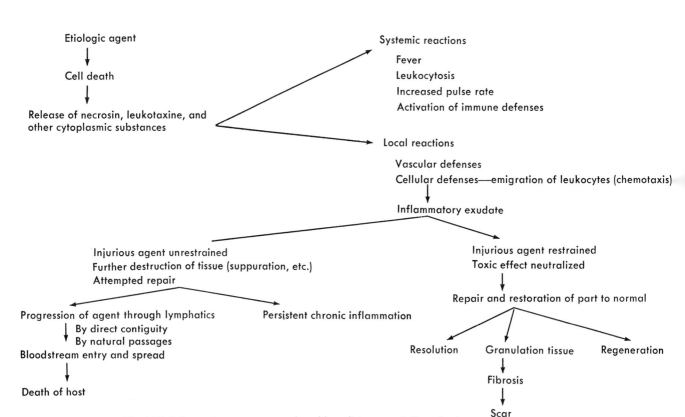

**Fig. 44-5.** Inflammatory process produced by a living agent, flow chart.

**Table 44-1**
Pathology of infectious diseases—the hallmark of some important infectious agents

| MICROORGANISM | PATHOGENICITY—TYPE LESION | DISEASE(S) |
| --- | --- | --- |
| **Bacteria** | | |
| *Staphylococcus* | Abscess (predilection for skin, also systemic) | Variety (p. 177) |
| *Streptococcus* | Spreading inflammation—cellulitis | Scarlet fever, puerperal sepsis, erysipelas |
| Pneumococcus | Exudate rich in fibrin | Lobar pneumonia, bronchopneumonia |
| Gonococcus | Catarrhal inflammation | Gonorrhea |
| Meningococcus | Purulent inflammation | Epidemic meningitis |
| Diphtheria bacillus | Pseudomembrane; no invasion at superficial site; toxemia from exotoxin | Diphtheria |
| Typhoid bacillus | Granulomatous inflammation | Typhoid fever |
| *Shigella* | Pseudomembrane—intestine | Bacillary dysentery |
| Tubercle bacillus | Granuloma—tubercle | Tuberculosis |
| Lepra bacillus | Granuloma; lepra cells | Leprosy |
| *Pseudomonas* species | Necrotizing inflammation | Variety (p. 258) |
| Spirochete of syphilis | Granuloma—gumma; fibrosis and vascular changes | Syphilis |
| *Rickettsias* | Vasculitis in small blood vessels, widespread | Variety (p. 268) |
| **Viruses** | Intracellular parasitism, sometimes inclusion bodies; little tissue reaction | Great variety (pp. 296-321) |
| **Fungi** | | |
| Systemic fungi | Granuloma plus suppuration; presence of etiologic agent important | Great variety (pp. 327-337) |
| **Protozoa** | | |
| *Plasmodium* of malaria | Hemolysis | Malaria |

infectious diseases they produce vary considerably. This may make difficult the recognition and treatment of an infectious disease.

Agents of infectious disease are commonly linked to the area of the animal body that they injure. On the one hand there are those that single out an organ or a system. The bacillus of dysentery primarily attacks the intestinal tract, and the pneumococcus primarily attacks the lungs. In infections in which the attack is directed primarily to a single organ, a generalized intoxication from some product released by the agent can contribute to disability and even cause death. On the other hand, certain organisms can and regularly do produce infection in a variety of tissues in widespread anatomic locations, for example, the microbes of wound infections, staphylococci, streptococci, and coliforms.

**Course.** Most acute febrile infections move through the different stages listed on p. 86.

**Pathologic findings.** There are certain pathologic changes found in nearly all infectious diseases, and in addition, each infectious disease has its own peculiar pattern. Among the general changes are some degree of anemia, degenerative lesions in vital organs, hyperplasia (cellular proliferation) of spleen and lymph nodes, stimulation of adrenal cortical activity, fluid and electrolyte imbalance, and digestive and nutritional disturbances. Practically all infectious diseases are accompanied by fever, and many are accompanied by leukocytosis. When fever or leukocytosis fails to occur in an infectious disease in which both should ordinarily be present, the situation is very serious.

**Important infectious diseases.** Table 44-1 gives the pathologic patterns for certain infectious disease–producing agents. Discussions of important infectious diseases are incorporated into the chapters devoted to the consideration of the various aspects of their etiologic agents.

## Questions for review

1 Define inflammation.
2 What are the three parts of the inflammatory process?
3 Classify causes of inflammation.
4 What is the purpose of the inflammatory exudate?
5 Describe the different types of inflammatory exudates.
6 Describe the vascular changes of localized inflammation.
7 What are the cardinal signs of inflammation? What causes each?
8 What are the differences between chronic and acute inflammation?

 9 What is pus? Why is the evacuation of pus beneficial?
10 What is granulation tissue? What are its functions? What is a granuloma?
11 Differentiate primary from secondary union of wounds.
12 Explain the formation of scar tissue. Why is old scar tissue white? Why are scars hairless and dry?

13 What two tissues does nature always use in repairing wounds?
14 Define abscess, boil, pseudomembrane, furuncle, carbuncle, phlegmon, ulcer, resolution, regeneration.
15 Outline the course of an infectious disease.

**References on pp. 503 and 504.**

# CHAPTER 45

# Injuries from nonliving agents

## Physical injuries

On occasion, the physical agents to be discussed produce significant injury to the human body.

**Trauma.** Trauma is often referred to as the "neglected disease of modern society." Under the heading of trauma (mechanical injury) are included blows, crushing injuries, cutting wounds (lacerations), falls, damage produced by foreign bodies (such as bullets, Fig. 45-1), and effects of pressure. Local complications of these injuries are damage to important organs, circulatory disturbances (including hemorrhage), and infection. The systemic condition of shock is often associated with trauma.

In this country trauma is the fourth leading cause of death. In persons up to 38 years old, it is the first. Automobile accidents are the most frequent cause of serious traumatic injury seen, and more persons have been killed on American highways since the turn of the century than have been killed in combat since the Revolutionary War.

**Extremes of temperature.** Disease may result from exposure to a moderate increase in heat or cold over a considerable period of time or from a shorter exposure to a much greater increase. In the first category from exposure to cold belong frostbite and chilblains, and from exposure to excess of heat belong heat cramps, heat exhaustion, and hyperpyrexia. In the second category belong the severe and often fatal effects from freezing, burns, and scalds.

Burns may be produced by hot air, steam, hot water, fire, or light and represent injury from heat at temperatures greater than those of the normal state. There are three kinds of burns pathologically (Fig. 45-2). The *first-degree burn* in the skin is a reddened area, minimally inflamed, with no destruction of tissue. This lesion is completely reversible. The *second-degree burn* is characterized by blister formation in the epidermis of the skin. There is some necrosis of the epithelium, but with the adequate regenerative capacity of the epidermis, healing occurs; that is, the tissues return to the normal state. The *third-degree burn* is characterized by necrosis of the epidermis, dermis, and underlying tissues. Destruction is severe in its extent; the tissues may even be charred. Healing of a third-degree burn can occur only with the formation of granulation tissue and scarring. If this is extensive, the contraction of the scar tissue in time produces considerable deformity of the part. Burns are often complicated by shock, which if severe enough, may cause death within 24 hours. Causes of death in burned patients at a later period are absorption of toxic substances from the burned area, bacterial (notably, *Pseudomonas aeruginosa*) infections, and severe malnutrition.

*Heat cramps* occur after prolonged exertion in a hot environment and are known as miner's cramps, fireman's cramps, and stoker's cramps. *Heat exhaustion* is characterized by collapse without elevation of body temperature during exposure to an excessively hot environment. *Heat hyperpyrexia* (heatstroke, sunstroke, thermic fever) is a syndrome with headache, vertigo, abdominal distress, delirium, and coma accompanied by an excessively high temperature (greater than 106° F.).

**Changes in atmospheric pressure.** Our bodies are accustomed to a certain atmospheric pressure, and any appreciable departure from this pressure, either above or below, gives rise to a distinct train of symptoms and signs. Increased pressure causes disturbances in deep-sea divers and caisson workers. Manifestations do not occur so long as the increased pressure is sustained but appear when the normal pressure is restored. Then gases that have been absorbed from the blood in increased amounts by the

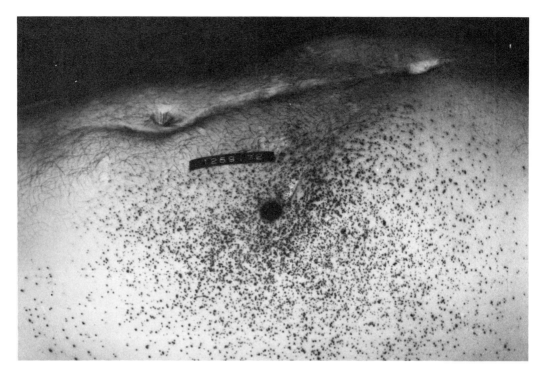

**Fig. 45-1.** Gunshot wound of abdomen. Bullet entrance wound is small and round, with abrasions about its margins; outlying areas are stippled by burned and unburned powder grains.

tissues during the period of increased pressure expand. The gaseous expansion tears the tissues and causes bleeding. The disturbances may be prevented by gradual restoration of the normal pressure. This condition is known as *decompression sickness* and is referred to by deep-sea divers and caisson workers as bends, chokes, itches, and staggers.

Among aviators, mountain climbers, or persons who are otherwise quickly transferred to an atmospheric pressure less than normal, a train of events ensues consisting of rapid respiration, weakness, dizziness, nosebleed, and vomiting. When an altitude of 35,000 feet or more is reached, the aviator suffers from decompression sickness that differs in no manner from that experienced by deep-sea divers and caisson workers. Decompression sickness at high altitude is independent of lack of oxygen.

At high altitudes—that is, above 15,000 to 20,000 feet—there is a significant decrease in the amount of oxygen available in the atmosphere. Persons so exposed may suffer severe anoxia, rapidly losing consciousness. Circulatory changes may lead to death. The people who live in mountainous areas at altitudes of from 10,000 to 15,000 feet have an increased number of red blood cells (polycythemia) to compensate for the low oxygen content of the air. More oxygen

bearers (red blood cells) are brought to the lungs to be aerated. When an altitude of more than 3 or 4 miles is reached, the oxygen content of the air is too low to be compatible with life.

Changes in the surrounding atmosphere may mean a deficiency in oxygen, as may conditions of the respiratory tract itself that obstruct the entry of air into the lungs. In drowning, water blocks the entrance of air and replaces it within the lungs. Death caused by obstruction of the flow of air through the air passages is known as *strangulation. Asphyxia* results from interference, in one way or another, with the pulmonary exchange of oxygen and carbon dioxide in the inspired air and the bloodstream.

A special form of injury related to a sudden and severe change in atmospheric pressure is *blast injury,* the most common cause of which is an explosion. Sudden changes in pressure may collapse the chest and tear or rupture the internal organs.

**Electric currents.** There is no essential difference between the results of contact with natural electric currents and the results of contact with artificial electric currents (Fig. 45-3). If death is not immediate, burns at the point of contact and shock are the usual findings. Immediate death is caused by inhibition of respiration and circulation.

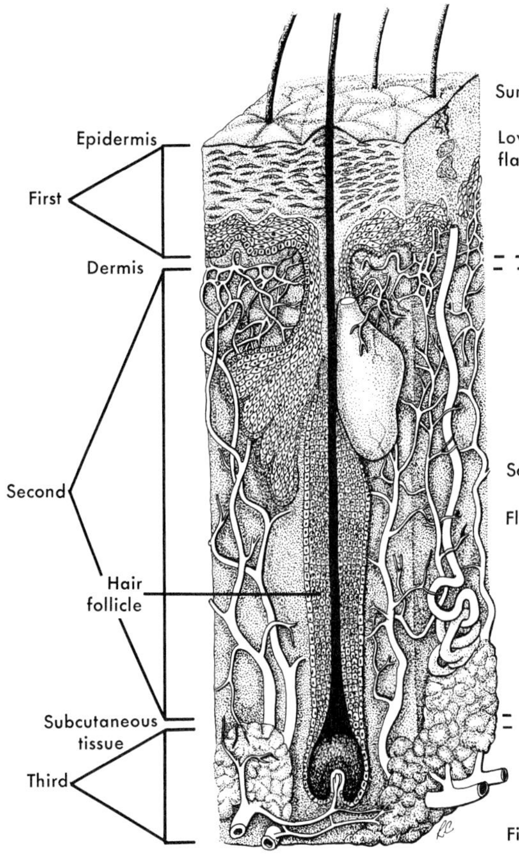

| Degree | | Nature of burn | Manifestations | Appearance of burned area | Outcome |
|---|---|---|---|---|---|
| First | Epidermis — Dermis | Sunburn  Low-intensity flash | Tingling  Hyperesthesia  Pain  Cooling relieves | Reddened  Blanches with pressure  Minimal edema | Complete recovery within days |
| Second | Dermis — Hair follicle | Scalds  Flash flame | Pain  Hyperesthesia  Sensitivity to cold | Blistered, mottled red base; weeping surface  Edema | Recovery within weeks  Scarring  Depigmentation  Infection converts to third degree |
| Third | Subcutaneous tissue | Fire | No pain  Shock  Hematuria and hemolysis of blood | Dry; pale white or charred  Skin broken with exposed fat  Edema | Grafting necessary  Eschar sloughs  Scarring  Loss of tissue and function |

**Fig. 45-2.** Burns of skin.

**Ultraviolet rays.** It must be remembered that ultraviolet light is responsible for the conversion of ergosterol in the skin to vitamin D, but long exposure to ultraviolet light may produce death of the tissue. An irritating exposure produces sunburn.

**Radiation.** We can feel heat radiating from a hot stove, and if we touch a hot object, we have the disagreeable sensation of being burned; but the kind of radiation about which we are now thinking is energy streaming from a source that we cannot feel, see, or sense in any way. At the time of contact we cannot tell that it is present or that it will injure. This energy, also called *radiant energy,* which the human senses do not detect, has been described as a stream of waves or particles thrown off from atoms whose nuclei are attempting to stabilize.

Atoms are the fundamental building blocks of all matter, living or nonliving; they are the smallest chemically reactive units to which elements can be reduced; and the nucleus of the atom is the inner core of that atom. With the development of atomic energy for military purposes and with its increasing importance in industry, radiation effects on the living human body become of the utmost concern. So-called radiation hazards are one of the major medical problems of the atomic age.

Most of what is known about the biologic effects of radiation has been learned in approximately the last two or three decades. Radiation is an important form of treatment of cancer, being used to treat cancers on the skin and deep within the body. Within Atomic Energy Commission installations there is occasionally an accidental exposure of varying severity, sometimes a fatal one. The study of the radiation effects in cancer patients, in accidentally exposed victims, and in survivors of the atomic bombing of Hiroshima and Nagasaki, together with a vast number of laboratory experiments on animals, has greatly added to our store of information concerning this form of energy and what it does to living cells and tissues.

*Ionization.* Radiation energy can injure because of its ability to penetrate to the atoms of the elements of which the cell is composed and change their structure. This kind of change is ionization. Because of ionization, exceedingly small, electrically charged particles are produced, and in the process body cells and tissues may be injured, distorted, and even destroyed. Cell nuclei are especially vulnerable. As with other injurious agents, certain factors modify the damage produced by ionizing radiation, such as the dose, penetration, and absorption of the radiant energy. There are three kinds of radiation that cause ionization (Table 45-1): (1) alpha radiation, possessing the greatest capacity to ionize but with little power to penetrate the body coverings, (2) beta radiation, more penetrating than alpha but not ionizing so strongly, and (3) gamma rays and x rays, ionizing poorly but able to penetrate deeply into the tissues of the body. Ionizing radiations may be obtained either from machines or from isotopes. X rays produced in certain high-voltage machines familiar in medical clinics and hospitals are manmade.

*Radioisotopes.* Two chemical elements, each having the same number of atoms but atoms of different weights (or mass), are *isotopes.* Isotopes behave exactly alike chemically, but there are important differences, as, for example, some are *radioactive.* This

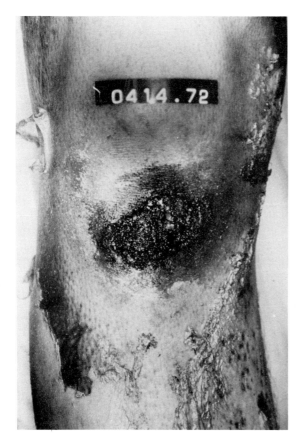

**Fig. 45-3.** Electrocution, electrical burn at contact point.

**Table 45-1**
Comparison of three forms of ionizing radiation

| NAME | SYMBOL | WHAT IT IS | PENETRATION IN AIR | PENETRATION IN TISSUE | WHAT STOPS IT |
|---|---|---|---|---|---|
| Alpha | $\alpha$ | Nucleus of helium atom | 5 cm. | 0.005 cm. (first layer of skin) | Paper; clothing |
| Beta | $\beta$ | High-speed electron | 200 cm. | 0.125 cm. ($\frac{1}{2}$ inch of soft tissue) | Paper; clothing; wood |
| Gamma | $\gamma$ | Electromagnetic wave like visible light | Thousands of meters (very penetrating) | Very penetrating; 60% of entrance dose equals exit dose (through several inches of soft tissue and bone) | Several feet of concrete or earth |

means that one form of the atom may possess an unstable nucleus and therefore be constantly discharging radiant energy. Radiation from a radioisotope is unlike that from an x-ray machine, which no longer produces radiation when the electric current is turned off. The term *half-life* is the length of time that it takes a given quantity of radioisotope to lose one-half its activity; it is a measure of the radioactivity of an isotope. A given radioactive chemical gives out a characteristic kind of radiation, and each has its own characteristic half-life. Loss of activity is *decay*. Of 1200 known isotopes, about 900 are radioactive.

Some radioisotopes are found in nature. Radioisotopes may be made in a complicated structure called a *nuclear reactor* (the atomic pile, cyclotron). This is a sort of atomic firing range into which the material to be activated is placed and then subjected to an intense bombardment, which penetrates to the nuclei of the atoms of the material.

*Nuclear medicine.* There are numerous well-established uses to which radioisotopes have been put in biology and medicine. Radioactive iodine has been the most widely used. Iodine is an important part of the thyroid hormone. Since the radioactive isotope behaves just as the normal element in the body, it is possible to trace the course of iodine in the body and its incorporation into hormone in the thyroid gland by substituting the radioactive substance for the normal one. Practically, this has proved to be an extremely valuable way of determining the function of the thyroid gland, and as a laboratory procedure it has certain advantages over the determination of the basal metabolic rate (p. 598). Other uses of radioisotopes in medicine include the use of radioactive vitamin $B_{12}$ in the diagnosis of pernicious anemia (p. 541), the use of a radioactive dye, rose bengal, to study the function of the liver, and the use of such chemicals as radioactive cobalt and radioactive gold in the treatment of certain advanced cancers. Table 45-2 gives a short listing of radioisotopes with their tissue affinities. .

**Table 45-2**
Radioisotopes related to tissues

| ISOTOPE | TISSUE AFFINITY |
|---------|-----------------|
| Iodine 131 | Thyroid gland |
| Phosphorus 32 | Bone marrow |
| Yttrium 90 | Pituitary gland |
| Carbon 14 | Total body |
| Strontium 90 | Bone |
| Iron 59 | Red blood cells |
| Lanthanum 140 | Gastrointestinal tract and liver |
| Molybdenum 99 | Kidney |

*Biologic effects.* Young actively growing cells are more susceptible to radiation than are mature cells. This is the basis of the x-ray and radium treatment of cancer, since in many instances the cancer cells are not fully mature cells. This means, too, that the growing and developing fetus in the uterus of a pregnant woman is especially liable to be damaged severely by radiation. Any cell, mature or otherwise, is peculiarly vulnerable if radiated while it is in the process of dividing. The injury to cells and tissues is basically the same regardless of the kind of radiant energy.

Cells especially susceptible to the injurious effect of radiation and said to be *radiosensitive* are lymphoid cells, bone marrow cells, lining cells of the alimentary tract, and the sex cells of the testis and ovary (Fig. 45-4). Radiation suppresses immune mechanisms in the body largely because the reticuloendothelial cells playing such an important part in these mechanisms are among the most radiosensitive tissues of the body. Cells and tissues somewhat less vulnerable but still affected are termed *radioresponsive*. These include lining cells of the skin and skin appendages, lining cells of blood vessels, salivary glands, growing bone, growing cartilage, tissues of the eye, and mature connective tissue. *Radioresistant* tissues are affected only by fairly high doses of radiation and include kidneys, liver, thyroid gland, pancreas, pituitary gland, adrenal glands, mature bone, mature cartilage, muscle, brain, and nervous tissue.

*Acute radiation sickness* follows the exposure of all the body to a sizable dose of penetrating radiation. It is seen in modified form in connection with localized radiation treatment, especially of certain cancers. As a complete disorder it is usually seen as the result of an atomic bomb explosion or of an accident in an installation that handles large quantities of radioactive material. Acute radiation sickness occurs in three phases. The initial phase, on the day of exposure, is characterized by nausea, vomiting, and weakness. The second phase, in which the person seems to be completely free of manifestations indicating any injury at all, follows; this asymptomatic phase lasts about 2 to 3 days. One of the most curious phenomena about radiant energy is this delayed or lag effect. A period of time free of any indications of the exposure is present between exposure and injury. The third phase is a severe one and relates to the damage produced by the radiation, which is primarily death of the cells in the blood-forming organs, the gastrointestinal mucous membrane, and the lymphoid tissue of the spleen and lymph nodes. The temperature rises, and there are constitutional symptoms. Because the bone marrow has been damaged, bleeding occurs into the skin and on the inside of the body. The hair falls out. The mucous membranes of the gum, mouth, throat,

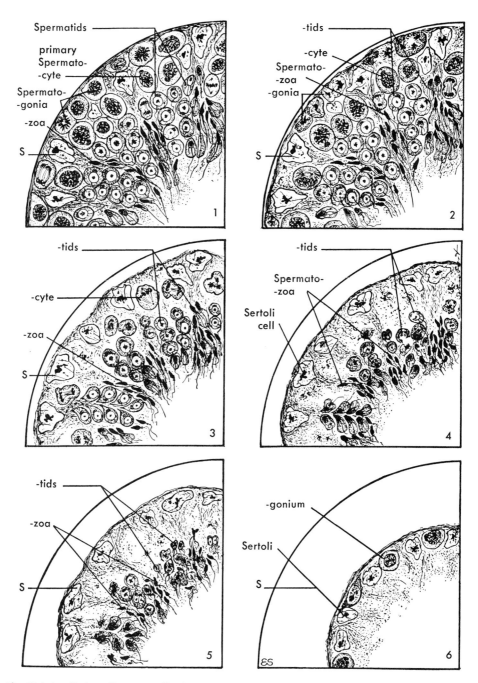

**Fig. 45-4.** Irradiation effects on cells of testis, diagrams. *1,* Normal seminal tubule, with cells in different stages of spermatogenesis as they mature from the periphery to center of tubule, for comparison with testicular tissue made at postirradiation intervals of 2 hours, *2;* 4 days, *3;* 8 days, *4;* 21 days, *5;* and 34 days, *6.* Note conspicuous loss of cells beginning at 2 hours postirradiation, *2,* and progression to almost complete depletion by 34-day interval, *6.* Abnormal mitoses are encountered as early as 2 hours, *2,* and remain in diagrams for 8 days, *3* and *4.* The more immature cells at periphery of tubule are first affected with relative sparing of more mature ones. By end of 21 days, *5,* however, more mature cells are taking abnormal shapes. (From Ackerman, L. V., and del Regato, J. A.: Cancer, ed. 4, St. Louis, 1970, The C. V. Mosby Co.)

and alimentary tract become ulcerated. The victim is vulnerable to generalized infection associated with severe anemia. Death may result from bleeding, anemia, infection, or sheer weakness.

We know much about the effects of acute exposure to radiation, but there are many unanswered questions as to the effects of long-continued exposures to radiation from various sources. There is good reason to believe that cancers may come as a late complication of prolonged exposure. Cancers of the skin were especially numerous on the hands of the early physicians who first used x rays right after they were discovered and before proper precautions were stressed. Leukemia is said to be more frequent in persons who constantly work with x rays, and it has appeared with increased frequency among the survivors of the atomic bomb explosion on Hiroshima and Nagasaki.

**Atomic bomb injury.** Atomic weapons are comparable to ordinary weapons except, of course, that they are more powerful and the explosion releases radiant energy. It is estimated that radiation is responsible for 15% to 20% of the deaths following the explosion of such a bomb. The radiation effect is both an immediate and a delayed one. The explosion may distribute radioactive dust over a widespread geographic area. This is called the *radioactive fallout*. One of the great dangers of exposure to radiation produced by an atomic bomb is that the radiation is applied to the whole body instead of to a restricted area, as it is in the treatment of cancer. For this reason a lethal dose of atomic bomb radiation may be no more than one-twentieth the dose used in the treatment of cancer. After the explosion of a hydrogen bomb radioactive dust in sufficient amount to produce death may fall over an area of 7000 square miles. Other effects of atomic bomb injury are burns and the impact or blast of the explosion.

## Other physical disturbances

**Foreign bodies.** A foreign body is a concrete object introduced into a part of the body where it would not normally be found. Foreign bodies may come from the outside (exogenous), or they may be formed within the body as a consequence of some unusual event (endogenous). The most important endogenous foreign bodies are stones, which are found in the urinary tract, biliary tract, pancreatic ducts, and respiratory tract (p. 561). Foreign bodies enter from the outside through the normal body openings or through traumatic breaks in the body coverings. Examples of exogenous foreign bodies are splinters, bullets, pieces of steel, dirt, and dust. The pathologic changes in the pneumoconioses are directly related to dusts breathed into the lungs, such as carbon, silica, asbestos, and beryllium.

What disposal the tissues will make of a foreign body depends on the size and digestibility of the particle. If it is very small, such as a particle of soot, it is taken up by phagocytic cells and carried away. If it is large, soft, and digestible, it is surrounded and digested by phagocytic cells. If it is large but not digestible, it is approached by cells that attempt to form a wall around it.

Foreign bodies obstruct, cause secondary infection, and incite granulomatous inflammation.

**Obstruction to hollow organs.** The principles are the same when obstruction occurs in an organ occupied by a central cavity as when it occurs in a solid gland with an excretory duct. The pathologic changes from obstruction are influenced by the kind, degree, and anatomic location of the anatomic obstruction and by the length of time present.

In a hollow organ or duct, obstruction is caused by stones (or other foreign bodies) in the lumen, disease or muscular paralysis of the wall, and tumors from surrounding areas that encroach on and compress the area. The effects are fourfold: (1) dilatation, (2) hypertrophy of smooth muscle, (3) infection, and (4) atrophy of secreting cells. The fluid or semifluid material usually contained within the lumen of a hollow organ collects behind the point of obstruction, distending and dilating the segment just before the obstruction. The smooth muscle of the wall hypertrophies to increase the strength of contraction in an effort to push the luminal contents past the obstructing point. If the situation is acute, the increased force of muscular contraction may produce intense cramping pain. One of the most serious consequences is infection. Pooled secretions in any obstructed passageway soon become infected. Stagnant urine in the lumen of an obstructed urinary bladder provides a good culture medium for bacteria, and the infection soon spreads to the wall to cause inflammation or a cystitis. Glandular cells of a secretory organ cannot elaborate more of their product if the material is accumulating in an obstructed outlet duct. The functioning cells soon cease their activities, and if the pressure is unrelieved, they atrophy and, in time, drop out.

Return to the normal state is closely associated with the amount of smooth muscle and elastic tissue in the wall of the involved organ. If these tissues are scant, the dilatation of the lumen may persist long after the events concerned with blockage are over. Pathologic changes following obstruction are important in many organ systems of the body, including the genitourinary tract, the alimentary tract, the respiratory tract, the biliary tract, a portion of the central

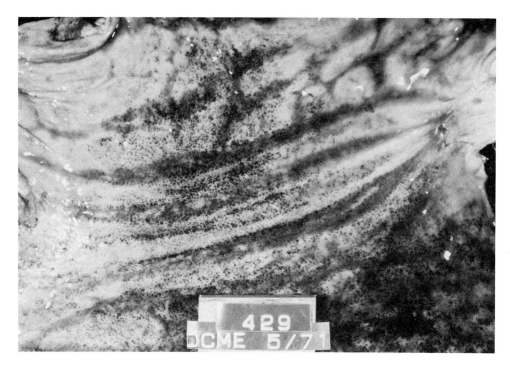

**Fig. 45-5.** Chemical gastritis. The injured mucosal surface of stomach shows many small hemorrhages.

nervous system, the salivary glands, and the circulatory system.

## Chemical injuries

Practically any chemical substance, if contacted or absorbed in large enough quantity, is capable of producing injury. A chemical harmful to the human body in fairly small amounts is spoken of as a poison.*

**General considerations.** Factors influencing the action of a chemical agent are dosage, susceptibility of the involved tissue, and nature and mode of action of the agent iself. Chemicals injurious to the human body may be classified as follows:

1. *Corrosives* destroy cells and tissues more or less immediately on direct contact. Examples are acids, alkalies, lye, phenolic compounds, and formaldehyde. The skin, lungs, and mucous membranes of the mouth, esophagus, and stomach (Fig. 45-5) are especially vulnerable.
2. *Heavy metal compounds* containing mercury, arsenic, lead, and phosphorus are selectively destructive to the internal organs.

*Lead poisoning* (usually chronic) is either an occupational hazard to adults or a disorder of environmental contamination in children. One of the main sources in the environment is lead paint peeling from houses built before 1950, since small children, especially, are prone to eat the paint chips. More than one half of patients are less than 2 years of age, and the mortality for them is high. Lead, a nonessential trace element, is largely deposited in bone (Fig. 45-6) when ingested, although it is found in brain, liver, and kidney. Its accumulation in the central nervous system leads to severe degenerative changes in brain (encephalopathy) and peripheral nerves (neuropathy). Associated with a secondary anemia is stippling of the red blood cells, a diagnostic feature for plumbism. A fingertip sample of blood can be analyzed for lead by an atomic absorption method.

3. *Gases* cause asphyxia by interfering with respiration and the intake of sufficient amounts of oxygen for life. The war gases are irritating to the skin, eyes, and lining of the respiratory tract.

*Carbon monoxide is a colorless, tasteless, odorless, and nonirritating gas* with an affinity

---

*At this point, it may be well to do away with the antidote myth, the widespread belief that there is an antidote for every known poison. In fact, there are but a few. Without specific antidotes, treatment of poisoning is mainly designed to eliminate the toxic agent before it can be absorbed.

*See also p. 472.

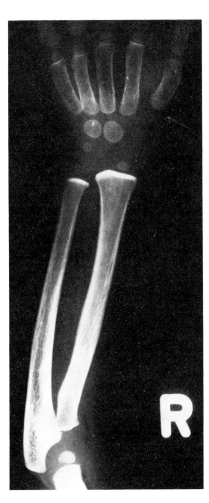

**Fig. 45-6.** "Lead line" at wrist and radiopacities produced by lead deposited in shafts of long bones near elbow. (Courtesy Dr. Jack Reynolds, University of Texas Health Sciences Center at Dallas.)

for hemoglobin 200 times that of oxygen, so that when it is inhaled, hemoglobin combines with it to form carboxyhemoglobin rather than with oxygen to form oxyhemoglobin. The pathologic changes that follow relate to the state of anoxia produced. With death in acute poisoning, blood, tissues, and organs of the body are colored a striking cherry red color. Carbon monoxide is a well-known poisonous gas for which there are numerous sources in our environment. Smokers tend to have elevated blood levels of carboxyhemoglobin.

4. *Volatile organic compounds* include alcohols, cyanides, chloroform, and well-known agents such as ether and nitrous oxide that in safe, controlled, and physiologic amounts are used for producing anesthesia during surgery. Chloroform and carbon tetrachloride are classic hepatotoxins. Methyl alcohol has an interesting affinity for the optic nerve and the cells of the retina; acute insult may be followed by atrophy of the optic nerve, with resultant blindness.

5. *Nonvolatile organic compounds,* like the group of volatile organic compounds, include several chemicals that in restricted amounts are safe valuable medical compounds to be used in treatment but that in larger or excessive amounts are dangerous to life. This is certainly true of the barbiturates and the opiates.

6. *Industrial poisons*—beryllium, silica, aniline dyes, fluorides, and DDT—represent major hazards in certain kinds of industry. Particles of silica and beryllium cause granulomas in body tissues, notably in the lungs. Aniline dyes may predispose the exposed person to the development of a malignant neoplasm.

7. *Bacterial toxins* cause diphtheria, tetanus, and botulism. In these diseases there is limited direct invasion by the bacteria themselves. In this category are included also the chemicals that produce food poisoning, such as the toxic products of staphylococci and other bacteria, and certain mushrooms.

8. *Animal venoms* from snakes, spiders, jellyfish, scorpions, and insects have varied effects on the human body. These poisons are usually injected into the body by a sting or bite and are disseminated over the body after absorption from the local site of contact. Some animal venoms are quite potent and are rapidly fatal if absorbed by the body.

9. *Therapeutic drugs* such as the antibiotics and the sulfonamides may injure the body if the person taking the drug has become sensitized to it. Reactions to this kind of injury are allergic.

**Effects.** The effects of chemical agents vary from slight local ones, when these agents contact the external surface of the body, to profound systemic ones, when they are absorbed into the body. The local changes are destructive at the site of contact and cause what are sometimes called chemical burns.

The systemic changes do not fall into any set pattern. The internal organs most commonly involved are the liver, brain, and kidneys. It would be expected that the liver would be affected. Physiologically the liver detoxifies or neutralizes poisonous substances gaining entrance to the body from the outside or forming as a result of normal metabolic processes. In poison cases degenerative changes and even necrosis are often seen in the liver cells.

Changes in the brain may be either organic (from

destruction of the nerve cells) or functional. Barbiturates and opiates in excessive amounts depress activity in the central nervous system, and if the vital centers that control the vital activities of respiration or heart action are sufficiently depressed, death ensues. This type of functional depression may be associated with no demonstrable pathologic change in brain tissue.

The kidney is also an excretory organ, and the highly specialized cells lining the proximal convoluted tubules are peculiarly susceptible to the toxic action of compounds of mercury and bismuth and to certain organic solvents. Tissues other than the three just mentioned that are not uncommonly altered by poisons are the heart, peripheral nerves, and blood cells. There may be degeneration of heart muscle, pathologic changes in the sheaths of peripheral nerves, and hemolysis of the red blood cells.

**Pathology of drug abuse.** The use of a variety of hallucinogens, opiates, stimulants, and sedatives rose to pandemic levels by the beginning of the 1970's. Human values at stake are more serious than illnesses provoked, but pathologic complications are worth noting. Complications are many and varied. Sudden death is one. Major hazards are found in the administration of the drugs with contaminated equipment and the sharing of dirty syringes and needles indiscriminately, as is common among addicts. There is the factor of the quality or purity of the drug preparation, the question of what might be contained in the drug sample. Consequently a whole gamut of infectious processes is seen. In the skin there are abscesses, ulcers, edema, lymphangitis, excoriations, drug rashes, pigmentations, burns, and scars. The systemic infections are grave: septicemia, bacterial endocarditis, mycotic endocarditis, septic thrombophlebitis with septic pulmonary infarcts, osteomyelitis, tetanus, malaria, and, one of the main complications, serum hepatitis.

**Alcoholism.** The most prevalent and serious type of drug addiction in the western world today is alcoholism. Alcohol (ethanol) the drug slows the activities of the central nervous system and is a sedative, tranquilizer, hypnotic or anesthetic, depending on the dose.

The pathology of alcoholism has many ramifications influenced by the amount consumed, the type of alcoholic beverage, the habit pattern of intake, the duration and frequency of ingestion, the adequacy of diet, and the interaction of constitutional factors. From the stomach and intestine alcohol diffuses directly and quickly into the bloodstream to move into body water. Every cell in the body receives a share proportional to its water content. Ethanol is eliminated biochemically in the liver, where better than 90% ingested is metabolized preferentially with priority over other substances handled by the liver. In general terms, pathologic changes relate to direct toxicity, alcohol injuring many body cells, and to indirect effects coming out of the alterations in behavior occasioned by the effect on neurones. Of grave concern is the association of alcoholic intoxication with auto accidents; it is a factor in better than one half of highway fatalities. Impairment of judgment and motor ability (Fig. 45-7) lead to other serious forms of trauma as well.

Direct cell injury from ethanol is best seen in the liver. Alcohol is an experimentally proved hepatotoxin,

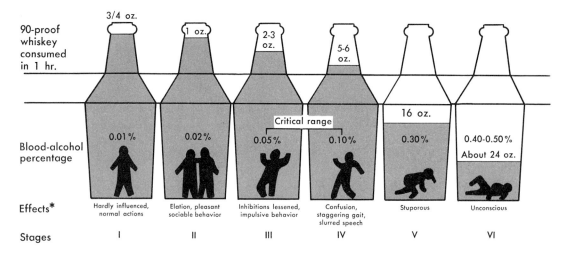

**Fig. 45-7.** Stages of alcoholic intoxication. *As indicated in text, no two persons react exactly the same to the drug.

and prolonged contact with it can mean fatty metamorphosis of liver cells (p. 470), development of alcoholic hepatitis, and progression on to the end-stage of portal cirrhosis. Associated with long-standing alcoholism are vitamin deficiencies, nutritional deficits, cardiomyopathy, pancreatitis, and gastritis. Because the resistance to bacterial infections is weakened, the addict is vulnerable to tuberculosis, lobar pneumonia, lung abscess, and the like.

## Immunologic injuries

Unfortunately, the immunologic response of the body is not always favorable and in fact may be quite harmful. *Immunopathology* is the study of tissue lesions and alterations consequent to immune reactions.

**Immunologic inflammation.** In certain forms of inflammation the precipitating injury is the result of an antigen-antibody reaction (or its equivalent). Although such a broad field as immunologic inflammation cannot be strictly categorized, four patterns of inflammatory response can be defined; anaphylactoid, necrotizing (also called cytolytic or cytotoxic), granulomatous, and fibrinoid.

In allergic states such as hay fever, allergic rhinitis, bronchial asthma, eczema, urticaria, angioneurotic edema, and others, there is a considerable outpouring of edema fluid and exudate, often into a mucous membrane. The exudate may be serous, fibrinous, hemorrhagic, or purulent, but almost invariably it contains a generous number of eosinophils. This cell is so regularly found in allergic states as to be designated the reacting cell of allergy or hypersensitivity. This inflammatory response is the *anaphylactoid* one, and except for the number of eosinophils, it is not unlike inflammation on a nonallergic basis.

Immunopathologic mechanisms may be responsible for cell and tissue death. The *necrotizing* response may be limited to given cells or may include the whole of a tissue, such as an area of skin or the cortex of the kidney (graft rejection). When it is limited to cells, the blood cells are often the ones. Transfusion reactions characterized by destruction of large numbers of red blood cells, hemolytic disease of the newborn based on an Rh incompatibility, and other forms of hemolytic anemia are examples of this response limited to cells.

Tuberculosis and fungous diseases are examples of the *granulomatous* response in immunologic inflammations; lesions are classic (p. 485).

There are a number of disease states wherein the basic immunologic disturbance postulated results in a degeneration or even a necrosis of collagen, the ground substance of connective tissue. The microscopic appearance is altered so that collagen stains more intensely and somewhat in the manner of fibrin,

hence the term *fibrinoid*. Since connective tissue is everywhere in the body and since this involvement may be more or less generalized, the signs and symptoms are many and varied. Diseases in which this type of change occurs in connective tissue are spoken of as the *collagen diseases*. The list of collagen diseases includes severe serum sickness, rheumatic fever, rheumatoid arthritis, polyarteritis nodosa, scleroderma, and disseminated lupus erythematosus.

**Autoimmunization.** Generally the immunologic mechanisms in the body protect. Microbes or substances that would enter and injure are attacked. Because the body recognizes its own cells, it differentiates between the protein of the foreign invader and that belonging to itself. "Unfortunately," as William Boyd says, "the immune system is a two-edged sword which can be turned against the body in that biological paradox nicknamed autoimmunity. The same forces that normally reject foreign material act in reverse and reject the cells and tissues of the body itself with unpleasant consequences."[*]

Many potentially antigenic substances exist in or on the surface of a person's own cells, but before these can induce an immune response, it is thought that they must be altered in some way, possibly by the action of bacteria, viruses, chemicals, or drugs. Once that change has been made, these antigens, now *autoantigens,* stimulate the body of the individual in whom they occur, in certain instances, to form the corresponding antibodies, or *autoantibodies.* The process by which antibodies are made by the body against its own cellular constituents is referred to as *autoimmunization.* The importance of autoimmunization lies in the unfavorable and disease-producing effects of certain of the immune responses to the autoantigen. The category of human disease resulting is that of the *autoimmune diseases.*

**Autoimmune diseases.** Autoantibodies can exist without disease. Under certain conditions, however, the reaction of autoantibodies (or sensitized immunocytes of the lymphoid series) with the specific tissues (the autoantigens) does result in disease, the clinical and pathologic picture of which is determined by the particular tissue attacked immunologically, its distribution in the body, and the extent of the damage done by the reaction. Autoimmunity (autoallergy) is seen in disorders of the thyroid gland, brain, eye, skin, joints, kidneys, and blood vessels.

Six features are emphasized in discussions of autoimmune disease: (1) the elevation of serum globulin, (2) the presence of autoantibodies in the serum, (3) the deposition of denatured protein in tis-

---

[*]Boyd, W.: A textbook of pathology, Philadelphia, 1970, Lea & Febiger.

**Table 45-3**
Examples of disease and antigen in autoimmunity

| AUTOIMMUNE DISEASE | AUTOANTIGEN |
| --- | --- |
| Acquired hemolytic anemia | Antigens on surface of red blood cells |
| Idiopathic thrombocytopenic purpura | Platelet antigens |
| Rheumatoid arthritis | Denatured gamma globulin |
| Systemic lupus erythematosus | Nuclear material including DNA; certain cytoplasmic substances |

sues, (4) the infiltration of lymphocytes and plasma cells in damaged tissues, (5) the benefit of treatment with corticosteroids, and (6) the coexistence of multiple autoimmune disorders.

In some autoimmune disorders the autoantigens involved are known, and circulating autoantibodies can be demonstrated in the patient's serum, especially when there is an associated elevation of gamma globulin (Table 45-3). In lupus erythematosus, for example, factors are present in the patient's serum that are active against nuclear material and certain cytoplasmic substances of cells. As a group the autoimmune diseases often give a history of preceding infection, tend to run in families, and are relieved by steroid hormones (ACTH and cortisone); the patient's serum gives a false positive test for syphilis. Virus particles have been associated with autoimmune diseases, but the relationship is unclear at this time.

Examples of autoimmune diseases include allergic (demyelinating) encephalomyelitis, Hashimoto's struma (chronic thyroiditis), rheumatoid arthritis, acquired hemolytic anemia (both warm- and cold-antibody types), and idiopathic thrombocytopenic purpura.

*Disseminated (systemic) lupus erythematosus.* One of the most interesting of the collagen and autoimmune diseases is disseminated lupus erythematosus (its name is derived from the Latin word for wolf). Disseminated lupus erythematosus is considered the prototype of the collagen diseases, and yet it is the autoimmune disease par excellence. A disease primarily of women,* it runs an acute or subacute course interspersed with periods of improvement. Although the mechanisms are obscure, immunologic injury is implicated in pathogenesis. It is postulated that disease-producing complexes are formed when the autoantibodies, the antinuclear globulins, react with breakdown products of nuclei in the normal wear and tear of cells. (See Fig. 45-8.) Anatomically, connec-

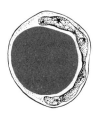

**Fig. 45-8.** Lupus erythematosus (LE) cell, drawing. This distinctive cell is found in blood and bone marrow of patient with lupus. It is a mature neutrophil that has phagocytized a homogeneous mass of nuclear material (degraded DNA) in presence of antinuclear autoantibody in serum.

tive tissue, a tissue widely distributed over the body, is destroyed. Therefore lesions can occur anywhere but select the kidney (wire loop lesion in glomeruli), heart, spleen (onion skin lesion), and skin (butterfly rash on the face). With the connective tissue changes are joint pains, fever, malaise, and anemia.

**Immune complex disease.** *Immune complex disease* is a term of recent origin to indicate a pathologic lesion and disease present because soluble antigen combines with circulating antibody in a given immunologic setting. Complement is fixed as a consequence, and the complex of antigen-antibody-complement is deposited on an endothelial wall. Once deposition takes place, a number of interrelated events follow that cumulate in tissue injury and inflammation at the site. The best example is found in the glomerulus of the kidney in some forms of glomerulonephritis.

## Questions for review

1 Briefly distinguish first-degree, second-degree, and third-degree burns.
2 What is the effect of high altitudes?
3 Briefly discuss ionizing radiation. What is its biologic effect?
4 What are isotopes? Radioisotopes? What is meant by nuclear medicine?
5 Explain what is meant by radiosensitive tissues. Radioresponsive tissues. Radioresistant tissues. Give examples of each.

---

*Polyarteritis (periarteritis) nodosa, another collagen disease basically similar to lupus, primarily involves men. An inflammatory disease of medium-sized arteries, it is sometimes involved with drug sensitivities.

6 What is radiation sickness? Briefly characterize the three stages.

7 How do foreign bodies produce disease?

8 Give the effects of an obstructing lesion on a hollow organ.

9 What are corrosive poisons? Name four.

10 What is the poisonous effect of methyl alcohol? Of lead? Of ethanol?

11 What three organs are usually most involved in chemical poisonings?

12 Give the four patterns for immunologic inflammation. List examples.

13 Explain autoimmunity.

14 Briefly characterize systemic lupus erythematosus.

## REFERENCES (Chapters 44 and 45)

Anderson, W. A. D., and Scotti, T. M.: Synopsis of pathology, ed. 8, St. Louis, 1972, The C. V. Mosby Co.

Arena, J. M.: Nine ways to reduce poisoning in children, Resident Staff Physician 17:46, May, 1971.

Cherubin, C. E.: Urban tetanus; the epidemiologic aspects of tetanus in narcotic addicts in New York City, Arch. Environ. Health 14:802, 1967.

Cherubin, C. E.: Clinical severity of tetanus in narcotic addicts in New York City, Arch. Intern. Med. 121:156, 1968.

Child, P. L.: An indepth look at drug abuse, Lab. Med. 2:11, July, 1971.

Chisolm, J. J., Jr.: The continuing hazard of lead poisoning, Hosp. Pract. 8:127, Nov., 1973.

Cohen, M. M.: The history of opium and the opiates, Tex. Med. 65:76, March, 1969.

Croft, H., and Frenkel, S.: Children and lead poisoning, Am. J. Nurs. 75:102, 1975.

Crosby, W. H.: Those two martinis before dinner every night, J.A.M.A. 231:509, 1975.

Day, S. B.: Severe burn as total body injury, Hosp. Pract. 5:110, April, 1970.

Deeths, T. M., and Breeden, J. T.: Poisoning in children— a statistical study of 1,057 cases, J. Pediatr. 78:299, 1971.

DeGross, J.: Emergency treatment of drug abuse and poison ingestion, Resident Staff Physician 16:43, Feb., 1970.

Dimijian, G. G.: Clinical evaluation of the drug user: current concepts, Tex. Med. 66:42, Jan., 1970.

Dinman, B. D.: Environment: carbon tetrachloride, J.A.M.A. 213:691, 1970.

Drug abuse: pandemic (editorial), J.A.M.A. 214:2327, 1970.

Drug abuse: where to find the facts, Today's Health 49:57, March, 1971.

Federal Source Book: Answers to the most frequently asked questions about drug abuse (compiled by the National Clearinghouse for Drug Abuse Information, operated by National Institute of Mental Health), Washington, D.C., 1971, Government Printing Office.

Finck, P. A.: Exposure to carbon monoxide, review of the literature and 567 autopsies, Milit. Med. 131:1513, 1966.

Force, E. E., and Millar, J. W.: Liver diseases in fatal narcotism, Arch. Pathol. 97:166, 1974.

Frisancho, A. R.: Functional adaptation to high altitude hypoxia, Science 187:313, 1975.

Graham, A., and Graham, F.: Lead poisoning and the suburban child, Today's Health 52:38, March, 1974.

Graham, D. Y.: Alcohol and alcoholism: acute and chronic sequelae, Tex. Med. 71:71, Feb., 1975.

Hamilton, A., and Hardy, H. L.: Industrial toxicology, Acton, Mass., 1974, Publishing Sciences Group, Inc.

Hansen, J. E., and others: Influence of elevation of origin, rate of ascent, and a physical conditioning program on symptoms of acute mountain sickness, Milit. Med. 132:585, 1967.

Helfer, R. E., and Kempe, C. H., editors: The battered child, ed. 2, Chicago, 1974, University of Chicago Press.

Hoeprich, P. D., editor: Infectious diseases, New York, 1972, Harper & Row Publishers.

Johnston, D. G., and Burger, W. D.: Injury and disease of scuba and skin divers, Postgrad. Med. 49:134, April, 1971.

Klonoff, H.: Marijuana and driving in real-life situations, Science 186:317, 1974.

Kolansky, H., and Moore, W. T.: Toxic effects of chronic marihuana use, J.A.M.A. 222:35, 1972.

Kolata, G. B.: Autoimmune diseases in animals; useful models for immunology, Science 184:1360, 1974.

Kowalewski, E. J.: The automobile—the greatest killer, Tex. Med. 66:92, June, 1970.

Land, H. W.: How a parent can reach his child about drugs, Today's Health 49:42, Aug., 1971.

Lepow, I. H., and Ward, P. A.: Inflammation: mechanisms and control, New York, 1972, Academic Press, Inc.

Lewis, H. E.: How man survives the cold, Sci. J. 7:29, Jan., 1971.

Long, K. R.: Pesticides—an occupational hazard on farms, Am. J. Nurs. 71:740, 1974.

Louria, D. B., and others: The human toxicity of certain trace elements, Ann. Intern. Med. 76:307, 1972.

Mason, J. K., and Reals, W. J., editors: Aerospace pathology, Chicago, 1973, College of American Pathologists Foundation.

Maugh, T. H., II: Marihuana: the grass may no longer be greener, Science 185:683, 1974.

Michaelson, M.: How safe are x-rays? Today's Health 46:12, June, 1968.

Michaelson, M.: Time to tame the abominable snowmobiler, Today's Health 48:47, Dec., 1970.

Moore, F. D.: The burn-prone society, J.A.M.A. 231:281, 1975.

Moritz, A. R., and Morris, R. C.: Handbook of legal medicine, ed. 4, St. Louis, 1975, The C. V. Mosby Co.

Moser, R. H.: Ruminations: heroin addiction, J.A.M.A. 230:728, 1974.

Parker, B. M.: The effects of ethyl alcohol on the heart, J.A.M.A. 228:741, 1974.

Pillari, G., and Narus, J.: Physical effects of heroin addiction, Am. J. Nurs. 73:2105, 1973.

Pollack, H., and Sheldon, D. R.: The factor of disease in the world food problems, J.A.M.A. 212:598, 1970.

Rose, J. B.: Tobacco, Tex. Med. 68:60, July, 1972.

Rosenow, E. C., III: The spectrum of drug-induced pulmonary disease, Ann. Intern. Med. 77:977, 1972.

Social disease: a new genre (editorial), Hosp. Trib. **4:**11, Oct. 5, 1970.

Stewart, R. D.: Poisoning from chlorinated hydrocarbon solvents, Am. J. Nurs. **67:**85, 1967.

Stone, O. J.: The effect of arsenic on inflammation, infection, and carcinogenesis, Tex. Med. **65:**40, Oct., 1969.

Teare, D., and Knight, B.: Death in the cot, Sci. J. **7:**71, Jan., 1971.

Thornton, W. E., and Thornton, B. P.: Adverse reactions to heroin use, South. Med. J. **67:**707, 1974.

Trice, H. M., and Roman, P. M.: Alcoholism and the job, Ithaca, N.Y., 1972, Cornell University Press.

Vaughan, J. H.: What we know about autoallergic diseases, Resident Staff Physician **17:**60, Feb., 1971.

Warm-water immersion foot (editorial), J.A.M.A. **200:**716, 1967.

Wetli, C. V., and others: Immunologic abnormalities in heroin addiction, South. Med. J. **67:**193, 1974.

Wiesseman, G. J., and others: *Pseudomonas* vertebral osteomyelitis in heroin addicts, J. Bone Joint Surg. **55-A:** 1416, 1973.

Wilson, R.: Acute high-altitude illness in mountaineers and problems of rescue, Ann. Intern. Med. **78:**421, 1973.

X-ray examinations . . . a guide to good practice, Rockville, Md., 1971, U.S. Department of Health, Education and Welfare, Public Health Service.

Young, A. W., Jr., and Rosenberg, F. R.: Cutaneous stigmas of heroin addiction, Arch. Dermatol. **104:**80, 1971.

# CHAPTER 46

# Neoplasms

## Concept of neoplasm

A neoplasm (Greek, *neo,* new, + *plasma,* formation) is a special but abnormal type of excessive tissue
growth of a destructive nature that serves no useful
purpose and that has a predisposition toward increasing in size, progressing and persisting at the expense
of the body. This excludes purposeful limited growths
caused by hypertrophy or inflammation. Neoplasms
are not controlled, limited, or regulated by any of the
factors normally restraining growth and multiplication of cells in the body. They are a society of cells
unto themselves. Physicians often use the word *tumor*
to designate any abnormal growth or mass that can
be felt in the body, regardless of whether it is a true
neoplasm. Actually *tumor* is derived from the Latin
word meaning a swelling and in its exact sense refers
simply to a mass of unusual or abnormal proportions
(not necessarily neoplastic). However, the word is
very commonly used so as to be interchangeable in
its meaning with the word *neoplasm.* True tumor
formation may occur in man, lower mammals, birds,
insects, fishes, reptiles, and even plants.

Before we enter into a discussion of neoplasms,
it is well to call the student's attention to three nonneoplastic processes: (1) hypertrophy, (2) hyperplasia,
and (3) metaplasia. These three reflect changes in
cells; two of them result from cellular proliferation.

*Hypertrophy* is a symmetric enlargement of an
organ or part of the body related to an increase in
the size of its component cells. It is the result of an
increase in the functional demands made on the tissue and may be either physiologic or pathologic.
Physiologic hypertrophy occurs in the parturient
uterus and disappears with termination of the pregnancy. Pathologic hypertrophy occurs in the urinary
bladder if the outflow of urine is obstructed. If one
kidney is surgically removed, the other hypertrophies.
This process is limited and controlled by the body.
It is generally thought that if the lesion causing pathologic hypertrophy is removed, the process is reversible.

*Hyperplasia* is an increase in the number of cells
of an organ or a part thereof because of irritation,
inflammation, or increased functional demands. The
organ usually enlarges, and an increase in functional
activity accompanies the enlargement. For example,
a physiologic demand for an increased amount of
the thyroid hormone causes hyperplasia of the thyroid gland, to produce this added amount. Under
certain abnormal circumstances the thyroid gland
may become hyperplastic, and the resultant condition is hyperthyroidism. The cells proliferate in hyperplasia, but it is to be emphasized that the proliferation is a simple and orderly one, of limited extent,
and well controlled by the body. (See Table 46-1 and
Fig. 46-1.)

*Metaplasia* is the replacement of one type of normal tissue by another type of normal tissue in an
area of the body where the second tissue does not
normally occur. The abnormality is that of location.
Metaplasia never oversteps the boundaries of the primary groups of tissue (epithelium or connective tissue); that is, one type of epithelium may be replaced
by another type of epithelium but not by connective
tissue, and one type of connective tissue may change
into another type of connective tissue but not into
epithelium. Examples of metaplasia are the replacement of the columnar epithelium of the gallbladder
by the squamous variety in the presence of gallstones
and the replacement of the laryngeal and tracheal
cartilages by bone in the elderly. The causes of epithelial metaplasia are inflammation, extremely rapid
growth, or vitamin A deficiency. Connective tissue
metaplasia may be caused by chronic inflammation,
necrosis, or the aging process. Metaplasia in itself
is not a neoplastic process, but in certain areas of
the body its presence is thought to predispose to the
subsequent development of true neoplasms.

*Hamartoma* is the term applied to a tumorlike
malformation composed of an *abnormal mixture* of
the *normal* constituents of an organ or tissue. The
constituents may be abnormal in amount, arrangement, degree of maturation, or in all respects, but

**Table 46-1**
Hyperplasia versus neoplasia

| POINT OF DIFFERENCE | HYPERPLASIA | NEOPLASIA |
|---|---|---|
| Cause and effect | Usually well defined; extrinsic stimulus physiologic or pathologic<br>Predictable effect | Not well defined—number of variables |
| Course | Purposeful | Meaningless |
| Progression | Limited (removal of stimulus means regression) | Unlimited to death of host |
| Type cell | That of tissue of origin<br>Reproduction in kind | That of tissue of origin<br>Reproduction—atypical to anaplastic* (completely unrecognizable) |
| Extent | Diffuse | Single focus (sometimes multicentric) |
| Spread from site | Contained | Metastases (spread from site) |

*Anaplasia is a quality displayed by neoplastic cells wherein they take on the appearance and arrangement of the embryonal stages of the cells from which they are derived. In such cells function is either absent or diminished, and identification of precise cell type may be difficult.

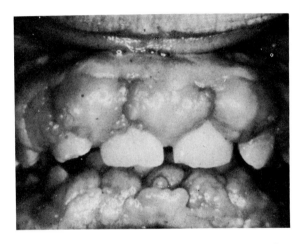

**Fig. 46-1.** Hyperplasia caused by the drug Dilantin (phenytoin). Note enlargement with distortion of gums. (From Bhaskar, S. N.: Synopsis of oral pathology, ed. 4, St. Louis, 1973, The C. V. Mosby Co.)

they lack the capacity of true neoplasm for uncontrolled growth and proliferation. They may be mistaken for neoplasm.

## General characteristics

**Causes.** The last quarter of a century has seen an enormous amount of thought and research directed toward the solution of the riddle of the cause of cancer, but it must be admitted that the riddle still remains unsolved. To add to the difficulty is the fact that the term cancer encompasses more than 100 medically distinct entities, each with its own unique pattern of expression. Investigators in this field have found themselves diverted at an early stage to basic studies in virology, microbiology, genetics, and immunology. Although thought and research have failed to reveal the exact etiology of tumor growth, they have brought forth many facts of wide application to the control of neoplasms. This is of inestimable importance because neoplasms in the United States now occupy second place as cause of death in man. The leading cause of death is cardiovascular disease. It is estimated that one out of four Americans now living will eventually develop cancer.

A given tumor arises from certain normal cells of one type (its tissue of origin) that have undergone a series of changes influenced by intrinsic or extrinsic factors (Fig. 46-2). By *intrinsic* or inherent factors are meant factors within the cells or within the body as a whole. Among these are heredity, age, sex, endocrine influences, and a natural predisposition to tissue overgrowth. By *extrinsic* or exciting factors are meant agents that originate without the body.

*Hereditary factors.* There seems to be some degree of inherited predisposition to the development of neoplasms because, for more than a hundred years, recorded histories of certain families have shown that the incidence of one group of neoplasms is greater in these families than in the population as a whole. Often the neoplasms affecting the members are of the same type and affect the same organ. In identical twins tumor growths may occur at about the same time.

Applying the technics of cytogenetics to the study of tumor cells, one can demonstrate abnormalities in the chromosomes of tumor cells. Changes in chromosomal number seem to be almost constant. Structurally abnormal chromosomes, called marker chromosomes, are found in many types of tumor cells. The best example is the *Philadelphia chromosome.*

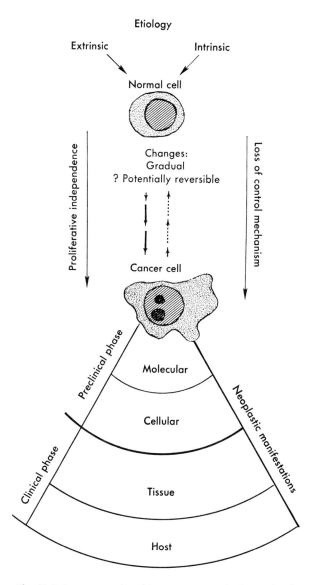

Etiology

Extrinsic          Intrinsic

Normal cell

Proliferative independence

Changes:
Gradual
? Potentially reversible

Cancer cell

Loss of control mechanism

Preclinical phase

Molecular

Neoplastic manifestations

Cellular

Clinical phase

Tissue

Host

**Fig. 46-2.** Stages postulated in cancerogenesis. Normal cell interreacts with etiologic (carcinogenic) factors in environment (extrinsic, intrinsic). Because of this, normal cell is changed to cancer cell (probably a gradual process). Once cancer has come into being, stage is set for development of mass of tumor cells and for it to produce signs and symptoms in host in which it developed. (From Talso, P. J., and Remenchik, A. P., editors: Internal medicine—based on mechanisms of disease, St. Louis, 1968, The C. V. Mosby Co.)

Specifically related to chronic granulocytic leukemia, it can be found in leukemic cells from nearly 95% of the typical cases. It cannot be found in other leukemias or in lymphoma. The risk of leukemia is about 20 times greater in Down's syndrome (p. 444), a disease with a known and characteristic chromosomal defect. (See Fig. 46-3.)

A number of agents known to produce cancer in man and animals (x rays, alkylating compounds, viruses) cause changes in chromosomes of normal cells, and the altered cells behave as malignant ones. However, chromosomally normal cells may behave as cancerous ones. The relationship of chromosomal damage to cancer is uncertain.

*Influence of environment.* The influence of the environment is quickly apparent in any study of the how and why of cancer. Cancer epidemiologists stress its importance and emphasize its role. Much valuable knowledge concerning cancerous growths of one kind or another has come from analysis of cancers in their natural settings. Numerous examples could be given from the geographic studies of cancer.

Many workers believe that in the development of 80% to 85% of all neoplasms, some factor in the surroundings has interacted over a period of time with a susceptible individual in the course of his daily life. The factors implicated (Table 46-2) relate to food eaten, air breathed, tobacco smoked, dust inhaled, climate, occupation, general working conditions, and many other things.

*Age and sex incidence.* Sarcomas are more common in young persons. Carcinomas are more common in persons past middle life. Males are more susceptible than females to certain tumors (cancer of the stomach, mouth, lip, and lung), whereas females are more susceptible to certain other kinds (cancer of the thyroid gland and gallbladder). On the whole, males are somewhat more susceptible than females to neoplasms when the organs peculiar to sex are excluded.

*Oncogenesis.* Agents that bring about the transformation of normal cells into tumor cells are known as *carcinogens* or *oncogens* (Table 46-3), regardless of the type of tumor produced. The process is carcinogenesis or oncogenesis. The study of tumors is *oncology.* Among the important oncogens are (1) chemical agents, (2) physical agents (ultraviolet rays, ionizing radiation, radioactive substances), (3) hormones, and (4) viruses.

Important chemical carcinogenic agents are some members of the coal tar group and their derivatives. Cigarette smoking is related to 80% of lung cancers because of this group. Certain of these compounds can produce cancer in a suitable experimental animal such as a rabbit if repeatedly applied to the skin

## Table 46-2
Some examples of environmental neoplasms

| FACTOR IN ENVIRONMENT | INDIVIDUALS INTERACTING WITH ENVIRONMENTAL FACTOR | ANATOMIC AREA AFFECTED; LOCATION OF RESULTANT NEOPLASM |
|---|---|---|
| Ionizing radiation | | |
| Radon and radioactive dust | Miners of uranium and cobalt ore | Lungs (inhalation) |
| Atomic bombings | Survivors of explosions in Japan | Blood-forming organs |
| Nonionizing radiation | | |
| Sun (ultraviolet rays) | Fair-skinned persons working out of doors, especially in southwestern United States—farmers, ranchers, soldiers, and others | Skin (direct penetration from exposure) |
| Heat | Persons in contact with heating devices | |
| | 1. Persons in Kashmir warming abdomen with kangri | Skin (direct contact) |
| | 2. Persons in China sleeping on kang (heated brick) | |
| | 3. Persons in Kashmir and Central America smoking chutta, with burning end of cigar in mouth | Mouth (direct contact) |

## Table 46-3
Examples of oncogenic agents

| AGENT | ANATOMIC NEOPLASM |
|---|---|
| **Chemical** | |
| Polycyclic hydrocarbons | Experimental skin tumors and sarcomas |
| 1. 9, 10-dimethylbenz(a)anthracene (potent) | |
| 2. Methylcholanthrene (potent) | |
| 3. Benz(a)anthracene (weak) | |
| Soot | Skin carcinoma (scrotal cancer of chimney sweeps) |
| Benzene | Leukemia |
| Tobacco | Cancer of lung and mouth |
| Azo dyes | |
| Dimethylaminoazobenzene (butter yellow) | Experimental liver tumors |
| Aromatic amines | |
| Beta-naphthylamine | Bladder cancer in man—occupational hazard in certain industries where there is contact with aniline dyes |
| Urethane | Lung adenomas in mice |
| Arsenic | Skin cancer in man |
| Uranium and chromates | Lung cancer in man |
| **Physical** | |
| X rays | Skin cancer |
| | Leukemia (bone marrow) |
| | Thyroid cancer |
| Ultraviolet irradiation | Skin cancer |
| **Biologic** | |
| Aflatoxin from common mold *Aspergillus* | Liver cancer in fish |
| *Schistosoma*—metazoan parasite producing nonneoplastic lesion that is premalignant | Cancer of bladder and liver |
| Chronic irritation—poorly defined role in oncogenesis | |
| 1. Gallstones | Carcinoma of gallbladder |
| 2. Ill-fitting dentures, other manifestations of poor oral hygiene | Cancer of gums and oral mucous membrane |

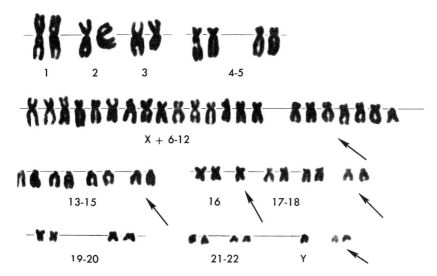

**Fig. 46-3.** Abnormal karyotype with abnormal number of chromosomes (aneuploidy) in bone marrow of patient with acute leukemia in relapse. The number of chromosomes is sixty, and arrows indicate supernumerary ones. A variety of chromosomal abnormalities is possible in acute leukemia relative to number and morphology but without any specificity. (From Reisman, L. E., and Matheny, A. P., Jr.: Genetics and counseling in medical practice, St. Louis, 1969, The C. V. Mosby Co.)

or appropriate tissue of the animal. Chemical agents are responsible for a number of occupational tumors in man. Among these are cancer of the skin in workers whose clothing is constantly soaked with mineral oil containing coal-tar derivatives (mule spinners) and cancer of the bladder in persons who work with aniline dyes.

Vinyl chloride in the plastics industry is responsible for a very rare angiosarcoma of the liver in workers exposed to it. It is emphasized as an industrial carcinogen, but vinyl chloride plastics are all about us in a variety of consumer goods such as aerosol sprays, cosmetic products, food wraps, phonograph records, and even in some medicated vaporizers.

Chemical carcinogens are numerous and varied. In fact, some 600 of them are known to be *man-made* organic compounds.

Marie Curie and her daughter Irene died of leukemia induced by a phenomenon to which Madame Curie gave the name "radioactivity." Carcinoma of the skin is very common in persons such as farmers, stockmen, and sailors whose skin, by reason of their occupation, is constantly exposed to sunlight (ultraviolet rays), wind, and dust. Leukemia seems to be more common among persons who are constantly exposed to slight overdoses of radiation than among the general population.

The role of hormones in the production of cancer is being given considerable study at the present time.

Cancer of the breast has been experimentally produced in mice by the injection of estrogenic substances, and cases of cancer of the breast in human beings in which there appeared to be some relation between the tumor growth and the injection of female sex hormones have been reported. The effect of reducing male sex hormones either by castration or by the injection of female sex hormones is used in the treatment of prostatic cancer to produce dramatic but temporary regression of the cancer. Diethylstilbestrol (DES) was used at one time to prevent miscarriage but discontinued because of its ineffectiveness. The transplacental carcinogenic effect of the hormone was realized when the rare vaginal adenocarcinoma appeared in the female offspring of such mothers.

Experimental evidence definitely indicates that filtrable viruses do cause several kinds of cancerous growths in lower animals, that is, in rabbits (Fig. 46-4), mice, chickens, hamsters, rats, dogs, frogs, monkeys, horses, squirrels, and deer (Table 46-4). There are more than sixty known viral oncogens. Cancer is induced in all major groups of animals (including subhuman primates). Table 28-6 emphasizes certain patterns in viral oncogenesis.

Leukemia is an important form of virus-induced neoplasm in animals. Within the last decade the polyoma virus has been shown to cause many different solid cancers in the skin, breast, lungs, gastrointestinal tract, and salivary glands of several species

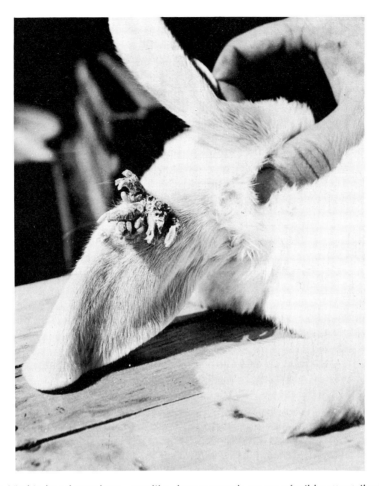

**Fig. 46-4.** Viral-induced neoplasm—wartlike, horny growth on ear of wild cottontail rabbit. Ears and eyelids are common sites for such tumors. An enzootic disease of wild rabbits, rabbit papillomatosis, is also seen in domestic ones. The virus is transmitted in nature by rabbit tick and in laboratory by mosquito. (From Hagen, K. W.: Bull. Pathol. **8:**308, 1967.)

**Table 46-4**
Some examples of viral neoplasms in animals

| ANIMAL SPECIES | DATE REPORTED | NEOPLASM |
|---|---|---|
| Chicken | 1908 | Chicken leukemias |
| Chicken | 1910 | Rous sarcoma |
| Rabbit | 1933 | Shope papilloma-carcinoma |
| Mouse | 1936 | Breast carcinoma* |
| Frog | 1938 | Kidney carcinoma |
| Mouse | 1951 | Spontaneous leukemia |
| Mouse | 1957 | Salivary gland tumors of polyoma virus |
| Hamster, rat, and rabbit | 1958 | Great variety of solid tumors produced by polyoma virus |
| Hamster | 1962 | Chest and liver tumors (adenovirus responsible isolated from human cancer) |

*This most common form of cancer in the most commonly used laboratory animal was shown by John Bittner to be related to a virus. The agent has been long referred to as Bittner's milk factor. Since Bittner's discovery the role of viruses in the induction of cancerous growths has been increasingly emphasized.

of laboratory animals. Oncogenic viruses are known to lie dormant for a long time in animals before they are activated. It is postulated that either external factors such as x rays and other forms of radiant energy or internal factors of metabolic or hormonal nature trigger the mechanism of neoplasia (new growth). John Bittner demonstrated that breast cancer in mice is caused by an interplay of the virus (milk factor), hormones, and hereditary background.

The role of viruses in human neoplasms is unknown, but recent experimental reports strongly suggest that viruses are indeed involved. In man, the common wart, verruca vulgaris, a benign or harmless tumor, has been clearly demonstrated to be caused by a virus. Viruslike particles have been isolated from human cancers, most recently from human breast cancer and from the milk of breast cancer patients. The particles closely resemble those producing breast tumors in mice. Table 46-5 presents viruses indicted as oncogens in man.

*Burkitt's lymphoma.* Burkitt's African lymphoma is a malignant disease of the jaw and abdomen affecting children between the ages of 2 and 14 years. The striking feature of the disease is its sharp geographic distribution. It is found in Central Africa limited to a malarious belt where the conditions of rainfall, temperature, altitude, vegetation, and humidity are the same. It also appears to be a geographic equivalent of lymphomas of children in other parts of the world. But, unlike lymphomas elsewhere, it has a pattern for a specific infectious disease, strongly suggesting that it is caused by an agent such as a virus, and the case for the viral etiology is getting stronger. Several viruses have been found in tumor tissue and in cell culture made of tumor. The Epstein-Barr virus was first isolated from such a cell culture.

At first it was postulated that the viral agent causing Burkitt's lymphoma was spread by a vector mosquito. The disease is prevalent in areas where malaria is endemic and is rare outside tropical Africa. Now it is thought that the mosquito is not more implicated than in the transmission of malaria, for it is believed that the damage to the lymphoid system from chronic malaria is the factor that determines in some way the oncogenic potential of a virus. The EB virus implicated here is also found in nonneoplastic disease elsewhere in the world.

*Chronic irritation.* An important factor in tumor growth seems to be prolonged chronic irritation. Apparently it is a contributing factor in cancer of the lip in pipe smokers and cancer of the cervix in women with unrepaired cervical lacerations of long standing. It is said that cancer rarely occurs in a normal tissue. Perhaps repeated efforts at repair after prolonged injury set the stage for the transition in normal cells.

**Resemblance to normal cells.** The tissue or group of cells in which a neoplasm arises is the *tissue of origin*. The cells of some neoplasms closely resemble their normal cells of origin, whereas in others there is little similarity. Tumor cells are permanently altered cells, with the power to multiply more rapidly than normal cells. As a rule, the more the cells of a neoplasm differ from the cells of the tissue from which they arise, the more dangerous will be the tumor.

### Table 46-5
Viruses indicted for oncogenicity in man

| VIRUS OR VIRUSLIKE PARTICLE | TUMOR |
| --- | --- |
| Type C and related particle* | Leukemia |
| | Lymphoma |
| | Sarcomas |
| | Bowen's disease (a precancerous skin change) |
| Type B particle (RNA particle) (mouse mammary tumor virus) | Breast cancer |
| EB virus (Epstein-Barr virus, herpes type virus) | Burkitt's lymphoma |
| | Hodgkin's disease |
| | Leukemia |
| | Lymphoma |
| *Herpesvirus hominis* type 2 (genital strain of herpes) | Carcinoma of cervix uteri |
| Reovirus type 3 | Burkitt's lymphoma |

*Leukoviruses with RNA core and double membrane, a complex of oncogenic viruses, the first ones isolated from animal neoplasms. Referred to as oncogenic RNA viruses, or oncornaviruses, they have been divided into three classes, A, B, and C (the most important). Crucial to their oncogenic potential is their relatively large genome as compared with other viruses and their possession of an RNA-directed (-dependent) DNA polymerase (reverse transcriptase). This enzyme mediates the synthesis of DNA from an RNA template and indicates a biochemical mechanism for the perpetuation of viral genome when the host cell divides.

When examined under the microscope, the cells of highly malignant neoplasms are usually found to stain deeply, to vary greatly in size and shape, and to have many mitotic figures (cells of normal tissues or benign tumors show none or relatively few).

**Autonomy of neoplasms.** The cells normally formed in the body are under its complete control. In neoplasms the cells are not, and they multiply repeatedly in an irregular and abnormal manner. If they have any function at all, it is abnormal and perverted and may be harmful to their host. Tumors of the parathyroid gland may cause severe disturbances of calcium metabolism and disease of the bones, and certain tumors of the ovary may give women a masculine appearance.

As Spencer has well said, cancer cells may be likened to ruthless gangsters who run amuck among the cells of an orderly functioning human economy.

**Nourishment.** While forming a part of the body, tumors are dependent on it only for nourishment, which they obtain regardless of the hardships that they impose. Tumor cells seem to have a curious priority on the nutrients of the host. Lipomas (tumors composed of fat) continue to grow after the body fat has been almost depleted, and other tumors continue to develop even though the body is starved. The end

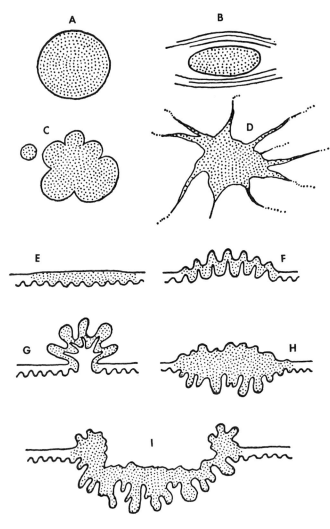

**Fig. 46-5.** Different shapes of neoplasms, sketch. **A** to **D,** Shapes in solid tissues; **E** to **I,** shapes and outlines on surfaces. **A,** Encapsulated spherical tumor. **B,** Encapsulated tumor compressed to an ovoid shape by surrounding tissues. **C,** Lobulated tumor formed by coalescence of several tumor foci. **D,** Malignant neoplasm with infiltrating outrunners. **E,** Intraepithelial tumor. **F,** Broad based papilloma. **G,** Papilloma with a stalk. **H,** Nonulcerated carcinoma. **I,** Ulcerated neoplasm.

stage for the host is a generalized emaciation and state of ill health designated a tumor cachexia.

The blood supply of neoplasms is obtained from the general circulation, and there may be an over-development of vessels in the neighborhood of a neoplasm to meet the demands that it makes. Occasionally growth is so rapid that the blood supply is incapable of sustaining it, and the neoplasm undergoes necrosis. This can be followed by infection, sloughing, and hemorrhage.

**Mode of growth.** Tumor growth may be of two kinds. If the tumor grows from its center and pushes the surrounding tissues aside but does not directly invade them, growth is *expansive*. If it grows from its periphery and strands of cells grow into the surrounding tissues and destroy them, it is *infiltrative*. Neoplasms growing by expansion are circumscribed, encapsulated, and sharply separated from the surrounding tissues. Those growing by infiltration are nonencapsulated and grade off imperceptibly into the surrounding tissues. Such neoplasms will recur after surgical removal unless they are so widely excised that all cells which have infiltrated the surrounding tissues are removed. The method by which a neoplasm grows bears crucially on its benign or malignant qualities. Clinically neoplasms may appear as (1) masses or nodules in the tissues, (2) areas of diffuse hardness, (3) elevated or smooth growths on a surface, (4) papillary outgrowths from a surface, and (5) ulcers. (See Fig. 46-5.)

**Resistance.** The cells of neoplasms have little resistance to destructive influences and little reparative ability. For this reason tumors, especially those of the skin, often show early ulceration and extensive necrosis. Ulceration may involve large blood vessels and lead to severe hemorrhage.

**Immunity in cancer.** The most significant advances in oncology today focus on the immunologic aspects of neoplasms.

In man and animals there have been many reasons for thinking that a relationship existed between an individual's immunologic system and his cancer, and such a relationship is generally accepted today. Some of the convincing evidence stems from the abundance of experimental work and the many interesting observations made on patients with organ transplants. The incidence of cancer after organ transplant is about 100 times that observed in the same age group of the general population. (Immune mechanisms must be tampered with dramatically for organ transplantation.) Malignancies complicate immunosuppression in many clinical settings, and in congenital immunologic deficiencies as well, there is a high incidence of cancer.

The immunology of cancer is complex, and a lot of work is being done on it. Most and maybe all neoplasms contain tumor-associated antigens new and "foreign" to the host. Tumor antigens are tumor-specific and provoke an antitumor response either in the host animal or upon transplantation of the tumor into a comparable animal. The immune response in the host is a function of cell-mediated immunity, the T cell system recognizing the antigens as foreign to the host and destroying them. The reaction is comparable to that of graft rejection. Tumor antigens arise because the cancer cell differs from the normal cell (not because of differences between donor and recipient animal). They probably result from the initial transformation of the normal cell into a cancerous one. At this early time a neoplasm is most vulnerable to the immune response. Undoubtedly many incipient ones are completely and quietly destroyed.

As to be expected, there are different kinds and degrees of tumor immunity. A special kind is found with tumors induced by viruses. Surface antigens appear as a direct effect of viral activity, and these are consistent for the same viral oncogen in other circumstances. Not so if the oncogenic mechanism is nonviral. That neoplasm has its own distinct antigen, it is true, but even though the same carcinogen is applied in exactly the same way to other anatomic areas in the same animal, that tumor antigen is not repeated. As a result of this effect, many antigenic types become possible with varying immunologic potential. If tumor cells are highly antigenic, they may immunize against themselves so efficiently that tumor growth is blocked.

In view of the existence of an immune mechanism, how does one explain the prevalence of clinical cancer? One can only surmise. It may be that the bulk of experimental cancers and cancers in human beings arise at a time when immunologic defenses are down. It may be that the tumoricidal T cell cannot contact the tumor antigen bound to the membrane of the tumor cell; its action is in some way blocked. It may be that a small fraction of starter growths can make the clinical scene because they combine the least in antigenicity with the highest in proliferative activity

**Fetal antigens.** Many human tumors express themselves as tumor antigens, proteins, glycoproteins, or polysaccharides that are normally present during the very early phases of embryonic and fetal life but are depressed to trace amounts in adults. Two such fetal antigens can be detected by radioimmunoassay. *Carcinoembryonic antigen* is related especially to cancer of the colon; *alpha fetoglobulin*, to cancer of the liver. Fetal antigens cannot be used for cancer screening, but testing for them is of value in the medical

## Table 46-6
Essential differences between benign and malignant tumors

| CHARACTERISTIC | BENIGN | MALIGNANT |
| --- | --- | --- |
| Growth | By expansion; push aside surrounding tissue; as a rule, growth slow | Infiltrate surrounding tissues; growth rapid |
| Limitation | Often encapsulated | Nonencapsulated, poorly defined |
| Recurrence | Do not recur after removal | Often recur after removal |
| Morphology | Resemble tissue of origin | Hardly resemble tissue of origin; appearance variably abnormal |
| Differentiation | Well differentiated | Less well, poorly differentiated, or undifferentiated |
| Mitotic activity | Slight | Usually great |
| Tissue destruction | Little | Extensive |
| Spread | Do not spread | Spread to different parts of body |
| Effect on body | Usually do not kill* | Always kill if not treated |

*Benign neoplasms at times may have serious consequences because of a particular anatomic location or because they elaborate excess hormone.

management and follow-up of patients known to have certain tumors.

## Classification

To classify neoplasms satisfactorily is very difficult. For anything like comprehensive coverage it is necessary to classify them from both the clinical and the histologic standpoints. (The latter refers to the origin and nature of the cells composing the neoplasm.)

From the clinical standpoint tumors are classified as *malignant* and *benign* (innocent or nonmalignant). In Table 46-6 are given the essential differences between malignant and benign tumors. In histologic classification a neoplasm is designated by adding the suffix *oma* to the name of the tissue from which the tumor originates. For example, myoma means a tumor originating from muscle. In neoplasms derived from connective tissue or muscle the suffix *oma* is reserved for nonmalignant tumors, whereas malignant tumors are designated by the suffix *sarcoma*. A fibroma is a benign tumor originating from fibrous tissue, whereas a fibrosarcoma is the malignant counterpart. The term *cancer* was formerly used to designate malignant tumors of epithelial origin (carcinomas) only, but it is used today in a broader sense to indicate any malignant tumor regardless of kind.

The classification as given in Table 46-7 includes most of the important neoplasms. In classification it should be remembered that fat, cartilage, bone, and vascular tissue are but specialized types of connective tissue.

## Benign neoplasms

Seven outstanding characteristics of benign neoplasms are as follows:

1. They grow by expansion and do not infiltrate the surrounding tissues; they are usually encapsulated.
2. They do not spread to other parts of the body, that is, do not metastasize.
3. They do not recur when removed surgically.
4. They do not cause extensive destruction of tissue.
5. They do not directly effect such changes in the body as anemia, weakness, or loss of weight.
6. They resemble closely the normal cells of the parent tissue, as a rule.
7. They do not kill except when located so as to press on or obstruct vital organs.

The slow expansive growth of the benign tumor, with its pressure on surrounding tissues, leads to the formation of a *capsule*. The capsule represents a reaction on the part of the surrounding tissues and is not directly a part of the tumor. Benign neoplasms are made up of tissue closely resembling normal adult tissue. They do not undergo degenerative changes so often as do malignant ones. Although benign neoplasms seldom produce serious illness or death, they may occasionally do so because of (1) position, (2) complications, or (3) production of an excess of hormone.

Benign tumors whose position interferes with the activities of vital organs are spoken of as being *malignant by position*. For example, a tumor of even small size, regardless of its nature, growing in the cranial cavity will eventually lead to death of the host if it presses on the brain.

Benign neoplasms may produce complications in remote organs by impinging on their vessels or nerves of supply. Among the dangerous complications are hemorrhage from an ulcerated surface and

**Table 46-7**
Classification of tumors

| | BENIGN | MALIGNANT |
|---|---|---|
| I. Neoplasms arising from epithelium | | |
|    1. Pavement epithelium (squamous, transitional) | Papilloma | Squamous cell carcinoma<br>Basal cell carcinoma<br>Transitional cell carcinoma |
|    2. Glandular epithelium | Adenoma<br>Cystadenoma<br>Polyp | Adenocarcinoma |
| II. Neoplasms arising from connective tissues | | |
|    1. Fibrous | Fibroma | Fibrosarcoma |
|    2. Embryonic fibrous tissue | Myxoma | Myxosarcoma |
|    3. Fat | Lipoma | Liposarcoma |
|    4. Cartilage | Chondroma | Chondrosarcoma |
|    5. Bone | Osteoma<br>Osteochondroma | Osteosarcoma (osteogenic sarcoma) |
|    6. Synovial membrane | Synovioma | Synovial sarcoma |
| III. Neoplasms of muscle | | |
|    1. Smooth muscle | Leiomyoma | Leiomyosarcoma |
|    2. Striated muscle | Rhabdomyoma | Rhabdomyosarcoma |
| IV. Neoplasms arising in nervous system | | |
|    1. Peripheral nerve sheaths | Neuroma<br>Neurofibroma<br>Neurilemoma (neurinoma) | Neurogenic sarcoma (neurofibrosarcoma) |
|    2. Sympathetic nervous system | Ganglioneuroma | Neuroblastoma |
|    3. Neuroglia | | Glioma<br>Retinoblastoma |
|    4. Meninges | Meningioma | |
| V. Neoplasms of endothelium and structures in which it functions | | |
|    1. Blood vessels | Hemangioma | Hemangioendothelioma<br>Angiosarcoma |
|    2. Lymph vessels | Lymphangioma | Lymphangiosarcoma<br>Lymphangioendothelioma |
|    3. Bone marrow | | Multiple myeloma<br>Ewing's tumor<br>Leukemia |
|    4. Lymphoid tissue | | Malignant lymphoma<br>Lymphosarcoma<br>Reticulum cell sarcoma |
| VI. Pigmented neoplasm (melanocytes, cells producing melanin) | Nevus | Malignant melanoma |
| VII. Neoplasm of trophectoderm (trophoblasts of placental villi) | Hydatidiform mole | Chorionepithelioma (choriocarcinoma) |
| VIII. Complex neoplasms occurring in | | |
|    1. Ovary | Dermoid cyst | Teratoma |
|    2. Testis | | Teratoma<br>Choriocarcinoma |
|    3. Kidney | | Mixed tumor |
|    4. Salivary glands | Mixed tumor | |

infection. A tumor that is joined to a surface or organ by a pedicle may twist on its pedicle, causing gangrene of the tumor since the pedicle carries the blood supply.

Most of the important neoplasms of the endocrine glands are benign, but they gain considerable clinical significance. This is because the cells of which they are composed may continue to elaborate in excess the hormone with which their normal cell counterpart is associated. Such hormone-producing tumors are designated as functional, and because the neoplasm provides an additional source, these growths may precipitate clinical states related to excess circulating hormone. For instance, benign tumors of the islands of Langerhans in the pancreas may produce insulin as do the normal island cells, even a small tumor sometimes releasing insulin into the bloodstream in generous quantities. The physiologic effects are very dramatic, since the insulin acts to lower the blood sugar to a hypoglycemic state, with its characteristic features.

## BENIGN EPITHELIAL TUMORS

Benign epithelial tumors may arise from any location where epithelium is found.

*Papillomas** are cauliflower-like projections that spring from the skin or mucous membrane. Those that are covered with stratified squamous epithelium are sometimes known as *hard papillomas* or *warts*. The wart seen on the hands of children is known as *verruca vulgaris*, the viral etiology of which is accepted. Papillomas of the larynx often occur in children and tend to disappear at puberty, but they may become malignant (Fig. 46-6). *Acuminate condylomas* (pointed or venereal warts of viral etiology) are moist papillomatous processes that occur around the genitals as a result of irritating discharges. They are especially common in gonorrhea. *Cutaneous horns* are epithelial overgrowths seated on a papillary base.

Papillomas covered with epithelium other than the stratified squamous type are sometimes known as *soft papillomas*. They occur most often in the intestinal canal and bladder. (See Fig. 46-7.) Soft papillomas, especially those of the bladder, are likely to become malignant.

*Adenomas* are tumors made up of glands and derived from glandular tissues such as the breast or prostate gland. *Cystadenomas* result when one or more of the glands of an adenoma enlarges and becomes cystic. This is usually caused by retention

---

*Referring simply to a growth protruding from a mucous membrane, the term *polyp* is sometimes used interchangeably with papilloma. Papilloma is a tumor not only projecting from the surface but derived from its epithelium.

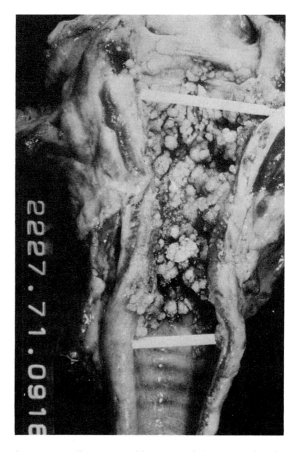

**Fig. 46-6.** Papillomatosis of larynx. Both benign and malignant papillomas present. Voice box has been opened to show abundant tumor growth.

within the glands of their own secretion. Cystadenomas are important in the ovary (p. 608) and in the breast, where they are papillary.

## BENIGN CONNECTIVE TISSUE TUMORS

*Fibromas* are benign neoplasms made up of fibrous connective tissue. In spite of the wide distribution of fibrous tissue, fibromas are relatively infrequent. They occur most often in the skin and mucous membranes. They are usually round or nodular, encapsulated, and frequently attached to the point of origin by a pedicle. *Nasal polyps* are soft pedunculated nonneoplastic fibrous masses in a patient with an allergic background.

*Keloids* are not true neoplasms but consist of overgrowths of the dense connective tissue of scars. They occur most often following burns and are said to be confined to certain races.

*Lipomas* are tumors composed of fat. In the ordinary sense they are the most benign of all tumors,

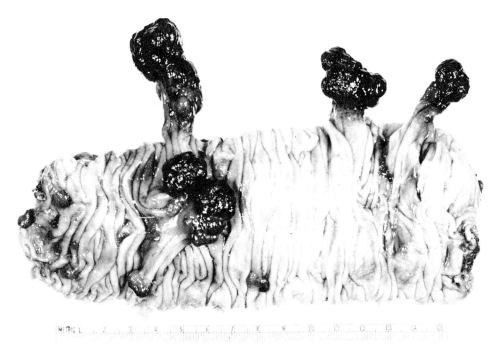

**Fig. 46-7.** Papillomas projecting from mucous membrane of opened segment of large bowel. Note stalks to papillomas and their hemorrhagic character. (From Anderson, W. A. D., editor: Pathology, ed. 6, St. Louis, 1971, The C. V. Mosby Co.)

but they may cause serious disturbances because of their large size. Lipomas occur chiefly in the subcutaneous tissues of the neck, shoulders, and buttocks, but they may occur wherever adipose (fat) tissue is found. They are usually round, lobulated, and surrounded by a thin capsule. They are removed with ease.

*Chondromas* are neoplasms composed of cartilage. Chondromas occur most often in connection with bones, especially the long bones and the bones of the hands and feet.

*Osteomas* are benign tumors composed of bone. It is often difficult to differentiate true osteomas, which are comparatively rare, from certain inflammatory or traumatic bony overgrowths, which are rather common. True osteomas usually occur in connection with the bones of the face, most often those of the nasal sinuses and orbit. Tumors such as fibromas, lipomas, and certain sarcomas may undergo secondary ossification.

*Angiomas* are tumors composed of newly formed blood or lymph vessels. If composed of blood vessels, they are *hemangiomas;* if composed of lymph vessels, they are *lymphangiomas.* Angiomas are to be differentiated from *telangiectases,* which are dilatations of capillaries or small veins already present.

*Capillary* hemangiomas consist of a network of capillaries. *Cavernous* hemangiomas consist of large communicating blood spaces that share adjacent thin walls. The most common site of capillary hemangiomas is the skin, especially the skin of the face. They may cover a considerable area and are spoken of as birthmarks, strawberry marks, or port-wine stains. Hemangiomas may ulcerate and be replaced by scar tissue. Cavernous hemangiomas are most often found in the liver and muscle. They are elevated, have a bluish color, and may be emptied by pressure. Marked hemorrhage may attend attempts to remove them. (See Fig. 46-8.)

Capillary lymphangiomas occur on the skin as colorless moles. The cavernous lymphangioma (cystic hygroma) may produce a diffuse enlargement of the tongue (macroglossia) or lip (macrocheilia) or it may occur in the soft tissues of the neck, from which it is removed with difficulty.

**OTHER BENIGN TUMORS**

*Myomas* are tumors composed of muscle. There are two types: *leiomyomas,* derived from smooth muscle, and *rhabdomyomas,* derived from striated or skeletal muscle. The former is one of the most common tumors, the latter one of the rarest. *Leiomyomas* are important in the uterus but may occur in the smooth muscle of the alimentary tract.

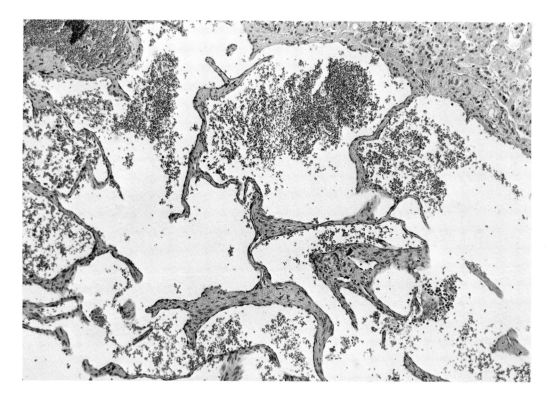

**Fig. 46-8.** Cavernous hemangioma of liver, microscopic section. Note wide vascular spaces separated by thin, poorly supported walls of connective tissue and containing red blood cells. (×120.)

*Pigmented nevi* (pigmented moles) are small dark or brown pedunculated or nonpedunculated structures that occur especially about the neck and face. Nevi are often covered with coarse hair. In a few cases the nevus covers a considerable area (example: the bathing trunk nevus). Nevi are composed of aggregations of peculiar cells, known as nevus cells, which lie beneath the epithelium. These cells contain a brown pigment, melanin, that gives the nevus its color. Nevi are usually congenital, but they may not be noticed until some time after birth. As a rule, they grow to a certain point and become stationary or regress, but occasionally they develop marked growth capacities and give rise to a highly malignant neoplasm, the malignant melanoma.

**MALIGNANT DEGENERATION**

Although the transformation of benign into malignant tumors is often discussed, how often it actually occurs is not known. In fact, it is more likely that a malignant tumor will arise from the heretofore normal tissues of an organ than it is that a benign neoplasm in the same location will become malignant. It must be admitted, however, that certain benign neoplasms or tumorlike growths do tend to become malignant

because of their location or the fact that they are subject to repeated injury. For instance, certain polypoid tumors of the alimentary tract are considered precancerous lesions, since it can be determined that a definite percentage of them will eventually be associated with frank cancer. Leukoplakia, a lesion occurring in the mouth and benign at first, is regularly associated with malignancy if the lesion is allowed to persist. So likely are tumors of the bladder to become malignant that pathologists tend to regard *all* such as potentially malignant.

**Malignant neoplasms**

There are certain characteristics that identify a neoplasm as malignant:

1. Malignant neoplasms are rather poorly separated from normal tissues. From the periphery, where growth is active, infiltrating processes extend out to impinge on and destroy the surrounding tissues.
2. They *metastasize;* that is, they spread to different parts of the body, where metastases (foci of secondary growth) are set up.
3. They tend to recur when removed surgically because the tumor cells have widely infiltrated

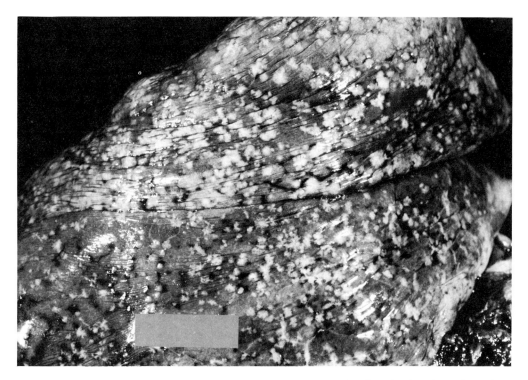

**Fig. 46-9.** Metastatic carcinoma (small ovoid, grayish white areas) distributed in lymphatic channels beneath pleural membrane of lung. Primary carcinoma was in breast.

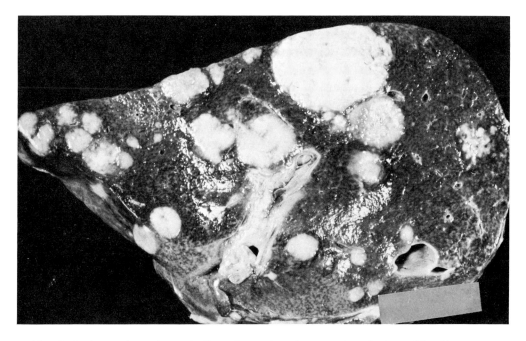

**Fig. 46-10.** Metastatic carcinoma in liver. Cut surface shows varying-sized, grayish white masses of secondary tumor replacing much of liver. Primary tumor was in tail of pancreas.

the surrounding tissue and the borders are poorly outlined.

4. They cause extensive destruction of tissue.
5. They produce such effects in the body as anemia, weakness, and loss of weight.
6. They have little resemblance to the normal cells of the parent tissue.
7. They kill, regardless of location, unless properly and vigorously treated.

The cells of malignant neoplasms are usually immature, with a capacity to multiply rapidly. This is why they grow faster than benign neoplasms. The arrangement of the cells in the malignant tumor does not conform to that of any normal tissue.

The two important groups of malignant neoplasms are the *carcinomas* of epithelial origin and the *sarcomas* of nonepithelial origin.

**Spread.** Malignant neoplasms spread by direct invasion of the surrounding tissues. Occasionally they spread by contact or implantation. By *metastasis* is meant the transfer of cells that have broken off from the parent tumor to other parts of the body, where they lodge, multiply, and produce secondary neoplasms similar to the primary focus. Metastasis may occur by the lymphatic system, the bloodstream, and transplantation across a serous cavity. Metastasis by the lymph stream is usually regional, that is, to the lymph nodes draining the area (Fig. 46-9). The lungs and liver are the most common sites of secondary growths when metastasis occurs by the bloodstream (Fig. 46-10). Sarcomas are said to metastasize by the bloodstream and carcinomas to metastasize by the lymph stream, but this is by no means invariable.

When metastasis occurs by way of the lymph stream, the tumor cells first lodge in the lymph nodes draining the tumor site. These nodes hold the cells in check for a time, but finally the cells gain the upper hand and by their multiplication destroy the nodes and replace them with tumor. Tumor cells then escape to the next set of nodes, and the process is repeated. This continues until the last lymphatic barrier has been overcome and the cells can pass directly into the bloodstream by way of the thoracic duct to be spread to remote parts of the body. When a malignant growth that metastasizes by the lymphatics is surgically excised, it is necessary to remove the regional lymph nodes as completely and extensively as possible.

In metastasis by transplantation, malignant cells break away from a tumor in a serous cavity (example: certain malignant tumors of the ovary) or invade a serous cavity (example: carcinoma of breast invading the pleural cavity) to be conveyed mechanically by the fluid of that cavity to different parts of the serous membrane, where they lodge, attach, and set up new foci of growth.

To a great extent, metastatic tumors retain the characteristics of the parent tumor. Some tumors metastasize early in their course, whereas others metastasize late. Occasionally metastasis may be far advanced before the primary neoplasm is clinically perceptible. In Table 46-8 are listed the important sites of metastasis of the more frequently encountered neoplasms. With the exception of the lungs, in which both primary and secondary malignant neoplasms are common, organs that are often the site of primary

**Table 46-8**

Patterns of metastases

| TUMOR | POINTS OF METASTASIS |
|---|---|
| Carcinoma of stomach and large intestine | Liver, peritoneum |
| Carcinoma of lung | Regional lymph nodes, other lung, liver, bones, and brain |
| Carcinoma of breast | Regional lymph nodes, lungs, and bones |
| Carcinoma of skin | Regional lymph nodes |
| Carcinoma of mouth and lip | Lymph nodes of neck |
| Carcinoma of prostate gland | Bones |
| Carcinoma of uterus | Cervix: body of uterus, vagina, pelvic lymph nodes, adnexal organs, bladder, and rectum<br>Body: regional lymph nodes, cervix, adnexal organs, and peritoneum |
| Carcinoma of ovary | Peritoneum, opposite ovary, uterine tubes, and uterus |
| Carcinoma of kidney | Bones |
| Carcinoma of thyroid gland | Bones, lungs, and regional lymph nodes |
| Sarcomas (soft tissue, bone, others) | Lungs and liver |
| Melanoma of eye | Liver |

malignant neoplasm are seldom the site of the metastatic one and vice versa.

In Table 46-9 is shown the susceptibility of organs to primary and secondary malignancies.

The complete removal of a malignant neoplasm is extremely difficult. From a practical standpoint a neoplasm may be considered cured if it does not recur within 5 years after treatment.

## MALIGNANT EPITHELIAL NEOPLASMS

We now come to the most interesting of all neoplasms, the carcinomas, which are among the most common ones affecting persons past 35 years of age. They are by no means rare in younger persons and when occurring in young people are more highly malignant than in older persons. Since epithelial cells form the superficial layers of the skin and mucous membranes as well as the active tissues of many organs and the lining of glands, it follows that carcinomas may occur in almost any part of the body.

A carcinoma occurs as a cauliflower-like growth, as a diffuse hardening of the tissues, or as an ulcer. The induration produced by certain internal carcinomas may be apparent on the surface, for example, the retraction of the nipple seen in cancer of the breast. Carcinomas often undergo ulceration. They usually spread by invasion of the lymphatics and by the outgrowth of branching extensions from the primary tumor that invade and destroy the surrounding tissues. A simple classification is as follows:

1. *Squamous cell carcinoma* (epidermoid carcinoma, epithelioma), arising from stratified squamous (pavement) epithelium—Squamous cell carcinoma may occur in any area where stratified squamous epithelium is found. Squamous cell carcinomas are most common on the skin and the lip and in the lung, mouth, and cervix uteri. Normally the downgrowth of pavement epithelium is limited by a struc-

ture known as the basement membrane. In squamous cell carcinoma the cells break through this barrier, invade the underlying tissues, and destroy them. *Basal cell carcinoma* (rodent ulcer), a variety of squamous carcinoma occurring in the skin, differs in structure from squamous cell carcinoma, does not grow so rapidly, and does not metastasize. It occurs most often in the regions of the face bordered by the ears, upper lip, and hairline as an ulcerative lesion that locally at times can be quite destructive, not only of soft tissues but also of regional bone. (See Fig. 46-11.)

2. *Adenocarcinoma,* arising from glands and producing glands or gland-like structures—This tumor is composed of cells whose cytoplasm possesses secretory functions. Adenocarcinomas* are found where glandular tissue is present normally. They are especially common in the alimentary tract, lung, female breast, and uterus.

3. *Transitional cell carcinoma,* arising from the stratified pavement epithelium lining the passages of the urinary tract—This type of carcinoma occurs in the renal pelvis, ureter, urinary bladder, and urethra.

## MALIGNANT CONNECTIVE TISSUE NEOPLASMS

Sarcomas are malignant neoplasms of connective tissue origin. The cells of sarcomas seem to have the quality of lawless multiplication more highly developed than any other tumor. Sarcomas are usually highly malignant because of both their widely invasive growth and the formation of distant metastases at an early stage.

---

*The more important adenocarcinomas and certain other neoplasms are discussed with diseases of the given organ system in subsequent chapters.

## Table 46-9

Occurrence of primary and secondary neoplasms

| FREQUENTLY SITE OF PRIMARY MALIGNANT NEOPLASM; SELDOM SITE OF SECONDARY | FREQUENTLY SITE OF SECONDARY MALIGNANT NEOPLASM; SELDOM SITE OF PRIMARY | SELDOM SITE OF MALIGNANT NEOPLASM; EITHER PRIMARY OR SECONDARY |
|---|---|---|
| Stomach | Lymph nodes | Spleen |
| Tongue | Liver | Heart |
| Breast | Pleura | Skeletal muscle |
| Uterus | Bone marrow | |
| Pancreas | | |
| Thyroid gland | | |
| Prostate gland | | |

Being of connective tissue origin, sarcomas are likely to occur in any part of the body (Fig. 46-12). They are more common in early life but may occur in elderly persons. Growth may be slow at first and then rapid, or it may be rapid from the beginning. Sarcomas are soft, bulky tumors of a white, gray, or pink color, with an abundant blood supply. They are usually single but may be multiple. Growth of the tumor may be so rapid that its blood supply is outstripped, which results in degenerative changes and hemorrhage. This is so frequent that a hemorrhage in a tumor suggests a sarcomatous nature. The cells of sarcomas are often round or spindle shaped and show marked variation in size and shape. Sarcomas differ from carcinomas in that they metastasize widely by way of the bloodstream at an earlier time in their course.

## OTHER MALIGNANT NEOPLASMS

*Gliomas* arise from neuroglia, the supporting tissue of the central nervous system. They occur in the brain and the retina. They do not metastasize but kill by local invasion and destruction. *Neuroblastomas* are rare tumors of childhood, composed of primitive and undeveloped nerve cells. Peculiarly they occur more often in the adrenal glands than in the nervous system.

*Malignant melanomas* (Figs. 46-13 and 46-14) are highly malignant brown or black pigmented tumors that usually arise from certain kinds of pigmented nevi in the skin but that may arise in other locations, especially in the eye. Most pigmented nevi remain

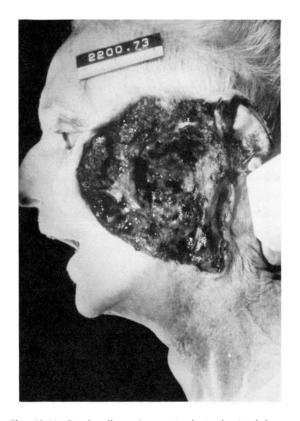

**Fig. 46-11.** Basal cell carcinoma (rodent ulcer) of face.

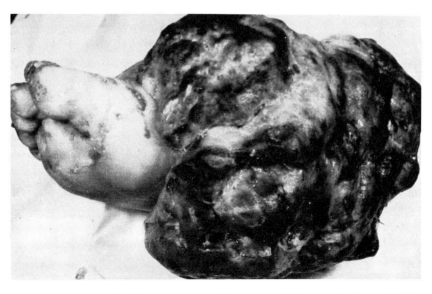

**Fig. 46-12.** Large fungating rhabdomyosarcoma of foot. (From Ackerman, L. V., and del Regato, J. A.: Cancer, ed. 4, St. Louis, 1970, The C. V. Mosby Co.)

quiescent throughout life, but a few give rise to these highly malignant tumors. Secondary melanotic foci appear in the skin. The spread continues rather rapidly until the lungs, kidneys, and other organs are studded with black tumor growths. Metastasis is widespread and destructive. Melanin, the pigment that gives the tumors their color, may appear in the urine.

*Malignant lymphomas* are tumors composed of lymphoid cells (the cells of which lymph nodes are composed) and occur in lymph nodes, spleen, and areas of the body, such as the bowel, where there are concentrations of lymphoid tissue. Lymphatic leukemia, a disease in which abnormal numbers of lymphocytes are seen in peripheral blood and bone marrow, is closely related to malignant lymphoma. An alternate term sometimes used for malignant lymphoma is *lymphosarcoma*.

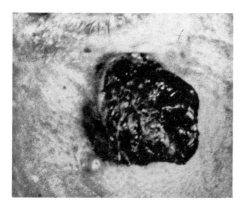

**Fig. 46-13.** Typical elevated black malignant melanoma of cheek, clinical photograph. (W. U. Neg. 52-4098; from Ackerman, L. V., and Rosai, V.: Surgical pathology, ed. 5, St. Louis, 1974, The C. V. Mosby Co.)

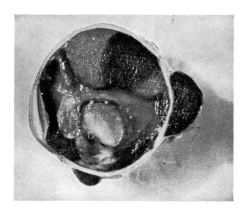

**Fig. 46-14.** Malignant melanoma of eye. Black tumor mass almost fills interior of eye and is also seen outside globe. (From Anderson, W. A. D.: Surgery **9**:425, 1941.)

## ESTIMATING THE MALIGNANCY OF A NEOPLASM

In estimating the malignancy of a neoplasm the following characteristics must be considered: (1) kind of neoplasm, (2) location, (3) extent of local growth and occurrence of metastasis, (4) rate of growth, (5) age of patient, and (6) microscopic appearance.

Some tumors are more likely to cause death than others. Malignant melanomas usually cause death regardless of treatment, whereas a basal cell carcinoma may exist for years without causing death, even if no treatment is given. Tumors in some locations are more dangerous than the same kind of tumor occurring in other locations. For example, a squamous cell carcinoma arising from a keratosis of the face is much less likely to cause death than is one arising on the hand or foot.

When a tumor has metastasized, the prognosis is unfavorable and increasingly poor with the extent of the metastases. As a rule, fast-growing tumors are more deadly than are slow-growing ones, but this is not always true. With some tumors the young succumb more quickly than the elderly. Broders, formerly of the Mayo Clinic, devised a method of grading tumors based on microscopic features in which, in order of malignancy, the tumor is placed in grade 1, 2, 3, or 4. This method is of distinct value.

## ECONOMIC IMPORTANCE AND VALUE OF EARLY DIAGNOSIS IN MALIGNANT NEOPLASMS

When we realize that in the registration area of the United States there are more than 1 million Americans being treated for malignant tumors, with an annual death rate of around 368,000, and that about 671,000 new cases are diagnosed each year, the economic importance of malignant neoplasm becomes apparent. More than 53 million Americans now living, at least one in four, will eventually have cancer according to present rates. At the present time malignant neoplasms are the second most important cause of death, and the death rate given above is increasing annually. The idea that cancer is primarily a disease of later life has done much to prevent its early recognition. Let us remember that although cancer pervades the later decades, it is by no means uncommon in early life. Its frequency during this period is increasing.

Since the cause of cancer is unknown, any discussion of it must deal with unknown factors. The practical weapons to stem the rising tide of malignant tumors now at our command are prevention, early recognition, correct diagnosis, and proper treatment applied early. The close relation that nurses and other members of the health care team bear to the physician, the patient, and the patient's family often places them in such a position that they can do a great deal. For this reason they should possess the general facts on cancer control and should be familiar with signs and symptoms that indicate beginning malignancy in the different organs.

**General facts.** Statistics show that the average patient waits 8 months after first suspecting a malignant condition before consulting a physician. With some tumors each month of delay decreases the chances of cure 16%. About half the number of cancer victims each year could be saved by early diagnosis and proper treatment. Many tumors appear to bear a definite relation to one of the various types of chronic irritation to which the body is continually exposed. To prevent this exposure or clear up the focus of irritation is to prevent cancer. The method that, more than any other, will bring to light beginning tumors is a periodic physical examination by a competent physician. It should be carried out at least once a year, and in women it should include a pelvic examination with a Pap (Papanicolaou) smear.

**Danger signals of cancer.** The American Cancer Society, Inc., considers the following the important danger signals of cancer:

1. Any sore that does not heal
2. A lump or thickening, in the breast or elsewhere
3. Unusual bleeding or discharge from a body orifice
4. Any change in a wart or mole
5. Persistent indigestion or difficulty in swallowing
6. Persistent hoarseness or cough
7. Any change in normal bowel habits

**Cancer of the skin.** The most prevalent type of cancer is that of the skin, but when detected early, it has a better than 90% cure rate. Lesions that show an increase in growth or other signs of activity should be treated to prevent their becoming malignant. Signs of early malignancy in pigmented moles are increase in size and increase in amount of pigment. Scaly small pigmented patches about the face of elderly persons are likely to become malignant. Weeping sores and those that continuously break down, scab, and heal may be malignant. An ulcer that does not heal after some 3 weeks should be studied to determine its malignant or nonmalignant nature.

## TUMORS IN CHILDREN

Tumors of childhood are by no means rare. Cancer kills more children in the 1 to 14 age group than any other disease. Benign tumors are more common than malignant ones. In children the common areas where malignancies originate are the central nervous system, eye, kidney, adrenal gland, and hematopoietic system. Only a small number are present in the endocrine glands, but when such tumors do occur, striking functional changes appear clinically because of the relationship of the endocrines to normal growth and development. Organs such as the breast, uterus, ovary, prostate gland, and gastrointestinal tract, commonly involved in adults, are rarely involved in children. Carcinoma of the skin is almost unheard of in young children. Metastatic tumor involvement of lung is fairly common, but primary lung neoplasm is rare. Although nevi are universally present even at birth, malignant melanoma is relatively rare. Many neoplasms of childhood seem to be peculiar to this age group and are not seen to any considerable extent in later life. The first sign of a tumor in a child is usually a mass.

Other neoplasms are discussed in the chapter dealing with diseases of the given organ system.

## CANCER THERAPY

Malignant neoplasms are treated by surgery, radiation, chemotherapy, and immunotherapy.

**Surgical treatment.** Surgical procedures are designed to remove the primary focus, enough normal tissue to include the ill-defined extensions into neighboring tissues, and, in some instances, the path of spread and lodgment in the regional lymph nodes.

**Radiation therapy.** The fundamental principle of radiation (x-ray and radium) therapy of malignant neoplasms is that the cells of malignant neoplasms are poorly differentiated cells and are therefore destroyed by radiation doses that have little effect on the normal cells of the body. Certain types of tumor cells are more easily destroyed by radiation than others. Although rapidly growing tumors composed of actively proliferating cells are more sensitive to radiation than slowly growing ones, it is not necessarily true that the more malignant a tumor is, the more sensitive it is to radiation. For instance, certain melanomas are highly malignant but not sensitive to radiation, whereas lymphomas are less malignant than melanomas but much more sensitive to radiation.

**Chemotherapy.** The use of drugs and other chemicals for treating cancer is still a research activity. The following are listed as kinds of agents with which results are encouraging: (1) cytotoxic agents, (2) antimetabolites, (3) steroid hormones, (4) selected antibiotics, and (5) radioactive isotopes.

Nitrogen mustards, which are highly toxic and with action comparable to radiation (radiomimetic), are examples of cytotoxic agents. They are used in the treatment of lymphomas and leukemias. The antimetabolites can interfere with metabolic processes of malignant cells because of their deceptive chemical similarity to certain essential vitamins or other metabolites. The widely used folic acid antagonists (example: amethopterin) produce good clinical remissions in children with acute leukemia. Steroid hormones are used with cancer of the breast and prostate gland. Estrogens provide temporary but dramatic relief to the patient with cancer of the prostate gland. Corticosteroid hormones are effective in lymphomas and leukemias. At least two antineoplastic antibiotics, actinomycin D and mitomycin C, both elaborated by Streptomycetes, and vinblastine, an alkaloid from the periwinkle plant, have an unfavorable effect on tumor growth. Examples of radioactive isotopes used are radioactive phosphorus ($^{32}$P) and radioactive gold ($^{198}$Au).

**Immunotherapy.** Immunotherapy refers to the mobilization of the body's own resources. The fact that the immune system of the cancer patient is inefficient as compared to that of the healthy noncancerous person has started a search for ways to bolster those protective immune responses in cancer patients. There are two approaches being given considerable thought today. One involves the use of BCG vaccine. BCG seems to stimulate and strengthen the cellular immunity of the body in an overall way. There is also interest in transfer factor. The administration of transfer factor supposedly confers a kind of "instant" cellular immunity. Immunotherapy has been somewhat successful on occasions, and the long-range prospects are encouraging.

## CAUSE OF DEATH

The death of a person with a malignant neoplasm is often caused by the associated or intercurrent complications rather than by the primary effects of the neoplasm. Among these are bronchopneumonia (most common cause), cachexia, spread of the tumor to vital organs, dissemination of the tumor over the body, obstruction of the natural passages of the body (as with tumors of the intestine or bladder), hemorrhage, and renal failure.

## Teratomas

Teratomas are complex tumors composed of irregularly arranged tissues that represent a conglomeration of several different organs. They are caused by errors in development and may be regarded as attempts to form a new individual within the tissues (usually the sex organs) of the host. A study of fetal development will show that there is a descending relation existing between identical twins, double monsters, parasitic fetuses, and teratomas. Teratomas occur chiefly in the ovary and testicle.

Closely related to the teratomas but of a simpler nature are the mixed tumors of the salivary glands and kidneys.

## Cysts

Cysts are saccular spaces walled off by connective tissue whose contents are liquid or semifluid. Cysts composed of one compartment are *unilocular* cysts; those composed of several compartments are *multilocular* cysts. Cysts have no special relation to tumors other than that certain tumors may be cystic or the walls of certain cysts may give rise to tumors. If a cyst forms part of a neoplasm, it is referred to as a neoplastic cyst.

Some cysts are congenital and may be caused by the persistence of ducts that normally disappear after embryonic life or to other errors of development. Such cysts may be found in the neck (branchial cleft cysts and thyroglossal duct cysts) or in the genitourinary tract (polycystic disease of the kidneys). Congenital cysts may also occur in the liver and lungs.

*Retention cysts* result from the occlusion of the duct of a gland with retention of secretions. A good example is the sebaceous cyst or wen, which is caused by the occlusion of the mouth of a sebaceous gland. Follicular cysts are the result of the oversecretion of glandular structures that do not have an outlet duct. The best example is the follicular cyst of the ovary.

Localized necrosis and softening in solid organs may lead to the formation of cystlike structures known as *pseudocysts.* Cysts may be associated with the growth of certain parasites. One of this type important in man is the echinococcus cyst, caused by a type of tapeworm, *Echinococcus granulosus* (p. 360).

## Questions for review

1 Define *neoplasm.* Explain how the word tumor is used in relation to neoplasms. What is the true and exact meaning of *tumor?*
2 What are the predisposing causes of tumors?
3 How are tumors classified from a clinical standpoint? From a histologic standpoint?
4 What are the outstanding characteristics of benign tumors?
5 Briefly describe keloid, chondroma, teratoma, retention cyst, hypertrophy, hyperplasia, metaplasia, osteoma, pigmented nevus, malignant melanoma.
6 What are the outstanding characteristics of malignant tumors?
7 What is meant by metastasis? How does it occur?
8 List oncogenic agents and their tumors.
9 Name the three classes of carcinomas.
10 Give three ways in which nonmalignant tumors may cause death.
11 What are the basic differences between a sarcoma and a carcinoma?
12 Give the seven danger signals of cancer.

**REFERENCES** (Chapter 46)

Ackerman, L. V., and del Regato, J. A.: Cancer: diagnosis, treatment, and prognosis, ed. 4, St. Louis, 1970, The C. V. Mosby Co.

Bhaskar, S. N.: Synopsis of oral pathology, ed. 4, St. Louis, 1973, The C. V. Mosby Co.

Booth, S. N., and others: Carcinoembryonic antigen (CEA) in management of colorectal carcinoma, Br. Med. J. **4:**183, 1974.

Bray, G. T.: Sign of the crab, Lab. Med. **1:**9, April, 1970.

Brooks, S. M.: The cancer story, Totowa, N.J., 1973, Littlefield, Adams & Co.

Bryan, W. R., and Endicott, K. M.: The problem of viral oncogenesis (editorial), Ann. Intern. Med. **67:**453, 1967.

Burger, M. M.: Surface properties of neoplastic cells, Hosp. Pract. **8:**55, July, 1973.

'75 cancer facts and figures, New York, 1974, American Cancer Society, Inc.

Carter, L. J.: Cancer and the environment. I. A creaky system grinds on, Science **186:**239, 1974.

Cole, J. W.: Carcinogens and carcinogenesis in the colon, Hosp. Pract. **8:**123, Sept., 1973.

Commoner, B.: Cancer as an environmental disease, Hosp. Pract. **10:**82, Feb., 1975.

Dean, A. G., and others: Clinical events suggesting Herpessimplex infection before onset of Burkitt lymphoma, Lancet **2:**1225, 1973.

Etiology of Burkitt's lymphoma (editorial), J.A.M.A. **198:**77, 1966.

German, J.: Oncogenic implications of chromosomal instability, Hosp. Pract. **8:**93, Feb., 1973.

Glemser, B.: The great "tumor safari," Today's Health **46:**44, Sept., 1968.

Gold, P.: Tumor-specific antigen in GI cancer, Hosp. Pract. **7:**79, Feb., 1972.

Gottlieb, S. K.: Chromosomal abnormalities in certain human malignancies, J.A.M.A. **209:**1063, 1969.

Gross, L.: Oncogenic viruses, ed. 2, Elmsford, N.Y., 1970, Pergamon Press, Inc.

Gross, L.: The role of viruses in the etiology of cancer and leukemia, J.A.M.A. **230:**1029, 1974.

Haagensen, C. D.: The lymphatics in cancer, Philadelphia, 1972, W. B. Saunders Co.

Hellström, K. E., and Hellström, I.: Immunologic defenses against cancer, Hosp. Pract. **5:**45, Jan., 1970.

Hersh, E. M., and others: Immunotherapy of cancer in man; scientific basis and current status, Springfield, Ill., 1973, Charles C Thomas, Publisher.

Holleb, A. I., and Ross, W. S.: Using the cancer cures we have now, Today's Health **48:**48, April, 1970.

Hussey, H. H.: Cancer immunotherapy (editorial), J.A.M.A. **227:**435, 1974.

James, A. G.: U.S. cancer death rate leveling . . . except for soaring lung cancer, Lab. Med. **1:**56, March, 1970.

Joncas, J., and others: Epstein-Barr virus infection in neonatal period and in childhood, Can. Med. Assoc. J. **110:**33, 1974.

Lilienfeld, A. M., and others: Cancer in the United States, Cambridge, Mass., 1972, Harvard University Press.

Lo Gerfo, P., and others: Studies on tumor-associated antigen: TAA, J. Surg. Res. **15:**290, 1973.

Macintyre, E. H.: Oncogenic viruses and human neoplasia, J. Am. Med. Wom. Assoc. **23:**520, 1968.

Marx, J. L.: Biochemistry of cancer cells: focus on cell surface, Science **183:**1279, 1974.

Marx, J. L.: Drinking water: another source of carcinogens? Science **186:**809, 1974.

Marx, J. L.: Tumor immunology. I. The host's response to cancer, Science **184:**552, 1974.

Marx, J. L.: Tumor immunology. II. Strategies for cancer therapy, Science **184:**652, 1974.

Marx, J. L.: Viral carcinogenesis: role of DNA viruses, Science **183:**1066, 1974.

Maugh, T. H., II: Cancer chemotherapy: now a promising weapon, Science **184:**970, 1974.

Maugh, T. H., II: Chemical carcinogenesis; a long-neglected field blossoms, Science **183:**940, 1974.

Maugh, T. H., II: RNA viruses: the age of innocence ends, Science **183:**1181, 1974.

Maugh, T. H., II: Vitamin A: potential protection from carcinogens, Science **186:**1198, 1974.

Maugh, T. H., II: Leukemia: a second human tumor virus, Science **187:**335, 1975.

McKerns, K. W., editor: Hormones and cancer, New York, 1974, Academic Press, Inc.

Melnick, J. L., and Rawls, W. E.: Herpesvirus in the induction of cervical carcinoma, Hosp. Pract. **4:**37, Feb., 1969.

Moore, C.: A synopsis of clinical cancer, ed. 2, St. Louis, 1970, The C. V. Mosby Co.

Moore, D. H.: Evidence in favor of existence of human breast cancer virus, Cancer Res. **34:**2322, 1974.

Moore, G. E.: Cancer: 100 different diseases, Am. J. Nurs. **66:**749, 1966.

Moore, G. E.: Cancer immunity: fact or fiction? Tex. Med. **64:**54, Oct., 1968.

Rapp, F.: Viruses and neoplasia, Hosp. Pract. **6:**49, May, 1971.

Rous, P.: The challenge to man of the neoplastic cell, Science **157:**24, 1967.

Rubin, P.: The cancer syndrome, J.A.M.A. **229:**1651, 1974.

Ryser, H. J.-P.: Special report: chemical carcinogenesis, CA **24:**351, 1974.

Schanche, D. A.: Cancer countdown to a significant advance, Today's Health **51:**44, July, 1973.

Schanche, D. A.: Vinyl chloride: time bomb on the production line, Today's Health **52:**16, Sept., 1974.

Silverstein, M. J., and Morton, D. L.: Cancer immunotherapy, Am. J. Nurs. **73:**1178, 1973.

Stevens, D. P., and Mackay, I. R.: Increased carcinoembryonic antigen in heavy cigarette smokers, Lancet **2:**1238, 1973.

Sutow, W. W., and others, editors: Clinical pediatric oncology, St. Louis, 1973, The C. V. Mosby Co.

Svoboda, E. H.: The child under treatment, Am. J. Nurs. **68:**532, 1968.

Talso, P. J., and Remenchik, A. P., editors: Internal medicine—based on mechanisms of disease, St. Louis, 1968, The C. V. Mosby Co.

Turner, M. D.: Carcinoembryonic antigen, J.A.M.A. **231:**756, 1975.

Vaisrub, S.: Immunotherapy for melanoma (editorial), J.A.M.A. **225:**1242, 1973.

Weiss, K.: Epidemiology of vaginal adenocarcinoma and adenosis: current status, J. Am. Med. Wom. Assoc. **30:**59, 1975.

Whitmore, W. F.: Wilms' tumor and neuroblastoma, Am. J. Nurs. **68:**527, 1968.

Willis, J., and Willis, M.: ". . . But there are always miracles," New York, 1974, Viking Press, Inc.

Willis, R. A.: Pathology of tumors, New York, 1967, Appleton-Century-Crofts.

Wilson, R. E., moderator: Horizons in tumor immunology, a seminar, Arch. Surg. **109:**17, 1974.

Wood, D. A.: New concepts in cancer control—preventable and avoidable cancer, CA **20:**140, 1970.

# Diseases of

# Cardiovascular system

## Heart

When one realizes that at the present time the most common cause of disability and death is heart disease, its importance becomes apparent. With our increased life-span the incidence of heart disease is rising steadily. If we include associated kidney disease in the use of the term *cardiovascular renal disease,* we can account for nearly one half of all deaths.

The physiologic pump that maintains the circulation of blood in the body is the heart. A strong organ primarily composed of striated muscle, it contracts and relaxes continuously around seventy to eighty times per minute for all the years of a person's life. It is made up of four chambers—two atria and two ventricles. On one side the right atrium opens into the right ventricle through the tricuspid valve. On the other side the left atrium communicates with the left ventricle through the mitral valve. From the large veins of the systemic circulation, blood drains into the right atrium. The right ventricle pumps it into the pulmonary vasculature to be oxygenated. From the pulmonary circuit the pulmonary veins collect blood for the left atrium. The left ventricle pumps blood into the intricate network of arteries, capillaries, and veins that comprise the systemic circulation (Fig. 47-1).

**Hypertrophy and dilatation.** There are two terms that enter into any discussion of cardiac pathology: (1) *hypertrophy,* meaning an increase in the size of the individual cardiac muscle fibers, and (2) *dilatation,* indicating an increase in the length (stretching) of the fibers. Either hypertrophy or dilatation causes enlargement of the heart, one of the most important clinical signs of heart disease.

In cardiac hypertrophy the increase in the size and strength of the heart muscle is a response to an increased work load. The important causes of hypertrophy are (1) obstruction to the flow of blood through the peripheral blood vessels, (2) disease conditions involving the heart valves, and (3) inflammatory and de-

generative changes in the heart muscle. Seldom does hypertrophy affect both sides of the heart equally, the chamber of the heart chiefly affected determined by the cause of the hypertrophy. Because of their thin muscular walls, the atria do not hypertrophy to the extent that the ventricles do. When there is an increased resistance to the flow of blood through the systemic vessels (as with hypertension), the left ventricle hypertrophies; when there is an increased resistance in the pulmonary circulation (as in emphysema), the right ventricle hypertrophies. There is a limit to the hypertrophy that the heart may undergo, and when this limit is passed, the patient goes into heart failure.

When a heart chamber is filled with more blood than normal, there is stretching of the cardiac muscle fibers and an increase in the volume capacity of that chamber. The chamber dilates. Physiologically this stretching of the muscle fibers results in increased strength of muscular contraction. For this reason dilatation of the heart is considered to precede the development of hypertrophy. In certain infectious diseases such as diphtheria, dilatation of the heart may be the result of a toxic effect on the muscle fibers, destroying their power to contract effectively. Acute toxic dilatation of the heart may be the cause of death in a severe infectious disease.

## MAJOR DISORDERS

In heart disease today the big five are congenital heart disease, coronary artery disease, hypertensive heart disease, rheumatic heart disease, and valvular disease. Coronary artery disease and hypertensive heart disease are the most frequent.

### Congenital heart disease

The list of malformations that have been described in the heart and great blood vessels is a long one. Generally the malformations involve (1) the position or size of the heart, (2) some rearrangement of the valves, or (3) the failure of development of a complete

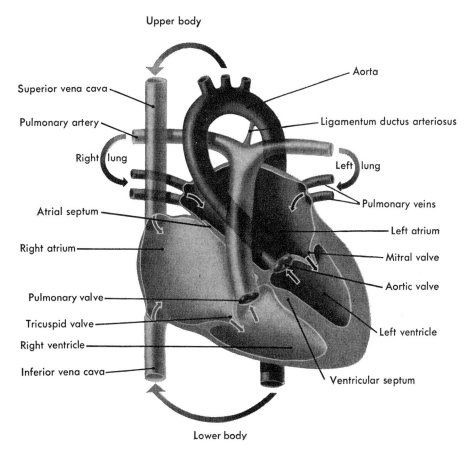

**Fig. 47-1.** The heart. Section to show *normal* flow of blood. Arrows indicate route through four chambers and great vessels. (From Ross clinical education aid no. 7, Ross Laboratories, Columbus, Ohio. In Young, C. G., and Barger, J. D.: Introduction to medical science, ed. 2, St. Louis, 1973, The C. V. Mosby Co.)

muscular partition to separate the right and left sides of the heart (Figs. 47-2 and 47-3).

Certain congenital cardiac defects, especially those in either the interauricular or interventricular septum, allow venous blood to be shunted from the *right* to the *left* side of the heart. The presence of venous blood in the arteries in sizable amounts produces *cyanosis*. Infants who are affected with congenital heart disease of such a nature that this mixing of venous and arterial blood occurs are cyanotic at birth and are known as blue babies.

The exact cause of congenital defects of the heart is largely unknown (Chapter 40). Most such defects are believed to form during the fifth to eighth week of intrauterine life, the time when the single-chambered tubular heart is undergoing a complicated stage of development to form a structure with four chambers.

Minor congenital anomalies may not have any effect on the heart other than to make it more sus-

ceptible to bacterial infection *(endocarditis)*, but extensive defects may seriously impair the capacity of the heart to perform work and may make postnatal life of any duration impossible. In addition to cyanosis the imperfect circulation accompanying congenital heart disease causes proliferative changes in the tissues, prominent among which are thickening of the lips and nose and clubbing of the ends of the fingers.

Congenital heart disease is receiving an increased amount of attention in recent years, for with greatly improved and newly developed technics of cardiac surgery, it is now possible to remedy certain defects and greatly to improve the physiologic effects of others that do not lend themselves to surgical elimination. For example, a *patent ductus arteriosus*, an abnormal communication between the aorta and the pulmonary artery, if it persists into postnatal life, can be completely obliterated. The physiologic disorders occasioned by a tetralogy of Fallot can be greatly improved

**529**

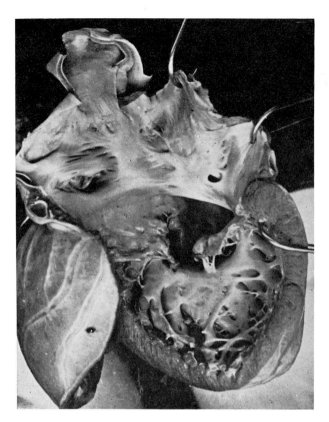

**Fig. 47-2.** Congenital defect of interventricular septum of heart (ostium atrioventriculare commune). You see the interior of left ventricle. The defect is large darkened area just to left of lower metal hook. (Courtesy Dr. V. Moragues, Omaha, Neb.; from Anderson, W. A. D., and Scotti, T. M.: Synopsis of pathology, ed. 8, St. Louis, 1972, The C. V. Mosby Co.)

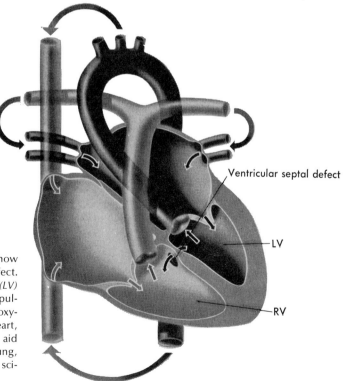

Ventricular septal defect

LV

RV

**Fig. 47-3.** Ventricular septal defect. Section to show *abnormal* flow of blood through congenital defect. Arrows indicate shunt of blood from left ventricle *(LV)* to right ventricle *(RV)* to overload right heart and pulmonary circulation (left-to-right shunt). Since oxygenated blood flows from left to right side of heart, there is no cyanosis. (From Ross clinical eduation aid no. 7, Ross Laboratories, Columbus, Ohio. In Young, C. G., and Barger, J. D.: Introduction to medical science, ed. 2, St. Louis, 1973, The C. V. Mosby Co.)

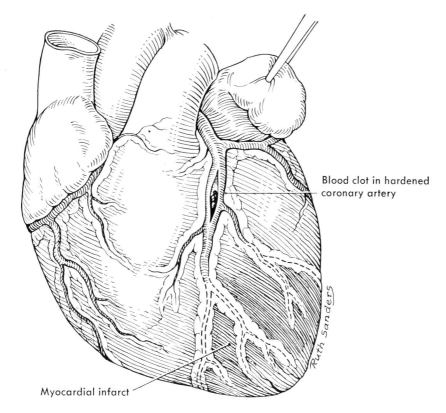

Blood clot in hardened coronary artery

Myocardial infarct

**Fig. 47-4.** Coronary occlusion secondary to coronary atherosclerosis, sketch. Anterior left descending branch of left coronary artery has been opened near its origin to show thrombus formed on an atherosclerotic plaque. The darkened area at apex is an infarct. Here, a nonfatal occlusion is portrayed, as evidenced by early vascular anastomoses about apex.

by cardiac surgery. As its name implies, there are four cardinal manifestations of the fairly common *tetralogy of Fallot:* (1) interventricular septal defect, (2) pulmonary artery stenosis, (3) a shift in the position of the aorta to the right, and (4) hypertrophy of the right ventricle.

**Coronary artery disease**

By coronary artery disease is meant pathologic change in the walls of the coronary arteries and its consequences. Right and left coronary arteries and branches supply nourishment and oxygen to the musculature of the heart.

The disease is especially prevalent among doctors and other professional men.

**Coronary occlusion** (Fig. 47-4). The most common cause of sudden death is heart failure, and the most common cause of heart failure is interference with coronary blood flow. The blood supply of a portion of the heart wall is suddenly cut off by an occlusion of one of the larger branches of the coronary arteries,

usually the anterior descending branch of the left coronary. This happens in 40% of sudden and unexpected deaths. Coronary occlusion may occur as a result of (1) arteriosclerosis, with narrowing of the lumen of the coronary arteries, (2) thrombosis of an already arteriosclerotic artery, (3) syphilitic involvement of the mouths of the coronaries, and (4) blockage of one of the arteries by an embolus. The effects of coronary occlusion depend on the location in the coronary circuit, the rate at which the blockage develops, and the extent to which blood is available through anastomotic connections with parts of the coronary circulation not so crucially involved.

**Myocardial infarction.** Although coronary heart disease is an important cause of sudden death, impairment of coronary blood flow may have other less severe consequences. When heart muscle dies as a result of interference with its blood supply, a myocardial infarct is formed. Infarcts may be large or small, depending on the size of the coronary vessel occluded. They are commonly located in the interventricular

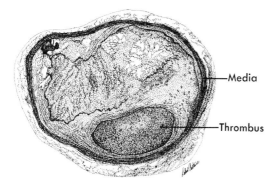

**Fig. 47-5.** Coronary occlusion in cross section of coronary artery, sketch. Circulation through this vessel is blocked as result of intimal thickening with thrombosis. Dark rim at periphery is compressed media (musculature). Changes in the thickened intima (fibrosis, lipid deposits, calcification) fill the great part of diseased vessel shown here.

septum (that part of the heart separating the right and left ventricles) and in the wall of the left ventricle. Sometimes infarction is massive and involves most of the heart muscle, in which case death is imminent. Soon after it is produced, a myocardial infarct begins to heal. For a large infarct, repair processes may require around 2 months. The end stage is a fibrous scar corresponding to the size of the infarcted area.

When interference with coronary blood flow is mild in degree and only slowly progressive, the heart muscle succumbs over small dispersed areas, referred to as *miliary infarcts* because of their minute dimensions. Healing in these results in patchy myocardial fibrosis and scarring of diffuse nature.

Coronary heart disease is most often the result of coronary arteriosclerosis (Fig. 47-5) and its complications, a process as a rule more severe in the left coronary artery. Embarrassment of its circulation generally means that the heart is less able to perform the work required of it. The clinical manifestations of cardiac insufficiency may be either the chest pain of *angina pectoris* or the systemic changes of *congestive heart failure.*

*Diagnostic enzymology.* As we learn more of the role of enzymes in complex biochemical processes going on in the body, certain of their properties suggest a practical application. The following characteristics of enzymes make them adaptable to clinical medicine. (1) Many are found only in precise anatomic areas. (2) They are relatively inert away from their usual biochemical environment. (3) They can be detected in trace amounts because of their catalytic nature. As a result the laboratory assay of certain enzymes has been standardized, and their relation to given diseases studied.

In myocardial infarction enzyme assay is very helpful in diagnosis and treatment. There are four enzymes specifically related to heart muscle and released with its injury. They are glutamic oxaloacetic transaminase (GOT), lactic dehydrogenase (LDH), creatine phosphokinase (CPK), and alpha hydroxybutyric acid dehydrogenase (HBDH). Table 47-1 shows the pattern of serum levels in two commonly used enzyme assays following the acute event of myocardial infarction.

### Hypertensive heart disease

Hypertensive heart disease reflects the pathologic changes in the heart and heart muscle that occur when the heart must pump blood into the peripheral circuits against a pressure head greater than normal. Since the left ventricle is most affected by the increased work load, the striking feature of this type of heart disease is the well-marked left ventricular hypertrophy, which may be associated with diffuse myocardial fibrosis.

**Variations in blood pressure.** By blood pressure is meant the pressure in millimeters of mercury that the blood exerts against the wall of the arteries. It depends on the strength of the heart action, elasticity of the arterial walls, capillary resistance to the blood flow, and the amount and viscosity of the blood. The maximum pressure (*systolic* blood pressure) occurs when the left ventricle reaches its greatest state of contraction, and the minimum (*diastolic* blood pressure) occurs when it is completely relaxed. The dif-

**Table 47-1**

Two serum enzymes important in myocardial infarction

| ENZYME IN SERUM | NORMAL VALUES (standard milliunits [mU]/ml.) | INCREASE AFTER ACUTE MUSCLE INJURY (hours) | PEAK (hours) | VALUES AT MAXIMUM (× normal) | RETURN TO NORMAL (days) |
|---|---|---|---|---|---|
| Serum glutamic oxaloacetic transaminase (SGOT) | 3 to 20 | 4 to 6 | 24 to 48 | 5× to 10× | 4 to 8 |
| Lactic dehydrogenase (LDH) | 40 to 60 | 8 to 24 | 24 to 72 | 3× to 5× | 8 to 14 |

ference between the two is the *pulse* pressure. An increase in the blood pressure is *hypertension,* a decrease *hypotension.* Hypotension occurs acutely in shock and as a more or less chronic condition in wasting diseases such as cancer, tuberculosis, and adrenal insufficiency.

*Hypertension.* In terms of a specific individual, normal blood pressure would be hard to define. From statistical studies on large populations, life insurance companies have evolved the limits of 140 mm. Hg for systolic pressure and 90 mm. Hg for diastolic pressure, above which hypertension is said to exist. In terms of grave consequences it is the *diastolic,* not the systolic, which is significant. Stated simply, hypertension is *increased peripheral resistance* in the cardiovascular circuit, and it is the diastolic pressure that indicates the level of that resistance.

Hypertension may be classified as essential (90% of the cases) and secondary. *Essential* hypertension, so named when no cause can be given for its occurrence, is now known to be significantly related to arteriosclerosis involving very small arteries (arterioles) in the kidneys. Clinically, essential hypertension is divided into the *benign* type, which is of slow evolution among persons in older age groups, and the *malignant* type, which usually occurs in young adults, progresses rapidly, and quickly proves fatal.

Heredity plays a part in the development of hypertension, as do body build (more common in short, stockily built persons) and obesity. Among contributing causes in a genetically susceptible person may be an excessive intake of sodium chloride over a period of time. Hypertension is more common in men than in women and in the black American than in the white. The malignant form is more prone to involve blacks than whites. Death in benign hypertension comes from heart failure, coronary occlusion, or cerebral hemorrhage. Death in malignant hypertension is from acute kidney failure.

The *secondary* type of hypertension complicates known disease, most often that of the vasculature or parenchyma of the kidney, an organ related to regulation of blood pressure. One renal mechanism is through the renin-angiotensin-aldosterone system, a system that may play an etiologic role in hypertension.

Renin is an enzyme formed by the kidney because of a reduction in the effective blood volume or pressure. It acts on angiotensinogen in plasma to convert it to angiotensin I, which is changed to angiotensin II in the lung. Physiologically angiotensin II constricts arterioles and induces secretion of aldosterone by the adrenal cortex. Aldosterone promotes the expansion of the extracellular fluid volume by enhancing sodium reabsorption and potassium excretion by the kidney. This adjustment, coupled with vasoconstriction, tends to elevate blood volume and pressure and depress output of renin. About one fourth of patients with essential hypertension have a low renin-plasma activity.

### Rheumatic heart disease

**Rheumatic fever.** Acute rheumatic fever, the forerunner of rheumatic heart disease, has a clinical course similar to an acute infection. In its acute phase there are fever, an increased pulse rate (tachycardia), and a characteristic type of polyarthritis (p. 638). Rheumatic fever is more common in northern than southern climates and is infrequent in the tropics. It is most common between the sixth and twelfth years of life.

More than 50% of the attacks of acute rheumatic fever are preceded by tonsillitis or severe sore throat caused by hemolytic streptococci. At this time the events of rheumatic fever are interpreted as an allergic reaction to the previous streptococcal infection. An important diagnostic feature is a rise in the serum titer of antistreptolysin O, which occurs in more than 80% of the cases.

The lesion in rheumatic fever is the injury to collagen. Small granulomatous nodules form in the connective tissues of the endocardium, the myocardium, and the pericardium* about foci of degeneration and fibrinoid necrosis of collagen. These nodules are called *Aschoff bodies.* As the inflammatory process subsides, there is healing, and the Aschoff body is converted into a fibrous scar. Similar nodules occur in serous and synovial membranes in other parts of the body and in the brain.

**Organic disease.** The most serious effects of rheumatic fever stem from the lesions in the heart. The increased heart rate reflects the inflammation. Rheumatic fever tends to be a disease of long standing, with repeated acute attacks. This favors the development of complications that add up to serious heart disease. With the buildup of repeated injury to the valves and layers of the heart, there is a corresponding buildup of the fibrous tissues of repair. The repair process greatly affects the valves. Over a period of time they are changed from thin, normally pliable membranes into rigid, thickened, even calcified masses contracted down on their orifices. Visible scarring and deformity mark the pathologic condition of *rheumatic heart disease.*

Important manifestations of rheumatic heart dis-

---

*The pericardium is the outer serous lining of the heart. The myocardium is the cardiac musculature, the functioning element. The endocardium lines the interiors of the four chambers. It is continuous with the endothelium of blood vessels and is folded on itself to form valves interposed between the atrium and ventricle of the same side or positioned at the exits of the ventricles.

ease are: (1) mitral stenosis—scarring of the mitral valve, which by closing off the valvular orifice blocks the flow of blood from the left atrium to the left ventricle, (2) dilatation of the left atrium—enlargement of the left atrium to contain the blood that collects behind the blocked valve (alterations of blood flow in the dilated chamber favor the development of thrombi there), and (3) cardiac arrhythmias—disturbances in the rhythm and rate of the heart.

Prevention of the harmful effects of rheumatic heart disease means stopping the recurrent attacks of acute rheumatic fever. Patients are protected as much as possible from streptococcal infections and are even given antibiotics prophylactically at times of the year when the incidence of such infections is high.

### Valvular disease

**Endocarditis.** Endocarditis is inflammation of the endocardium, including the reduplications thereof that are the heart valves. It is important because of its immediate effects and the permanent injury it produces. The term *endocarditis* without qualification means valvular endocarditis. As a rule, the process selects one or more valves, but it may include the endocardium of the ventricular wall (mural endocarditis). In adults the valves of the left side of the heart are mainly attacked, the mitral valve more often than the aortic. In fetal life those of the right side are more frequently involved.

When bacteria are deposited on a valve, they injure the surface and cause the valve to swell. Fibrin, platelets, and blood cells collect at the site to form thrombi known as *vegetations* (Fig. 47-6). With severe injury, necrosis leads to ulceration of one or more cusps of the valve. Vegetations, ulcerations, the associated reparative changes, and the actual destruction of parts of a valve result in changes (thickening, retraction, and adhesions) incompatible with normal function. Scarred and deformed, the valve is a leaky one. Blood passing through the deformed orifice produces an abnormal blowing sound known as a *murmur*.

*Classification.* Endocarditis may be classified as (1) acute simple or vegetative endocarditis, in which there is little tendency for the vegetations to ulcerate, (2) acute ulcerative endocarditis, in which ulceration and destruction of the valve are the distinguishing features, (3) subacute bacterial endocarditis, in which there are friable vegetations, septic embolism, and a slow clinical course, and (4) chronic endocarditis, or chronic valvular disease.

Acute fulminating endocarditis is most often caused by *Streptococcus pyogenes*. Subacute bacterial endocarditis (SBE) is usually caused by the viridans category of *Streptococcus* species, notably *Streptococcus mitis.** Both may be caused by other orga-

---

*Alpha hemolytic (viridans) streptococci also responsible for SBE include *Strep. salivarius* and *Strep. sanguis*. Although *Strep. viridans* is still used in clinical medicine for the causative streptococcus, this designation is not a true species name.

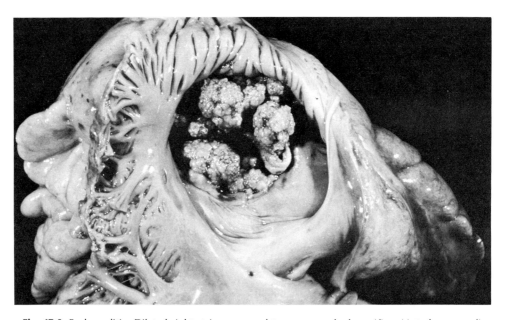

**Fig. 47-6.** Endocarditis. Dilated right atrium opened to expose valvular orifice. Note large, cauliflower-like excrescences (vegetations) on leaflets of tricuspid valve. Causative organism, *Candida albicans*. Patient was a drug addict and, as such, a person prone to involvement of tricuspid valve.

nisms. Many patients with subacute bacterial endocarditis give a history of dental extractions just before the onset of disease. Such dental procedures provide occasion for the transient release of bacteria into the bloodstream, where they precipitate onto a heart valve. The bacteria injure the valve and trigger the formation of a vegetation. The vegetation may fragment and send small infected emboli into the systemic circulation if the thrombus is located on the aortic or mitral valves. These small emboli containing bacteria lodge in the organs of the body and produce infected infarcts.

**Chronic valvular disease.** Chronic valvular disease is associated with end-stage deformities of two types. In one type the cusps of the valve become shortened, thickened, curled, or otherwise deformed, so that the valve cannot close properly. Blood leaks back into the cavity behind the lesion when the chamber in front contracts. For instance, when the mitral valve is diseased, blood leaks back into the left atrium during contraction of the left ventricle. This results in an *insufficiency* or *incompetency* of the valve or a *regurgitation* of blood. In the second type of deformity, *stenosis*, the orifice becomes closed off because of contraction of the supporting valve ring, projection of stiffened cusps, and adhesions between the edges of the cusps. A normal volume of blood cannot be pumped through it. Insufficiency and stenosis are frequently associated.

Acquired valvular deformities are usually a result of chronic rheumatic endocarditis. With rheumatic valvulitis the mitral valve and then the aortic valve are most frequently involved. Syphilis is occasionally a cause of chronic valvular disease affecting the aortic valve. The process usually represents an extension of syphilitic aortitis.

When a valve becomes stenosed, the cavity forcing the blood through the opening hypertrophies to overcome the obstruction to the blood flow. In regurgitation the cavity behind the affected valve dilates and hypertrophies to take care of the normal amount of blood plus that which is regurgitated. As long as the hypertrophied heart furnishes sufficient blood to the body, the defect is said to be *compensated*. When the hypertrophied heart can no longer do this, heart failure occurs, and the defect is said to be *decompensated*. Decompensation is characterized by dyspnea, edema, cyanosis, ascites, and enlargement of the liver.

## Blood vessels
### ARTERIES

**Arteriosclerosis** (Fig. 47-7). Arteriosclerosis is a degenerative process that produces a hardening, thickening, and inflexibility of the arterial side of the circulation. Its most important effect is to interfere with the blood flow and therefore to impair the blood supply to crucial areas of the body. When the degenerative process involves the large elastic arteries such as the aorta and the coronary and cerebral arteries, it is a change primarily concentrated in the lining (intima) of these vessels, designated *atherosclerosis*. Fibrous tissue proliferation associated with a deposition of fatty substances and calcific salts results in the formation of intimal plaques. In advanced cases calcification may be so extensive that the vessel crackles between the fingers when it is crushed. Atheromatous plaques may break down and ulcerate, and the surface may be covered by a thrombus.

The form of arteriosclerotic degeneration that thickens the entire wall and further narrows the lumen of that smallest unit of the arterial circulation, the arteriole, is spoken of as *arteriolar sclerosis*. Arteriolar sclerosis is notable in the kidney, where it is related to hypertension, but it is also seen in other areas of the body.

Arteriosclerosis has been attributed to various causes, but we are yet ignorant as to its exact cause. Age, diet, blood pressure, hormones, cholesterol metabolism, and many other factors have been implicated.

**Aneurysm.** An aneurysm is a localized dilatation of an arterial wall, most often occasioned by the combined effects of a weakened vessel wall and increased blood pressure. The common types are fusiform, in which there is a spindle-shaped dilatation of the whole circumference of the artery, and saccular, in which there is a bulging saclike dilatation of a limited area.

Syphilis is an important factor in the production of aneurysms in the thoracic aorta. Arteriosclerosis is the most common cause of aneurysms of the abdominal aorta. Aneurysms develop slowly and may reach a diameter of 3 or 4 inches. Thrombi form within the sac. As the sac enlarges, the surrounding tissues are eroded or pushed aside. An aneurysm of the ascending arch of the aorta may erode the ribs and sternum and appear beneath the skin as a pulsating mass. Aneurysms ultimately rupture, and in the case of the larger ones the rupture causes sudden death by exsanguinating hemorrhage. The rupture of saccular aneurysms of the cerebral arteries is one of the causes of cerebral hemorrhage (apoplexy).

### VEINS

**Varicose veins (varices).** When the amount of blood that veins have to support is increased by obstruction of the return flow to the heart and when their poorly supported walls are weakened, veins dilate and become tortuous. The action of gravity intensifies the condition in the lower extremities. Factors that

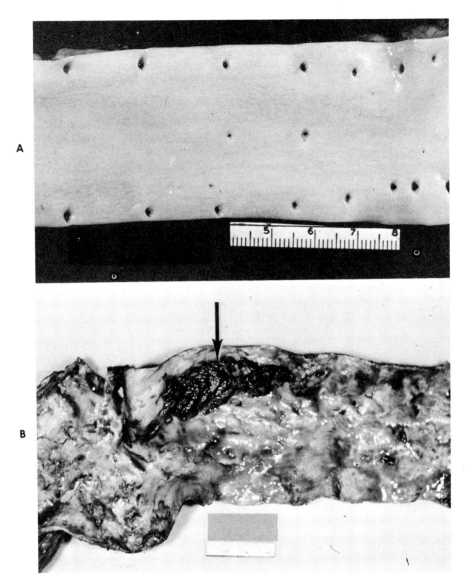

**Fig. 47-7.** Arteriosclerosis, effects on lining surface or intima of blood vessel. **A,** Normal aorta (with smooth surface). **B,** Atherosclerosis of aorta with typical thrombus attached (arrow). Note roughened, granular appearance. Thin eggshell layer found in lining results from calcification accompanying advanced arteriosclerosis.

may produce obstruction to the venous return and predispose to varix formation are heart failure, overwork, standing for long periods of time, pregnancy, and abdominal tumors. Loss of support from the surrounding soft tissues, as occurs in generalized weight loss, may contribute.

The most frequent site of varicose veins is the inside of the lower extremities. Other types are esophageal varices, varicocele (varices of the spermatic cord), and hemorrhoids (varices of the perianal veins). Vari-

cose veins are especially liable to mechanical injury, inflammation, and hemorrhage. The tissues drained by varicose veins are liable to infection and then heal poorly.

## Questions for review

1 What tissue changes may occur as a result of the altered circulation in congenital heart disease?
2 Name the most important causes of hypertrophy of the heart.

3 What is meant by dilatation of the heart?

4 What changes occur in the heart as a result of endocarditis? How may endocarditis be classified?

5 What is stenosis? Regurgitation? How does the heart react to stenosis or insufficiency of one of its valves?

6 What are the causes of coronary occlusion?

7 Give the results of coronary occlusion.

8 What are varicose veins? What are some predisposing causes?

9 What is an aneurysm? Where do aneurysms most commonly occur?

10 Describe the changes that take place in the arterial wall in arteriosclerosis.

11 Briefly discuss enzymes and myocardial infarction.

**References on pp. 552 and 553.**

# CHAPTER 48

# Diseases of
# Blood

Blood consists of an aqueous solution of proteins and salts, known as plasma, in which are suspended *erythrocytes* (red blood cells), *leukocytes* (white blood cells), and *platelets*. (See Figs. 48-1 and 48-2 and Table 48-1.) The function of the erythrocytes is to transfer oxygen to the body cells. This property resides in *hemoglobin,* the iron-bearing pigment of the cell. The leukocytes destroy bacteria by phagocytosis, and the platelets play a part in the coagulation of blood. The plasma gathers and transports food material to the body cells and conveys their waste products to the kidneys, lungs, intestine, and skin to be excreted. (Plasma minus fibrinogen is serum.)

## Red blood cells and hemoglobin

Throughout life red blood cells (erythrocytes) are constantly being produced and destroyed. (See Fig. 48-3.) In early fetal life, formation of erythrocytes (*erythropoiesis*) takes place largely in the liver and spleen while the bone marrow is developing. Shortly before birth the bone marrow has become the main site for production of red blood cells, white blood cells, and platelets and is actively functioning in all bones in the body. When adult life is reached, *hematopoiesis* (blood cell formation) is limited to the marrow of the ribs, sternum, pelvis, vertebrae, and skull. When red cells have outlived their period of usefulness (about

## Table 48-1
Formed elements of the blood

| CELL | DIAMETER in μ (μm.) | NUMBER PER CUBIC MILLIMETER OF BLOOD | FUNCTION | PRIMARY SOURCE | PLACE OF DESTRUCTION |
|---|---|---|---|---|---|
| Red cell (erythrocyte) | 7.5 to 8 | 4.5 to 5 million | Contains hemoglobin; transport of oxygen and carbon dioxide | Bone marrow | Spleen and other areas of reticuloendothelial system |
| White cell (leukocyte) | | 5000 to 9000 | Role in body's defense including immune mechanisms | | Reticuloendothelial system and various other sites, as lung and alimentary tract |
| Granulocyte Neutrophil Eosinophil Basophil | 10 to 15 | 1500 to 8000 0 to 700 0 to 150 | | Bone marrow | |
| Lymphocyte | 7 to 18 | 1000 to 4500 | Immune system | Lymphoid tissues over body | |
| Monocyte | 12 to 20 | 40 to 800 | Immune system | Reticuloendothelial system | |
| Platelet (thrombocyte) | 2 to 3 | 260,000 ± 115,000 | Role in coagulation of blood | Bone marrow | ? |

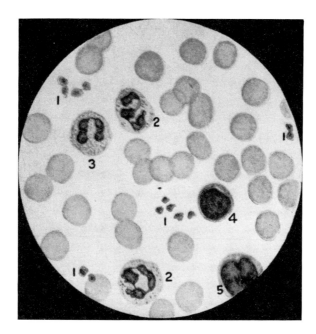

**Fig. 48-1.** Wright-Giemsa–stained smear (see Glossary) of normal blood as seen through the microscope, showing the blood cells—erythrocytes, leukocytes, and platelets. *1*, Platelets; *2* to *5*, leukocytes—of which there are the following: *2*, polymorphonuclear neutrophilic leukocyte; *3*, eosinophilic leukocyte (large red granules of eosinophil do not stand out in black and white photograph); *4*, lymphocyte; *5*, monocyte. Nonnucleated cells are erythrocytes. In preparation of this illustration an area showing a large number of leukocytes was selected, which leaves the impression that the blood contains a higher proportion of leukocytes in relation to the number of blood cells than it actually does. The normal proportion is 1 leukocyte to between 500 and 700 red cells. (Photograph of color plate from Frankel, S., and Reitman, S., editors: Gradwohl's clinical laboratory methods and diagnosis, ed. 6, St. Louis, 1963, The C. V. Mosby Co.)

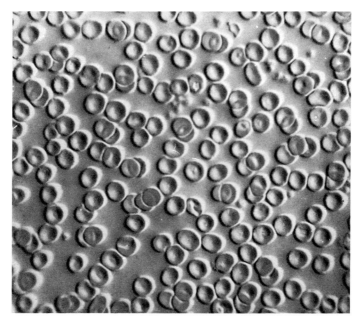

**Fig. 48-2.** Red blood cells in thin film of blood upon which vaporized chromium was shadow-cast at fixed angle. Note biconcave shape. (From Mountcastle, V. B., editor: Medical physiology, ed. 12, St. Louis, 1968, The C. V. Mosby Co.)

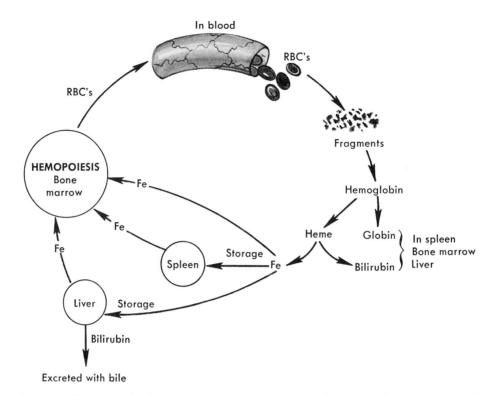

**Fig. 48-3.** Life history of red blood cell, diagram. Red blood cell is formed in bone marrow, circulated in peripheral blood, and degraded in reticuloendothelial system. Note conservation of iron. (From Tuttle, W. W., and Schottelius, B. A.: Textbook of physiology, ed. 16, St. Louis, 1969, The C. V. Mosby Co.)

120 days), they are destroyed by the phagocytic cells of the reticuloendothelial system, particularly those of the spleen, and their hemoglobin is converted into bile pigment. When there is an extreme demand for erythrocytes, as may happen as a result of excessive destruction or failure of normal production, the marrow of bones ordinarily not concerned in erythrocyte production may resume that activity, and even the liver and spleen may attempt again to discharge their embryonic erythrocyte-producing functions.

Under normal conditions erythrocyte production and destruction are so evenly balanced that a level of around 4.5 to 5 million red cells per cubic millimeter* of blood is constantly maintained. Stained smears of the blood show the red cells to be all very much alike. These red cells are known as *normocytes*. When for some reason red cell destruction is greatly increased, immature cells such as *reticulocytes* (cells showing a skein in their cytoplasm) and *normoblasts* (nucleated red blood cells) appear in the bloodstream. The bone marrow compensates for the loss of red

*Normal variations from the values given for blood cell elements exist, of course.

blood cells by increasing its production of the immature nucleated cells that develop into the nonnucleated erythrocytes. (Normal red blood cells do not possess nuclei.)

Physiologically hemoglobin is responsible for gaseous transport in the body. Oxygen is carried by the hemoglobin molecule in the red cell container to the tissues, where it is released; carbon dioxide is taken up in the tissues by hemoglobin and is also carried in the red cell bucket to the lungs to be released. The hemoglobin content of the blood is usually expressed in grams per 100 milliliters (gm./100 ml.) or sometimes as a percentage of normal. The normal hemoglobin content of the blood is about 14.5 to 15 gm./100 ml. Hemoglobin is the only means by which oxygen can travel to the tissues, and when the amount of hemoglobin is reduced, all the organs of the body suffer. The *hematocrit* is an important measurement of red blood cell concentration. It is important as a test for the presence of an anemia. Defined, the hematocrit is the volume of red cells obtained when blood subjected to centrifugal force is packed tightly in a tube. The normal values are around 47% for men and 42% for women.

# ANEMIA

Anemia is an impoverishment of the blood caused by a decrease in red cells, hemoglobin, or both. In most instances both red cells and hemoglobin are decreased, at times in the same proportion but not necessarily so. Generally an anemia is caused by blood loss, by an interference with production of red cells in the bone marrow, by accelerated destruction of red cells, or by combinations of these factors.

**Classification.** If anemias are classified on the basis of etiology, there are two general groups: (1) anemias of decreased production and (2) anemias of increased destruction. The first occurs when the bone marrow fails to produce erythrocytes in sufficient numbers. The second occurs when, as a result of certain abnormal factors, the erythrocytes are destroyed before they have lived their normal span of life in the circulation.

## Decreased-production anemias

I. Deficiencies
   A. Iron deficiency (examples: loss of blood, hookworm disease, milk anemia of infancy)
   B. Deficiency of antipernicious anemia principle—vitamin $B_{12}$ (example: pernicious anemia)
   C. General nutritional deficiencies
II. Injury to bone marrow and blood-forming organs
   A. Destruction of bone marrow by physical or chemical agents (examples: action of x rays, lead poisoning)
   B. Mechanical replacement of marrow—myelophthisis (examples: leukemia, malignant tumors in bones)
   C. Aplastic and hypoplastic anemia (secondary to known factor or primary and of unknown etiology)

## Increased-destruction anemias

I. Acute excessive blood loss or hemorrhage
II. Disintegration of blood cells (hemolysis)
   A. Hemolytic anemias associated with hereditary defects of the red blood cells (examples: congenital hemolytic anemia, sickle cell anemia, Mediterranean anemia)
   B. Hemolytic effects of living agents (examples: malaria, infections with hemolytic streptococci)
   C. Hemolytic effects of physical and chemical agents (examples: severe thermal burns, benzene, sulfonamides, animal and vegetable poisons)
   D. Immune body reactions (examples: blood transfusion reactions, erythroblastosis fetalis)
III. Overactivity of spleen (hypersplenism) (p. 552)
   A. Primary and of unknown origin
   B. Secondary to diseases of spleen

Another classification of anemia is based on the size of the red blood cells and their hemoglobin content. This is not an etiologic classification but a practical one in that by following the laboratory procedures on which it is based, the anemias are often correctly diagnosed and a definite mode of therapy suggested. When this classification is used, the anemias are divided first into *macrocytic, normocytic,* and *microcytic,* the erythrocytes being larger than normal, of normal size, or smaller than normal, and second into *hyperchromic, normochromic,* and *hypochromic,* the cell containing more hemoglobin than normal, a normal amount, or less than normal. Using this classification, we have the following types:

1. *Macrocytic hyperchromic* (the red blood cells are larger than normal and contain more hemoglobin than normal)
2. *Macrocytic normochromic* (the red blood cells are larger than normal but contain only the normal amount of hemoglobin)
3. *Macrocytic hypochromic* (the red blood cells are larger than normal but contain less than the normal amount of hemoglobin)
4. *Normocytic normochromic* (the cells are of normal size and contain a normal amount of hemoglobin)
5. *Normocytic hypochromic* (the red blood cells are of normal size but contain less than the normal amount of hemoglobin)
6. *Microcytic hypochromic* (the red blood cells are both smaller than normal and contain less than the normal amount of hemoglobin)

**Decreased-production anemias.** There are several clinically important decreased-production anemias. *Pernicious anemia* (addisonian anemia) is a macrocytic hyperchromic anemia of late adult life. Untreated, it always ends in death. It is characterized clinically by its peculiar blood picture, the absence of free hydrochloric acid in the stomach, a lemon yellow color of the skin, and gastrointestinal disturbances. So regularly does the absence of free hydrochloric acid from the stomach accompany pernicious anemia that most hematologists refuse to make a diagnosis of pernicious anemia when hydrochloric acid is present. A smooth, red, painful tongue is conspicuous, and spinal cord changes leading to neurologic disturbances are classic (Fig. 48-4).

The red blood cell count per cubic millimeter of blood may be reduced to 1 million or less, but the hemoglobin is not reduced in proportion. As a whole, the cells are larger than normal

Vitamin $B_{12}$ must be present for the normal development, division, and maturation of cells. In its absence abnormalities appear. As a result of a deficiency of vitamin $B_{12}$, in pernicious anemia certain large red blood cells called *megaloblasts* become very prominent, especially in the bone marrow but also in the peripheral blood. Within a matter of hours after an injection of vitamin $B_{12}$, maturation of the red cell series in the marrow reverts to normal and megaloblasts disappear. Deficiency of this factor also affects normal cell maturation in the leukocytes and platelets

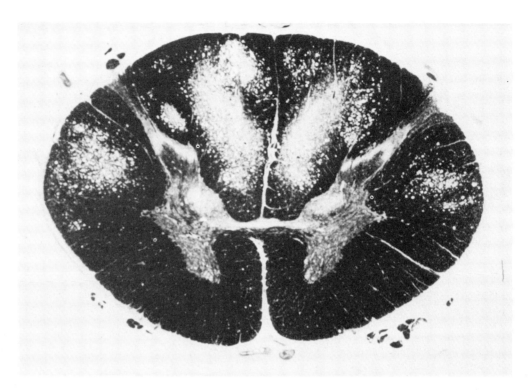

**Fig. 48-4.** Pernicious anemia, degenerative changes in spinal cord. A special stain has demonstrated the myelin of fiber tracts making up the normal *white matter* of the cord. Where myelin is present and the architecture preserved, the microsection above is black. Note mottling near sides and in upper part of cord, reflecting loss of tissue (whitish areas). (The staining should be uniform about the central H-shaped gray matter.)

of the bone marrow and in the epithelial cells of the alimentary tract. Recently circulating antibodies to gastric parietal cells have been demonstrated in pernicious anemia by indirect immunofluorescence.

*Megaloblastic anemias,* similar to pernicious anemia, are seen in patients with carcinoma of the stomach, disease of the small bowel, and total surgical removal of the stomach. In disease of the stomach the source of intrinsic factor, which is necessary for the absorption of vitamin $B_{12}$, is gone. Disease of the small bowel impairs absorption of vitamin $B_{12}$. Some of these anemias related to pernicious anemia are satisfactorily treated with folic acid, a substance also required for the normal maturation of blood cells. Although folic acid is comparable to vitamin $B_{12}$ in its activity, the two are not interchangeable.

An anemia similar in many respects to pernicious anemia may appear in the latter months of pregnancy, but the changes in the blood picture are not so severe, and these patients have free hydrochloric acid in the gastric juice. Usually labor is uncomplicated by anemia, and the anemia spontaneously disappears after delivery.

*Iron-deficiency anemia* (p. 481) is microcytic hypochromic. The amount of hemoglobin is reduced greatly within a very small cell. The bone marrow, in an attempt to compensate for the loss of oxygen-carrying capacity of the peripheral blood, undergoes a furious type of hyperplasia. Iron deficiency is very commonly caused by chronic blood loss from either open or concealed bleeding. Manifestations include weakness, fatigability, and nervous irritability. Pallor is present.

*Aplastic anemia* is a rare disease in which the erythrocyte-producing activity of the bone marrow virtually ceases, and the natural destruction of the red cells eventually leads to a fatal anemia. The blood shows no abnormality other than a great reduction in red cells, in hemoglobin, and often in white blood cells and platelets. A bone marrow inactivity of greater or lesser degree may be caused by certain drugs, notably benzene and certain other coal-tar products, but why aplastic anemia occurs with no predisposing factor is not known. Aplastic anemia is a normocytic normochromic anemia. The clinical findings relate to the bone marrow shutdown, notable bleeding (because of few platelets), and infection (because of scarce leukocytes).

**Increased-destruction anemias.** Anemias of increased destruction are *hemolytic* anemias. Anemias caused by blood loss are discussed in this category, although chronic iron loss of repeated hemorrhage leads to an iron-deficiency anemia.

*Hemorrhage* may be acute or chronic. Chronic hemorrhage, especially the hidden (occult) one, is the more likely to be associated with severe anemia. Immediately after an acute hemorrhage, the cell count of the blood is unaffected because all the constituents of the blood have been lost in their normal proportions. After a very short while, nature begins to make up for the loss in volume by transferring fluids from the tissues to the blood vessels, and the cell count begins to fall. At a later period, replacement begins, with a more rapid delivery of red cells than hemoglobin.

*Sickle cell anemia* (p. 446) is a hemolytic anemia affecting 1 out of 500 black Americans. It is associated with a basic abnormality of the red cell.

*Erythroblastosis fetalis* (see also p. 113), or hemolytic disease of the newborn, attacks the fetus before it is born or within the first few days of postnatal life. It is characterized by destruction of erythrocytes and a great increase in nucleated red blood cells (erythroblastosis). Other signs that may be present are edema, jaundice, pallor, and enlargement of the liver and spleen.

Depending on which symptoms and signs predominate, hemolytic disease of the newborn occurs in three clinical forms: hydrops fetalis, icterus gravis neonatorum, and congenital anemia of the newborn. With the extreme edema of *hydrops fetalis* or universal edema, the child is born dead or dies within a few hours. In *icterus gravis neonatorum,* characterized by jaundice at birth or appearing soon thereafter, death usually does not occur until the first or second week of extrauterine life. About one fourth of these patients recover. *Congenital anemia of the newborn* is the least severe of the three conditions. There is usually a rather profound anemia without jaundice or edema.

Chronic anemia may be found with a number of subacute and chronic inflammatory diseases such as tuberculosis, malaria, syphilis, and pellagra. When renal function is impaired in chronic kidney disease, anemia is part of the clinical picture. In hemopoietic disorders such as Hodgkin's disease, chronic lymphatic leukemia, and lymphosarcoma, anemia is secondary. The pathogenesis of anemia in these diseases is not always well understood. Perhaps it comes about as a result of both decreased production and increased destruction.

Contact with certain chemicals such as lead, mer-

cury, arsenic, and benzene or the taking of acetanilid, an important constituent of many patent headache remedies, may lead to a profound secondary anemia of the hemolytic type.

*Idiopathic acquired hemolytic anemia* is an entity associated with no preexisting disease or etiologic factor. It is considered the best example of a hematologic disorder on an autoimmune basis. The Coombs test, which is positive, demonstrates the attachment of the patient's antibody globulin to his own red blood cells, which can be so hemolyzed by the autoantibodies. The hematologic features of the disease are in keeping with a hemolytic state and include jaundice, an enlarged spleen, signs of compensatory hematopoiesis in the bone marrow, and a variably severe anemia.

## POLYCYTHEMIA

The disorder opposite in its meaning to anemia is polycythemia. Here there is a great increase in the blood volume, number of red blood cells, hemoglobin, white cells, and platelets. *Polycythemia vera (erythremia)* is a slowly progressive disease in which the manifestations stem directly from the fact that blood of increased viscosity is generally congested in the organs and tissues of the body. There is a peculiar dusky appearance to the face, and the extremities are cyanotic. The spleen is enlarged.

An increase in the number of circulating erythrocytes alone may occur as *secondary polycythemia* in a person living at a high altitude or in a person with congenital heart disease, chronic pulmonary disease, or Cushing's syndrome.

## Leukocytes

Unlike the red blood cells, which in their mature stage are of a single type, there are several varieties of white blood cells that differ in their origin, appearance, and function. With their percentages expressed in a *differential count,* the following are the leukocytes (white blood cells) as encountered in normal blood:

| | |
|---|---|
| Polymorphonuclear neutrophilic leukocytes | 55% to 65% |
| Lymphocytes | 25% to 35% |
| Monocytes | 3% to 6% |
| Eosinophils | 1% to 3% |
| Basophils | 1/2% to 1% |

The polymorphonuclear neutrophilic leukocytes, eosinophils, and basophils are known as *granulocytes* because of the prominent granules in their cytoplasm (demonstrated in Wright-stained blood smears). The granulocytes are formed in the bone marrow. The lymphocytes are formed in the lymph nodes, spleen, and other areas of lymphoid tissue from the fixed reticuloendothelial cells, and the monocytes are derived from the reticuloendothelial system. Leukocytes are destroyed largely in the reticuloendothelial system of the body. As a result of disease the normal percentage relation existing among the different types of leukocytes is profoundly disturbed.

## LEUKOCYTOSIS

Normally the number of leukocytes ranges from 5000 to 9000 per cubic millimeter of blood. As a result of disease the number may be increased or decreased. A more or less transient increase in number in response to an infectious agent is known as leukocytosis. A permanent and in most cases a considerably greater increase associated with malignant disease of the leukocyte-producing tissues themselves is known as *leukemia*. Leukocytosis is a protective mechanism, whereas leukemia is a destructive malignant neoplasm. When leukocytosis occurs, there is not a proportional increase in all types of leukocytes, but as a rule only one or two types are affected.

In leukocytosis total counts of 20,000 to 30,000 per cubic millimeter are frequent; more than 50,000 is not uncommon, but 100,000 is seldom exceeded. With counts such as these, from 85% to 90% of the total leukocytes are polymorphonuclear neutrophils. Leukocytosis is most often associated with acute suppurative conditions such as acute appendicitis, salpingitis, peritonitis, and meningitis. Septicemia and certain acute infectious diseases such as pneumonia, erysipelas, and smallpox are also accompanied by leukocytosis.

Certain infectious diseases show either no change in the number of leukocytes or *leukopenia* (decrease in the number of leukocytes). The most important of these are typhoid fever, tuberculosis, measles, German measles, mumps, and influenza. They may, however, be complicated by conditions that cause leukocytosis, as is the case when perforation or hemorrhage complicates typhoid fever. *Agranulocytic angina* is characterized by ulceration of the mouth and throat related to a marked reduction in the polymorphonuclear neutrophilic leukocytes. Counts from typical cases may show the total leukocytes to be reduced to less than 1000 and the percentage of neutrophils to less than 10%. The prognosis is very grave.

*Lymphocytosis* (increase in the number of lymphocytes) accompanies typhoid fever, whooping cough, Malta fever, and syphilis. Lymphocytosis may occur without an increase in the total number of leukocytes, because the polymorphonuclear neutrophilic leukocytes may be reduced concurrently. The presence of a high leukocyte count (20,000 to 30,000) and a marked increase in lymphocytes (50% to 70%) together are strongly suggestive of whooping cough in a susceptible child.

*Eosinophilia* (increase in eosinophils above 5%) occurs in malaria, asthma, certain skin diseases, scarlet fever, and granulocytic leukemia. It also frequently indicates the presence of intestinal parasites, particularly hookworms and tapeworms.

The monocytes are increased (*monocytosis*) in typhoid fever, malaria, amebic dysentery, and the recovery stage of many acute infections.

An increase in basophils occurs in granulocytic leukemia and may follow the injection of therapeutic serums.

## LEUKEMIA

Leukemia is a malignant tumor of the blood-forming tissues, a cancer of the blood, or a cancer in solution. It is characterized by an overproduction of white blood cells and the presence of great numbers of immature and abnormal forms in the bone marrow and hemopoietic organs. The white blood cells in the marrow may fail to develop and remain abnormally immature. Many of the immature and abnormal leukemic cells gain access to the circulating bloodstream. These proliferating leukemic cells fill the bone marrow spaces, prevent the immature red cells from maturing, and interfere with the formation of platelets by crowding out the megakaryocytes, the cells from which platelets are derived. The leukemic cells spill into widely scattered areas of the body and accumulate, even in organs with no inherent blood-forming capacity. The spleen, liver, and lymph nodes (organs of the hematopoietic system), however, are strikingly involved.

There are three types of leukemia: granulocytic (myelogenous), lymphatic, and monocytic, designated according to the particular white cell that is involved in the proliferative process. Leukemias are also classified as acute, subacute, or chronic, depending on the clinical course, duration of disease, and prominence of immature and abnormal cell types in blood and bone marrow. Acute leukemias are characterized by sudden onset, fever, profound anemia, and rapid course. Chronic leukemias pursue a protracted course, often over a period of many years, and usually the clinical symptoms are less severe in nature.

*Granulocytic (myelogenous) leukemia* (Plate 2, *A*) is characterized by the appearance in the blood of an excessive number of granulocytes and precursors (the myeloblasts and myelocytes of the bone marrow from which granulocytes are derived). The total number of leukocytes may reach 800,000 per cubic millimeter. Remissions, during which the number of leukocytes returns to normal, may occur, but the disease finally progresses to a fatal end. Characteristics of the

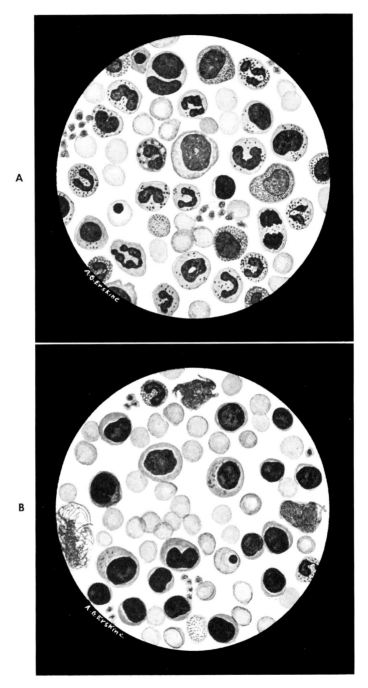

**Plate 2.** Leukemia, microscopic appearance of stained blood smears. **A,** Granulocytic (myelogenous) leukemia. Note both large number and many different kinds of leukocytes present. **B,** Lymphatic leukemia. Note large number of lymphocytes. (From Frankel, S., and others, editors: Gradwohl's clinical laboratory methods and diagnosis, ed. 7, St. Louis, 1970, The C. V. Mosby Co.)

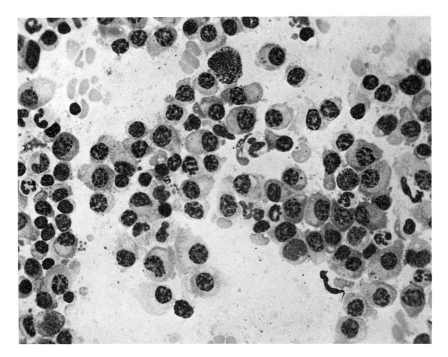

**Fig. 48-5.** Plasma cell (multiple) myeloma in bone marrow aspirate from sternum of patient. Note encroachment of large number of abnormal plasma cells (myeloma cells) on normal marrow cells. (Wright's stain; ×200.) (From Lichtenstein, L.: Bone tumors, ed. 4, St. Louis, 1972, The C. V. Mosby Co.)

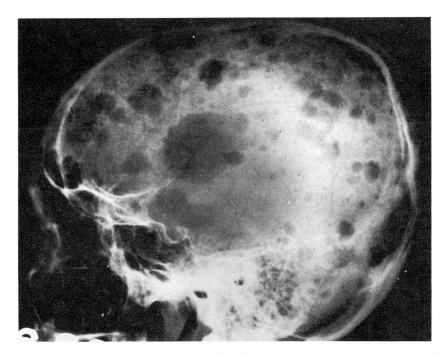

**Fig. 48-6.** Plasma cell (multiple) myeloma in skull, radiograph. Note punched-out areas produced by aggregations of abnormal plasma cells (myeloma cells) in marrow cavity of skull bones. (From Lichtenstein, L.: Bone tumors, ed. 4, St. Louis, 1972, The C. V. Mosby Co.)

disease are high white cell count, anemia, secondary hemorrhages, and marked splenic enlargement.

*Lymphatic* leukemia (Plate 2, *B*) is characterized by enlargement of the spleen and lymph nodes and the appearance in the blood and bone marrow of an abnormal number of lymphocytes and precursors (lymphoblasts and lymphoid cells from which the lymphocytes are derived). The leukocytes may reach 200,000 or more per cubic millimeter, and of this number, from 90% to 95% may be lymphocytes and lymphoblasts. The associated anemia is usually not so severe in lymphatic leukemia as in granulocytic. Like the granulocytic type, lymphatic leukemia is subject to remissions during which the leukocyte count may return to normal, but eventually it is fatal. Acute lymphoblastic leukemia is the most common form in children. Its incidence peaks at age 3 to 4 years.

*Monocytic* leukemia is usually rapidly fatal but is infrequent.

## PLASMA CELL (MULTIPLE) MYELOMA

The plasma cell is included with the white blood cells although it does not circulate in the bloodstream. It is important as the cell that synthesizes antibody globulin. Normally present in tissues and held to be derived from the lymphocyte, it is prominent in subacute and chronic inflammation. Plasma cell myeloma (*multiple myeloma*), a disease often insidious in onset, presents clinically with pain, pathologic fractures, anemia, hemorrhagic tendencies, and kidney disease. Abnormal plasma cells, called *myeloma cells*, aggregate in multiple discrete cellular foci in the marrow of the skull, ribs, sternum, and clavicles to produce a typical punched-out appearance as seen on x-ray examination. (See Figs. 48-5 and 48-6.) In keeping with their normal prototype, the abnormal plasma cells elaborate globulins but of abnormal quality and quantity. The abnormal globulins in myeloma can be easily detected by serum electrophoresis, a physical technic used in the laboratory to separate and identify the various

## Table 48-2

Examples of drugs commonly related to hematologic disorders

| CLASS OF DRUG | HEMATOLOGIC DISORDER | | |
| | ANEMIA (APLASTIC) | LEUKOPENIA OR GRANULOCYTOPENIA | THROMBOCYTOPENIA |
| --- | --- | --- | --- |
| Antimicrobials, antibiotics, and chemotherapeutics | Chloramphenicol Sulfonamides | Chloramphenicol Sulfonamides | Chloramphenicol Sulfonamides Streptomycin Quinine |
| Analgesics | Phenylbutazone (Butazolidin) | Aminopyrine Dipyrone | Phenylbutazone (Butazolidin) |
| Anticonvulsants | Mephenytoin (Mesantoin) Trimethadione (Tridione) | | Mephenytoin (Mesantoin) Trimethadione (Tridione) |
| Organic solvents | Benzene | | |
| Insecticides | DDT Chlorodane | | |
| Antithyroid compounds | | Thiouracil Methimazole (Tapazole) Propylthiouracil | Potassium perchlorate |
| Tranquilizers | | Chlorpromazine (Thorazine) Promazine (Sparine) Prochlorperazine (Compazine) | Meprobamate (Miltown) |
| Diuretics | Acetazolamide (Diamox) Chlorothiazide (Diuril) | | Acetazolamide |
| Hypoglycemics | Tolbutamide (Orinase) Chlorpropamide (Diabinese) | | Tolbutamide Chlorpropamide |
| Heavy metal compounds | Gold salts | | |
| Antiarthritic | | | Colchicine |
| Miscellaneous | | | Quinidine |

protein fractions of the serum. The diagnosis is made by identifying the abnormal plasma cells in the bone marrow. When they spill into the peripheral blood, *plasma cell leukemia* exists.

## Platelets

Platelets *(thrombocytes)* are colorless objects about one-third the size of a red blood cell. Their chief function ties in with the coagulation of blood. Normally the blood contains about 145,000 to 375,000 platelets per cubic millimeter. When the count falls below 60,000, a distinct hemorrhagic tendency is present. A reduction in the number of platelets is spoken of as *thrombocytopenia*, and when it causes hemorrhage, the condition is spoken of as *thrombocytopenic purpura*. Thrombocytopenia is regularly secondary to the various types of leukemia and certain anemias, such as aplastic anemia. It is also secondary to drug sensitivities, chickenpox, and radiation exposure.

*Idiopathic thrombocytopenic purpura*, a primary disease of persons in younger age groups, has a more or less sudden onset of hemorrhagic phenomena in the skin and mucous membranes, with easy bruising. Although *megakaryocytes*, the parent cells of platelets, are active in the bone marrow, the peripheral platelet count is greatly reduced. Splenectomy in most instances alleviates the condition.

## Adverse drug reactions

The rapid expansion of knowledge in medicine today includes a wide application in the field of drugs and similar therapeutic agents, many of which are invaluable. At times, however, a reaction both unpredictable and unfavorable occurs in a patient receiving a given drug. A common manifestation of such an adverse drug reaction is a decrease in the number of red blood cells (anemia, usually an aplastic one, though it can be hemolytic), white blood cells (leukopenia or granulocytopenia), platelets (thrombocytopenia), or a combination of all three (pancytopenia). The listings in Table 48-2 cite important examples of offending drugs.

## Questions for review

1  Where are red blood and white blood cells produced in the body?
2  Briefly define erythrocytes, leukocytes, thrombocytes, leukocytosis, leukopenia, erythroblastosis, anemia.
3  What is the importance of vitamin $B_{12}$ in blood disease?
4  Classify anemias as to cause.
5  What is the hematocrit?
6  What is an adverse drug reaction?
7  What is meant by a differential blood count? What is its clinical value?
8  Name the different types of white blood cells. Which type represents the largest percentage of white blood cells?
9  List diseases in which there is leukocytosis.
10  Name two types of leukemia and give the findings in each.
11  What is the function of blood platelets?
12  Briefly characterize polycythemia, thrombocytopenic purpura, plasma cell myeloma, pernicious anemia.

**References on pp. 552 and 553.**

# CHAPTER 49

# Diseases of
# Lymphoid tissues

## Lymph nodes

Fortunately the human body is well provided with lymphoid tissue including masses (solitary and conglomerate nodules) incorporated into the major organ systems (alimentary, respiratory, and genitourinary) and many lymph nodes, both superficially and deeply placed. Some of the lymph nodes are clinically significant because of their accessibility for evaluation and their anatomic relation to a given disease. Important groups are found internally in the tissues in front of the backbone, in the mesentery of the bowel, and along the trunk and branches of the tracheobronchial tree and externally in the neck, armpit, and groin.

### ENLARGEMENT

If a lymph node is diseased, in all likelihood it is enlarged. Often spoken of as *lymphadenopathy,* lymph node enlargement is very important in diagnosis. Strictly speaking, the term lymphadenopathy has a wider meaning and indicates simply disease of the lymph nodes. The most common causes of lymphadenopathy are classified as follows:

I. Generalized enlargement
   A. Leukemia
   B. Acute generalized infections such as measles, scarlet fever, rubella, smallpox, and bubonic plague
   C. Malignant lymphoma (lymphosarcoma and reticulum cell sarcoma)
   D. Infectious mononucleosis
   E. Serum sickness
   F. Syphilis (secondary stage)
   G. Certain generalized skin diseases
   H. Generalized metastases of certain carcinomas
II. Localized enlargement
   A. Nodes discrete
      1. Acute or chronic nonsuppurative lymphadenitis
      2. Tuberculosis
      3. Gumma
      4. Tularemia

      5. Fungous diseases
      6. Filariasis
      7. Trauma
      8. Metastases from malignant tumors
      9. Early stages of Hodgkin's disease
   B. Nodes matted together
      1. Late stages of tuberculosis of nodes
      2. Advanced stages of Hodgkin's disease (Fig. 49-1)
      3. Suppurative lymphadenitis
      4. Malignant lymphoma

The location of enlarged nodes and the degree of involvement are important considerations in the evaluation of lymphadenopathy. Generalized lymphadenopathy of slight degree is probably caused by infection, whereas generalized or localized involvement with very large nodes may well represent malignancy.

*Enlargement of the cervical nodes* may be caused by infections of the scalp, ear, teeth, mouth, or throat; by tuberculosis, infectious mononucleosis, leukemia, malignant lymphoma, and Hodgkin's disease; and by metastatic tumors arising in areas drained by these nodes.

*Enlargement of the axillary nodes* may be caused by acute infections and trauma of the hand, metastatic carcinoma (especially of the breast in women), leukemia, tuberculosis, metastatic melanoma, and Hodgkin's disease.

*Enlargement of a small node (Virchow's node) or a group of nodes* above the inner end of the left clavicle may be the first indication of a carcinoma of the lung or stomach. Biopsy of the *scalene* lymph node aids in the diagnosis of chest diseases.

*Enlargement of the inguinal nodes* may be caused by venereal diseases or other infections of the genitals, infections of the lower extremities, metastasis from melanoma or carcinoma, leukemia, tuberculosis, or Hodgkin's disease.

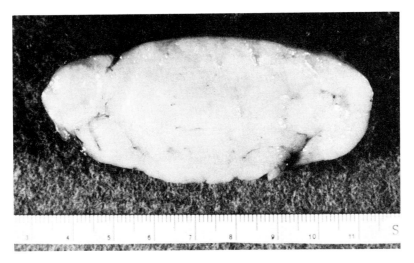

**Fig. 49-1.** Hodgkin's disease of lymph nodes. Mass of enlarged, confluent lymph nodes sectioned. Note loss of normal architecture.

## PIGMENTATION-CALCIFICATION

The lymph nodes store pigment that they pick up in the lymph vessels of the body. Carbon particles from dust in the air are regularly deposited in the chest nodes draining the lungs. Tattoo pigment may be deposited in lymph nodes adjacent to the skin site. Calcium deposits in lymph nodes are usually caused by healed tuberculosis, except in the mesenteric nodes where they may follow typhoid fever.

## INFLAMMATION

**Lymphadenitis.** Lymphadenitis, or inflammation of lymph nodes, is caused by irritants filtered out of the lymph in the afferent vessels. By far the most common and important ones are bacteria and bacterial products. Lymphadenitis may be acute or chronic. Acute lymphadenitis may be simple (nonsuppurative) or suppurative. It is observed near bacterial infections, as in the neighborhood of abscesses, acutely infected gallbladders, and inflamed appendices. Systemic diseases causing acute lymphadenitis are typhoid fever, tularemia, and bubonic plague. With suppurative lymphadenitis the lymph vessels passing to the node become infected (lymphangitis). This is indicated by red lines in the skin along the course of lymphatics to the node. A sinus tract may form to the skin from suppurating superficial lymph nodes.

**Tuberculosis.** Tuberculosis of the lymph nodes occurs in adults, but it is primarily a disease of childhood. The affected nodes are at first firm and discrete. Later they mat together, and the tubercles within the nodes fuse and become caseous (Fig. 49-2). From cervical nodes the caseous material may be discharged onto the skin surface through a sinus tract. If there is

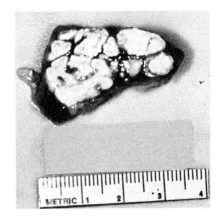

**Fig. 49-2.** Caseous lymph nodes.

healing, the nodes are converted into fibrous masses and calcified. Tuberculosis of the cervical lymph nodes is often referred to as *scrofula*. During the Middle Ages scrofula was known as the king's evil, and it was believed that a king could cure the disease by touching the patient.

**Syphilis.** The nodes draining the site of a chancre are enlarged, hard, and painless. Suppuration does not occur. In secondary syphilis there is a generalized enlargement of the lymph nodes, especially evident in the epitrochlear and the superficial nodes of the back of the neck.

## NEOPLASM

**Hodgkin's disease.** Hodgkin's disease is a chronic disease of lymphoid tissue (the exact cause of which

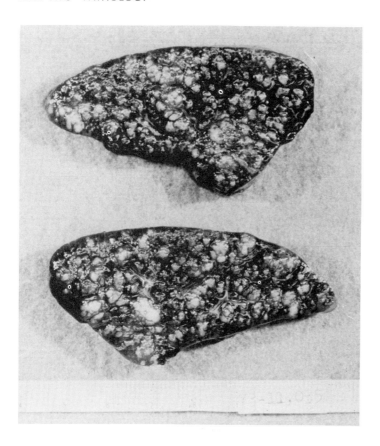

**Fig. 49-3.** Hodgkin's disease of spleen, sectioned surface. Scattered, varying-sized foci of disease distort normal structure.

is not known). Although generally considered a malignant neoplasm, it shows some of the pathologic features of chronic granulomas. It preferentially strikes young adult males. Beginning as a painless enlargement of a group of lymph nodes, usually on one side of the neck, the disease runs its downhill course over several years. Untreated, it is invariably fatal.* As a rule, one member after another of a group of nodes becomes involved, after which the process extends to adjoining nodes or to other sites of lymphoid tissue, such as the spleen (Fig. 49-3) and bowel. Eventually many organs of the body are included. At first the lymph nodes are discrete, but they later mat together, and the masses reach disfiguring proportions.

Eosinophilia, anemia, and other changes in the peripheral blood picture may be present. A large bizarre cell of characteristic appearance, the Reed-Sternberg cell, in the granulomatous reaction is diagnostic.

**Malignant lymphoma.** Malignant lymphoma (lymphosarcoma), the malignancy derived from lymphoid cells, is the most important primary tumor of the lymph nodes and lymphoid tissue elsewhere. A disease of middle life, it is characterized by progressive enlargement and fusion of lymph nodes until nodes throughout the body are involved. Often the alimentary tract is incorporated. The outcome is invariably fatal (without treatment).* Pathologically a malignant overgrowth of lymphocytes or precursor cells blots out the normal architecture of the lymph node.

**Metastatic malignancy.** Metastatic neoplasms are more common to the lymph nodes than are primary ones. In the nodes these secondary neoplasms are more likely to be carcinomas than sarcomas. Because of the frequency with which carcinomas involve the lymph nodes draining the site of the primary tumor, it is often imperative that these nodes be removed routinely when the tumor is eradicated surgically. If tumor cells have destroyed this first barrier and passed to more remote areas, surgical removal of the tumor may be impossible. A lymph node that is the site of a metastatic tumor may not be enlarged, and nodes draining a tumor site may be enlarged without being invaded by tumor cells.

## Spleen

The spleen is a large encapsulated mass of lymphoid tissue adapted to a peculiar circulation

---

*Modern-day therapy has greatly improved the prognosis of lymphoid neoplasms.

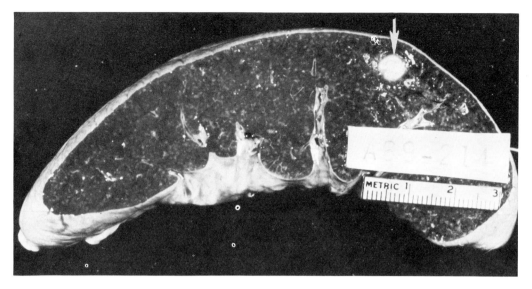

**Fig. 49-4.** Spleen, tuberculosis. Sectioned surface shows rounded gray-white focus of caseation (arrow).

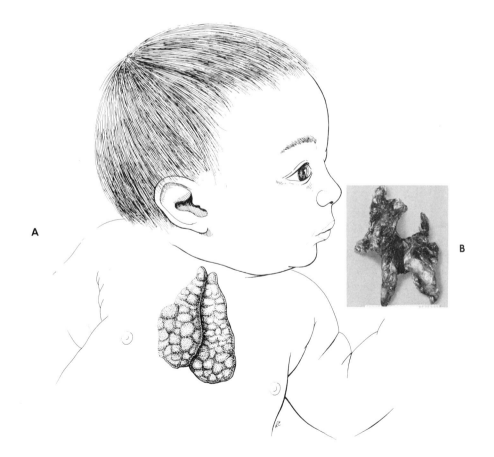

**Fig. 49-5. A,** Thymus gland near time of birth. Note size (larger than baby's fist) and position in upper chest. **B,** Thymus gland of adult—an atrophic, shriveled, ill-defined mass of tissue.

of blood (p. 98). The normal spleen may occasionally be ruptured by blows and falls and in automobile accidents. Enlarged spleens may be ruptured by more trivial injuries. Rupture leads to serious hemorrhage.

Since enlargement of the spleen, *splenomegaly,* forms an important physical sign, it is well to keep in mind its most important causes. Acute splenomegaly occurs in malaria, typhoid fever, endocarditis, septicemia, pyemia, typhus, and plague. Chronic enlargement of the spleen may be caused by passive congestion, chronic malaria, syphilis, portal hypertension, leukemia, or hemolytic anemia. Granulomatous disease may involve the spleen with or without enlargement (Fig. 49-4).

In addition to its role in immunologic processes in the body (p. 101), the spleen is an important hematologic organ. Although not necessary for normal living, the spleen as a component of the reticuloendothelial system functions in the breakdown of hemoglobin and the formation of bile pigment and acts as a reservoir of blood.*

If its role in the destruction of blood cells is exaggerated because of primary or secondary disease processes involving the spleen, the condition of *hypersplenism* results. In hypersplenism too many red blood cells, platelets, or white blood cells—or increased numbers of all these—are eliminated from the circulation. Anemia, thrombocytopenia, leukopenia, or pancytopenia results. Neoplasms, either primary or metastatic, rarely involve the spleen, except malignant lymphomas and the leukemias.

## Thymus

The thymus (see also p. 98) is a lobular, partly epithelial, and partly lymphoid organ. Present at birth (Fig. 49-5, *A*), it continues to enlarge until puberty, after which it atrophies and is replaced by fatty tissue in the adult (Fig. 49-5, *B*). This has always suggested that the thymus plays a significant role in the individual's development (p. 101).

Pathologic atrophy of the thymus is seen in severe illnesses and injuries and with large doses of steroid hormones. Hyperplasia is seen in hyperthyroidism. The neoplasm is the *malignant thymoma. Myasthenia gravis* is a condition of abnormal muscular weakness and fatigability that appears related to the thymus in a poorly understood way. In more than half the patients the thymus is hyperplastic, and in many there is a thymoma.

---

*Physiologically it has been said that the spleen acts as a combination manufacturing shop, filtration unit, waste disposal, salvage plant, and reservoir.

## Questions for review

1 Enumerate six common causes of enlarged lymph nodes.
2 Give causes of lymphadenitis.
3 Why are the lymph nodes of the axillary region often removed when radical breast amputation for cancer is done?
4 What are some diseases characterized by enlargement of the spleen?
5 Characterize Hodgkin's disease and malignant lymphoma.
6 What is hypersplenism?
7 Briefly discuss the thymus.

**REFERENCES** (Chapters 41, 47 to 49)

Aagaard, G. N.: Treatment of hypertension, Am. J. Nurs. **73:** 620, 1973.

Abramson, H., and others, editors: Sickle cell disease: diagnosis, management, education, and research, St. Louis, 1973, The C. V. Mosby Co.

Aisenberg, A. C.: Updated Hodgkin's disease; value of immunologic testing, J.A.M.A. **222:**1301, 1972.

American Heart Association Cookbook, New York, 1973, David McKay Co., Inc.

Anderson, W. A. D., editor: Pathology, ed. 6, St. Louis, 1971, The C. V. Mosby Co.

Aronow, W. D.: Tobacco and the heart, J.A.M.A. **229:**1799, 1974.

Ascari, W. Q., and others: $Rh_0$ (D) immune globulin (human), J.A.M.A. **205:**1, 1968.

Baldini, M. G., and Ebbe, S., editors: Platelets: production, function, transfusion, and storage, New York, 1974, Grune & Stratton, Inc.

Bauer, J. D., and others: Clinical laboratory methods, ed. 8, St. Louis, 1974, The C. V. Mosby Co.

Bauke, J.: Chronic myelocytic leukemia, Lab. Med. **2:**43, Jan., 1971.

Bennett, I., and Simon, M.: The prudent diet, New York, 1972, David White, Inc.

Blumenthal, S., and Jesse, M. J.: Prevention of atherosclerosis: a pediatric problem, Hosp. Pract. **8:**81, April, 1973.

Bolin, R. H., and Auld, M. E.: Hodgkin's disease, Am. J. Nurs. **74:**1982, 1974.

Bowie, E. J. W., and others: Mayo Clinic laboratory manual of hemostasis, Philadelphia, 1971, W. B. Saunders Co.

Brodie, J. L.: Sickle cell anemia—the disease of challenge, J. Am. Med. Wom. Assoc. **27:**411, 1972.

Brown, B. A.: Hematology: principles and procedures, Philadelphia, 1973, Lea & Febiger.

Brown, M. S., and Alexander, M. M.: Physical examination. Part II. Examining the heart, Nursing '74 **4:**41, Dec., 1974.

Clark, C. A.: The prevention of Rh isoimmunization, Hosp. Pract. **8:**77, Jan., 1973.

Cole, P.: Epidemiology of Hodgkin's disease, J.A.M.A. **222:** 1636, 1972.

Crosby, W. H.: Sickle cell trait, J.A.M.A. **229:**1105, 1974.

Culter, C.: Haute cuisine for your heart's delight: a low-cholesterol cookbook for gourmets, New York, 1973, Clarkson N. Potter, Inc.

Dawson, R. B., Jr.: Drug induced blood dyscrasias, Resident Staff Physician **15:**50, Aug., 1969.

DelBueno, D. J.: Electrolyte imbalance: how to recognize and respond to it, RN **38**:54, March, 1975.

Deutsch, P., and Deutsch, R.: The heart attack you didn't know you had, Today's Health **47**:42, July, 1969.

Dougherty, W. M.: Introduction to hematology, ed. 2, St. Louis, 1976, The C. V. Mosby Co.

Elves, M. W.: The lymphocytes, ed. 2, Chicago, 1972, Year Book Medical Publishers, Inc.

Frankel, S., and others: Gradwohl's clinical laboratory methods and diagnosis, ed. 7, St. Louis, 1970, The C. V. Mosby Co.

Freda, V. J.: The control of Rh disease, Hosp. Pract. **2**:54, Jan., 1967.

Freese, A. S.: The useful organ we can live without, Today's Health **47**:65, Nov., 1969.

Freese, A. S.: Yes, you're a "blue blood," Today's Health **48**:46, Aug., 1970.

Friedman, N. J.: Mechanisms of disseminated intravascular coagulation and its rapid laboratory diagnosis, Lab. Med. **2**:46, Jan., 1971.

Gaston, M.: Screening for sickle cell gene (editorial), South. Med. J. **67**:257, 1974.

Goldberger, E.: A primer of water, electrolyte and acid-base syndromes, ed. 4, Philadelphia, 1970, Lea & Febiger.

Halberstam, M.: Heart scares, Today's Health **52**:36, April, 1974.

Hardison, C. S.: The leukocyte count, J.A.M.A. **204**:377, 1968.

Hardison, C. S.: The sedimentation rate, J.A.M.A. **204**:257, 1968.

Harper, T. A.: Laboratory guide to disordered haemostasis, New York, 1971, Appleton-Century-Crofts.

Johnston, R. B., Jr.: Increased susceptibility to infection in sickle cell disease: review of its occurrence and possible causes, South. Med. J. **67**:1342, 1974.

Kannel, W. B.: The Framingham study and chronic disease prevention, Hosp. Pract. **5**:78, March, 1970.

Kiester, E., Jr.: Life blood for young Cliff Watson, hemophiliac, Today's Health **51**:42, Dec., 1973.

King, G. E.: Taking the blood pressure, J.A.M.A. **209**:1902, 1969.

Laragh, J. H.: An approach to the classification of hypertensive states, Hosp. Pract. **9**:61, Jan., 1974.

"Leukemia houses" (editorial), Ann. Intern. Med. **67**:674, 1967.

Lukes, R. J.: Prognosis and relationship of histologic features to clinical stage (Hodgkin's disease), J.A.M.A. **222**:1294, 1972.

Maugh, T. H., II: Leukemia: much is known, but the picture is still confused, Science **185**:48, 1974.

Mayer, G. G.: Disseminated intravascular coagulation, Am. J. Nurs. **73**:2067, 1973.

McCombs, R. P.: Fundamentals of internal medicine, ed. 4, Chicago, 1971, Year Book Medical Publishers, Inc.

McCurdy, P. R.: "$B_{12}$ shots," flip side, J.A.M.A. **231**:289, 1975.

Miale, J. B.: Laboratory medicine—hematology, ed. 4, St. Louis, 1972, The C. V. Mosby Co.

Million, R. R.: Hodgkin's disease in 1974, J.A.M.A. **228**:328, 1974.

Mollison, P. L.: Clinical aspects of Rh immunization, Am. J. Clin. Pathol. **60**:287, 1973.

Morse, E. E.: Platelet transfusions, Lab. Med. **1**:37, Nov., 1970.

Mountcastle, V. B., editor: Medical physiology, ed. 13, St. Louis, 1974, The C. V. Mosby Co.

Nalbandian, R. M.: The molecular basis for the pathogenesis, diagnosis, and treatment of sickle cell disease, Lab. Med. **2**:12, May, 1971.

Nour-Eldin, F.: Blood coagulation simplified, New York, 1971, Appleton-Century-Crofts.

Rheingold, J. J.: Acute leukemia, its smoldering phase, or leukemia never starts on Thursday, J.A.M.A. **230**:985, 1974.

Robinson, M. G., and Halpern, C.: Infections, *Escherichia coli*, and sickle cell anemia, J.A.M.A. **230**:1145, 1974.

Rosenbaum, D. L.: The diagnosis and management of Hodgkin's disease: current concepts, CA **20**:286, 1970.

Ross, W. S.: Leukemia: "we're starting to use the word cure," Today's Health **48**:49, Oct., 1970.

Rubin, P.: Comment: the reclassification of Hodgkin's disease, J.A.M.A. **222**:1303, 1972.

Rubin, P.: Updated Hodgkin's disease. A. Introduction, J.A.M.A. **222**:1292, 1972.

Schechter, P. J., and others: Sodium chloride preference in essential hypertension, J.A.M.A. **225**:1311, 1973.

Schmidt, R. M.: Laboratory diagnosis of hemoglobinopathies, J.A.M.A. **224**:1276, 1973.

Schumann, D., and Patterson, P.: Multiple myeloma, Am. J. Nurs. **75**:78, 1973.

Seiverd, C. E.: Hematology for medical technologists, ed. 4, Philadelphia, 1972, Lea & Febiger.

Silberstein, E. B.: The Schilling test, J.A.M.A. **208**:2325, 1969.

Smith, C. H.: Blood diseases of infancy and childhood, ed. 3, St. Louis, 1972, The C. V. Mosby Co.

Stern, P.: APA: insidious foe of an aging Swede . . . Addison's pernicious anemia, Am. J. Nurs. **75**:78, 1975.

Stude, C.: Cardiogenic shock, Am. J. Nurs. **74**:1638, 1974.

Tharp, G. D.: Shock: the overall mechanisms, Am. J. Nurs. **74**:2208, 1974.

Viola, M. V.: Acute leukemia and infection, J.A.M.A. **201**:923, 1967.

Ward, F. A.: A primer of haematology, New York, 1971, Appleton-Century-Crofts.

White, C. A., and others: $Rh_0$ (D) immune globulin to prevent Rh hemolytic diseases, Am. Fam. Physician **3**:85, Feb., 1971.

Wiley, L.: Shock, Nursing '74 **4**:43, May, 1974.

Williams, W. J.: Blood coagulation, Resident Staff Physician **15**:39, Nov., 1969.

Wissler, R. W.: Development of atherosclerotic plaque, Hosp. Pract. **8**:61, March, 1973.

Zane, P.: The Jack Sprat cookbook (or good eating on a low cholesterol diet), New York, 1973, Harper & Row, Publishers.

Zimmerman, D. R.: Rh—the intimate history of a disease and its conquest, New York, 1973, The Macmillan Co.

# CHAPTER 50

# Diseases of
# Respiratory tract

The respiratory system comprises a number of anatomic passageways through which the air we breathe travels to the delicately structured central organ of the tract, the lung. During inspiration, air containing oxygen passes through the nose, the pharynx (throat), the larynx (voice box), the trachea (windpipe), and down into the successively smaller divisions of the bronchial tree that terminate in myriads of tiny air sacs, the pulmonary alveoli. Each of these air spaces is bounded by blood-filled capillaries of the pulmonary circulation, the thinnest sort of membrane separating the air in the alveolus from the blood of the capillary lumen. This is an ideal arrangement for the physiologic exchange of gases occurring at the site. The oxygen of the air diffuses across the membrane into the lumen of the blood vessel to be carried to the cells of the body. At the same time carbon dioxide, the waste product of body metabolism, is given up by the blood; it diffuses in the reverse direction, travels up the respiratory tract, and with expiration of air is released from the body. The total surface area for diffusion of oxygen and carbon dioxide between blood and air space is about half the size of a tennis court. The energy needed to sustain pulmonary function is equivalent to that supplied by two lumps of sugar a day. (See Fig. 50-1.)

## Nose

**Rhinitis.** Acute rhinitis may be caused by the inhalation of irritating fumes or large quantities of dust, but it occurs most often in the form of the common cold or as an accompaniment of such infectious diseases as measles and whooping cough. The acute rhinitis of hay fever is an allergic condition.

Chronic rhinitis may be caused by repeated attacks of the acute disease, chronic sinus infections, or continued inhalation of irritating fumes or dust. It occurs in two forms: hypertrophic and atrophic. In the hypertrophic form the nasal mucosa is thickened, drainage

is obstructed, and polypoid outgrowths may occur. Atrophic rhinitis may follow the hypertrophic form or occur as a primary disease. In atrophic rhinitis the nasal mucosa atrophies, and the glands become inactive. When ulceration, crust formation, and a fetid discharge are present, the disorder is known as *ozena*.

**Tumors.** The most common tumorlike growth of the nose is the nasal polyp. We have used the term *tumorlike* because polyps are inflammatory (not neoplastic) overgrowths of the nasal mucosa that project into the nasal passages, obstructing respiration and interfering with the drainage of the nasal sinuses. Carcinomas or sarcomas of the nose occur.

**Adenoids.** The pharyngeal tonsil is a collection of lymphoid tissue on the posterior wall of the nasopharynx. Ordinarily it increases in size until about the third year of life, after which it remains stationary until about the age of puberty; it gradually decreases in size thereafter. If the lymphoid tissue hypertrophies and obstructs the nasal passages, it is referred to as adenoids. This is a well-known type of obstruction of the respiratory passages.

## Larynx

**Laryngitis.** Acute laryngitis and acute rhinitis have common causes and often occur together. Like acute rhinitis, acute laryngitis accompanies many infectious diseases. Acute laryngitis may result from prolonged or excessive use of the voice, as in singing, speaking, or shouting. It commonly extends to the trachea. In children swelling of the laryngeal mucosa may lead to spasmodic constriction of the laryngeal muscles, producing the paroxysmal dyspnea and cyanosis of *spasmodic croup,* which must be differentiated from diphtheritic laryngitis.

Chronic laryngitis may follow repeated attacks of acute laryngitis, or it may result from the constant abuse of the voice or from the continued inhalation of irritating substances.

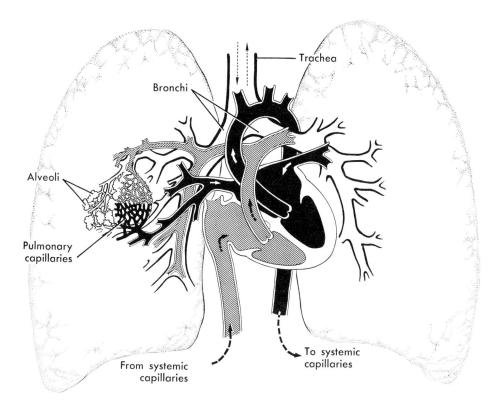

**Fig. 50-1.** Lung, with connections to cardiovascular system, schematic representation. On left, pulmonary alveoli without their covering of capillary blood vessels are shown. The capillary network is indicated just to their right. From 5 to 7 liters of air moves in and out of these air sacs each minute with respiratory movements of chest wall. In contact with this volume of air is blood high in carbon dioxide and low in oxygen. The right ventricle of heart pumps 70 to 100 ml. of this blood into pulmonary circulation with each beat. From lungs, the blood, with its carbon dioxide content lowered and its oxygen replenished, is drained into left ventricle, which pumps it into systemic circulation to contact body cells.

**Tumors.** The serious lesions of the larynx are the neoplasms. The benign *papilloma* is found about the vocal cords. The malignant *squamous cell carcinoma* originates in a vocal cord, mainly in older men, and makes up 2% to 4% of human malignancies.

## Lungs

**Bronchitis.** Acute bronchitis may involve one or both sides of the bronchial tree and occur as a superficial inflammation limited to the larger bronchi or as an extensive inflammation involving the smaller bronchi and the bronchioles *(bronchiolitis)*. Acute bronchitis is dangerous in infants, the elderly, and the debilitated.

Chronic bronchitis is a rather common disease that follows influenza, bronchopneumonia, or repeated attacks of acute bronchitis. It accompanies pulmonary tuberculosis, asthma, or passive congestion of the lungs. Continued exposure to irritating dusts or fumes may cause primary chronic bronchitis. An important feature of this disorder is the chronic cough. The patient must cough frequently to partially clear an accumulation of mucus produced in excess by the enlarged and hyperactive mucous glands lining the respiratory tract.

**Bronchiectasis.** Bronchiectasis is a chronic disease characterized by dilatation of one or more bronchi and inflammation in the bronchial walls as well as in the adjacent pulmonary tissues. Dilatation, which may be extensive, is usually cylindrical or saccular. Bronchiectasis is brought about by disease processes in the lungs that destroy the tissues of the bronchial wall. Infection and increased intrabronchial pressure such as occurs with coughing and bronchial obstructions are aggravating factors. Because the normal mechanisms for drainage are damaged, secretions stagnate, and an infectious process already present is intensified. Staphylococci, streptococci, pneumococci,

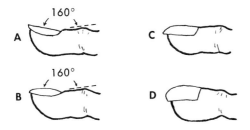

Fig. 50-2. Clubbing of fingers in heart and lung disease. **A** and **B,** Normal straight and curved nails for comparison with clubbed fingers of **C** and **D.** (From Egan, D. F.: Fundamentals of inhalation therapy, ed. 2, St. Louis, 1973, The C. V. Mosby Co.)

and sometimes anaerobic organisms are the culprits.

Bronchiectasis most often complicates bronchopneumonia, but it may figure in various pulmonary disorders—tuberculosis, lung abscess, influenza, foreign body aspiration, and neoplasm. In this common disease, chronic cough, profuse sputum, and hemoptysis (blood in the sputum) are classic. In fact, bronchiectasis is a more frequent cause of bloody sputum than is tuberculosis. Clubbing of the fingers (Fig. 50-2) and toes may be seen as for any heart or lung ailment in which there is chronic impairment of the oxygenation of the blood (anoxemia).

**Inflammation.*** The term *pneumonia* means inflammation of the lung. As used, it refers to the consolidation or solidification (Figs. 18-9 and 50-3) of the air sacs with inflammatory exudate. The pulmonary alveoli, bronchioles, and smaller bronchi are filled with inflammatory cells (p. 188).

The term *pneumonitis* is an alternate for pulmonary inflammation and is sometimes used when the inflammatory changes are concentrated in the interstitial supporting tissues rather than in the air sacs. A review of infectious agents in the light of pulmonary inflammation is given in Table 50-1.

**Pneumoconioses.** The dust diseases are occupational and occur in industries in which workers breathe inorganic dust particles over long periods of time. The tissue reaction in the lung depends on the chemical nature of the dust, but the type lesion is chronic granulomatous inflammation of the foreign body type, with marked fibrosis. Needless to say, residual scarring means loss of respiratory function. Tuberculosis easily complicates the condition, and if pulmonary fibrosis is severe, failure of the right heart occurs. Important examples of pneumoconioses are anthracosis, silicosis, and asbestosis. *Anthracosis* is the benign form, since inhalation of carbon particles

---

*The pathology of tuberculous inflammation is discussed on p. 249.

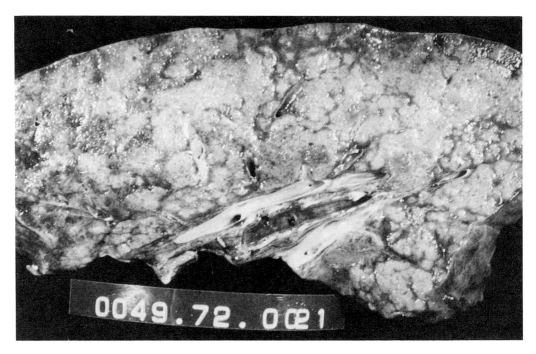

**Fig. 50-3.** Pneumonia (solidification of air spaces with exudate), sectioned surface (of lung). Note wide, irregularly outlined, grayish white area of involvement.

**Table 50-1**
Relation of pulmonary inflammation to injurious agent

| CAUSE | DISEASE |
| --- | --- |
| Infective (living) agents | |
| Bacteria | Lobar pneumonia and bronchopneumonia (pneumococcal) |
| | Staphylococcal and streptococcal pneumonia; tuberculosis |
| | Tularemic pneumonia; actinomycosis |
| | Primary atypical pneumonia (*Mycoplasma pneumoniae*) |
| Fungi | Candidiasis; histoplasmosis; coccidioidomycosis |
| Rickettsias | Q fever; interstitial pneumonitis of typhus and Rocky Mountain spotted fever |
| Chlamydiae (bedsoniae) | Pneumonitis of psittacosis |
| Viruses* | Viral pneumonias; pneumonitis of influenza |
| Nonliving agents | |
| Chemical | Pneumoconiosis; lipoid pneumonia; byssinosis (cotton fiber dust disease) |
| Physical | Radiation pneumonitis |
| Immunologic | Rheumatic pneumonia; pneumonitis of serum sickness |

*Viruses of the childhood exanthemas (rubella, varicella) as well as respiratory viruses can produce viral pneumonia or pneumonitis.

does not disturb pulmonary function; the accumulation of pigment is striking but of no consequence. *Silicosis* is the severe form, representing a hazard to miners and rock workers, who must breathe particles of free silica. *Asbestosis* is caused by inhalation of asbestos dust in certain industries (Fig. 50-4).

**Lung abscess.** Abscess of the lung is caused by the inhalation of infectious material or the deposit of bacteria from the bloodstream within the lung. Infectious material may be aspirated during operations about the nose and mouth. Abscesses complicate pneumonias caused by the pyogenic bacteria. When saprophytic fusiform bacilli and spirochetes from the mouth either initiate or invade secondarily the necrotic focus, the lesion becomes *pulmonary gangrene.*

**Circulatory disturbances.** When blood from an injured or diseased area enters a bronchus, hemorrhage from the lungs takes place. Chronic passive hyperemia accompanies heart disease. Edema may result from impairment of the circulation or be inflammatory. Thrombi in the veins of the extremities and pelvis may release emboli that lodge in the lungs. Small pulmonary emboli produce infarcts in a congested or edematous lung. A large pulmonary embolus occluding the pulmonary artery or one of its main branches causes death within minutes.

**Bronchial obstruction.** Obstruction to a bronchus may be either complete or incomplete. A foreign body in the lumen, an intrinsic disease of the wall, or an extrinsic lesion that presses on the bronchus may each obstruct it. Important causes are neoplasms, pressure from enlarged lymph nodes, bronchitis, and bronchial asthma.

*Atelectasis* is a state of collapse in which the air sacs of the lungs are completely airless. Involving a portion of a lung, a whole lung, or both lungs, it may occur as a congenital condition or develop during postnatal life. In congenital atelectasis the lung fails to expand and to aerate; in postnatal atelectasis expanded air sacs collapse. Collapse is caused by complete obstruction of a bronchus and also by accumulation of fluid or air in the pleural cavity, which presses against the lung. When a bronchus is completely obstructed, the air beyond the obstruction is absorbed by the blood, and the lung collapses.

*Emphysema,* the consequence of *incomplete* or *partial* bronchial obstruction, is characterized by overdistention of the lungs with air (Fig. 50-5). The air sacs enlarge, and the intervening septa stretch and break down. The lungs are bloodless, soft, and pillowlike. Large blebs project on poorly supported margins of the lungs. The chest is barrel shaped. Emphysema is seen in the lungs of persons who play wind instruments, of glassblowers, of asthmatics, and of certain patients with chronic bronchitis. Emphysema and chronic bronchitis considered together are referred to as *chronic obstructive pulmonary disease* (COPD).

Chronic obstructive emphysema is one of the most important and most crippling of pulmonary diseases. It is progressive and may be generalized or localized. Prone to occur in men over the age of 50 years, it is associated clinically with marked dyspnea (shortness of breath), cough, and wheezing. Although the lungs are supercharged with air, the difficulty lies in moving it. There is increased resistance to the flow of air in the lung. Vital capacity is decreased, and expiration of air is work for the patient.

The term *senile* (small lung) *emphysema* is used to indicate an enlargement of the alveoli resulting from

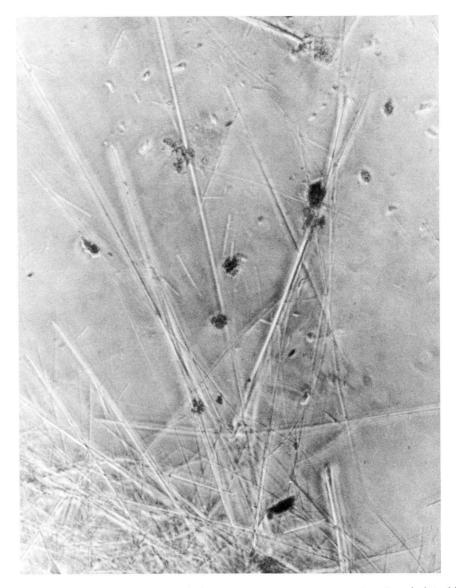

**Fig. 50-4.** Asbestos fibers, greatly magnified. (Courtesy Dr. E. Press, Oregon State Board of Health, Portland; from Oregon Health Bull. **47:**1-10, Feb., 1969.)

atrophy of their walls. The disease occurs frequently in elderly persons and gives rise to few or no symptoms. It is not true emphysema.

One form of emphysema is attributed to a deficiency of a plasma protein, alpha-1-antitrypsin. This genetic defect involving an enzyme is inherited as an autosomal recessive trait.

**Bronchial asthma** (p. 131). In asthmatic attacks there is spasm of the bronchial muscle, with hypersecretion of mucus by the glands. The lungs are emphysematous. The cell of allergic inflammation,

the eosinophil, participates in the inflammation of the bronchial wall.

**Cor pulmonale.** Cor pulmonale is hypertrophy of the right ventricle of the heart in response to the strain thrown on it by chronic pulmonary disease. With the increased pressure in the pulmonary circulation, the right heart may fail. Before the death of the patient there is hyperemia of systemic veins, enlargement of the liver, edema, and cyanosis.

**Respiratory distress syndrome.** Nearly half the deaths in infants under 1 year of age are caused by

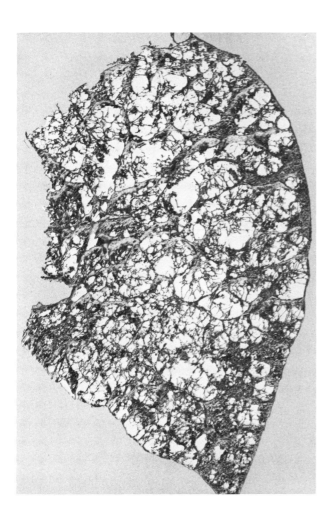

**Fig. 50-5.** Severe emphysema in thin slice of lung. Note marked enlargement of air spaces, with rupture of alveolar walls in many areas. (From Rodman, T., and Sterling, F. H.: Pulmonary emphysema and related lung diseases, St. Louis, 1969, The C. V. Mosby Co.)

respiratory disease. One important form causing death in the first few days of life is respiratory distress syndrome, also known as *hyaline membrane disease*. As indicated by the name, there is a characteristic type of difficult breathing beginning shortly after birth. The baby breathes very rapidly, the chest is caved in, and the abdomen is protuberant. With each breath the baby whines or grunts. As the disorder progresses, the baby turns blue. Most likely to develop this syndrome is a small premature baby born by cesarean section to a diabetic mother. Pathologically the dark red airless lung tissue looks like liver. Microscopically the hyaline membranes are brightly staining and line the pulmonary alveoli (Fig. 50-6).

**Neoplasms.** The lung is a common site for both metastatic and primary neoplasms. Among the tumors that metastasize to the lungs are carcinomas, sarcomas, and malignant melanoma. Primary neoplasm of the lung is quite common, and its frequency is increasing. More common in males, it is found at all ages, but especially between the ages of 50 and 60 years. The primary neoplasm of the lung is *bronchogenic carcinoma*, which may be either a squamous cell carcinoma (Fig. 50-7) or an adenocarcinoma. Squamous cell carcinoma metastasizes widely in the body. The pathologic picture of a neoplasm in the lung relates to the extent of bronchial obstruction produced.

**Air pollution and lung disease.** One of the primary effects of air pollution is the aggravation of preexisting respiratory ailments, notably bronchitis, emphysema, asthma, and lung cancer. The increase of chronic pulmonary disease is correlated with the industrialization of modern society.

## Sputum
### GENERAL CHARACTERISTICS

**Amount.** Any appreciable amount of sputum is abnormal, but a small amount may be raised by normal persons living in a dust-laden atmosphere. Excep-

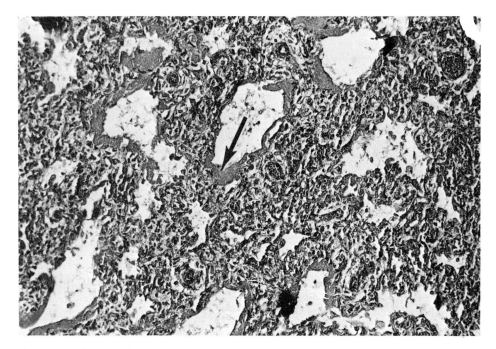

**Fig. 50-6.** Hyaline membranes (arrow) in microsection of lung. Note several air spaces wholly or partly lined by a homogeneous band of material. Intervening lung tissue is collapsed and airless. (×140.)

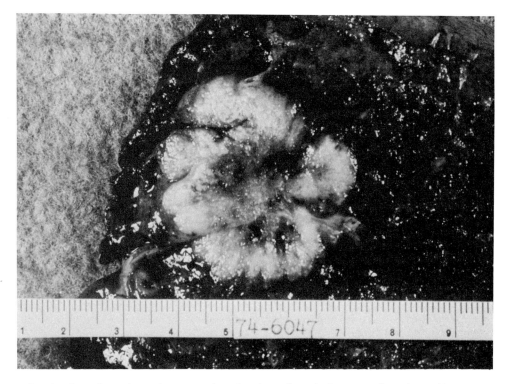

**Fig. 50-7.** Bronchogenic carcinoma, sectioned surface of surgically resected specimen. Note grayish white tumor with serrated margins.

tionally large amounts are expectorated in bronchiectasis, pulmonary edema, gangrene of the lungs, rupture of an abscess into a bronchus, and far-advanced pulmonary tuberculosis.

**Consistency.** Sputum may be of a watery or a gelatinous consistency. The tenacious character of sputum is the result of its content of mucus. In lobar pneumonia the sputum is often so tenacious that it will not pour.

**Color.** Purulent sputum is usually yellow, gray, or green. Green sputum is found in the presence of *Pseudomonas aeruginosa.* A reddish or reddish brown color indicates the presence of blood or products derived from blood. The rusty color of sputum in pneumonia results from the presence of decomposing hemoglobin.

**Character.** Sputum may be serous, mucoid, purulent, or mucopurulent. Serous sputum is thin and watery and is most often seen in pulmonary edema, in which it may be admixed with air to produce a froth. Mucoid sputum is clear, sticky, and tenacious. It is most often seen in bronchitis. Thick purulent sputum usually accompanies bronchial ulceration. Mucopurulent sputum occurs in many conditions. Frothy sputum containing fat may be caused by the lodgment of fatty emboli in the lungs.

The causes of bloody sputum are chronic passive hyperemia of lungs with mitral stenosis, pulmonary tuberculosis with cavity formation, bronchiectasis, pulmonary abscess, and bronchogenic carcinoma.

**Content.** Masses of necrotic tissue or inspissated exudate that have become impregnated with calcium salts are *lung stones.* They are most frequently expectorated by persons with tuberculosis of long duration. Lung stones may be very small, or they may reach a diameter of 1 cm. Stones originating in the bronchi are *broncholiths;* those originating in the lung tissue are *pneumoliths.*

Cheesy, pea-sized objects may occur in the sputum of acute progressive or far-advanced tuberculosis. These objects contain myriads of tubercle bacilli.

Bakers may expectorate doughy masses; cotton mill workers may expectorate cottony masses. Foreign bodies, such as bits of cloth or shot, may accidentally gain access to the lung and subsequently be coughed up.

## SPUTUM IN DISEASE

**Tuberculosis.** In tuberculosis the sputum shows wide variations. In the incipient stage of the disease no sputum may be expectorated, or it may be very scanty and of a grayish yellow or white color. As the disease progresses, the amount of sputum increases until in the far-advanced stages great quantities are produced.

The failure to find tubercle bacilli in the sputum does not necessarily mean that the disease does not exist, because the bacilli may be sparse or absent even though the disease is far advanced. One specimen of sputum may show the bacilli in abundance, and few or no bacilli may be found in a specimen taken a few days later. Tuberculous lesions not communicating with a bronchus will not yield tubercle bacilli to the sputum. Such are known as closed lesions, in contrast to open lesions.

**Other conditions.** The sputum in *lobar pneumonia* is scanty and tinged with blood (rusty). It is highly tenacious and is often expectorated with difficulty. Many pneumococci are usually present.

The sputum in *pulmonary gangrene* is a dirty brown color and has a foul and offensive odor.

The sputum in *bronchial asthma* is at first scanty, clear, and grayish in color. Later it is mucoid and microscopically shows the structures known as Curschmann's spirals and Charcot-Leyden crystals.

## Pleura

**Hydrothorax, hemothorax, and pneumothorax.** The occurrence of fluid, blood, or air in the pleural cavity is known as hydrothorax, hemothorax, and pneumothorax, respectively. Hydrothorax may be a part of the generalized dropsy of heart or kidney disease. Hemothorax may be caused by wounds of the chest, malignant tumors of the lungs or pleura, tuberculous pleurisy, or the rupture of an aneurysm into the pleural cavity. Pneumothorax may be caused by penetrating wounds of the chest wall or a communication between the pleural sac and a bronchus. When air enters a pleural sac, the negative pressure maintained in the sac is released, and the lung collapses. So much air can enter the sac that neighboring organs are pushed aside and the opposite lung is compressed.

**Pleuritis.** Pleuritis or *pleurisy,* as it is commonly called, is inflammation of the pleura. It may be caused by generalized infections or by the extension of local infections. Among the generalized infections are septicemia or pyemia. Among the local conditions, the extension of which leads to pleuritis, are pneumonia, tuberculosis, influenza, gangrene of the lung, pericarditis, and, less often, hepatitis. Pleuritis may also occur as a result of penetrating wounds of the chest. The most frequent causative organisms are streptococci, pneumococci, and tubercle bacilli.

Pleurisy occurs in three major forms: fibrinous, serofibrinous, and purulent. The second form often represents a progression of the first and the third a progression of the second, but each may possess its own distinctive features from the beginning.

## Questions for review

1  What is rhinitis?
2  Discuss bronchiectasis. What causes this condition?
3  Describe the changes in the lungs in emphysema.
4  Briefly define pneumonia and pneumonitis. List causative agents.
5  Give causes of hemoptysis.
6  What is the importance of the pneumoconioses?

7  Describe the sputum in lobar pneumonia, tuberculosis, and bronchial asthma.
8  What is the most common primary pulmonary neoplasm?
9  What are lung stones? How are they formed?
10  Define hydrothorax, hemothorax, pneumothorax.
11  What are some common causes of pleurisy?
12  Give causes and types of bronchial obstruction.

**References on p. 582.**

# CHAPTER 51

# Diseases of
# Digestive system

The digestive system comprises the mouth, pharynx, esophagus, stomach, small intestine, large intestine, rectum, and anus. The oral cavity at the beginning of this hollow tract and the stomach are expanded areas. The esophagus is a short straight tube. The small and large bowel, although of different diameters, together make up a tortuous tube some 30 or more feet in length.

Food taken into the mouth is broken up and mixed with the secretions of the oral cavity by a process of chewing. From here it is moved to the stomach, where the complex processes of digestion and absorption more properly begin. These are continued in the three parts of the small intestine—the duodenum, jejunum, and ileum. The large bowel removes water from a residue of unabsorbed material that is eliminated through the anus as feces.

## Lips, mouth, and tongue
### INFLAMMATION

The terms *stomatitis, glossitis*, and *gingivitis* indicate an inflammation of the mouth, tongue, and gums, respectively. These conditions are closely related, both etiologically and clinically. Inflammation of the lips is *cheilitis*.

**Catarrhal stomatitis or gingivitis.** Catarrhal stomatitis or gingivitis (if the gums are markedly involved) is a superficial nonulcerative inflammation of the mouth. It may be caused by mechanical, thermal, chemical, or bacterial irritants. Possibly some cases occurring when body resistance is lowered are infectious. This explains why catarrhal stomatitis appears during the course of typhoid fever, measles, gastric disorders, and diabetes.

**Aphthous stomatitis.** In aphthous stomatitis small white spots lying on an inflamed base occur on the lower lips and gums. In layman's terminology, these are canker sores. The etiology of this type of stomatitis is not known, but it is very common in teething chil-

dren who live in unhygienic surroundings or who are suffering from debilitating diseases. In adults aphthous stomatitis may be associated with digestive disturbances, and in women it may occur at each menstrual period or during pregnancy or the puerperium.

**Ulceromembranous stomatitis or gingivitis.** Ulcerative stomatitis or gingivitis may be the result of many different causes. It is found in unclean mouths with neglected teeth. It is characterized by profuse salivation, offensive breath, and the presence of areas of ulceration that most often begin on the margins of the gums and spread to the adjacent mucosa. The ulcers soon become covered with a dirty grayish pseudomembrane. In some cases the ulceration may be so extensive as to cause loosening of the teeth. Other names for this disorder include trench mouth, Vincent's angina, and fusospirochetal gingivostomatitis.

The disease may occur during acute exanthematous diseases, in grave nutritional disturbances, and in poorly nourished children. One important form of ulceromembranous gingivostomatitis is mercurial; it follows the taking of mercury compounds or affects persons whose occupation exposes them to mercury. The gingivitis and stomatitis are produced by the elimination of mercury in the saliva.

**Thrush.** Thrush is discussed on p. 332.

**Syphilis.** The lip is the most common site of extragenital chancres, and occasionally a chancre occurs within the oral cavity. Chancres of the lip and oral cavity are usually contracted by kissing and extremely rarely by the use of infected eating utensils. Mucous patches occur almost exclusively in the mouth and throat and are among the most infectious of all syphilitic lesions. During the secondary stage of the disease they are well-circumscribed, whitish, slightly raised lesions, most numerous on the inside of the lips and along the edges and on the surface of the tongue. White, star-shaped scars at the angles of the mouth (rhagades) are strong evidence of syphilis, especially the congenital type.

### NEOPLASM

In addition to the malignant neoplasms various benign tumors such as angiomas, papillomas, and fibromas may occur in the mouth.

**Epulis or giant cell tumor.** Giant cell tumor arises from the alveolar process of the jaw. It is a hard, slowly growing, benign tumor seen as a projecting mass from the gingiva, usually located in the region of the incisor teeth.

**Cancer of the lip and mouth.** Cancer of the lip and mouth often occurs at sites of chronic irritation, as caused by dental irregularities, chronic infections, tobacco, and hot pipe stems. Broken, out of line, and sharp-edged teeth and ill-fitting dentures are often at fault.

*Squamous cell carcinoma of the lip* occurs in males over 40 years of age, beginning as a thickened, pearly gray nodule, warty outgrowth, or ulcer, almost always on the lower lip. As a rule, the point of origin is the mucocutaneous junction about halfway between the midpoint of the lower lip and the angle of the mouth. In untreated cases death usually occurs within 1 to 3 years. In cancer of the lip and mouth, metastasis tends to come early.

*Squamous cell carcinoma of the tongue* begins on the edge of the anterior two-thirds of the tongue. The disease is characterized by its rapid course and high mortality, since the mobility of the tongue favors early spread to regional tissues.

*Leukoplakia* (white spot disease), a hyperplastic change in squamous epithelium of the mouth associated with chronic irritation, is an important precancerous lesion.

## Throat
### INFLAMMATION

**Pharyngitis.** Pharyngitis, inflammation of the pharynx, often represents the extension of rhinitis and nasopharyngitis. From the pharynx infection may extend to the larynx. Like rhinitis and nasopharyngitis, pharyngitis may be acute or chronic.

**Tonsillitis.** Tonsillitis is a frequent accompaniment of inflammation in other parts of the upper respiratory tract and is similar to that seen in the pharynx and larynx, except that exudate composed of exfoliated epithelial cells, white blood cells, and bacteria accumulates within the depths of the tonsillar crypts in the masses of lymphoid tissue. The bacteria may even colonize the crypts. Plugs of exudate project from the mouths of crypts and appear on the reddened surface of the tonsil as many small white patches. With repeated acute inflammation the lymphoid tissue of the tonsils and adenoids becomes hyperplastic. Ulceration or extensive necrosis of the tonsils is uncommon with the usually occurring acute low-grade upper respiratory infections, especially those related to the common cold.

**Retropharyngeal abscess.** By the term *retropharyngeal abscess* is meant an abscess in the loose tissues between the posterior pharyngeal wall and the vertebral column. Such may be acute or chronic. An acute abscess usually represents the extension of a phlegmonous pharyngitis, whereas a chronic one usually complicates tuberculosis of the cervical vertebrae. Acute retropharyngeal abscess is characterized by marked prostration, extensive swelling, pain on swallowing, loss of voice, and inability to open the mouth. The mortality is high, and death occurs as a result of suffocation.

**Diphtheria.** Diphtheria is discussed on pp. 241 and 489.

**Septic sore throat.** Septic sore throat is discussed on p. 187.

## Esophagus
### STENOSIS—STRICTURE

Stenosis or stricture of the esophagus results from (1) swallowing of hot liquids or corrosive chemicals, (2) tumors within the lumen, (3) the lodging of foreign bodies within the lumen, and (4) external pressure from tumors, enlarged lymph nodes, pericardial effusion, or an enlarged heart. When the esophagus is injured to such an extent that ulceration occurs, there is healing but with the formation of a scar, and if the ulceration has been extensive enough, the contraction of the scar produces a stricture, an abnormal narrowing of the lumen. Strictures may be single or multiple and are particularly extensive after the swallowing of corrosive poisons. The accidental swallowing of commercial lye is the most common cause of esophageal stricture in children (who mistake it for milk). In the beginning of its course esophageal stenosis is characterized by slight difficulty in swallowing solids. As the stenosis progresses, the difficulty increases until at last the patient is unable to swallow either solids or liquids, and death from starvation can occur.

### NEOPLASM

Benign tumors of the esophagus are comparatively rare. Squamous cell carcinoma of the esophagus is among the most hopeless of diseases. The first symptom is difficulty in swallowing. Unfortunately the disease is usually well advanced before symptoms occur. Death is most often caused by tumor perforation of a respiratory passage that leads to aspiration pneumonia, pulmonary gangrene, or lung abscess.

## Stomach and duodenum
### CONGENITAL DEFECTS

**Pyloric stenosis.** Congenital hypertrophic stenosis is the most important congenital defect of the stomach. The hypertrophy of the ring of muscle fibers surrounding the pylorus may be so great that the pyloric passage is almost completely occluded. The mass of hypertrophied muscle can be palpated through the abdominal wall. The cause of the disease is not known, but it affects firstborn males. As a rule, no changes are present at birth, and the infant does well for the first 2 to 4 weeks of life. Then, without apparent cause, vomiting begins. The child vomits after eating, and the vomiting ceases as soon as the stomach is empty. As the stenosis progresses, the vomiting becomes worse. The stomach dilates and hypertrophies to four or five times its normal size, and the muscular contractions to force food through the pyloric opening may be so intense that the peristaltic waves can be seen passing across the abdominal wall. Unless relieved, the child dies of starvation.

### GASTRIC HEMORRHAGE

Sizable hemorrhages are usually caused by carcinoma, ulcer, or intense passive congestion secondary to cirrhosis of the liver. The coffee-ground vomitus of partially digested blood is particularly significant in gastric carcinoma, but it may also occur in gastric ulcer or other diseases of the stomach. Exsanguinating hemorrhages secondary to portal vein obstruction may occur from a ring of varicose veins at the cardiac end of the stomach.

It is sometimes necessary to determine whether bloody material was vomited (hematemesis) or came from the lungs (hemoptysis). In hematemesis the reaction of the material is usually acid, and hydrochloric acid may be detected by chemical tests, whereas material from the lungs is alkaline in reaction and does not contain hydrochloric acid. By contrast with the coffee-ground appearance of blood of gastric origin, blood of pulmonary origin is usually frothy and bright red. However, gastric blood stemming from traumatic injury is also bright red in color and streaks the vomitus. Blood in gastric contents may be that swallowed from bleeding gums.

### PEPTIC ULCER

Peptic ulcers (Figs. 51-1 and 51-2) occur most commonly in the stomach (especially the pyloric part) and the first portion of the duodenum. They are four times as common in the duodenum. Because of the part accorded the gastric juice in the production of these ulcers, they have been called peptic, in recogni-

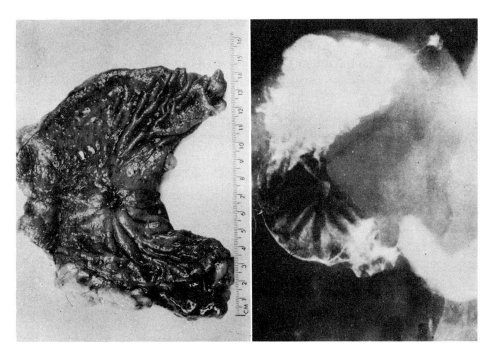

**Fig. 51-1.** Benign peptic ulcer of stomach, surgical specimen correlated with radiograph. Note typical way in which mucosal folds radiate from edge of ulcer crater. (From Kirsch, I. E.: Radiology **64:**357, 1955.)

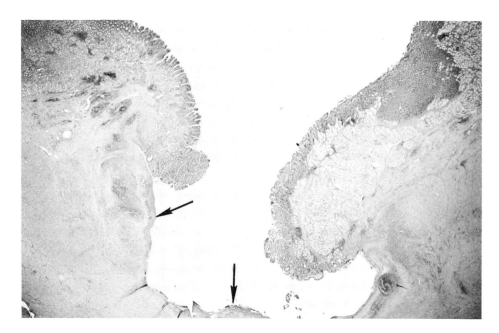

**Fig. 51-2.** Chronic peptic ulcer of stomach in microsection. Area of ulceration is concave (arrows), with mucous membrane overhanging the excavation on each side. Lumen and lining mucosa of stomach are in upper part of photograph. (×8.)

tion of the action of pepsin, the most important enzyme of the gastric juice.

Most theories of the causation of peptic ulcers are based on the assumption that in some manner a circumscribed portion of mucosa becomes devitalized and is subsequently digested by the gastric juice. Just how devitalization occurs is not known. Peptic ulcers occur as primary lesions or complicate extensive burns and acute septicemia.

Acute gastric ulcers are usually multiple and vary from pinhead size to 1 inch in diameter. In many cases no signs are present, and the ulcer heals without leaving a scar, but in other cases serious complications develop.

Chronic peptic ulcers are usually single and are most often from 1 to 2 inches in diameter. Hemorrhage is frequent and perforation can occur, although perforation is largely prevented by adhesions formed between the base of the ulcer and adjacent organs and tissues. Contraction of the scar of a healed ulcer may lead to pyloric stenosis. Chronic peptic ulcers are much more important than acute ones in both stomach and duodenum.

Hemorrhage from a chronic peptic ulcer may be fatal. In hemorrhages of moderate severity the patient feels a sudden pain and becomes faint and after a few hours passes one or more tarry stools. Perforation is indicated by sudden intense pain, shock, and rigidity of the abdominal muscles. Without immediate treatment the patient dies of generalized peritonitis within 24 to 48 hours. Gastric ulcers may be malignant neoplasms, but chronic duodenal ulcers are practically always noncancerous.

**Duodenal ulcer.** Ulcers of the duodenum are confined almost entirely to the portion receiving the acid gastric chyme. They may be acute or chronic. Like gastric ulcers, acute duodenal ulcers may be multiple. The clinical picture of chronic duodenal ulcer is much like that of chronic gastric ulcer, and the clinical differentiation of the two is often difficult.

### NEOPLASM

**Carcinoma.** For reasons undetermined, gastric carcinoma is on the decline in the United States, although the stomach is still an important site. Carcinoma of the stomach is more common in men than women and usually occurs after the fortieth year. The disease seems to be especially prevalent in certain families. Napoleon and members of his family suffered with this disorder.

The first signs of cancer of the stomach are persistent unexplained indigestion and lack of appetite, especially for meats, with a peculiar disturbance of taste.

Carcinoma usually affects the pyloric end of the stomach, occurring as (1) a large fungating mass

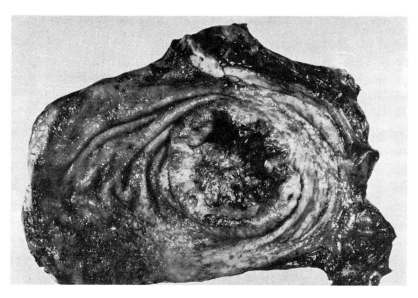

**Fig. 51-3.** Ulcerating carcinoma of stomach. Note raised, rolled edges of ulcer crater (compare orientation of mucosal folds to lesion in Figs. 51-1 and 51-4). (From Ackerman, L. V., and del Regato, J. A.: Cancer, ed. 4, St. Louis, 1970, The C. V. Mosby Co.)

projecting into the cavity of the stomach, (2) an ulcerated area with a craterlike appearance (Fig. 51-3), or (3) a diffuse infiltration of the stomach wall. The first type is the least dangerous because it does not invade the stomach wall deeply or metastasize early, and because of its large size it is rather easily discovered. Generalized invasion of the wall of the stomach by tumor with marked proliferation of connective tissue leads to the production of *linitis plastica* or leather-bottle stomach.

Among the local effects of carcinoma of the stomach are hemorrhage, perforation, and pyloric stenosis. The latter lesion, aided by fermentation of the stagnated stomach contents, leads to marked dilatation of the stomach. Gastric carcinoma metastasizes to the regional lymph nodes, liver, peritoneum, lungs, and bones.

## GASTRIC ANALYSIS

For testing and evaluation in the clinical laboratory (gastric analysis), gastric contents are aspirated through a tube passed into the stomach.

**Amount.** In normal persons the amount of gastric juice secreted each day is probably between 1500 and 3000 ml. The rate of secretion and the composition of the juice depend on several factors, important among which are the health of the person, neurogenic stimuli, action of hormones, presence of food in the stomach, and certain psychic influences such as hunger, fear, and mental anxiety.

**Composition.** At the height of digestion the stomach contains (1) water, (2) pepsin (protein-splitting enzyme), (3) hydrochloric acid, (4) mucin, (5) other electrolytes, (6) products of digestion, and (7) undigested food. In addition to these, gastric lipase (fat-splitting enzyme), cathepsin (proteolytic enzyme), and organic acids may be present. The stomach also secretes the *intrinsic factor*, a glycoprotein, which binds to *extrinsic factor*, now known to be vitamin $B_{12}$, present in meat and other foods. The interaction of the two factors aids the absorption of the large molecule of vitamin $B_{12}$ from the small intestine.

**Acidity.** Hydrochloric acid is of special importance in gastric physiology because it promotes the digestive action of pepsin, the most important digestive enzyme of the stomach. Hydrochloric acid occurs in two forms: combined and free. When food is in the stomach, a portion of the hydrochloric acid secreted enters into combination with the protein portion of the food to form protein salts of hydrochloric acid. This is known as combined acid. When the affinities of the proteins of the food have been satisfied, the excess acid appears in the free or uncombined state. In gastric analysis therefore we speak of *combined hydrochloric acid, free hydrochloric acid,* and *total acidity.* The last represents the total of the combined hydrochloric acid, free hydrochloric acid, and all other acids and acid salts that may be present. Free and total acidity are measured in terms of the amount of 0.1N alkali required to neutralize the acid in 100 ml.

of gastric contents, using two different indicators with color changes at two different pH values. The results are spoken of as *degrees* of acidity. The pH of gastric contents can also be measured electrometrically. The amount of free hydrochloric acid carries the greatest diagnostic significance.

An increased amount of free hydrochloric acid in the stomach contents is *hyperchlorhydria;* a decreased amount, *hypochlorhydria;* and an absence, *achlorhydria.* Hyperchlorhydria is almost always present in early cases of chronic peptic ulcer but may occur in other conditions such as chronic gastritis and gallstones. In carcinoma of the stomach and pellagra free hydrochloric acid is usually reduced in amount or is absent. In pernicious anemia it is absent in every case.

**Fasting state.** The average volume of the fasting stomach contents is around 50 ml. If the volume is more than 150 ml., a hypersecretion of gastric juice or an inability of the stomach to empty itself is indicated. Normal fasting contents are said to have an average total acidity of around 10 to 50 degrees and an average free hydrochloric acid content around 5 to 25 degrees. Ordinarily from 50 to 100 ml. of gastric contents may be removed at the end of 1 hour after a test meal. At this time the total acidity normally ranges around 50 to 70 degrees, the free hydrochloric acid around 25 to 50 degrees, and the combined around 10 to 15 degrees.

*However, it must be noted that wide normal variations exist.* *

**Bacterial content.** Normal acidity in the stomach inhibits the growth of microbes. The gastric juice destroys important bacterial toxins except the toxin of *Clostridium botulinum.* The Boas-Oppler bacillus, which is a *Lactobacillus* species and the only organism of significance encountered in the gastric contents, occurs in most cases of cancer of the stomach but is seldom found in other conditions.

**Tubeless gastric analysis.** Since the passage of the gastric tube is not always relished by the patient, technics have been developed to circumvent intubation. When an exchange resin such as the commercial product, Diagnex Blue, is taken orally, chemical reactions occur in the stomach with free gastric acidity, the results of which can be determined in the urine. With this resin a dye, azure A, is eluted in the stomach but passed to the kidneys for elimination, where it is

___

* A precise range of gastric acidity has not been established because of the variable stimulation of the different test meals and technics. A stomach in the *fasting* state has not received food for a period of at least 8 hours.

easily measured in the urine. This is *tubeless gastric analysis* and indicates the ability of the stomach to form acid.

**Application.** Gastric analysis is often resorted to when either gastric ulcer or carcinoma is suspected. The gastric findings may help to differentiate these two common conditions. In chronic peptic ulcer the gastric acidity is usually high. In gastric carcinoma, it is usually below normal or absent, uncommonly is normal, and rarely is above. The Boas-Oppler bacillus is found with malignancy, not with ulcer. Blood may be associated with either.

## Intestines
### ABNORMALITIES OF SHAPE AND POSITION

**Diverticula.** Diverticula may be congenital or acquired. Acquired diverticula may arise from either the small or large intestine but are more common and larger in connection with the latter (especially in the descending colon).

The most important congenital diverticulum is *Meckel's diverticulum,* which is caused by an incomplete obliteration of the primitive yolk stalk. It arises from the ileum about 18 inches above the cecum. Showing considerable variation in size and shape, it occurs most of the time as a thumblike process extending from the intestine and measuring from 1 to 3 inches in length. When Meckel's diverticulum is inflamed, it simulates appendicitis. It may ulcerate and even perforate.

**Hernia.** The term *hernia* * in its broadest sense means protrusion of a viscus through an opening in the body cavity that contains it. The term often refers to the protrusion of a part of the intestine (usually the small intestine) or some other abdominal viscus through an opening in the abdominal wall. A hernia is produced when an abdominal viscus passes through (1) an opening that has not closed completely or a completely closed one that is congenitally weak (inguinal, femoral, and umbilical hernias), (2) openings occasioned by injuries to the abdominal wall, or (3) a weakened area in a healed surgical incision of the abdominal wall.

A typical hernia in the abdomen consists of the *sac,* which represents a pouchlike protrusion of the peritoneum, and the *contents,* which usually are intestine or omentum or both.

*Kinds.* Inguinal, femoral, and umbilical hernias are the most common kinds. *Inguinal* hernias are of two types: (1) the *indirect,* in which the components of the hernia enter the inguinal canal through the internal abdominal ring and leave by way of the exter-

___

* The lay term for hernia is *rupture.*

nal abdominal ring to descend into the scrotum, and (2) the *direct,* in which the viscus passes directly through the abdominal wall and emerges from the external abdominal ring, where it appears under the skin or passes to the scrotum. In women inguinal hernias pass to the labia majora. In *femoral* hernias the hernia protrudes from the femoral ring and presents on the inside of the thigh. *Umbilical* hernias occur in infants as a result of imperfect closure of the abdominal wall at the umbilicus.

A *diaphragmatic hernia* represents an upward displacement of an abdominal viscus through an acquired or congenital opening in the diaphragm. The diaphragm is a flat sheet of muscle fibers, important in respiration, that forms a partition between the abdominal area and the chest cavity. A special kind of diaphragmatic hernia is the *hiatal hernia,* occurring at the opening through which the esophagus passes to the stomach. A small part of the wall of the stomach may protrude through this opening into the chest cavity near its connection to the esophagus. Oftentimes this is of no consequence, but in a few persons acid from the stomach regurgitates into the esophagus to induce inflammatory changes and sometimes even ulceration.

In a general way it may be said that a hernia results when increased intra-abdominal pressure forces certain structures in the abdominal cavity into the hernial opening. The hernia may come on suddenly, as after a strain, or more gradually. When the hernial contents can be returned to their normal position within the abdominal cavity, the hernia is said to be *reducible.* Inflammatory adhesions between the hernia and surrounding structures may make the hernia *irreducible,* as may a collection of feces in the lumen of the portion of intestine entering the hernial sac. An irreducible hernia without any disturbance of blood supply is said to be *incarcerated.* When the blood supply is cut off, the hernia is said to be *strangulated.* Incarcerated hernias can quickly become strangulated. Strangulation, an ever-present danger in all hernias, is quickly followed by congestion, swelling, and paralysis of the bowel, with resulting gangrene and peritonitis.

## TRAUMA

**Perforation.** Perforation of the intestine may be produced directly (by blows or blunt injury to the abdomen) or indirectly (from blows to the back or from a fall). In many cases little sign of external injury is present. The signs of intestinal perforation are profound shock, abdominal rigidity, vomiting, and pain. If the patient survives the initial shock, peritonitis follows.

## INFLAMMATION

Of importance are the communicable diseases caused by bacteria—typhoid fever and salmonelloses (p. 203), bacillary dysentery (p. 207), and tuberculosis (p. 251)—and those caused by intestinal parasites, including amebic dysentery (Chapter 31).

## OBSTRUCTION

By intestinal obstruction is meant a partial or complete occlusion of the bowel lumen or the effect of occlusion produced by an interference with the passage of its contents. Obstruction may be acute or chronic and may affect the large or small intestine. The large intestine tolerates obstruction much better than the small intestine, and complete obstruction of the large bowel may exist for several days without causing symptoms.

**Causes.** The causes of intestinal obstruction may be classified as mechanical and paralytic. Mechanical causes include (1) changes involving the intestinal wall (strangulation of hernias, intussusception, volvulus, and the contraction of scars from ulcers), (2) outside pressure (from bands, adhesions, tumors, or misplaced organs), and (3) obstruction within the lumen (tumors, polyps, calculi, intestinal parasites, and foreign bodies). Paralytic obstruction or *paralytic ileus* is caused by blocking of the blood or nerve supply of the intestine. This effects paralysis of the given segment. Since the paralyzed segment is unable to pass its contents, the bowel is just as truly obstructed as if it were mechanically obstructed. Paralytic ileus, which is always acute, is caused by peritonitis and complicates fractures of the ribs and infectious conditions such as pneumonia. Sometimes it results from mesenteric thrombosis or occurs as a postoperative complication, especially when the intestine has not been gently manipulated. Rarely, it occurs without known cause.

*Intussusception.* Intussusception means the slipping or telescoping of a portion of intestine into the succeeding portion. Intussusception is said to be brought about by increased peristalsis of the segment that becomes invaginated or by atony of the portion that receives it.

As the upper segment slips into the lower, the bowel is obstructed, and the mesentery is pulled between the two layers of intestine and pinched so that from the very beginning, both obstruction and interference with blood supply exist. When acute intussusception occurs, the classic features of obstruction appear. A chronic form of intussusception that may end in acute obstruction occasionally occurs in adults.

*Volvulus.* By volvulus is meant the twisting of a loop of intestine on its long axis or the rotation of a loop of intestine to such an extent that its mesentery becomes twisted. In either case interference with the blood supply of the affected segment leads to paralytic ileus, gangrene, and peritonitis. The disease occurs most often in elderly persons, and the pelvic colon is the most common site.

**Kinds.** Strangulated hernias, constrictions by fibrous adhesions, intussusception, or volvulus most often cause *acute mechanical obstruction* of the intestine. A coil of intestine may be obstructed if it slips into an opening or pocket formed by a fibrous band extending from the bowel to the mesentery or an adjacent segment of bowel.

Acute intestinal obstruction can occur with lightning rapidity and practically never without interference in the blood supply of the affected segment; many of its features come from the involvement of the blood supply. In fact, blocking of the blood supply to a segment of intestine may, within itself, cause obstruction. At first, there is violent peristalsis above the obstruction, giving rise to most intense pain. Shock, vomiting, and abdominal rigidity follow, with paralysis and dilatation of the bowel. Serum pours into the distended bowel, and bacteria multiply in its stagnated contents; these combine to increase the distention. The vomiting increases and becomes fecal. The pa-

tient soon goes into collapse. The intestinal wall blackens and becomes gangrenous. If actual rupture does not occur, bacteria permeate the intestinal wall. Violent peritonitis speedily develops and rapidly proves fatal. The higher the obstruction in the intestinal tract, the more severe and rapidly fatal it is.

*Chronic intestinal obstruction* differs from acute obstruction in that there is no interference with the blood supply. If the blood supply becomes blocked, the chronic obstruction becomes acute. Chronic obstruction may be caused by the growth of tumors in the intestinal wall and the gradual contraction of scars. Chronic obstruction is always incomplete. When it becomes complete, the manifestations of acute obstruction develop. In the large bowel the obstruction may be complete several days before there is any indication.

## MALABSORPTION SYNDROME

If because of disease there is an interference in the process of absorption of food from any part of the gastrointestinal tract, the malabsorption syndrome may develop. The clinical features of this disorder are diarrhea, abdominal distention, weight loss, weakness, pigmentation of the skin, presence of fat in the stools (steatorrhea), various signs of vitamin and min-

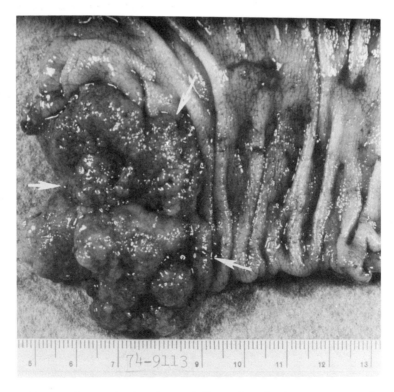

**Fig. 51-4.** Adenocarcinoma of colon. Arrows indicate ulcerating tumor on mucosal surface.

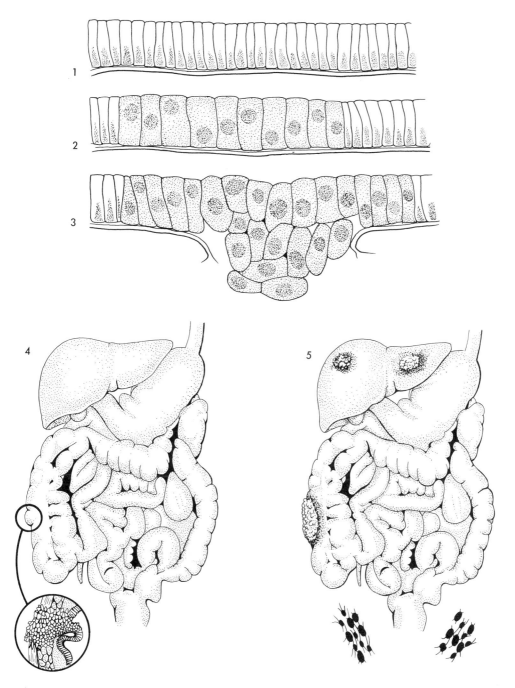

**Fig. 51-5.** Natural history of cancer of the large bowel. **1,** Segment of normal bowel. **2,** Focus of carcinoma-in-situ (noninvasive). **3,** Early invasion—disruption of basement membrane but cancer localized. **4,** Invasive carcinoma—penetration of muscle layer of bowel wall to serosa. **5,** Metastases to regional lymph nodes and to distant organs—liver, lung, brain, and bone. (Redrawn from Berlin, N. I.: Hosp. Pract. **10:**83, Jan., 1975.)

eral deficiencies, and, in a young individual, retardation of growth and development. Malabsorption syndrome may be either primary or secondary. It is secondary to any pathologic process that cuts down on the effective surface area for absorption, as for example, extensive surgical resection of bowel, malignancies, intestinal obstruction, or heavy parasitic infection. Examples of the primary form are celiac disease and sprue, which are biochemical disorders characterized by enzymatic deficits in the mucosal cells of the small intestine. (Most of the food that we eat is absorbed from the small intestine.)

### NEOPLASM

Neoplasms are rare in the small bowel and common in the large bowel. In more than one-half the cases the site of the tumor is in the descending colon, sigmoid, and rectum. Cancer of the colon and rectum are among the most common internal cancers today. The important benign tumor is the *adenomatous polyp,* which may occur as a single lesion or as multiple ones *(polyposis).* For the most part, it is considered to be a precancerous lesion.

The malignant tumor of the colon is the *adenocarcinoma* (Fig. 51-4). In the left colon it is an annular constricting lesion that produces a napkin ring obstruction. In the right colon a fungating mass projects into the lumen. Secondary ulceration associated with bleeding may give rise to severe anemia.

At first, carcinoma of the colon may be symptomless. A vague abdominal distress may appear that increases to pain, at first intermittent, then constant. When obstruction is brought about by the tumor, there are changes in bowel habits. Alternating episodes of diarrhea and constipation characterize the disease. Carcinoma of the colon eventually leads to acute intestinal obstruction. Metastases are to the regional lymph nodes, the peritoneum, and the liver (Fig. 51-5).

## Vermiform appendix
### INFLAMMATION

Appendicitis (inflammation of the appendix) usually begins in the mucosa and spreads to the other layers of the appendix. The bacteria that most often cause appendicitis are *Escherichia coli,* staphylococci, and streptococci. The bacteria reach the wall of the appendix by way of its lumen, occasionally by way of the bloodstream. Certain anaerobic bacteria that are normal inhabitants of the intestine may act as secondary invaders. Obstruction to the lumen of the appendix is considered the single most important factor in the development of acute appendicitis. Fecaliths may lodge in the lumen and impinge on the wall in such a way as to interfere with the blood supply. Obstruc-

tion can also be produced by inflammatory swelling of the mucosa and sometimes in children by marked hyperplasia of the lymphoid tissue, which is normally so abundant in the appendiceal mucosa of a young person. When occlusion of the lumen from any cause occurs, the tissues of the wall are more vulnerable to bacterial invasion. This factor along with the rather poor blood supply of the appendix predisposes it to gangrene.

Appendicitis is confined almost exclusively to civilized races. Evidence strongly indicates that its great frequency in civilized man is in some way connected with his diet. Appendicitis can be classified as acute and chronic. Acute appendicitis includes diffuse, suppurative, and gangrenous forms of inflammation plus the complication of perforation.

**Acute appendicitis.** The diffusely inflamed appendix is greatly swollen, soft, and bright or dark red in color; the serous surface may be covered with fibrin; and the lumen may be filled with exudate. There is a diffuse inflammation of all layers of the wall of the appendix. When the inflammation is so intense as to cause widespread suppuration of the wall, the process is spoken of as *suppurative* appendicitis. When the inflammatory process reaches the serous surface of the appendix, localized peritonitis produces adhesions about the appendix that may later save the patient's life.

If during the course of diffuse appendicitis there is thrombosis of vessels or the appendix is swollen, bent, and twisted on itself, the interference in the blood supply may result in gangrene. The gangrene may be confined to the tip of the appendix, may occur in multiple foci, or may involve the whole organ. When gangrene occurs, perforation is imminent.

Perforation comes from the pressure exerted on the inflamed and weakened wall by a fecalith in the lumen. It most often affects the tip of the appendix but may occur at any point. If perforation takes place after adhesions have formed about the appendix, the adhesions may act as a wall to prevent the generalized dissemination of the infectious material, and a localized collection of pus limited by a wall of adhesions is found surrounding the appendix. This is an *appendiceal abscess.* If the perforation takes place before adhesions have formed or, if the contents of the appendix are under such tension that the adhesions are broken when the perforation occurs, the infectious material is widely disseminated, and generalized peritonitis follows. Appendiceal abscesses may enlarge and break into the general peritoneal cavity. They may evacuate their contents through a fistulous opening into the intestine. Small abscesses may be absorbed, leaving the appendix bound in a mass of adhesions.

**Chronic appendicitis.** When a patient complains of vague abdominal pain, backache, flatulence, and slight tenderness over the appendix, a diagnosis of chronic appendicitis is often made. That many of these patients have true chronic appendicitis is doubtful. True chronic inflammation of the appendix is rare, but because of previous acute attacks the appendix may become thickened, constricted, kinked, and bound by adhesions to such an extent that it is predisposed to recurrent acute attacks, and in rare instances the vague symptoms just enumerated may be produced.

In the condition known as *obliterative appendicitis* the appendix is shrunken, firm, and pale, and the lumen is completely or partially obliterated by an ingrowth of connective tissue. In some cases the obliterative process is confined to the end of the appendix. Appendiceal obliteration may result from the atrophy of old age, or it may be of inflammatory origin. Such appendices probably never give rise to symptoms in the absence of acute inflammation.

## Rectum and anus
### INFLAMMATION

**Proctitis.** Proctitis or inflammation of the rectum may be caused by bacterial infections, parasites, toxic agents, irritating injections, or irritation from fecal material. It may be secondary to such conditions as hemorrhoids or rectal tumors. In acute proctitis the mucosa is swollen and edematous. Mucus, blood, and pus may be present. Ulceration may occur, or the inflammation may diffuse through the rectal wall and involve the perirectal tissues, producing *periproctitis*.

**Abscess.** The most important abscess connected with the rectum is the *ischiorectal* abscess, which occurs in the loose tissue of the ischiorectal fossa and is caused by the extension of an infection arising about the anal canal. An ischiorectal abscess may open just into the rectum or into the rectum and onto the skin. The latter produces a fistulous tract connecting the lumen of the rectum with the outside of the body.

**Fissure.** An anal fissure is a painful linear ulcer that occupies one of the furrows between the longitudinal folds of the anal margin. It results from trauma or overstretching of the anal canal by the passage of hard fecal masses. The fissure becomes infected and because of repeated infection and stretching fails to heal. It produces agonizing pain and may lead to ischiorectal abscess.

**Fistula.** A rectal fistula (fistula in ano) is a discharging sinus (or sinuses) with one or more openings into the anal canal and one or more openings onto the surface of the body or into some body cavity such as the vagina or bladder. It is usually formed in the following manner. The mucosa of the anus becomes infected, and the infection burrows into the surrounding tissues, especially into the ischiorectal fossa, leav-

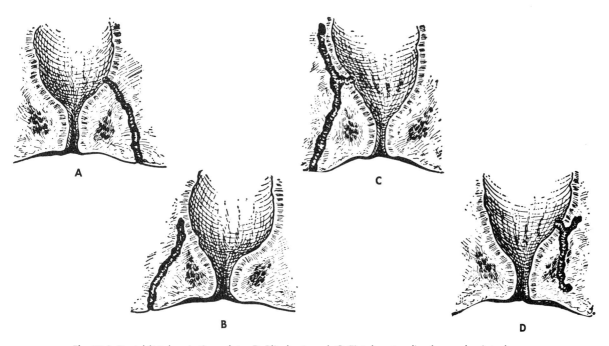

**Fig. 51-6.** Rectal fistulas. **A,** Complete. **B,** Blind external. **C,** Fistula extending beyond point of opening into gut. **D,** Blind internal.

ing a fistulous tract behind it; an abscess develops and opens on the surface of the body or into the vagina or bladder. When the tract reaches the surface of the body or a body cavity, the fistula is said to be complete; until this has occurred, the fistula is said to be incomplete. (See Fig. 51-6.)

## HEMORRHOIDS

Hemorrhoids or *piles* are varicosities and dilatations of the veins that form a plexus beneath the mucosal lining of the rectum and anus. If the lower end of the plexus is affected, the hemorrhoids are covered by the anal skin; if the upper end, the rectal mucous membrane covers them. Hemorrhoids that are covered by skin are known as external hemorrhoids; those covered by mucous membrane, as internal hemorrhoids.

Any condition that interferes with the return of blood from the plexus or in any way throws an increased burden on it predisposes to hemorrhoids. Among the general causes of hemorrhoids are failing heart action and cirrhosis of the liver with obstruction of the portal circulation. Among the local causes are constipation, pressure from a pelvic tumor, a pregnant or misplaced uterus, carcinoma of the rectum, and an enlarged prostate gland. Constipation is by far the most important local cause.

Uncomplicated external hemorrhoids have the same appearance as varicose veins in other parts of the body. Internal hemorrhoids occur as elongated, soft, dark purple masses that arise in the first 3 or 4 cm. of rectal mucosa above the anorectal line.* The oozing of blood from hemorrhoids may cause anemia.

## STRICTURE

Benign strictures of the rectum may be congenital or acquired. Acquired strictures may be caused by external pressure from bands or adhesions or by narrowing of the lumen resulting from contraction of scar tissue following inflammations or operations. An infectious cause is lymphopathia venereum (p. 274). Benign strictures are usually located from 1 to 1½ inches above the anus. They are commoner in blacks than in whites.

## PROLAPSE

Prolapse of the rectum is a pathologic descent of one or more layers of the rectum through the anus.

## NEOPLASM

Adenocarcinoma of the rectum forms about 5% of all carcinomas and about three fourths of all intes-

tinal tumors. It occurs more often in men than in women and is rare in blacks. Certain rectal tumors usually considered to be benign, notably adenomas and papillomas, have a tendency to become carcinomatous.

Carcinoma of the rectum usually begins in the mucosa and gradually invades the muscular wall, producing a stricture. The most constant manifestations are bleeding, pain, and constipation or alternating diarrhea and constipation. Pain indicates that the growth has extended beyond the confines of the rectum, since the rectum itself has no pain sensation. Probably the most constant early sign of carcinoma of the rectum is a feeling of discomfort in the rectum not relieved by defecation.

Carcinoma of the rectum may spread to the prostate gland, bladder, vagina, and uterus by direct extension, to the neighboring lymph nodes by the lymphatic system, and to the liver by the bloodstream.

## FECES

Feces are a mixture of (1) undigested food remains, (2) partially digested food and products of digestion, (3) products added by the activity of the digestive tract, such as bile and pancreatic enzymes, (4) decomposition products, (5) epithelial cells, (6) bacteria, and (7) water. The normal offensive odor of the stool is caused by the decomposition products, indole and skatole.

**Color.** Normally the stool is of a light or dark brown color because of the presence of hydrobilirubin, which is derived from bilirubin, one of the bile pigments. Changes in color may be caused by diet, drugs, disease, or hemorrhage. A meat diet gives a dark color; milk gives a yellow color; with a vegetable diet, the stool is of a greenish brown color. After the ingestion of bismuth salts or drugs containing iron, the stool is black or greenish black. Clay- or putty-colored stools occur when the amount of bile or pancreatic juice delivered to the intestine is deficient. The clay color is the result of an abnormally large amount of undigested fat. Green stools occur in the diarrheas of children but may occur in apparently healthy persons. Stools containing large amounts of pus or mucus may be gray in color.

**Mucus.** Mucus may occur intimately mixed with the stool, may be on the outside of it, or may form casts of the intestine. An excessive amount is always abnormal and indicates an irritation or inflammation. In dysentery, ileocolitis, and intussusception the stools may consist entirely of blood-streaked mucus. Mucus casts may be mistaken for tapeworms.

**Melena.** Blood may occur in feces as a result of disease in any part of the alimentary tract. In some

---

*The line that marks the junction of the rectal mucosa and the skin.

cases it can be detected by gross observation, whereas in others its detection depends on chemical tests for *occult blood*. Macroscopic blood may occur as streaks on the surface of the stool. A sizable quantity of blood intimately mixed with the stool gives it a tarry black, red-brown, or red color. Tarry stools are caused by the digestive action of intestinal enzymes on the blood and indicate that the hemorrhage originated high in the alimentary tract (throat, esophagus, stomach, or small intestine). A red or red-brown color indicates that the hemorrhage probably originated in the lower bowel. If diarrhea is present, blood from high intestinal hemorrhages may be red in color because it is swept along so swiftly as to be little affected by the digestive enzymes. Blood streaks on the outside of the stool indicate rectal or anal lesions such as ulcers, fissures, or hemorrhoids. The serious causes of blood in the feces are cancer or ulcer of the stomach or intestine.

## Liver

The liver, placed in the right upper quadrant of the abdomen and partly attached to the diaphragm, is the largest gland in the body and one of the most complex organs biochemically. Its functions are many, complex, and divergent. Its most important anatomic connection is to the portal vein, from which it receives the blood collected by the tributaries draining the gastrointestinal tract.

### DEGENERATIONS

The liver is subject to practically all the degenerative lesions such as cloudy swelling, amyloid infiltration, fatty changes, and pigmentation.

**Fatty metamorphosis.** Fatty metamorphosis is discussed on p. 469.

**Acute necrosis.** The term *acute yellow atrophy* is sometimes applied to a condition characterized by widespread and diffuse necrosis of the liver. There are many causes of this severe type of liver disease.

Chemicals called hepatotoxins are especially toxic for liver cells and may produce necrosis. Examples are phosphorus, carbon tetrachloride, chloroform, and arsenicals. Diffuse necrosis of the liver may also be caused by viruses (the viruses of yellow fever and hepatitis) and by metabolic disorders (severe hyperthyroidism).

The liver is enlarged at first and quite yellow; in the later stages it is shrunken, reddish in color, and covered by a wrinkled capsule. The course of clinical disease is short and characterized by fever, marked jaundice, coma, and other manifestations of acute hepatic insufficiency. Acute yellow atrophy is misnamed because the lesions are essentially necrotic instead of atrophic.

## CIRCULATORY DISTURBANCE— PORTAL OBSTRUCTION

In portal obstruction there is an interference with the passage of blood through the portal vein into the liver. It may be caused by thrombosis of or pressure on the portal vein outside the liver or its branches within the liver. When the portal vein becomes obstructed, its tributaries dilate. Dilatation of the veins around the umbilicus leads to the formation of a *caput medusae*. Dilatation of the hemorrhoidal veins causes hemorrhoids, and fatal hemorrhage may result from varices formed in the esophagus and stomach. Ascites and edema of the lower extremities occur.

### INFLAMMATION

Viral hepatitis is discussed on p. 316.

**Abscess.** Abscess of the liver may be caused by (1) extension of an inflammation from the gallbladder and bile ducts (cholangitis), (2) the transfer of infectious material to the liver by the portal vein or hepatic artery, and (3) amebic dysentery.

Pyogenic abscesses are most often secondary to ulcerative conditions of the intestine, suppurative appendicitis, or infected hemorrhoids but may occur as a part of septic endocarditis or generalized pyemia. Amebic abscesses are caused by *Entamoeba histolytica* carried from the intestinal ulcers of amebic dysentery to the liver by the portal vein (Fig. 31-4).

Pyogenic abscesses are often small and multiple. Amebic abscesses are usually single and often reach a large size; they are filled with a curdy, brown, foul-smelling material that is partly pus and partly disintegrated liver cells.

A liver abscess may be absorbed, become encapsulated and calcified, or rupture into the peritoneal or pleural cavity. Occasionally an abscess opens on the outside of the body.

### CIRRHOSIS

Cirrhosis, the end stage of chronic liver disease, is increasing in importance and becoming one of the leading causes of death in this country. It is a chronic disorder of the liver characterized by an increase in the supporting connective tissue of the organ, with degeneration of its parenchymatous cells. A characteristic feature of the disease pertains to the scattered nodules of regenerating liver tissue, which give the gross nodularity and contribute to the distortion of connections among liver cells, blood vessels, and bile ducts. There are three main types of the disease: portal, postnecrotic, and biliary.

**Portal cirrhosis (alcoholic cirrhosis, hobnail liver).** Portal cirrhosis is the most common form of cirrhosis of the liver and is twice as common in males as in females. Alcohol, dietary deficiencies, and diges-

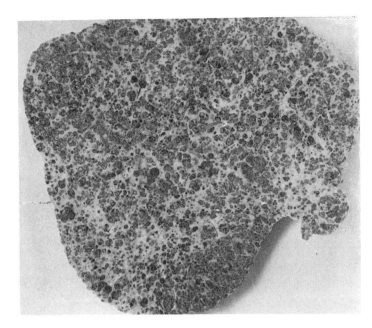

**Fig. 51-7.** Nodular liver of portal cirrhosis, cut surface.

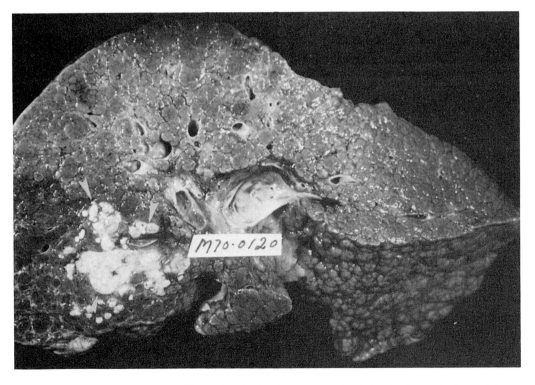

**Fig. 51-8.** Primary carcinoma of liver developing in postnecrotic cirrhosis. Tumor in lower left corner (arrows). Note multicentric sites of origin.

tive disturbances are important etiologic factors, although the pathogenesis of the disease is not clear. The fibrosis, the degeneration and loss of parenchymal tissue, plus the nodules of regenerating liver cells, all give the liver a very particular gross and microscopic appearance. (See Fig. 51-7.) The liver is smaller than normal, hard, and finely nodular. Portal obstruction is a regular accompaniment of portal cirrhosis, with passive hyperemia of the abdominal viscera. Splenic enlargement is an important sign. Massive recurrent ascites is related to the portal obstruction and to a reduction of the plasma protein levels in the blood (*hypoproteinemia*).

Of the three plasma proteins, albumin and fibrinogen are formed in the liver. Globulin, the third, is built up in the reticuloendothelial organs, of which the liver is one. These proteins can be measured chemically in the plasma, and deviations from normal values are important changes related to liver disease. The lowered amount of albumin, which is associated with failure of the liver to synthesize this protein in normal amounts, contributes to the development of the ascites and peripheral edema seen in the cirrhotic patient.

**Postnecrotic cirrhosis (coarse nodular cirrhosis, toxic cirrhosis, healed yellow atrophy).** Postnecrotic cirrhosis is the end stage, usually months or years later, of a diffuse necrosis of liver such as results from the action of chemical hepatotoxin or drug, or from the injury of viral hepatitis. The pattern of scarring and nodular regeneration is an uneven one, and the liver is considerably distorted. The nodules may be fairly large (Figs. 51-8 and 44-4), and in scattered focal areas, normal liver tissue may have even been spared. The medical effects are comparable to those of portal cirrhosis.

**Obstructive biliary cirrhosis.** In obstructive biliary cirrhosis the pathologic changes occur as a result of obstruction to outflow of bile. The obstruction may be in the biliary system outside the liver or within the intrahepatic system of ducts. The bile stagnates and collects within the lumina of the bile ducts, which dilate considerably. There are an increase in fibrous connective tissue and a degeneration of parenchymal tissue. Especially striking is the pigmentation of liver tissue seen in the well-advanced condition. The large, hard liver is a deep green in color, and bile pigment is seen microscopically within the cytoplasm of the liver cells. Jaundice is marked in the patient.

In infancy a congenital anomaly of the bile duct system may be the cause of this type of cirrhosis, the child usually succumbing to the disorder some time before the end of the first year of life. Important causes of biliary cirrhosis in older persons include strictures in the biliary ducts, gallstones, or a malignant neoplasm growing in the head of the pancreas in such a way as to obstruct the common bile duct just before it enters the duodenum.

## NEOPLASM

Benign tumors of the liver are comparatively rare. Of these, hemangiomas are most important. Of the malignant tumors, metastatic carcinomas and sarcomas are most significant. Primary carcinoma of the liver is quite rare in the United States, but when it does occur, it usually complicates preexisting cirrhosis (Fig. 51-8). In fact, carcinoma is sometimes listed as an important complication of portal cirrhosis. In Africa and the Orient primary carcinoma of the liver is prevalent. Carcinoma is unusual in that when present, it can almost invariably be demonstrated to arise in several scattered foci within the liver substance, that is, from *multicentric* sites of origin. The neoplasm originates in the liver cells as a parenchymal cell carcinoma or in the bile ducts as an adenocarcinoma.

## LIVER FUNCTION

One of the vital organs, the liver is a very complex structure, and the list of normal physiologic functions it regularly performs is a lengthy and imposing one. A given physiologic function may lend itself rather easily to measurement chemically in blood or urine, and as a result a number of tests on blood and urine have been devised that relate rather specifically to certain metabolic processes carried out in the liver. From this it would seem that evaluating the status of the liver in disease would be an easy matter in the clinical laboratory. Such is not the case, however. One reason why this is so is that the liver possesses an enormous reserve, estimated at 85% to 90%. This means that we have much more liver tissue than we absolutely need for normal living. In fact, it can be demonstrated in a suitable experimental animal that easily 75% of the total amount of liver tissue present may be surgically removed and yet the animal will continue to be well and free of symptoms. Practically, then, the vast liver reserve means that extensive disease present in the liver may not give any measurable indication of its activity.

We also know that the various functions the liver performs are not necessarily interrelated and that hepatic physiology is irregularly and inconsistently involved even in the same pathologic process in different patients. Although it is often impossible to determine exactly the amount of damage to liver cells in a given situation, we can nevertheless gain useful information by using not a single chemical determination but several, that is, a *battery* of tests. Let us consider a few.

Since the liver functions in bile pigment metabolism, serum bilirubin and urinary urobilinogen may be helpful. Since the plasma proteins are synthesized in the liver, deviations from normal values relate to liver disease. The total amount of blood cholesterol and the amount altered or esterified may be significant because the chemical alteration, the esterification, is done in the liver. There are many other important tests of liver function, such as those that relate to excretion of injected dyes, detoxification activities, and carbohydrate metabolism.

## Gallbladder and bile ducts

The gallbladder is a pear-shaped, hollow organ closely attached to the back surface of the liver. The neck continues into the cystic duct, which joins the common hepatic duct to become the common bile duct, emptying into the duodenum.

The gallbladder is a reservoir for bile and actively concentrates it by removing some of the water.

### JAUNDICE (ICTERUS)

The yellow color of plasma and bile is caused by the bile pigment bilirubin, which is derived from hemoglobin liberated by the destruction of red blood cells and excreted in bile by the liver. If the liver loses its ability to excrete the bilirubin normally formed or if the destruction of red blood cells becomes so great that more bilirubin is formed than the liver can excrete, the pigment content of the blood rises to a high level, and the tissues of the body take on a yellow color—the condition known as icterus or jaundice. Icterus may be accompanied by an intense itching of the skin, prolonged clotting time of the blood, and a tendency to hemorrhage. In many cases bile appears in the urine.

Jaundice resulting from interference with the excretion of bile by the diseased or damaged liver cells is known as *hepatocellular* or *hepatogenous* jaundice. If jaundice is produced by an obstruction in the biliary passages blocking the outflow of bile into the intestine, it is *obstructive*. Jaundice caused by an overproduction of bilirubin is known as *hematogenous* jaundice.

The most important causes of obstructive jaundice are inflammatory swellings of the mucosa occluding the excretory bile ducts, gallstones in the ducts, outside pressure on the ducts, and occlusion of the bile ducts within the liver by cirrhosis. If occlusion affects only the cystic duct, jaundice will not occur. Hepatocellular injury associated with jaundice is produced by severe anoxemia, viruses, and hepatotoxins. Among the important causes of hematogenous jaundice are those diseases characterized by an increased destruction of red blood cells (certain hemolytic anemias), severe infections, certain instances of poison-

ing, and the disease entity known as hereditary spherocytosis or congenital hemolytic anemia (p. 446).

### INFLAMMATION

Inflammation of the bile ducts is known as *cholangitis*, inflammation of the gallbladder as *cholecystitis*. Both may be acute or chronic.

**Acute cholecystitis.** Acute cholecystitis may be catarrhal or suppurative and begins in the gallbladder as a result of the irritation caused by gallstones or retained bile. It may represent the extension of cholangitis. Suppuration may be so extensive that the gallbladder becomes filled with a purulent exudate (*empyema of the gallbladder*), and peritonitis may occur because of rupture of the gallbladder or direct extension of the infection through its wall. Acute cholecystitis may also be gangrenous, with a chemical type of necrosis of the gallbladder wall. Either gangrenous or suppurative cholecystitis is an acute surgical emergency.

**Chronic cholecystitis.** Chronic cholecystitis follows the acute form, or it may be more or less chronic from the beginning. The condition of the gallbladder depends on the relation existing between infection and obstruction. If infection is the principal feature and obstruction is slight, the wall is thickened, elasticity is lost, and the size of the cavity is reduced. If infection plays an insignificant part and obstruction plays the major role, the wall is thin and the organ is markedly dilated and filled with a viscid fluid.

Chronic cholecystitis is important in the production of gallstones, and gallbladders containing stones are often the site of acute or chronic cholecystitis.

### CHOLELITHIASIS

**Gallstones.** Gallstones are calculi that ordinarily form in the gallbladder but that may form in the larger bile ducts. They are composed of certain constituents of the bile that have precipitated onto a nucleus of bacteria and dead cells derived from the epithelium of the gallbladder or duct in which they are situated. In some cases the nucleus is composed of inspissated mucus.

*Causes.* The causes of gallstones are conditions that precipitate the constituents of bile. Important among these are inflammation of the gallbladder or bile ducts, obstruction to the outflow of bile, and an increase in the cholesterol content of the blood. Of these, inflammation is most active. Gallstones frequently follow typhoid fever, in which two important etiologic factors (infection and increased cholesterol content of the blood) are present. In such cases typhoid bacilli form the nuclei of the stones. Other bacteria that have been found inside the nuclei of gall-

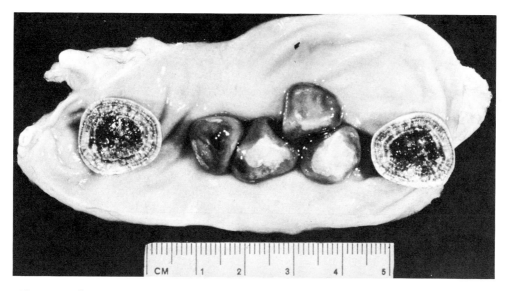

**Fig. 51-9.** Gallstones lying within gallbladder (cholelithiasis and cholecystitis). Note size of smooth-surfaced, faceted calculi. Two stones have been sectioned to show internal structure. Note concentric rings of cholesterol in relation to darker bile pigment.

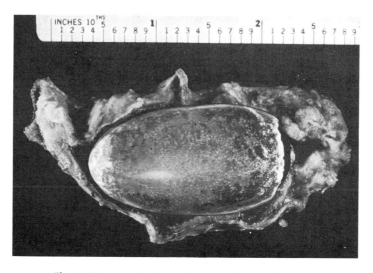

**Fig. 51-10.** Large cholesterol stone within gallbladder.

stones are colon bacilli, streptococci, and staphylococci.

*Kinds.* Gallstones may be single or multiple. (See Figs. 51-9 and 51-10.) In multiple stones the number may run into the hundreds. Single stones are usually large and round or oval. Multiple stones are faceted. Gallstones may be composed of cholesterol, calcium bilirubinate, or combinations of the two (mixed stones). Cholesterol stones are large, single, oval, and comparatively smooth and seldom cause trouble. Ty-

phoid fever and pregnancy predispose to this type of stone. Mixed stones (the most common type) are multiple and composed of concentric layers of cholesterol and bile salts. Calcium bilirubinate stones are small, black, and granular in appearance.

*Effects.* Stones may exist for many years without causing symptoms other than vague abdominal distress, and this is especially true of the larger smooth stones because they do not enter the bile passages to produce obstruction. If a small stone attempts to leave the gallbladder or enter a duct, an attack of gallstone colic is triggered. The attack terminates suddenly when the stone passes through the duct or drops back into the gallbladder, and it terminates gradually when the stone becomes impacted in a duct. When a gallstone lodges in the common duct, the patient becomes jaundiced, and the stool clay colored. If a stone is in the cystic duct, jaundice does not occur unless the end of the stone obstructs the common duct, but bile does not enter the gallbladder. The gallbladder wall thins out, and the lumen becomes distended with mucus. The condition is known as *hydrops* of the gallbladder. If infection occurs, the hydrops changes to *empyema* of the gallbladder. Gallstones may cause ulceration and perforation of the wall of the gallbladder.

### NEOPLASM

Adenocarcinoma is the most important tumor of the gall bladder and constitutes from 1% to 2% of all carcinomas. It is about four times as common in women. The average age of patients with carcinoma of the gallbladder is in the neighborhood of 60 years, and in 75% of the cases gallstones are present. On the other hand, around 3% of all gallbladders containing stones show carcinoma also. The tumor extends directly to the liver.

## Pancreas

The pancreas is a pink-white organ lying behind the peritoneum and intimately bound to the duodenum. It is the second largest gland connected to the alimentary tract. One set of cells in the pancreas elaborates digestive ferments, carried to the lumen of the intestinal tract through a series of ducts. Another set of cells elaborates the hormone insulin, released directly into the bloodstream.

### FAT NECROSIS

When the pancreas is injured to such an extent that the pancreatic juice escapes, the fatty tissue that the juice contacts undergoes a peculiar type of digestion known as fat necrosis, caused by the action of the pancreatic lipase on the fat cells. The fatty tissues most often affected are those of the pancreas itself, the omentum, and the mesentery. The causes of pancreatic fat necrosis are acute and chronic pancreatitis, obstruction of the pancreatic duct, and neoplasms.

### INFLAMMATION

*Pancreatitis* may be acute or chronic, and the acute type may be hemorrhagic or suppurative. If the ampulla of Vater is blocked by a stone and bile is prevented from entering the duodenum, the bile may be regurgitated into the pancreatic duct system. Bile acts as a strong chemical irritant in the pancreatic tissues and may produce not only pancreatitis but necrosis of tissue as well. Pancreatitis often leads to jaundice and fat necrosis.

In pancreatic disease enzymes of pancreatic function such as lipase and amylase may be released in large amounts. The laboratory determination of the levels of these enzymes in serum and urine is important in the diagnosis of pancreatic disorders.

### NEOPLASM

Adenomas are of rare occurrence and in some cases involve the islands of Langerhans. An adenoma of the island cells is a functional tumor that leads to *hyperinsulinism* (overproduction of insulin); the characteristic train of events is caused by the lowering of blood sugar. Cysts of the pancreas may occur.

Carcinoma of gland cell type is the most common neoplasm of the pancreas. It usually occurs in the head of the pancreas but may occur throughout the organ. When the head of the pancreas is involved, the common bile duct is compressed, and intense jaundice ensues. If the head is not involved, jaundice does not occur. Carcinoma of the body and tail of the pancreas, with generalized metastases, is associated with widespread venous thromboses.

## Peritoneum

The peritoneum is the delicate serous membrane lining the abdominal cavity. The mesothelial cells on the surface are lubricated by a very small amount of a thin, straw-colored fluid.

### ASCITES

By ascites is meant the accumulation of serous fluid in the peritoneal cavity. It may occur as part of a generalized edema induced by failing heart action or impaired kidney function, but the most pronounced cases are caused by portal obstruction, especially when the obstruction results from cirrhosis of the liver.

The collection of fluid in the abdominal cavity displaces the abdominal organs, and the upward pressure of the diaphragm embarrasses respiration. Pressure on the abdominal veins may lead to passive congestion of the lower extremities.

### INFLAMMATION

*Peritonitis* is inflammation of the peritoneum. Usually acute, it may be chronic. It occurs most often as a localized process but may become generalized. The most likely type of chronic peritonitis is tuberculous peritonitis. On the other hand, tuberculous peritonitis may develop with such rapidity as to give rise to acute manifestations.

**Acute peritonitis.** Acute peritonitis may be the result of mechanical irritation (as occurs when the peritoneum is unduly traumatized surgically or when sterile foreign bodies such as sponges are left in the peritoneal cavity) or of chemical injury (as occurs when antiseptics are applied to the peritoneum), but most cases are caused by bacterial infection. The bacterial culprits are colon bacilli, streptococci, staphylococci, and pneumococci.

Bacteria may reach the peritoneal cavity (1) through perforations in the walls of abdominal viscera, (2) by passing directly through the gangrenous wall of an abdominal viscus, (3) by extending through a fallopian tube, (4) from the outside by penetrating accidental or surgical wounds, and (5) by the bloodstream. The last method is infrequent, but it may occur in septicemia.

Ordinarily, acute peritonitis begins as a local condition and may remain localized because of the prompt formation of adhesions about the site of infection, but many times the infection spreads rapidly to become generalized peritonitis. If localized peritonitis does not spread, it resolves or forms an abscess. Peritonitis caused by the rupture of a gastric or duodenal ulcer and peritonitis resulting from streptococci or pneumococci both rapidly become generalized and, untreated, quickly cause death of the patient.

Peritonitis caused by the colon bacillus is the most frequent form and fortunately is sometimes comparatively benign. The organisms reach the peritoneum from the intestinal tract, most often as a complication of appendicitis. Streptococcal peritonitis usually results from penetrating wounds of the abdomen or an extension of puerperal sepsis. Pneumococcal peritonitis may be secondary to a pneumococcal infection in some other part of the body. As a primary lesion (no relation to other infections in body), peritonitis is pneumococcal and complicates chronic nephrosis. In primary peritonitis the pneumococci reach the peritoneum through the vagina, uterus, and fallopian tubes in females.

**Tuberculous peritonitis.** Tuberculous peritonitis is most common in children and young adults. It ordinarily occurs secondary to tuberculosis in some other part of the body. It may occur rather acutely as a part of generalized miliary tuberculosis or as a chronic process secondary to tuberculosis of the fallopian tubes, ovaries, or mesenteric lymph nodes. Less often it is secondary to tuberculosis in distant foci. The manifestations of generalized miliary tuberculosis may be so prominent that the abdominal aspects are entirely overlooked.

Tuberculous peritonitis may be moist or dry. In the former the peritoneum is studded with small tubercles, and a voluminous thin yellow exudate is present; in the latter the coils of intestines are matted together by adhesions, and the omentum is greatly thickened. Tubercles may or may not be present.

## ABDOMINAL ADHESIONS

The contraction of abdominal adhesions may produce mild discomfort or intestinal obstruction.

## NEOPLASM

The most important tumor of the peritoneum is metastatic carcinoma originating in the abdominal organs. The stomach is the most common site of the primary growth, and the ovary is next. Peritoneal cancer is frequently accompanied by ascites and hemorrhage.

A peculiar tumor growth of the peritoneum is *pseudomyxoma peritonei,* which follows rupture of pseudomucinous cysts of the ovary or less frequently mucoceles (mucous cysts) of the appendix. In this condition the peritoneum is plastered with masses of soft gelatinous material. These masses may occur in every part of the abdominal cavity and cause extreme distention. In a few cases removal of the primary growth checks the peritoneal spread, but as a rule, the disease proves difficult to manage.

## Questions for review

1  What is the most common site of extragenital chancre?
2  Discuss carcinoma of the lip.
3  Give causes of retropharyngeal abscess.
4  What are the causes of gastric hemorrhage? Differentiate hematemesis from hemoptysis.
5  What is the importance of peptic ulcers?
6  What is the composition of gastric contents during digestion?
7  Give the causes of an esophageal stricture.
8  What is meant by cirrhosis? Discuss types.
9  Of what significance is the presence of free hydrochloric acid in the gastric contents?
10  How is tubeless gastric analysis performed?
11  What is Meckel's diverticulum? What is its origin? Why is it important?
12  What is a hernia? Name the different kinds and discuss each.
13  What is meant by the following terms when applied to hernias: reducible, obstructed, strangulated?
14  What is the difference between mechanical and paralytic obstruction of the intestine?
15  Define intussusception, volvulus.
16  Briefly discuss appendicitis.
17  How is an anal fistula formed?
18  Give the kinds and some of the causes of hemorrhoids.
19  What is the most common sign of carcinoma of the rectum?
20  Give some of the causes of portal obstruction.
21  Discuss jaundice—its origin and significance.
22  What is the origin of gallstones?

**23** How may bacteria reach the peritoneum?
**24** Discuss tuberculous peritonitis.

**REFERENCES** (Chapters 50 and 51)

Ackerman, L. V., and Rosai, J.: Surgical pathology, ed. 5, St. Louis, 1974, The C. V. Mosby Co.

Asbestos and the public health (editorial), J.A.M.A. **210:**966, 1967.

Asbestos dust—a community hazard (editorial), J.A.M.A. **209:**1216, 1969.

Berland, T.: Coping with emphysema, Today's Health **50:**54, Nov., 1972.

Burdette, W. J.: The continuing challenge of colorectal carcinoma, Hosp. Pract. **8:**146, May, 1973.

Burkitt, D. P.: Epidemiology and etiology, J.A.M.A. **231:**517, 1975.

Carper, J.: Cirrhosis: a growing threat to life, Today's Health **48:**26, Feb., 1970.

Chang, T-W.: Respiratory viral infections, factors influencing their clinical spectrum, Med. Sci. **18:**43, Feb., 1967.

Cherniack, N. S.: Abnormal breathing patterns, their mechanisms and clinical significance, J.A.M.A. **230:**57, 1974.

Cole, W.: Hypoglycemia: shortage of body fuel, Today's Health **46:**40, Nov., 1968.

Comroe, J. H., Jr.: The lung, Sci. Am. **214:**56, Feb., 1966.

Comroe, J. H., Jr., and others: The lung: clinical physiology and pulmonary function tests, ed. 2, Chicago, 1962, Year Book Medical Publishers, Inc.

Eastridge, C. E., and others: What we've learned from 1,284 cases of lung cancer, Resident Staff Physician **15:**58, Sept., 1969.

Environment: a death of air, J.A.M.A. **212:**25, 1970.

Fenoglis, C. M., and Lane, N.: The anatomic precursor of colorectal carcinoma, J.A.M.A. **231:**640, 1975.

Fishman, A. P.: Chronic cor pulmonale, Hosp. Pract. **6:**101, May, 1971.

Foley, M. F.: Pulmonary function testing, Am. J. Nurs. **71:**1134, 1971.

Gall, E. A., and Mostofi, F. K.: The liver, Baltimore, 1973, The Williams & Wilkins Co.

Gambill, E. E.: Pancreatitis, St. Louis, 1973, The C. V. Mosby Co.

Goldsmith, J. R.: Air pollution and disease, Hosp. Pract. **5:**63, May, 1970.

Heitzman, E. R.: The lung: radiologic-pathologic correlations, St. Louis, 1973, The C. V. Mosby Co.

Kazemi, H.: Pulmonary function tests, J.A.M.A. **206:**2302, 1968.

Kerr, L. E.: The environment: coal workers' pneumoconiosis (black lung), J.A.M.A. **216:**1361, 1971.

Key, M. M., and others: Pulmonary reactions to coal dust, New York, 1971, Academic Press, Inc.

Kilburn, K. H.: Pathogenesis and treatment of chronic bronchitis, Resident Staff Physician **14:**62, Jan., 1968.

Lazar, H. P.: Explaining your stomach pains, Today's Health **52:**34, May, 1974.

Levine, R.: Hypoglycemia, J.A.M.A. **230:**462, 1974.

Lorber, B., and Swenson, R. M.: Bacteriology of aspiration pneumonia, Ann. Intern. Med. **81:**329, 1974.

Lyons, H. A.: Obstructive emphysema, Hosp. Med. **7:**56, Jan., 1971.

MacGregor, I. L.: Carcinoma of the colon and stomach, a review with comment on epidemiologic associations, J.A.M.A. **227:**911, 1974.

Marx, J. L.: Air pollution: effects on plants, Science **187:**731, 1975.

Massion, C. G.: The elusive pancreatic lipase, Lab. Med. **2:**26, Feb., 1971.

Medical News: more smoking: worse malignancy, J.A.M.A. **211:**2081, 1970.

Painter, N. S.: Diseases of the colon and diet, Nurs. Mirror **136:**26, June 29, 1973.

Popper, H.: The problem of hepatitis, Am. J. Gastroenterol. **55:**355, 1971.

Reid, L.: Research strengthens link between air pollution, disease, Today's Health **47:**18, Jan., 1969.

Reid, L.: Cor pulmonale, Nurs. Mirror **136:**26, June 1, 1973.

Rodman, T., and Sterling, F. H.: Pulmonary emphysema and related lung diseases, St. Louis, 1969, The C. V. Mosby Co.

Rubin, P.: Current concepts in cancer, cancer of GI tract: colon, rectum, anus: introduction, J.A.M.A. **231:**513, 1975.

Sasahara, A. A., and Foster, V. L.: Pulmonary embolism: recognition and treatment, Am. J. Nurs. **67:**1634, 1967.

Schaffner, F., and others, editors: The liver and its diseases, New York, 1974, Intercontinental Medical Book Corp.

Spain, D. M., and others: Emphysema in apparently healthy adults, J.A.M.A. **224:**322, 1973.

Stuart-Harris, C.: Chronic bronchitis, Nurs. Mirror **137:**26, Aug. 10, 1973.

Talso, P. J., and Remenchik, A. P., editors: Internal medicine—based on mechanisms of disease, St. Louis, 1968, The C. V. Mosby Co.

Walker, A. R. P.: Dietary fibre and the pattern of disease (editorial), Ann. Intern. Med. **80:**663, 1974.

Wepler, W., and Wildhirt, E.: Clinical histopathology of the liver, New York, 1972, Grune & Stratton, Inc.

Whatley, J. L.: Battle for breath, Today's Health **45:**42, Feb., 1967.

Wynder, E. L., and others: The epidemiology of lung cancer, J.A.M.A. **213:**2221, 1970.

# CHAPTER 52

# Diseases of
# Urinary tract

The urinary system consists of the kidneys, ureters, bladder, and urethra.

## Kidneys

The kidneys are a pair of almost symmetrical organs that rid the body of practically 85% of its waste products. In addition, they help maintain the normal volume, composition, and pH of the blood.

Each kidney consists of myriads (over a million per kidney) of structural units, known as *nephrons*, which are held together by connective tissue stroma. Each nephron consists of an epithelial-lined uriniferous tubule about 35 mm. in length that begins near the surface of the kidney as a closed bulbous expansion *(Bowman's capsule)*, containing a small tuft of capillaries known as a *glomerulus*. (See Fig. 52-1.) The capsule with its enclosed glomerulus is known as a *malpighian* body or renal corpuscle. In pursuing their tortuous course through the kidney the uriniferous tubules vary widely in diameter. After forming many convolutions they open into the collecting tubules, which pass to the hilus of the kidney and drain into the *kidney pelvis*. This is the collecting basin formed by the expanded portion of the upper end of the ureter.

The glomerulus within Bowman's capsule is formed in the following manner. A minute branch of the renal artery *(afferent artery)* enters the capsule and divides into many branches of capillary size that entwine to form a knot-like mass but that join to form a single vessel *(efferent artery)* before leaving the capsule. Outside the capsule this vessel again breaks up into capillaries distributed to the tubule draining the malpighian body. The points at which the afferent and efferent arteries penetrate the capsular wall are rather close to each other so that the glomerulus is attached to only a limited portion of the wall. The space that separates the unattached portion of the glomerulus from the capsular wall is known as the *space of Bowman*. The afferent vessel is slightly larger than the efferent, which increases the filtering capacity of the glomerulus.

As the blood flows through the glomerulus, water and certain of the nonprotein constituents of the plasma filter through the glomerular wall into the space of Bowman. This filtrate then passes to the lumen of the tubule draining the space. The volume of filtrate passing through the glomeruli of the kidneys is more than 100 times greater than the volume of urine excreted. If there were not some mechanism whereby the glomerular filtrate were concentrated, the loss of such large amounts of fluid in the filtrate would effect a fatal dehydration of the individual in a matter of only a few minutes. This concentration is accomplished by the resorption of water, salts, and organic substances from the filtrate as it passes through the length of the tubules.

The rate at which plasma filters through the glomeruli depends on: (1) the rate at which the blood flows through the glomeruli, (2) the pressure under which the blood flows, (3) the presence of any disease condition that might obstruct the free flow of blood through the patent capillary lumina of the glomeruli, (4) the presence of disease that scars and obliterates the capillary loops, and (5) the rate at which filtrate flows from the space of Bowman.

### CLASSIFICATION OF RENAL DISEASE

The following outline gives the major disease processes of importance in the kidney:

1. Congenital disorders (p. 445)
2. Circulatory disorders such as infarction, hyperemia, hemorrhage
3. Renal disease related to systemic metabolic disease: lesions in kidney associated with
   a. Diabetes
   b. Gout
   c. Hyperparathyroidism

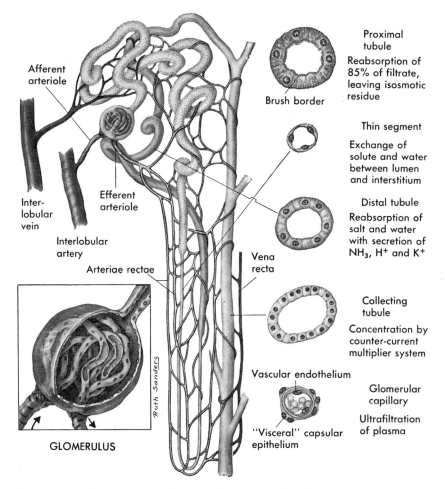

Afferent
arteriole

Efferent
arteriole

Inter-
lobular
vein

Interlobular
artery

Arteriae rectae

Vena
recta

GLOMERULUS

Proximal
tubule

Brush border

Reabsorption of
85% of filtrate,
leaving isosmotic
residue

Thin segment

Exchange of
solute and water
between lumen
and interstitium

Distal tubule

Reabsorption of
salt and water
with secretion of
$NH_3$, $H^+$ and $K^+$

Collecting
tubule

Concentration by
counter-current
multiplier system

Vascular endothelium

Glomerular
capillary

Ultrafiltration
of plasma

"Visceral" capsular
epithelium

**Fig. 52-1.** Anatomy of the nephron. (From Grollman, A., and Grollman, E. F.: Pharmacology and therapeutics, Philadelphia, 1970, Lea & Febiger.)

4. Inflammatory disease of glomerulus
   a. Diffuse glomerulonephritis: acute, subacute, and chronic
   b. Focal embolic glomerulonephritis: one of the important complications of subacute bacterial endocarditis; infected emboli from heart valves lodge in glomeruli
5. Nephrosis (toxic, chemical, bile)
6. Interstitial nephritis
7. Nephrosclerosis: fibrosis and scarring of kidney tissue produced by blood vessel disease
   a. Arteriosclerotic nephrosclerosis: arteriosclerosis of larger vessels, with resultant scarring of fairly large areas of renal parenchyma
   b. Arteriolar nephrosclerosis: arteriolar sclerosis with resultant scarring of multiple small areas of renal tissue; this is the lesion peculiarly related to essential hypertension
8. Infection
   a. Pyelonephritis
   b. Abscess
   c. Tuberculosis
9. Neoplasms

## CIRCULATORY DISORDER— RENAL HEMORRHAGE

Punctate hemorrhages may occur in glomerulonephritis, intense passive congestion of the kidneys, malignant nephrosclerosis, and certain blood dyscrasias. The important causes of massive renal hemorrhage are neoplasms, blood dycrasias (including leukemia), severe hemolytic states, and stones.

## NEPHRITIS

The term *nephritis* or *Bright's disease* has been applied to conditions that affect both kidneys diffusely and are associated with inflammatory or degenerative changes in the renal tubules, glomeruli, or blood vessels. The important feature of nephritis is its diffuse bilateral nature, which distinguishes it from localized affections of the kidneys, such as abscesses.

**Forms.** Depending on its varied etiology, pathology, and manifestations, there are many forms of nephritis, and elaborate classifications of the disease have been proposed. The following separation is based on the anatomic part of the kidney primarily involved: (1) *glomerulonephritis,* referring to disease of the glomeruli, (2) *nephrosis* or *tubular nephritis,* designating primary disease of the tubular system of the kidney, (3) *interstitial nephritis,* referring to disease processes concentrated in the interstitial connective tissues, and (4) *nephrosclerosis,* indicating diseases affecting large and small blood vessels and their effects on the kidney. This classification, like most others, is weakened by the fact that these entities seldom occur in pure form; that is, although one component of the kidney is primarily attacked, all others are more or less involved.

Glomerulonephritis and interstitial nephritis are mainly inflammatory changes that may be present in acute, subacute, or chronic stages. Glomerulonephritis is thought to be an allergic reaction that follows infections with hemolytic streptococci. Nephrosis almost invariably means degenerative or retrogressive changes in the epithelium of the tubular system. In the majority of cases it is caused by the effect of bacteria or their metabolic by-products, by certain toxic substances resulting from disturbed metabolism within the body, or by certain chemical poisons such as mercury bichloride, carbon tetrachloride, or potassium bichromate.

**Effects.** When the kidneys become diseased, they often lose their ability to concentrate nitrogenous waste products (uric acid, urea, creatinine), chlorides, and other substances brought to them by the bloodstream for excretion. Therefore these waste products accumulate in the blood. Along with the loss of their power to excrete wastes, the kidneys fail to excrete certain inert dyes such as phenolsulfonphthalein, which may be used to test kidney function. If a disease process involves the glomerulus so as to interfere with its normal filtering mechanism, red blood cells and the albumin of the plasma proteins may pass into the tubular system and be present in the urine.

When the tubules of the kidneys become diseased, albuminous material collects in them and coagulates, forming molds or *casts* of the tubules. The pressure of the fluid forming behind the casts sweeps them out of the tubules with the urine. The material of which the casts are composed may pass from the blood through diseased glomeruli and tubules, or it may be derived from the degeneration of the epithelium of the tubules. Casts made up of coagulated albuminous ma-

terial alone are known as *hyaline* casts and are the least significant of all. Granules, pus cells, red blood cells, fat droplets, waxy substances, or epithelial cells may become incorporated in the casts, giving rise to granular, pus, blood, fatty, waxy, and epithelial casts, respectively. Granular casts indicate a comparatively mild degeneration of the tubules, fatty and waxy casts a moderately severe change, and epithelial casts a still more severe degeneration. Blood and pus casts indicate hemorrhage and suppuration, respectively, of one or both kidneys.

High blood pressure resulting from changes in the minute arterioles of the kidneys is a frequent accompaniment of nephritis. Many cases are accompanied by edema, which may be caused by changes in the kidneys themselves or by cardiac failure brought about by the high blood pressure.

As a rule, glomerulonephritis is characterized by high blood pressure, retention of nitrogenous waste products, and a tendency toward uremia, whereas nephrosis or tubular nephritis is characterized by little or no increase in blood pressure, no retention of nitrogenous waste products, and little tendency toward uremia.

Cases of acute glomerulonephritis may recover without leaving any marked alteration of the kidneys, heal with scar formation, become chronic, or cause immediate death. Death in acute glomerulonephritis may result from cardiac failure or cerebral hemorrhage, both of which are caused by high blood pressure, or it may be caused by uremia. In chronic glomerulonephritis death may result from any of those conditions that cause death in acute glomerulonephritis, or it may be brought about by intercurrent infection.

*Uremia.* Uremia indicates the condition in which severely diseased kidneys are no longer able to excrete waste products (urea, uric acid, creatinine) from the body or to save for the body certain essential substances such as sodium. Therefore the components containing nitrogen ordinarily eliminated in the urine tend to accumulate in excess in the blood and body fluids, and certain needed substances (water, sodium, chloride) tend to decrease. Complete loss of function by the kidneys is usually designated as *renal insufficiency.* The clinical signs and symptoms most often manifested are headache, convulsions, drowsiness, and stupor, deepening into a coma that ends in death. In other cases nausea, vomiting, and diarrhea are prominent features.

## THE KIDNEY IN HYPERTENSION

**Nephrosclerosis.** The kidney lesion that is constantly associated with benign essential hypertension of any significant duration is *benign arteriolar* nephrosclerosis, although the exact relation of the two disorders is as yet undetermined. This is a diffuse process affecting both kidneys. The degenerative change comes first in the arterioles, with a slowly developing thickening of the vessel wall that results in a well-marked narrowing of the lumen. At the same time there is gradual impairment of the blood supply to the areas supplied by the affected arterioles. Glomeruli and tubules slowly shrink, finally succumb, drop out, and are replaced by scar tissue. Because of the small size of the arteriole, the area of scar is also small. The presence of many small scars in both kidneys produces a characteristic granularity especially noted on the outer surfaces of these organs.

*Malignant* nephrosclerosis, the kidney lesion of malignant hypertension, is in some ways comparable to the benign form; but here the associated hypertension is quite severe. The arterioles become necrotic, and the areas of supply are infarcted as a result of the rapid progression of the disorder. The necrotic arterioles may rupture, causing small hemorrhages in the renal tissue. Malignant nephrosclerosis is uncommon, but when it does happen, the acute renal insufficiency is fatal.

## INFECTION

**Pyelonephritis.** Pyelonephritis (Fig. 52-2), or inflammation of both the kidney parenchyma and the kidney pelvis, occurs most often in childhood, during pregnancy, or as a complication of kidney stones. This is the condition commonly referred to as pyelitis, and it is said to be the most common kidney disease.

The organisms most often responsible for pyelonephritis are the enteric bacilli, staphylococci, and streptococci. They may reach the kidney by the bloodstream or ascend from an inflammatory condition of the lower urinary tract. Inflammation is often suppurative in character, and multiple abscess formation is common. Pyelonephritis may be unilateral or bilateral; however, the right kidney often shows greater involvement than the left.

**Tuberculosis.** Tuberculosis of the kidney may occur acutely as part of a generalized miliary tuberculosis or as a chronic local condition. Chronic tuberculosis of the kidney is secondary to tuberculosis of the lungs, bones, or lymph nodes, and the bacilli reach the kidney by way of the bloodstream.

Chronic renal tuberculosis begins as one or more tubercles that fuse together. As the condition progresses, the tubercles are converted into cheesy foci that discharge their contents into the renal pelvis. The kidney is left more or less honeycombed with cavities that continue to enlarge and coalesce until all that remains of the kidney is a shell surrounding multiple cavities. In the beginning, chronic renal tuberculosis is unilateral, but after a time the other kidney

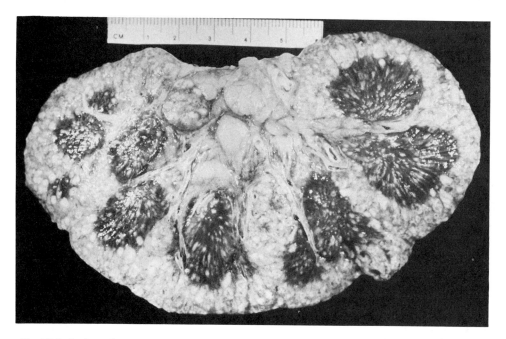

**Fig. 52-2.** Pyelonephritis, sectioned surface of kidney. Note multiple small, grayish foci of suppuration in cortex and medulla.

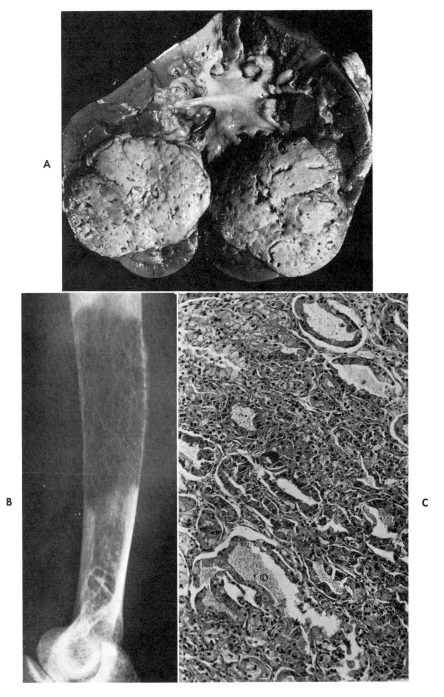

**Fig. 52-3.** Hypernephroma. **A,** Primary growth in kidney (sectioned surface). **B,** Radiograph of metastatic focus in humerus. Metastases of this tumor may be discovered before primary growth suspected. **C,** Microscopic appearance of the tumor. Note glandular spaces. (From Lichtenstein, L.: Bone tumors, ed. 4, St. Louis, 1972, The C. V. Mosby Co.)

becomes involved. If the renal pelvis or ureter is closed off by spread of the disease, no urinary abnormalities can be found.

### NEOPLASM

Benign and malignant neoplasms occur in the kidneys. Important ones are the hypernephroma, a tumor of adults, and the Wilms' tumor of the kidney, one of the common tumors of childhood. Both are malignant.

*Hypernephroma* (Grawitz tumor; renal cell carcinoma) (Fig. 52-3) arises from kidney tissue and occurs as yellowish, greasy masses that often show areas of hemorrhage and small cysts. Hypernephromas may be small and remain so throughout their course, or they may suddenly grow rapidly, quickly form bulky tumors that destroy the kidney substance, and extend into the kidney pelvis, renal veins, and inferior vena cava. On the other hand, apparently quiescent tumors may give rise to distant fatal metastases. Metastasis occurs most often to the lungs and bones. About 20% of hypernephromas have already metastasized when first observed by the physician. Most hypernephromas occur in persons more than 45 years of age, and the most common early symptom is hematuria.

*Wilms' tumor* (embryoma; mixed tumor; embryonal adenosarcoma) usually shows clinical manifestations before the third year of life. These tumors are composed of epithelial cells admixed with muscle fibers, cartilage, bone, or fatty tissue; they often grow rapidly and to a large size. Metastasis is by way of the bloodstream to the lungs and brain. The first sign in over half the children is a tumor mass that can be palpated in the abdomen (Fig. 52-4).

## Pelvis and ureters

The urine as formed by the kidney is little changed in the excretory passages, the walls of which contain a well-developed musculature. The muscular contractions are important in moving the urine along the tract. From the thin-walled, funnel-shaped pelvis at the hilus of each kidney the urine is passed in the narrow lumen of the ureter to the urinary bladder. The thick-walled ureter is some 10 inches in length.

### URINARY TRACT OBSTRUCTION

**Hydronephrosis.** Hydronephrosis is a dilatation of the kidney pelvis, with compression of the kidney tissue caused by an obstruction to the outflow of urine. Obstruction of both ureters, the urethra, or the bladder causes bilateral hydronephrosis, whereas obstruction of one ureter causes unilateral hydronephrosis. Obstruction of the ureter may be caused by congenital atresia, strictures, kinks, stones, or outside pressure from tumors. Obstruction in the bladder may be caused by stones, tumors, or diseases of the spinal cord that cause paralysis of the bladder muscles. Obstruction of the urethra may be caused by strictures, prostatic enlargement, or congenital malformations. Bilateral hydronephrosis is regularly associated with secondary infection.

**Pyonephrosis.** In pyonephrosis there is dilatation of the kidney pelvis, but it is filled with thick purulent material instead of clear urine as in hydronephrosis. Pyonephrosis may be caused by tuberculosis, infection around a calculus, or infection of a hydronephrosis. Often there is so much destruction of tissue that the kidney is converted into a thin-walled sac of pus.

**Nephrolithiasis (kidney stones).** Renal calculi are formed in the kidney pelvis by the precipitation of normal or abnormal constituents of the urine. They may be large or small; sandlike, smooth, or rough; and regular or irregular in contour. They are usually single but may be multiple. As a rule, the larger calculi form more or less complete casts of the kidney pelvis and have projections that extend within the calyces. These are known as dendritic or coralliform stones, and in some cases the branching may be so extensive

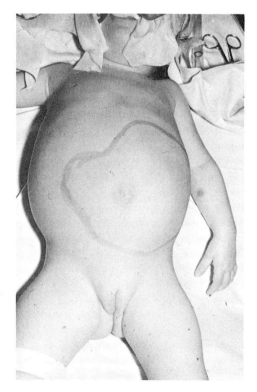

**Fig. 52-4.** Wilms' tumor in a young child. The extent of palpable tumor is outlined on skin of abdomen.

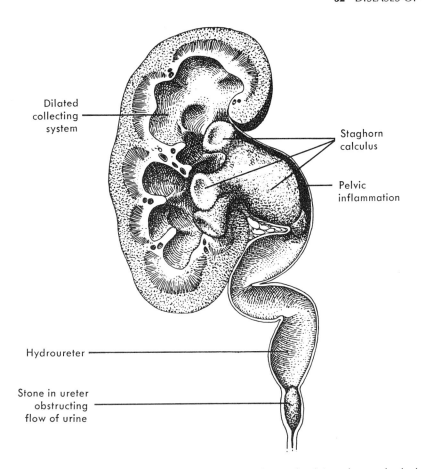

Dilated
collecting
system

Staghorn
calculus

Pelvic
inflammation

Hydroureter

Stone in ureter
obstructing
flow of urine

**Fig. 52-5.** Stones in urinary tract. Staghorn calculus is seen in renal pelvis and second calculus in ureter. Resultant pathology: marked dilatation of renal pelvis and ureter, compression atrophy of kidney, and secondary inflammation. (From Winter, C. C.: Practical urology, St. Louis, 1969, The C. V. Mosby Co.)

as to remind one of the antlers of a deer (staghorn calculus). Kidney stones may enter the ureter, where they may become arrested or pass to the bladder. (See Fig. 52-5.)

Just why renal calculi form is not known, but among the predisposing factors are infection of the kidney pelvis, interference with the outflow of urine, and vitamin A deficiency.

The clinical features of renal calculi show marked variation, depending on the size and shape of the calculus and the presence or absence of complicating infection. If the kidney pelvis is not infected and the stone is smooth and too large to enter the ureter, symptoms are slight or absent. If a stone enters the ureter, it brings on an attack of renal colic. In most cases the stone passes on to the bladder. If it is arrested in the ureter, hydronephrosis develops unless the stone is surgically removed. Ulceration and stricture formation often occur at the point of lodgment.

Large irregular stones of the kidney pelvis may cause extensive ulceration of tissue. Stones in any location predispose to infection; therefore pyelonephritis is a common complication, and hydronephrosis following the impaction of a stone in the ureter is soon converted into pyonephrosis.

## Bladder

The urinary bladder is the hollow muscular reservoir for the temporary storage of urine.

### MALFORMATIONS

**Congenital.** The most important congenital malformation of the bladder is *exstrophy,* in which the abdominal wall is divided and the anterior wall of the bladder is absent, so that the mucosa of the bladder and the ureteral openings are exposed to the outside of the body. Other malformations are often associated with exstrophy of the bladder. Sometimes the small intestine discharges into the bladder, and the large intestine is absent.

Occasionally the bladder may be double, small, or absent. Congenital diverticula may be found in infants and young children, but they are rare.

**Acquired.** Dilatation of the bladder may be caused by paralysis of the bladder muscles from disease of the spinal cord, or it may result from congenital or acquired obstruction of the neck of the bladder or of the urethra. In acute dilatation the wall of the bladder is thinned, but when dilatation comes slowly, the wall is hypertrophied.

Acquired diverticula of the bladder wall result from pockets of the mucosa that are pushed through the muscular coat by increased intravesical pressure. Diverticula usually occur in men over 60 years of age and are associated with some form of chronic obstruction of the urethra such as stricture or prostatic enlargement.

As a rule, diverticula are small, but in exceptional cases they may be as large as the remainder of the bladder. They may communicate with the bladder by an opening as large as the diverticulum or one scarcely larger than the lead of a pencil. Because of their lack of muscle, diverticula cannot empty themselves, and the stagnant urine soon becomes contaminated with bacteria.

Cystocele is a bulging of the bladder and anterior vaginal wall into the vagina. It is caused by a relaxation of the anterior vaginal wall brought about by a weakening of the pelvic floor.

### INFLAMMATION

**Cystitis.** The healthy bladder is remarkably resistant to infection, but a bladder weakened by injury or disease is as liable to infection as any other organ. The conditions that weaken the bladder and predispose to cystitis are obstruction to the outflow of urine, paralysis of the bladder muscles, vesical calculi, and neoplasms. Like most other inflammatory conditions, cystitis may be acute or chronic.

Although cystitis may be brought about by the excretion of highly concentrated urine or irritating drugs, it is almost always caused by bacterial infection, and the bacteria most often responsible are the enteric bacilli, staphylococci, streptococci, the typhoid bacillus, and gonococci. The causative organisms may reach the bladder by way of the urethra, or they may descend from the kidney pelvis and ureter, and in a few cases they are brought to the bladder by the bloodstream or lymph stream. They may reach the bladder from the urethra by the extension of a posterior urethritis, or they may be introduced through the urethra by the use of contaminated instruments.

In acute cystitis all the signs of an active inflam-

mation are present. There may be hemorrhage. In some cases the bladder wall may become so soft that it is easily penetrated by a catheter.

Chronic cystitis follows acute cystitis or occurs as a primary process. Some degree of chronic cystitis almost always accompanies vesical calculi. As a rule, the bladder wall is thickened, and in some cases the mucosa may show polypoid outgrowths. Portions of its transitional epithelium may be converted into stratified squamous epithelium.

**Tuberculosis.** Tuberculosis of the bladder is most often secondary to tuberculosis of the kidney, but it may be secondary to tuberculosis of the prostate gland, seminal vesicles, or epididymis. It begins in the form of small tubercles that break down and form shallow ulcers that, in turn, coalesce to form an extensive ulcer.

### OBSTRUCTION

**Vesical calculi (bladder stones).** Vesical calculi may occur in the form of fine particles ("gravel" in voided urine) or as stones of considerable size. They are formed from constituents of the urine that ordinarily remain in solution but that have precipitated because of supersaturation or other chemical changes in the urine. The constituents of the stone are deposited on a nucleus that may be a stone that has descended from the kidney pelvis, a foreign body, or a clump of epithelial cells, mucus, and pus or bacteria. Vesical calculi often form with low-grade inflammation of the bladder or stagnation of urine. Vesical calculi are usually single and spherical but may be multiple and faceted. They promote inflammation and may ulcerate and perforate the bladder wall. If the stone becomes engaged in the urethra, the patient is seized with a paroxysm of pain and may pass blood.

**Retention.** Retention of urine may be caused by urethral obstruction incident to lesions in the bladder or by paralysis of the bladder muscles resulting from diseases of the spinal cord. Retention sometimes occurs in shock, peritonitis, and infectious diseases. Postoperative retention often follows pelvic operations or operations about the rectum. Paralytic retention results from either inhibition of the expulsive muscles or stimulation of the sphincter muscles of the bladder. Retained urine decomposes, becoming a vesical irritant as well as an ideal culture medium for bacterial growth.

**Incontinence.** By incontinence of urine is meant an inability to retain urine. It may be caused by hyperesthesia of some portion of the urinary tract, some disease of the central nervous system, great bodily weakness, or malformations of the urinary tract. Among the diseases of the spinal cord that may cause incontinence are locomotor ataxia, tumors, and gum-

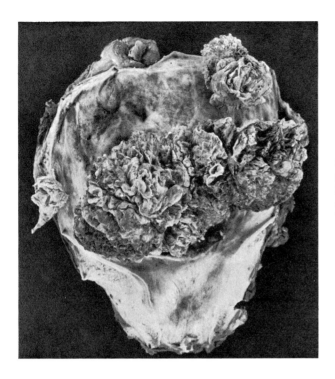

**Fig. 52-6.** Malignant neoplasm of urinary bladder. On inside lining surface of bladder is seen elongated, projecting tumor, composed of numerous papillary folds. (From Anderson, W. A. D., editor: Pathology, ed. 6, St. Louis, 1971, The C. V. Mosby Co.)

mas. In the paralytic form, urine continually dribbles from the bladder and is expelled in spurts during the muscular activity of laughing, coughing, or severe exercise.

*Nocturnal enuresis* is a peculiar type of incontinence that occurs in nervous children. The child voids while sleeping, usually during the early hours of the night, and has no knowledge of the act until he awakes.

## NEOPLASM

The most common tumor of the bladder is the papilloma, appearing as a soft shaggy tumor, which grows from the bladder wall (Fig. 52-6). It is most common in men between 30 and 50 years of age. Painless hematuria is the chief feature. Because of their tendency to become malignant, all such tumors of the bladder should be considered malignant until proved innocent. The malignant neoplasm of the bladder is a transitional carcinoma that may either be a papillary tumor or one that diffusely infiltrates the bladder wall.

## Urethra

In the urethra urine passes from the bladder to the outside of the body. A short channel in the female, the urethra is a more extended one in the male, carrying not only the urine but also the seminal products and the secretions of the glands accessory to the male genital system.

## INFLAMMATION

**Urethritis.** Urethritis is of two types: specific, caused by gonococci, and nonspecific, from other causes. Both types may be either acute or chronic.

*Nonspecific* urethritis may be caused by highly irritating injections or bacteria introduced by nonsterile instruments. The organisms most often responsible for this form of urethritis are staphylococci and streptococci.

*Gonorrheal* urethritis begins in the male as anterior urethritis; with proper care it remains limited, but when improperly treated, it extends to the posterior urethra. Infection in the various crypts and glands connected with the posterior urethra may spread to the prostate gland, bladder, epididymis, and seminal vesicles. The posterior urethra may also act as a focus of infection from which gonococci are spread to the joints. The inflammatory changes in the male urethra are likely to lead to strictures. Other important complications of gonorrheal urethritis are abscess of the periurethral glands in both sexes and abscess of Bartholin's glands in the female. In both male and female the periurethral glands may shelter infectious gonococci.

*Stricture.* Stricture of the urethra results from contraction of scar tissue within the urethral wall. Strictures may be congenital or traumatic, but the great majority occur as an aftermath of gonorrhea. As a rule, strictures develop slowly, and signs of obstruction may not appear until long after the primary condition has

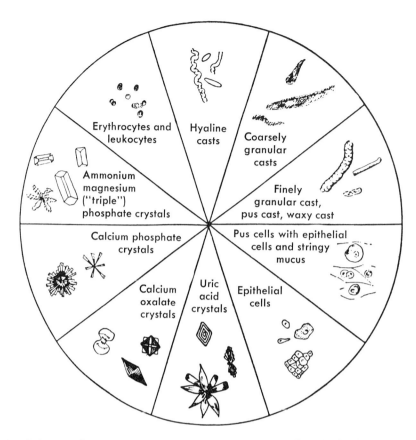

**Fig. 52-7.** Urinary sediment, important constituents. (Courtesy Alma Elizabeth Morrow, Sacramento, Calif.)

subsided. Stricture of the urethra is rare in women.

Ulceration behind the stricture as well as perforation of the urethra by the false passage of sounds (instrumentation*) may lead to urinary extravasation involving the external genitals, perineum, and the skin of the thighs and lower abdomen.

### TUMOR

**Urethral caruncle.** A urethral caruncle is a peculiar growth of vascular granulation tissue that arises within or near the orifice of the female urethra. Usually it is single, sessile or pedunculated, of a bright red color, and extremely tender. It has a tendency to occur in elderly women and is troublesome because of the pain it causes, especially on urination.

## Urine

**General characteristics.** Urine is essentially an aqueous solution of waste products. Important constit-

uents normally excreted are water, uric acid, urea, ammonia, creatine, chlorides, sulfates, and phosphates. (See Fig. 52-7.)

The amount of one of these substances in the urine may be decreased by (1) a decrease in the amount in the blood or (2) diseases of the kidneys that reduce the excretory capacity. It may be increased by (1) an increase in the amount in the blood or (2) an increased permeability of the glomeruli of the kidneys.

There is a definite relation between the amount of these substances in the blood and urine; for example, when the kidneys fail to excrete urea, uric acid, or creatinine, the amount in the blood increases.

*Amount.* The amount of urine excreted by normal adults varies from 1200 to 1500 ml. per day. An increase in amount is known as *polyuria,* a decrease as *oliguria,* and a complete suppression as *anuria.* Polyuria is most often seen in diabetes and chronic nephritis. Oliguria is most often seen in acute nephritis, fevers, and severe diarrheas.

*Color.* As a rule, urine is of an amber color, and the more highly concentrated it is, the deeper its color.

---

*A sound is an instrument designed to be introduced into a body cavity or passageway, often to dilate it.

Bloody urines are often brown, black, or smoky in color. In phenol poisoning the urine is a brownish black color. Ingestion of methylene blue turns the urine green. In certain cases of melanoma the urine turns black.

*Appearance.* Normal urine is clear when passed. On standing, it forms a faint cloud that settles to the bottom. This is known as a *nubecula* and consists of epithelial cells, mucus, and leukocytes. A turbidity when urine is passed is caused by the precipitation of phosphates or urates or by the presence of blood, pus, or bacteria.

*Specific gravity.* The normal specific gravity ranges from 1.013 to 1.023. Usually the smaller the amount of urine passed, the higher the specific gravity; and the more urine passed, the lower it is. Diabetes mellitus is an exception to this rule because in this condition a large amount of urine of high specific gravity is passed. The high specific gravity results from the large amount of sugar (glucose) in the urine.

*Reaction.* Normal urine is acid in reaction but becomes alkaline on standing. Alkalinity of freshly voided urine may be caused by the ingestion of certain foods and drugs or by the decomposition of urea by bacterial action. The latter indicates an infection in some part of the urinary tract.

**Abnormal constituents.** Certain constituents abnormal in the urine may be normally present in the blood and appear in the urine not as a result of kidney disease but because the amount in the blood has increased to such a degree that the kidneys allow a spillover into the urine. A good example is glucose. Other substances appear in the urine as a result of disease of the kidney. Among these are sugar, albumin, bile, hemoglobin, indican, acetone, diacetic acid, and such microscopic elements as casts, pus, and red blood cells. (See Fig. 52-7.)

*Albuminuria.* Albumin in the urine (albuminuria) is found in many disease conditions. Albuminurias may be divided into (1) true albuminurias, in which albumin is released from the kidney either because it escapes from an altered glomerulus or because it is liberated from damaged tubular cells, and (2) false albuminurias, in which materials containing albumin (blood, pus, bile) gain access to the urine at some point along the urinary tract. True albuminurias may be caused not only by primary disease of the kidneys but also by secondary effects on the kidneys from disease elsewhere in the body. These secondary effects are quite important in acute infectious disease and in chemical poisoning. So-called physiologic albuminurias may follow prolonged exercise or cold baths.

*Glycosuria.* Sugar in the urine is glycosuria. Sugar does not indicate a particular compound but is a term applied to a group of related compounds that show considerable variation in characteristics. When we speak of sugar in the urine, we usually refer to glucose (dextrose), which is the one most frequently found and the one that appears in the urine of diabetes mellitus. It should be remembered that normal urine contains an amount of glucose too small to be detected by ordinary laboratory tests. Lactose (milk sugar) may sometimes occur in the urine of nursing mothers.

*Acetone bodies.* Acetone, diacetic acid, and beta-hydroxybutyric acid (collectively spoken of as acetone bodies) are often found in association because they have the same origin. They are normally formed in the liver during fat metabolism and are carried to the tissues for utilization. If glycogen is depleted in the liver as a result of deficient carbohydrate metabolism, the liver metabolizes a greater amount of fat, thus releasing acetone bodies to the tissues in greater amounts than they can be utilized. Excessive formation of acetone bodies is therefore related to diseases of carbohydrate metabolism. Diabetes mellitus is the most important example. A marked increase of acetone bodies in the urine of a diabetic person may be a sign of impending coma, and their narcotic action explains at least some of the features of diabetic coma. Acetone bodies also occur with pernicious vomiting of pregnancy, with starvation, and in the diarrheas of children.

*Blood.* Hemoglobin may appear in the urine with or without red blood cells. *Hemoglobinuria* means the presence of hemoglobin in the urine, and *hematuria* means the presence of red blood cells. Hemoglobinuria is most often associated with substances or conditions producing rapid and marked blood destruction, such as certain poisons, bites of certain snakes, malaria, and transfusion of incompatible blood. *Malarial hemoglobinuria* is spoken of as blackwater fever. *Paroxysmal hemoglobinuria* is a condition in which the patient has paroxysms of hemoglobinuria without known cause. The paraoxysms often follow exposure to cold, and the condition is most frequent in persons who have syphilis.

Red blood cells occur in the urine most often with glomerulonephritis, tumors of the urinary tract, blood dyscrasias, tuberculosis, kidney stones, and bladder stones. Hematuria is an important sign in tumors of the urinary tract. Menstrual blood in a female must be excluded before one can say that a true hematuria exists.

*Others.* Bile appears in the urine in obstructive jaundice.

Casts never appear in a strictly normal urine, but their presence does not necessarily indicate permanent disease. The casts most often seen are the hyaline and granular types. (See Fig. 52-7.)

Pus in the urine (pyuria) occurs most often in

cystitis, pyelonephritis, urethritis, and tuberculosis of the kidney.

Important pathogenic bacteria that may be found in the urine are the enteric bacilli, staphylococci, streptococci, tubercle bacilli, and typhoid bacilli.

**Urine in diabetes.** There are two kinds of diabetes: diabetes mellitus and diabetes insipidus. The term *diabetes* as commonly used refers to diabetes mellitus. This is a disease of metabolism brought about by a failure of the pancreas to produce enough of its internal secretion, insulin, which controls sugar metabolism.

Two erroneous ideas concerning glycosuria and diabetes are prevalent. (1) The presence of glucose in the urine means that the patient has diabetes mellitus. (2) Diabetes mellitus is a disease of the kidneys. Although persistent glycosuria is most often caused by diabetes mellitus, such is not necessarily the case, and transient glycosurias are frequently the result of other causes.

Normally the blood contains from 90 to 120 mg. of glucose per 100 ml., and a small amount, but not enough to be detected by the tests ordinarily used, passes into the urine. When the amount in the blood reaches a certain point, the threshold, the kidneys are no longer able to hold the glucose back, and enough to be detected by ordinary tests spills over into the urine. The threshold point in normal persons lies between 160 and 180 mg. per 100 ml. of blood. When kidney function is impaired, the threshold point is higher. Therefore, with the exception of one condition (renal glycosuria), the appearance of glucose in the urine indicates that the amount in the blood exceeds the threshold level. This may result from increased intake (alimentary glycosuria) or impaired utilization, as occurs in diabetes mellitus.

In untreated *diabetes mellitus* the high sugar content of the blood is associated with the excretion of large quantities of pale urine that contains sugar and is of a high specific gravity. Acetone is usually present in moderately severe cases, and diacetic acid and beta-hydroxybutyric acid are present in very severe cases. It should be remembered that just as the diseased kid-

ney loses its ability to excrete the waste products of the body, it also loses its ability to excrete sugar. For this reason the quantitative estimation of the amount of glucose in the blood is of more value than is the estimation of the amount in the urine.

In renal glycosuria the amount of sugar in the blood is not above normal, but sugar is found in the urine. The cause of this condition is not known.

In *diabetes insipidus* (p. 598) large quantities of pale urine of a low specific gravity are excreted. The urine contains neither sugar nor albumin.

## Questions for review

1 Discuss briefly the anatomy of the kidney and explain how urine is formed.
2 Name some of the malformations of the kidney.
3 What are three important causes of massive renal hemorrhage?
4 Briefly discuss nephritis.
5 Differentiate hydronephrosis from pyonephrosis.
6 Name three metabolic diseases that produce changes in the kidneys.
7 Discuss the formation of casts and give the significance of each type.
8 Mention two diseases in which the term *diabetes* is used as a part of the name and answer the following questions about each:
   (a) What changes occur in the amount of urine?
   (b) Does the urine contain sugar?
   (c) Is the specific gravity of the urine low, normal, or high?
   (d) Name the organ in which abnormality is responsible for the disease.
9 What is the renal neoplasm of childhood? What is usually the first sign of this tumor?
10 Differentiate benign from malignant nephrosclerosis.
11 What is focal embolic glomerulonephritis?
12 What is meant by uremia? By renal insufficiency?
13 What organisms are the most commonly encountered in pyelonephritis? How do they reach the kidney? What is pyelitis?
14 List the abnormal constituents of urine. What pathogenic bacteria are most often found in the urine?

**References on pp. 619 and 620.**

# CHAPTER 53

# Diseases of
# Endocrine glands

Instead of passing out of the gland by a duct, the secretory products of certain glands are absorbed directly into the bloodstream. Such secretions, known as *internal secretions* or *hormones*, are substances formed in one part of the body but carried in the blood to another organ or tissue whose physiologic activity they influence. Glands such as the thyroid, parathyroid, pituitary, and adrenal glands release their secretions in this manner and are known as *ductless* or *endocrine* glands. Other glands having an endocrine function are the gonads (ovary and testis) and the islands of Langerhans in the pancreas.

A complicated interrelation exists between the endocrine glands, and the action of one is often profoundly influenced by the secretion of another. This interaction of the endocrine glands as well as the functional activity of the individual glands is, at best, imperfectly understood. The physiologic action of one gland may be increased or suppressed by changes within the gland itself or by the influence of the secretions of other glands acting on it. Secretory disturbances in one gland may produce secondary changes in another endocrine gland—for example, the hyperplasia of the pituitary gland secondary to the decreased activity of the thyroid gland in primary hypothyroidism. The total pathologic picture of an endocrine disorder represents the sum of the effects in the gland primarily affected plus certain effects from other glands whose physiologic function is affected by the primary disorder. The gland that exercises the greatest influence over other glands is the pituitary. It is known as the master gland.

Diseases of the endocrine glands fall into two major categories: (1) those related to the fact that the gland is producing too much of its hormone, result, a state of *hyperfunction,* and (2) those caused by the fact that the gland is elaborating a considerably reduced amount of its hormone, result, a state of *hypofunction.* The causes for the two disturbances may be varied, but generally a state of hyperfunction is related to either hyperplasia of the glandular cells or a true neoplasm.

Most cases of hyperfunction of the thyroid gland are caused by hyperplasia; hyperfunction in the pituitary, adrenal, and parathyroid glands is usually the result of neoplasm. The causes of hyperplasia or neoplasm in endocrine glands are unknown.

Hypofunction may be caused by anything that destroys glandular tissue or injures it so that its output of hormone is sharply reduced.

To emphasize the pathologic disorders of hyperfunction and hypofunction is to stress the physiologic significance of hormones, their far-reaching effects in the body, and the importance of a proper balance for normal well-being.

Another point serving to emphasize the special features of the endocrine disorders is the fact that certain glands play such an important role in the normal growth and development of the individual—notably the thyroid, pituitary, and adrenal glands and the gonads. A deviation from normal in an infant or a growing child gives certain changes that are quite distinct from those in the adult with the same basic disorder. A separation is made between infantile and adult disorders. For instance, cretinism is infantile hypothyroidism; myxedema is the adult disease. If the anterior lobe of the pituitary gland is destroyed in early life, a pituitary dwarf results. In the adult, Simmonds' disease or pituitary cachexia develops. If there is hyperfunction of the pituitary gland in early life, the individual grows into a giant (Fig. 53-1). After full growth has been obtained, the hyperfunction produces acromegaly, and the excess growth is not nearly so marked.

## Pituitary gland (hypophysis)

The pituitary gland, the size and shape of a bean, is tucked in a sheltered bony recess on the undersurface of the brain, to which it is connected by a stalk. This master gland consists of an anterior lobe and a smaller posterior lobe that differ in development, structure, and function. The anterior lobe is a glandular structure, and the posterior lobe is made of neuroglial tissue.

The anterior lobe has a number of functions, among which are (1) control of skeletal growth,* (2) regulation of the activity of the thyroid gland (thyrotropic or thyrotropin-stimulating hormone) and the adrenal glands (adrenocorticotropic hormone, ACTH),

---

*The human growth hormone (HGH) has been synthesized. Some 191 amino acids had to be strung together in just the right sequence.

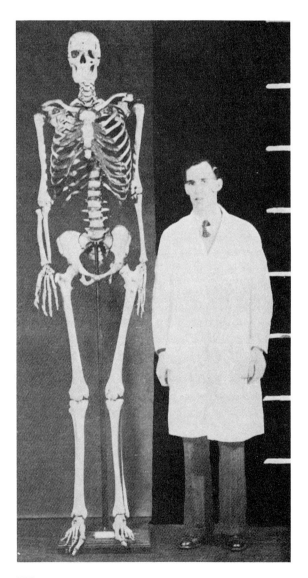

596

(3) regulatory action on the metabolism of carbohydrates and fats, and (4) influence on sexual development (gonadotropic hormones). The anterior lobe secretes at least two hormones that in the female have a maturing action on the graafian follicles of the ovary and stimulate the production of ova; the corresponding hormones in the male stimulate the development of the germinal epithelium of the tubules of the testis and act on the interstitial cells in the testis that produce the male sex hormone.

The lactogenic hormone initiates a flow of milk in the breast of a woman following the birth of her baby.

Pituitrin, an extract of the posterior lobe, causes contraction of smooth muscle fibers of the pregnant uterus at term, increases peristalsis, retards the flow of urine, slows heart action, and raises blood pressure. It is frequently used in obstetrics and surgery.

Overfunction and underfunction of the pituitary gland give rise to *hyperpituitarism* and *hypopituitarism,* respectively.

## HYPERPITUITARISM

Excessive activity of the anterior lobe of the pituitary gland occurs as two prominent clinical forms: gigantism and acromegaly.

**Gigantism.** Gigantism results when excessive activity of the pituitary is congenital or sets in during the active growth periods of childhood, before ossification of the skeleton is complete. The pituitary giant is abnormally tall, especially because of excessive length of the lower extremities. Lesions of other endocrine glands are present. Pituitary giants are often sexually impotent and frequently die of diabetes. In many cases the hyperactivity of the anterior lobe is found to result from an adenoma or, rarely, from hyperplasia of certain cells.

Adenomas are most often benign, although some progress locally. Some of the effects of tumors result from the pressure that the expanding lesion exerts on neighboring cells confined in the bony pocket. If functional cells are destroyed, the patient may show not only signs of increased hormone production but also indications of loss of hormonal activity.

**Acromegaly.** When anterior pituitary hyperactivity sets in after ossification of the skeleton is complete, acromegaly develops. The bones of the hands, feet, and lower jaw thicken and enlarge (Fig. 53-2). The

---

**Fig. 53-1.** Skeleton of Irish giant, an example of pituitary hyperfunction during early life. The markings in feet on right emphasize difference in height between normal man nearly 6 feet tall and the pituitary giant nearly 8 feet tall. (From Willis, R. A.: The principles of pathology, St. Louis, 1950, The C. V. Mosby Co.)

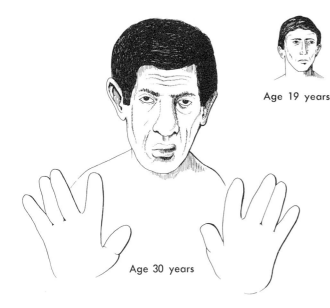

Age 19 years

Age 30 years

**Fig. 53-2.** Acromegaly (before and after disease). Note changes in facial features and the enlargement and thickening of hands.

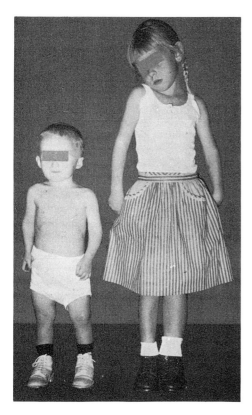

**Fig. 53-3.** Pituitary dwarfism. Both children are 4 years old. The dwarf on left stands 25 inches tall and normal child on right 39 inches tall. The dwarf has perfectly formed features with normal proportions. (From Raney, R. B., Sr., and Brashear, H. R., Jr.: Shands' handbook of orthopaedic surgery, ed. 8, St. Louis, 1971, The C. V. Mosby Co.)

enlargement of the lower jaw gives rise to the highly characteristic lion face appearance. In addition, there is considerable enlargement of the nose, lips, ears, and internal organs. Some degree of gigantism may be present. Diabetes mellitus, refractory to insulin, is often present. The mentality may be normal or impaired. After a long period of time pituitary hyperfunction is followed by a loss of function, indicated by sexual impotence, drowsiness, and a tendency toward obesity. As in gigantism, the hyperactivity of the anterior lobe is in many cases found to result from growth of an adenoma.

## HYPOPITUITARISM

Hypoactivity of the anterior lobe of the pituitary results when destruction of the gland is produced by pressure from tumors, vascular changes, inflammations, and metastases from systemic malignancies.

**Dwarfism.** When there is a congenital absence or great diminution in the secretion of the anterior lobe of the pituitary gland in early life, dwarfism results (Fig. 53-3). There is an almost complete lack of growth and sexual development. The pituitary dwarf old enough to be fully grown has the physical development and proportions of a small child and no secondary sex characters.

**Pituitary cachexia (Simmonds' disease).** On rare occasions, especially after childbirth, a generalized wasting away without apparent cause occurs in women. Weight loss is marked, internal organs atrophy, there is loss of sexual function, and the hair and teeth fall out. There are mental changes, and the affected woman seems to age prematurely. The destructive lesion of the whole pituitary gland or of the anterior lobe is necrosis, which further complicates a delivery already associated with severe hemorrhage and shock.

## DIABETES INSIPIDUS

Diabetes insipidus is produced by disease of the posterior lobe of the pituitary gland or injury to the adjoining hypothalamus in the brain. As a consequence the antidiuretic hormones are not elaborated, and the patient passes large quantities of urine (polyuria). At the same time he experiences an excessive and extraordinary thirst (polydipsia).

# Thyroid gland

The thyroid gland is a bilobed mass in the neck occupying either side of the windpipe. It is made up of closed sacs or follicles normally filled with a storage material (colloid) that contains the thyroid hormone. The thyroid hormone is a combination of iodine with amino acid to form *thyroxine*. (The thyroid hormone is unique in the body in that it is an amino acid.) In the thyroid gland the hormone is stored in a protein containing iodine. The combination is known as *thyroglobulin*. When an excessive amount of thyroid hormone is absorbed into the blood, *hyperthyroidism* develops. When an insufficient amount is absorbed, the result is *hypothyroidism*.

The thyroid gland controls the rate of basal and general metabolism, influences body growth and development, and exerts an influence over the nervous system and the development of the sex glands. It undergoes hypertrophy at puberty and also during menstruation and pregnancy. It undergoes atrophy in old age.

The amount of iodine present influences the activity of the thyroid gland, which is regulated by the thyrotropic hormone of the pituitary gland. The content of *protein-bound iodine* in the blood (the PBI test) is an index of the amount of thyroid hormone circulating in the blood. It is a test that can be closely correlated with hyperfunction and hypofunction of the thyroid gland.

## GOITER

The term *goiter* or *struma* does not refer to a specific disease but merely indicates an increase in the size of the thyroid gland. This increase may result from several causes and may be associated with normal, decreased, or increased secretion of thyroid hormone. The goiter may be a diffuse enlargement of the gland or an irregular one, forming a nodular goiter. Important causes of goiter are chronic iodine deficiency, hyperplasia of the gland, certain rare degenerative and inflammatory conditions, and neoplasm.

Iodine is most important to the elaboration of thy-

roid hormone. The gland traps most of the iodine in the bloodstream and incorporates it into hormone. Goiter that results from iodine deficiency is endemic, simple, or colloid and is often a nodular involvement of the gland. Such goiters are endemic in certain geographic districts such as Switzerland and the Great Lakes and the Mississippi and Ohio Valley regions of the United States, where the food and water are naturally deficient in iodine. They may be prevented by addition of a sufficient amount of iodine to the food supply or to the supply of salt (iodized salt). Iodine also has some curative action, but the goiter returns when iodine is discontinued. Endemic or colloid goiters commonly appear in girls shortly before or at the time of puberty and during pregnancy. Endemic goiters are more common in women than men and are often associated with hypothyroidism. The word *colloid* refers to an increased amount of colloid that fills and distends the follicles microscopically.

## HYPOTHYROIDISM

A deficiency of thyroid secretion present before the baby is born leads to *congenital myxedema* or *cretinism,* a pathetic state characterized by a number of abnormalities of growth and development. These include slow development of bones, late closure of the fontanels and cranial sutures, dwarfism, and delayed dentition. The baby's lips and tongue are thick; the skin is pasty. Body temperature is low, and mental activity is retarded. In addition, there are lack of hair, extreme susceptibility to cold, low basal metabolism, and decrease in protein-bound iodine of the blood. The clinical picture is full blown about the sixth month. Cretinism of this type is also known as *endemic cretinism* and is common among the offspring of mothers who themselves have endemic goiter. Cretins may have simple goiters, or their thyroids may be hypoplastic or even absent.

Hypothyroidism occurring in early life as a result of infection or in a child of a healthy mother is known as *sporadic* cretinism. Sporadic cretinism is, in truth, myxedema of the very young, or *juvenile myxedema*. Administration of thyroid extract has some curative effect on cretinism, but the child is seldom completely restored to normal either physically or mentally. Response to treatment is better in juvenile myxedema than in the congenital form. Congenital myxedema may be prevented by the administration of iodine to the mother during pregnancy.

When thyroid deficiency develops in adult life, *myxedema* follows. The skin becomes puffy and dry, the eyelids swell (Fig. 53-4), the tongue and lips thicken, the hair falls out, the sexual functions decline, and nervous symptoms develop. So-called myxedema madness may be present. The body temperature and

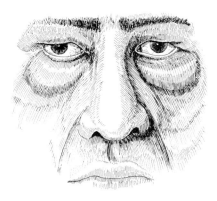

**Fig. 53-4.** Hypothyroidism. Note puffiness of eyelids.

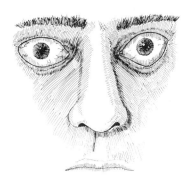

**Fig. 53-5.** Hyperthyroidism with associated exophthalmos. Note the white of the scleral coat of the eye seen above the pupil.

basal metabolism fall below normal, the patient becomes extremely susceptible to cold, and there is a marked slowing and sluggishness of thought, perception, and motion. The function of practically every part of the body is diminished.

*Myxedema* is caused by a loss of thyroid function brought about by disease or surgical removal of the thyroid gland. Myxedema resulting from surgical removal is known as *cachexia strumipriva*. Myxedema shows marked improvement with thyroid medication, but the hypothyroid state returns if medication is discontinued. The thyroid gland may be enlarged in myxedema, but the enlargement results from the accumulation of nonfunctional tissue.

## HYPERTHYROIDISM

Hyperthyroidism results when the thyroid gland becomes overactive and releases into the circulation excessive amounts of the thyroid hormone. The overactive gland may be diffusely hyperplastic or a nodular goiter (example: toxic adenoma). Hyperthyroidism is characterized by an increased rate of general and basal metabolism, tachycardia (fast heart rate), profound nervous disturbances, tremor, weight loss, weakness, intolerance to heat, and attacks of profuse sweating. The protein-bound iodine is increased in the bloodstream. Disturbances of menstruation are common in women. (Thyroid disease is more prevalent in women than in men.) A special and the most severe form of the disease in which, in addition to the above manifestations, exophthalmos (Fig. 53-5) is present is known as *exophthalmic goiter* or *Graves' disease*. The end stage of the hyperactive gland of Graves' disease is exhaustion, at which time a state of hypothyroidism appears.

The causes of the hyperthyroid state are not completely worked out. In Graves' disease the administration of iodine leads to a temporary reaccumulation

of colloid in the gland, which disappeared with the development of hyperplasia, and a temporary abatement of manifestations. Thiouracil and thiourea derivatives are also used in the treatment of hyperthyroidism, especially Graves' disease. The diffusely hyperplastic gland or the hyperplastic nodule may have to be surgically removed.

**Laboratory diagnosis.** The laboratory diagnosis of hyperthyroidism and thyroid disorders generally depends on tests determining the following: (1) the basal metabolic rate, (2) the level of the protein-bound iodine in the serum, (3) the uptake of radioactive iodine by the thyroid gland, and (4) the rate of conversion of radioactive iodine into iodine bound by protein. Radioactive iodine (iodine 131) has been more widely and effectively used than has any other radioisotope and has proved most valuable in the evaluation of thyroid gland disorders. With the radioactivated compounds of iodine it is possible to trace and follow the course of iodine in the body and into the thyroid tissue. Radioiodine ($^{131}$I) is also being successfully used today in the treatment of hyperthyroidism.

## INFLAMMATION

The thyroid gland appears to be immune to the effect of many of the living agents producing acute infections in other parts of the body. *Thyroiditis* (inflammation of the thyroid) refers to two special forms.

A prolonged, self-limited disease of acute onset is *subacute (de Quervain's) thyroiditis*, occurring in women, the cause of which is unknown. Pathologically degenerative changes in the follicles are associated with a granulomatous inflammation, which seems to be of foreign-body type. *Hashimoto's struma*, a disease of women at about the time of menopause, is characterized by enlargement of the gland and mild hypothyroidism in the late stages. The excessive accumulation of lymphoid tissue in the thyroid gland makes the pathologic picture a striking one. This is currently considered one of the autoimmune diseases. Although a few normal persons have antithyroid antibodies and patients with any type of thyroid disease have a greater than normal incidence, the presence of autoantibodies in this disease is considered significant. Autoantibodies that can be demonstrated in the patient's serum are formed against the patient's own thyroglobulin (or a part of it).

### NEOPLASM

Neoplasms of the thyroid gland may be either benign or malignant. The clinical manifestations of malignant neoplasms may be quite unusual. Carcinoma of the thyroid is most common in women in their sixties and sometimes grows very slowly over a period of years. It can be rapidly fatal, however. It often arises in a previously benign adenoma. Metastases occur to the lymph nodes of the neck and to the lungs and bones. If the metastatic tumor tissue is well-differentiated thyroid tissue, it will take up radioactive iodine. The poorly differentiated tumor tissue will not do so.

## Parathyroid glands

The parathyroid glands are four small organs usually attached loosely to the thyroid gland posteriorly but which may be included within its capsule. They produce internal secretions that regulate calcium and phosphorus metabolism and help to maintain the normal level of blood calcium (9 to 11 mg. per 100 ml. or 4.5 to 5.5 mEq. per liter).

There are at least two parathyroid gland hormones, *parathormone* and *calcitonin,* with three physiologic activities regulating the level of calcium in the bloodstream (maintenance of calcium homeostasis). Parathyroid hormones pull calcium out of the bones if needed and increase the absorption of calcium from the intestinal tract. By their action on the kidney they can control the amount of phosphorus lost in the urine, which regulates the amount of phosphorus in the blood and hence the amount of calcium (the level of calcium is directly related to that of phosphorus).

### HYPOFUNCTION

In *hypoparathyroidism,* the state wherein the parathyroid glands fail to release a normal amount of parathormone, the calcium level in the blood is sharply reduced to produce the clinical state of calcium deficiency known as *tetany.* Tetany is a condition of heightened neuromuscular irritability in which spasmodic muscular twitchings, abnormal reflexes, and even convulsive seizures appear. It is quickly relieved by the administration of calcium. The accidental removal of the parathyroid glands was one of the causes

of unexplained death in the early days of thyroid surgery, for unless parathyroid extract is given, complete removal of the parathyroid glands is quickly followed by tetany, ending in death.

### HYPERFUNCTION

Increased activity of the parathyroid glands (*hyperparathyroidism*) is caused by an adenoma of one of the glands or by diffuse hyperplasia of all four. When the parathyroid tissue is overactive, calcium in excess is withdrawn from the bones and is lost to the body. The bones soften and lose their strength, and there is marked rarefaction with cyst formation (*osteitis fibrosa cystica* or *von Recklinghausen's disease*). (See Fig. 53-6.) With hypercalcemia there is a predisposition to stone formation in the kidneys, and calcium salts are deposited in soft tissues, especially in the kidneys, lungs, and stomach.

Diffuse hyperplasia of the parathyroid glands may be secondary to advanced kidney disease because of the role of the kidney in maintaining the level of phosphorus in the blood. If phosphorus is abnormally retained in the blood, the level of calcium falls, and the parathyroids are stimulated to increased hormone production. When this alteration of calcium and phosphorus metabolism occurs in young children, it leads to bone changes known as *renal rickets.*

## Adrenal glands

Like caps atop the kidneys, the adrenal glands are paired organs consisting of two portions, an outer zone (cortex) and a central portion (medulla), which differ in origin, structure, and function. Complete extirpation of both adrenal glands experimentally in animals produces no significant symptoms for about 1 week. Then suddenly the animals begin to lose large amounts of salt and water in the urine; they become very weak and prostrated. The blood sugar drops sharply, the temperature and basal metabolic rate fall, the appetite is poor, diarrhea may be present, and death comes on in 1 to 3 days after the onset of this disorder. Extirpation experiments have shown that the cortex, not the medulla, is the part of the gland that is essential to life.

**Adrenal cortex.** The endocrine influence of the adrenal cortex is exerted on salt and water metabolism and on protein and carbohydrate metabolism. It also affects the establishment of the secondary sex characters, body pigmentation, vitamin C metabolism, and the level of the blood pressure.

About thirty steroid compounds have been isolated experimentally from the adrenal cortex, but only six have been found to be active physiologically. Of these, two especially have incited much clinical interest because of their therapeutic value in modifying the

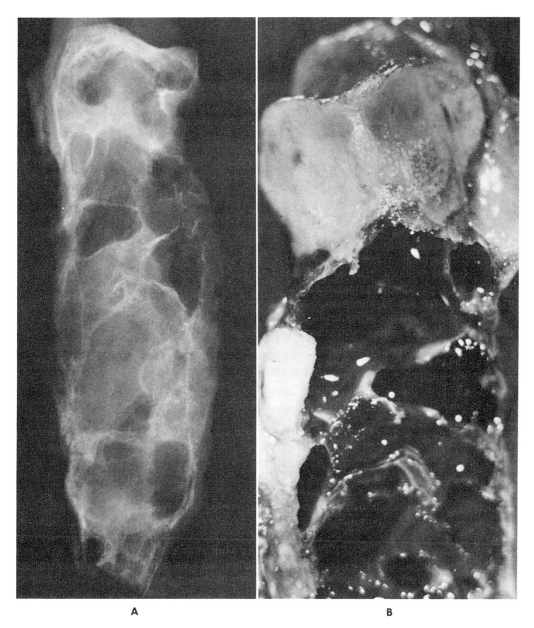

A                                    B

**Fig. 53-6.** Hyperparathyroidism causing bone disease in a 57-year-old woman. Serum calcium level 14.5 mg./100 ml. Parathyroid adenoma was removed surgically. **A,** Radiograph of bone. Note thinning of bone cortex and rarefaction. **B,** Gross appearance of bone. Note cystic change. (From Lichtenstein, L.: Diseases of bone and joints, ed. 2, St. Louis, 1975, The C. V. Mosby Co.)

symptoms of chronic rheumatism, acute rheumatic fever, and certain other unrelated disorders. The two steroids are *cortisone* (compound E) and *hydrocortisone* (compound F). They exert their effect even when adrenal insufficiency does not exist, and although the mechanism of their action is unknown, it is not thought that these compounds correct a hormone deficiency in the usual sense.

Physiologically there are three groups of steroid hormones: (1) *mineralocorticoids* (example: aldosterone), which control salt and water metabolism, (2) *glucocorticoids* or sugar hormones (examples: hydrocortisone and cortisone), which regulate metabolism of sugar and also of fat, and (3) *sex hormones* (androgens), whose action on the male of the species is of low physiologic potency. (A small amount of estrogen is also produced.)

The output of adrenal cortical hormones is regulated by the adrenocorticotropic hormone (ACTH), which is released by the anterior lobe of the pituitary gland under the proper stimulation. This hormone appears to stimulate all the known functions of the adrenal cortex and because of this fact has itself come into wide clinical use. It has been found to have similar beneficial effects in diseases that respond to cortisone, hydrocortisone, and related compounds, such as the following:

1. Collagen diseases: rheumatoid arthritis, acute rheumatic fever, periarteritis nodosa
2. Allergic states: bronchial asthma, allergic rhinitis, contact dermatitis
3. Disorders of the blood-forming organs: leukemia, lymphosarcoma, thrombocytopenia
4. Others: chronic nephrosis, ulcerative colitis, hepatitis

It must be remembered that the prolonged therapeutic use of the potent steroid hormones leads to toxic effects. There are changes in facial features, a characteristic type of obesity, hirsutism, decreased carbohydrate tolerance with an elevated blood sugar, elevation of blood pressure, and mental changes. Also, cortisone has a decided anti-inflammatory action; it not only interferes with the formation of antibodies but also suppresses the basic changes in the inflammatory process.

In the adrenal cortex, lesions related to functional states are either regressive or proliferative. Injuries to the cortex may come from hemorrhage, vascular disturbances, infections, and carcinomatous metastases. Atrophy of the cortex may be produced by extended dosage of cortisone.

**Adrenal medulla.** The adrenal medulla produces *epinephrine,* or adrenaline as it is often called, which causes contraction of the blood vessels, raises blood pressure, slows the heart, and suppresses fatigue. The output of epinephrine is increased by emotional disturbances such as anger and in periods of stress. This hormone helps the body in times of danger.

## HYPOFUNCTION—ADDISON'S DISEASE

Addison's disease, chronic insufficiency of the adrenal cortex, is a peculiar disease in which autopsy reveals a bilateral destructive lesion of the adrenal glands. Tuberculosis, idiopathic atrophy or necrosis, and neoplastic involvement of the glands are three causes.

The disease is most common in males who have reached the later years of life. It begins rather insidiously with digestive disturbances and loss of appetite. These are followed by vomiting, diarrhea, decrease in blood pressure, progressive emaciation and weakness, and a peculiar splotchy, grayish brown pigmentation of the skin. After a time the untreated patient becomes so weak that he takes to his bed, from which he never rises. The time elapsing between the onset of the disease and death is usually about 1 year.

## HYPERFUNCTION

**Adrenal cortex.** Hyperfunction of the adrenal cortex is associated with diffuse hyperplasia, adenomas, and carcinoma of the cortex, although these lesions are found without functional effects. Three clinical disorders are related to excess hormonal production: (1) Cushing's syndrome, (2) adrenogenital syndrome, and (3) primary aldosteronism.

One of these, *Cushing's syndrome,* may also be produced clinically by large doses of adrenocortical steroids, as in the treatment of leukemias. This disorder, found in young adult women, is a composite of weakness, ease of tiring, diminished sexual function, and high blood pressure in a moon-faced individual whose obesity is marked off in the head, neck, and trunk. A growth of facial hair and purplish markings on the skin of the abdomen and buttocks complete the picture. A characteristic pathologic change in the pituitary gland accompanies a lesion of the adrenal cortex.

In *adrenogenital syndrome (adrenal virilism)* an excess of male sex hormone dominates. This is dramatic when seen in a female of any age. If the condition is congenital, a pseudohermaphrodite is born. Before masculinization in the adult female is complete, secondary sex characters must regress. Then the body hair pattern changes to that of a male, the voice deepens, and the clitoris hypertrophies.

The features related to the biochemical disturbance of *primary aldosteronism* are periodic muscular weakness of severe grade, high blood pressure, and excessive thirst and urine flow. The amount of potassium in the blood is quite low and that in the urine elevated.

**Adrenal medulla.** A consequence of its high epinephrine and norepinephrine content, the *pheochromocytoma (chromaffinoma),* a rare tumor of the adrenal medulla, is associated with hypertension severe in its paroxysms.

# Pancreas

Although we have found that the pancreas has an important external secretion that contains digestive enzymes, we must not forget that it has an important internal secretion that regulates carbohydrate metabolism. This hormone, known as *insulin,* is produced by the islands of Langerhans.

## DIABETES MELLITUS

When there is an absolute or relative deficiency of the action of insulin at the surface of or within certain body cells, the metabolic disorder known as diabetes mellitus results. This is an inherited disease. In the absence of insulin, glucose is not changed to glycogen and stored within the liver but accumulates in the blood *(hyperglycemia)* and escapes into the urine *(glycosuria).* Insulin also affects the metabolism of fats and proteins. As the disease progresses, the derangements related to these two foodstuffs become apparent.

The nature of the metabolic defect in diabetes is not determined. The impairment of insulin activity may be that the body does not produce enough or that the action of available insulin is blocked from its primary task of facilitating the entry of glucose into the cells of the body.

Various lesions of the pancreas have been found related to diabetes, but no lesion has been called *the* lesion of diabetes mellitus. Although the clinical and physiologic disturbances may be profound, the pathologic findings are not specific. The disease is a functional disorder.

There are two clinical types of diabetes: juvenile diabetes and maturity-onset diabetes. In these the underlying metabolic defect, the treatment, and the outlook are different.

Juvenile diabetes, the severe form, begins early in life—childhood or adolescence—and usually progresses rapidly. Because of damage to small blood vessels, there are many serious complications—blindness (diabetic retinopathy), kidney failure (diabetic glomerulosclerosis), heart disease, and gangrene of the limbs as a result of circulatory embarrassment. Amputation may have to be done.

Maturity-onset diabetes, representing at least 75% of cases of this prevalent disease, usually begins after the age of 40 and is generally less severe than juvenile diabetes. The former does not move so quickly, and the incidence of serious complications is less.

The biochemical derangements occasioned by the lack of insulin in a diabetic patient are dramatic ones. There are severe fluid and electrolytic disturbances, acidosis develops, and death may occur in diabetic coma. Infection is a hazard for the diabetic person. The hardening of the arteries, often a regular feature, leads to cardiovascular complications.

In diabetes mellitus, carbohydrate metabolism may be restored to normal, and practically all the manifestations of the disease can be controlled by the administration of insulin. With regular injections, many juvenile diabetics can be maintained over a long period of time. The older diabetics may stay regulated with just weight loss, diet, and the oral antidiabetic drugs.

Insulin must be carefully administered. Overdosage triggers a train of events resulting from low blood sugar *(hypoglycemia)* and consisting of weakness, fatigue, profuse sweating, mental disturbances, and convulsions. This condition, known as *hyperinsulinism,* may be of gradual or sudden onset. It demands immediate treatment. Manifestations usually appear when the blood sugar falls to a level of around 45 to 50 mg. per 100 ml. of blood.

## Questions for review

1 What are the manifestations of myxedema? What is a cretin?
2 What are the manifestations of hyperthyroidism? What is Graves' disease?
3 What is the laboratory diagnosis of hyperthyroidism? What is the importance of radioiodine?
4 Give the findings in hyperinsulinism.
5 Characterize hyperparathyroidism.
6 What endocrine disturbance causes each of the following: gigantism, acromegaly, Simmonds' disease, dwarfism, tetany, Addison's disease, Cushing's syndrome, diabetes insipidus?
7 List six diseases that are favorably affected by treatment with cortisone or related compounds. What are the complications of such therapy?
8 What is ACTH? Name three steroid hormones.
9 Briefly explain the following: goiter, struma, hormone, parathormone, mineralocorticoid, thyroxine, glucocorticoid, autoimmune disease, calcitonin.

**References on pp. 619 and 620.**

# CHAPTER 54

# Diseases of
# Male reproductive organs

The reproductive system of the male comprises the testes, the complex excretory duct system with its auxiliary glands, and the penis. In transit through the ducts the male sex cells are mingled with secretions from the accessory structures to form the semen.

## Testis and epididymis

The nearly symmetrical oval testes contain a highly convoluted system of seminiferous tubules lined by a complex epithelium. Most of this epithelium is made up of germinal or spermatogenic cells that proliferate and mature characteristically to form the mature male germ cells. The principal hormone of the testis is testosterone.

The comma-shaped epididymis, on the back of each gonad, is the much-twisted duct of the testis.

### INFLAMMATION

Inflammation of the body of the testis is known as *orchitis*. Inflammation of the epididymis is known as *epididymitis* (Fig. 54-1). Inflammations of the testis may be classified as (1) those confined to the epididymis, of which gonorrhea is the best example, (2) those confined to the body of the testis, of which mumps and syphilitic orchitis are examples, and (3) those affecting both epididymis and body.

**Acute epididymitis.** Gonorrheal epididymitis is the most common type of acute epididymitis and the usual complication of gonorrhea in the male. It is generally secondary to posterior urethritis. Mostly unilateral, it may be bilateral. Properly treated, acute gonorrheal epididymitis may be cured without any permanent defect, but in some cases scarring may be so great as to obstruct the passage of spermatozoa. Bilateral epididymitis of this type leads to sterility. As a rule, the body of the testicle is not involved.

**Acute orchitis.** Acute orchitis frequently complicates mumps or acute infectious diseases and may result from trauma. In many cases it leads to atrophy and fibrosis of the testis with loss of spermatogenesis. Bilateral orchitis with atrophy, fibrosis, and loss of function causes sterility. In certain types of acute orchitis suppuration with abscess formation occurs.

**Chronic orchitis.** Chronic orchitis may be a continuation of the acute form, but many cases arise without antecedent attacks. Many cases are caused by syphilis.

**Tuberculosis.** In the great majority of cases tuberculosis of the testis is secondary to tuberculosis in some other organ, especially the lungs. It usually begins in one epididymis, from which it spreads to the other epididymis and to other parts of the genital system. As a rule, the body of the testis is not involved until the disease is far advanced.

**Syphilis.** Syphilis of the testis occurs as a diffuse inflammation or as single and multiple gummas (Fig. 54-2), and the process is usually confined to the body of the testis. Diffuse inflammations are more frequent, but gummas are more easily recognized. Gummas cause testicular enlargement, whereas diffuse inflammation has little effect on the size and shape of the testis until far advanced, at which time testicular atrophy is produced.

### NEOPLASM

Practically all tumors of the testicle are malignant, and some highly so. Fortunately, they are rare. The majority occur between the ages of 20 and 45 years. One important neoplasm is the *teratoma,* which may form such a bulky mass as to destroy the gonad completely. It contains a hodgepodge of tissue types not ordinarily found in the testicle (muscle, bone, cartilage, mucous glands, brain tissue). *Choriocarcinoma* of the testis shows an irregular arrangement of cells normally belonging to the human placenta. These trophoblastic cells behave in a most malignant fashion.

Most malignant neoplasms of the testicle produce

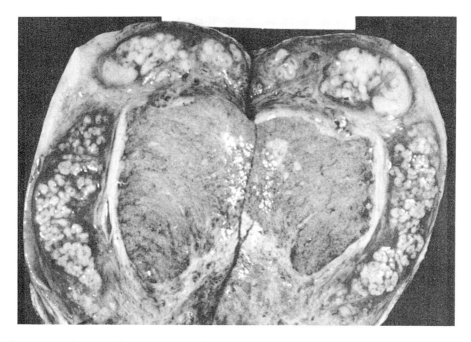

**Fig. 54-1.** Purulent epididymitis. Sectioned surface of testis and epididymis shows tortuous course of pus within canal of epididymis. Testis not inflamed.

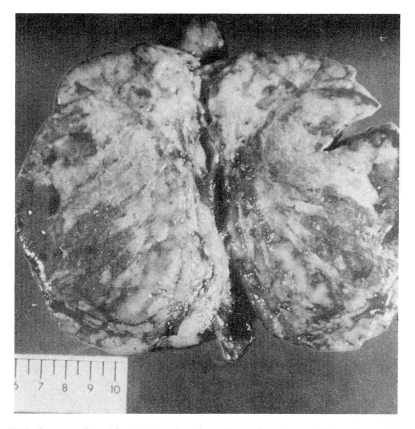

**Fig. 54-2.** Gumma of testicle. Sectioned surface shows distortion and loss of normal tissue.

pituitary-like hormones (chorionic gonadotropins) similar to those produced by the placenta in a pregnant female. This means that the Aschheim-Zondek test, a test for pregnancy, is strongly positive in a male with choriocarcinoma of the testis. The test is of considerable value in diagnosis and in following the course of treatment. If the tumor is completely removed, the Aschheim-Zondek test becomes negative. If the tumor recurs or foci of metastasis enlarge, the test becomes strongly positive again.

Undescended or misplaced testes are more often the site of tumors than are normal ones. *Cryptorchism* is the term designating failure of the testicle to descend into the scrotum.

## HYDROCELE

During its descent to the scrotum in early life the testis becomes invested with a peritoneal sac known as the tunica vaginalis. Normally the sac separates from the peritoneal cavity, but sometimes a communication between the two remains. This sac can fill with a large amount of clear, pale yellowish fluid, a condition spoken of as a hydrocele. When the opening between the peritoneal cavity and tunica vaginalis has not closed, the fluid is derived from the peritoneal cavity. In acute hydrocele the amount of fluid seldom exceeds 100 ml., and it may be turbid or frankly purulent. In chronic hydrocele the amount of clear, yellow fluid ranges from 100 to 300 ml. or more. Acute hydrocele most often means tuberculous or gonorrheal involvement of the testis. Chronic hydrocele may follow the acute form or come on without apparent cause. Hydrocele causes enlargement and deformity of the scrotum, and in long-standing cases pressure causes atrophy of the testis.

As a result of trauma, such as kicks, blows, or surgical manipulation, blood may escape into the hydrocele sac, converting the hydrocele into a *hematocele*.

## VARICOCELE

Varicocele is the varicose dilatation of the veins of the spermatic cord. It is most common in young men and usually occurs on the left side. The veins become irregularly dilated, producing a large, twisted, tortuous mass. Although there are many theories as to causation, none is generally accepted. A few cases result from pressure exerted on the spermatic vein by an abdominal tumor.

Varicocele is characterized clinically by reflex dis-

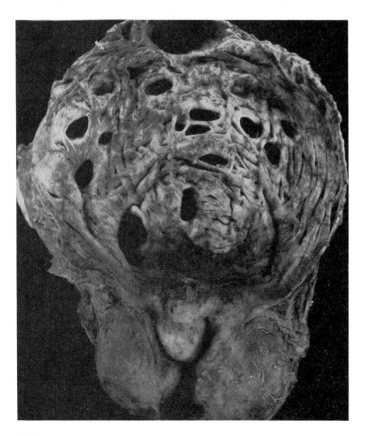

**Fig. 54-3.** Hyperplasia of prostate gland with obstruction to urethra. The urinary bladder is opened. Cut surfaces of the two lateral lobes of prostate gland are seen in lower part of photograph. These are enlarged as is middle lobe, a nodular projection into lumen of urethra. The obstruction to urinary outflow led to thickening (hypertrophy) of bladder wall with diverticula (indicated as many small black areas in bladder wall). (From Anderson, W. A. D., editor: Pathology, ed. 6, St. Louis, 1971, The C. V. Mosby Co.)

turbances and a sensation of weight and pain. These features may incapacitate a patient who has a nervous temperament.

## Prostate gland

Both a glandular and a muscular organ, the dark brown–red prostate gland surrounds the first part of the male urethra. Its secretion is a component of semen.

### INFLAMMATION

**Acute prostatitis.** Acute prostatitis is often the extension of gonorrheal posterior urethritis but may result from other causes such as infection of the posterior urethra following catheterization. Much less frequently, small abscesses form from blood-borne infection in septicemia or pyemia.

Acute prostatitis occurs as diffuse inflammation or with suppuration. Small abscesses occurring in suppurative prostatitis become encapsulated, and larger ones point into the perineum or rupture into the urethra. Swelling of the prostate leads to considerable pain and compresses the urethra, interfering with urination.

**Chronic prostatitis.** Chronic prostatitis is a continuation of the acute form and a common accompaniment of prostatic hyperplasia.

**Tuberculosis.** Tuberculosis of the prostate often extends from the prostate gland to the other genital organs. Typical caseous foci are formed.

### HYPERPLASIA

Hyperplasia, which produces an enlargement of the prostate gland (often referred to as *benign prostatic hypertrophy*), usually occurs in men past their fiftieth year. In some cases the enlargement results from an increase in the number of glandular structures of the prostate gland; in others it is caused by hypertrophy of the fibromuscular stroma, but in most cases both glands and stroma are involved. The enlargement may be smooth or nodular, generalized or localized. The most important localized form is an enlargement of the middle lobe that projects into the posterior urethral wall as a rounded elevation or obstructing bar.

Prostatic hyperplasia interferes with urination, and this is especially true when the middle lobe is enlarged. Obstruction to urination leads to hypertrophy and dilatation of the bladder (Fig. 54-3), cystitis, and ascending infection. When the middle lobe projects upward, a depression in the floor of the bladder is formed behind the enlarged lobe. This depression contains a small amount of *residual urine* that cannot be expelled during urination. Residual urine decomposes and becomes infected, which leads to cystitis. Repeated catheterization, often necessary in prostatic enlargement, also favors bladder infection. Obstruction in the lower urinary tract interferes with normal renal function.

### CARCINOMA

More than 15% of enlarged prostate glands contain an adenocarcinoma. Carcinoma may be present with hyperplasia, but the two conditions are not considered related. Carcinoma is also a disease of men past 50 years of age. After the carcinoma becomes well established, it progresses rapidly, with extension locally to the bladder and seminal vesicles and metastases to the bones and regional lymph nodes. The results of the treatment of carcinoma of the prostate gland with stilbestrol (female sex hormone) and by castration indicate that the secretions of certain endocrine glands are a factor in the production of the disease.

The level of serum acid phosphatase is an important laboratory determination in the evaluation of cancer of the prostate gland. Acid phosphatase is a normal intracellular component of many cells in the body. In the prostate gland it is found extracellularly in the prostatic secretions. With metastasis of cancer of the prostate, the amount of the serum acid phosphatase is strikingly elevated.

## Questions for review

1 What is epididymitis? Orchitis?
2 Give causes and results of acute epididymitis and acute orchitis.
3 What is a hydrocele? Give some of the causes.
4 What is a varicocele?
5 Discuss prostatic hyperplasia. Is it related to carcinoma?
6 To what locations does carcinoma of the prostate gland spread?
7 How is the Aschheim-Zondek test used in persons with testicular tumors?

**References on pp. 619 and 620.**

# CHAPTER 55

# Diseases of

# Female reproductive organs

The reproductive system of the female comprises external and internal genitalia and the mammary glands (breasts). The structures of the external genitalia, on the surface of the body, are referred to collectively as the vulva. The internal genitalia, found within the body, are the ovaries, the fallopian tubes (oviducts, uterine tubes), the uterus (womb), the cervix (mouth of the womb), and the vagina. In the mature female the response of the internal genitalia and breasts to ovarian hormones is patterned in characteristic cycles.

## Ovaries

The size and shape of large almonds, the ovaries incorporate within their substance the developmental sequences of the graafian follicle, which contains the female sex cell, and a complement of hormone-producing cells about it known as granulosal cells. The ovum is released (ovulation) from a fully matured follicle, which may be as large as 0.8 cm. in diameter. Afterward the follicle collapses, there is an accumulation of fat in the granulosal cells, and because of this transformation a new structure, the corpus luteum, emerges. Fully formed, the corpus luteum may be 1 to 1.5 cm. in diameter. If pregnancy does not supervene, the transformed follicle regresses. Its end stage is a scar in the ovarian stroma.

### CYSTS

**Follicular cyst.** When a graafian follicle develops but fails to rupture, its ovum often degenerates and more fluid is poured into the follicle, distending it to form a follicular cyst (Fig. 55-1). These may be single or multiple and are the most common cysts of the ovary. Seldom more than 3 cm. in diameter, follicular cysts are filled with a clear, colorless fluid.

**Corpus luteum cyst.** If cyst formation occurs after the ovum has been expelled and the processes leading to the formation of a corpus luteum have begun, a corpus luteum cyst results. These cysts are usually single, with a thick yellow lining. They may be several centimeters in diameter, sometimes much larger, and are thought to arise from a previously existing corpus luteum hematoma.

**Dermoid cyst.** A dermoid cyst (Fig. 55-2) is a benign neoplasm that may occur in fetal life or childhood but usually does not reach full development until after puberty. Dermoid cysts form 20% of all ovarian tumors and in some cases are bilateral. It is a rather thick-walled cyst filled with a yellow, putty-like greasy material that is secreted by sebaceous glands and often contains hair. Structures common in the wall of a dermoid cyst are sebaceous glands, rudimentary teeth, cartilage, bone, thyroid tissue, and poorly developed eyes. At one point on the lining of the cyst cavity a small nipple-shaped mass, known as the *mammilla,* may be seen. This tumor belongs to the group known as teratomas (tumors made up of tissues derived from two or more of the embryonic germ layers). It rarely exceeds the size of an orange and seldom causes symptoms.

### CYSTADENOMAS

About 60% of the benign tumors of the ovary are glandular tumors in which so much fluid is secreted by the glandular epithelium that the glands dilate into cysts. Such tumors are cystadenomas. Cystadenomas of the ovary are of two types: pseudomucinous and serous (the terms referring to the gross contents of the cysts).

**Pseudomucinous cystadenoma.** A pseudomucinous cystadenoma is a round or oval, multiloculated tumor containing many cystic spaces filled with a thick, yellow, stringy mucoid material, pseudomucin. These tumors are usually unilateral and pedunculated and unless surgically removed may reach almost unbelievable size. They are not malignant in the ordinary sense, but spilling of their contents into the abdominal cavity gives rise to the condition known as *pseudomyxoma peritonei* (p. 581).

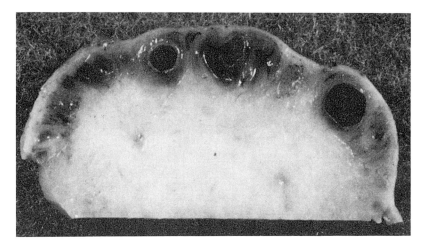

**Fig. 55-1.** Follicular cysts in cortex of ovary (sectioned surface).

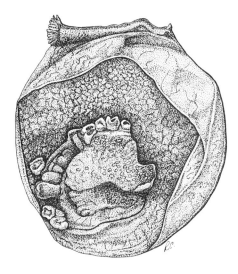

**Fig. 55-2.** Dermoid cyst of ovary that has been opened. Note teeth in rudimentary jaw. Fallopian tube overlies large cyst.

**Serous cystadenoma.** A serous cystadenoma is usually a unilocular, thick-walled cyst with papillary projections extending from the lining into the cyst cavity (Fig. 55-3). It is filled with a serous fluid. In many cases the papillary growths perforate the wall of the cyst and appear on the outside, from which they spread to the peritoneum to cause widespread secondary growths. Ascites rapidly develops as a consequence. Papillary serous cystadenomas are often bilateral and seldom of greater size than a large orange. Because of their marked tendency to spread to the peritoneum and the fact that more than 50%

recur after surgical removal, papillary cystadenomas should be considered potentially malignant.

### CARCINOMA

The pseudomucinous and serous cystadenomas just mentioned have their *malignant* counterparts in the ovary. These malignant tumors are cystic neoplasms known as pseudomucinous and serous cystadenocarcinomas, respectively. The two forms of cystic carcinoma are the most common types of malignant tumor primary to the ovary. They involve one ovary, then the other, and metastasize to the uterus, peritoneum, and lumbar lymph nodes, producing early ascites. They may be rapidly fatal. Secondary carcinoma of the ovary is more common than primary carcinoma and is usually bilateral. It is most often secondary to carcinoma of the intestine, stomach, or uterus.

## Fallopian tubes

The fallopian tubes are paired ducts attached to the uterus. The ovary on each side is near the opposite and free extremity. After its release from the ovary, the ovum traverses this anatomic passageway to the uterus.

### INFLAMMATION

*Salpingitis* or inflammation of the fallopian tubes is usually caused by organisms that reach the lumen of the tubes through the uterine cavity, but some cases result from organisms that penetrate the outer portions of the tube wall from the broad ligament and extend through to the lumen. Like other inflammations, salpingitis may be acute or chronic.

**Acute salpingitis.** Fully 70% of the cases of acute

**609**

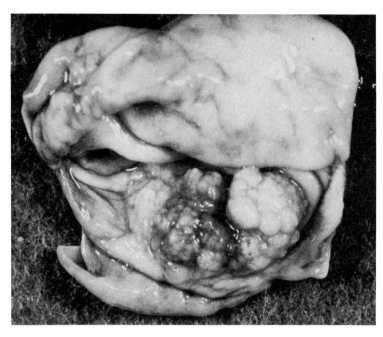

**Fig. 55-3.** Papillary serous cystadenoma of ovary (benign). Cyst opened and collapsed to show focus of papillary growth below and smooth inner lining above.

salpingitis are caused by gonococci that reach the tubes across the uterine cavity. Nongonorrheal salpingitis is usually caused by streptococci, staphylococci, or *Escherichia coli.* Streptococcal salpingitis follows a streptococcal infection of the puerperal uterus or an attempt to produce an abortion. As a rule, both tubes are involved in acute salpingitis, and the infectious material may escape from the extremities of the tubes to produce localized peritonitis.

Gonococci produce an acute catarrhal inflammation in the mucous membrane of the tube, with little destruction of tissue at first. If infections are repeated, however, there is a cumulative effect. Minor degrees of injury to the epithelial lining of the tube lead to numerous adhesions of the mucosal folds, and the acute stage merges into the subacute and chronic forms, characterized by damage and distortion of the tubes.

**Chronic salpingitis.** Chronic salpingitis, usually the sequel to an acute gonococcal infection, is characterized by marked scarring of the tubes with the formation of numerous and extensive adhesions involving the rugae, the fimbriae of the tubes, and surrounding structures. By the time that the disease has become chronic, the adhesions of the fimbriae have closed the peritoneal extremity of the tube. Inflammatory thickening in the mucosa of the uterine end has also helped to convert the lumen of the tube

into a closed cavity. The inflammation being of a purulent character, the cavity fills with pus, producing a *pyosalpinx* or pus tube. Purulent material may remain in such tubes for a long time. After many years, when the original inflammation has become quiescent, there may be resorption of the purulent material of the pus tube, so that the lumen comes to contain a thin watery fluid. A *hydrosalpinx* is then said to be present.

The chronic inflammatory process in the tube may spread to involve the ovary, which becomes adherent to the tube. A *tubo-ovarian abscess* may be formed. Chronic salpingitis is important because of its tendency to cause adhesions, sterility, and tubal pregnancy.

**Tuberculous salpingitis.** Tuberculosis attacks the fallopian tubes more often than any other female generative organ. It is always secondary to tuberculosis in some other part of the body, usually the lungs, and is complicated by tuberculous endometritis.

### ECTOPIC PREGNANCY

Normally the ovum is fertilized in the fallopian tube (the lovers' lane of the genital tract), and the fertilized ovum passes to the uterus where the fetus develops. Sometimes (about once in 300 pregnancies) the progress of the fertilized ovum is arrested in the tube, and it attaches to the tube wall. This constitutes a tubal pregnancy. Less often the ovum is fertilized outside of the fallopian tube and instead of entering the tube becomes attached to some abdominal structure, where a placenta is formed and the fetus starts to develop. This is known as a *primary abdominal pregnancy*. Pregnancies occurring outside the uterus are ectopic or extrauterine pregnancies. Of these, tubal pregnancies are by far the most important.

Chronic salpingitis is a common (but not the only) cause of tubal pregnancy, since in this condition the thickened and matted folds of the tubes form pockets and recesses that entrap the fertilized ovum on its way to the uterus. According to some investigators tubal pregnancy is related to small areas of endometrial tissue in the mucosa of the fallopian tube into which implantation of the fertilized ovum accidentally occurs. It is a well-known fact that endometrium does grow in places other than its normal location.

When the fertilized ovum is arrested in the tube, development begins, and chorionic villi of the placenta burrow into the tubal wall. Because of the anatomy of the tubes with their thin walls, it is practically impossible for a tubal pregnancy to go to full term. It will end either by tubal abortion or by tubal rupture. In *tubal abortion* the erosion of the wall of the tube caused by the growth of the chorionic villi leads to hemorrhage into the gestational sac, and at the same time the lumen of the tube fills with blood. If the fimbriated extremity of the tube is open, the contractions of the tube may expel the pregnancy into the abdominal cavity. *Tubal rupture*, occurring in about 25% of tubal pregnancies, results from the destruction of a portion of the tubal wall by the erosive action of the chorionic villi. Rupture may be accompanied by enough hemorrhage and shock to cause the death of the patient within a short period of time. As a rule, the fetus is destroyed when the tube ruptures, but in rare instances the fetus is slowly extruded and remains alive; the placenta may become attached to the abdominal organs, producing a secondary abdominal pregnancy.

In abdominal pregnancy the placenta may be so poorly developed that the fetus does not reach maturity but dries up and becomes infiltrated with lime salts, forming a *lithopedion*.

## Uterus

The pear-shaped uterus is a hollow thick-walled muscular organ in the midregion of the pelvis. Here the fertilized ovum undergoes its development into a new individual. The uppermost part is the fundus of the uterus, the main part the corpus or body, and the lowermost part (one third of the total organ) a prolongation into the upper vagina, the neck or cervix.

The passageway of the cervix extends through the endocervix and opens onto the vaginal portion or ectocervix. The lining of the ectocervix is squamous epithelium (pavement, nonsecretory type epithelium) unlike the lining of the endocervix and the endometrium of the uterus, which are glandular. There are also differences in function and reaction to disease between the endometrial lining of the uterus and the epithelial linings of the endocervix and ectocervix.

### HEMORRHAGE

Increased menstrual bleeding is known as *menorrhagia,* and uterine hemorrhage not related to menstruation is *metrorrhagia* or intermenstrual bleeding. Either form of hemorrhage accompanies certain generalized diseases or localized disorders of the reproductive organs. The systemic diseases include bleeding diseases, certain anemias, leukemia, cirrhosis of the liver, nephritis, and syphilis. Localized lesions include those produced by trauma, inflammation, complications of pregnancy, and tumors. Uterine bleeding may also occur as a result of ovarian dysfunction or an imbalance of ovarian hormones, in which instance it is referred to as *functional* bleeding.

The most important lesions responsible for uterine hemorrhage are benign and malignant neoplasms that occur in the reproductive organs. Any woman with unexplained uterine bleeding should be carefully examined for cancer, especially if the bleeding begins after menopause. *Postmenopausal bleeding* should be assumed to be caused by cancer until proved otherwise. Rarely, a girl will menstruate long before the age of puberty. This is known as *precocious menstruation*. Postpartum hemorrhage, occurring after detachment of the placenta at childbirth, should cease when the uterus contracts; it can continue indefinitely if the uterus does not contract properly or if a portion of the placenta fails to be expelled.

### INFLAMMATION

**Acute endometritis and endocervicitis.** Acute inflammation of the endometrium follows childbirth or attempts at abortion and is usually caused by streptococci of the hemolytic type.

In gonorrheal infections the cervix and endocervix are chiefly involved. The inflammation begins as a catarrhal process and progresses to suppuration, with the production of a large amount of greenish yellow pus. Acute gonorrheal cervicitis and endocervicitis often become chronic.

**Chronic endometritis and endocervicitis.** Chronic endometritis may result from retained placental tissue. Unrelated to a pregnancy, it is rare because such an inflammatory process is nearly always eliminated by the regular monthly desquamation of the endometrium. Chronic cervicitis and endocervicitis may be continuations of the acute form, or they may arise without previous acute attack. Gonococcal inflammation may be very resistant to treatment, the cervix remaining infected long after the disease has been eradicated elsewhere. The exposed position of the cervix and the frequency with which it is lacerated during childbirth make it a frequent site of chronic nonspecific inflammation.

Frequently the mouths of the inflamed endocervical glands become blocked. Accumulation of secretion and cystic distention results in *nabothian (retention) cysts*.

### NEOPLASM

**Leiomyomas.** Uterine leiomyomas, spoken of as fibroids, are benign tumors made up of bundles of smooth muscle fibers separated by varying proportions of connective tissue. They may occur beneath the endometrium (submucosal leiomyomas), in the uterine wall (interstitial or intramural leiomyomas), or projecting from the outer surface of the uterus (subserosal leiomyomas). In their beginning, submucosal and subserosal leiomyomas occupy an intra-

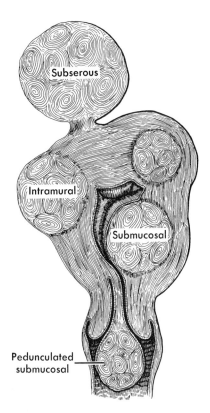

**Fig. 55-4.** Leiomyomas of uterus. Uterus sectioned to show placement and swirling pattern of well-defined tumors.

mural position. Uterine leiomyomas are among the most common of all tumors. They occur between the ages of puberty and menopause and are more common in women who have not had children. They seldom arise in the cervix. (See Fig. 55-4.)

Leiomyomas of the uterus are sharply encapsulated. If they have not undergone degenerative changes, they are white and glistening in appearance. Those containing a large amount of connective tissue are extremely hard. Benign in the pathologic sense, they may cause marked deformity of the uterus, give rise to pressure symptoms (constipation and malposition of the uterus), interfere with conception, produce abortion, obstruct labor, and cause extensive bleeding.

Submucosal fibroids can cause almost continuous bleeding from the endometrium and in some cases may produce an increase in size of the uterus that is easily mistaken for pregnancy. Subserosal fibroids are usually multiple and may be enormous. They may project from the uterus as knob-like processes or be attached to it by a distinct pedicle. They cause marked deformity and displacement of the uterus but ordinarily do not interfere with menstruation and conception.

Leiomyomas undergo atrophy or hyaline degeneration, and portions become liquefied, producing cysts. Calcification and sarcomatous degeneration sometimes occur. Leiomyomas sometimes undergo a rapid necrosis, the onset of which is announced by sudden pain and tenderness, and on section the tumor has the appearance of a beefsteak. This is known as *red degeneration*. Sometimes a tumor will grow rapidly during pregnancy. After childbirth the leiomyoma may remain large or return to its former size.

**Polyps.** Based more on shape than microscopic structure, the term *polyp* is applied to a heterogeneous group of benign growths. Included under this term are pedunculated leiomyomas, polyploid masses of endometrium, and papillomas of the endometrium and cervix. Polyps are especially important as a cause of abnormal bleeding.

**Hydatidiform mole.** A hydatidiform mole (Fig. 55-5) is a characteristic cluster of vesicular grape-like masses that was once presumably a normal placenta but is not associated with a living fetus. A mole has pathologic features of a degenerative process in the placenta because of the cystic change which the chorionic villi undergo, but because of proliferative changes displayed by the chorionic epithelium, it must be regarded as a true neoplasm.

**Carcinoma of the cervix.** On a worldwide basis carcinoma of the cervix is the commonest site of cancer in women. In the United States, as a result of

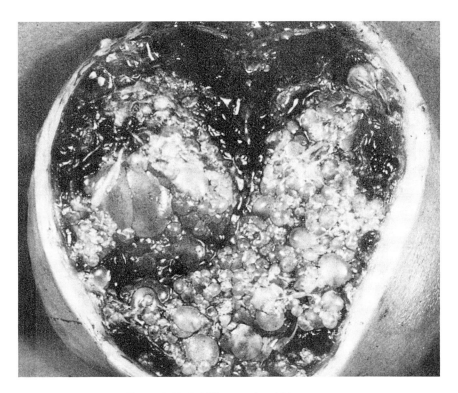

**Fig. 55-5.** Hydatidiform mole within uterus.

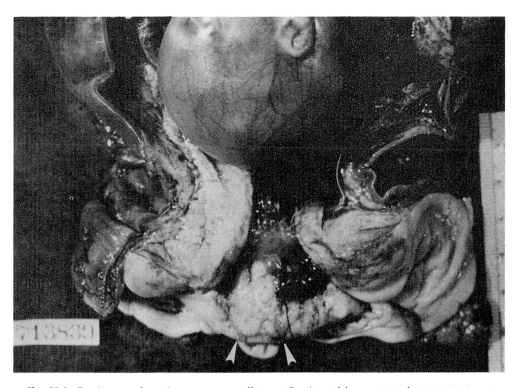

**Fig. 55-6.** Carcinoma of cervix, squamous cell type. Cervix and lower part of pregnant uterus opened to show whitish, cauliflower-like growth (arrows) at cervical os and extending up into endocervix.

613

cytologic screening of large segments of the population, the incidence has been reduced to a third of that in the prescreening era.

Fully 95% of cases of cancer of the cervix arise in women who have had children, and the disease traditionally occurs in women in their mid-forties.

Carcinoma of the cervix is usually of the squamous cell type and occurs grossly as (1) an induration of the cervix, (2) an ulceration, or (3) a cauliflower growth protruding from the cervix (Fig. 55-6). Carcinoma of the cervix grows more rapidly than carcinoma of the body of the uterus, and growth is more rapid in comparatively young women than in older women. It often begins on the surface of the cervix but invades the deeper tissues, after which the cervix becomes converted into a funnel-shaped ulcer with its apex pointing toward the body of the uterus.

The first sign of carcinoma of the cervix is either a watery, blood-tinged discharge or contact bleeding. Unfortunately when such signs appear, ulceration has already occurred. As the disease progresses, bleeding increases and the discharge becomes fetid. Extension to the bladder, rectum, vagina, and pelvic lymph nodes draining the cervix occurs early, and secondary bacterial infection of the carcinomatous mass is common. The presence of pain means that the carcinoma has already spread beyond the confines of the cervix. Secondary growths in the lungs and liver may occur. Death ordinarily takes place within 12 to 18 months after the carcinoma is recognized, unless proper treatment is instituted. It is often caused by disease of the kidneys, produced when the cancerous growth encircles and obstructs the ureters in their course through the pelvis. Profuse, even exsanguinating, hemorrhage is a common complication.

*Carcinoma in situ.* Although it does occur in the skin and elsewhere in the body, carcinoma in situ (intraepithelial carcinoma) is especially important in the cervix. It might be considered the pathologic prologue to the story of cancer, for it is a lesion that represents all the changes in cells that fix their malignant destiny short of all-out invasion. In the cervix it is the early and *confined* manifestation of carcinoma. In fact, the cervix may appear normal grossly; yet microscopically it will show a malignant transformation of its lining squamous epithelium, which for a time is held back by natural tissue barriers. At this stage, the disease is easily treated and readily cured.

The safeguard against cancer of the cervix uteri is the periodic pelvic examination, including cytologic study of the Pap smear taken of the cervix. This is important in all women, particularly in women who have had children. With universal screening of women, this cancer could virtually be eliminated.

**Carcinoma of the body of the uterus** (Fig. 55-7). Carcinoma of the body of the uterus forms approximately 10% of the uterine carcinomas. It occurs about 10 years later in life than carcinoma of the cervix, often after the menopause. At this time any bleeding from the uterus is abnormal, and because this neoplasm is associated with abnormal bleeding from the first, it is usually recognized earlier than is carcinoma of the cervix.

Carcinoma of the corpus uteri usually begins in the fundus and grows into the cavity of the uterus as a soft cauliflower mass that fills the entire cavity. It then invades the wall of the uterus, which it may penetrate and thus spread to the peritoneum. When metastasis occurs, it is to the pelvic lymph nodes and the ovaries. In structure, carcinoma of the

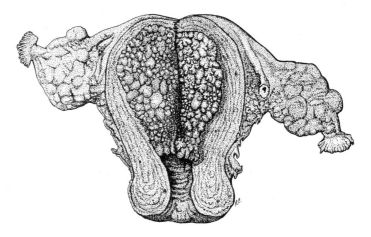

**Fig. 55-7.** Carcinoma of body of uterus in cross section.

body of the uterus is an adenocarcinoma. Carcinoma of the body of the uterus grows more slowly than does carcinoma of the cervix and has much less tendency to ulcerate and invade the surrounding organs. This, with its earlier recognition, makes it a much less formidable disease than carcinoma of the cervix.

**Chorionepithelioma.** The malignant counterpart to hydatidiform mole, chorionepithelioma (choriocarcinoma) is a peculiar tumor that arises from the covering cells of the chorionic villi of the placenta and occurs at the placental site in the uterus. It not only may occur after the expulsion of a hydatidiform mole, which is considered in itself a benign tumor, but may also occur after an abortion, after a normal delivery, or even during pregnancy. Chorionepithelioma is a soft mass, somewhat resembling placental tissue, that infiltrates the uterine wall and projects into the uterine cavity. In most cases growth is rapid and metastasis to the pelvic organs and lungs comes early. Abnormal bleeding or severe hemorrhage often leads to a diagnosis.

## Exfoliative cytology

**Pap (Papanicolaou) smear.** We have continuously emphasized the fact that changes associated with disease take place in the cell. Exfoliative cytology has applied this fact to the identification of malignant tumor cells that have an appearance microscopically quite different from that of normal cells. Malignant tumor cells lend themselves well to a smear technic, for they do not stick to each other as do normal cells but tend to separate, and if the tumor is located on a mucosal surface, they tend to be desquamated therefrom, usually into a lumen to be admixed with whatever fluid is normally present. It is then possible to take some of this fluid containing desquamated cells, smear it on a slide, fix it in 95% alcohol (immediately), stain it, and examine the cells under the microscope. If the body surface is accessible, greater numbers of cells may be obtained by a gentle scraping of the area with a flat wooden tongue blade.

The *cytologic smear test* is used to study desquamated cells from the uterus and cervix, but exfoliated cells from other body areas may also be studied in this way: those in sputum and bronchial secretions from the respiratory tract, urine from the urinary tract, stomach secretions and other fluids from the alimentary tract, and secretions from the breast. George Papanicolaou (1883-1962) was the first to call attention to the fact that malignancies of the uterus and cervix could be accurately diagnosed by microscopic examination of desquamated cells in vaginal secretions. He also devised the special staining technic for cytologic smears. As a result of his work in

the field of exfoliative cytology these smear preparations are universally referred to as Pap smears.

The advantages of the Pap smear are several. To obtain the specimen usually entails very little if any inconvenience; there is no surgery or anesthesia. Secretions may contain cells from the entire exposed surface and therefore sample a wider area than would a random tissue biopsy. It must be emphasized, however, that the smear does not replace the very important tissue biopsy but is a valuable preliminary step. The final and ultimate diagnosis of a malignant neoplasm is made only after suitably taken tissue has been subjected to microscopic examination. The cytologic smear test has its greatest usefulness in the detection of very early cancers, especially of the cervix of the uterus. In many cases carcinomas in situ and very early carcinomas of the cervix have been found by smears before the growth could be detected by clinical inspection. Cervical smears taken successively are used as follow-up measures when a carcinoma of the cervix has been treated by irradiation; the earliest recurrence of the growth may be first detected in the smear.

Cytologic smears are studied by either a pathologist or by a *cytotechnologist,* a person specially trained in the microscopic study of cells and working under the supervision of a pathologist.

## Pregnancy tests

**Biologic tests.** During pregnancy the placenta elaborates hormones that are like certain hormones produced by the anterior lobe of the pituitary gland, and these chorionic gonadotropic hormones are found in large amounts in the blood and urine of a pregnant woman. If pregnant urine is injected into the body of a sexually immature female animal, the gonadotropic hormones act on the graafian follicles of the ovary to induce maturation. This phenomenon is the basis of the highly reliable *Aschheim-Zondek* and *Friedman* tests for pregnancy. In the former the white mouse is used as the test animal, and in the latter the rabbit is used. Recently developed tests use the family of frogs and toads, both males and females. It is a peculiar fact that the mature South African clawed toad carries eggs throughout the year but extrudes them only after mating or when injected with these chorionic gonadotropic hormones. Chorionic gonadotropins injected into a male frog cause the detachment and excretion of spermatozoa contained in the tubules of the testis.

**Immunologic tests.** A number of immunologic tests have been devised, most being a modification of the basic principle that human chorionic gonadotropin as antigen is neutralized by antihuman chorionic gonadotropin. The reaction can be measured in several ways. In one test the end point is agglutination inhibition. Latex particles are coated with human chorionic gonadotropin. Under the conditions of the test, if these particles are not clumped, the test is positive. This means that the chorionic gonadotropin in the test urine was neutralized by the antiserum with no antibody left over to react with the sensitized latex particles. If the reverse of this situation occurs, antibody, not being utilized in the test urine, is available to clump the latex—a negative test. Immunologic tests are more rapid and technically sidestep certain aspects of animal maintenance and testing; they also give reliable results that correlate well with those of the biologic procedures.

**Importance.** Chorionic gonadotropic hormones are secreted normally with a pregnancy and abnormally in the presence of a hydatidiform mole. They may also be secreted abnormally with a chorionepithelioma in the female and with a malignant neoplasm of the testis in the male. Therefore the pregnancy tests are positive and especially useful in evaluating these conditions. They are also important in the study of menstrual irregularities that are common with gynecologic disease and in the diagnosis of ectopic pregnancy, in which early surgery may be lifesaving.

## Vagina

The vagina is the flattened musculomembranous passage from cervix to vulva.

### INFLAMMATION

**Acute catarrhal vaginitis.** Acute catarrhal vaginitis may be caused by gonococcal infections, mechanical or chemical irritations, and highly irritating uterine discharges. Primary gonococcal vulvovaginitis is common in children, but the gonococcal vaginitis of adults is usually secondary to gonococcal urethritis or cervicitis, and even when both of these are present, the adult vagina may show little involvement.

**Trichomonal vaginitis.** In certain intractable cases of vaginitis with a copious, cream-colored, foamy discharge, the organism *Trichomonas vaginalis* is found in abundance.

**Monilial vaginitis.** Vaginitis caused by *Candida (Monilia) albicans* is frequent in diabetes and pregnancy.

## Breasts

The breasts are accessory organs of the female reproductive system. Covered with skin and placed on the front of the chest, each of the two mammary glands is a conical mass of glandular tissue traversed and supported by bands of fibrous tissue and much fat. Only at the end of pregnancy do they reach their full development for physiologic function during the period of lactation.

### CONGENITAL ABNORMALITIES

Abnormalities of the breasts are discussed on p. 444.

### INFLAMMATION

**Acute mastitis.** Inflammation of the breast is known as *mastitis*. Acute mastitis may occur in the form of an abscess or less commonly as a diffuse process. Abscesses are caused by staphylococci, whereas diffuse inflammation is usually caused by streptococci. Fully 90% of the cases of acute mastitis occur during the first few weeks of lactation; the causative bacteria gain access to the breast through fissures in the nipple. When an abscess forms, only one may be present, or there may be several that are discrete or communicating.

Occurring less often are mastitis of the newborn and the hematogenous mastitis complicating typhoid fever, scarlet fever, and mumps. Expression of the secretion of the breast of newborn infants, at one time a practice of midwives, often led to acute purulent mastitis. Breast abscess in newborn infants is seen today as an important manifestation of disease resulting from antibiotic-resistant staphylococci.

**Fibrocystic disease of the breast.** Ovarian hormones are known to influence breast tissue to proliferate or to involute in a somewhat cyclic manner. Fibrocystic disease of the breast designates a group of related conditions that basically represent a perversion of these hormonal effects on breast tissue because of an imbalance of the ovarian hormones. Because the nature of these disturbances in breast tissue was poorly understood by the early observers, the term *chronic cystic mastitis* was one of the first used, and it has persisted. The designation *mastitis*, however, is a misnomer, since this group of disorders in the breast is not inflammatory in origin; nor is it considered neoplastic. Other terms that have been applied reflect the varied manifestations of the disease: mammary dysplasia, cystic disease of the breast, mazoplasia, Schimmelbusch's disease, and cystiphorous desquamative epithelial hyperplasia of Cheatle and Cutler. (True chronic mastitis, meaning chronic inflammation of the breast, is quite rare and usually is seen as tuberculosis or fungous disease.)

Fibrocystic disease begins near the time of menopause, and the patient may complain of a lump or pain in the breast that is slightly worse at menstruation. More than one lump may be present, and both breasts may be involved. The breast has a granular, indurated feel, and when it is incised, a great increase in connective tissue with cysts of varying size is found. The larger cysts have papillomatous processes growing from their walls. Most authorities insist that fibrocystic disease is so frequently a forerunner of carcinoma of the breast that it should be considered precancerous.

## DISCHARGES FROM THE NIPPLE

Almost half the bloody discharges from the nipple are caused by carcinoma. The remainder result from trauma, benign tumors, and cysts associated with chronic cystic mastitis. A chocolate discharge may occur in chronic cystic mastitis, and a purulent discharge occurs when an abscess breaks into a milk duct.

## TUMORS

**Cysts.** Cysts of the breast are caused by retention of secretions, inflammation, tumor growths, or abnormal involution. Encapsulation of abscesses or hemorrhages may lead to the formation of pseudo-

cysts. Obstruction of a milk duct leads to the formation of a cyst filled with a liquid resembling milk, known as a *galactocele*. Cyst formation is an important feature of fibrocystic disease wherein multiple cysts of all sizes are prominent in the breast.

**Fibroadenoma.** Fibroadenoma is the most common benign tumor of the breast. It occurs as a freely movable, circumscribed, well-encapsulated mass of glandular and connective tissue, growing slowly and giving rise to few symptoms, often being discovered only by accident. Fibroadenomas seldom exceed a size greater than 3 cm. in diameter and rarely become cancerous.

**Carcinoma.** Carcinoma of the breast is one of the most frequent forms of malignant neoplasm as well as one of the commonest in women. (In the United States it is the number one cancer, but over the

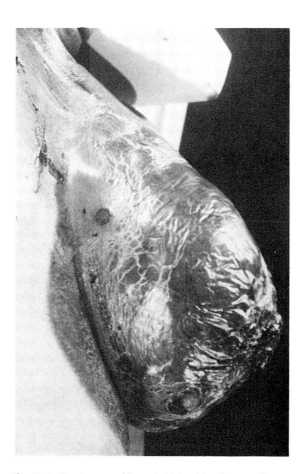

**Fig. 55-8.** Carcinoma of breast. Note skin changes ("peau d'orange").

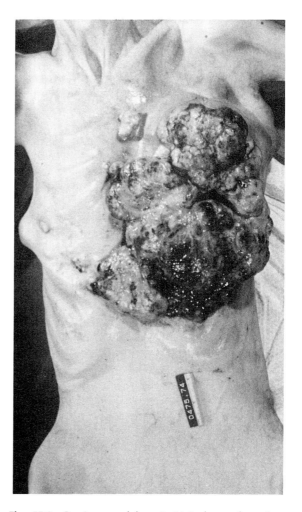

**Fig. 55-9.** Carcinoma of breast. Note large, fungating, ulcerated growth over chest wall of emaciated woman.

world, cancer of the cervix uteri is said to be.) When recognized late and improperly treated, it is rapidly fatal. The fact that 85% of women who receive early treatment for cancer of the breast are alive at the end of 5 years whereas only 4% of those who are treated late are alive at that time is proof of the importance of early diagnosis and treatment. Carcinoma of the breast occurs after the age of 30 years and is present with increasing frequency through the successive decades of life. Female relatives of breast cancer patients are at a 2 to 3 times greater risk. The first sign of cancer is usually a painless lump, often found by accident. In a few cases the first sign is bleeding from the nipple.

The theory that a virus is in some way directly implicated in the causation of breast cancer is getting stronger. A type-B RNA particle is suspect and has been found in the milk of women with breast cancer. Hormones are also implicated.

Carcinoma of the breast (Figs. 55-8 and 55-9) infiltrates the surrounding breast tissue, overlying skin, and underlying muscles. Involvement of the skin leads to ulceration, and involvement of the underlying muscles anchors the tumor to the chest wall. Carcinoma spreads early into blood vessels and lymphatics, which are plentiful in the breast. Metastases occur to the axillary, supraclavicular, and mediastinal lymph nodes. When the lymph nodes become involved, it is only a short time until secondary growths occur in distant points such as lungs, liver, and bones. Carcinomas of the medial portion of the breast are more dangerous than those in the outer part of the breast because they metastasize directly to the mediastinal lymph nodes and to the internal organs.

Nearly all carcinomas of the breast originate in the cells that line the duct system of the breast and are therefore termed *duct cell* carcinomas. There are three commonly occurring forms: (1) scirrhous, so

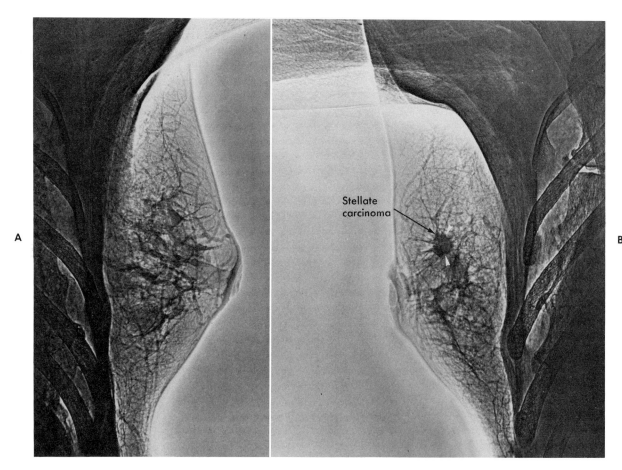

Stellate carcinoma

A

B

**Fig. 55-10.** Xeroradiographic technic for mass screening. **A,** Xeroradiograph of normal breast. **B,** Xeroradiograph showing breast cancer. Note stellate mass in upper part of breast (arrow) and nipple retraction. (Xeroradiographs supplied by Xerox Corp., Xeroradiography, Pasadena, Calif.)

called because of the firm gritty consistency of the gross tumor, (2) medullary (encephaloid), a grossly soft and cellular tumor, so called because of its resemblance to brain tissue, and (3) papillary cystadenocarcinoma, a tumor arising as a papillary growth projecting from the lining of a duct or a cyst within the breast. Two or even all of these forms may be found in a single tumor. In addition, Paget's disease of the nipple is frequent enough to be clinically important.

*Scirrhous* carcinoma, the most common form of breast carcinoma, begins as a hard, fixed, poorly circumscribed nodule, usually in the upper, outer quadrant. It extends and infiltrates irregularly and involves the underlying muscles and overlying skin. Involvement of the large milk ducts leads to retraction of the nipple. Involvement of the axillary and supraclavicular lymph nodes occurs in late cases. The tumor grows rather slowly, and the breast becomes small, hard, and flattened. When sectioned, the white, glistening cancerous area cuts with gritty resistance. There are poorly defined extensions into the surrounding tissue. Microscopically, scirrhous carcinoma of the breast is characterized by the presence of few carcinoma cells and a superabundance of connective tissue. The overgrowth of connective tissue gives the tumor its characteristic gross consistency.

*Medullary (encephaloid)* or soft carcinoma of the breast grows rapidly, quickly invades the skin, ulcerates, and appears externally as a fungating mass. Lymph node involvement occurs early. Microscopically, medullary carcinoma is characterized by the presence of wide strands of rapidly growing carcinoma cells and a small amount of connective tissue. This tumor quickly kills. An acute inflammatory form of medullary carcinoma of the breast sometimes develops during lactation.

*Papillary cystadenocarcinomas* are commonly associated with discharge from the nipple, usually bloody.

*Paget's disease of the nipple* begins as a red, unruly eczematous condition of the nipple. It is followed by carcinoma of the breast, often at a distance from the nipple. The relation of carcinoma to irritation produced by the eczema is controversial.

**Early detection.** Regular breast self-examination as promoted by the American Cancer Society is important. Some 95% of women discover the lump in the breast themselves. However, by the time a cancerous lump is palpable, in around 60% of women the cancer has already spread to the regional lymph nodes, thus defining a stage in which the 5-year survival rate is only 40% to 45%. (Fortunately, in many instances the lump in the breast is not malignant, but it should always be evaluated by the physician.)

The detection of the very early, occult lesion is the prime goal of mass screening projects, which are appearing over this country. Three diagnostic procedures generally considered more sensitive than palpation are used. (1) Thermography is a technic based on the determination of infrared emissions from the surface of the breast. Cancer may produce a focal increase in such emissions. (2) Mammography is a safe, simple technic for soft tissue radiography. (3) Xeroradiography, another method of soft tissue radiography, gives excellent contrast between fat and soft tissues (Fig. 55-10).

## Questions for review

1 Name three benign ovarian cysts.
2 Explain the formation of a pyosalpinx.
3 What is the pathogenesis of an ectopic pregnancy?
4 What are fibroids? Name three varieties.
5 What are the early signs of carcinoma of the cervix?
6 Give important causes for uterine bleeding.
7 Differentiate carcinoma of the body of the uterus from that of the cervix.
8 Briefly discuss chorionepithelioma, hydatidiform mole.
9 Discuss the prevalence and importance of carcinoma of the breast.
10 What is the Pap smear?
11 List the areas of the body in which the cytologic smear technic may be of value.
12 Name two reliable tests for pregnancy.
13 What is the clinical importance of carcinoma in situ?
14 Give the pathologic features of carcinoma of the breast.

**REFERENCES** (Chapters 52 to 55)

Ackerman, L. V., and Rosai, J.: Surgical pathology, ed. 5, St. Louis, 1974, The C. V. Mosby Co.
Anderson, W. A. D., and Scotti, T. M.: Synopsis of pathology, ed. 8, St. Louis, 1974, The C. V. Mosby Co.
Barber, H. R. K., and others: Cancer of endometrium, Tex. Med. **70:**41, July, 1974.
Beacham, D. W., and Beacham, W. D.: Synopsis of gynecology, ed. 8, St. Louis, 1972, The C. V. Mosby Co.
Bell, J. L.: Immunologic tests for pregnancy, Lab. Med. **1:**45, July, 1970.
Block, L. H., and Lamy, P. P.: These drugs discolor the feces or urine, Resident Staff Physician **15:**47, Feb., 1969.
Bloodworth, J. M. B.: The pathology of diabetes mellitus, Lab. Med. **1:**33, July, 1970.
Blythe, W. B.: Hemodialysis—in lieu of the artificial kidney, Lab. Med. **1:**29, Oct., 1970.
Brandt, N.: Your son has diabetes, Today's Health **51:**35, June, 1973.
Breast cancer: fear and facts, Time, Nov. 4, p. 107, 1974.
Brodie, B., and von Haam, J.: Children born with adrenogenital syndrome, Am. J. Nurs. **67:**1018, 1967.

Bugg, R.: Your body's silent partners, Today's Health **47:** 54, Jan., 1969.

Burton, B. T.: Artificial kidneys: where we stand, Today's Health **45:**26, July, 1967.

Burton, B. T.: Whither dialysis and renal transplantation? J.A.M.A. **230:**1403, 1974.

Catt, K. J.: An ABC of endocrinology, Boston, 1972, Little, Brown & Co.

Davidson, E. H.: Hormones and genes, Sci. Am. **212:**36, June, 1965.

Dunea, G., and Freedman, P.: Proteinuria, J.A.M.A. **203:** 973, 1968.

Early detection of breast cancer with mammography, RN **37:**36, Dec., 1974.

Egan, R. L.: Mammography, Am. J. Nurs. **66:**108, 1966.

Fusaro, R. M., and Goetz, F. C.: Common cutaneous manifestations and problems of diabetes mellitus, Postgrad. Med. **49:**84, June, 1971.

Gardner, H. L., and Kaufman, R. H.: Benign diseases of the vulva and vagina, St. Louis, 1969, The C. V. Mosby Co.

Germuth, F. G., Jr., and Rodriguez, E.: Immunopathology of the renal glomerulus; immune complex deposit and antibasement membrane disease, Boston, 1973, Little, Brown & Co.

Gharib, H.: Triiodothyronine, J.A.M.A. **227:**302, 1974.

Gordan, G. S., and Roof, B. S.: Laboratory tests for hyperparathyroidism, J.A.M.A. **206:**2729, 1968.

Heptinstall, R. H., with contributions from J. M. Kissane, R. T. McCluskey, and K. A. Porter: Pathology of kidney, ed. 2, Boston, 1974, Little, Brown & Co.

Horwitz, C. A., and others: A comparative study of five immunologic pregnancy tests: an analysis of 1,863 cases, Am. J. Clin. Pathol. **58:**305, 1972.

Jay, A. N.: Hypoglycemia . . . symptoms—diagnosis—treatment, Am. J. Nurs. **62:**77, 1962.

Kashgarian, M., and Burrow, G. N.: The endocrine glands, Baltimore, 1974, The Williams & Wilkins Co.

Kaufman, S. A.: From a gynecologist's notebook: questions women ask, New York, 1974, Stein & Day, Publishers.

Kincaid-Smith, P., and others, editors: Glomerulonephritis: morphology, natural history, and treatment, New York, 1973, John Wiley & Sons, Inc.

Kissane, J. M., editor: Pathology of infancy and childhood, ed. 2, St. Louis, 1975, The C. V. Mosby Co.

Kraus, F. T.: Gynecologic pathology, St. Louis, 1967, The C. V. Mosby Co.

Lamont-Havers, R. W.: Surprising findings about diabetes, Today's Health **46:**66, April, 1968.

Lancaster, R. G., and Marsh, H. H.: Urinalyses can be interesting, Med. Lab. Observer **3:**35, March-April, 1971.

Landau, R. L.: Tests of testicular function, J.A.M.A. **207:** 353, 1969.

Levine, R.: Hypoglycemia, J.A.M.A. **230:**462, 1974.

Lippman, R. W.: Urine and the urinary sediments: a practical manual and atlas, ed. 2, Springfield, Ill., 1973, Charles C Thomas, Publisher.

McLennan, C. E., and Sandberg, E. C.: Synopsis of obstetrics, ed. 9, St. Louis, 1974, The C. V. Mosby Co.

Miller, J. E., and others: Mammography, Dallas Med. J. **60:**478, 1974.

Muehrcke, R. C.: Acute renal failure—diagnosis and management, St. Louis, 1969, The C. V. Mosby Co.

Nelson, J. H., Jr., and Hall, J. E.: Detection, diagnostic evaluation, and treatment of dysplasia and early carcinoma of cervix, CA **20:**150, 1970.

Nordyke, R. A.: The overactive and the underactive thyroid, Am. J. Nurs. **63:**66, May, 1963.

Novak, E. R.: Ovarian tumors, Hosp. Med. **7:**60, March, 1971.

Novak, E. R., and Woodruff, J. D.: Novak's gynecologic and obstetric pathology, ed. 7, Philadelphia, 1974, W. B. Saunders Co.

Potter, E. L.: Malformations of the kidney, Wom. Physician **25:**357, 1970.

Potter, E. L.: Normal and abnormal development of the kidney, Chicago, 1974, Year Book Medical Publishers, Inc.

Prien, E. L., Sr.: The riddle of urinary stone disease, J.A.M.A. **216:**503, 1971.

Prout, G. R., Jr.: Chemical tests in the diagnosis of prostatic carcinoma, J.A.M.A. **209:**1699, 1969.

Ratliff, J. D.: I am Joe's hypothalamus, Reader's Digest **96:**124, March, 1970.

Ross, W. L.: Breast cancer: past, present, and future, South. Med. Bull. **59:**7, Feb., 1971.

Rubin, P.: Cancer of the urogenital tract: Wilms' tumor and neuroblastoma, J.A.M.A. **204:**981, 1968.

Sanford, J. P.: Management of urinary tract infections, Resident Staff Physician **15:**70, Jan., 1969.

Scott, R., Jr.: Needle biopsy in carcinoma of the prostate, J.A.M.A. **201:**958, 1967.

Schanche, D. A.: Medical help for children who grow too little, Today's Health **53:**16, March, 1975.

Strax, P.: Early detection: breast cancer is curable, New York, 1974, Harper & Row, Publishers.

Sutherland, E. W.: Studies on the mechanism of hormone action, Science **177:**401, 1972.

The thyroid: your energy gland, Today's Health **45:**14, April, 1967.

Wakeley, C.: Tumours occurring in the male breast, Nurs. Mirror **137:**26, Aug. 17, 1973.

Weindling, H., and Henry, J. B.: Laboratory test results altered by "The Pill," J.A.M.A. **229:**1762, 1974.

William, D. G.: Glomerulonephritis, Nurs. Mirror **138:**50, June 14, 1974.

Williams, H. T. G., and others: Gangrene of the feet in diabetics, Arch. Surg. **108:**609, 1974.

Winter, C. C.: Practical urology, St. Louis, 1969, The C. V. Mosby Co.

Yolles, S. F.: The mystery gland, Today's Health **44:**76, March, 1966.

# CHAPTER 56
# Diseases of
# Central nervous system

The central nervous system comprises the brain and spinal cord. Here impulses from over the body are integrated with impulses originating from environmental stimuli. It is a central clearinghouse presiding over the biologic activities of the individual.

## Meninges

The brain and spinal cord are covered by three membranes or meninges. The dura mater is a dense and fibrous membrane. The arachnoid mater is a thin, transparent one. The pia mater is a delicate and vascular membrane. The cerebrospinal fluid circulates in the subarachnoid space existing between the arachnoid and pia mater.

### HEMORRHAGE

Hemorrhage may be extradural (between the dura and bone), subdural (between the dura and arachnoid, that is, in the subdural space), or subarachnoid (between the pia and arachnoid membranes in the subarachnoid space).

*Extradural* hemorrhages are caused by direct or indirect injuries that separate the dura from the bone and rupture blood vessels. Unrelieved, severe extradural hemorrhages cause death.

*Subdural* hemorrhage (Fig. 56-1) is usually caused by mechanical blows with or without fracture of the skull and is the most common type of traumatic intracranial hemorrhage. The hemorrhage comes from the large venous sinuses, the large arteries, or the cerebral veins. Bleeding is much more rapid in subdural than in extradural hemorrhage, and in severe cases death is quick.

*Subarachnoid* hemorrhages (Fig. 56-2) are the result of laceration of the brain (traumatic) or rupture of a malformed or diseased blood vessel in the subarachnoid space (spontaneous).

## INFLAMMATION

**Meningitis.** The formation of pus accompanies *purulent* meningitis. (See Fig. 56-3.) In this disease the blood shows a marked increase in polymorphonuclear neutrophilic leukocytes, and lumbar punc-

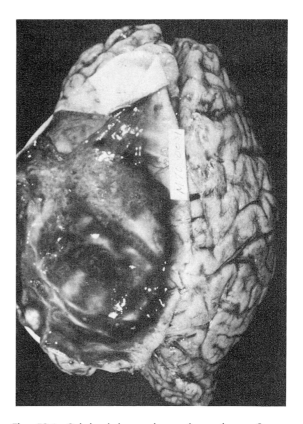

**Fig. 56-1.** Subdural hemorrhage, from above. Space-occupying mass of blood impinging on left cerebral hemisphere.

621

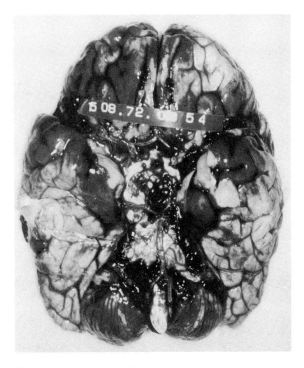

**Fig. 56-2.** Subarachnoid hemorrhage from undersurface of brain. Diffuse distribution of blood with some accumulation about brainstem.

ture reveals turbid or frankly purulent cerebrospinal fluid. The causative microbes are demonstrated in smear and culture. Organisms producing purulent meningitis are meningococci, pneumococci, influenza bacilli, staphylococci, streptococci, colon bacilli, and typhoid bacilli. Of these, meningococci, pneumococci, and influenza bacilli are the most important. (See Table 56-1.) Meningococci are responsible for the epidemic form of meningitis. *Nonepidemic* meningitis is produced by the other organisms.

Bacteria reach the meninges in several ways; the most important are (1) by the bloodstream, (2) by penetrating wounds, (3) by passage from the nasopharyngeal mucosa through the lymph spaces, and (4) by extension of regional infections from the middle ear, mastoid process, bony sinuses, or cranial bones. Purulent meningitis is a frequent complication of cavernous sinus thrombosis.

*Pneumococcal* meningitis may result from the extension of a pneumococcal infection of the middle ear or mastoid process, or it may complicate lobar pneumonia. *Streptococcal* meningitis may be a complication of such systemic diseases as measles, endocarditis, septicemia, or facial erysipelas, or it may be caused by the extension of a neighboring infection. Meningitis resulting from *Salmonella typhi* occurs as a rare complication of typhoid fever.

*Tuberculous* meningitis is a well-marked acute allergic inflammation of the meninges associated

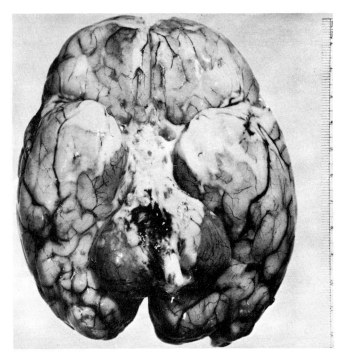

**Fig. 56-3.** Purulent meningitis. Shown is undersurface of brain. Note whitish areas like an icing irregularly spread out on it. This is appearance of characteristic fibrinopurulent exudate. (From Anderson, W. A. D., and Scotti, T. M.: Synopsis of pathology, ed. 8, St. Louis, 1972, The C. V. Mosby Co.)

with the formation of tubercles. It is usually a disease of childhood but may occur in adults. It may follow generalized miliary tuberculosis or result from bacilli brought to the meninges by the bloodstream from distant foci. Tubercle bacilli may extend directly to the meninges from adjacent tuberculous foci in the brain or the bones of the skull and spinal column.

As a rule, the tubercles are more numerous on the meninges covering the base of the brain, but the meninges of the entire brain may be involved, and tubercles may be found on the lining of the ventricles and within the substance of the brain. An accumula-

tion of excess fluid in the ventricles in tuberculous meningitis is so common that the disease has been called *acute hydrocephalus.*

Tuberculous meningitis differs from purulent meningitis in that it lasts longer and the cerebrospinal fluid is seldom frankly purulent. The disease was uniformly fatal until the advent of tuberculocidal drugs. Now some patients recover.

*Syphilitic* meningitis, more properly called *meningovascular syphilis,* is a syphilitic involvement of the meninges and vessels of the central nervous system, with or without involvement of the brain itself.

**Table 56-1**

Microbes related to meningitis

| | ORGANISM | COMMENT |
|---|---|---|
| A. Primary meningitis | | |
| 1. Common offenders | Neisseria meningitidis | Cause of epidemic cerebrospinal fever |
| | Haemophilus influenzae | Most frequent cause of meningitis in infants and children when meningococci not implicated |
| | Streptococcus pneumoniae | Common cause of endemic meningitis in adults, less so in children |
| 2. Less common offenders | Mycobacterium tuberculosis | Cause of purulent or nonpurulent meningitis— singly or in combination |
| | Other Neisseria species | |
| | Coliforms | |
| | Listeria monocytogenes | |
| | Streptococcus pyogenes | |
| | Klebsiella-Enterobacter-Serratia organisms | |
| | Salmonella species | |
| | Bacteroides species | |
| | Pseudomonas species | |
| | Proteus species | |
| | Nocardia asteroides | |
| | Escherichia coli | Cause of purulent meningitis in newborn infants |
| B. Secondary meningitis | | Organisms are introduced directly into meninges |
| 1. Common offenders | Staphylococcus aureus | because of recent trauma, surgical procedure, |
| | Pseudomonas species | lumbar puncture, or congenital malformation |
| | Escherichia coli and other coliforms | (example: spina bifida) |
| | Proteus species | |
| 2. Less common offenders | Any pathogenic microbe with capacity to invade human tissue | |
| C. Meningitis part of generalized infection | | |
| 1. Common offenders | Neisseria meningitidis | Part of fulminating meningococcal septicemia |
| | Streptococcus pneumoniae | |
| | Mycobacterium tuberculosis | Part of miliary tuberculosis |
| 2. Less common offenders | Neisseria gonorrhoeae | Almost any generalized infection with bacteremia may be associated with meningitis |
| | Salmonella typhi | |
| | Brucella species | |
| | Staphylococcus aureus | |
| | Bacillus anthracis | |
| | Nocardia asteroides | |
| | Cryptococcus neoformans (fungus) | |

It is the most common of the manifestations of neuro-syphilis.

Although not all patients with syphilis develop meningovascular involvement, many do, usually within the first 5 or 6 years after infection. It may develop as early as 2 months or as late as 40 years. The meninges are variably thickened. The vascular changes consist of fibrosis, thickening of the walls, and perivascular accumulation of chronic inflammatory cells. Thrombosis or vascular rupture leading to hemiplegia may occur.

## Brain

The brain is the expanded and intricately elaborate upper part of the cerebrospinal nervous axis. It almost completely fills the cranial cavity.

### INJURIES

**Cerebral concussion.** When a person receives an injury to the head, he may be groggy for a time and quickly recover, or he may sink into a state of unconsciousness with subnormal temperature and scarcely perceptible respiration and pulse. On rare occasions, he dies from respiratory failure. Widespread loss of cerebral control following injury without organic lesion (such as fracture of the skull, hemorrhage, or laceration of the brain) is known as cerebral concussion.

Various theories have been proposed to explain concussion of the brain. One is that concussion results from a molecular disturbance in the brain. Another is that it is caused by suddenly induced cerebral anemia. Still another is that the jar accompanying the injury drives the cerebrospinal fluid from the lateral and third ventricles into the fourth ventricle with such force that it paralyzes the cardiac and respiratory centers.

After concussion the patient may show signs of cerebral irritability for a long time (4 or 5 years in some cases). Damage incurred as a result of the concussion may be permanent. In most cases memory of the injury and the events immediately preceding it are completely wiped out.

**Compression.** Any condition that (1) reduces the capacity of the skull, (2) increases the volume of the brain, or (3) increases the amount of fluid in the cranial cavity raises intracranial pressure and compresses the brain. Among such are hemorrhage, inflammation, edema, tumors, and fractures with marked depression of the inner and outer bony tables of the skull. The most common cause is hemorrhage.

The rapidity with which symptoms develop depends on the rapidity with which the compression develops. In some cases it is a matter of seconds and in others a matter of months. The first clinical changes to develop are headache, projectile type vomiting (unrelated to the taking of food), drowsiness, slow pulse, high blood pressure, increased spinal fluid pressure, and choked disks. As the pressure increases, the patient convulses, becomes stuporous and comatose, develops Cheyne-Stokes respiration, and is incontinent of feces and urine. The deepening coma may end in death from respiratory failure.

### CIRCULATORY DISTURBANCES

**Hydrocephalus.** Situated on the walls of the lateral ventricles of the brain are tufts of delicate capillaries known as the choroid plexuses, through which the components of the cerebrospinal fluid are filtered from the plasma to the ventricles. Here cerebrospinal fluid is formed. From the ventricles the fluid flows through three small openings in the roof of the fourth ventricle to the subarachnoid space.

When the passage of fluid from the ventricles to the subarachnoid space is blocked, the ventricles become widely dilated, and the overlying brain tissue becomes reduced to a thin layer—the condition known as hydrocephalus (water on the brain). From the clinical standpoint, hydrocephalus is classified as congenital (occurring at birth or before bony union of the skull bones is complete) and acquired (occurring after the skull is completely ossified).

In congenital hydrocephalus the enlargement of the head may be so great during intrauterine life that normal birth is impossible. More often the head is a little larger than normal at birth but enlarges rapidly after birth, and the child dies weeks, months, or years later. (See Figs. 56-4 and 56-5.)

Acquired hydrocephalus is caused by an obstruction of the circulation of the cerebrospinal fluid by adhesions (especially those caused by septic or tuberculous meningitis) or by the growth of tumors. Since bony union of the skull bones is complete or nearly so before acquired hydrocephalus begins, the skull does not show the marked enlargement seen in the congenital form, and, of course, the ventricles are not so widely dilated, but the increase in intracranial pressure is equally terrific.

Extreme degrees of hydrocephalus are incompatible with life. In moderate degrees the patient may be able to lead a fairly active life, and sometimes the mentality remains unaffected. Frequently, mental deterioration is complete in the individual, whose intact vital centers in the brainstem allow only a continuing miserable and vegetative existence.

**Stroke.** *Stroke* (cerebrovascular accident, CVA) is an umbrella term used to indicate changes in the brain brought about by a local circulatory embarrassment of nontraumatic (spontaneous) character. Since

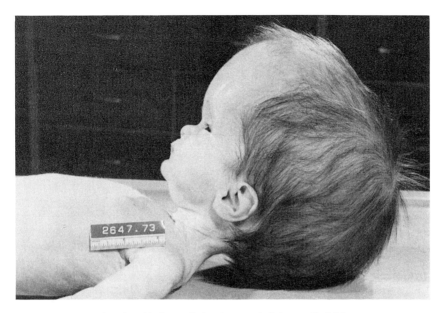

**Fig. 56-4.** Hydrocephalus (congenital) in small child.

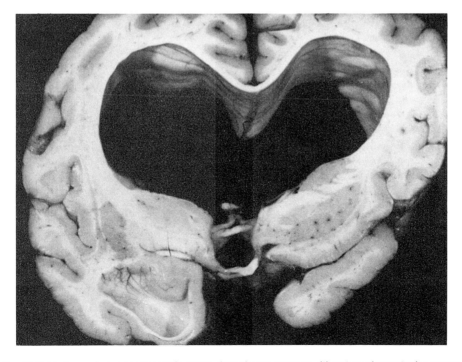

**Fig. 56-5.** Hydrocephalus (congenital). Brain slice shows extreme dilatation of ventricular system.

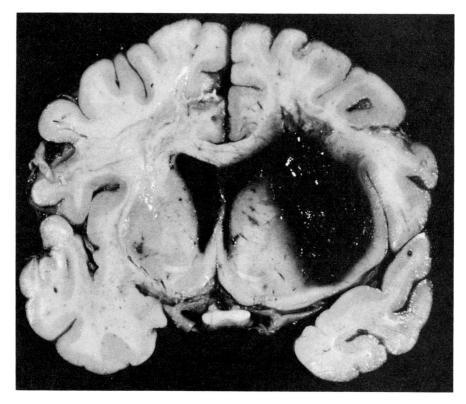

**Fig. 56-6.** Intracerebral hemorrhage, from patient with apoplexy. Note asymmetry of two sides of brain as seen in this slice. A large fresh hemorrhage (darkened area on right) has burst into ventricle.

the proportion of elderly persons in our population is growing larger, there is a renewed interest in the problems associated with stroke.

Pathologically strokes are related to three basic processes (with a few exceptions): (1) thrombosis, (2) hemorrhage, and (3) embolism.

The clinical features of stroke vary widely. The cerebrovascular accident may be precipitous, with the stricken patient deprived of all sense and motion. This is the familiar pattern and has usually been called stroke or apoplexy. It is most likely to be caused by massive cerebral hemorrhage. (See Fig. 56-6.)

However, more frequently what is known as a stroke is less dramatic. There may be only slight defects in speech, thought, motion, sensation, and vision. Consciousness is not lost or necessarily affected. Some degree of recovery is nearly invariable. This is the type related to thrombosis. It is the most common type, accounting for half of cerebrovascular accidents. An arteriosclerotic change in an artery comes first. Subsequently an occluding thrombus is added to the picture to produce the ischemic change in the brain.

As would be expected, the neurologic disturbances depend on the extent of brain tissue damaged or destroyed and may be focal or diffusely distributed.

Clinical technics have been advanced to estimate cerebral blood flow, visualize the blood vessels, and determine the availability of oxygen to brain cells. Therapeutic procedures have been devised involving the use of anticoagulants and certain surgical technics.

**Hemorrhage.** Among the many types of intracranial hemorrhage of diverse cause, the one of greatest importance is the spontaneous hemorrhage in the brain substance caused by vascular disease.

The manifestations of brain hemorrhage depend on the size of the hemorrhage, the rapidity of formation, and the location. Even small hemorrhages that involve the vital centers may cause immediate death. In the event of apoplexy, the patient gradually or suddenly becomes unconscious and may have convulsions. He may be in profound coma, with flushed face, stertorous breathing, and incontinence of feces and urine. If coma does not end in death, consciousness gradually returns after hours or days, but the patient is usually left with one or more disabling aftereffects, the most important of which is paralysis. Whatever the outcome of a given episode, the underlying cause remains, and the hemorrhages may recur until one proves fatal.

**Thrombosis and embolism.** Emboli derived from the left side of the heart in acute endocarditis or chronic valvular disease or from thrombotic lesions of the lungs lodge in the cerebral vessels. Thrombosis of the cerebral vessels may result from arteriosclerotic or syphilitic changes, or it may accompany certain infectious diseases and blood dyscrasias.

In both thrombosis and embolism the mass of brain supplied by the occluded vessel dies and rapidly disintegrates. This condition is known as *encephalomalacia* or softening of the brain. The functional disturbances are similar to those of brain hemorrhage. Like cerebral hemorrhage, both thrombosis and embolism are usually followed by paralysis. Fat embolism may cause generalized convulsions and quickly prove fatal.

## INFLAMMATION

**Encephalitis.** The term *encephalitis* indicates an inflammation of the brain substance. It is used practically to indicate conditions either inflammatory or degenerative. If the meninges are involved, the condition is spoken of as *meningoencephalitis*. If the spinal cord is also involved (as it commonly is), the process is referred to as *encephalomyelitis*. The following classification is based on etiology:

1. Encephalitis (and encephalomyelitis) caused by demonstrable organisms—bacteria, spirochetes, fungi, rickettsias, animal parasites
2. Encephalitis (and encephalomyelitis) caused by filtrable viruses
3. Encephalitis (and encephalomyelitis) of unknown cause (acute disseminated, postinfectious, postvaccinal, or allergic) (p. 313)

The viral group of encephalitides is the most important (p. 312). Encephalitis is a prominent complication of typhus fever, diphtheria, scarlet fever, measles, whooping cough, influenza, typhoid fever, or malaria. In some of these diseases the encephalitis may not appear until the primary infection has subsided. In cerebral malaria the encephalitis results from plugging of the cerebral capillaries by agglutinated parasites.

The onset of encephalitis (brain fever) is usually sudden, with hyperexcitability or stupor, stiffness of the neck, localized paralysis, and in some cases convulsions. If recovery occurs, the patient may be left with residual paralysis, epileptiform convulsions, and mental changes.

**Neurosyphilis.** General paresis (general paralysis of the insane, paralytic dementia), a diffuse meningoencephalitis caused by *Treponema pallidum*, is characterized by progressive mental deterioration, insanity, and generalized paralysis terminating in death. One of the three important forms of neurosyphilis, it occurs in about 3% of patients who have syphilis. It is more common in highly civilized than in primitive races, and in civilized races it is more common in better educated than in less well-educated persons. Its frequency in males is about five times as great as in females. Excessive mental strain and alcoholism are predisposing factors.

Juvenile paresis, which ordinarily begins between the twelfth and eighteenth years, is a rather common complication of congenital syphilis and usually lasts from 2 to 5 years after the onset of symptoms.

**Brain abscess.** Brain abscesses are most often caused by pyogenic bacteria, colon bacilli, and *Pseudomonas aeruginosa*. The causative organisms reach the brain through penetrating wounds or by extension from neighboring foci of suppuration in the middle ear, mastoid process, or bony sinuses. They may be brought to the brain by the bloodstream, especially from suppurative foci in the lungs. The most common cause of brain abscess in civilian life is extension from suppurative otitis media or mastoiditis. Brain abscesses are usually single but may be multiple. Multiple abscesses are usually of embolic origin.

The manifestations may develop with such great rapidity as to endanger the patient's life, or the abscess may lie dormant for months or years. The most common findings of chronic brain abscess are loss of weight, decrease in appetite, and signs of cerebral compression. Slight fever and moderate leukocytosis are often present. Most brain abscesses ultimately end fatally.

## BRAIN TUMORS

Included within the term *brain tumor* are all neoplasms arising within the cranial cavity, both those that are primary in the brain substance, bone, or other intracranial structures and those that are metastatic. The majority, however, arise within the brain, and more than half are *gliomas*, that is, tumors arising from the supporting glial tissue of the nervous system.

In children brain tumors are found in the cerebellum and are most frequently *astrocytomas, medulloblastomas,* and *ependymomas.* In adults the predominant one is the highly malignant *astrocytoma* (glioblastoma multiforme) that occurs in the cerebrum. *Meningiomas,* second to gliomas in frequency, arise in the meninges, are comparatively benign, grow slowly, but encroach on the brain substance.

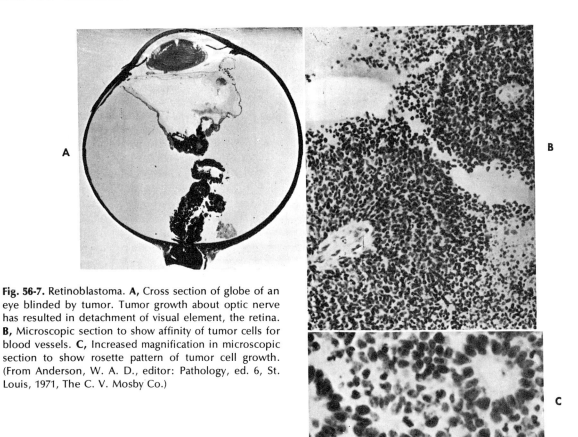

**Fig. 56-7.** Retinoblastoma. **A,** Cross section of globe of an eye blinded by tumor. Tumor growth about optic nerve has resulted in detachment of visual element, the retina. **B,** Microscopic section to show affinity of tumor cells for blood vessels. **C,** Increased magnification in microscopic section to show rosette pattern of tumor cell growth. (From Anderson, W. A. D., editor: Pathology, ed. 6, St. Louis, 1971, The C. V. Mosby Co.)

Metastatic tumors are usually from primary neoplasms in the lungs but may come from other organs of the body.

Brain tumors show no tendency to metastasize to distant parts of the body, and some have little tendency to invade the surrounding tissue. Extreme danger lies in the increase in intracranial pressure that they produce. Some brain tumors kill within a few months, whereas others allow the patient to live for several years.

Closely related to brain tumors are the *retinoblastomas* (retinal gliomas of the eye) of childhood, which are locally destructive. They have a familial incidence and occur before the child is 4 years old. In 20% of the cases tumors occur in both eyes. The outcome is usually fatal. (See Fig. 56-7.)

### EPILEPSY

Epilepsy is not a definite disease entity but, like jaundice and dropsy, is a condition that may result from several different causes. The dominant feature is the recurrent seizure.

The typical epileptic seizure begins with loss of consciousness associated with extreme pallor of the face and hands. A phase of generalized muscular rigidity follows during which respiration ceases, the tongue is bitten, and the normal color of the face returns but progresses to cyanosis. Muscular rigidity then abates and violent convulsive movements of the body begin. During the convulsive attacks the patient makes peculiar sounds, and a clear or bloody froth exudes from the mouth. After the attack is over, the patient remains in a condition of stupor or complete exhaustion for a variable period of time. An attack such as this is known as *grand mal* epilepsy. When the patient merely loses consciousness for a few seconds, it is *petit mal* epilepsy. The epileptic patient may show mental deterioration and be despondent, hypersensitive, disagreeable, or suspicious. Memory of the attack is usually completely effaced.

### CEREBRAL PALSY

The term *cerebral palsy* is used to include a certain group of neurologic disorders occurring in children. These, in most instances, represent a disturbance of the motor system of the brain as a result of a lesion incurred during intrauterine life or in early infancy. However, there is no characteristic type of brain involvement pathologically. Contributory causes are developmental defects in the central nervous system, trauma at birth, neonatal asphyxia, kernicterus associated with erythroblastosis fetalis, mechanical injury to the head, vascular anomalies, and prematurity.

The clinical patterns are fairly consistent. The most characteristic finding is that of weakness and spasticity of the extremities. Secondary, slow, irregular, and purposeless movements are seen in the fingers and toes (athetosis). Sometimes the lower extremities are more involved than the upper extremities. The walk may be characteristic. The child tends to walk on his toes, the knees rub together, and the legs cross in progression so that the walk is called a scissors gait. Neurologic manifestations are, of course, variable, depending on the nature and extent of the brain damage. There may be some degree of mental impairment, although many of these children are brighter than they appear since their

difficulty presents a handicap to self-expression. Cerebral palsy is distinguished from other diseases of the central nervous sytem occurring in children by its nonprogressive nature.

If the disorder is severe, it may manifest itself in nursing or feeding difficulties, irritability, and even convulsive seizures in the small infant. Rigidity of extremities may be apparent. The patients who show disturbances early in life usually do poorly, and many of them succumb in infancy. Milder cases may go unrecognized for the first 6 to 8 months of life. They are detected only when it is noted that the child is not developing properly; that is, he fails to sit up or cannot hold his head up. Many of these children finally learn to walk around 4 to 5 years of age.

## SYNCOPE

Syncope, or fainting, means loss of consciousness for only a short period of time. The commonest type of fainting is psychogenic in origin and is related to an emotional disturbance. Fainting is also present in situations in which there is either some interference in blood flow to the brain, usually as a result of heart

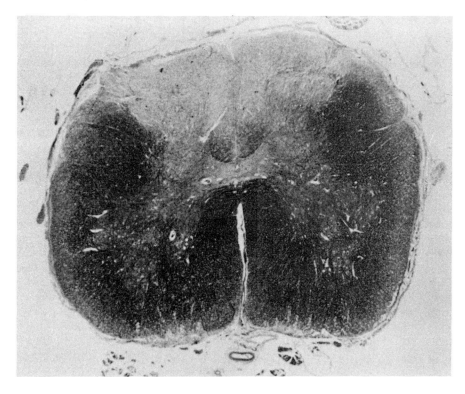

**Fig. 56-8.** Tabes dorsalis. Degeneration of posterior columns of spinal cord reflected in asymmetry of upper part of cord (upper part of photograph) with loss of staining quality. Compare with degenerative changes in Fig. 48-4.

disease or some chemical change in the blood, such as hypoglycemia. There are forms of heart disease that result in diminution of cerebral blood flow because of pronounced disturbances in cardiac rate and rhythm. Attacks of syncope are associated with the rare presence of a ball valve thrombus in the left atrium. This is a movable thrombus so attached to the wall of the atrium that it can fall over the mitral valve, occluding it and temporarily blocking the flow of blood through the valvular opening. Primary disorders of the brain may produce repeated episodes of unconsciousness.

## Spinal cord

The spinal cord is the cylindric portion of the central nervous system found in the upper two thirds of the backbone (the vertebral canal). It is 43 to 45 cm. in length.

### INFLAMMATION

Poliomyelitis is discussed on p. 313.

### DEGENERATION

**Tabes dorsalis.** Tabes dorsalis or locomotor ataxia is a degeneration of the posterior columns of the spinal cord (Fig. 56-8) and the posterior nerve roots and ganglia caused by *Treponema pallidum*. Since the disease attacks the sensory pathways of the cord, its manifestations are chiefly those of muscular incoordination and disturbances in sensation. Among the common ones are pain, ataxic gait, visceral crises, loss of sensation and reflexes, optic atrophy, and disturbances of rectal and bladder sphincters.

**Multiple sclerosis.** Multiple sclerosis is a chronic degenerative disease of unknown etiology. It seems to have a predilection for a young person between the ages of 20 and 35 years, and in the next 25 years or more of that person's life there will be multiple recurrent episodes, reflecting a scattered patchy type of degeneration and progressive destruction throughout the central nervous system. The spinal cord, especially, is involved.

The lesion is a type of liquefaction of the fatty coverings (myelin sheaths) of nerve fibers at focal points anywhere in the brain or spinal cord. As a result of it there is a reaction in the supporting tissues of the nervous system, and scar tissue is formed. The name *multiple sclerosis* derives from the deposition of the dense, firm sclerotic tissue (scar) in plaques at the multiple sites of involvement. Although the disease strikes the myelin sheath initially, in the end stages the nerve fiber is lost as well. With it is lost sensory or motor function.

As the unknown injury comes and goes, so the neurologic manifestations emerge and remit, although each time recovery tends to be less and less complete. Motor changes that are seen include paralyses, tremors, and partial or complete loss of coordination. Sensory changes include numbness, tingling, nystagmus, double vision, even blindness. Mental states are variable. In advanced cases there is loss of bladder or bowel control.

## Cerebrospinal fluid
### CHARACTERISTICS

Normal cerebrospinal fluid is a crystal clear, colorless, sparkling liquid with a specific gravity of about 1.001 to 1.008. The normal cell count is up to five cells per cubic millimeter. More than ten cells per cubic millimeter is abnormal. The protein content of normal spinal fluid is 15 to 45 mg. per 100 ml. of fluid. Cerebrospinal fluid contains about one-half as much sugar and slightly more chloride than does blood. The pressure exerted by the cerebrospinal fluid is influenced by so many factors that pressure readings made on different subjects or the same subject at different times show considerable variation. With the patient in the recumbent position the cerebrospinal fluid pressure in children ranges from 45 to 90 mm. water, and in adults from 130 to 150 mm.

### PATHOLOGIC CHANGES

**Color and appearance.** The cerebrospinal fluid in disease may be yellow or blood-tinged. Yellow fluids are found in certain types of tumors of the spinal cord or may be a late result of hemorrhage.

*Turbid fluids* usually indicate purulent meningitis and call for immediate microbiologic investigation. The fluid is clear or, at the most, only slightly opalescent in tuberculous meningitis, neurosyphilis, encephalitis, and poliomyelitis.

In acute purulent meningitis the cerebrospinal fluid pressure is greatly increased, but the fluid sometimes contains so much pus that it will scarcely flow through the needle. The fluid is opalescent or distinctly turbid and often has a green or yellow hue. In most cases of purulent meningitis the causative organisms may be easily demonstrated by smears made from the fluid, but occasionally cultures are necessary.

In the early stages of brain abscess the cerebrospinal fluid is clear. At a later stage the abscess may give rise to meningitis or may rupture and its contents be mixed with the fluid.

*Blood* is found in the cerebrospinal fluid as a result of old or recent hemorrhage, or it may be accidentally introduced during the lumbar puncture. If the blood imparts a dark red or brown color to the fluid, an old hemorrhage is indicated. Fresh blood suggests a recent hemorrhage or a bloody tap. If blood results from hemorrhage, it will be uniformly mixed with the fluid. If blood is accidentally introduced, it will be more abundant in the first few drops of fluid removed. Fractures of the skull do not give bloody spinal fluid unless the meninges are torn, and a cerebral hemorrhage does not cause bloody fluid unless it breaks into a ventricle or opens on the surface of the brain.

**Cells.** An increase in cells in the cerebrospinal fluid accompanies almost any inflammatory condition of the central nervous system. When the cell count reaches 200 per cubic millimeter, a distinct turbidity is present. An increase in cells is most marked in the acute types of meningitis, and the majority of the cells are polymorphonuclear neutrophilic leukocytes. Thousands may be present. In tuberculous meningitis, poliomyelitis, encephalitis, and syphilitic involvement of the central nervous system, there is some increase in cells, and the lymphocyte is the predominating cell.

**Chemical changes.** The amount of *sugar* in the fluid is decreased in meningitis, increased in encephalitis, and normal in poliomyelitis.

*Chlorides* are decreased in meningitis, especially the tuberculous type, and are within normal limits in poliomyelitis and encephalitis.

The amount of *protein* in cerebrospinal fluid is variably increased in the majority of diseases of the central nervous system.

**Other pathologic features.** All types of neurosyphilis give a positive Wassermann test on the cerebrospinal fluid, and in most cases a positive test is also obtained on the blood. The colloidal gold test gives a characteristic curve in paresis.

When tumors of the spinal cord completely obstruct the flow of cerebrospinal fluid, the fluid shows one or more of the changes characteristic of *Froin's syndrome:* (1) yellow coloration of the fluid, (2) high protein content with slight or no increase in cells, and (3) massive coagulability.

Even a painstaking study of slides carefully prepared from the cerebrospinal fluid rarely reveals tubercle bacilli. The organisms may be more easily recovered by culture.

## Questions for review

1 By what routes may the bacteria causing purulent meningitis reach the meninges?
2 What causes cerebral compression? Give some of the features.
3 List the anatomic locations for hemorrhage in the central nervous system.
4 Give causes of encephalitis.
5 What organisms are most often the cause of brain abscess? How may they reach the brain?
6 What is the difference between grand mal and petit mal epilepsy?
7 What are the three important forms of neurosyphilis? Discuss each briefly.
8 What does fresh blood in the cerebrospinal fluid indicate?
9 Name three types of meningitis in which the cerebrospinal fluid is turbid. Name three conditions affecting the central nervous system in which the cerebrospinal fluid is clear.
10 Give the characteristics of normal cerebrospinal fluid. How and where is it formed?
11 What are some of the characteristics of brain tumors? What is Froin's syndrome?
12 Briefly discuss cerebral palsy.
13 List three causes of syncope.
14 What is meant by cerebral concussion?

**References on p. 641.**

# CHAPTER 57

# Diseases of
# Bones and joints

The skeletal system, that framework about which the body is built and by which it is supported, may be divided into two major parts, the bony elements and the articulations or joints.

## Bones

Bone is a specialized connective tissue. Its characteristic hardness fits it to be the mechanical support for the skeleton of the body. It also houses the bone marrow and is a body store for calcium. The periosteum is the specialized fibrous tissue covering for bone.

### INFLAMMATION

**Osteomyelitis.** Inflammation of the bone may primarily involve cancellous bone and marrow, compact bone, or periosteum, giving rise to osteomyelitis, osteitis, and periostitis, respectively. In most cases the inflammation spreads from the primary focus until cancellous bone, marrow, compact bone, and periosteum are all involved. The mechanisms of inflammation in bone are the same as in inflammation elsewhere; the difference in results are caused by the peculiar structure of bone.

*Acute hematogenous* osteomyelitis, a disease primarily of childhood, is most often caused by bacteria that have been carried to the cancellous bone and marrow by the bloodstream. The bacteria may be deposited during the course of septicemia or bacteremia. In some cases osteomyelitis is traced to the ingress of bacteria from the periosteum or from contaminated gunshot wounds, compound fractures, or amputations. Infections of the middle ear can spread to the mastoid process and cause fulminating osteomyelitis. Staphylococci are the organisms most often responsible for acute osteomyelitis.

Acute hematogenous osteomyelitis begins in the end of a long bone, especially the upper end of the tibia or the lower end of the femur. From the point

of origin the infection spreads along the marrow cavity of the bone until the whole shaft is filled with purulent material. The infection may then extend by the blood vessels to the periosteum. The exudate commonly perforates the bone to produce a sinus that discharges on the surface. Fragments of bone become necrotic in osteomyelitis; the dead bone is known as the *sequestrum*. It acts as a foreign body to aggravate in some

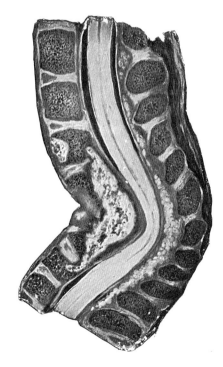

**Fig. 57-1.** Pott's disease of spine. In this cross section of a deformed spine, note destruction and collapse of bone and accumulation of grayish white exudate compressing spinal cord (the elongated smooth structure seen centrally).

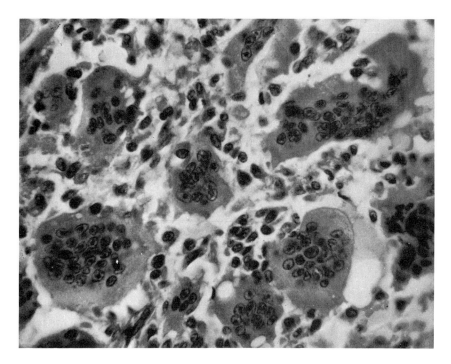

**Fig. 57-2.** Characteristic multinucleated giant cells of giant cell tumor in the fibula. (×420.) (From Lichtenstein, L.: Bone tumors, ed. 4, St. Louis, 1972, The C. V. Mosby Co.)

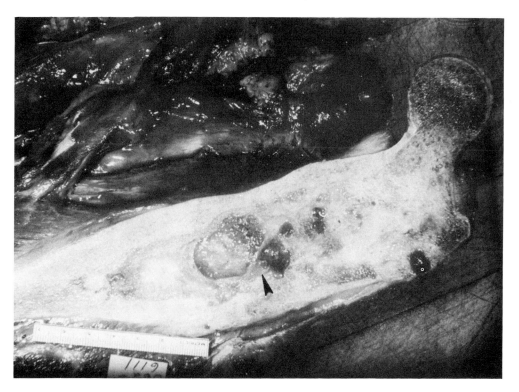

**Fig. 57-3.** Chondrosarcoma of femur, sectioned. Note extension of tumor outward, cystic spaces (arrow), and overall destruction. Globular head of femur is to the upper right.

way the inflammatory process. In fulminating cases of osteomyelitis the joint may be involved, but in most cases the epiphyseal cartilage protects the joint against invasion. Before the days of modern antibiotic therapy, acute fulminating osteomyelitis was a serious condition with a dismal outlook; for when a bone became infected, the bacteria could remain for years, giving rise to *chronic* osteomyelitis with recurrent, more or less acute attacks.

**Tuberculosis.** Tubercle bacilli reach the bones from distant foci via the bloodstream or by direct extension from a joint. Tuberculosis of the bones is seen in childhood and usually begins in the cancellous tissue of the vertebrae or in the ends of the long bones, particularly the tibia and femur. The disease is primarily an osteomyelitis.

At first one or more caseous foci are formed, and tubercles aggregate around them. With caseation there is softening, and the involved area gradually forms a tuberculous abscess. The destructive process spreads along the length of the medullary cavity of a long bone, and the abscess discharges on the surface. With destruction of bone the periosteum is stimulated to form new osseous tissue, which greatly expands the affected bone. Since tuberculosis of the bone often extends to the joint and vice versa, bone and joint tuberculosis are associated.

Tuberculosis of the spine (Pott's disease) is a disease of childhood but may occur in adults. (See Fig. 57-1.) The vertebrae involved are the last three dorsal, or thoracic, and the first two lumbar. As a rule, two or more vertebrae are involved. In children the centers of the vertebrae are primarily attacked, in adults the periphery. When the central portion is attacked, the bone is destroyed and replaced by tuberculous granulation tissue, which becomes converted into softened caseous material. Finally the affected vertebrae are crushed by the weight that they support, resulting

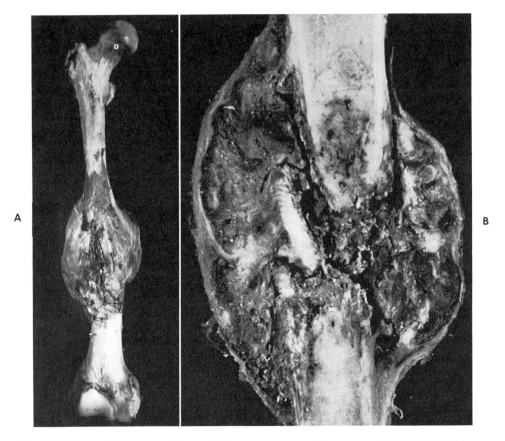

**Fig. 57-4.** Osteogenic sarcoma of femur. **A,** Gross appearance of tumor at midpart of shaft of bone. Note destruction. The unsuspected cancer caused a pathologic fracture 1 month before operation. **B,** Cross section of same tumor showing cancerous bone formation in gap between severed ends of bone shaft and outward into soft tissues. (From Lichtenstein, L.: Bone tumors, ed. 4, St. Louis, 1972, The C. V. Mosby Co.)

in an anterior curvature of the spinal column. When the peripheral portion of the bone is attacked, there is not so much bone destruction and deformity is less.

Tuberculous exudate has a remarkable tendency to burrow, and the exudate from tuberculous vertebrae may approach the surface at a considerable distance from the diseased bone, the point of approach depending to a great extent on the location of the involved vertebrae. In tuberculosis of the cervical vertebrae the exudate may collect between the vertebral column and the posterior pharyngeal wall, forming a retropharyngeal abscess. In the vertebrae of the thoracic region the exudate may enter the sheath of the psoas muscle, forming a psoas abscess that reaches the skin surface in the groin. Such a cold abscess may be mistaken for a hernia. A collection of tuberculous exudate is not a true abscess, but the word *abscess* is commonly applied.

**Syphilis.** The lesions of congenital syphilis may be present at birth or appear later. The most characteristic is *osteochondritis* that affects the area of growth between the diaphysis (shaft) and epiphysis

(end of the shaft) of the long bones. Since the osteochondritis interferes with growth, the bones do not reach their normal length. The epiphyses may become separated from the shafts of the bones and the child be unable to walk. When the tibia is thickened and curved forward, the so-called saber blade tibia or saber shin is formed. The destructive action of gummas in the nasal bones and palate may give rise to saddle nose and perforation of the palate. Gummas of the skull are not infrequent, and bossing of the skull and craniotabes are common.

In late congenital syphilis and in acquired syphilis the periosteum is most often involved, the medulla of the bone may be also, but the joints seldom are. The periosteal involvement, usually of the shin bones, takes the form of periostitis with marked fibrosis, and gummas may occur. In fibrous periostitis the formation of bony nodules gives the shins a roughened, uneven appearance. The involvement of the underlying bone is more extensive in gummas of the periosteum than in fibrous periostitis. In either case extensive rarefaction or sequestrum formation (sequestration) may occur.

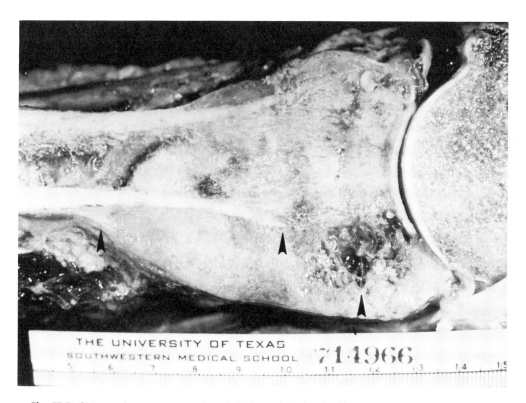

**Fig. 57-5.** Osteogenic sarcoma, sectioned. Follow white band of bone cortex into tumor (center arrow), noting extension of tumor out and down shaft of bone (left arrow). Cystic area of tumor (arrow) in lower right of photograph. Joint cartilage and space to right of expanded end of cancerous bone.

## OSTEOPOROSIS

The loss of bone density after a 2-weeks mission was an unexpected complication of space travel for the astronauts, but under other circumstances *osteoporosis* or rarefaction of bone is one of the most common of bone ailments. In varying degree it is an almost constant feature of advancing age *(senile osteoporosis)*. The bones especially affected are those of the spine, the pelvis, and the long bones of the extremities. Since the brittle bones crack easily, spontaneous fractures with deformity and resultant incapacity are the hazards. The reasons for this condition are not always clear-cut. Gonadal hormones affect the bone formation. As would be expected, the condition is prominent in the female after menopause. It is also found in endocrine disorders and in severe nutritional deficiencies.

## NEOPLASM

**Benign neoplasms.** The most important benign neoplasms of bone are osteomas, chondromas (tumors derived from cartilage), fibromas, myxomas, and giant cell tumors.

*Osteomas* are benign, comparatively rare tumors composed of bone. True osteomas may be confused with certain common bony overgrowths, among which are calluses (which form at the site of fractures) and exostoses.

True osteomas usually occur in connection with the bones of the face, most often in the nasal sinuses or orbit. Secondary ossification may occur in fibromas, lipomas, and certain sarcomas.

*Giant cell tumors* (Fig. 57-2), which are comparatively benign, are thought by some authorities to represent a peculiar reaction to an inflammatory condition and not to be neoplasms at all. Giant cell tumors affect the lower jaw, where they are known as *epulides* (plural of *epulis*), and they may occur in other locations, notably the ends of long bones, where they are not quite so benign. The growth usually arises near the periosteum and forms a firm, slowly enlarging mass, but in a few cases it arises in the medullary por-

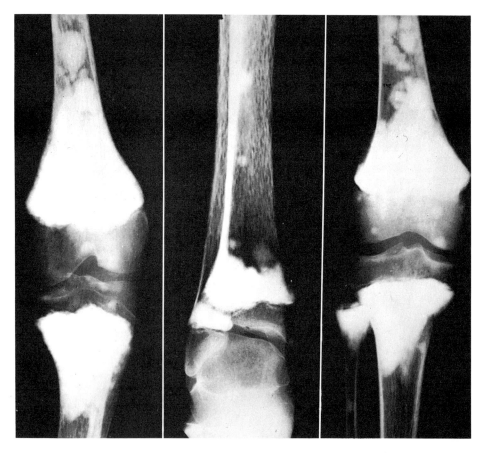

**Fig. 57-6.** Radiographs to best demonstrate by increased radiodensity in tumor foci the enhanced bone-forming capacity of sclerosing osteogenic sarcoma. Long bones of lower extremities are involved. (From Lichtenstein, L.: Bone tumors, ed. 4, St. Louis, 1972, The C. V. Mosby Co.)

tion of the bone and is soft and jellylike in consistency. Epulis is the former type of growth. As a rule, giant cell tumors require no treatment other than adequate local excision.

Giant cell tumors should not be confused with certain highly malignant sarcomas that contain true tumor giant cells thought to be osteoclasts.

**Primary malignant neoplasms.** Primary malignant neoplasms of bone are sarcomas. Osteogenic sarcoma, Ewing's tumor, and periosteal fibrosarcoma are the most important ones. A malignant tumor arising in bone made up principally of cartilage is a *chondrosarcoma* (Fig. 57-3). *Periosteal fibrosarcoma* is a com-

paratively rare tumor arising from the periosteal connective tissue and may reflect the osteogenic capacity of the periosteum in the formation of new bone. *Osteogenic sarcoma* (Figs. 57-4 and 57-5), the most frequent primary bone tumor, usually begins about the knee in the end of one of the long bones of an adolescent or young adult. Producing enlargement and much distortion of bone, the tumor is an irregular admixture of bone-forming (sclerosing or osteoblastic, Fig. 57-6) and bone-destroying (osteolytic) elements. *Ewing's tumor* (Fig. 57-7) is a soft grayish cellular tumor that involves the shaft of a long bone in a child.

A causative relation between trauma and tumor

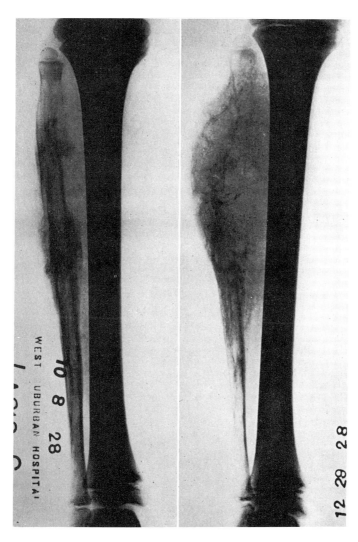

**Fig. 57-7.** Radiographs of fibula to show bone-destroying (osteolytic) nature of Ewing's tumor. Radiograph on left was taken less than 3 months earlier than one on right. Note progression of tumor. (Radiologic appearance of tibia, bone to the right of fibula, is unchanged.) (From Lichtenstein, L.: Bone tumors, ed. 4, St. Louis, 1972, The C. V. Mosby Co.)

growth is more strongly suggested in bone tumors than in any other neoplasm. However, bone tumors seldom follow such extensive injuries as fracture.

**Metastatic malignancies.** The important metastatic tumors to bone are carcinomas, the most serious of which are primary in the breast, lung, thyroid gland, kidney, prostate gland, and stomach. The bones most often affected are the vertebrae, ribs, sternum, skull, pelvis, femur, and humerus, and it is the cancellous portion that is invaded. Pain, swelling, or fracture of a long bone frequently calls attention to the metastatic site before the primary tumor has been discovered. A fracture occurring at the site of a tumor metastasis is called a *pathologic* fracture. Widespread carcinomatous involvement of the bone marrow is rarely a cause of a profound anemia.

## Joints

Joints are the connective tissue structures that connect bones one to the other so as to permit varying degrees and kinds of motions between them.

### CLASSIFICATION OF JOINT DISEASE

During the course of illness in a number of widely divergent disease states there will be an involvement of the joints or related tissues adjoining. Joint disease (loosely referred to as arthritis) may be only a small part of the total picture, or it may be the most significant finding. The following classification* indicates its patterns:

| | |
|---|---|
| Polyarthritis of unknown etiology | Rheumatoid arthritis<br>Juvenile rheumatoid arthritis<br>  (Still's disease) |
| Connective tissue disorders (collagen diseases) | Polyarteritis nodosa<br>Systemic lupus erythematosus |
| Rheumatic fever | |
| Degenerative joint disease (osteoarthritis) | |
| Arthritis associated with known infectious agents<br>Bacteria | *Brucella*<br>Gonococcus<br>Pneumococcus<br>*Salmonella*<br>*Staphylococcus*<br>*Treponema* (congenital syphilis)<br>Tubercle bacillus |
| Virus | Rubella virus |
| Fungus | *Coccidioides immitis* |
| Traumatic or neurogenic or both | Traumatic (direct injury)<br>Tertiary syphilis (Charcot joint<br>  in tabes dorsalis) |

*Modified from a classification of arthritis and rheumatism accepted by the American Rheumatism Association.

| | |
|---|---|
| Arthritis with known biochemical (or endocrine) abnormalities | Gout<br>Hemophilia<br>Sickle cell disease<br>Hyperparathyroidism<br>Scurvy<br>Acromegaly<br>Hypothyroidism |
| Allergy and drug reactions | Serum sickness |
| Tumors | Leukemia<br>Synovioma<br>Metastatic tumors<br>Plasma cell myeloma |
| Miscellaneous disorders | Amyloidosis |

In the following paragraphs some of the more important forms of joint disease are discussed.

### INFLAMMATION

**Acute arthritis.** Acute arthritis (inflammation of a joint) may be of infectious or noninfectious origin and may be suppurative or nonsuppurative. One of many joints may be involved. Acute arthritis of infectious origin may be caused by streptococci, staphylococci, pneumococci, or, less often, other bacteria. One of the less common causes of acute arthritis is the gonococcus, but in many cases gonorrheal arthritis is chronic rather than acute. In infectious arthritis the causative bacteria may reach the joint through penetrating wounds or by extension from a nearby site of infection in one of the bones composing the joint, but in the majority of cases they are conveyed to a joint or joints by the bloodstream. Arthritis of bloodstream origin may occur during the course of septicemia, subacute bacterial endocarditis, and certain infectious diseases, especially pneumonia, scarlet fever, typhoid fever, epidemic meningitis, and undulant fever. Noninfectious arthritis may result from injuries of the joints or may be of allergic origin.

In a few cases of purulent arthritis caused by pyogenic organisms, recovery with a fairly useful joint occurs, but in most cases the destruction of tissue is so great that the reparative processes lead to fibrous and bony adhesions and the joint is fixed and immobilized. This is ankylosis of the joint.

**Rheumatic fever.** One of the most characteristic features of rheumatic fever occurring in late childhood or early adult life is the accompanying polyarthritis, which is acute and nonsuppurative. The process migrates from one area of the body to another; as the inflammatory reaction subsides in one joint, it develops in another. The joints most often involved are the knee, ankle, shoulder, wrists, elbow, hip, hand, and foot. Affected joints are distended with fluid and extremely painful. When the inflammation subsides,

**Table 57-1**

Comparison of two forms of chronic arthritis

|  | RHEUMATOID ARTHRITIS | OSTEOARTHRITIS |
|---|---|---|
| Sex incidence | Women | Men |
| Age of onset | Under 40 years | Over 40 years |
| Clinical onset | Gradual; sometimes acute | Always gradual |
| Pathologic change | Inflammatory condition of synovial membrane | Degenerative condition of bone and cartilage |
| Joints involved | Bilateral symmetrical involvement of hand and wrist joints | Unilateral asymmetrical involvement of large weight-bearing joints |
| General body reactions | Toxicity with fever; weight loss; anemia | None |
| Local reactions | Local signs of inflammation; marked deformity; ankylosis | No local reaction; deformity not marked; no true ankylosis; bony spurs present |

the joint returns to normal, and residual deformity is rare.

**Chronic arthritis.** There are two forms of chronic arthritis of obscure etiology in which classification is made on the basis of clinical manifestations of the disease and structural changes occurring in the affected joints. They are rheumatoid arthritis* and degenerative joint disease. (See Table 57-1.)

*Rheumatoid* arthritis is a common type of chronic arthritis occurring in women between 20 and 40 years of age. It is infrequent in adult males. The onset may be gradual, or it may be acute, with fever and painful joints. As a rule, the process is polyarticular but symmetrical. Beginning in the joint capsule, it involves the joints of the hands and feet, with one or more of the larger joints, particularly the knee and shoulder, also being affected. The hip joint is seldom affected. There may be fluid in the involved joints (hydrarthrosis), and in a few cases hard, freely movable, painless subcutaneous nodules form about the joints (Fig. 57-8). The end stage is fibrous and bony fixation of the joint (ankylosis). This disease is characterized by its progressive course, and the resultant deformity and interference with function may render the patient hopelessly crippled for life. (See Fig. 57-9.)

Rheumatoid arthritis often follows severe physical strain, injuries, and exposure to bad weather, and in many cases a hereditary factor seems to be present. Many patients give a history of antecedent infections. The chronic nature of this disease, the ups and downs of the clinical course, and the presence of factors in the serum that behave like antibodies against body antigens all strongly point to a background of autoimmunity. A specific agglutination test using particles of polystyrene latex coated with gamma globulin identifies an immunoglobulin (IgM) in the blood, the *rheumatoid factor*. The rheumatoid factor, although not specific for rheumatoid arthritis, is significantly related to it.

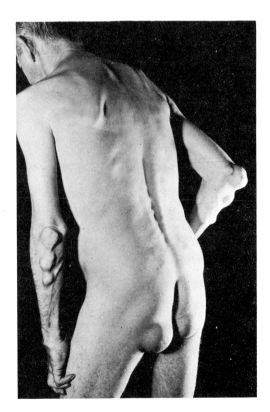

**Fig. 57-8.** Rheumatoid nodules of arms. Note two synovial cysts over buttocks (cystic accumulations of fluid over ischial tuberosities). (Courtesy Dr. A. M. Lefkovits, Memphis, Tenn.)

---

*Rheumatoid arthritis is also known as atrophic arthritis and arthritis deformans. Some authors prefer to include any type of arthritis accompanied by marked deformity and crippling under the term *arthritis deformans*. Degenerative joint disease is known also as osteoarthritis and hypertrophic arthritis.

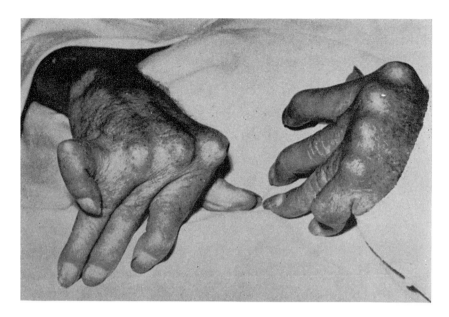

**Fig. 57-9.** Rheumatoid arthritis. Note deformity associated with enlargement of knuckles and atrophy of small muscles in hands. (From Prior, J. A., and Silberstein, J. S.: Physical diagnosis—the history and examination of the patient, ed. 4, St. Louis, 1973, The C. V. Mosby Co.)

*Degenerative joint disease* differs from rheumatoid arthritis in being degenerative rather than inflammatory and more common in males than in females. It is usually insidious in onset and occurs most often in middle life and old age.

The articular cartilage is attacked primarily, and the large weight-bearing joints are affected, often only a single joint. Although the disease produces cartilaginous and bony overgrowths, it is not followed by ankylosis. Bony nodules known as *Heberden's nodes* are formed around affected joints of the fingers and toes. Portions of the synovial membrane may undergo calcification, become separated from the site or origin, and occur as freely movable objects in the joint cavity, known as joint mice. The bones about joints affected with this type of arthritis have little tendency to repair. The exact cause of degenerative joint disease is not known. In some cases it follows an injury; it is commonly associated with marked arteriosclerosis.

**Gonorrheal arthritis.** Gonorrheal arthritis formerly complicated or followed 2% to 5% of the cases of gonorrhea, but since the advent of antimicrobial drugs, it is rare. Gonorrheal arthritis occurs more often in men than in women and usually affects the larger joints, especially the knee. As a rule, only a few joints are attacked, and in many cases the infection is confined to a single joint.

Acute gonorrheal arthritis often begins suddenly with chills, fever, swelling of the affected joint or joints, and intense pain. There is usually serofibrinous exudation into the joint, which is red, swollen, and painful. The process may end by resolution or progress to chronic arthritis with hydrops or suppuration.

Chronic hydrops of gonorrheal origin is comparatively painless and most often is monarticular, attacking one of the larger joints. Ordinarily, constitutional symptoms are absent. Chronic hydrops may end spontaneously or resist all forms of treatment. Chronic suppurative arthritis is associated with fever, constitutional symptoms, pain, and destruction of the joint.

**Tuberculous arthritis.** Pyogenic infections of the bones seldom involve the joints, whereas tuberculosis of the joints is usually caused by the extension of a tuberculous process from an adjacent end of one of the bones of the joint. However, in some cases it begins as a primary process in the synovial membrane without involvement of the bone. The latter mode of origin is more common in adults. The tuberculous focus in the bone or synovial membrane may be secondary to some other focus in the body, such as pulmonary tuberculosis, but in many cases a primary focus cannot be detected. Injury to a joint seems to render it more susceptible to invasion by tubercle bacilli.

Tuberculous arthritis usually occurs before the sixth year of life, but no age is exempt. As a rule, the infection is confined to a single joint, and the joints most often affected, in order of frequency, are the hip, knee, elbow, shoulder, and ankle. Excluding tuberculosis of the spine, tuberculosis of the hip is more common than tuberculosis of all other joints combined. When the arthritis is caused by extension of a tuberculous process from an adjacent bone, any part of the joint may be attacked, but the synovial membrane is ultimately involved, and caseous foci beginning in the synovial membrane finally destroy the articular cartilage and invade the regional bone.

Although a spontaneous cure may occur in all but the more advanced cases of tuberculous arthritis, such is not the usual outcome, and surgery has to be done to effect a cure. Even then the patient may be left with a stiff or completely ankylosed joint. Secondary infection of the sinuses from a tuberculous joint may lead to suppuration within the joint cavity. Amyloid infiltration of the liver, spleen, and kidneys follows long-standing cases.

**Syphilitic arthritis.** Syphilis of the joints may complicate either congenital or acquired syphilis. Congenital syphilis of the joints may occur in the form of *syphilitic epiphysitis* in infants or *syphilitic synovitis* in older children and young adults. In the former the involvement of the epiphysis leads to swelling, tenderness, and pain in the joint. Separation of the epiphysis may occur. In syphilitic synovitis the knee is most often affected, and the condition is usually bilateral. It may take the form of simple effusion or gummatous synovitis.

The joint manifestations of acquired secondary syphilis are not of a destructive nature, and the only symptom may be rheumatic pains that are worse at night and that are not aggravated by motion. In most cases, however, there are moderate tenderness of the joint, swelling, and limitation of motion. The knees are most often affected, and the condition is frequently bilateral.

In acquired tertiary syphilis there is a gummatous or diffuse inflammatory infiltration of the synovial membrane, and the articular ends of the bones may be affected. The affection is usually monarticular, and the knee joint is most often involved. There is considerable swelling but no redness of the joint.

## METABOLIC ABNORMALITY

**Gout.** See p. 472.

## Questions for review

1 Define osteomyelitis, osteitis, periostitis, osteoporosis, epulis, Herberden's node.
2 What organisms are most often responsible for acute osteomyelitis? How do they reach the bones? What portion of the bone is most often the site of origin? What bones are most often involved?
3 How do tubercle bacilli reach the bones? Give the sequence of events in tuberculosis of bone.
4 What is Pott's disease? How does it differ in children and adults?
5 Give the causes of acute arthritis.
6 How does syphilis affect bones?
7 Briefly contrast rheumatoid arthritis with degenerative joint disease.
8 Name three primary tumors of bone. Give the most common primary sites for metastatic malignancies in bone.
9 What is a pathologic fracture?

## REFERENCES (Chapters 56 and 57)

Anderson, W. A. D., editor: Pathology, ed. 6, St. Louis, 1971, The C. V. Mosby Co.

Bauer, J. D., and others: Clinical laboratory methods, ed. 8, St. Louis, 1974, The C. V. Mosby Co.

Braney, M. L.: The child with hydrocephalus, Am. J. Nurs. **73:**828, 1973.

Forster, F. M.: Clinical neurology, ed. 3, St. Louis, 1973, The C. V. Mosby Co.

Heaney, R. P.: Pathophysiology of osteoporosis: implications for treatment, Tex. Med. **70:**37, Dec., 1974.

Jaffe, H. L.: Metabolic, degenerative and inflammatory diseases of bone and joints, Philadelphia, 1972, Lea & Febiger.

Johnson, J. S., and others: Rheumatoid arthritis, 1970-1972, Ann. Intern. Med. **78:**937, 1973.

Lichtenstein, L.: Bone tumors, ed. 4, St. Louis, 1972, The C. V. Mosby Co.

Lichtenstein, L.: Diseases of bone and joints, ed. 2, St. Louis, 1975, The C. V. Mosby Co.

Maddox, M.: Subarachnoid hemorrhage, Am. J. Nurs. **74:** 2199, 1974.

Mazzola, R., and Jacobs, G. B.: Brain tumors: diagnosis and treatment, RN **38:**42, March, 1975.

Raney, R. B., Sr., and Brashear, H. R.: Shands' handbook of orthopedic surgery, ed. 8, St. Louis, 1971, The C. V. Mosby Co.

Sharp, J. T.: Infectious agents in the arthritides: current status, Hosp. Pract. **6:**142, May, 1971.

Soffer, A.: What you should know about strokes, Today's Health **46:**40, Aug., 1968.

Stehbens, W. E.: Pathology of the cerebral blood vessels, St. Louis, 1972, The C. V. Mosby Co.

Walike, B. C., and others: Rheumatoid arthritis: personality factors, Am. J. Nurs. **67:**1427, 1967.

Whedon, G. D.: Battling the bone-thinner, Today's Health **45:**66, Sept., 1967.

Ziff, M.: Viruses and the connective tissue diseases, Med. Coll. Va. Q. **10**(2):57, 1974.

# Glossary

**abscess**  Circumscribed collection of pus.

**acetone bodies**  Term used to denote acetone, diacetic acid, and beta-hydroxybutyric acid, collectively.

**achlorhydria**  Absence of hydrochloric acid from gastric juice.

**acidosis**  Condition characterized by a decrease in alkalinity of the blood.

**acquired immunity**  Immunity person acquired after birth.

**active carrier**  Person or animal that becomes carrier after recovery from given disease.

**active immunity**  Immunity brought about by activity of certain body cells of the person becoming immune on direct exposure to an antigen.

**acuminate**  Pointed, tapering.

**acute disease**  Disease that runs a rapid course with more or less severe manifestations.

**adenocarcinoma**  Gland cell carcinoma.

**adenoma**  Benign tumor of glandular origin.

**adenopathy**  Disease of glands; often used to indicate lymph node enlargement.

**adhesion**  Adherence or knitting together of two surfaces.

**adjuvant**  Substance mixed with an antigen to enhance antigenicity and antibody response.

**aerobe**  Organisms whose growth requires presence of atmospheric oxygen.

**afferent**  Bringing to or into.

**agammaglobulinemia**  Deficiency or absence of gamma globulin in the blood usually associated with increased susceptibility to infection.

**agar**  Gelatinous substance prepared from Japanese seaweed; use as base for solid culture media.

**agenesis**  Defective development or absence of body part.

**agglutination**  Visible clumping of cells suspended in a fluid.

**agglutinins**  Antibodies that cause agglutination.

**agglutinogen**  Any substance that, acting as an antigen, stimulates production of agglutinins.

**air pollution**  Dust, smoke, or chemical fumes in air.

**albinism**  Congenital absence of pigment from the skin and other structures.

**albuminuria**  Increase of albumin in urine.

**algid**  Cold; an algid fever is one in which patient goes into state of collapse.

**alkaloid**  Basic substance found in plants that is usually the part of the plant with medicinal properties.

**alkalosis**  Condition characterized by increased alkalinity of the blood.

**allergen**  Substance that can induce allergic state when introduced into body of susceptible person.

**allergy (hypersensitivity)**  State in which affected person exhibits unusual manifestations in contact with allergen.

**alum toxoid**  Toxoid treated with aluminum compound.

**alveolar process**  Portion of the jaw in which teeth embedded.

**alveolus** (pl., **alveoli**)  Cavity or sac; small air sac at end of bronchial tree in which gas exchange occurs in lung.

**amboceptor**  Substance that combines with cells and complement to dissolve cells (example: hemolysin).

**ambulatory**  Not confined to bed.

**ameba, amoeba** (pl., **amebas, amoebae**)  Protozoon moving by extruding fingerlike processes (pseudopods).

**amebiasis**  Infection with pathogenic amebas; acute amebiasis is amebic dysentery.

**amino acids**  Organic chemical compounds containing amino ($NH_2$) group and carboxyl (COOH) group, which form chief structure of proteins.

**aminoaciduria**  Excess of one or more amino acids in urine.

**ampulla**  Normal, saccular widening of a canal.

**anaerobe**  Organism that grows only or best in absence of atmospheric oxygen.

**anaphylactoid**  Like anaphylaxis.

**anaphylaxis**  State of hypersusceptibility to a protein resulting from previous introduction of the protein into the body.

**anaplasia**  Condition of neoplastic cells indicating their loss of differentiation or their reversion to more primitive forms.

**anasarca**  Generalized edema.

**anastomosis**  Communication between two blood vessels.

**anemia**  Impoverished condition of the blood caused by reduction in red blood cells, hemoglobin, or both.

**aneurysm**  Pathologic dilatation of artery resulting from weakness of its wall.

**angioma**  Tumor composed of blood or lymph vessels.

**angstrom** (Å)  One tenth of a nanometer (millimicron) or one 254-millionth of an inch.

**ankylosis**  Stiffening or fixation of a joint.

**anoxemia**  Physiologic lack of oxygen in the blood.

**anoxia**  Physiologic deficiency of oxygen in body tissues.

**antagonism**  Mutual resistance.

**antibacterial serum**  Antiserum that destroys or prevents growth of bacteria.

**antibiotic**  Agent produced by one organism that destroys or inhibits another organism.

**antibody**  Agent in body that destroys or inactivates certain foreign substances that gain access to body, particularly microbes and their products.

**anticoagulant**  Agent that prevents coagulation.

**antigen**  Substance that when introduced into body, causes production of antibodies.

**antiluetic**  Antisyphilitic.

**antiseptic**  Substance that prevents growth of bacteria.

**antiserum**  Immune serum.

**antitoxin**  Immune serum that neutralizes or prevents action of a toxin.

**antivenin**  Antitoxic serum for snake venom.

**anuria**  Complete suppression of urine.

**aphthous**  Characterized by presence of small ulcers.

**aplasia**  Incomplete or defective development of tissue.

**apoplexy**  Sudden loss of consciousness followed by paralysis resulting from cerebrovascular lesion.

**arachnoid mater**  Middle of three membranes covering brain and spinal cord.

**arbovirus (togavirus)**  Virus borne by and isolated from arthropods.

**Argyll Robertson pupil**  Pupil that reacts to distance but not to light.

**arteriole**  Small artery that ends in a capillary.

**arthritis**  Inflammation of a joint.

**Aschheim-Zondek test**  Pregnancy test utilizing the mouse.

**ascites**  Abnormal collection of fluid in abdominal cavity.

**aseptic**  Free from living microorganisms.

**asphyxia**  Condition that results from interference, in one way or another, with the exchange of oxygen and carbon dioxide between inspired air and the bloodstream by way of the lungs.

**aspirate**  To draw by suction as when fluid is removed with syringe, or material is drawn into the lungs during inspiration.

**ataxic gait**  Gait characterized by lack of muscular coordination.

**atelectasis**  Collapse of lung tissue.

**atony**  Lack of tone or tension; flaccidity.

**atopy**  Human allergy with hereditary background.

**atresia**  Congenital absence or abnormal closure of normal opening or passage.

**atrium (pl., atria)**  Upper chamber of each half of heart.

**atrophy**  Decrease in size of part, organ, tissue, or cell, once of normal size.

**attenuated**  Weakened.

**autoantibody**  Antibody formed against autoantigens.

**autoantigen**  Antigens present in same individual as antibody-forming cells and not "foreign" to body.

**autoclave**  Apparatus for sterilizing by steam under pressure; pressure steam sterilizer.

**autogenous vaccine**  Vaccine made from culture of bacteria obtained from given patient.

**autoimmune disease**  Disease wherein autoimmunization against certain body proteins is pathogenetic mechanism.

**autoimmunity**  Unusual state resulting from production (*autoimmunization*) by body of antibodies against its own proteins.

**autoinfection**  Infection of one part of body by bacteria derived from some other part of body.

**autolysis**  Disintegration of tissues and cells after death; caused by action of autogenous enzymes.

**autopsy**  Examination of internal organs of dead body.

**autotrophic**  Organisms that can form their proteins and carbohydrates out of inorganic salts and carbon dioxide.

**avitaminosis**  Vitamin deficiency disease.

**B lymphocytes**  Thymus-independent lymphocytes (B cells).

**bacteremia**  Condition in which bacteria are in bloodstream but do not multiply there.

**bactericide**  Agent lethal to bacteria.

**bacteriology**  Science that treats of bacteria.

**bacteriolysins**  Antibodies that cause solution of bacteria in presence of complement.

**bacteriophages (phages)**  Bacterial viruses.

**bacteriostasis**  Inhibition of bacterial growth; bacteria, however, not directly killed.

**Bang's disease**  Contagious abortion of cattle.

**BCG (bacillus of Calmette-Guérin)**  Vaccine against tuberculosis made from bovine strain of tubercle bacilli attenuated through long culturing: name derived from the two French scientists developing the strain.

**benign**  Mild in character; not malignant.

**biologic transfer of infection**  Mode of transfer of infection from host to host by animal or insect in which agent causing disease undergoes cycle of development.

**biopsy**  Removal and examination, usually microscopic, for diagnosis of tissue from living body.

**biotherapy**  Treatment of disease with living agent or its products.

**blastogenesis**  Morphologic transformation of small lymphocytes into larger cells appearing like blast cells when exposed to antigens to which they are sensitized.

**blood dyscrasia**  Disease of blood or blood-forming organs.

**blood serum**  *see* **serum.**

**boil**  Abscess of skin and subcutaneous tissue.

**bossing**  Formation of knoblike protuberances.

**Bowman's capsule**  Double-walled vesicle surrounding renal glomerulus.

**broad-spectrum**  Term used to indicate that an antibiotic is effective against large array of microorganisms.

**bronchiectasis**  Disease in which enlarged, damaged bronchial tubes gather mucus and fluid and become infected.

**bronchiolitis**  Inflammation of bronchioles (terminal branches of the tracheobronchial system).

**bronchopneumonia**  Small focal areas of inflammatory consolidation in lungs.

**bubo**  Inflammatory enlargement of lymph node, often with pus formation.

**buffer**  Substance or system of substances in body fluids to lessen effect of addition of acids or alkalies.

**bulla (pl., bullae)**  Large holes in lungs like balloons holding stale air, formed by breakdown of walls of several adjacent alveoli.

**cachexia**  Generalized wasting of the body.

**calcification**  Deposition of calcium salts in tissues.

**calculus**  Abnormal mass of mineral salts within lumen of hollow organ or channel in human body.

**callus**  Plastic exudate deposited at site of fracture; takes part in healing of fracture and then gradually disappears.

**calyces** (sing., **calyx**)  Recesses in pelvis of kidney into which openings of pyramids project.

**cancellous bone**  Inner spongy portion of bone.

**cancer**  Lay term for neoplasm.

**capnophilic**  Growing best in presence of $CO_2$.

**capsule**  Envelope that surrounds certain bacteria; membranous structure surrounding a joint, organ, or tumor.

**carbohydrates**  Class of organic chemical compounds composed of carbon, hydrogen, and oxygen, the latter two in the proportion to form water; to this class belong sugars, starches, and cellulose.

**carcinogenesis**  Induction of cancer.

**carcinogenic**  Applied to agent capable under suitable circumstances of inducing cancer.

**carcinoma**  Malignant neoplasm of epithelial origin.

**carcinoma in situ**  Preinvasive or intraepithelial carcinoma; an epithelial neoplasm showing all expected features of malignancy except invasion and metastasis.

**carditis**  Inflammation of the heart.

**caries**  Decay of bone; caries in teeth (dental caries) are the layman's cavities.

**carrier**  Person in apparent health who harbors pathogenic agent in his body.

**caseous**  Cheeselike.

**cast**  Mold of tubular structure, particularly of kidney tubule.

**catabolism**  Metabolic breakdown of complex bodies into products of more simple composition.

**cataract**  Opacity of the crystalline lens of eye.

**catarrhal**  Characterized by outpouring of mucus.

**cell**  Minute protoplasmic structure, the anatomic and physiologic unit of all animals and plants; that is, all animals and plants are made up of one or more cells, and their activities depend on combined activities of those cells.

**cell (tissue) culture**  Cultivation of tissue cell away from human or animal body.

**cellulitis**  Diffuse inflammation of connective tissue.

**Celsius**  Inventor of the temperature scale setting 100° between the freezing point at zero and the boiling point of water.

**centigrade thermometer**  Temperature scale with 100° between the melting point of ice at zero and the boiling point of water at 100.

**centrioles**  Two or more structures contained in centrosome and prominent during cell division.

**centrosome (cell center)**  Condensed portion of cytoplasm of certain cells containing centrioles; plays an important part in cell division.

**cervical**  Pertaining to the neck.

**chain reaction**  Series of successive reactions in which each succeeding reaction depends on preceding one and that, when once begun, continues until one or more of the chemicals taking part in reaction are exhausted.

**chancre**  Primary lesion of syphilis.

**Charcot-Leyden crystals**  Crystals found in the sputum in bronchial asthma.

**cheilitis**  Inflammation of the lips.

**cheilosis**  Condition marked by cracking and scaling of surface of lips and corners of the mouth as result of vitamin B deficiency.

**chemotaxis**  Reaction to a chemical whereby cells are attacted (positive chemotaxis) or repelled (negative chemotaxis) by chemical.

**chemotherapy**  Treatment of disease by administration of drugs that destroy the causative organism of the disease but do not injure patient.

**Cheyne-Stokes respiration**  Type of respiration in which respiratory movements increase in depth to certain point and then decrease, after which all respiratory movements cease for 5 to 40 seconds; then cycle is repeated.

**chilblain**  Burning, itching, and redness of hands, feet, nose, and other parts of body caused by repeated exposure to damp cold.

**choked disk**  Edema of optic nerve at point where it enters retina.

**cholangitis**  Inflammation of the bile ducts.

**cholecystitis**  Inflammation of the gallbladder.

**cholelithiasis**  Presence or formation of gallstones (choleliths).

**cholesterol**  Fatlike alcohol ($C_{27}H_{45}OH$), occurring as crystals with notched corners; found in blood, bile, egg yolk, and animal fats.

**chorea**  Disorder that usually occurs in childhood and is characterized by involuntary spasmodic movements of limbs and facial muscles; St. Vitus' dance.

**chorionic villi**  Vascular processes on outer layer of fetal membrancs during early stages of development that become part of placenta.

**chromatin**  Stainable part of nucleus of a cell forming network of fibrils; it is deoxyribonucleic acid attached to protein base and is carrier of genes in inheritance.

**chromogenic**  Color-producing.

**chromosomes**  Rod-shaped masses of chromatin that appear in cell nucleus during mitosis; play important part in cell division and transmit hereditary characteristics of cell.

**chromatography**  Method of chemical analysis whereby certain compounds of a mixture are separated by use of their solubility and absorptive properties.

**chronic**  Long-continued.

**chyme**  Partially digested food that passes from the stomach to duodenum.

**cicatrix**  Scar.

**cilia** (sing., **cilium**)  Hairlike processes that spring from certain cells and by their action create currents in liquids; if cells are fixed, liquid is caused to flow, but if cells are unicellular organisms suspended in the liquid, they move.

**ciliates**  Unicellular organisms that move by cilia.

**cirrhosis**  Disease of liver; progressive destruction of liver cells is associated with regeneration of cells and a marked increase in fibrous tissue.

**clinical**  Founded on actual observation.

**clinical case**  Person ill and showing signs of a disease.

**clinical pathology**  Pathology applied to the solution of clinical problems, especially with the use of laboratory methods in clinical diagnosis.

**clone**  Progeny of single cell.

**coagulase**  Enzyme that hastens coagulation.

**coagulation**  Formation of a blood clot.

**coliform bacteria**  Group of bacteria consisting of *Escherichia coli* and related intestinal inhabitants.

**collagen diseases**  Group of diseases characterized by pathologic changes in collagen of the connective tissue of body (examples: rheumatic fever, lupus erythematosus, scleroderma).

**collateral circulation**  Circulation maintained by way of small anastomosing vessels when a main vessel is obstructed.

**colon bacillus**  *Escherichia coli.*

**colony**  Visible growth of bacteria on culture medium; all the progeny of single preexisting bacterium.

**color index**  Amount of hemoglobin in a red blood cell as compared with normal.

**coma**  State of profound unconsciousness from which patient cannot be aroused.

**commensalism**  Symbiosis in which one organism benefited and other not affected.

**communicable**  Capable of being transmitted from one person to another.

**compensation**  Counterbalance to defect of structure or function; for example, in heart disease such as valvular defect, circulation may be maintained by increased work done by heart muscle, and if patient shows no ill effects, heart failure is said to be compensated.

**complement**  Lytic substance found in normal blood that can destroy bacteria or other cells when combined with antigen-antibody complex.

**complement fixation**  Destruction or inactivation of complement by combination of antigen, antibody, and complement, the basis of complement fixation tests for syphilis and other diseases.

**complication**  Disease state concurrent with another disease.

**conception**  Fertilization of ovum.

**concretion**  Calculus.

**condyloma**  Wartlike growth.

**congenital**  Existing at time of birth or shortly thereafter.

**congestion**  Hyperemia.

**consolidation**  Solidification, as of lung in pneumonia.

**constitutional**  Relating to makeup of body as a whole.

**consumption**  Wasting away; lay term for pulmonary tuberculosis.

**contagious**  Highly communicable; in common parlance, a disease easily "caught."

**contamination**  Soiling with infectious material.

**convalescent carrier**  Person or animal that harbors organisms of a disease during recovery from the disease.

**convalescent serum**  Serum of person recently recovered from a disease; in a few cases injection of convalescent serum seems to be of value in treatment or in prevention of the disease in others.

**Coombs' test**  Test to detect the presence of globulin antibodies on surface of red blood cells; used to detect sensitized red cells in hemolytic diseases.

**coproantibodies**  Antibodies formed in the colon.

**coprophilic**  Having affinity for feces and filth.

**coprozoic**  Living in or found in feces.

**corpus luteum**  Yellow body at surface of ovary formed after rupture of graafian follicle with release of ovum.

**counterstain**  Second stain of different color applied to smear to render effects of first stain more distinct.

**craniotabes**  Areas of thinning and softening of the bones of an infant's skull.

**Credé's method**  Instillation of 2% silver nitrate solution in each eye of newborn infants to prevent ophthalmia neonatorum.

**crisis**  Sudden change in course of a disease; diseases that terminate by sudden change for better are said to end by crisis.

**cryobiology**  Science that treats of effects of low temperatures on biologic systems.

**cryostat**  Equipment wherein temperature can be kept at low level; can contain microtome for sectionizing frozen tissue.

**crypt**  Simple gland or minute cul-de-sac.

**culture**  Growth of microorganisms on nutrient medium; to grow microorganisms on such a medium.

**culture media** (sing., **medium**)  Artificial food material on which microorganisms are grown (cultured).

**cutaneous**  Pertaining to skin; cutaneous inoculation is carried out by rubbing infectious material on abraded skin.

**cyanosis**  Blue or purple color of skin and mucosae resulting from reduction of oxygen in blood.

**cycle**  Series of changes leading back to starting point.

**cyst**  Abnormal saccular structure containing liquid, air, or solid; stage in history of certain protozoa during which time encysted organism protected by surrounding wall.

**cystadenoma**  Benign tumor of glandular tissues associated with cystic dilatation of glandular lumina.

**cysticercus**  Larval form of tapeworm in tissues of intermediate host; develops into adult worm on entry into intestinal canal of definitive host.

**cystitis**  Inflammation of the urinary bladder.

**cytogenetics**  Branch of genetics devoted to study of chromosomes, with special reference to visualization, examination, and counting of chromosomes.

**cytology**  Science treating of study of cells, their origin, structure, and function.

**cytolysin**  Antibody that dissolves cells.

**cytopathogenic (cytopathic) effect**  Pathologic changes in cells of given cell (tissue) culture referable to action of some injurious agent, especially those caused by viruses grown in the cell culture.

**cytoplasm**  Protoplasm of cell other than that of nucleus.

**dactylitis**  Inflammation of finger or toe.

**Dakin's solution**  Neutral solution of sodium hypochlorite; once used in disinfection of wounds.

**decidual**  Pertaining to decidua, the altered mucous membrane of pregnant uterus.

**decompensation**  Failure of compensation in heart disease; with inability of heart to maintain adequate circulation, patient shows consequent ill effects.

**dedifferentiation**  Reverse differentiation of a tissue to more primitive stage.

**defibrinate**  To remove fibrin of blood.

**definitive** Final; ending.

**degenerate** To undergo progressive deterioration.

**degeneration** Deterioration; change from higher to lower form.

**degerm** To remove bacteria from skin by mechanical cleaning or application of antiseptics.

**dementia** Insanity characterized by loss of such mental faculties as reason and memory.

**deoxyribonucleic acid** *see* **DNA.**

**dermatitis** Inflammation of skin.

**dermatomycoses** Superficial fungous infections of skin and its appendages.

**dermatophytes** Fungi parasitic for the skin.

**dermotropic** Affinity for skin.

**desensitization** Condition wherein an organism does not react to specific antigen to which it previously did; process of bringing about this state.

**desquamation** Shedding of superficial layer of skin in scales or shreds.

**DEV** Duck embryo vaccine for rabies.

**diaphysis** Shaft of a long bone.

**diarrhea** Abnormal frequency or fluidity of bowel movements.

**diathesis** Condition of the body wherein tissues are more than usually susceptible to certain disease processes.

**diatomaceous earth** Earth made up of petrified bodies of diatoms (unicellular algae).

**Dick test** Skin test to determine susceptibility to scarlet fever.

**differential blood count** Determination of percentage of different types of leukocytes in blood.

**differential stain** Stain distinguishing between different groups of organisms.

**differentiation** Process whereby cells and tissues of embryo acquire completely individual characteristics during stages of growth and maturation of the organism.

**diplococci** Cocci occurring in pairs.

**direct contact** Spread of disease more or less directly from person to person.

**disinfectant** Substance that disinfects.

**disinfection** Destruction of all disease-producing organisms and their products.

**dissociation** Separation, dissolution of relations.

**diurnal** Occurring during day.

**diverticulum** Pouch or sac opening out from tubular organ.

**DNA** Deoxyribonucleic acid; one of the two nucleic acids that have been identified; essential for biologic inheritance.

**dominance** Supremacy in specific situation of one of two or more competitive or mutually antagonistic factors.

**droplet infection** Infection conveyed by spray thrown off from mouth and nose in talking or coughing.

**dropsy** Excessive accumulation of fluid in tissues or cavities of body.

**drug-fast** Resistance to action of drugs; microbes able to withstand harmful action of given drug.

**DTP** Diphtheria-tetanus-pertussis vaccine.

**dyscrasia** Diseased condition marked by general ill health and debility.

**dysentery** Diarrhea plus blood and mucus in stool from inflammation of alimentary tract.

**EBV** Epstein-Barr virus.

**ecchymoses** Purple or blue areas caused by hemorrhagic extravasation of blood into skin.

**eclampsia** Convulsions of toxic origin occurring during latter part of pregnancy or during labor.

**ecology** Science of organisms as affected by factors of their environments.

**ecosystem** Basic unit in ecology derived from interaction of living and nonliving elements in a given area.

**ectoenzyme** Enzyme excreted into surrounding medium through plasma membrane of cell forming it.

**ectopic** Out of place; for example, ectopic pregnancy occurs outside cavity of uterus.

**ectoplasm** Outer clear zone of cytoplasm of unicellular organism.

**edema** Abnormal accumulation of fluid in tissues.

**efferent** Bearing away from.

**effusion** Escape of fluid from blood vessels or lymphatics into tissues or body cavities.

**electrolyte** Substance that in solution conducts an electric current.

**electrophoresis** Application of an electric current to separate substances that move faster in an electric field from those that move more slowly.

**elementary bodies** Virus particles.

**embedding** Fixation of tissue specimen in firm medium to hold it in place as very thin slices are cut.

**embolism** Obstruction of a vessel by an object (embolus) floating in bloodstream; most common emboli are portions of thrombi, agglutinated bacteria, tumor cells, and fat.

**embryonic layers** *see* **germ layers.**

**emphysema** Overdistention of pulmonary air sacs with air; presence of air in the tissues.

**empirical** Based on experience or observation.

**empyema** Collection of pus in a cavity; when used without qualification, collection of pus in pleural cavity.

**encephalitis** Inflammation of brain.

**encephalomyelitis** Inflammation of brain and spinal cord.

**endemic** More or less continuously present in a community.

**endocarditis** Inflammation of endocardium or lining membrane of heart including that of the valves.

**endoenzyme** Enzyme liberated only when cell that produces it disintegrates.

**endogenous** Originating within the organism.

**endometriosis** Occurrence of endometrium in locations other than lining of uterus.

**endometritis** Inflammation of endometrium.

**endoplasm** Zone of granular cytoplasm found near nucleus of many unicellular organisms.

**endoplasmic reticulum** Membrane-limited, canalicular organelle in cytoplasm of cells.

**endothelium** Flattened epithelium lining heart, blood vessels, and lymph vessels.

**endotoxin** Toxin liberated only when cell producing it disintegrates.

**enteric bacteria**  Bacteria isolated from gastrointestinal tract.

**enterotoxin**  Toxin that brings about diarrhea and vomiting, usually following ingestion of contaminated food.

**enteroviruses**  Viruses isolated from the gastrointestinal tract.

**enuresis**  Bed wetting.

**enzyme**  Catalytic substance secreted by a living cell capable of changing other substances without undergoing any change itself.

**eosinophil**  Granular leukocyte whose granules stain with eosin.

**epicardium**  Layer of the pericardium immediately enveloping the heart.

**epidemic**  Disease that attacks a large number of persons in a community at same time.

**epidemiology**  Science that treats of epidemics.

**epiphysis**  Portion of a long bone developed from a center of ossification distinct from that in shaft and separated from shaft at first by a layer of cartilage; the ends of the long bones of the limbs are formed in this manner.

**epiphysitis**  Inflammation of an epiphysis.

**epistaxis**  Nosebleed.

**epitrochlear**  Relating to the epitrochlea or inner condyle of humerus.

**essential**  Disease of unknown cause; idiopathic.

**etiology**  Cause.

**eucaryote**  Protist with true nucleus.

**exacerbation**  Increase in severity of a disease.

**exanthem**  Febrile disease accompanied by skin eruption.

**exfoliate**  To come off in strips or sheets, particularly the stripping of the skin after certain exanthematous diseases.

**exfoliative cytology**  Study of cells cast off from a body surface.

**exogenous**  Coming from outside the body.

**exostosis**  Bony outgrowth springing from surface of a bone.

**exotoxin**  Toxin that is secreted by a microorganism into surrounding medium.

**extracellular**  Outside of cells.

**extradural**  On outside of dura mater.

**extragenital**  Outside of genital tract.

**extraneous**  Outside organism and not belonging to it.

**extrinsic**  From without.

**exudate**  Fluid and formed elements of the blood extravasated into tissues or cavities of body as part of inflammatory reaction.

**facultative**  Able to do a thing although not ordinarily doing it; for example, a facultative anaerobe is an organism that can live in absence of oxygen but does not ordinarily do so.

**familial**  Affecting several members of the same family.

**fecalith**  Intestinal concretion formed around center of fecal material.

**feedback**  Return of part of output of a system as input.

**ferment**  Enzyme.

**fermentation**  Breaking down of complex organic compounds, particularly carbohydrates by enzymes.

**fever**  Abnormally high body temperature, usually related to disease process.

**fibrinolysin**  Substance that dissolves or destroys fibrin.

**fibroma**  Nonmalignant tumor of fibrous connective tissue.

**filaria**  Long, threadlike roundworm living in circulatory or lymphatic system.

**filariform**  Resembling filariae.

**fimbriated**  Having fimbriae (fingerlike structures); fimbriated extremity of fallopian tube is fringed abdominal end of the tube.

**fistula**  Abnormal passage leading from body cavity or hollow organ to external surface or to another body cavity or hollow organ.

**fixation of tissues**  Hardening and preserving of fresh tissue or microbes by immersion in preservative solution; anatomic detail is so maintained that microscopic study may be made.

**fixed virus (rabies)**  Street or wild rabies virus adapted to rabbit and less virulent for man and dog.

**flagella** (sing., **flagellum**)  Long, hairlike processes that by their lashing activity cause the organism to move; one or more flagella may be attached to one or both ends of organism.

**flagellates**  Organisms that move by means of flagella.

**flatulence**  Presence of excessive amount of gas in stomach and intestines.

**flocculation test**  Test dependent on coalescence of finely divided or colloid particles into larger visible ones.

**fluid toxoid**  Toxoid not further treated with aluminum compounds.

**fluorescence**  Property of emitting light after exposure to light.

**fluorescent antibodies**  Antibodies that fluoresce.

**focal infection**  Localized site of more or less chronic infection from which bacteria or their products are spread to other parts of body.

**fomites**  Substances other than food that may transmit infectious organisms.

**foramen ovale**  Opening in septum between atria of the fetal heart; this foramen closes at birth or soon thereafter.

**fractional sterilization**  Heating of material at a low temperature for a given time on 3 or 4 successive days, with storage in interval under conditions suitable for bacterial growth; heating kills vegetative bacteria and any spores developing into vegetative bacteria during incubation periods.

**fracture, pathologic**  Fracture occurring spontaneously without previous trauma to bone; inherent disease destroys bone structure so that it yields to even minimal stress and strain.

**Friedman test**  Pregnancy test utilizing rabbit.

**fulminating**  Sudden, severe, overwhelming.

**fumigation**  Exposure to fumes of a gas that destroys bacteria or vermin.

**functional**  Pertaining to function but not to structure.

**fundus**  Portion of a hollow organ farthest removed from the outlet.

**fungating**  Growing exuberantly, like a fungus.

**Fungi Imperfecti**  Fungi lacking sexual spores; many important pathogens.

**fungicide**  Agent destructive to fungi.

**fungus** (pl., **fungi**)  Unicellular and multicellular vegetable organisms that feed on organic matter; molds, mushrooms, and toadstools.

**furunculosis**  Presence of a number of furuncles or boils.

**gamete**  One of two cells (either male or female) whose union is necessary for sexual reproduction.

**gamma globulin**  Fraction of globulin of blood with which antibodies associated.

**ganglion**  Aggregation of nerve cells within the brain or along the course of a nerve; a cystic swelling connected with a tendon sheath.

**gangrene**  Ischemic necrosis plus putrefaction.

**gastritis**  Inflammation of the stomach.

**gene**  Biologic unit of heredity, self-producing and located in definite position (locus) on a particular chromosome.

**generalized infection**  Infection that involves the whole body.

**genetic determinants**  Carriers of genetic information.

**genetics**  Study of heredity.

**genome**  Complete set of hereditary factors.

**germ**  Pathogenic microbe.

**germ cell**  Cell specialized for reproduction.

**germ layers**  Primary layers of cells formed early in development of embryo from which tissues and organs develop.

**germicide**  Agent that destroys germs.

**Giemsa stain**  Stain (azure and eosin dyes) used to demonstrate protozoa, viral inclusion bodies, and rickettsias.

**globulin**  Class of proteins characterized by being insoluble in water but soluble in weak solutions of various salts; globulin is one of the important proteins of blood plasma.

**glomerulus**  Small tuft of capillaries in a malpighian body of the kidney.

**glycosuria**  Excretion of sugar (glucose) in the urine.

**gnotobiosis**  Science of rearing and keeping animals either born germ-free or with limited known microbial flora.

**goiter**  Enlargement of thyroid gland.

**Golgi apparatus**  Organelle of cell cytoplasm made up of irregular network of canals or solid strands.

**graafian follicles**  Vesicular bodies in ovary, each of which contains an ovum.

**Gram stain**  Method of differential staining devised by Hans Christian Gram, Danish bacteriologist.

**gram-negative**  Bacteria decolorized by Gram's method but stained with counterstain (red or brown).

**gram-positive**  Bacteria not decolorized by Gram's method; retain original violet color of Gram stain and are not stained by counterstain.

**granulation tissue**  Youthful tissue composed of connective tissues cells and thin-walled blood vessels; plays an important part in healing of wounds and forms scar tissue.

**granulocyte**  Cell containing granules within its cytoplasm; granular leukocyte (polymorphonuclear neutrophil, eosinophil, or basophil).

**granuloma**  Circumscribed collection of reticuloendothelial cells surrounding point of irritation.

**granulomatous**  Inflammation with marked response by reticuloendothelial system.

**grouping**  Classification (*see also* **typing**).

**gumma**  Granuloma of late stages of syphilis.

**habitat**  Place where plant or animal found in nature.

**half-life**  Time in which radioactivity originally associated with an isotope will be reduced by one half through radioactive decay.

**halophile**  Salt-loving organism.

**heat stroke**  Syndrome of headache, vertigo, slight delirium, and fever caused by exposure to excessively high temperature.

**hectic fever**  Fever recurring daily; characterized by chills, sweating, and flushed countenance.

**hematemesis**  Vomiting of blood.

**hematocrit**  Volume percent of red blood cells in centrifuged oxalated blood; apparatus for determining this volume.

**hematogenous**  Originating in the blood or borne by the blood.

**hematology**  Science and branch of medicine treating of blood and disease of blood-forming organs.

**hematoma**  Circumscribed effusion of blood.

**hematuria**  Presence of blood in urine.

**hemiplegia**  Paralysis of one side of body.

**hemoconcentration**  Rapid increase in relative red cell content of the blood.

**hemoglobin**  Oxygen-carrying red pigment of red blood cell.

**hemoglobinopathy**  Disease resulting from abnormal chemical structure of hemoglobin molecule.

**hemoglobinophilic**  Applied to organisms growing especially well in culture media containing hemoglobin.

**hemoglobinuria**  Presence of hemoglobin in the urine.

**hemolysin**  Antibody that dissolves red blood cells in presence of complement.

**hemolysis**  Lysis of red blood cells.

**hemolytic**  Causing hemolysis.

**hemopericardium**  Blood in pericardial cavity.

**hemoperitoneum**  Blood in peritoneal cavity.

**hemophilia**  Hereditary blood dyscrasia resulting from a defect in clotting mechanism, characterized by a tendency to profuse and long-continued hemorrhage; affects males but is transmitted by females.

**hemophilic**  Blood-loving, hemoglobinophilic.

**hemoptysis**  Blood in sputum.

**hemorrhage**  Escape of blood from blood vessel.

**hemothorax**  Blood in pleural cavity.

**hepatitis**  Inflammation of liver.

**hepatogenous**  Arising in liver.

**hereditary**  Transmitted through members of family from generation to generation.

**hernia**  Protrusion of organ or part of organ through wall of cavity that contains it; most common type is protrusion of abdominal viscus through abdominal wall.

**heterologous**  Derived from animal of another species.

**heterophil**  Having affinity for antigens or antibodies other than one for which it is specific.

**heterotrophic**  Applied to organisms requiring simple form of carbon for metabolism.

**hilus**  Opening into an organ for the entrance or exit of vessels or ducts.

**Hinton test**  Precipitation test for syphilis.

**homeostasis**  Tendency to stability within internal environment or fluid matrix of an organism.

**homologous serum jaundice**  Type of viral jaundice following administration of human serum.

**hormone**  Chemical formed in one part of body and carried by blood to another part or organ that it stimulates to functional activity.

**host**  Animal or plant upon which a parasite lives.

**hyaline**  Glassy or transparent.

**hydrarthrosis**  Collection of fluid in a joint.

**hydrocele**  Collection of fluid in sacculated cavity, specifically in tunica vaginalis testis.

**hydrocephalus**  Condition, usually congenital, characterized by accumulation of fluid in cerebral ventricles, dilatation of ventricles, thinning of brain, separation of cranial bones, and enlargement of head.

**hydrolysis**  Decomposition caused by incorporation and splitting of water.

**hydrops**  *see* **dropsy.**

**hydrosalpinx**  Accumulation of serous fluid in fallopian tube.

**hydrothorax**  Collection of noninflammatory serous fluid in pleural cavity.

**hyperchlorhydria**  Presence of excess of hydrochloric acid in gastric juice.

**hyperchromic**  Containing more than a normal amount of pigment; refers especially to red blood cells.

**hyperemia**  Presence of an increased amount of blood in a part.

**hyperglycemia**  Excessive level of glucose (sugar) in the blood.

**hyperimmune**  Quality of possessing degree of immunity greater than that usually found under similar circumstances.

**hyperopia**  Farsightedness.

**hyperplasia**  Increase in size related to increase in number of component units.

**hyperpyrexia**  Very high fever; usually more than 106° F.

**hypersensitivity**  Allergy.

**hypersplenism**  Increased activity of spleen; may be associated with anemia, neutropenia, and thrombocytopenia.

**hyperthyroidism**  Train of events brought about by excessive activity of thyroid gland or the taking of too much thyroid extract.

**hypertonic**  Applied to solution with higher osmotic pressure than that of a reference one.

**hypertrophy**  Increase in size of cells of an organ brought about by increase in functional demands made on it.

**hypha** (pl., **hyphae**)  One of the filaments composing a fungus.

**hypochlorhydria**  Deficiency in hydrochloric acid of gastric contents.

**hypochromic**  Containing less than normal amount of coloring matter; refers especially to red blood cells.

**hypoglycemia**  Abnormally low concentration of glucose (sugar) in blood.

**hypokalemia**  Abnormally low potassium concentration in blood.

**hypoprothrombinemia**  Deficiency of prothrombin in blood.

**hypostatic congestion**  Stagnation of blood in lower parts of body because of weakness of heart action and effects of gravity; most often seen in dorsal portion of lungs of persons who have been in bed for long time.

**hypotension**  Low blood pressure.

**hypothyroidism**  Train of events caused by insufficient activity of the thyroid gland.

**hypotonic**  Applied to solution with lower osmotic pressure than that of reference one.

**iatrogenic**  Adverse condition resulting from physician's treatment.

**icterus**  Jaundice.

**idiopathic**  Of unknown cause.

**idiosyncrasy**  Individual and peculiar susceptibility or sensitivity to drug, protein, or other agent.

**ileocolitis**  Inflammation of mucous membrane of the ileum and colon.

**immune**  Exempt from given infection.

**immune bodies**  Antibodies.

**immune globulin**  Sterile preparation of globulin from blood; antibodies normally associated with gamma globulin fraction of blood proteins.

**immune serum**  Serum containing immune bodies.

**immunity**  Natural or acquired resistance to a disease.

**immunoglobulins**  Antibodies.

**immunohematology**  Branch of hematology treating of immune bodies in blood.

**immunologist**  One versed in immunity.

**immunology**  Science that deals with immunity.

**impetigo contagiosa**  Infectious vesicular and pustular eruption most often seen on face and other body areas of children.

**inclusion bodies**  Round, oval, or irregularly shaped particles in cytoplasm and nucleus of cells parasitized by viruses; colonies of viruses.

**incompatible**  Not capable of being mixed without undergoing destructive chemical changes or acting antagonistically.

**incompetency**  Incapability to perform required work; for example, an incompetent heart valve does not close completely, allowing blood to leak back through it when chamber in front contracts.

**incontinence**  Inability to prevent the discharge of the body excretions, particularly urine and feces.

**incubate**  To promote growth of microorganisms by placing them in an incubator.

**incubation period**  Period intervening between time of infection and appearance of the symptoms.

**incubator**  Cabinet in which constant degree of temperature is maintained for purpose of growing cultures of bacteria.

**indicator**  Something that renders visible the completion of a reaction.

**indirect contact**  Transfer of infection by means of inanimate objects, contaminated fingers, water, food, and the like.

**infarction** Death of tissue because of interference with circulation.

**infection** Invasion of body by pathogenic agents with their subsequent multiplication and production of disease; inflammation from living agents.

**infectious** Having qualities that may transmit disease.

**infestation** Invasion of body by macroscopic parasites such as insects; refers particularly to parasites on surface of the body.

**infiltration** Accumulation in a tissue of substance not normally found there.

**inflammation** Protective reaction on part of tissues brought about by presence of irritant; reaction to injury.

**inhibition** Diminution or arrest of function.

**inoculate** To implant microbes or infectious material onto culture media; to introduce artificially biologic product or disease-producing agent into body.

**inspissate** To thicken by evaporation or absorption of fluid.

**insufficiency** Condition of being inadequate, as with a vital organ that cannot, because of disease, perform its normal functions.

**insulin** Hormone arising in the islands of Langerhans of pancreas; regulates carbohydrate metabolism.

**intercurrent infection** Infection that attacks person already ill of another disease.

**interferon** Protein produced by cells infected with certain viruses; inhibits viral reproduction and spread.

**intermittent sterilization** *see* **fractional sterilization.**

**internal secretion** Hormone.

**intersex** Intermingling characteristics of each sex in one individual as a result of some flaw in embryonic development.

**interstitial** Relating to spaces or gaps between cells in a structure.

**intoxication** Poisoning.

**intracranial** Within the skull.

**intracutaneous** Intradermal.

**intradermal** Within the substance of skin.

**intraperitoneal** Within peritoneal cavity.

**intraspinal** Within vertebral canal.

**intrauterine** Within uterus.

**intravenous** Within a vein.

**intrinsic** From within.

**intussusception** Infolding or telescoping of one segment of intestine into another.

**involution forms** Abnormal forms assumed by microorganisms growing under unfavorable conditions.

**iodophors** Disinfectants with the germ-killing iodine carried by surface-active solvent.

**iris** Diaphragm in anterior portion of the eye that is perforated by pupil.

**iritis** Inflammation of the iris.

**ischemia** Local anemia caused by obstruction of arterial blood supply of part.

**isoantigens** Antigens from individual of same species.

**isolate** To close all avenues by which a person may spread infection to others; to separate from others.

**isologous** Pertaining to same species.

**isotonic** Having same osmotic pressure as that of standard reference solution.

**isotopes** Atoms of same element having different atomic weights but generally same chemical behavior.

**jaundice** Deposition of bilirubin in skin and tissues, with resultant yellowish discoloration in patient with hyperbilirubinemia.

**Kahn test** Precipitation test for syphilis.

**karyosome** Chromatin mass or knot on linin network of nucleus.

**karyotype** Chromosomal makeup of cell, individual, or species.

**keratitis** Inflammation of cornea.

**keratoconjunctivitis** Inflammation of cornea and conjunctiva.

**kernicterus** Cerebral manifestations of severe jaundice in newborn infant; degeneration of nerve cells caused by accumulation of bilirubin in brain.

**Kline test** Precipitation test for syphilis.

**Koch's postulates** Certain requirements that must be met before a given microorganism can be considered the cause of a certain disease.

**laceration** Wound made by tearing of tissue.

**lactation** Production of milk.

**lactiferous** Conveying milk (example: lactiferous ducts of breast).

**lag phase** Period of time between stimulus and resultant reaction.

**larva** (pl., **larvae**) Young of any animal differing in form from its parent.

**latent** Seemingly inactive, potential, concealed.

**leptospirosis** Diseased produced by leptospires.

**lesion** Specific pathologic structural or functional change (or both) brought about by disease.

**leukemia** Malignant disease characterized by marked increase in number of leukocytes and their precursors both in bloodstream and in blood-forming organs.

**leukocidin** Substance that destroys leukocytes.

**leukocyte** White blood cell.

**leukocytosis** Transient protective increase in leukocytes in blood brought about in response to injury.

**leukopenia** Pathologic decrease in leukocytes in blood.

**leukoplakia** Condition characterized by irregular white patches on tongue and inside of cheek.

**lipase** Fat-splitting enzyme.

**lithopedion** Calcified fetus; stone child.

**local infection** Infection confined to restricted area.

**lues venerea** Syphilis.

**lumbar** Pertaining to that part of back between ribs and pelvis.

**lumpy jaw** Actinomycosis in cattle.

**lymphadenitis** Inflammation of lymph node.

**lymphadenopathy** Disease of lymph node.

**lymphocyte** Nongranular white blood cell of lymphoid origin.

**lymphocytosis** Increase in lymphocytes in blood.

**lymphoid tissue** Delicate connective tissue lattice with lymphocytes and related cells in its meshes.

**lymphoma** Tumor of lymphoid tissue.

**lyophilization**  Creation of stable product by rapid freezing and drying of frozen product under high vacuum.

**macrocytic**  Applied to abnormally large cells, especially red blood cells.

**macromolecule**  Very large molecule having polymeric chain structure.

**macrophage**  Large mononuclear, wandering phagocytic cell that originates in reticuloendothelial system.

**macroscopic**  Visible to naked eye.

**macules**  Small flat reddish spots in skin.

**malignant**  Virulent, going from bad to worse; for example, a malignant tumor infiltrates surrounding tissues, spreads to distant parts of body, has tendency to recur after removal, and if left untreated always causes death.

**Mantoux test**  One of tuberculin skin tests.

**marker**  Something that identifies or is used to identify.

**Mazzini test**  Precipitation test for syphilis.

**mechanical transfer (of infection)**  Transfer of infection by insects in which infectious agent is spread mechanically and undergoes no cycle of development in body of particular insect.

**medical technologist**  Specialist in technics of performing tests vitally related to medicine.

**medulla**  Center of a part.

**medullary cavity**  Marrow cavity of bone.

**meiosis**  Special type of cell division during maturation of sex cells by which normal number of chromosomes is halved.

**membranous croup**  Lay term for diphtheria.

**meningitis**  Inflammation of meninges.

**menopause**  Time in a woman's life when menstruation terminates.

**menorrhagia**  Excessive menstrual flow.

**metabolism**  Sum total of chemical changes whereby nutrition and functional activities of body maintained.

**metachromatic granules**  Granules of deeply staining material found in certain bacteria.

**metastasis**  Spread of disease from primary focus to distant parts of body; in malignant tumors, appearance of secondary growths in parts of body at a distance from primary growth.

**metazoa**  Multicellular animals.

**metrorrhagia**  Excessive bleeding from uterus not associated with menstruation.

**microaerophilic**  Applied to microorganisms that require free oxygen for their growth, but in an amount less than oxygen of atmosphere.

**microbe**  Microscopic unicellular organism.

**microbiology**  Science that treats of microbes.

**microcytic**  Applied to cells of less than normal size; especially red blood cells.

**microgram**  One thousandth of a milligram or one millionth of a gram.

**microhematocrit**  Apparatus for determining volume percentage of red blood cells in small sample of blood centrifuged in capillary tube.

**micrometer**  One thousandth of a millimeter or one twenty-five thousandth of an inch.

**micron**  Micrometer.

**microorganism**  Organism of microscopic size.

**miliary**  Small, resembling a millet seed in size.

**minimum lethal dose (MLD)**  Smallest dose that will cause death.

**mitochondrion** (pl., **mitochondria**)  Small, spherical or rod-shaped cytoplasmic organelles.

**mitosis**  Indirect cell division.

**mixed culture**  Culture containing two or more kinds of organisms.

**mixed infection**  Infection with two or more kinds of organisms.

**mixed vaccine**  Vaccine containing two or more kinds of organisms.

**molds**  Multicellular fungi.

**mole**  Nevus.

**molt**  Act of shedding outer body covering (skin, cuticle, feathers).

**monarticular**  Relating to single joint.

**morbid**  Pertaining to or affected with disease.

**morbidity**  Departure (subjective or objective) from state of physiologic well-being (WHO definition).

**mordant**  Chemical added to a dye to make it stain more intensely.

**morphologic**  Pertaining to shape or form.

**multipara**  Woman who has given birth several times.

**murmur**  Soft, blowing heart sound most often caused by valvular lesion.

**mutagenesis**  Induction of genetic mutation.

**mutation**  Change or alteration in form or qualities; permanent transmissible change in characters of offspring from those of parents.

**mycelium**  Vegetative part of a fungus, consisting of many hyphae.

**mycobacteriosis**  Disease produced by certain unclassified members of the genus *Mycobacterium*.

**mycohemia**  Presence of fungi in bloodstream.

**mycology**  Science that deals with fungi.

**mycophage**  Fungal virus.

**mycosis**  Disease caused by fungi.

**mycotoxin**  Fungal toxin.

**myocarditis**  Inflammation of myocardium.

**myopia**  Nearsightedness.

**nanometer (millimicron)**  One millionth of a millimeter.

**natural immunity**  Immunity with which person or animal is born.

**necrosis**  Death of tissue while yet part of living body.

**negative staining**  Staining of background but not of organism.

**Negri bodies**  Inclusion bodies found in certain brain cells of animal with rabies; diagnostic for rabies.

**neoplasm (neoplasia)**  New growth of abnormal cells of autonomous nature (scientific term for layman's "cancer"); word *tumor* is used synonymously, although its true meaning is mass.

**nephrosis**  Degenerative disease of tubular system of kidney.

**neuralgia**  Severe throbbing pain along course of nerve.

**neuritis**  Inflammation of nerve.

**neurosyphilis**  Syphilis affecting central nervous system.

**neurotropic** Having affinity for central nervous system or nervous tissue.

**night blindness** Imperfect vision or blindness at night or in dim light, with good vision on bright days.

**NIH** National Institutes of Health.

**nonpathogenic** Not productive of disease.

**normal flora** Bacterial content of given area during health; reasonably constant as to quantity and proportions.

**normoblast** Nucleated red blood cell at certain developmental stage.

**normochromic** Containing normal amount of coloring matter; especially pertains to red blood cells.

**normocytic** Applied to cells of normal size; especially red blood cells.

**nosocomial** Pertaining to hospital or infirmary.

**nosology** Science of classification of disease.

**nuclear medicine** Use of radioisotopes in medicine.

**nucleic acids** Complex chemical substances closely associated with transmission of genetic characteristics of cells; the two identified are ribonucleic acid and deoxyribonucleic acid; cells of bacteria and higher organisms contain both RNA and DNA; viruses contain one or the other but not both.

**nucleolus** (pl., **nucleoli**) Body within nucleus of a cell that takes part in metabolic processes of the cell and plays part in its multiplication.

**nucleoprotein** Simple basic protein combined with nucleic acid.

**nucleus** (pl., **nuclei**) Central, compact portion of cell; functional center of the cell.

**occult** Concealed, not discernible to the senses; for example, occult blood can be detected only by chemical tests.

**old tuberculin (OT)** Special type of tuberculin.

**oligemia** Deficiency in volume of blood.

**oliguria** Decrease below normal in amount of urine excreted.

**oncogenic** Tumor-producing.

**ontogeny** Complete developmental history of individual organism.

**opalescent** Like an opal in display of colors.

**opportunists** Microbes that produce infection only under especially favorable conditions.

**opsonins** Substances in blood that render microorganisms most susceptible to phagocytosis.

**optimum temperature for growth** Temperature at which microbes grow best.

**OPV** Oral poliovirus vaccine.

**organelle(s)** Specialized part of protozoon that performs special function; specific particles of organized living substance present in almost all cells.

**ossification** Bone formation.

**osteitis** Inflammation of bone.

**osteochondritis** Inflammation of bone with its cartilage.

**osteogenic** Bone-producing.

**osteomyelitis** Inflammation of bone marrow.

**otitis media** Inflammation of middle ear.

**palsy** Paralysis, word used only with certain kinds.

**pancreatitis** Inflammation of pancreas.

**pandemic** Epidemic widespread, even of worldwide extent.

**Pap smears** Smears of various body secretions for study of exfoliated cells from particular anatomic site; introduced by George Papanicolaou; usually refers to smears of cervix uteri.

**papilloma** Circumscribed outgrowth from skin or mucous membrane (example: wart).

**paralytic ileus** Intestinal obstruction from inhibition of bowel motility; various causes, for example, peritonitis.

**parasite** Animal or plant organism that lives on another.

**parasitology** Science that treats of parasites and their effects on other living organisms.

**parenchyma** Specialized functioning tissue or cells of an organ.

**parenterally** In some manner other than by intestinal tract.

**parietal** Relating to wall of a cavity.

**paroxysm** Sudden attack of a disease or acceleration of manifestations of existing disease.

**passive carrier** Person or animal that harbors causative agent of disease without having had the disease.

**passive immunity** Immunity produced without body of person or animal becoming immune taking any part in its production.

**pasteurization** Heating of milk for a short time to a temperature that will destroy pathogenic bacteria but will not affect its food properties and flavor.

**pathogenesis** Sequence of events in development of given disease state.

**pathogenicity** Disease-producing quality.

**pathognomonic** Specifically characteristic or diagnostic of a disease.

**pathology** Branch of medicine treating of nature of disease, especially with reference to structural and functional changes in tissues and organs of human body.

**Paul-Bunnell test** Heterophil antibody test on serum; important in diagnosis of infectious mononucleosis.

**pepsin** Digestive enzyme occurring in gastric contents and acting on proteins.

**peptic** Pertaining to digestion.

**pericardium** Saclike structure surrounding heart.

**periosteum** Thick fibrous membrane covering surface of bone.

**periostitis** Inflammation of periosteum.

**peripheral** Related to or situated at periphery, outer part or surface of body.

**periproctitis** Inflammation of tissue about rectum.

**peritonitis** Inflammation of peritoneum.

**permanent carrier** Person or animal that harbors disease-producing agent for months or years.

**petechia** (pl., **petechiae**) Pinpoint hemorrhage.

**Petri dish** Round glass dish with cover, used for growing bacterial cultures.

**Peyer's patches** Collection of lymphoid nodules packed together to form oblong elevations of mucous membrane of small intestine, their long axis corresponding to that of intestine.

**phage typing** Use of bacteriophages and their lytic properties to classify bacteria.

**phagocyte** Cell capable of ingesting bacteria or other foreign particles.

**phagocytosis** Process of ingestion by phagocytes.

**phenol coefficient** Measure (ratio) of the disinfecting property of a chemical compared with that of phenol (carbolic acid).

**phlebitis** Inflammation of vein.

**phlegmon** Acute diffuse inflammation of subcutaneous connective tissue.

**photosynthesis** Elaboration of glucose from carbon dioxide and water by sunlight in presence of chlorophyll.

**phylogeny** Complete developmental history of a race or group of animals.

**piles** Hemorrhoids.

**pinocytosis** Cell-drinking, imbibition of liquids by cells; minute invaginations on surface of cells close to form fluid-filled vacuoles.

**Pirquet's test (von Pirquet)** One of tuberculin skin tests.

**plaques** Visible areas of cellular damage caused by virus inoculated into susceptible tissue culture cells; analogous to colonies of bacteria on agar plate.

**plasma** Fluid portion of circulating blood; fluid portion of clotted blood is *serum*.

**plasma membrane** Outer membrane encasing protoplasm of cell.

**plasmids** Generic term for intracellular inclusions considered to have genetic functions; extrachromosomal genetic elements.

**plasmolysis** Shrinking of a cell suspended in hypertonic solution.

**plasmoptysis** Swelling and bursting of a cell suspended in hypotonic solution.

**plastids** Small bodies found in cytoplasm of cells; have to do with cell nutrition and contain the chlorophyll of green plants.

**pleomorphism** Existence of different forms in same species.

**plethora** Excessive amount of circulating blood.

**pleurisy** Inflammation of pleura.

**pleuritis** Inflammation of pleural membrane.

**pleuropneumonia** Infectious pneumonia and pleurisy of cattle.

**pneumoconiosis** Chronic disease and scarring of lung tissue caused by prolonged inhalation of certain dusts.

**pneumonia** Inflammatory consolidation or solidification of lung tissue; presence of exudate blots out air-containing spaces.

**pneumonitis** Inflammation of supporting framework of lung.

**pneumothorax** Air in pleural cavity.

**pneumotropic** Having affinity for the lungs.

**polar bodies** Deeply staining bodies found in one or both ends of certain species of bacteria.

**pollution** State of being unclean; as used in bacteriology, containing harmful substances other than bacteria.

**polyarticular** Affecting many joints.

**polyp (polypus)** Pedunculated swelling or outgrowth springing from skin or a mucous membrane.

**polyuria** Excessive excretion of urine.

**precancerous** Applied to condition likely to develop into cancer.

**precipitation** Clumping of proteins in solution by addition of specific precipitin.

**precipitins** Antibodies that cause precipitation.

**pregnancy tests** Tests to determine presence of products of conception.

**prehension** Grasping.

**preservative** Substance added to product to prevent microbial growth and consequent spoiling.

**primary** First; especially the first focus of disease.

**primary infection** First of two infections, one occurring during course of other.

**procaryote** Protist without true nucleus.

**proctitis** Inflammation of rectum.

**prognosis** Forecast of outcome of disease.

**properdin** Protein component of globulin fraction of blood playing role in immunity.

**prophylaxis** Prevention of disease.

**proprietary** Referring to fact that a given item is a commercial one.

**prostration** Great depression of vital activities.

**protein** One of group of complex organic nitrogenous compounds, widely distributed in plants and animals; form principal constituents of protoplasm; are essentially combinations of amino acids and their derivatives.

**proteolytic** Bringing about digestion or liquefaction of proteins.

**protist** Member of kingdom Protista that includes all single-celled organisms (bacteria, algae, slime molds, fungi, protozoa); some plantlike, some animal-like, some neither.

**protoplasm** Living material of which cells are composed.

**protozoology** Science that treats of protozoa.

**protozoon** (pl., **protozoa**) Unicellular animal organism.

**proud flesh** Exuberant growth of granulation tissue that protrudes from a wound and shows no immediate tendency to undergo scar formation.

**provocative dose** Dose stimulating appearance of given effect.

**pseudomembrane** Fibrinous exudate forming tough membranous structure on surface of skin or mucous membrane.

**pseudomucin** Protein resembling mucin found in certain cysts, especially those of ovary.

**pseudopod** Temporary protoplasmic process put forth by protozoon for purposes of locomotion or obtaining food.

**psoas abscess** Abscess in sheath of the psoas major muscle; usually results from tuberculosis of spinal column; usually points on inner side of thigh.

**psychosis** Disorder of the mind.

**psychrophile** Cold-loving organism, growing best at low temperatures.

**ptomaines** Basic substances resembling alkaloids formed during decomposition of dead organic matter.

**pure culture** Culture containing only one species of organism.

**purpura** Hemorrhages in skin and mucous membranes.

**purulent** Containing pus.

**pus** Fluid product of inflammation, consisting of leukocytes, bacteria, dead tissue cells, foreign elements, and fluid from the blood.

**pustule**   Circumscribed elevation on skin containing pus.

**putrefaction**   Decomposition of proteins.

**pyelitis**   Inflammation of kidney pelvis.

**pyelonephritis**   Inflammation of renal parenchyma and pelvis.

**pyemia**   Form of septicemia in which organisms in bloodstream lodge in organs and tissues and set up secondary abscesses.

**pyogenic**   Pus-forming.

**pyosalpinx**   Collection of pus in fallopian tube.

**quiescent**   Not active.

**quinsy**   Layman's term for peritonsillar abscess.

**racial immunity**   Immunity peculiar to race.

**radiant energy**   Energy from radioactive source.

**radiation therapy**   Treatment by radium or x ray.

**radioactive decay**   Loss of radioactivity.

**radioactivity**   Spontaneous breakdown of atoms of a substance with release of alpha, beta, or gamma rays.

**radioimmunoassay**   Determination of antigen or antibody concentration (also of other proteins) by means of radioactive-labeled substance reacting with test substance in a prescribed way.

**radioisotope**   Isotope form of element that is radioactive.

**radioresistant**   Applied to cells or tissues resistant to, or little affected by, radiation.

**radioresponsive**   Applied to cells or tissues affected only by high doses of radiation.

**radiosensitive**   Applied to cells or tissues easily injured or destroyed by radiation.

**raw milk**   Unpasteurized milk.

**receptors**   Precise chemical groupings on surface of target cell; those on immunologically competent cell can combine specifically with antigen.

**recessive**   Not exerting controlling influence; genetically incapable of expression unless carried by both members of a set of homologous chromosomes.

**recrudescent**   Recurrence of symptoms of a disease after a period of days or weeks.

**recurrent**   Reappearing, as symptoms after an intermission.

**reduction**   Removal of oxygen from, or addition of hydrogen to, a compound.

**regeneration**   Natural replacement of lost parts.

**regurgitation**   Backward flowing.

**remission**   Temporary cessation of manifestations of disease.

**remittent**   Characterized by remissions.

**rennin**   Milk-curdling enzyme.

**replication**   Process by which genetic determinants are duplicated during cell multiplication, so that identical genetic characters are passed on to next generation.

**resident bacteria**   Bacteria normally occurring at given anatomic site.

**resistance**   Inherent power of body to ward off disease.

**resolution**   Subsidence of inflammation.

**retention**   Keeping in the body of material normally excreted; in the case of urine, secretion continues, but the urine is not passed.

**reticuloendothelial system**   System of phagocytic cells scattered through various organs and tissues, particularly spleen, liver, bone marrow, and lymph nodes; plays important part in immunity.

**Rh factor**   Blood factor, agglutinogen, found on red blood cells of most persons; so named because of its occurrence on red blood cells of rhesus monkeys.

**rhinitis**   Inflammation of nose.

**ribosomes**   Ribonucleoprotein granules in cell cytoplasm.

**rickettsias**   Minute microorganisms that must live within cells; members of genus *Rickettsia;* animal reservoirs of infection important, and organisms transmitted to man by arthropod vectors. Members of Bergey's Part 18 that includes chlamydiae and 16 other genera besides *Rickettsia.*

**ringworm**   Fungous disease of skin.

**RNA**   Ribonucleic acid; when of viral origin, infectious for susceptible cells.

**rodent**   Gnawing mammal (examples: rat, mouse).

**Romberg's sign**   Swaying of the body when subject stands with feet together and eyes closed.

**rose spots**   Characteristic spots in skin over lower portion of trunk and abdomen in typhoid fever.

**rudimentary**   Imperfectly developed.

**ruga** (pl., **rugae**)   Fold, ridge, or wrinkle.

**Sabin vaccine**   Live poliomyelitis oral vaccine, developed by Dr. Albert Sabin.

**Salk vaccine**   Poliomyelitis vaccine containing formalin-inactivated virus, developed by Dr. Jonas Salk.

**salmonellosis**   Infection with organism of the genus *Salmonella;* manifestations may be varied.

**salpingitis**   Inflammation of fallopian tube (salpinx).

**sanitary**   Conducive to health.

**sanitize**   To reduce number of bacteria to safe level as judged by public health standards.

**sapremia**   Condition in which products of action of saprophytic bacteria on dead tissues are absorbed into body and produce disease.

**saprophyte**   Organism that normally grows on dead matter.

**sarcoma**   Malignant neoplasm of nonepithelial origin.

**Schick test**   Skin test to detect susceptibility to diphtheria.

**sciatica**   Neuralgia of sciatic nerve.

**scirrhous**   Indicating quality of hardness caused by abundance of connective tissue.

**scrofula**   Tuberculosis of lymph nodes, particularly those of neck.

**secondary infection**   Infection occurring in host already suffering from primary infection.

**section**   Segment or portion; tissue sections for microscopic study are exceedingly thin slices.

**sedimentation**   Settling of solid matter to bottom of liquid.

**selective action**   Tendency on part of disease-producing agents to attack certain parts of the body.

**Semple vaccine**   Rabies vaccine prepared from rabbit brain treated with phenol.

**sensitivity**   Quality or state of being sensitive.

**sensitization**   Process of rendering sensitive.

**sepsis**   Poisoning by microorganisms or their products.

**septic**  Relating to presence of pathogenic organisms or their poisonous products.

**septicemia**  Systemic disease caused by invasion of bloodstream by pathogenic organisms, with their subsequent multiplication therein.

**sequestrum**  Portion of dead bone that has become separated from healthy bone.

**serology**  Branch of science that deals with serums, especially immune serums.

**serum**  Fluid that exudes when blood coagulates; portion of plasma left after the plasma protein fibrinogen is removed.

**sessile**  Having broad base of attachment.

**signs**  Objective disturbances produced by disease; observed by physician, nurse, or person attending patient.

**simian viruses**  Viral contaminants in tissue (cell) cultures of normal monkey cells.

**simple stain**  Stain using only one dye.

**sinus**  Tract leading from an area of disease to body surface.

**skin test dose (STD)**  Unit of measurement of scarlet fever toxin, amount required to produce positive reaction on skin of person susceptible to scarlet fever.

**slough**  A separation of dead tissue from living tissue.

**smear**  Very thin layer of material spread on a glass microslide.

**species immunity**  Immunity peculiar to species.

**specific gravity**  Weight of a substance as compared with weight of equal volume of distilled water.

**spirilla** (sing., **spirillum**)  Bacteria of corkscrew shape.

**spontaneous**  Occurring without external stimulation.

**sporadic**  Occurring separately or apart from others of its kind.

**sporadic disease**  Disease that occurs in neither endemic nor epidemic form.

**spore**  Highly resistant form assumed by certain species of bacteria when grown under adverse influences; the reproductive cells of certain types of organisms.

**sporulation**  Production of spores or division into spores.

**squamous**  Platelike or scaly.

**stain**  Dye used in bacteriologic and histologic technics.

**staining**  Coloring cells or tissues with dyes.

**staphylococci** (sing., **staphylococcus**)  Cocci that occur in irregular, grapelike clusters.

**stenosis**  Narrowing or closure of canal or passage.

**sterile**  Free of living microorganisms and their products.

**sterilization**  Process of making sterile.

**stock vaccine**  Vaccine made from cultures other than those from patient who is to receive vaccine.

**strain**  Subdivision of species.

**strangulation**  Cutting off air or blood supply by constriction.

**streptococci**  Cocci that divide in such a manner as to form chains.

**streptolysins O and S**  Hemolysins produced by streptococci.

**stricture**  Narrowing or closure of tubular structure.

**stroma**  Supporting connective tissue framework of organ or gland.

**stupor**  Unconsciousness.

**subacute**  Referring to disease between acute and chronic in time.

**subcutaneous**  Beneath skin.

**subdural**  Beneath dura matter.

**substrate**  Substance on which enzyme acts.

**sulfur granules**  Small yellow granules found in pus from lesions of actinomycosis.

**sunstroke**  Heatstroke caused by action of sun rays.

**superinfection**  New (superimposed) infection with drug-resistant microbes as a complication of antimicrobial therapy for a preexisting infection.

**suppression**  Sudden cessation of normal discharge, as when kidneys suddenly stop excreting urine.

**suppuration**  Formation of pus.

**supraclavicular**  Above clavicle.

**susceptibility**  State or quality of being vulnerable.

**sycosis barbae**  Folliculitis of beard.

**symbiosis**  Mutually advantageous association of two or more organisms.

**symptoms**  Subjective disturbances caused by disease that are felt or experienced by patient but not directly measurable; for example, pain is definitely felt by the patient but cannot be seen, heard, or touched.

**syncope**  Fainting.

**syndrome**  Set of symptoms and signs found together in a pattern; etiologic factors are variable.

**synovitis**  Inflammation of synovial membrane.

**system**  Group of organs concerned in performing same general function; the entire organism.

**systemic**  Relating to a system; relating to entire organism instead of a part.

**T lymphocytes (T cells)**  Thymus-dependent lymphocytes.

**taxon**  Particular group into which related organisms are classified.

**taxonomy**  Branch of biology treating of arrangement and classification of biological organisms.

**technic**  Method of performing an operation, test, or other procedure.

**template**  Pattern, mold, guide, blueprint.

**teratogenesis**  Production of physical defects in offspring in utero.

**teratology**  Study of abnormal development and congenital malformations.

**teratoma**  Complex tumor whose substance represents several different tissues.

**terminal disinfection**  Disinfection of room after it has been vacated by patient.

**terminal infection**  Infection with streptococci or other pathogenic bacteria that occurs during course of chronic disease and causes death.

**Thallophyta**  Division of plant kingdom to which the fungi belong.

**therapy**  Treatment.

**thermal death point**  Degree of heat necessary to kill liquid culture of a given species of bacteria in 10 minutes.

**thrombocytopenia**  Deficiency of platelets in blood.

**thrombosis**  Formation of a thrombus, a blood clot within lumen of cardiovascular system during life.

**tinea**  Dermatomycosis.

**tissue** Collection of cells forming a definite structure.

**tissue culture** *see* **cell culture.**

**tissue of origin** Tissue in which neoplasm arises and therefore the tissue that neoplasm attempts to reproduce.

**titer** Measure of minimal amount of given substance needed for precise result in titration; standard strength of a solution established by titration.

**titration** Determination of concentration of contained substance by measuring least amount of another substance that, when added to test solution, produces precise reaction.

**tolerance** Ability to endure without ill effect.

**toxemia** Presence of toxins in the blood.

**toxin** Poisonous substance elaborated during growth of pathogenic bacteria.

**toxoid** Toxin treated in such a manner that its toxic properties are destroyed but its antibody-producing properties are unaffected.

**tracheotomy** Surgical opening into trachea or windpipe.

**transduction** Transmission of genetic factor from one bacterial cell to another by viral agent.

**transformation** Artificial conversion of bacterial types within a species by transfer of DNA from one bacterium to another.

**transudate** Noninflammatory collection of fluid.

**trauma** Wound or injury.

**trephine** Instrument for removing a circular disk of bone from the skull.

**trophozoite** Active, motile, feeding stage of a protozoon.

**tubercle** Nodule or granuloma that forms the unit specific lesion of tuberculosis.

**tuberculin** Toxic protein extract obtained from tubercle bacilli.

**tuberculous** Affected with tuberculosis.

**tumor** Mass; by common usage, word designates neoplasm, or a lesion to be differentiated from neoplasm.

**turgid** Swollen.

**typing (classification)** Determination of category to which an individual, object, microbe, or the like belongs with respect to given standard of reference.

**ulcer** Circumscribed area of inflammatory necrosis of epithelial lining of a surface.

**ulceration** Process of ulcer formation.

**unicellular** Composed of but a single cell.

**unilateral** Confined to one side.

**unit** Standard of measurement.

**uremia** Toxic state produced by retention of certain chemicals normally eliminated in urine.

**vaccination** Introduction of a vaccine into the body.

**vaccine** Causative agent of a disease so modified that it is incapable of producing disease but retains its power to cause antibody formation.

**vaccinia** Cowpox.

**vaginitis** Inflammation of vagina.

**variation** Deviation from the parent form.

**varix** (pl., **varices**) Enlarged and tortuous vein, artery, or lymph vessel.

**VDRL (Venereal Disease Research Laboratory) test** Precipitation test for syphilis.

**vector** Carrier of disease-producing agents from one host to another, especially an arthropod (fly, mosquito, flea, louse, or other insect).

**vegetation** Growth or excrescence; clot adherent to diseased heart valve.

**vegetative bacteria** Nonsporeforming bacteria or sporeforming bacteria in their nonsporulating state.

**venereal** Transmission of disease by intimate sexual contact.

**ventricle** Small cavity, especially of heart or brain.

**vertigo** Sensation of going round and round, either of oneself or of external objects.

**vesicle (blister)** Small circumscribed elevation of skin containing thin, nonpurulent fluid.

**viremia** Presence of virus in bloodstream.

**virilism** Masculinity; development of masculine physical and mental traits in the female.

**virology** Science that treats of viruses and viral diseases.

**virucide** Agent destroying or inactivating virus.

**virulence** Ability of organism to produce disease.

**virus** Submicroscopic agent of infectious disease that requires living cells for its proliferation.

**virus-neutralizing antibodies** Antibodies that inactivate viruses.

**viscerotropic** Having affinity for internal organs of chest or abdomen.

**viscus** (pl., **viscera**) Internal organ, especially one of abdominal organs.

**vital functions** Functions necessary for maintenance of life.

**vitamins** Certain little-understood food substances whose presence in very small amounts is necessary for normal functioning of body cells.

**Wassermann test** Complement fixation test for syphilis; devised by August von Wassermann.

**Weil-Felix reaction** Nonspecific but highly valuable agglutination test for typhus fever; uses a member of *Proteus* group as the organism agglutinated.

**wheal** Circumscribed elevation of skin caused by edema of underlying connective tissues.

**Widal test** Agglutination test for typhoid fever.

**wild virus** Virus found in nature.

**Wright's stain** Mixture of eosin and methylene blue; used to demonstrate blood cells and malarial parasites.

**x rays (roentgen rays)** Highly penetrating form of ionizing radiation produced in special high-voltage equipment.

**xerophthalmia** Dry, lusterless eyeball resulting from vitamin A deficiency.

**yeasts** Unicellular fungi.

**zoology** Science that treats of animal life.

**zoonosis** (pl., **zoonoses**) Disease of animals that may be secondarily transmitted to man.

# Index

INDEX